# NELSON
# ESSENTIALS OF
# PEDIATRICS

# NELSON

# ESSENTIALS OF PEDIATRICS

*Third Edition*

## RICHARD E. BEHRMAN, M.D.

Managing Director
Center for the Future of Children
The David and Lucile Packard Foundation
Clinical Professor of Pediatrics
Stanford University and University of California, San Francisco
Attending Physician
Lucile Salter Packard Children's Hospital at Stanford
Stanford, California

## ROBERT M. KLIEGMAN, M.D.

Professor and Chairman
Department of Pediatrics
Medical College of Wisconsin
Pediatrician-in-Chief
Children's Hospital of Wisconsin
Milwaukee, Wisconsin

## W.B. SAUNDERS COMPANY
*A Division of Harcourt Brace & Company*
Philadelphia London Toronto Montreal Sydney Tokyo

**W.B. SAUNDERS COMPANY**
*A Division of Harcourt Brace & Company*

The Curtis Center
Independence Square West
Philadelphia, Pennsylvania 19106

**Library of Congress Cataloging-in-Publication Data**

Nelson essentials of pediatrics / [edited by] Richard E. Behrman, Robert M. Kliegman.—3rd ed.

p.    cm.

Includes bibliographical references and index.

ISBN 0–7216–7229–9

1. Pediatrics.    I. Nelson, Waldo E. (Waldo Emerson).    II. Behrman, Richard E.
   III. Kliegman, Robert.    [DNLM: 1. Pediatrics.    WS 100 N425 1998]

RJ45. N418 1998    618.92—dc21

DNLM/DLC                                                        97–15484

NELSON ESSENTIALS OF PEDIATRICS                    ISBN 0–7216–7229–9

Printed in the United States of America.

Last digit is the print number:    9    8    7    6    5    4    3    2

*This book is dedicated to Waldo E. Nelson. His lifelong commitment to the physical and emotional health of children and to the education of those who care for children embodies the essential goals toward which we aspire.*

# Contributors

**Herbert T. Abelson, M.D.**

George M. Eisenberg Professor and Chairman, Department of Pediatrics, University of Chicago, Pritzker School of Medicine. Physician-in-Chief, University of Chicago Children's Hospital, Chicago, Illinois.
*Oncology*

**R. Stephen S. Amato, Ph.D., M.D.**

Clinical Professor, Department of Pediatrics, University of Maryland Medical Center. Lecturer, Department of Pediatrics, Johns Hopkins University School of Medicine. Chairman of Pediatrics and Director, Division of Medical Genetics, Department of Medicine, Greater Baltimore Medical Center, Baltimore, Maryland.
*Human Genetics and Dysmorphology*

**Ira Bergman, M.D.**

Professor of Pediatrics and Neurology, Department of Pediatrics, University of Pittsburgh School of Medicine. Attending Physician, Division of Child Neurology, Children's Hospital of Pittsburgh, Pittsburgh, Pennsylvania.
*Neurology*

**Dennis D. Black, M.D.**

Professor, Department of Pediatrics, University of Arkansas College of Medicine. Attending Physician, Arkansas Children's Hospital, Little Rock, Arkansas.
*The Gastrointestinal Tract*

**Michael M. Brook, M.D.**

Assistant Professor, Department of Pediatrics (Cardiology), and Associate Director, Pediatric Echocardiography, University of California, San Francisco, School of Medicine. Attending Pediatric Cardiologist, The Medical Center at the University of California, San Francisco, and Moffett-Long Hospitals, San Francisco, California.
*The Cardiovascular System*

**Aaron L. Friedman, M.D.**

Professor, Department of Pediatrics, University of Wisconsin Medical School. Chairman, Department of Pediatrics, University of Wisconsin Hospital and Clinics, Madison, Wisconsin.
*Nephrology: Fluids and Electrolytes*

**Nicole S. Glaser, M.D.**

Fellow in Pediatric Endocrinology, University of California, Davis, School of Medicine, Davis, California.
*Endocrine Disorders*

**Carolyn M. Kercsmar, M.D.**

Associate Professor, Department of Pediatrics, Case Western Reserve University School of Medicine. Director, Children's Asthma Center, Rainbow Babies and Children's Hospital, Cleveland, Ohio.
*The Respiratory System*

**Barbara S. Kirschner, M.D.**

Professor, Department of Pediatrics, University of Chicago, Pritzker School of Medicine. Attending Physician, University of Chicago Children's Hospital, Chicago, Illinois.
*The Gastrointestinal Tract*

**Robert M. Kliegman, M.D.**

Professor and Chairman, Department of Pediatrics, Medical College of Wisconsin. Pediatrician-in-Chief, Children's Hospital of Wisconsin, Milwaukee, Wisconsin.
*Fetal and Neonatal Medicine*

Richard E. Kreipe, M.D.

Associate Professor of Pediatrics and Chief, Division of Adolescent Medicine, University of Rochester School of Medicine and Dentistry, Rochester, New York.
*Adolescent Medicine*

Steven E. Krug, M.D.

Associate Professor, Department of Pediatrics, Northwestern University Medical School. Head, Division of Pediatric Emergency Medicine, Children's Memorial Hospital, Chicago, Illinois.
*The Acutely Ill or Injured Child*

Elizabeth R. McAnarney, M.D.

Professor and Chair, Department of Pediatrics, University of Rochester School of Medicine and Dentistry, Rochester, New York.
*Adolescent Medicine*

John F. Nicholson, M.D.

Associate Professor of Pediatrics and Pathology, Columbia University College of Physicians and Surgeons. Associate Attending Pediatrician, Babies and Children's Hospital, New York, New York.
*Inborn Errors of Metabolism*

Judyann C. Olson, M.D.

Associate Professor, Department of Pediatrics, Medical College of Wisconsin. Pediatric Rheumatologist, Children's Hospital of Wisconsin, Milwaukee, Wisconsin.
*Rheumatic Diseases of Childhood*

Michael J. Painter, M.D.

Professor of Neurology and Pediatrics, University of Pittsburgh School of Medicine. Chief, Division of Child Neurology, Children's Hospital of Pittsburgh, Pittsburgh, Pennsylvania.
*Neurology*

Alice Prince, M.D.

Professor, Department of Pediatrics, Columbia University College of Physicians and Surgeons. Attending Pediatrician, Babies and Children's Hospital, Columbia–Presbyterian Medical Center, New York, New York.
*Infectious Diseases*

J. Paul Scott, M.D.

Professor, Department of Pediatrics, Medical College of Wisconsin. Head, Department of Pediatric Hematology, Children's Hospital of Wisconsin, Milwaukee, Wisconsin.
*Hematology*

Virginia A. Stallings, M.D.

Associate Professor, Department of Pediatrics, University of Pennsylvania School of Medicine. Senior Physician, Children's Hospital of Philadelphia, Philadelphia, Pennsylvania.
*Pediatric Nutrition and Nutritional Disorders*

Dennis M. Styne, M.D.

Professor, Department of Pediatrics, University of California, Davis, School of Medicine, Davis, California.
*Endocrine Disorders*

Stephen B. Sulkes, M.D.

Associate Professor of Pediatrics, University of Rochester School of Medicine and Dentistry. Pediatric Discipline Coordinator, The Strong Memorial Hospital, Center for Developmental Disabilities, Children's Hospital at Strong, Rochester, New York.
*Developmental and Behavioral Pediatrics*

Andrew M. Tershakovec, M.D.

Assistant Professor, Department of Pediatrics, University of Pennsylvania School of Medicine. Associate Physician, Children's Hospital of Philadelphia, Philadelphia, Pennsylvania.
*Pediatric Nutrition and Nutritional Disorders*

George H. Thompson, M.D.

Professor, Department of Orthopaedic Surgery and Pediatrics, Case Western Reserve University. Director, Department of Pediatric Orthopaedics, Rainbow Babies and Children's Hospital, Cleveland, Ohio.
*Common Orthopaedic Problems of Children*

Dale T. Umetsu, M.D.

Associate Professor and Chief, Division of Allergy and Clinical Immunology, Department of Pediatrics, Stanford University School of Medicine. Director, Center for Allergy, Asthma, and Immunology, Lucile Salter Packard Hospital at Stanford, Stanford, California.
*Immunology and Allergy*

# Preface

The exponential expansion of the scope and content of pediatrics during the 20th century has been reflected in the 15 editions of *Nelson Textbook of Pediatrics*. Thus, it has continued to serve as the major reference text for those who care for children, incorporating progress in clinical care and biomedical science and technology. However, the explosion in information and understanding about normal growth and development and about the diagnosis, management, and prevention of the diseases and disorders of childhood has made it difficult for many medical students to read the entire text during a core pediatric clerkship. In publishing *Nelson Essentials*, we have addressed this issue by focusing on essential aspects of pediatric health and illness within the context of the special educational needs of the medical student and starting house officer.

*Nelson Essentials* is primarily intended to introduce important pediatric problems and diseases, representing both the common illnesses of childhood and the less common disorders of special educational importance that exemplify pathophysiologic mechanisms and disease processes. This book is not a "primer," and it is not a synopsis of or a companion to the *Nelson Textbook of Pediatrics*. The term "essential" does not mean "superficial" or "outlined." Rather, in a readable text with a simplified format and an array of tables and figures, *Nelson Essentials* provides students with sufficient information to improve their understanding of representative pediatric problems and clinical decisions, enabling them to gain a basic understanding of the particular disease process and to develop a clinical approach to a child's problem. In addition, the relatively short text can be digested during the usual length of a core pediatric clerkship.

The contents of this third edition have been significantly updated and incorporate many helpful suggestions made by students and faculty who used the second edition. We have organized each chapter in a way that reflects the clinical approach to patients. The student or house officer first should learn to generate a broad differential diagnosis based on the data obtained by taking a history and performing a physical examination; second, to perform an initial analysis of this information, which is facilitated by thinking in terms of the course of the illness (acute or chronic), the organ system involved, and the evidence suggesting that a particular pathophysiologic process may be present (e.g., infection or neoplasm); and third, to use this clinical information and its analysis to determine the kind of laboratory data that will further modify and narrow the list of diagnostic possibilities and lead to more specific diagnostic testing.

Besides organizing the chapters to reflect this logical process, we have emphasized the physiologic and pathophysiologic aspects of pediatric disease and, when applicable, the genetic bases, since the understanding of this biology is critical for clinical decision making. Each new contact the student has with a sick child and the family should reinforce the understanding of the pathophysiologic basis of disease and the psychosocial dynamics of illness.

Presenting the essentials of pediatric medicine does not always permit detailed discussion of the range of variations of each pediatric illness or disease or coverage of all of the less common disorders. To facilitate a student's interest in obtaining additional knowledge, cross-references to the relevant chapters in the 15th edition of *Nelson Textbook of Pediat-*

*rics* as well as selected references to other literature are provided.

The editors especially wish to express their gratitude and appreciation to the hard-working and dedicated authors of the individual chapters. In addition, we thank the many medical students, house staff, and faculty who provided constructive criticism that has improved the final text.

RICHARD E. BEHRMAN
ROBERT M. KLIEGMAN

# Contents

# Chapter 1

# DEVELOPMENTAL AND BEHAVIORAL PEDIATRICS

Stephen B. Sulkes

## GROWTH AND DEVELOPMENT

Knowledge of the normal growth and development of children is essential for preventing and detecting disease by recognizing overt deviations from normal patterns. Although the processes of growth and development are not completely separable, it is convenient to refer to "growth" as the increase in the size of the body as a whole or the increase in its separate parts, and to reserve "development" for changes in function, including those influenced by the emotional and social environments. The development of the human organism is a very large, complex topic, but in order to identify and treat underlying disorders, it is important for all who care for children to be familiar with normal patterns of growth and development so that they can recognize abnormal variations.

Within the broad limits that characterize normal development, every individual's path of growth and development through the life cycle is unique, with a range of complex, interrelated changes occurring from the molecular to the behavioral level. One goal of pediatrics is to help each child achieve his or her individual potential for growth and development, thus becoming a mature adult. An important means of accomplishing this goal involves periodically monitoring each child for the normal progression of growth and development and screening for abnormalities (Fig. 1–1).

### NORMAL GROWTH PATTERNS

Deviations in growth patterns are nonspecific but very important indicators of serious medical disorders. They often provide the first clue that something is wrong, occasionally even when the parents do not suspect a problem. An accurate measurement of height, weight, and head circumference should be obtained at every health supervision visit. Serial measurements are much more useful than single measurements because deviations from a particular child's growth pattern can be detected even if the value remains within arbitrarily defined normal limits (e.g., between the 3rd and the 97th percentiles).

Normal growth patterns have spurts and plateaus, so one can expect some shifting on percentile graphs, but large shifts warrant attention. Large discrepancies among height, weight, and head circumference percentiles also deserve attention. For example, when caloric intake is inadequate the weight percentile falls first, then the height, and last the head circumference. Similarly, an increasing weight percentile in the face of a falling height percentile suggests hypothyroidism. A head circumference that is disproportionately large may occur when there is familial megalencephaly, hydrocephalus, or merely "catch-up" growth in a neurologically normal premature infant. Serial measurement of head circumference along with the history (knowing the size of the parents' heads is essential) and the current physical examination helps to distinguish among these possibilities.

Whenever possible, growth should be assessed by plotting accurate measurements on growth charts (Figs. 1–2 to 1–14), and comparing them with previous measurements. The most common reasons for deviant measurements are technical (faulty equipment and human errors in measurement or plotting), so the first step in investigating a deviant measurement should be to repeat it. It is also helpful to know some rough rules of thumb, as presented in Table 1–1 (see p. 16).

1

Each child and family is unique; therefore, these **Recommendations for Preventive Pediatric Health Care** are designed for the care of children who are receiving competent parenting, have no important health problems, and are growing and developing in satisfactory fashion. **Additional visits may become necessary** if circumstances suggest variations from normal.

## Committee on Practice and Ambulatory Medicine

These guidelines represent a consensus by the Committee on Practice and Ambulatory Medicine in consultation with national committees and sections of the American Academy of Pediatrics. The Committee emphasizes the great importance of **continuity of care** in comprehensive health supervision and the need to avoid **fragmentation of care.**

A **prenatal visit** is recommended for parents who are at high risk, for first-time parents, and for those who request a conference. The prenatal visit should include anticipatory guidance and pertinent medical history. Every infant should have a newborn evaluation after birth.

| AGE[4] | NEWBORN[1] | 2–4d[2] | By 1mo | 2mo | 4mo | 6mo | 9mo | 12mo | 15mo | 18mo | 24mo | 3y | 4y | 5y | 6y | 8y | 10y | 11y | 12y | 13y | 14y | 15y | 16y | 17y | 18y | 19y | 20y | 21y |
|---|---|---|---|---|---|---|---|---|---|---|---|---|---|---|---|---|---|---|---|---|---|---|---|---|---|---|---|---|
| | | | | INFANCY[3] | | | | | | | | EARLY CHILDHOOD[3] | | | MIDDLE CHILDHOOD[3] | | | ADOLESCENCE[3] | | | | | | | | | | |
| **HISTORY** Initial/Interval | • | • | • | • | • | • | • | • | • | • | • | • | • | • | • | • | • | • | • | • | • | • | • | • | • | • | • | • |
| **MEASUREMENTS** | | | | | | | | | | | | | | | | | | | | | | | | | | | | |
| Height and Weight | • | • | • | • | • | • | • | • | • | • | • | • | • | • | • | • | • | • | • | • | • | • | • | • | • | • | • | • |
| Head Circumference | • | • | • | • | • | • | • | • | • | • | | | | | | | | | | | | | | | | | | |
| Blood Pressure | | | | | | | | | | | | • | • | • | • | • | • | • | • | • | • | • | • | • | • | • | • | • |
| **SENSORY SCREENING** | | | | | | | | | | | | | | | | | | | | | | | | | | | | |
| Vision | S | S | S | S | S | S | S | S | S | S | S | O[5] | O | O | O | O | O | S | O | S | S | O | S | S | O | S | S | O |
| Hearing[6] | S/O | S | S | S | S | S | S | S | S | S | S | O | O | O | O | O | O | S | O | S | S | O | S | S | O | S | S | O |
| **DEVELOPMENTAL/ BEHAVIORAL ASSESSMENT[7]** | • | • | • | • | • | • | • | • | • | • | • | • | • | • | • | • | • | • | • | • | • | • | • | • | • | • | • | • |
| **PHYSICAL EXAMINATION[8]** | • | • | • | • | • | • | • | • | • | • | • | • | • | • | • | • | • | • | • | • | • | • | • | • | • | • | • | • |
| **PROCEDURES—GENERAL[9]** | | | | | | | | | | | | | | | | | | | | | | | | | | | | |
| Hereditary/Metabolic Screening[10] | •←—→ | | | | | | | | | | | | | | | | | | | | | | | | | | | |
| Immunization[11] | • | | • | • | • | • | | • | • | • | | | • | • | • | | | • | • | | | | | | | | | |
| Hematocrit or Hemoglobin | | | | | | | | • | | | • | | | | | | | | | | | | | | | | | |
| Urinalysis | • | | | | | | | | | | • | | | • | | | | | | | | | | | | | | • |
| **PROCEDURES—PATIENTS AT RISK** | | | | | | | | | | | | | | | | | | | | | | | | | | | | |
| Lead Screening[12] | | | | | | | | • | | | • | | | | | | | | | | | | | | | | | |
| Tuberculin Test[15] | | | | | | | | ★ | ★ | ★ | ★ | ★ | ★ | ★ | ★ | ★ | ★ | ★ | ★ | ★ | ★ | ★ | ★ | ★ | ★ | ★ | ★ | ★ |
| Cholesterol Screening[16] | | | | | | | | | | | | | | | | | | ★ | ★ | ★ | ★ | ★ | ★ | ★ | ★ | ★ | ★ | ★ |
| STD Screening[17] | | | | | | | | | | | | | | | | | | ★ | ★ | ★ | ★ | ★ | ★ | ★ | ★ | ★ | ★ | ★ |
| Pelvic Exam[18] | | | | | | | | | | | | | | | | | | ★ | ★ | ★ | ★ | ★ | ★ | ★ | ★ | ★ | ★ | ★ |
| **ANTICIPATORY GUIDANCE[19]** | • | • | • | • | • | • | • | • | • | • | • | • | • | • | • | • | • | • | • | • | • | • | • | • | • | • | • | • |
| **INJURY PREVENTION[20]** | • | • | • | • | • | • | • | • | • | • | • | • | • | • | • | • | • | • | • | • | • | • | • | • | • | • | • | • |
| **INITIAL DENTAL REFERRAL[21]** | | | | | | | | | | | | • | | | | | | | | | | | | | | | | |

1. Breastfeeding encouraged and instruction and support offered.
2. For newborns discharged in less than 48 hours after delivery.
3. Developmental, psychosocial, and chronic disease issues for children and adolescents may require frequent counseling and treatment visits separate from preventive care visits.
4. If a child comes under care for the first time at any point on the schedule, or if any items are not accomplished at the suggested age, the schedule should be brought up to date at the earliest possible time.
5. If the patient is uncooperative, rescreen within six months.
6. Some experts recommend objective appraisal of hearing in the newborn period. The Joint Committee on Infant Hearing has identified patients at significant risk for hearing loss. All children meeting these criteria should be objectively screened. See the Joint Committee on Infant Hearing 1994 Position Statement.
7. By history and appropriate physical examination; if suspicious, by specific objective developmental testing.
8. At each visit, a complete physical examination is essential, with infant totally unclothed, older child undressed and suitably draped.
9. These may be modified, depending upon entry point into schedule and individual need.
10. Metabolic screening (eg, thyroid, hemoglobinopathies, PKU, galactosemia) should be done according to state law.
11. Schedule(s) per the Committee on Infectious Diseases, published periodically in *Pediatrics.* Every visit should be an opportunity to update and complete a child's immunizations.
12. Blood lead screen per AAP statement "Lead Poisoning: From Screening to Primary Prevention" (1993).
13. All menstruating adolescents should be screened.
14. Conduct dipstick urinalysis for leukocytes for male and female adolescents.
15. TB testing per AAP statement "Screening for Tuberculosis in Infants and Children" (1994). Testing should be done upon recognition of high risk factors. If results are negative but high risk situation continues, testing should be repeated on an annual basis.
16. Cholesterol screening for high risk patients per AAP "Statement on Cholesterol" (1992). If family history cannot be ascertained and other risk factors are present, screening should be at the discretion of the physician.
17. All sexually active patients should be screened for sexually transmitted diseases (STDs).
18. All sexually active females should have a pelvic examination. A pelvic examination and routine pap smear should be offered as a part of preventive health maintenance between the ages of 18 and 21 years.
19. Appropriate discussion and counseling should be an integral part of each visit for care.
20. From birth to age 12, refer to AAP's injury prevention program (TIPP®) as described in "A Guide to Safety Counseling in Office Practice" (1994).
21. Earlier initial dental evaluations may be appropriate for some children. Subsequent examinations as prescribed by dentist.

Key: • = to be performed   ★ = to be performed for patients at risk   S = subjective, by history   O = objective, by a standard testing method   ←—→ = the range during which a service may be provided, with the dot indicating the preferred age.

NB: Special chemical, immunologic, and endocrine testing is usually carried out upon specific indications. Testing other than newborn (eg, inborn errors of metabolism sickle disease, etc.) is discretionary with the physician.

The recommendations in this publication do not indicate an exclusive course of treatment or serve as a standard of medical care. Variations, taking into account individual circumstances, may be appropriate.

FIGURE 1–1. Recommendations for preventive pediatric health care. (From Committee on Practice and Ambulatory Medicine, American Academy of Pediatrics. Pediatrics, 96[2], 1995. Copyright American Academy of Pediatrics, 1995.)

FIGURE 1–2. Length by age percentiles for girls, ages birth to 36 mo. (From Hamill PVV, Drizd TA, Johnson CL, et al: Physical growth: National Center for Health Statistics percentiles. Am J Clin Nutr 32:729, 1979. © American Society for Clinical Nutrition.)

*Variability in body proportions* occurs from fetal to adult life (Fig. 1–15). There is also considerable variation in body form among normal children, often following familial patterns. Differences in body proportions depend on variations in the growth rates of parts of the body or organ systems. Certain growth disturbances result in characteristic changes in the proportional sizes of trunk, extremities, and head.

There are distinctive patterns of proportionate growth rates for several body systems that correlate closely with function. Growth of the nervous system is most rapid in the first 2 yr, whereas the growth rate for lymphoid tissue peaks at about 12 yr. Osseous maturation (bone age) is determined from roentgenograms on the basis of (1) the number and size of epiphyseal centers; (2) the size, shape, density, and sharpness of outline of the ends of bones; and (3) the distance separating the epiphyseal center from the zone of provisional calcification. Functional correlations also exist between growing systems. Thus, bone age corresponds more closely to sexual maturity, which is dependent on the growth and development of the endocrine system, than to chronologic age. The heart is relatively large at birth, and a pubertal growth spurt in its size parallels the general growth spurt. Pulse rate and blood pressure vary with age and growth, as do a great many metabolic and nutritional changes.

## References

Behrman RE, Kliegman RM, Arvin AM (eds): Nelson Textbook of Pediatrics, 15th ed. Philadelphia, WB Saunders, 1996, Chapters 9–13.

FIGURE 1–3. Weight by age percentiles for girls, ages birth to 36 mo. (From Hamill PVV, Drizd TA, Johnson CL, et al: Physical growth: National Center for Health Statistics percentiles. Am J Clin Nutr 32:729, 1979. © American Society for Clinical Nutrition.)

Hall D: Monitoring children's growth, BMJ 311:583, 1995.
Lowrey GH: Growth and Development of Children, 8th ed. Chicago, Year Book Medical Publishers, 1986.

## DEVELOPMENTAL MILESTONES AND THEORIES

The use of developmental milestones to assess development focuses on discrete behaviors that can be observed by the clinician or accepted as present by parental report. The approach is based on comparing the patient's behavior with that of many normal children whose behaviors evolve in a uniform sequence and within specific age ranges. A behavior is the response of the neuromotor system to a specific situation, and the development of this system, like that of other organ systems, is determined largely by genetic endowment. Environment influences development mainly by distorting the normal pattern.

Norms for discrete behaviors provide a convenient way to monitor development (Fig. 1–16 and Assessment later in the chapter), but they provide an incomplete picture. Although a sequence of specific, easily measured behaviors can adequately represent some areas of development (e.g., gross motor, fine motor, language), other areas, particularly social and emotional development, are not adequately assessed by this means. In addition, easily measured developmental milestones are only well established through age 6 yr. Many other types of assessment, including intelligence tests, achievement tests, personality profiles, and neurodevelopmental assessments that expand the developmental milestone approach beyond age 6 yr, are available for all ages, but they generally require

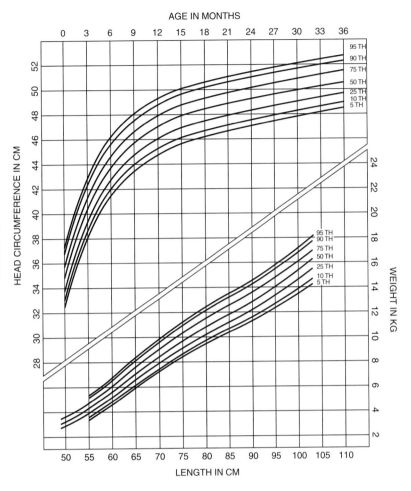

FIGURE 1–4. Head circumference and weight by length percentiles for girls, ages birth to 36 mo. (From Hamill PVV, Drizd TA, Johnson CL, et al: Physical growth: National Center for Health Statistics percentiles. Am J Clin Nutr 32:729, 1979. © American Society for Clinical Nutrition.)

time and expertise in administration and/or interpretation that are not available in the primary care medical setting.

Pediatricians therefore need to supplement their screening of developmental milestones with less precise but possibly more important screening of psychosocial issues that are pertinent at each age. The following brief presentation of some developmental theories is intended as an introduction to these important areas.

## Piaget

Piaget's theory is the major theory of cognitive development. *Cognition* is defined as the process of knowing in the broadest sense, including perception, memory, judgment, and reasoning. Piaget contended that the development of cognitive ability occurs in a fixed sequence of qualitatively different stages; that is, a child's mind works in different ways in each stage. Table 1–2 presents a brief outline of the major characteristics of each stage

(see p. 18). Unrealistic parental expectations often result from lack of understanding about how a child's logic differs from that of an adult. A behavioral problem often can be improved by helping the parent see an episode of problem behavior from the child's perspective.

Piagetian theory also includes the concept of **equilibration**, the mechanism for the formation of knowledge. Equilibration involves two processes that are set in motion when a person is confronted with a new situation that he or she does not fully understand: (1) **assimilation** involves attempts to reshape the new experience to make it fit with accustomed ways of thinking, and (2) **accommodation** involves revisions in the accustomed ways of thinking to fit with the new experience. When the disequilibrium produced by the new experience is resolved by using both processes, a new equilibration is achieved at a higher level of cognitive organization. Disequilibrium, thus, is a necessary stimulus for development. Avoidance of new or unfamiliar experiences will limit the chances for

FIGURE 1–5. Stature by age percentiles for girls, ages 2–18 yr. (From Hamill PVV, Drizd TA, Johnson CL, et al: Physical growth: National Center for Health Statistics percentiles. Am J Clin Nutr 32:729, 1979. © American Society for Clinical Nutrition.)

cognitive growth. An important related concept is *cognitive dissonance*, the degree to which a new stimulus differs from familiar stimuli. Novelty attracts children, but if the cognitive dissonance is too great, they will be frightened or frustrated and will not achieve a new equilibrium (cognitive growth).

### Freud

Freudian theory contains a number of concepts helpful in understanding child development. The principle of *psychic determinism* holds that no psychic event happens in a chance or random way but instead is determined by preceding psychic events. "Freudian slips" (e.g., forgetting a meeting that is expected to be stressful) illustrate this principle. At a conscious level, these seem to be simple mistakes with no apparent explanation, but the theory contends that unconscious mental processes are responsible for their occurrence. A patient's explana-tion for a behavior or recounting of an event taps only the conscious level; probing questions may bring more information to the conscious level. The concept of innate sexual and aggressive drives that provide "psychic energy" also is central to Freudian theory. Freud proposed five stages of psychosexual development, with different parts of the body serving as the focus of gratification of the sexual drive at different ages (Table 1–3) (see p. 19).

One of Freud's most enduring contributions is his hypothesis about the organization of mental processes into id, ego, and superego. The **id** is the source of the person's impulses and drives and is dominant at birth. The **ego** is the pragmatic, rational part of the mind, consisting of those functions that have to do with the individual's relationship to the environment (sensory perception, motor control, memory, affect, thinking). Initially the ego is the servant of the id, finding ways to achieve gratification of the id impulses. Gradually, the ego exerts increasing control over the id in the service

FIGURE 1–6. Weight by age percentiles for girls, ages 2–18 yr. (From Hamill PVV, Drizd TA, Johnson CL, et al: Physical growth: National Center for Health Statistics percentiles. Am J Clin Nutr 32:729, 1979. © American Society for Clinical Nutrition.)

of greater long-term gratification and avoidance of discomfort. The **superego**, or "conscience," comprises the moral precepts of an individual's mind and his or her ideal aspirations.

*Identification* is one of the hypothesized processes by which the ego gains mastery over the id; it is manifested by a child's identifying with people or things that are highly charged with psychic energy. Identification is apparent in the observation that children behave according to what they see and experience rather than what they are told. Fantasized gratification is another process by which the ego gains mastery over the id. A *fantasy* (dream or daydream) in which the wishes of the id are represented as fulfilled results in partial gratification of id impulses. The id impulse may be so nearly satisfied that it is easy for the ego to control the impulse afterward. This is the idea behind play therapy.

The most important factor in the control of id impulses is *anxiety*. "Automatic anxiety" develops whenever a child's psyche is overwhelmed by a flood of stimuli too great to be mastered or discharged. These stimuli may be external, but most often they are internal, arising from the id. This type of anxiety is characteristic of infancy because of the immaturity of the ego, but it also is found in adult life in cases of anxiety neurosis. In the course of development, the ego acquires the capacity to produce "signal anxiety" when a potential danger situation arises (i.e., the threat of a traumatic situation), which enables the ego to inhibit id impulses. Freud proposed the following sequence of danger situations in early and later childhood that persist unconsciously to some degree throughout life:

1. Loss of the object—separation from a person or thing that is an important source of gratification.
2. Loss of the object's love.
3. Loss of the penis (or analogous genital injury in females).

STATURE IN INCHES

FIGURE 1–7. Weight by stature percentiles for prepubertal girls. (From Hamill PVV, Drizd TA, Johnson CL, et al: Physical growth: National Center for Health Statistics percentiles. Am J Clin Nutr 32:729, 1979. © American Society for Clinical Nutrition.)

4. Guilt, or disapproval of the superego.

**Defense mechanisms** are unconscious ego processes that focus narrowly on the reduction of anxiety by the control of id impulses. *Repression* occurs when the ego bars from consciousness the unwanted id impulse. *Suppression* is the conscious equivalent of repression. *Reaction formation* occurs when one of a pair of ambivalent attitudes is made unconscious and kept unconscious by an overemphasis on the other (e.g., love/hate, cruelty/gentleness, and stubbornness/compliance). Reactions to a new sibling may include the use of defense mechanisms such as *repression* (of hostile wishes toward the sibling) and *reaction formation* (love instead of hate) as well as other ego processes such as *identification* with the mother (imitating caregiving). Other common defense mechanisms include *denial*—the disavowal of an unpleasant or unwanted piece of external reality (repression involves internal impulses), and *projection*—the attribution of one's own wish or impulse to another person (e.g., the imaginary friend in early childhood).

Defense mechanisms are evidence of healthy coping as well as a sign of anxiety. Therefore, in the treatment of anxiety, the aim is not to attack the defense mechanism directly but, rather, to understand the source of the anxiety that creates the need for the defense mechanism and to work toward the removal of the source.

According to Freud, resolving the *Oedipus complex* between the ages of 3 and 6 yr results in development of the superego. The Oedipus complex involves an ambivalent attitude toward both parents regardless of the gender of the child (e.g., a wish to eliminate the jealously hated father and take his place in a sensual relationship with the mother). Such wishes arouse fears of retaliation and the loss of love, resulting in the formation of the superego to control the impulses. Subsequently, the superego becomes the principal source of anxiety, guilt, and unconscious feelings of inferiority but may also produce feelings of joy and self-satisfaction.

### Erikson

Erikson revised and expanded Freud's psychosexual stages into psychosocial stages that span the life cycle. His theory emphasized the development of the ego within a social context rather than on the instinctual drives of the id. Erikson's stages start from a focus on a particular part of the body and then expand to a consideration of the social context of the child's behavior (see Table 1-3). For example, in Freud's oral stage, the major mode of gratification includes sucking and feeding. In Erikson's parallel stage, the major psychosocial issue involves the development of "basic trust versus basic mistrust" that the mother will meet the infant's needs. Similarly, in the next stage Erikson

goes beyond Freud's narrow focus on bowel control (anal stage) and proposes "autonomy versus shame and doubt" as the central psychosocial issue. Specific behaviors that may serve as the focus of the child's struggle with this psychosocial issue include toilet training but may be generalized to other behaviors that involve control of the body and the environment.

Normal resolution of each psychosocial issue involves the development of a balance between the positive and negative attitudes that characterize the issue, with a ratio favoring the positive. Each issue is never completely resolved but becomes part of the developmental history of the individual, which influences the resolution of each subsequent stage. The sequence of issues proposed by Erikson coincides with the widening circle of societal exposures and demands that are common to all human cultures. Individuals may **regress** to an earlier stage when a previously attained balance is disrupted by new events and stresses (e.g., birth of a sibling, starting school, illness, separation from

FIGURE 1–9. Weight by age percentiles for boys, ages birth to 36 mo. (From Hamill PVV, Drizd TA, Johnson CL, et al: Physical growth: National Center for Health Statistics percentiles. Am J Clin Nutr 32:729, 1979. © American Society for Clinical Nutrition.)

loved ones, moves, family turmoil). Puberty and adolescence frequently upset balances achieved in preceding stages and require a reworking of the issues to achieve new balances.

### References

Behrman RE, Kliegman RM, Arvin AM (eds): Nelson Textbook of Pediatrics, 15th ed. Philadelphia, WB Saunders, 1996, Chapters 8, 11–15.

Brenner C: An Elementary Textbook of Psychoanalysis. Garden City, NY, Doubleday, 1973.

Erikson EH: Childhood and Society, 2nd ed. New York, WW Norton, 1963.

Ginsburg H, Opper S: Piaget's Theory of Intellectual Development, 2nd ed. Englewood Cliffs, NJ, Prentice-Hall, 1979.

### BONDING AND ATTACHMENT

Bonding and attachment are terms that describe the affectional relationships between parents and infants. **Bonding** occurs rapidly, shortly after birth and reflects the feelings of the parents toward the newborn (unidirectional); **attachment** involves reciprocal feelings between parent and infant and develops gradually over the first year. Effective bonding in the postpartum period may enhance the development of attachment. An increased awareness of the importance of bonding has led to significant improvements in routine birthing procedures and postpartum parent-infant contact.

Attachment to a specific, stable parent figure is crucial for a child's normal mental and physical development. Beyond mere feeding and protection, attachment to a primary caregiver also serves to promote exploration of the environment and learning.

Between 9 and 18 mo, children normally become insecure about separation from the primary caregiver. This insecurity coincides with the child's increasing cognitive and motor abilities. The child is beginning to understand simple, immediate, cause-and-effect relationships and thus can anticipate separations (e.g., after Mommy gets her coat) but still has an inadequate appreciation of time

FIGURE 1–10. Head circumference and weight by length percentiles for boys, ages birth to 36 mo. (From Hamill PVV, Drizd TA, Johnson CL, et al: Physical growth: National Center for Health Statistics percentiles. Am J Clin Nutr 32:729, 1979. © American Society for Clinical Nutrition.)

and delayed gratification. In addition, the child's new motor skills and attraction to novelty may lead to headlong plunges into new adventures that result in fright or pain followed by frantic efforts to find and cling to the primary caregiver. This often results in dramatic swings from stubborn independence to clinging dependence that can be frustrating and confusing to parents. With a secure attachment, the period of ambivalence may be shorter and less tumultuous.

### References

Ainsworth M: The development of infant-mother attachment. *In* Caldwell BM, Ricciuti HN (eds): Child Development and Social Policy. Review of Child Development Research Series. Vol 3. New York, Russell Sage Foundation, 1973, 1–94.

Behrman RE, Kliegman RM, Arvin AM (eds): Nelson Textbook of Pediatrics, 15th ed. Philadelphia, WB Saunders, 1996, Chapters 8–12.

Crittenden PM: Attachment and risk for psychopathology: The early years. J Dev Behav Pediatr 16(3 Suppl):S12, 1995.

## LEARNING THEORY

Learning theory postulates that behavior is primarily a product of external environmental determinants and that manipulation of the environmental antecedents and consequences of behavior can be used to modify maladaptive behavior and to increase desirable behavior. **Conditioning** is the process through which behavior is modified by environmental manipulations.

*Respondent (classic) conditioning* is illustrated by Pavlov's famous experiment in which a dog's salivary response was conditioned to occur at the sound of a bell. The experiment starts with an automatic stimulus-response relationship—food (unconditioned stimulus) stimulating salivation (unconditioned response). Conditioning occurs when another stimulus (bell ringing in Pavlov's experiment) is presented just before or with the unconditioned stimulus (food). After many presentations of the two stimuli together, the bell (conditioned stimulus) alone will elicit the response:

FIGURE 1–11.  Stature by age percentiles for boys, ages 2–18 yr. (From Hamill PVV, Drizd TA, Johnson CL, et al: Physical growth: National Center for Health Statistics percentiles. Am J Clin Nutr 32:729, 1979. © American Society for Clinical Nutrition.)

salivation (conditioned response). Respondent conditioning has been used to explain **phobic behavior,** in which a previously unfeared object or stimulus now arouses fear because it is associated with the occurrence of an unconditioned fearful stimulus (e.g., an episode of falling off a diving board leads to a fear of all swimming). Phobias can be treated by *desensitization,* a process involving training in relaxation techniques, later coupled with gradual exposure to stimuli associated more and more closely with the feared stimulus. The most effective treatment currently available for nocturnal enuresis involves respondent conditioning (see Enuresis).

*Operant conditioning* modifies behavior by manipulating the antecedents or the consequences of the behavior. The four major methods for operant conditioning are positive reinforcement, negative reinforcement, extinction, and punishment. Many common behavioral problems of children can be helped by these methods.

**Positive reinforcement** occurs when there is an increase in the frequency of a behavior because it is followed by a favorable event (e.g., the child who eats vegetables more often after being rewarded with dessert). **Negative reinforcement** occurs when there is an increase in the frequency of a behavior because it is followed by the removal or avoidance of an unpleasant event (e.g., a parent's wrath is avoided by staying away from the stove). Conversely, reinforcement also may occur unintentionally, increasing the frequency of an undesirable behavior. **Extinction** occurs when there is a decrease in the frequency of a previously reinforced behavior because the reinforcement is withheld. This is the principle behind the common advice to ignore such behavior as crying at bedtime or temper tantrums that parents may unwittingly reinforce through attention and comforting. **Punishment** occurs when there is a decrease in the frequency of a behavior because it is followed by an unpleasant consequence.

FIGURE 1–12. Weight by age percentiles for boys, ages 2–18 yr. (From Hamill PVV, Drizd TA, Johnson CL, et al: Physical growth: National Center for Health Statistics percentiles. Am J Clin Nutr 32:729, 1979. © American Society for Clinical Nutrition.)

## References

Behrman RE, Kliegman RM, Arvin AM (eds): Nelson Textbook of Pediatrics, 15th ed. Philadelphia, WB Saunders, 1996, Chapter 8.

Graziano AM, Diament DM: Parent behavioral training: An examination of the paradigm. Behav Modif 16(1):3, 1992.

Hirsh DLO, Russo DC: Behavior management. In Levine MD, Carey WB, Crocker AC, Gross RT (eds): Developmental-Behavioral Pediatrics. Philadelphia, WB Saunders, 1983, pp 1068–1099.

## INDIVIDUAL DIFFERENCES

Normal children differ widely in behavior. Failure to appreciate this fact may result in labeling behavior as abnormal or pathologic when the problem may be simply that the behavior does not fit into an expected pattern that is too narrowly defined. Although there are always gray areas between clearly normal and clearly abnormal behavior, in clinical situations the differentiation between abnormal and normal (although perhaps unusual) behavior frequently rests on a judgment of whether the behavior is adaptive. This judgment must be made in the context of the environment in which the individual functions as well as in the context of the unique physical and mental characteristics of the individual. Alternatively, the physician must avoid explaining away serious problems by attributing them to individual variations in behavior.

There are significant individual differences in the normal development of **temperament** (behavioral style). There are three common constellations of temperamental characteristics:

1. The "easy child" (40%) is characterized by regularity of biologic functions (consistent, predictable times for eating, sleeping, and elimination), positive approach to new stimuli, high adaptability to change, mild or moderate intensity in responses, and a positive mood.

FIGURE 1–13. Weight by stature percentiles for prepubertal boys. (From Hamill PVV, Drizd TA, Johnson CL, et al: Physical growth: National Center for Health Statistics percentiles. Am J Clin Nutr 32:729, 1979. © American Society for Clinical Nutrition.)

2. The "difficult child" (10%) is characterized by irregularity of biologic functions, negative withdrawal from new stimuli, poor adaptability, intense responses, and a negative mood.
3. The "slow-to-warm-up child" (15%) is characterized by a low activity level, withdrawal from new stimuli, slow adaptability, mild intensity in responses, and somewhat negative mood.

The remaining children have more mixed temperaments. The individual temperament of a child has important implications for parenting and for the advice a pediatrician may give in anticipatory guidance or behavior problem counseling (see Management of Developmental and Behavioral Problems).

Although temperament may be to some degree "hard wired" (nature) in each child, the environment (nurture) in which the child grows has a strong impact on the child's adjustment ("goodness of fit"). Social and cultural factors can have marked effects on the child through differences in parenting style, educational approaches, and behavioral expectations. Although we are only beginning to understand the multitude of ways in which the environment can influence development, aspects of the environment clearly play an important role in the etiology and management of many behavioral problems of children.

Gardner noted variable patterns in cognitive processes described as "multiple intelligences." Based on observations of geniuses and individuals with unique skills, this theory suggests that most people have unique mixes of innate strengths and

FIGURE 1–14. Changes in head circumference with age for boys and girls. (From Nellhaus G: Composite international and interracial graphs. Pediatrics 41:106, 1968.)

TABLE 1–1.  Rules of Thumb for Growth

**Weight**
1. Weight loss in first few days: 5–10% of birth weight
2. Return to birth weight: 7–10 days of age
   Double birth weight: 4–5 mo
   Triple birth weight: 1 yr
   Quadruple birth weight: 2 yr
3. Average weights: 3.5 kg at birth
   10 kg at 1 yr
   20 kg at 5 yr
   30 kg at 10 yr
4. Daily weight gain: 20–30 g for first 3–4 mo
   15–20 g for rest of the first yr
5. Average annual weight gain: 5 lb between 2 yr and puberty (spurts and plateaus may occur)

**Height**
1. Average length: 20 inches at birth, 30 inches at 1 yr
2. At age 3 yr, the average child is 3 ft tall
3. At age 4 yr, the average child is 40 in tall (double birth length)
4. Average annual height increase: 2–3 inches between age 4 yr and puberty

**Head Circumference (HC)**
1. Average HC: 35 cm at birth (13.5 inches)
2. HC increases: 1 cm/mo for first yr (2 cm/mo for first 3 mo, then slower)
   10 cm for rest of life

weaknesses. Recognizing the strengths and weaknesses of an individual can be useful in planning for school, career, and recreational aspects of life.

### References

Behrman RE, Kliegman RM, Arvin AM (eds): Nelson Textbook of Pediatrics, 15th ed. Philadelphia, WB Saunders, 1996, Chapter 8.
Bronfenbrenner U: The Ecology of Human Development. Cambridge, MA, Harvard University Press, 1979.
Carey WB: Temperament issues in the school-aged child. Pediatr Clin North Am 39(3):569, 1992.
Gardner H: Multiple Intelligences: The Theory in Practice. New York, BasicBooks, 1993, p xvi.

## ADOLESCENCE

Early, middle, and late adolescence are characterized by different behavioral and developmental issues (see Table 7–3). The age at which each issue becomes manifest and the importance of these issues vary widely among individuals, as do the rates of cognitive, psychosexual, psychosocial, and physical development.

During *early adolescence*, a young person experiences maximal somatic and sexual growth. Thinking is focused on the present and on the peer group. Identity is focused primarily on the physical changes, and concern is about normality. Exploratory, undifferentiated sexual behavior resulting in physical contact with same-sexed peers is normal during early adolescence, although heterosexual interests can also develop. Strivings for independence are ambivalent.

*Middle adolescence* can be a most difficult time for both adolescents and the adults who have contact with them. Cognitive processes are more sophisticated. Through formal operational thinking, middle adolescents can experiment with ideas, consider things as they might be, develop insight, and reflect on their own feelings and those of others. As they mature cognitively and psychosocially, these adolescents focus on issues of identity not limited solely to the physical aspects of the body. As middle adolescents socialize with peers, experiment sexually, engage in risk-taking behaviors, and develop employment and interests outside the home, they augment their unique, developing identities. As a result of experimental, risk-taking behaviors, they may experience unwanted pregnancies, drug addiction, or motor vehicle accidents. The strivings of the middle adolescent for independence, testing of limits, and need for autonomy are maximal and often distressing to their families, teachers, or other authority figures.

*Late adolescence* is usually marked by full formal operational thinking, including thoughts about the future (educationally, vocationally, and sexually). Late adolescents are usually more committed to their sexual partners than are middle adolescents. Unresolved separation anxiety from previous developmental stages may emerge at this time as the young person begins to move physically away from the family of origin to college or vocational school, a job, or military service.

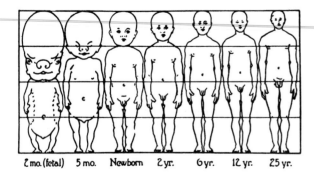

FIGURE 1–15.  Changes in body proportions from second fetal month to adulthood. (From Robbins WJ, et al: Growth. New Haven, Yale University Press, 1928, by permission of the publisher.)

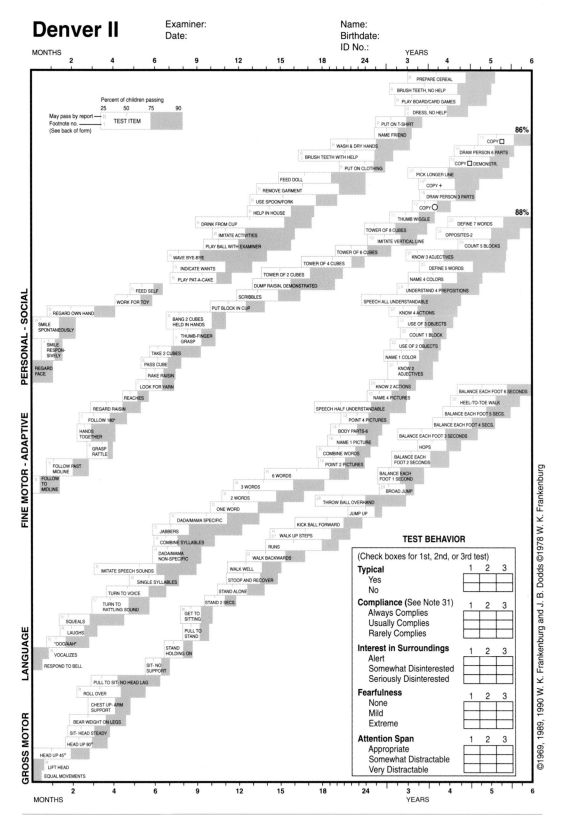

FIGURE 1–16. Scoring form for Denver II (Denver Developmental Screening Test, 2nd ed). (From Frankenburg WK, Dodds JB: Denver, Denver Developmental Materials, Inc. Copyright 1990 by W. K. Frankenburg and J.B. Dodds.)

**TABLE 1–2.** Jean Piaget's Stages of Cognitive Development

| Stage | Description | Major Developments |
|---|---|---|
| *Sensorimotor*<br>Birth to 2 yr | Learning occurs through activity, exploration, and manipulation of the environment. Motor and sensory impressions form the foundation of later learning. | Learns to differentiate self from world—beginning sense of self-identity.<br>Formation and integration of schemes—as in learning that sucking on a nipple produces milk or that shaking a rattle produces a noise.<br>Achieves object permanence—that things exist even when not visible. Simple tool use. |
| *Preoperational*<br>2 to 6 or 7 yr | Child capable of symbolic representations of world, as in use of language, play, and deferred imitation. Still not capable of sustained, systematic thought. | Engages in symbolic play—can represent something with something else.<br>Some decline in egocentricity—can take greater account of others' points of view.<br>Develops language and drawing as modes of representing experience. |
| *Concrete Operations*<br>6 or 7 to 11 yr | Child becomes capable of limited logical thought processes, as in seeing relationships and classifying, as long as manipulable, concrete materials are available. | Becomes aware that some aspects of things remain the same despite changes in appearance (conservation).<br>Can mentally reverse a process or action (reversibility).<br>Can focus on more than one aspect of a situation at a time (decentration).<br>Can deduce new relationships from sets of earlier ones (transitivity).<br>Can order things in sequence (seriation).<br>Can group objects on the basis of common features (classification). |
| *Formal Operations*<br>12 yr through adulthood | Can reason logically and abstractly. Can formulate and test hypotheses. Thought no longer depends on concrete reality. Can play with possibilities. | Can deal with abstract ideas.<br>Can manipulate variables in a scientific situation.<br>Can deal with analogies and metaphors.<br>Can reflect on own thinking.<br>Can work out combinations and permutations. |

Adapted from Stone LJ, Church J: Childhood and Adolescence. New York, Random House, 1979, pp 42–43.

## References

Behrman RE, Kliegman RM, Arvin AM (eds): Nelson Textbook of Pediatrics 15th ed. Philadelphia, WB Saunders, 1996, Chapters 15, 102–115.

Litt IF: Pubertal and psychosocial development implications for pediatricians. Pediatr Rev 16(7):243, 1995.

McAnarney E, Kreipe R, Orr DP, Comerci G. (eds): Textbook of Adolescent Medicine. Philadelphia, WB Saunders, 1992.

# ASSESSMENT

## THE PRIMARY CARE SETTING

### Initial History and Observations

Developmental and behavioral problems are more common than any category of problems in pediatrics except acute infections and trauma. Parents often neglect to mention these problems because they think the physician is uninterested or cannot help. Therefore, there is a need to screen for the presence of such problems in every health supervision visit, particularly in the preschool years when the pediatrician may be the only professional to evaluate the child. The limited time allotted to each health supervision visit will not allow a detailed assessment, but it is essential that a few questions be asked to supplement observations of the child's behavior during the visit. This also will encourage parents to express behavioral and developmental concerns about the child that then can be the focus of anticipatory guidance or early problem solving. Table 1–4 suggests an outline of topics for screening in health supervision visits.

The environment in which the child grows and

TABLE 1–3.  Stage Theories of Socioemotional Development

| | Birth–18 mo | 18 mo–3 yr | 3–6 yr | 6–12 yr | Adult |
|---|---|---|---|---|---|
| Erikson (psychosocial development) | **Trust versus Mistrust** Infants learn to trust, or mistrust, that their needs will be meet by the world, especially by the mother. | **Autonomy versus Shame, Doubt** Children learn to exercise will, to make choices, to control themselves, or they become uncertain and doubt that they can do things by themselves. | **Initiative versus Guilt** Children learn to initiate activities and enjoy their accomplishments, acquiring direction and purpose. If they are not allowed initiative, they feel guilty for their attempts at independence. | **Industry versus Inferiority** Children develop a sense of industry and curiosity and are eager to learn, or they feel inferior and lose interest in the tasks before them. | **Identity versus Role Confusion** Adolescents come to see themselves as unique and integrated persons with an ideology, or they become confused about what they want out of life. |
| Freud (psychosexual development) | **Oral Stage** Infants obtain gratification through stimulation of the mouth, as they suck and bite. | **Anal Stage** Children obtain gratification through exercise of the anal musculature during elimination or retention. | **Phallic Stage (Oedipal)** Children develop sexual curiosity and obtain gratification through masturbation. They have sexual fantasies about the parent of the opposite sex and guilt about their fantasies. | **Latency Stage** Children's sexual urges are submerged; they put their energies into acquiring cultural skills. | **Genital Stage** Adolescents have adult heterosexual desires and seek to satisfy them. |
| Piaget (see Table 1–2) | *Sensorimotor* | *Preoperational* | | *Concrete* | *Formal* |

Adapted from Clarke-Stewart A, Koch JB: Children: Development through Adolescence. New York, John Wiley, 1983, p 11; and Stone LJ, Church J: Childhood and Adolescence. New York, Random House, 1979, pp 42–43.

19

TABLE 1–4.    Topics for Health Supervision Visits

**Focus on the Child**
    Concerns (parent's or child's)
    Past problem follow-up
    Immunization and screening test update
    Routine care (eating, sleeping, elimination, health habits)
    Developmental status
    Behavioral style and problems

**Focus on the Child's Environment**
    Family
        Caregiving schedule for caregiver who lives at home
        Parent-child and sibling-child interactions
        Extended family role
        Family stresses (work, move, finances, illness, death, marital and other interpersonal relationships)
        Family supports (relatives, friends, groups)

    Community
        Caregivers outside the family
        Peer interaction
        School and/or work
        Other activities

    Physical environment
        Appropriate stimulation
        Safety

develops is a crucial component of the causes and manifestations of problems, especially behavioral and developmental problems. Furthermore, appropriate approaches to managing these problems depend on the environmental context. Ignorance of the context will result in ineffective and perhaps inappropriate management suggestions from the physician. Table 1–5 lists some of the contextual factors that should be considered in the etiology of a child's behavioral problem.

Building rapport with the parents and the child is a prerequisite for obtaining the often sensitive information that is essential for understanding a behavioral or developmental problem. Rapport usually can be quickly established if the parents sense that the clinician respects them and is genuinely interested in listening to their concerns. Rapport with the child can be developed by engaging him or her in developmentally appropriate conversation or play, providing toys while interviewing the parents, and being sensitive to the fears the child may have. Too often the child is ignored until it is time for the physical examination. Like their parents, children will feel more comfortable if they are greeted by name and involved in pleasant interactions before they are asked sensitive questions or threatened with examinations. Young children can be engaged on the parent's lap, which provides security and places the child at the eye level of the examiner.

With adolescents, emphasis should be placed on

building a doctor-patient relationship that is distinct from the relationship with the parents. This does not mean the parents should be excluded; however, the adolescent should have the opportunity to express concerns to and ask questions of the clinician in confidence. This confidence can be achieved by meeting with the adolescent alone for at least part of each visit. However, confidentiality has limits, and parents must be informed when the clinician has concerns about the health and safety of the child. Often the clinician can convince the child to inform the parents directly of a problem or can reach an agreement with the child about how the parents will be informed.

### Expanded History and Observations

Because the initial health supervision visit is brief, it is best to explore developmental and behavioral problems during subsequent visits when more comprehensive information and observations can be obtained, unless the problem is simple and the clinician knows the family well.

Specific interviewing practices will enhance the collection of behavioral information. Responses to open-ended questions often provide clues to underlying, unstated problems and identify the appropriate direction for further, more directed questions. Sensitivity to the way something is said, not just to what is said, provides important clues for content areas to pursue. The interviewer unintentionally may restrict the scope of the discussion

TABLE 1–5.    Context of Behavioral Problems

**Child Factors**
    Health (past and current)
    Developmental status
    Temperament (e.g., difficult, slow to warm up)
    Coping mechanisms

**Parental Factors**
    Misinterpretations of stage-related behaviors
    Mismatch of parental expectations and characteristics of child
    Parental characteristics (e.g., depression, disinterest, rejection, overprotectiveness)
    Coping mechanisms

**Environmental Factors**
    Stress (e.g., marital discord, unemployment, personal loss)
    Support (e.g., emotional, material, informational, child care)

**Parent-Child Interactions**
    The common pathway through which the listed factors interact to influence the development of a behavior problem
    The key to resolving the behavior problem

by prematurely using directed questions. Because histories about developmental and behavioral problems are often vague and confusing, to reconcile apparent contradictions the interviewer frequently must request clarification (to ascertain the meaning of a word to the patient), more detail, or mere repetition. By summarizing an understanding of the information at frequent intervals and by recapitulating at the close of the visit, the interviewer and patient can ensure that they understand each other. To build trust and to encourage the patient to talk about difficult issues, the physician must convey respect and empathy for the patient. Empathy is apparent when the physician recognizes the emotions that underlie the patient's responses and communicates this understanding both verbally and nonverbally.

Other techniques for improving the quality of information include the detailed description of a typical day (including parental responses to problem behaviors), and discussion of the physician's observations of the child's behavior and of parent-child and physician-child interactions during the visit. Although the child's behavior during the visit is likely to be unrepresentative of his or her typical behavior, the physician's observations will serve as a springboard for discussion.

A very useful technique is to ask the parents to keep a diary of the occurrence and duration of problem behaviors as well as the antecedents and parental responses, if possible. This practice often reveals a pattern to the behavior that was not previously apparent to the parents. Projective techniques may provide additional useful information (e.g, "What are your happiest, saddest, and maddest moments?" or "If you could have any three wishes, what would they be?"). Third-person techniques (e.g., "Most boys your age are concerned about . . ." or asking about the drinking behavior of friends) may permit a child to talk about an issue that would be too difficult to handle if confronted directly.

If the clinician's impression of the child differs markedly from the parent's description, there may be a crucial parental concern that has not yet been expressed because it may be very difficult for the parent to talk about (e.g., marital problems), or it may be unconscious, or its relevance to the child's behavior may be overlooked by the parent. Alternatively, the physician's observations may be atypical, even with multiple visits. The observations of teachers, relatives, and other regular caregivers may be crucial in sorting out this possibility. The parent also may have a distorted image of the child, rooted in parental psychopathology. A sensitive, supportive, and noncritical approach to the

parent may facilitate referral for appropriate therapy.

## References

Behrman RE, Kliegman RM, Arvin AM (eds): Nelson Textbook of Pediatrics, 15th ed. Philadelphia, WB Saunders, 1996, Chapters 5, 7, 18.

Boyle WE, Hoekelman RA: The pediatric history. *In* Hoekelman RA, Friedman SB, Nelson NM et al (eds): Primary Pediatric Care, 3rd ed. St. Louis, CV Mosby, 1997, pp 45–54.

## Screening Tests

Developmental milestone screening has the advantages of relative ease, continuity of parental observation, and objectivity of professional observation; however, it also suffers from several weaknesses. Clinicians using such criterion-based approaches may think of development as a stepwise rather than continuous process and erroneously assume a child to be normal once a particular milestone has been achieved, even in the face of a larger pattern of delay. Cultural differences, inadequacy of memory, wishful thinking, or simply misunderstanding the clinician's question may affect the quality of information gleaned from parents or other caretakers. Direct observation is limited by the brevity of the clinician's interaction with the child, unfamiliarity and discomfort for the child with the medical environment, and observer biases based, for example, on the child's playfulness or physical attractiveness. Standardized screening tools can help to minimize such sources of error.

Many clinicians use formal screening tests to detect or better define developmental and/or behavioral problems. As in any screening test, a failed developmental screen implies the need for more conclusive "gold standard" evaluation.

**Denver Developmental Screening Tests.** The Denver Developmental Screening Test (DDST) assesses the development of children from birth to age 6 yr. Two common criticisms of the DDST include the paucity of language items in the first 2 yr and questions about its appropriateness for children in some ethnic and social class subgroups. The Denver II is the most recent revision (Fig. 1–17; see Fig. 1–16). It assesses the development of children from birth to age 6 yr with items in four categories: (1) Personal-Social, (2) Fine Motor-Adaptive, (3) Language, and (4) Gross Motor. Its items were carefully selected for their reliability and consistency of norms across subgroups. The Denver II is very useful as a screening instrument, but it cannot adequately assess the complexities of socioemotional development. In addition, the criteria for passing are set low to minimize labeling

1. Try to get child to smile by smiling, talking or waving.  Do not touch him/her.
2. Child must stare at hand several seconds.
3. Parent may help guide toothbrush and put toothpaste on brush.
4. Child does not have to be able to tie shoes or button/zip in the back.
5. Move yarn slowly in an arc from one side to the other, about 8" above child's face.
6. Pass if child grasps rattle when it is touched to the backs or tips of fingers.
7. Pass if child tries to see where yarn went.  Yarn should be dropped quickly from sight from tester's hand without arm movement.
8. Child must transfer cube from hand to hand without help of body, mouth, or table.
9. Pass if child picks up raisin with any part of thumb and finger.
10. Line can vary only 30 degrees or less from tester's line. ✓
11. Make a fist with thumb pointing upward and wiggle only the thumb.  Pass if child imitates and does not move any fingers other than the thumb.

12. Pass any enclosed form.  Fail continuous round motions.
13. Which line is longer? (Not bigger.)  Turn paper upside down and repeat. (pass 3 of 3 or 5 of 6)
14. Pass any lines crossing near midpoint.
15. Have child copy first.  If failed, demonstrate.

When giving items 12, 14, and 15, do not name the forms.  Do not demonstrate 12 and 14.

16. When scoring, each pair (2 arms, 2 legs, etc.) counts as one part.
17. Place one cube in cup and shake gently near child's ear, but out of sight.  Repeat for other ear.
18. Point to picture and have child name it.  (No credit is given for sounds only.)
    If less than 4 pictures are named correctly, have child point to picture as each is named by tester.

19. Using doll, tell child:  Show me the nose, eyes, ears, mouth, hands, feet, tummy, hair.  Pass 6 of 8.
20. Using pictures, ask child: Which one flies?... says meow?... talks?... barks?... gallops? Pass 2 of 5, 4 of 5.
21. Ask child: What do you do when you are cold?... tired?... hungry?  Pass 2 of 3, 3 of 3.
22. Ask child:  What do you do with a cup?  What is a chair used for?  What is a pencil used for?
    Action words must be included in answers.
23. Pass if child correctly places <u>and</u> says how many blocks are on paper. (1, 5).
24. Tell child: Put block **on** table; **under** table; **in front of** me, **behind** me.  Pass 4 of 4.
    (Do not help child by pointing, moving head or eyes.)
25. Ask child: What is a ball?... lake?... desk?... house?... banana?... curtain?... fence?... ceiling?  Pass if defined in terms of use, shape, what it is made of, or general category (such as banana is fruit, not just yellow).  Pass 5 of 8, 7 of 8.
26. Ask child: If a horse is big, a mouse is __?  If fire is hot, ice is __?  If the sun shines during the day, the moon shines during the __?  Pass 2 of 3.
27. Child may use wall or rail only, not person.  May not crawl.
28. Child must throw ball overhand 3 feet to within arm's reach of tester.
29. Child must perform standing broad jump over width of test sheet (8 1/2 inches).
30. Tell child to walk forward, ⟳⟳⟳⟳➡ heel within 1 inch of toe.  Tester may demonstrate.
    Child must walk 4 consecutive steps.
31. In the second year, half of normal children are non-compliant.

**OBSERVATIONS:**

FIGURE 1–17. Instructions for the Denver Developmental Screening Test. Numbers are coded to scoring form (Fig. 1–16). "Abnormal" is defined as two or more delays (failure of an item passed by 90% at that age) in two or more categories, or two or more delays in one category with one other category having one delay and an age line that does not intersect one item that is passed. A "suspect" or "questionable" score is given if one category has two or more delays or if one or more categories have one delay and in the same category the age line does not pass through one item that is passed. (From Frankenburg WK: Denver II Developmental Screening Test, 2nd ed. Denver, Denver Developmental Materials, Inc.)

TABLE 1–6. Rules of Thumb for Speech Screening

| Age (Yr) | Speech Production | Articulation (Amount of Speech Understood by a Stranger) | Following Commands |
|---|---|---|---|
| 1 | 1–3 words | | One-step commands |
| 2 | 2- to 3-word phrases | ½ | Two-step commands |
| 3 | Routine use of sentences | ¾ | |
| 4 | Routine use of sentence sequences; conversational give-and-take | Almost all | |
| 5 | Complex sentences; extensive use of modifiers, pronouns, and prepositions | Almost all | |

normal children as abnormal; this may result in failing to identify children with mild but significant developmental problems. Children with "suspect" or "questionable" scores, therefore, must be followed carefully.

An abbreviated Denver screen has been validated using only 12 items per subject (the three items in each category falling immediately to the left but not touching the age line). This abbreviated test is very helpful in busy clinical settings. A two-stage screening procedure can be used in which every child is given the abbreviated screen and only those with suspect or abnormal scores get a full Denver screen. Another adaptation of this screen is a parental questionnaire using 97 of the original DDST items (Prescreening Developmental Questionnaire, PDQ). There was a high agreement rate between parent responses and DDST scores in a largely middle-class sample.

**Speech and Language Screening.** Language screening is important because it correlates best with cognitive development in the early years. Table 1–6 provides some rules of thumb for language development that focus on speech production (expressive language). Receptive language is not assessed by these rules and only incompletely assessed by the Denver II. Although expressive language (speech) is the most obvious language element, the most dramatic changes in language development in the first years involve recognition and understanding (receptive language). Also, much language up to age 2 yr is visually mediated (e.g., pointing). Thus, language screening deserves focused attention. One useful tool is the Early Language Milestone (ELM) Scale (Fig. 1–18), which screens visual and auditory receptive and expressive skills.

Whenever there is a language delay, a hearing deficit must be considered (see Hearing Impairment). Conditions that have a high risk for an associated hearing deficit are listed in Table 1–7.

Early clues that indicate a need for audiologic and speech evaluation are listed in Table 1–8.

*Dysfluency* ("stuttering") is very common in 3 and 4 yr olds. Unless the dysfluency is severe, is accompanied by tics or unusual posturing, or occurs after age 4 yr, parents should be counseled that it is normal and to accept it calmly and patiently. Comments like "relax," "slow down," or "think before you speak" may be counterproductive for a child who already may be too anxious about a behavior over which he or she has little control.

**Temperament Questionnaires.** The Carey Infant Temperament Questionnaire is widely used to assess temperament in 4- to 8-mo olds. Questionnaires for assessing behavioral style at older ages are also available and can be very helpful in tailoring anticipatory guidance about behavioral issues or management plans for behavioral problems to the individual characteristics of the child.

**More Extensive Assessment Instruments.** Some pediatricians develop expertise in more ex-

TABLE 1–7. Conditions Considered High Risk for Associated Hearing Deficit

Congenital hearing loss in first cousin or closer relative
Bilirubin of 20 mg/dL or above
Congenital rubella or other nonbacterial intrauterine infection
Defects in the ear, nose, or throat
Birth weight of 1500 g or less
Multiple apneic episodes
Exchange transfusion
Meningitis
5-min Apgar* score of 5 or less
Persistent fetal circulation (primary pulmonary hypertension)
Treatment with ototoxic drugs (e.g., aminoglycosides, loop diuretics)

*Apgar = *a*daptability, *p*artnership, *g*rowth, *a*ffection, *r*esolve.

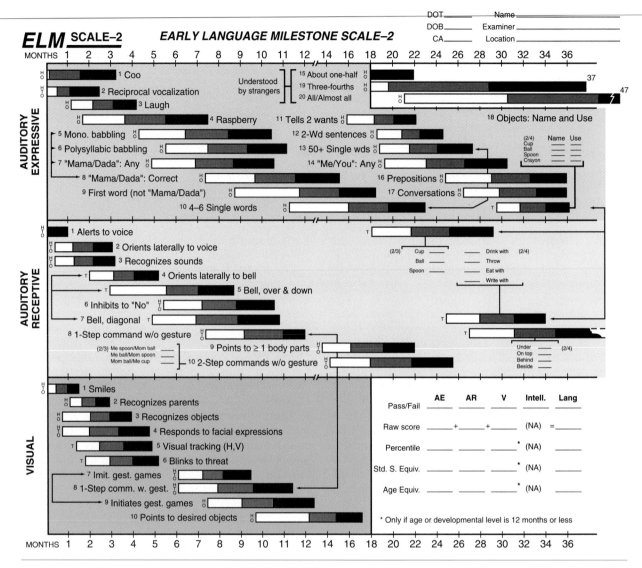

**FIGURE 1–18.** Early language milestone scales for auditory and visual development. (Early Language Milestone Scale—2 [ELM Scale—2]: A language screening instrument that covers auditory expressive, auditory receptive, and visual language development from birth to 36 mo, and intelligibility of speech up to 4 yr of age. Austin, TX, PRO-ED, 1987. Copyright 1983, 1993 by James Coplan, M.D. Reproduced by permission.)

tensive assessment instruments, including the Brazelton Neonatal Behavioral Assessment Scale, the Pediatrics Examination of Educational Readiness, and the Pediatric Early Elementary Examination. These assessments require training for expertise in administration and interpretation.

## TEAM ASSESSMENT OF COMPLEX PROBLEMS

When screening efforts suggest the presence of significant developmental lags, the pediatrician should take responsibility for coordinating the fur-

ther assessment of the child that is indicated and providing the continuity in the relationship that has developed with the child and family. The physician should become aware of the facilities and programs for assessment and treatment in his or her area. If the child was considered "high risk" because of prematurity or another identified illness that might have long-term developmental impact, a structured follow-up program already may exist to monitor the child's progress. Federal laws mandate that special education programs be provided for all children with developmental disabilities from birth through 21 yr.

TABLE 1–8.  Clues to When a Child with a Communication Disorder Needs Help

**0–11 Mo**

Before 6 mo, the child does not startle, blink, or change immediate activity in response to sudden loud sounds

Before 6 mo, the child does not attend to the human voice and is not soothed by his or her mother's voice

By 6 mo, the child does not babble strings of consonant + vowel syllables or imitate gurgling or cooing sounds

By 10 mo, the child does not respond to his or her name

At 10 mo, the child's sound-making is limited to shrieks, grunts, or sustained vowel production

**12–23 Mo**

At 12 mo, the child's babbling or speech is limited to vowel sounds

By 15 mo, the child does not respond to "no," "bye-bye," or "bottle"

By 15 mo, the child will not imitate sounds or words

By 18 mo, the child is not consistently using at least six words with appropriate meaning

By 21 mo, the child does not respond correctly to "Give me - - -," "Sit down," or "Come here" when spoken without gestural cues

By 23 mo, two-word phrases have not emerged that are spoken as single units ("Whatszit," "Thank you," "Allgone")

**24–36 Mo**

By 24 mo, at least 50% of the child's speech is not understood by familiar listeners

By 24 mo, the child does not point to body parts without gestural cues

By 24 mo, the child is not combining words into phrases ("Go bye-bye," "Go car," "Want cookie")

By 30 mo, the child does not demonstrate understanding of on, in, under, front, and back

By 30 mo, the child is not using short sentences ("Daddy went bye-bye")

By 30 mo, the child has not begun to ask questions, using where, what, why

By 36 mo, the child's speech is not understood by unfamiliar listeners

**All Ages**

At any age, the child is consistently dysfluent with repetitions, hesitations; blocks or struggles to say words. Struggle may be accompanied by grimaces, eye blinks, or hand gestures.

Adapted from Weiss CE, Lillywhite HE: Communication Disorders: A Handbook for Prevention and Early Detection. St. Louis, CV Mosby, 1976.

## Medical Assessment

The physician's main goals in team assessment are to identify the cause of the developmental dysfunction and to identify and interpret other medical conditions that have a developmental impact. The comprehensive history (Table 1–9) and physical examination (Table 1–10) should include a careful graphing of growth parameters and an accurate description of dysmorphic features (see Chapter 4).

## Motor Assessment

Although the traditional neurologic examination provides an excellent basis for evaluating motor function, it should be supplemented by an adaptive functional evaluation. Watching the child at play can aid in such assessment. In addition, standardized tools for evaluating gross and fine motor abilities are utilized by physical and occupational therapists to estimate age-appropriate functional levels.

## Psychologic Assessment

This includes the testing of cognitive ability (Table 1–11) and the evaluation of personality and emotional well-being by a skilled evaluator. The intelligence quotient (IQ) and mental age scores, taken in isolation, are only partially descriptive of a person's functional abilities, which are a combination of cognitive, adaptive, and social skills. Tests of achievement are subject to variability based on experience and must be standardized for social factors. Projective and nonprojective tests are useful in understanding the child's emotional status. Although a child should not be labeled as having a problem solely on the basis of a standardized test, such tests do provide important and reasonably objective data for evaluating a child's growth within a particular educational program.

## Educational Assessment

The educational assessment refers to the evaluation of areas of specific strengths and weaknesses in reading, spelling, written expression, and mathematical skills. Schools routinely screen children with group tests to aid in problem identification and program evaluation. For the child with special needs, this should ultimately lead to individualized testing and the development of an individualized educational plan (IEP) that will enable the child to progress comfortably in school. Diagnostic teaching, in which the child's response to various teaching techniques is assessed, also may be helpful.

## Social Environment Assessment

Assessment of the environment in which the child is living, working, playing, and growing is also important in understanding the child's development. A home visit by a social worker, community health nurse, or home-based intervention specialist can provide valuable information about the child's social milieu.

**TABLE 1–9.** Information to Be Sought During the History Taking of a Child with Suspected Developmental Disabilities

| Item | Possible Significance |
|---|---|
| *Parental Concerns* | Parents are quite accurate in identifying developmental problems in their children |
| *Current Levels of Developmental Functioning* | Should be used to monitor child's progress |
| *Temperament* | May interact with disability or may be confused with developmental delay |
| *Prenatal History* | |
| Alcohol ingestion | Fetal alcohol syndrome; an index of care-taking risk |
| Illegal drug, toxin, medication exposure | Developmental toxin (e.g., phenytoin); may be an index of caretaking risk |
| Radiation exposure | Damage to central nervous system (CNS) |
| Nutrition | Inadequate fetal nutrition |
| Prenatal care | Index of social situation |
| Injuries, hyperthermia | Damage to CNS |
| Smoking | Possible CNS damage |
| Human immunodeficiency virus (HIV) exposure | Congenital HIV infection |
| Maternal phenylketonuria (PKU) | Maternal PKU effect |
| Maternal illness | Toxoplasmosis, rubella, cytomegalovirus, herpesvirus infections |
| *Perinatal History* | |
| Gestational age, birth weight | Biologic risk from prematurity and small for gestational age |
| Labor and delivery | Hypoxia or index of abnormal prenatal development |
| Apgar scores | Hypoxia, cardiovascular impairment |
| Specific perinatal adverse events | Increased risk for CNS damage |
| *Neonatal History* | |
| Illness—seizures, respiratory distress, hyperbilirubinemia, metabolic disorder | Increased risk for CNS damage |
| Malformations | May represent syndrome associated with developmental delay |
| *Family History* | |
| Consanguinity | Autosomal recessive condition more likely |
| Mental functioning | Increased hereditary and environmental risks |
| Illnesses (e.g., metabolic disease) | Hereditary illness associated with developmental delay |
| Family member died young or unexpectedly | May suggest inborn error of metabolism or storage disease |
| Family member requires special education | Hereditary causes of developmental delay |
| *Social History* | |
| Resources available (e.g., financial, social support) | Necessary to maximize child's potential |
| Educational level of parents | Family may need help to provide stimulation |
| Mental health problems | May exacerbate child's conditions |
| High-risk behaviors (illicit drugs, sex) | Increased risk for HIV infection; index of care-taking risk |
| Other stressors (e.g., marital discord) | May exacerbate child's conditions or compromise care |
| *Other History* | |
| Gender of child | Important for X-linked conditions |
| Developmental milestones | Index of developmental delay; regression may indicate progressive condition |
| Head injury | Even moderate trauma may be associated with developmental delay or learning disabilities |
| Serious infections (e.g., meningitis) | May be associated with developmental delay |
| Toxic exposure (e.g., lead) | May be associated with developmental delay |
| Physical growth | May indicate malnutrition; obesity, short stature associated with some conditions |
| Recurrent otitis media | Associated with hearing loss and abnormal speech development |
| Visual and auditory functioning | Sensitive index of impairments in vision and hearing |
| Nutrition | Malnutrition during infancy may lead to delayed development |
| Chronic conditions like renal disease or anemia | May be associated with delayed development |

From Liptak G: Mental retardation and developmental disability. *In* Kliegman RM (ed): Practical Strategies in Pediatric Diagnosis and Therapy. Philadelphia, WB Saunders, 1996.

TABLE 1–10. Information to Be Sought During the Physical Examination of a Child with Suspected Developmental Disabilities

| Item | Possible Significance |
|---|---|
| *General Appearance* | May indicate significant delay in development or obvious syndrome |
| *Stature* | |
| Short stature | Williams syndrome, malnutrition, Turner syndrome; many children with severe retardation have short stature |
| Obesity | Prader-Willi syndrome |
| Large stature | Sotos syndrome |
| *Head* | |
| Macrocephaly | Alexander syndrome, Sotos syndrome, gangliosidosis, hydrocephalus, mucopolysaccharidosis, subdural effusion |
| Microcephaly | Virtually any condition that can retard brain growth (e.g., malnutrition, Angelman syndrome, de Lange syndrome, fetal alcohol effects) |
| *Face* | |
| Coarse, triangular, round, or flat face; hypo- or hypertelorism, slanted or short palpebral fissure; unusual nose, maxilla, and mandible | Specific measurements may provide clues to inherited, metabolic, or other diseases like fetal alcohol syndrome, *cri du chat* (5p- syndrome), or Williams syndrome |
| *Eyes* | |
| Prominent | Crouzon syndrome, Seckel syndrome, fragile X |
| Cataract | Galactosemia, Lowe syndrome, prenatal rubella, hypothyroidism |
| Cherry-red spot in macula | Gangliosidosis ($GM_1$), metachromatic leukodystrophy, mucolipidosis, Tay-Sachs disease, Niemann-Pick disease, Farber lipogranulomatosis, sialidosis III |
| Chorioretinitis | Congenital infection with cytomegalovirus, toxoplasmosis, or rubella |
| Corneal cloudiness | Mucopolysaccharidosis I and II, Lowe syndrome, congenital syphilis |
| *Ears* | |
| Pinnae, low set or malformed | Trisomies such as 18, Rubinstein-Taybi syndrome, Down syndrome, CHARGE association, cerebro-oculo-facial-skeletal syndrome, fetal phenytoin effects |
| Hearing | Loss of acuity in mucopolysaccharidosis; hyperacusis in many encephalopathies |

*Table continued on following page*

References

Behrman RE, Kliegman RM, Arvin AM (eds): Nelson Textbook of Pediatrics, 15th ed. Philadelphia, WB Saunders, 1996, Chapters 5, 17, and 40.
Coplan J: Normal speech and language development: An overview. Pediatr Rev 16(3):91, 1995.
Frankenburg WK, Dodds J, Archer P, et al: Denver II: A major revision and restandardization of the Denver Developmental Screening Test. Pediatrics 89:91, 1992.
McInerny TK: Children who have difficulty in school: A primary pediatrician's approach. Pediatr Rev 16(9):325, 1995.
Newton R, Wraith J: Investigation of developmental delay. Arch Dis Child 72:460,1995.

## MANAGEMENT OF DEVELOPMENTAL AND BEHAVIORAL PROBLEMS

### INTERVENTION IN THE PRIMARY CARE SETTING

After assessment, the clinician must decide whether a problem requires referral for further diagnostic work-up and/or management, or whether management in the primary care setting is appropriate. Some of the counseling roles required in caring for these children are listed in Table 1–12 and discussed below. In this context, the word "patient" refers to the child and/or parent. When a child is young, much of the counseling interaction takes place between the parents and the clinician; as the child matures, direct counseling shifts increasingly toward the child.

The assessment process (particularly that of expanded history and observations) may be therapeutic in itself. By assuming the role of a nonjudgmental, supportive listener, the clinician creates a climate of trust in which the patient feels free to express difficult or even painful thoughts and feelings. Ventilation of these feelings alone may be helpful; in addition, it may free the patient from a preoccupation with previously unexpressed emotions, allowing the patient to move on to the work of understanding and resolving the problem. Interview techniques also may facilitate clarifi-

TABLE 1–10.  Information to Be Sought During the Physical Examination of a Child with Suspected Developmental Disabilities *Continued*

| Item | Possible Significance |
| --- | --- |
| *Heart* | |
| Structural anomaly or hypertrophy | CHARGE association, CATCH-22, velo-cardio-facial syndrome, glycogenesis II, fetal alcohol effects, mucopolysaccharidosis I; chromosomal anomalies like Down syndrome; maternal PKU; chronic cyanosis may impair cognitive development |
| *Liver* | |
| Hepatomegaly | Fructose intolerance, galactosemia glycogenosis types I–IV, mucopolysaccharidosis I and II, Niemann-Pick disease, Tay-Sachs disease, Zellweger syndrome, Gaucher disease, ceroid lipofuscinosis, gangliosidosis |
| *Genitalia* | |
| Macro-orchidism | Fragile X syndrome |
| Hypogenitalism | Prader-Willi syndrome, Klinefelter syndrome, CHARGE association |
| *Extremities* | |
| Hands, feet, dermatoglyphics, and creases | May indicate specific entity like Rubinstein-Taybi syndrome or be associated with chromosomal anomaly |
| Joint contractures | Sign of muscle imbalance around joints—e.g., with meningomyelocele, cerebral palsy, arthrogryposis, muscular dystrophy; also occurs with cartilaginous problems such as mucopolysaccharidosis |
| *Skin* | |
| *Café au lait* spots | Neurofibromatosis, tuberous sclerosis, Bloom syndrome |
| "Eczema" | Phenylketonuria, histiocytosis |
| Hemangiomas and telangiectasia | Sturge-Weber syndrome, Bloom syndrome, ataxia-telangiectasia |
| Hypopigmented macules, streaks, adenoma sebaceum | Tuberous sclerosis, hypomelanosis of Ito |
| *Hair* | |
| Hirsutism | De Lange syndrome, mucopolysaccharidosis, fetal phenytoin effects, cerebro-oculo-facial-skeletal syndrome, trisomy 18 |
| *Neurologic* | |
| Asymmetry of strength and tone | Focal lesion, cerebral palsy |
| Hypotonia | Prader-Willi syndrome, Down syndrome, Angelman syndrome, gangliosidosis, early cerebral palsy |
| Hypertonia | Neurodegenerative conditions involving white matter, cerebral palsy, trisomy 18 |
| Ataxia | Ataxia-telangiectasia, metachromatic leukodystrophy, Angelman syndrome |

From Liptak G: Mental retardation and developmental disability. *In* Kliegman RM (ed): Practical Strategies in Pediatric Diagnosis and Therapy. Philadelphia, WB Saunders, 1996.

CHARGE = *c*oloboma *h*eart defects, *a*tresia choanae, *r*etarded growth, *g*enital anomalies, *e*ar anomalies (deafness); CATCH-22 = *c*ardiac defects, *a*bnormal face, *t*hymic hypoplasia, *c*left palate, *h*ypocalcemia-defects on chromosome No. 22; PKU = phenylketonuria.

cation of the problem for the patient as well as for the clinician. The patient's ideas about the causes of the problem and descriptions of attempts to deal with it can provide a basis for developing strategies for problem management that are much more likely to be implemented because they emanate in part from the patient. Furthermore, the respect shown by the clinician in endorsing the patient's ideas, when appropriate, can increase the patient's self-esteem and sense of competency. The provision of reassurance appropriate to the patient's concern is potentially of great additional benefit, but reassurance given too hastily and nonspecifically may suggest a lack of regard for the patient.

Educating parents regarding normal and aberrant development and behavior may prevent problems through early detection and anticipatory guidance. Such education also communicates the physician's interest in hearing parental concerns. Early detection is important because intervention can be started before the problem becomes entrenched and associated problems develop.

Many families expect and need specific, detailed parenting advice from the clinician. Other parents will work out the details if the clinician first provides some general principles and guidelines. When the parents or child play a relatively passive role in the development of the plan, it is particu-

**TABLE 1–11.   Tests of Cognition**

| Test | Age Range | Special Features |
| --- | --- | --- |
| *Infant Scales* | | |
| Bayley Scales of Infant Development (2nd ed.) | 2–42 mo | Mental, psychomotor scales, behavior record; weak intelligence predictor |
| Cattell Infant Intelligence Scale | Birth–30 mo | Used to extend Stanford-Binet downward |
| Gesell Developmental Schedules | Birth–3 yr | Used by many pediatricians |
| Ordinal Scales of Infant Psychological Development | Birth–24 mo | Six subscales; based on Piaget's stages; weak in predicting later intelligence |
| *Preschool Scales* | | |
| Stanford-Binet Intelligence Scale (4th ed.) | 2 yr–adult | Four area scores, with subtests and composite IQ score |
| McCarthy Scales of Children's Abilities | 2½–8 yr | 6–18 subtests; good at defining learning disabilities; strengths/weaknesses approach |
| Wechsler Primary and Preschool Test of Intelligence–Revised (WPPSI-R) | 3–6½ yr | 11 subtests; verbal, performance IQs; long administration time; good at defining learning disabilities |
| Merrill-Palmer Scale of Mental Tests | 2–4½ yr | General test for young children |
| Differential Abilities Scale | 2½ yr–adult | Special nonverbal composite; short administration time |
| *School-Age Scales* | | |
| Stanford-Binet Intelligence Scale (4th ed.) | 2 yr–adult | See above |
| Wechsler Intelligence Scale for Children (3rd ed.) (WISC III) | 6–16 yr | See comments on WPPSI-R |
| Leiter International Performance Scale | 2 yr–adult | No verbal abilities needed |
| Wechsler Adult Intelligence Scale–Revised (WAIS-R) | 16 yr–adult | See comments on WPPSI-R |
| Differential Abilities Scale | 2½ yr–adult | See above |
| *Adaptive Behavior Scales* | | |
| Vineland Adaptive Behavior Scale | Birth–adult | Interview/questionnaire; typical persons + blind, deaf, and retarded |
| American Association on Mental Retardation (AAMR) Adaptive Behavioral Scale | 3 yr–adult | Useful in retardation, other disabilities |

IQ = intelligence quotient.

larly important to give them a written copy of the plan to review and to be certain that the details are fully understood. Specific suggestions for changes in the family environment often are very useful. One helpful suggestion is to arrange for respite and increased emotional support for the primary caregiver, who usually is discouraged and ex-

**TABLE 1–12.   Primary Care Counseling Roles**

Allow ventilation
Facilitate clarification
Support patient problem solving
Provide specific reassurance
Provide education
Provide specific parenting advice
Suggest environmental interventions
Provide follow-up
Facilitate appropriate referrals
Coordinate care and interpret reports after referrals

hausted by the time the clinician hears about the problem. The clinician also may suggest other community services to relieve pressure and to improve the coping ability of the family (e.g., nursery school, tutors, recreational programs, and parent support and education groups).

Most developmental and behavioral problems appear simple when initially presented, and often a small amount of education, reassurance, and a few simple suggestions are sufficient. Follow-up is crucial, however, because complex problems often present as simple problems, and clinicians must be ready to accept failure of their suggestions without attributing the failure to inadequacy in the parents' application of the recommendations. Indications for referral to developmental disability or mental health specialists will vary according to the expertise of the primary care clinician, but children should not be followed for long periods of time in the hope that they will "outgrow" the problem.

After referral, the clinician is needed to help coordinate and interpret the evaluations and recommendations.

## COUNSELING PRINCIPLES

Behavioral change must be learned, not imposed. It is easiest to learn when the lesson is simple, clear, and consistent and presented in an atmosphere free of fear or intimidation. Parents often try to impose behavioral change in an emotionally charged atmosphere. Clinicians often try to "teach" parents with hastily presented advice when the parent is distracted by other concerns. The teacher (parent or clinician) must also remember that patient repetition is the basis of learning.

Apart from management strategies directed specifically at the problem behavior, regular times for *positive parent-child interaction* should be instituted. Frequent, brief, affectionate physical contact over the day will provide opportunities for positive reinforcement of desirable child behaviors and for building a sense of competence in the child and the parent. Parents should be reminded to "catch the child being good," and to criticize the child's *behavior*, rather than the child.

*Guilt* is felt by almost all parents when their child has a developmental-behavioral problem. This may be due to the assumption or fear that the problem was caused by inadequate parenting, or guilt about previous angry responses to the child's behavior (e.g., excessive physical punishment or derogatory comments). The clinician should not unwittingly contribute to parental guilt with insensitive comments that may be construed as criticism by the parents. The clinician should, if possible and appropriate, find ways to alleviate guilt. Guilt may be a serious impediment to problem solving and can be diffused by honestly pointing out how often other parents have similar problems and by empathizing with the difficulties of coping with the problem.

It is usually beneficial to find ways to increase support for the primary caregiver. A mother is better able to nurture a child well when she is well nurtured herself.

The clinician must be careful of using developmental or behavioral labels, even though they may be helpful in diagnosis and management. These labels can become self-fulfilling prophecies as the people in the child's environment treat the child as "difficult," which becomes part of the child's self-concept.

## INTERDISCIPLINARY TEAM INTERVENTION

In many cases, the breadth and quality of services needed to serve appropriately the child who has developmental problems require a team of professionals. This is commonly the case in follow-up programs for infants leaving intensive care nurseries. Although such Early Intervention Programs are now mandated across the United States, the physician may play a key role in guiding the child and family to these services. Once the child reaches school age, the public school system takes increasing responsibility for developmental and educational services, and the physician's role becomes primarily one of consultation on medically related issues.

*Educational intervention* for the young child begins as home-based infant stimulation, often using an early childhood educator, nurse, or occupational, speech, or physical therapist to provide direct stimulation for the child and to train the family to provide the stimulation. As the child matures, a center-based nursery program may be indicated. For the school-aged child, special services may range from extra attention given by the classroom teacher to a self-contained special educational classroom. Home-based tutoring or residential programs typically are reserved for only the most behaviorally or cognitively impaired children in this age range.

*Psychologic intervention* may take several forms. Therapy may be parent- or family-directed or may become, with the older child, purely child-directed. Therapeutic approaches include guidance therapies such as directive advice-giving, counseling the family or child in their own solutions to problems, psychotherapy, behavior management techniques, psychopharmacologic methods, and cognitive therapy.

*Motor intervention* may be performed by a physical or occupational therapist, or by another professional under his or her direction. Neurodevelopmental therapy (NDT), the most commonly used method, is based on the concept that nervous system development is hierarchical and subject to some plasticity. The focus is on gait training and motor development, including daily living skills and perceptual abilities to assist in the guidance of motor activity, such as eye-hand coordination, spatial relationships, and motor sequencing. Sensory integration therapy is sometimes used by occupational therapists to structure sensory experience from the tactile, proprioceptive, and vestibular systems to allow for adaptive motor responses.

*Speech and language intervention* by the speech

therapist is usually part of the overall educational program and is based on the tested language strengths and weaknesses of the child. Children requiring this type of intervention may demonstrate difficulties in reading and other academic areas as well as develop social and behavioral problems owing to their difficulties in being understood and in understanding others.

*Hearing intervention,* performed by the audiologist and otolaryngologist, includes monitoring hearing acuity, providing amplification when necessary via hearing aids, and treating ear infections.

*Social and environmental intervention* generally takes the form of nursing or social work involvement with the family. Frequently, the task of coordinating the services of other disciplines falls to these specialists.

*Medical intervention* for the child with a developmental disability involves providing primary care and specific treatment of conditions associated with disability. Although curative treatment often is not possible owing to the irreversible nature of many disabling conditions, functional impairment can be minimized through thoughtful medical management. Certain general medical problems are found more frequently in the mentally retarded and developmentally disabled population (Table 1–13).

### References

Behrman RE, Kliegman RM, Arvin AM (eds): Nelson Textbook of Pediatrics, 15th ed. Philadelphia, WB Saunders, 1996, Chapters 17, 30, 40, 510.

Liptak GS: The role of the pediatrician in caring for children with developmental disabilities: Overview. Pediatr Ann 24(5):232, 1995.

Sulkes SB: MD's DD Basics: Identifying common problems and preventing secondary disabilities. Pediatr Ann 24(5):245, 1995.

## CRYING

The compelling sound of an infant's cry makes it an effective distress signal and appropriate to the human infant's prolonged dependence on a caregiver. However, cries are discomforting and may be alarming to parents, many of whom find it very difficult to listen to their infant's crying for even short periods of time.

Many reasons for crying are obvious, such as hunger and discomfort due to heat, cold, illness, and lying position. These reasons, however, account for a relatively small percentage of infant crying and usually are recognized quickly and alleviated. In the absence of a discernible reason for the behavior, crying often stops when the infant is

**TABLE 1–13.** Recurring Medical Issues in the Developmentally Disabled

| Problem | Ask About or Check |
|---|---|
| Motor | Range of motion examination; scoliosis check; assess mobility; interact with orthopedist, physiatrist, and PT/OT as needed |
| Other syndrome-specific problems | Ongoing evaluation of other "physical" problems as indicated by known MR/DD etiology |
| Diet | Dietary history, feeding observation, growth parameter measurement and charting, supplementation as indicated by observations |
| Sensory impairments | Functional vision and hearing screening; interaction as needed with audiologist, ophthalmologist |
| Dermatology | Examine *all* skin areas for decubitis ulcers or infection |
| Dentistry | Examine teeth and gums; confirm access to dental care |
| Behavioral problems | Aggression, self-injury, pica; sleep problems; psychotropic drug levels and side effects |
| Advocacy | Educational program, family supports, financial supports |
| Seizures | Major motor, absence, other suspicious symptoms; monitor anticonvulsant levels and side effects |
| Infectious diseases | Ear infections, diarrhea, respiratory symptoms, aspiration pneumonia, immunizations (especially hepatitis B) |
| Constipation (GI problems) | Constipation, gastroesophageal reflux, GI bleeding (stool for occult blood) |
| Sexuality | Sexuality education, hygiene, contraception (when appropriate), ± genetic counseling |

GI = gastrointestinal; MR/DD = mental retardation/developmental disability; PT/OT = physical therapist/occupational therapist.

held. In most infants, there are frequent episodes of crying with no apparent cause, and holding or other soothing techniques seem ineffective. Infants cry and fuss for a mean of 1¾ hr/day at age 2 wk, 2¾ hr/day at age 6 wk, and 1 hr/day at 12 wk. Counseling about normal crying may relieve guilt and diminish concerns, but for some the distress caused by the crying cannot be suppressed by logical reasoning. For these parents, respite from exposure to the crying may be necessary to allow them to cope appropriately with their own distress. Without relief, fatigue and tension may result in an inappropriate parental response such as leaving the infant in the house alone or abusing the infant.

Acute pathologic crying is usually not relieved by holding and may be due to serious medical conditions (surgical abdomen, infections, trauma-abuse, testicular torsion), hair tourniquets, corneal abrasion, intussusception, or reactions to drugs or vaccines.

## COLIC

Colic is characterized by periods of unexplained irritability and crying in healthy, well-fed infants. The crying may be intense, and it may be brief or last for hours. The episodes typically recur in the late afternoon or evening but may occur at any time. The onset is usually in the first 2–3 wk with resolution by 3 mo, although it sometimes lasts much longer. Colic occurs in 10–20% of infants. Its etiology, although unknown, is probably multifactorial, with infant, parent, and environmental factors playing potentially important roles.

*Management* begins with sympathetic listening to the parents' frustration and concern, which should not be quickly dismissed with vague reassurance that lots of crying is to be expected. Education about normal crying patterns, specific reassurance about health concerns, suggestions about techniques for consoling the infant, and recommendations for increased support and respite for the primary caregiver often are helpful.

The most effective and appropriate intervention for a crying episode is to pick up and soothe the infant. Greater maternal responsiveness to cries in the first 3 mo is associated with decreased crying and increased use of other forms of communication by the infant later in the first year. For some, however, this is impractical, particularly if the infant must be carried virtually all the time to control crying. Also, when a crying episode does not respond to holding, prolonged attempts to soothe the infant may be counterproductive, serving only to increase parental fatigue and guilt. The interactions may become tense, abrupt, and even hostile, with resulting escalation of the infant's irritability. In order to optimize parental ability to be sensitive and responsive to their infant, parents need to be well rested and to have some time for themselves.

Other techniques that may work include gentle motion (e.g., automatic rockers, stroller or car rides), continuous monotonous noise or music (e.g., mechanical alarm clock, radio), pacifier, or a warm water bottle next to the abdomen. Although only a small percentage of colic cases may be caused by food intolerance, the practice of chang-

ing formulas remains popular because it allows time for the colic to resolve on its own. Sedatives may be indicated for a limited time to break the cycle of crying and loss of sleep when the family can no longer cope with the problem; choices include diphenhydramine (1 mg/kg) or chloral hydrate (25 mg/kg) 1 hr before the worst period of crying each day (or before the parents' bedtime) for 1–2 wk. An often effective alternative is to encourage the parents to arrange for a weekend away from the infant.

### References

Behrman RE, Kliegman RM, Arvin AM (eds): Nelson Textbook of Pediatrics, 15th ed. Philadelphia, WB Saunders, 1996, Chapters 11, 44.1, 44.4.
Mones RL, Asnes RS: The colicky baby: Helping parents cope. Contemp Pediatr April:86–98, 1986.

## DISCIPLINE

Discipline involves teaching, not merely punishment. The ultimate goal is the child's self-control. Overbearing punishment to control a child's behavior will interfere with the learning process and focus on external control at the expense of the development of self-control.

Commonly used and effective techniques to control the undesirable behavior of children include scolding, physical punishment, and threats. However, these techniques have potential adverse side effects on children's sense of security and self-esteem. The effectiveness of scolding diminishes the more it is used, and it should not be allowed to expand from an expression of displeasure about a specific event to derogatory statements about children that may be interpreted as loss of love for them. Scolding also may escalate to the level of psychologic abuse. Frequent mild physical punishment also may become less effective and tempt the parent to escalate the physical punishment, increasing the risk of child abuse. Threats by parents to leave or give up the child are perhaps the most powerful and psychologically damaging ways to control a child's behavior. Children of any age may remain fearful and anxious about loss of the parent long after the threat is made. An alternative common technique is positive reinforcement for desirable behavior. It is a powerful tool for molding a child's behavior, particularly when it is given immediately after the behavior occurs. It fosters self-control and self-esteem.

Parenting involves a dynamic balance between *setting limits* on the one hand and allowing and encouraging freedom of expression and exploration on the other. Children whose behavior is out of control improve when clear limits on their behavior are set and enforced. In general, children find comfort and security in clear limits. However, parents must agree on where the limit will be set and how it will be enforced. The limit and the consequence of breaking it must be clearly presented to the child. Enforcement of the limit should be consistent and firm. Too many limits will be hard to learn and may thwart the normal development of autonomy. The limit must be reasonable in terms of the child's age, temperament, and developmental level.

*Extinction* is a systematic way to eliminate a frequent, annoying, and relatively harmless behavior by ignoring it. First, parents record the frequency of the behavior in the baseline phase in order to appreciate realistically the magnitude of the problem and to evaluate progress in eliminating it. To determine what reinforces the behavior (and therefore what needs to be consistently eliminated), it is essential to record the consequences of the behavior before any changes are made in the parental response or in other environmental factors. An appropriate behavior is identified to give the child a positive alternative that the parents can reinforce. Parents should be warned that the annoying behavior usually increases in frequency and intensity (may last weeks) before it decreases when the parent ignores it (removes the reinforcement).

The *time-out procedure* is another very useful technique to modify inappropriate behaviors that cannot be ignored. It consists of a short period of isolation that interrupts the behavior and requires considerable effort by the parents initially. A simple isolation technique, such as making a child stand in the corner or sending a child to his or her room, may be effective. If such a technique is helpful, a more systematic procedure may be needed. For example, one very effective protocol for the time-out procedure involves interrupting the child's play when the behavior occurs and having the child sit in a dull, isolated place for a brief period, measured by a portable kitchen timer. This inescapable and unpleasant consequence of the undesired behavior motivates the child to learn to avoid the behavior. If done matter-of-factly and with a minimum of expressed anger by the parent, such a time-out procedure is a potent teaching tool with less chance for adverse side effects than other commonly employed discipline techniques.

### References

Behrman RE, Kliegman RM, Arvin AM (eds): Nelson Textbook of Pediatrics, 15th ed. Philadelphia, WB Saunders, 1996, Chapters 12–14, 26, 27.

Brayden RM, Poole SR: Common behavioral problems in infants and children. Prim Care 22(1):81, 1995.

Christophersen ER: Anticipatory guidance on discipline. Pediatr Clin North Am 33:789, 1986.

## ENURESIS

Enuresis is urinary incontinence at any age when urinary continence is considered normal. Enuresis is primary when the child has never been continent of urine for a prolonged period and secondary when incontinence recurs after a prolonged period of continence (6–12 mo). *Nocturnal enuresis* is the most common type. At least one episode of **bedwetting** per month occurs in 15–30% of 6 yr olds (higher in boys and blacks) and 4–16% of 12 yr olds. The prevalence of bedwetting is so common before age 6 yr that it is not called enuresis. About 20% of bedwetters after age 4 yr, however, have secondary enuresis, which warrants a more careful evaluation. *Daytime enuresis* has a prevalence rate of only about 1% in 6–12 yr olds, with no gender prevalence. Most children are continent of urine during waking hours by age 3–4 yr.

An organic *etiology* is present in fewer than 5% of children with primary enuresis and in only 1% of children with primary nocturnal enuresis. The reason for almost all primary enuresis is a delay in the maturation of urethral sphincter control. This immaturity may be prolonged by a psychologic overlay related to concerns about the problem on the part of parents and the child. Secondary enuresis usually is due to a psychologically stressful event or condition but also is more likely than primary enuresis to have an organic cause. A urinary tract infection is the most common organic etiology. Uncommon causes include chemical distal urethritis (e.g., from bubble bath), congenital anomalies (e.g., spina bifida), severe lower urinary tract obstruction (e.g., from posterior urethral valves, urethral cyst, or urethral duplication), ectopic ureter, diabetes mellitus or insipidus, and pelvic masses (e.g., presacral teratoma, fecal impaction, hydrocolpos).

In addition to incontinence, other related *clinical manifestations* of organic causes include dysuria, frequency, hematuria, straining on urination, dribbling, small-caliber stream, stress incontinence (with coughing, lifting, or running), gait disturbance, poor bowel control, and continuous dampness. A careful history and physical examination can rule out unusual causes. Urinalysis and a urine culture should be performed at the initial visit.

*Treatment* is usually not recommended before age 6 yr because spontaneous cure rates are high. Even after age 6 yr, the spontaneous cure rate for

**TABLE 1–14.  Enuresis Counseling**

Child assumes active, responsible role
  Keeps calendar of wet and dry nights
  Talks to physician
  Urinates just before bedtime
  Changes wet clothes and bedding

Fluids not given after dinner

Punishments and angry parental responses avoided

Positive reinforcement given for each dry night (star
  chart or other reward, depending on age)

Reassurance given about etiology and prognosis (aim is
  to remove blame and guilt)

primary enuresis is 15%/yr; for secondary enuresis without an organic cause, spontaneous cure rates are also high.

Three commonly used treatments are counseling (Table 1–14), enuresis alarms, and imipramine. Enuresis alarms are the most effective treatment currently available. Cure rates are about 70%, with relapse rates of 10–15% in 5–15 yr olds. Complete success often takes several months. Imipramine has a high rapid initial response rate within the first week, but the relapse rate after discontinuation of the drug is so high that the long-term cure rate when the patient is taken off the drug is barely above the spontaneous cure rate. The dose of imipramine is 50 mg before bedtime for 8–12 yr olds and 75 mg for children over age 12 yr. After 1 mo without enuresis, the drug should be tapered over 2–4 wk. Untoward effects include anticholinergic symptoms, bone marrow suppression, and life-threatening accidental ingestions. Blood counts should be taken every 2–4 wk while the patient is on therapy.

### References

Behrman RE, Kliegman RM, Arvin AM (eds): Nelson Textbook of Pediatrics, 15th ed. Philadelphia, WB Saunders, 1996, Chapters 21.3, 497.
Howe AC, Walker CE: Behavioral management of toilet training, enuresis, and encopresis. Pediatr Clin North Am 39(3):413, 1992.

## ENCOPRESIS

Encopresis is incontinence of fecal material at any age when fecal continence is considered normal. In the United States, bowel control is usually achieved between 2 and 3 yr of age, and encopresis usually refers to regular fecal incontinence after age 4 yr. It involves a continuum from mild fecal soiling of underwear to the passage of larger amounts of fecal material. Encopresis has a prevalence of about 1% in 1st and 2nd graders; about 80% of those with encopresis are boys.

The *pathogenesis* of encopresis is based on retention of stool. The retention may be intermittent or partial, with the child having regular but incomplete defecation. With increasing retention, sensory feedback from the bowel is reduced, the rectal wall is stretched and loses contractile strength, and water absorption from fecal material increases, resulting in larger and harder feces. The result is a vicious circle in which the child has less control of his or her bowel movements.

*Etiologic factors* that contribute to the development of encopresis include constitutional predisposition for inefficient intestinal motility, overly aggressive and prolonged medical management (laxatives, enemas, and suppositories), dietary manipulation for perceived constipation, anal fissures and rashes that cause pain on defecation, and surgical procedures for imperforate anus and other anorectal conditions. Parental overreaction to irregular frequency or form of bowel movements may result in inappropriate use of medications or diet changes and/or counterproductive demands on the child. Not only may demands be impossible for the child to meet (i.e., he or she may not yet be ready for toilet training), but parental coercion may stimulate the negativism and resistance that characterize the toddler's budding autonomy. Toileting may be perceived as a negative experience by the child, who may withhold stool out of a need to exercise control or out of fear for the consequences of soiling. The resulting increased retention exacerbates the problem. During the preschool years, irrational fears of the toilet also often result in withholding. During the school years, rigid or hurried schedules or reluctance to use the school bathroom may cause alterations in bowel habits. At any age, psychosocial stresses or illness may cause a regression in toilet training or a change in bowel habits that may potentiate encopresis.

Although encopresis may be more prevalent in children with severe behavioral and developmental disorders, it usually occurs in children and families without significant psychopathology. However, encopresis may result in ridicule and shame for the child and family and carries a significant risk of secondary isolation, depression, and low self-esteem. Because parents and children may not spontaneously mention this problem during the interview, it should be specifically inquired about.

*Diagnosis* is based on a comprehensive assessment, with particular emphasis on a description of bowel patterns since birth, the age of onset of bowel-related symptoms, the effects of attempts to manage the symptoms, associations of the onset or exacerbations of symptoms with psychosocial stresses in the family, and the effects of the problem on the child and other family members. The child should be talked to directly about his or her perception of the problem and feelings about management plans. Hirschsprung disease must also be considered in the differential diagnosis of encopresis (see Chapter 11).

A comprehensive approach to *treatment* is presented in Table 1–15. This approach involves reassurance about the commonness of the problem and an emphasis on the need for patience. Relapses are common, most often related to new or recurrent psychosocial stresses or illnesses. Refractory cases may involve complex underlying psychologic issues that warrant further investigation, organic disease that warrants re-evaluation, or inadequate evacuation of a chronic impaction.

TABLE 1–15. Management of Encopresis*

| Treatment Phase | Treatment Program | Comments |
| --- | --- | --- |
| Initial counseling | Education and "demystification" of the problem<br>Removal of blame<br>Establishment and explanation of treatment plan | Include diagram, review of colonic function, shared observation and x-ray views<br>Emphasize need for intestinal "muscle building" |
| Initial catharsis<br>Inpatient | High normal saline enemas (750 ml b.i.d.), 3–7 days<br>Bisacodyl (Dulcolax) suppositories b.i.d., 3–7 days<br>Use of bathroom for 15 min after each meal | Patient admitted when:<br>  Retention is very severe<br>  Home compliance likely to be poor<br>  Parents prefer admission<br>  Parental administration of enemas is inadvisable psychologically |
| At home | For moderate to severe retention, three–four cycles as follows:<br>  Day 1: hypophosphate enemas (Fleet's Adult) twice<br>  Day 2: bisacodyl (Dulcolax) suppositories twice<br>  Day 3: bisacodyl (Dulcolax) tablet once<br>For mild retention, senna or danthron, one tablet daily for one to two weeks<br>Follow-up abdominal x-ray examination to confirm adequate catharsis | Dosages or frequency may need alteration if child experiences excessive discomfort<br>Admission should be considered if there is inadequate yield<br>No lubricant during this phase |
| Maintenance regimen | Child sits on toilet twice a day at same times each day for 10 min each time<br>Light mineral oil (at least 2 tablespoons) twice a day, usually for at least 4–6 mo<br>Multiple vitamins, 2/day, between doses of mineral oil<br>High-roughage diet: bran, cereal, vegetables, fruits<br>Use of an oral laxative (senna or danthron) for 2–3 wk, then alternate days of mineral oil for 1 mo (given between doses); then laxative is discontinued; lubricant is continued | A kitchen timer can be helpful<br>A chart with stars for sitting may be good for children younger than 7 yr<br>Bathroom reading encouraged<br>Mineral oil can be put in juice, soft drinks, or any other medium<br>Vitamins to compensate for alleged problems with absorption secondary to mineral oil<br>Diet should be applied but not to the point of coercion |
| Follow-up pattern | Visits every 4–10 wk, depending on severity, need for support, compliance, and associated symptoms<br>Telephone availability to adjust doses when needed<br>In case of relapse:<br>  Check compliance<br>  Use of oral laxative (e.g., Senokot) for 1–2 wk<br>  Adjust dosage of mineral oil<br>Counseling or referral for associated psychosocial and developmental issues<br>Continuing use of demystification diagram to document progress | Duration of treatment can be as long as 2–3 yr or as short as 6 mo<br>Signs of relapse:<br>  Excessive oil leaks<br>  Large-caliber stools<br>  Abdominal pain<br>  Decreased frequency of defecation<br>  Soiling<br>Physician should spend time alone with child<br>In patients who are slow to respond, physician should sustain optimism; persistence cures almost all cases (eventually) |

Modified from Levine MD: Encopresis. *In* Levine MD, Carey WB, Crocker AC (eds): Developmental-Behaviorial Pediatrics, 2nd ed. Philadelphia, WB Saunders, 1992, p 394.

*All dosages and frequencies are for an average-sized 7-yr-old child. Appropriate adjustments should be made for smaller and larger patients.

### References

Behrman RE, Kliegman RM, Arvin AM (eds): Nelson Textbook of Pediatrics, 15th ed. Philadelphia, WB Saunders, 1996, Chapters 21.4, 252.
Nolan T, Oberklaid F: New concepts in the management of encopresis. Pediatr Rev 14(11):447, 1993.

## TOILET TRAINING

Toilet training involves the mastery of bowel and urinary control while a child is awake and asleep. The ages at which these tasks are mastered vary widely in different cultures as well as within cultures (see Enuresis and Encopresis). The decision about when to start toilet training should be based on the following readiness signals: (1) dry periods lasting several hours, (2) interest in the potty chair, (3) desire to be changed when wet or dirty, and (4) ability to carry out a series of simple commands. Some general principles about approaching toilet training are as follows:

1. Anger or punishment for lack of performance on the potty chair or for accidents off the potty chair is usually counterproductive and inappropriate.
2. When the child resists sitting on the potty chair, allow her or him to get up and try again after a meal.
3. If resistance is persistent, postpone training for at least several weeks.
4. Power struggles should be avoided. The result may be stool retention, chronic constipation, encopresis, and/or strained parent-child relations. It is almost impossible to win a battle of wills with a toddler, and imposing the will of the adult may interfere with the child's developing autonomy and increase feelings of shame and doubt.
5. A key to successful toilet training is to approach it so that the child sees it as his or her own accomplishment.
6. The age at which daytime training is likely to be successful varies according to individual characteristics of the child: predictability of the child's elimination schedule; ability of the child to anticipate elimination and to understand the steps involved in toileting (getting to the bathroom on time, undressing, sitting on the potty chair, eliminating, wiping, flushing, and redressing); and motivation of the child to toilet train.
7. Many children find it difficult to relax enough while on the potty chair to allow urine or stool to flow. Distracting the child by reading to him or her may be helpful.

**TABLE 1–16.** Timing Method for Toilet Training

After demonstrating readiness signals, child introduced to potty chair.

Child initially sits on potty chair briefly, fully clothed.

Child then sits on potty chair with pants down for gradually increasing lengths of time (1 min, up to a maximum of 10 min).

Simple explanations of toileting procedure given repeatedly and emphasized by placing wet or soiled diapers in the potty.

Parent attempts to anticipate child's need to go (hence "timing method"), puts child on potty chair, and provides positive reinforcement for successful elimination on potty chair (praise, hug, star chart, stickers, or some other sufficiently motivating reward that can be given repeatedly).

One of the many possible approaches to toilet training is the method presented in Table 1–16. This method works well for children with predictable elimination schedules. Children with irregular elimination schedules may have to be able to anticipate the need to go themselves before they can be trained. Complete daytime toilet training should be expected to take a long time. Success is sporadic initially, and occasional accidents are common long after toilet training is accomplished.

### References

Behrman RE, Kliegman RM, Arvin AM (eds): Nelson Textbook of Pediatrics, 15th ed. Philadelphia, WB Saunders, 1996, Chapters 12, 13.
Howe AC, Walker CE: Behavioral management of toilet training, enuresis, and encopresis. Pediatr Clin North Am 39(3):413, 1992.

## RECURRENT PAIN DISORDERS

Chronic, recurrent pain syndromes in childhood most commonly involve abdominal pain, headache, limb pain, or chest pain. It is unusual for children to present with more than one such pain syndrome at the same time, although they often may have had chronic, recurrent pain in a different location of the body in the past. An organic etiology is found in only about 10% of children. The diagnosis of psychogenic pain, however, should be based not only on the absence of adequate physical findings to explain the pain but also on evidence specific for the etiologic role of psychologic factors. Most chronic recurrent pain syndromes have no clear organic or emotional origin.
*Diagnosis* is based on a careful physical examination and history, including a comprehensive psy-

chosocial assessment. In addition to the location, quality, and chronology of the pain, attention must be focused on the circumstances in which the pain is experienced. Signs and symptoms that increase the likelihood of an organic etiology include constant pain, pain awakening the child from sleep, well-localized pain, and physical findings such as fever; weight loss; jaundice; changes in the color, consistency, or frequency of stools; and urinary tract symptoms.

It is important to distinguish between psychologic conditions that preceded and those that followed the onset of the recurrent pain syndrome, because evidence of psychologic stress usually is found by the time the child presents with a chronic problem. The nurturing responses of the family may provide secondary gain that prolongs the pain complaints. Alternatively, frustration with failure to find a specific cause may result in accusations of malingering and increased stress on the child that may create additional reasons for chronic pain. Diagnostic studies should be undertaken in response to specific findings that suggest an organic etiology.

Counseling with reassurance of the benign nature of the pain is the primary treatment for the nonorganic diagnosis. Symptom diaries (including the events that immediately precede and follow the pain episode) are very helpful in the ongoing management of the problem as well as in the initial assessment. It is important to minimize secondary psychologic consequences of recurrent pain syndromes.

### References

Behrman RE, Kliegman RM, Arvin AM (eds): Nelson Textbook of Pediatrics, 15th ed. Philadelphia, WB Saunders, 1996, Chapters 20, 62, 148, 252, 288.
Rickert VI, Jay MS: Psychosomatic disorders: The approach. Pediatr Rev 15(11):448, 1994.

## FAILURE TO THRIVE

Failure to thrive (FTT) is a term used to describe an inadequate growth rate in a young child. Although this may refer to weight below the 3rd percentile on a standard growth chart, many children below the 3rd percentile are normal and some above it may have fallen from a much higher percentile and are failing to thrive. Growth percentile changes demonstrated over time, although meaningful, can be misleading in the first year or two, when wide fluctuations in percentile position are not uncommon in normal children. For example, it is quite common for a child who is above the 75th percentile in weight in the first 6–9 mo to fall to

the 50th percentile or lower from 9 to 18 mo and then to maintain that percentile position. When the percentile drop is great, it is helpful to compare the child's weight percentile to height and head circumference percentiles. It is not a concern when the weight falls from a disproportionately high percentile position to a position consistent with height and head circumference. A fall to a disproportionately low weight is a cause for concern.

In the short term, a child who is failing to thrive as a result of inadequate caloric intake will drop in weight percentile before dropping in height and head circumference. Over time, the height percentile also will fall but the head circumference is usually spared, unless the FTT is severe. In comparison, the child with poor growth due to hypothyroidism will experience slowed height growth with sparing of weight growth. FTT also may be defined as weight less than 80% of the median weight for height. Weight-by-height charts (see Figs. 1–7 and 1–13) are particularly helpful when adequate serial measurements are unavailable.

An etiologic approach to the *differential diagnosis* of FTT is presented in Table 1–17 along with some of the common causes. Almost every chronic and/or serious condition in childhood may cause FTT. It is the diagnosis for 3–5% of children admitted to teaching hospitals. In most children with inadequate growth, both organic and nonorganic risk factors are present. Children with primarily environmental causes may present with physical signs and symptoms due to nutritional deficiency, unusual diets, recurrent infection, and perhaps neuroendocrine responses to stress (e.g., diarrhea, vomiting, depressed growth hormone levels, delayed bone age, iron or zinc deficiency, lead poisoning, elevated serum transaminase levels, and glucose intolerance). Conversely, the environmental stresses faced by the family of a child with a chronic illness may adversely affect the adequacy of nutritional and psychologic nurturing of the child, as in the parents of the child with recurrent vomiting who exhibit stress around feeding that further impedes intake. Infection with human immunodeficiency virus (HIV) often is associated with complex combinations of both organic and environmental factors resulting in poor growth.

In early infancy, feeding difficulties are the predominant cause of FTT, including lactation failure, inadequate feeding frequency or volume, and formula-mixing errors. A calorically inadequate diet at any age may be due to ignorance or neglect by the caregivers. It also may result from irregular caregiving arrangements that involve many caregivers, sometimes themselves children. Diet histories often do not coincide with actual diets, particu-

TABLE 1–17.  Etiology of Failure to Thrive

| Mechanism | Disorders |
| --- | --- |
| *Nonorganic* | |
| Psychosocial | Poor maternal-child interaction, poor feeding technique, psychologically disturbed mother, unusual maternal nutritional beliefs, errors in formula preparation, emotional deprivation (dwarfism), child neglect |
| *Organic* | |
| Inability to suck, swallow, or masticate | CNS pathology (psychomotor retardation), neuromuscular disease (Werdnig-Hoffmann, myotonia congenita, dysautonomia) |
| Maldigestion, malabsorption | Cystic fibrosis, celiac disease, Schwachman-Diamond syndrome, chronic diarrhea |
| Poor nutrient utilization | Renal failure, renal tubular acidosis, inborn errors of metabolism |
| Vomiting | CNS abnormality (tumor, infection, increased pressure), metabolic toxin (inborn errors of amino or organic acid metabolism), intestinal obstruction (pyloric stenosis, malrotation), renal tubular disease |
| Regurgitation | Gastroesophageal reflux, hiatal hernia, rumination syndrome |
| Elevated metabolic rate | Thyrotoxicosis, chronic disease (bronchopulmonary dysplasia, heart failure), cancer, inflammatory lesions (SLE, inflammatory bowel disease, chronic infection), immunodeficiency diseases, burns |
| Reduced growth potential | Chromosomal disorders, primordial dwarfism, skeletal dysplasia, specific syndromes (fetal alcohol) |
| Combinations | Human immunodeficiency virus infection |

CNS = central nervous system; SLE = systemic lupus erythematosus.

larly when there are multiple caregivers. Even a competent mother simply may not know the actual intake of the child unless a detailed diary is kept by all caregivers.

Among children with milder growth abnormalities, the ratio of environmental to organic causes shifts further toward environmental causes. The diagnosis of an environmental cause should be based on observations of caregiver-child interactions as well as on historic data from all important adults and from the child, if possible. Environmental contributors to nonorganic FTT include postpartum depression; maternal depression related to a significant loss (spouse or parent); a social environment characterized by many stresses and poor social support; and caregiver-child interactional patterns that are hostile, rejecting, or aloof.

History and observation are the most important aspects of the *diagnostic evaluation* of FTT. If possible, the attitudes and interactions of important caregivers with each other as well as with the child should be observed or obtained by history. The presence of behavioral problems of the child or siblings (e.g., excessive crying, discipline problems, sleep disturbances, and feeding problems) often is associated with family dysfunction. *Clinical manifestations* in children experiencing environmental deprivation include "frozen watchfulness," minimal smiling, decreased vocalization, resistance to being held, and self-stimulating rhythmic behaviors.

If a careful history and physical examination fail to identify a cause or clue that suggests specific diagnostic procedures, it is very unlikely that any tests will reveal a cause. In one study of children admitted to a teaching hospital with FTT of unknown etiology, fewer than 2% of tests performed during the hospitalization contributed to a diagnosis and all of the positive tests were associated with a positive finding in the initial history and physical examination. Still, it is standard procedure to obtain a few screening tests: a complete blood count, urinalysis, serum electrolytes, and perhaps an erythrocyte sedimentation rate. If even mild gastrointestinal symptoms are present, a stool culture, pH, reducing substances test, and guaiac test are indicated.

*Treatment* of FTT by hospitalization of the child may be particularly stressful when the parent-child attachment is insecure. If the cause appears to be inadequate caloric intake, a reasonable initial ambulatory plan may be to provide dietary advice and have caregivers keep a detailed diary of feedings and the frequency, volume, and consistency of stools and vomitus. If the picture remains unclear and the child fails to exhibit catch-up growth within several weeks, hospitalization is necessary because adequate nutrition is crucial for brain development during the first 2 yr of life.

One common approach to FTT of unknown etiology, after outpatient attempts to manage the problem have failed, is to admit the child to the hospital and to observe him or her for weight gain after demonstrating adequate caloric intake. Most children will grow if given 120 kcal times the median weight in kilograms for the child's measured length over each 24-hr period. If the child gains weight, FTT resulting from inadequate intake is assumed and steps are taken to monitor and support the environment as well as the child's nutrition after discharge. If the child fails to gain, an organic cause is more aggressively sought. However, as noted above, environmental and organic factors usually occur together. Table 1–18 presents data from one study demonstrating the time required in the hospital before catch-up weight gain was observed in children with calorie-deprivation FTT.

Table 1–19 presents a protocol for management in or out of the hospital. Deferment of investigations decreases the stress of hospitalization, which may shorten the time required to achieve adequate caloric intake and thereby to test the hypothesis that the FTT is due to inadequate caloric intake. Because catch-up growth must be demonstrated, more calories should be provided than the normal requirements for the child's current depressed weight. A positive change in the mood of a child usually is followed by accelerated weight gain in 1–2 days. The parents should be involved in the development and implementation of the management plan.

The *prognosis* for children hospitalized for nonorganic FTT in the first 2 yr of life shows a high percentage of retardation (15–67%), school learning problems (37–67%), and behavioral disturbances (28–48%) at 3–11 yr of age. Continued FTT is a much less frequent problem.

### References

Behrman RE, Kliegman RM, Arvin AM (eds): Nelson Textbook of Pediatrics, 15th ed. Philadelphia, WB Saunders, 1996, Chapters 38.2, 39.

TABLE 1–18. Time Required in Hospital for Accelerated Weight Gain in Children with Calorie-Deprivation Failure to Thrive

| |
| --- |
| Age younger than 6 mo<br>Most gaining by 2–3 days<br>All gaining by 9 days |
| Age 6–24 mo<br>Gaining by 2–17 days<br>2 of 25 required more than 2 wk |
| Age 2 yr or more<br>All gaining in 2–7 days |

Adapted from Ellerstein NS, Ostrov BE: Growth patterns in children hospitalized because of caloric-deprivation failure to thrive. Am J Dis Child 139:164–166, 1985. Copyright 1985, American Medical Association.

TABLE 1–19. Hospital Protocol for Failure to Thrive of Unknown Etiology

Defer all investigations for at least 1 wk (assuming no clues for organic etiology on comprehensive history and physical examination).

Aim to provide 120 kcal/24 hr times median weight (kg) for *measured* length.

Record the following data daily:
Weight before breakfast (unclothed)
Total calories consumed in the previous 24 hr
Calories/kg of *ideal weight* in the previous 24 hr
Output (stool, urine, vomitus)

Record observations of the child's behavior and interactions of the child with the parents and the staff.

Provide an organized program of stimulation, including regular affectionate interaction with adults.

Involve the parents from the start in the feeding and stimulation interventions.

Begin interdisciplinary evaluations on admission (e.g., social worker, nurse, nutritional support team or dietitian, behavioral/developmental specialist).

Frank D, Silva M, Needleman R: Failure to thrive: Mystery, myth, and method. Contemp Pediatr 10:114, 1993.

## CHILD ABUSE AND NEGLECT

Child abuse is a frequent, serious problem that every state and the federal government have addressed by laws. The Child Abuse Prevention and Treatment Act (Public Law 93–247) defines child abuse and neglect as "the physical or mental injury, sexual abuse, negligent treatment, or maltreatment of a child under the age of eighteen by a person who is responsible for the child's welfare under circumstances which indicate that the child's health and welfare is harmed or threatened thereby." In most cases, child abuse needs to be understood as a symptom of family dysfunction. Only by understanding the factors that contribute to its occurrence can a logical management plan be developed (Fig. 1–19).

Estimates of the *incidence* of child abuse and neglect vary widely, depending on the definition and the source. Approximately 1% of children are reported to be abused or neglected each year. Approximately two thirds of cases involved physical abuse, one fourth sexual abuse, 5% FTT due to underfeeding, and smaller percentages for other causes, including medical neglect, grossly inadequate supervision, intentional drugging or poisoning, and severe emotional abuse. Estimates of the

FIGURE 1–19.  Model for understanding child abuse. (From Bittner S, Newberger EH: Pediatric understanding of child abuse and neglect. Pediatr Rev 2:198, 1981. Copyright American Academy of Pediatrics, 1981.)

incidence of child abuse based on household surveys range from 1 to 4 million cases/yr. Abuse is less likely to be reported if it involves children from white, nonpoor families; if the mother is alleged to be responsible for the abuse; and if the abuse is emotional rather than physical.

Physicians may be reluctant to report cases because they are uncomfortable in the role of accuser, the antithesis of their usual role of compassionate helper, or because of time constraints, concern over possible court appearances, and lack of knowledge about the problem or how to proceed once child

abuse is suspected. Laws that govern reporting attempt to overcome this reluctance by mandating the report of "suspected" abuse, by making physicians immune from suits related to a report made in good faith, and by making it the responsibility of protection agencies (not physicians) to determine whether abuse has actually occurred. Physicians thus can attempt to maintain a helping relationship with the family by telling them that they are obligated by law to make a report but that their aim is to help find ways to prevent a recurrence of the injury or condition. Some families react with anger or hurt, but others welcome the opportunity to find help for their difficult situation.

To detect less obvious cases of child abuse, the physician must be sensitive to the more subtle signs and must take the time to obtain an expanded history and behavioral observations. Because a determination of whether a report is warranted may take more time or expertise than the physician has, the use of a social worker who specializes in child abuse or, preferably, a child abuse team may be invaluable.

### Physical Abuse

Conservative estimates indicate that 1–2% of children in the United States are physically abused at some time during childhood and that 10% of injuries seen in a hospital emergency room in children younger than 5 yr of age are due to abuse. About one third of physical abuse cases occur in children under 1 yr of age and another one third between ages 1 and 6 yr. Approximately 2000 deaths per year in the United States are a result of physical abuse. The abuser is a related caregiver in 90% of cases, a male friend of the mother in 5%, an unrelated babysitter in 4%, and a sibling in 1%. Physical abuse usually occurs in the context of increased social-environmental stresses and often is triggered by child behaviors such as persistent crying, wetting or soiling, spilling, or disobedience. Fewer than 10% of abusive parents have psychotic or criminal personalities.

Some *clinical manifestations* of physical abuse are unequivocal. Distinctive bruising patterns are often caused by blunt instruments, belts, cords, hand slaps, pinches, choke holds, and bites. Burn patterns from cigarettes, irons, hot plates, and forced submersion into scalding water are also distinctive. A circular burn limited to the buttocks and genitalia with no involvement of the hands or feet is incompatible with falling into or mistakenly entering a tub of hot water.

Usually, however, the presentation of child abuse is not as clear. Bruises, burns, and fractures may be accidental and often are dismissed as such without adequate consideration of other causes. Accidental bruises are most common over the forehead, anterior tibia, and bony prominences; bruises confined to the buttocks or lower back are most commonly caused by abuse. Anaphylactoid (Henoch-Schönlein) purpura may present with ecchymoses over the buttocks, but usually purpura from organic causes does not have the limited distribution of bruising characteristic of child abuse. Healing cigarette burns may be mistaken for impetigo or atopic or contact dermatitis.

Some presentations of serious child abuse may not suggest the diagnosis at all. Subdural hematomas may be caused by violent shaking leading to the tearing of bridging cerebral vessels, in the absence of injury to the skull or scalp. Serious abdominal injuries may be caused by striking or squeezing the abdomen (e.g., rupture of the liver, spleen, intestines, or blood vessels; traumatic pancreatitis; or intramural hematomas); children with these injuries may present with signs and symptoms of an acute abdomen but may not have evidence of external trauma to raise the suspicion of child abuse.

Table 1–20 outlines the *diagnostic evaluation* for suspected child abuse. The history is crucial when the injury is not pathognomonic for abuse. The interviewer should strive to be a supportive listener while avoiding judgmental statements that may arouse increased defensiveness. After beginning the interview with nonthreatening general conversation, the focus should be on concrete details about how the injury occurred. Key questions are whether the family's explanation for the injury is compatible with the physical findings and whether the explanation is consistent among family members, including the injured child, and subsequent interviews with the same family member. If old enough to be interviewed, the child should be interviewed alone. The interviewer must be very sensitive to the child's feelings of fear or guilt.

Description of the injury and identification of the probable cause are the relatively easy aspects of a child abuse work-up. A comprehensive evaluation of the family and social environment is essential to guide subsequent management decisions when the diagnosis is child abuse. Hospital admission may be necessary to treat the child's injuries and to ensure the child's safety until it can be determined that it is safe to return home or to an alternative setting.

### Sexual Abuse

This injury involves engaging a child in sexual activities that the child often does not understand, to which the child cannot give informed consent, or that violate the sexual social taboos. This definition includes a broad range of sexual activities (e.g., exhibitionism, fondling, child pornography, and oral, anal, and genital contact), both inside and outside the family. Some reserve the term "sexual abuse" to refer to forced sexual contact between a victim and perpetrator, while using the term "sexual misuse" for when a child is exposed to sexual stimulation inappropriate for the child's role in the family. **Incest** is sexual abuse by a close relative

**TABLE 1–20.**  Initial Diagnostic Evaluation for Suspected Child Abuse

**History**
  Obtain separate histories from parents, other adults, and child (if possible)

  Record history precisely
    Record direct quotations
    Clarify ambiguous statements
    Use qualifiers like "the mother alleges that . . ." rather than "the child was . . ."

  Record the following:
    Data and time of evaluation
    Date, time, and place of alleged abuse
    Informant
    How alleged abuse occurred and who allegedly caused it
    History of past abuse

**Physical Examination**
  Perform careful, complete examination

  List bruises by site, size, shape, and color

  Check the retina, eardrums, oral cavity, and genitalia for signs of occult trauma

  Check bones and joints for tenderness and range of motion

  Record height and weight percentiles

  Obtain color photographs of injuries (include paper with patient's name, date, and time in the photograph)

**Laboratory Test**
  Radiologic bone survey (skull, thorax, spine, long bones) for children under age 5 yr who are suspected victims of child abuse

  Bleeding studies when bruising present (platelet count, bleeding time, prothrombin time [PT], and partial thromboplastin time [PTT])

**Disposition**
  Consult immediately with social worker or child abuse team to arrange comprehensive multidisciplinary evaluation

  Report to mandated agency if indicated

  Inform parents of need to report and desire to be helpful

  Hospitalize the child if further investigation necessary to determine safety of home and/or to treat injuries

  Establish multidisciplinary follow-up plan (health and social services)

that involves intercourse. **Molestation** is sexual abuse by a stranger, with or without penetration. **Rape** involves forced genital contact. **Sexual assault** involves violent or nonviolent manual, oral, or genital contact with genitalia of the victim or the perpetrator. Activities that are considered to be normal sexual exploratory behavior among children of similar age may be considered sexual abuse

or misuse if the ages are discrepant. There are at least 250,000 cases of sexual abuse per year in the United States, with the more serious and chronic forms affecting 1–3% of children. Most recognized sexual offenders are male, of whom about 20% are adolescents.

The *clinical manifestations* of sexual abuse may be more difficult to recognize than those of physical abuse. Early warnings may include simulation of sexual acts with dolls, inclusion of genitalia in drawings, precocious flirtation, and verbalization of concern about sexual molestation in general. Direct statements from children about abusive behaviors should be taken seriously. Most sexually abused children are very reluctant to break the secrecy of the abuse because of fear and guilt; many who do make a statement recant it later. Many nonspecific behavioral problems may be associated with sexual abuse, including sleeping and eating disorders, school dysfunction, phobias, depression, acting out behaviors, conversion reactions, and suicide attempts.

The presence in prepubertal children of genital and anal trauma or diseases that are usually sexually transmitted (e.g., gonorrhea, syphilis, lymphogranuloma venereum, trichomoniasis, genital herpes, and chlamydial infections) should raise a strong suspicion of sexual abuse. Recurrent urinary tract infections, recurrent nonspecific vaginitis, genital warts, or early pregnancy may also be the result of sexual abuse.

The diagnostic evaluation in Table 1–20 may need to be modified for sexual abuse. If it is clear that others also will need to interview the child (e.g., social worker, child protective worker, or police), it may be best to arrange a single, joint interview to obtain the initial detailed history because multiple histories are often traumatic for the child. If possible, observation rooms and videotaped interviews should be used. Local authorities should be consulted regarding consent, confidentiality, and admissibility of evidence obtained using such techniques. Questions should be open ended and as nonjudgmental as possible. Dolls with body parts often involved in sexual abuse, drawings of a person or the family, and toys may help in the interview. Clarification of terminology frequently is necessary to be certain that the interviewer understands what the child means, and vice versa. If a girl is pubertal, a menstrual history should be obtained.

The physical examination often is easier for the child and the physician after a sensitive, supportive interview. If it must occur before the detailed history is obtained, the physician will need to obtain at least a brief history to guide the examination.

Particularly important points include the type and time of the alleged abusive act and subsequent events that may alter the presence of evidence (e.g., bathing, urinating, defecation, brushing teeth, or changing clothes). It is best to obtain this information from someone other than the child if there is not sufficient time to approach the sensitive questions gradually. The examination should proceed like a normal general one, with special attention to any evidence of physical abuse, trauma, or the presence of blood or semen on body parts or clothing. The knee-chest position may provide better visualization of the vagina and anus in prepubertal girls, although the lithotomy position is usually better as girls approach puberty. Wood lamp inspection of the body and clothing is indicated to look for the fluorescence of sperm. Laboratory evaluation for suspected sexual abuse is outlined in Table 1–21. Many hospital emergency departments have standardized protocols and kits for specimen collection developed in collaboration with law enforcement agencies.

Treatment of sexually transmitted diseases is discussed in Chapter 7. Pregnancy can be prevented within 72 hr of intercourse by giving two norgestrel and ethinyl estradiol (Ovral) tablets at the time of examination and two more 12 hr later. The physician will need the help of social workers and perhaps mental health professionals to immediately assess child and family functioning, the family's social environment, and their needs for services. A child victim will need extensive counseling. Hospital admission may be warranted for treatment of injuries, for mental health evaluation, or to ensure safety. Subsequently, the effectiveness of health and social services to which the child and family have been referred should be monitored and close communication maintained among the professionals involved in the evaluation and continuing care of the family. Medical follow-up must ensure adequate treatment of injuries and infections; serology for syphilis should be rechecked in 6 wk.

### References

Behrman RE, Kliegman RM, Arvin AM (eds): Nelson Textbook of Pediatrics, 15th ed. Philadelphia, WB Saunders, 1996, Chapters 13, 37, 38, 288, 551, 504.

Krugman RD: Recognition of sexual abuse in children. Pediatr Rev 8:25, 30, 1986.

Sirotnak AP, Krugman RD: Physical abuse of children: An update. Pediatr Rev 15(10):394, 1994.

## SEPARATION FROM ONE OR BOTH PARENTS

### Hospitalization

About 30% of children are hospitalized at least once during childhood, and about 5% have multiple hospital admissions. Along with separation from parents, hospitalization stresses include the illness itself (with discomfort, pain, fear, uncertainty, parental anxiety), separation from almost everything that is familiar (siblings, home, friends, school, customary routines), and exposure to many strange and threatening experiences (painful and uncomfortable procedures, many new people, sick or disabled people experiencing pain and emotional upset).

Hospitalization of a child can result in (1) distress during the hospitalization, (2) disturbance on return home, and (3) long-term sequelae. Distress during hospitalization is most marked between 6 mo and 4 yr of age. It is related to the degree of separation from all people to whom the child is attached, lack of opportunity to form new attachments (large numbers of frequently changing caregivers), and the strangeness of the environment. On returning home, many children exhibit regressive, withdrawn, ambivalent, or labile behavior.

Prolonged and serious illnesses in children place great stress on the parents (marital relationships,

TABLE 1–21.  Laboratory Evaluation of the Sexually Abused Child

---

*Motile sperm*
  Wet mount of vaginal specimen (mouth, rectum, if indicated)
  Cervical mucus aspirate

*Infection*
  Gonococcal cultures (vagina, cervix, rectum, throat)
  Gram stain of vaginal specimen for bacteria (e.g., gonococcus, *Gardnerella vaginalis*)
  KOH preparation of vaginal specimen for *Candida*
  Wet preparation of vaginal specimen for *Trichomonas*
  Other cultures of vagina or cervix (e.g., for *Chlamydia, Candida,* herpes)
  Syphilis serology (initially and 6 wk later)
  HIV tests

*Serum or urine pregnancy test (if child is pubertal)*

*Specimens for police report (if indicated)*
  Air-dried slide specimens from the vagina, cervix, rectum, and mouth (can be tested for sperm antibodies, blood, acid phosphatase)
  Fingernail scrapings for blood or fabric particles if a struggle took place
  Collection of loose hairs or threads of fabric from body and clothing

---

KOH = potassium hydroxide; HIV = human immunodeficiency virus.

parenting of siblings, and work performance) and siblings, who are often neglected to some degree while the parents are consumed by the care of and anxiety over the sick child. Even with conditions that are judged as relatively mild by health care providers, the behavior of the parents toward the sick child may be altered for a long time after the illness resolves. Common problems include difficulties with separations, infantilization, preoccupation with bodily functions, and decreased school achievement.

## Divorce

The problems associated with divorce are usually chronic and often devastating for both the children and the parents. Divorce is usually not a single event but a sequence of difficult changes and adjustments that span years. For years prior to divorce, children may be exposed to family turmoil that may include violent arguments and physical violence, including that between their parents, other family members, and perhaps themselves. Alternatively, some children, particularly young ones, may be completely unaware that a problem exists until one of the parents leaves. For the parents, the period between the separation and the formal divorce can be particularly acrimonious, making it very difficult for them to help the children cope with their losses, fears, and disruptions in the usual pattern of family life.

Complicating the family's emotional adjustment to the divorce are the untoward economic effects experienced by many of these families. Often ex-husbands fail to provide child support payments. Women, who are usually the custodial parents, may lack the education, job skills, or experience to get adequately compensated and secure jobs. When a mother who has remained in the home to care for a preschool child must start work, that child suffers a second loss. The custodial parent also must assume household responsibilities that previously were shared. In addition, relocation to cheaper housing often is necessary, frequently involving a loss of friends and familiar school and neighborhood. Worsening parent-child relations often result from these additional stresses. It is usually not until after the first year of divorce that reduced tension and an increased sense of well-being begin to emerge in the children of divorce. Because many divorced women and men remarry, there will be further periods of adjustment as stepparents and often stepchildren join the family.

The most important determinant of initial responses of children to divorce is the age of the child (Table 1–22). In the long term, more than one

**TABLE 1–22.** Assistance Related to the Age of the Child

| Age | Common Reactions of Child | Role of Physician |
|---|---|---|
| 2–5 yr | Regression, irritability, sleep disturbance | Encourage restabilization of household and bedtime routines; Reassure child; Urge restoration of contact with departed parent |
| 6–8 yr | Open grieving, feelings of rejection | Support maintenance of child's relationship to both parents; reassure child |
| 9–12 yr | Fear, anger at one or both parents | Express interest and availability to child |
| Adolescence | Worried about own future, depressed and/or acting-out behavior | Offer opportunity for private discussion |

From Wallerstein JS: Separation, divorce, and remarriage. *In* Levine MD, Carey WB, Crocker AC (eds): Developmental-Behavioral Pediatrics, 2nd ed. Philadelphia, WB Saunders, 1992, p 140.

third of children are psychologically troubled and distressed 5 yr after the divorce. The most frequent clinical finding is depression. Poor psychologic adjustment in children is more likely when parental fighting continues and when they remain in the custody of a lonely, depressed, or emotionally disturbed parent.

Children who are told about the divorce before the actual separation and who are reassured that they will continue to see both parents are calmer at the time of separation. Children should be told the details about what their living arrangements and daily routines will be after the separation. They also need to be told repeatedly that they did not cause the divorce and that their efforts cannot mend it. Young children may be told that the divorce is necessary to bring an end to fighting or unhappiness between the parents. Older children may have more specific questions that should be answered simply without going beyond a concrete, superficial response unless questioned further. Children need to be assured that neither parent expects them to take sides, and they need to be allowed to love both parents. They also need to be allowed to express and vent feelings of anger, sadness, and disappointment. There is a continuing need for reassurances after the separation. Children who receive additional attention from grandparents, family, and friends do better than those who do not.

## References

Behrman RE, Kliegman RM, Arvin AM (eds): Nelson Textbook of Pediatrics, 15th ed. Philadelphia, WB Saunders, 1996, Chapters 30.1, 32–36, 41.
Emery RE, Coiro MJ: Divorce: Consequences for children. Pediatr Rev 16(8):306, 1995.
Jellinek MS, Kearns ME: Separation anxiety. Pediatr Rev 16(2):57, 1995.

## SLEEP DISORDERS

Sleep patterns in children follow a typical developmental sequence, with the gradual increase of deep sleep and the development of regular sleep cycles. Sleep stages are defined by electroencephalographic (EEG), electromyographic, and electrooculographic characteristics, such as waking, rapid eye movement (REM), and non-REM sleep. Most infants (up to 70%) will sleep through the night (at least 5 hr at a stretch) by 3 mo post-term, at which time they have assumed schedules of about four sleep periods within 24 hr. Premature infants take longer to assume the patterns typical of full-term infants. Most children experience a point later in the first year of life, often associated with an intercurrent illness, when they begin to wake at night again, sometimes falling into patterns of night waking that persist for years and that require behavioral interventions for correction.

Common sleep disruption disorders may be organic in nature or related to environmental factors that usually are easily remedied once their features are recognized. Table 1–23 lists several common sleep disruption patterns and their treatments. When schedules need to be regularized, imposing a routine bedtime and naptime for the child, along with a usual presleep routine, and firmly but supportively maintaining it despite protests can be very successful. When parental work and lifestyles result in children being awakened early and going to bed late, the schedule must be arranged so that the child gets enough sleep. In children with delayed sleep phase onset, the circadian clock is probably set so that the child is not ready for sleep at the prescribed bedtime; treatment involves either gradually moving the bedtime backward 15–30 min/day or forward by 2–3 hr/night over a week.

*Obstructive sleep apnea* occurs in children as well as in adults and frequently is associated with a predisposing physical condition, such as tonsillar hypertrophy. It is characterized by snoring, may be associated with enuresis and/or obesity, and also may be associated with hyperactivity and school dysfunction in some children. Weight reduction and otolaryngologic surgery may be indicated.

*Night terrors* (pavor nocturnus), bedwetting (enuresis), and sleepwalking are common deep sleep phenomena that are developmentally normal and usually do not represent pathologic processes. Similarly, head rolling, head banging, and rocking are seen in many normal children between 9 mo and 3 yr of age and usually are benign, self-limited phenomena. If these behaviors persist or are associated with other developmental lags, they should be further evaluated.

## References

Adair RH, Bauchner H: Sleep problems in childhood. Curr Probl Pediatr 23(4):147; discussion, 142, 1993.
Behrman RE, Kliegman RM, Arvin AM (eds): Nelson Textbook of Pediatrics, 15th ed. Philadelphia, WB Saunders, 1996, Chapters 11, 21.5, 106.
Ferber R: Sleep disorders. In Levine MD, Casey WD, Crocker AC (eds): Developmental-Behavioral Pediatrics, 2nd ed. Philadelphia, WB Saunders, 1992, pp 398–406.

## MENTAL RETARDATION

Mental retardation (MR) is significantly subaverage general intellectual functioning for a child's developmental stage, existing concurrently with deficits in adaptive behavior. MR is defined statistically as tested cognitive performance that is 2 standard deviations below the mean (roughly below the 3rd percentile) of the general population. This implies that as many as 7.5 million persons in the United States can be characterized as having mental retardation; clinical estimates range from 2.2 to 10 million (the higher number includes persons with so-called borderline intelligence and poor social adaptation). About 60,000 individuals with cognitive impairment live in public residential facilities.

Levels of MR from IQ scores derived from two typical tests are shown in Table 1–24. These categories do not necessarily reflect the actual functional level of the tested individual. In school, a child with mild MR may, because of poor social (adaptive) abilities, be better served in a class for children defined as "trainable," whereas another child who tests in the moderate range of retardation but who has especially good language abilities may be more stimulated in a class for children defined as "educable." Current practice supports the position that persons who perform in the severe or profound ranges of MR are capable of responding to some educational interventions as well.

The etiology of the central nervous system (CNS) insult resulting in MR may relate to genetic

TABLE 1–23.   Childhood Sleep Disruption Disorders

| Type | Cause | Symptoms | Treatment |
|---|---|---|---|
| **_Organic_** | | | |
| Colic | Unknown | Crying, irritability | Rocking, pacifier, nursing Support until resolution |
| Medications | Stimulants Bronchodilators Anticonvulsants | Failure to fall asleep; restless sleep | Adjust dosage/timing; change medication |
| Illness | Any chronically irritating disorder (e.g., otitis, dermatitis, asthma, esophageal reflux) | Painful crying out | Treat disease symptomatically |
| Central nervous system disorders | Variable; rule out seizures | Decreased sleep | Evaluate environment Sedatives as last resort |
| **_Parasomnias_** | | | |
| Sleepwalking, sleep terrors | Stage IV (deep) sleep instability | Awakening 1–3 hr after falling asleep | Reassurance; protective environment |
| Confusional arousals | | Intense crying, walking, disorientation, talking | |
| Enuresis | ? Stage IV instability Metabolic disease (e.g., diabetes) Urinary tract infection Urinary anatomic anomaly | Bedwetting | Rule out medical conditions Fluid limitation Prebed voiding Behavioral approaches (bell and pad) Emotional support Medication (e.g., imipramine) Reassurance |
| **_Sleep-Wake Schedule Disorders_** | | | |
| Irregular sleep-wake pattern | No defined schedule | Variable waking and sleeping | Regularize schedule |
| Regular but inappropriate sleep-wake schedule | Napping at wrong times Prematurely eliminated nap | Morning sleepiness Night wakenings | Rework schedule |
| Delayed sleep phase | Late sleep onset with resetting of circadian rhythm | Late sleep onset Morning sleepiness Not sleepy at bedtime | Enforce wake-up time Gradually move bedtime earlier or keep awake overnight to create drowsy state |
| **_Environmental and Psychosocial Factors_** | | | |
| Inappropriate sleep-onset associations | No defined bedtime routine Child falls asleep in conditions different from those of the rest of the night | Night wakings requiring intervention | Regularize routine Minimize nocturnal parental response |
| Excessive nocturnal fluid | Child gets food/drink with each awakening | Night waking or wanting drink | Gradually decrease nocturnal fluid |
| Inconsistent limit setting | Parental anxiety | Delayed bedtime Excessive expression of "needs" by child | Modify parental behavior to improve limit setting Gradually increase limits |
| Anxieties; fears | Separation anxieties | Night waking Refusal to sleep | Reassurance when appropriate Counseling in severe cases |
| Social disruptions | Family stressors | Night waking Refusal to sleep | Family counseling Regularize routines |

TABLE 1–24.  Levels of Mental Retardation

| Level of Retardation | Stanford-Binet IQ Score | WISC-III IQ Score | Educational Label |
|---|---|---|---|
| Mild | 67–52 | 70–55 | "Educable (EMR)" |
| Moderate | 51–36 | 54–40 | "Trainable (TMR)" |
| Severe | 35–20 | 39–25 | |
| Profound | Below 20 | Below 24 | Severe-profound |

IQ = intelligence quotient; WISC-III = Wechsler Intelligence Scale for children (3rd ed).

disorders, teratogenic influences, perinatal insults, acquired childhood disease, and environmental/ social factors (Table 1–25). Although a single organic cause may be found, each individual's performance should be considered a function of the interaction of environmental influences on the person's organic substrate. Thus, it is common for a child with mental retardation to have behavioral difficulties resulting from both the retarding condition itself and the family's reaction to the child and his or her condition. In general, more severe forms of retardation can be traced to biologic factors, and the earlier the cognitive slowing is recognized, the more severe the deviation from normal is likely to be. The pattern of an individual's development can aid in making a diagnosis, but at any given point in time it may be very difficult to predict future performance accurately.

In an approach to the diagnosis of MR, the first step is to provide interdisciplinary evaluations to identify functional strengths and weaknesses. Expertise from several disciplines is needed to characterize the child functionally for purposes of medical and habilitative therapies (see earlier topics of Interdisciplinary Team Assessment and Intervention). Once the developmental lags have been identified, the history and physical examination may

TABLE 1–25.  Mechanisms of Developmental Disabilities*

| Disorder | Total in Group with Mental Retardation (%) |
|---|---|
| *Hereditary disorders:* preconceptual origin, variable expression, multiple somatic effects, frequently a progressive course<br>Inborn errors of metabolism (e.g., Tay-Sachs disease, Hurler disease, phenylketonuria)<br>Other single gene abnormalities (e.g., muscular dystrophy, neurofibromatosis, tuberous sclerosis)<br>Chromosomal aberrations, including translocation, fragile X syndrome<br>Polygenic familial syndromes | 5 |
| *Early alterations of embryonic development:* sporadic events affecting embryogenesis, phenotypic changes, usually a stable developmental handicap<br>Chromosomal changes, including trisomy (e.g., Down syndrome)<br>Prenatal influence syndromes (e.g., intrauterine infections, drugs, alcohol, unknown) | 32 |
| *Other pregnancy problems and perinatal morbidity:* impingement on progress of fetus during last two trimesters or on newborn, neurologic abnormalities frequent, handicap stable or occasionally worsening<br>Fetal malnutrition and placental insufficiency<br>Perinatal difficulties (e.g., prematurity, hypoxia, trauma) | 11 |
| *Acquired childhood diseases:* acute modification of developmental status, variable potential for functional recovery<br>Infection (e.g., encephalitis, meningitis)<br>Cranial trauma<br>Other (e.g., cardiac arrest, drowning, intoxications) | 4 |
| *Environmental and social problems:* dynamic influences, operational throughout development, commonly combined with other handicaps<br>Deprivation<br>Parental neurosis, psychosis<br>Childhood neurosis<br>Childhood psychosis | 18 |
| *Unknown causes:* no definite hereditary, gestational, perinatal, acquired, or environmental issues; or else multiple elements present | |

Adapted from Crocker AC, Nelson RP: Mental retardation. *In* Levine MD, Carey WB, Crocker AC (eds): Developmental-Behavioral Pediatrics, 2nd ed. Philadelphia, WB Saunders, 1992, p 502.
*Mental retardation, cerebral palsy, seizure disorders, and sensory handicaps.

suggest the point in development at which a CNS insult may have taken place and minimize the need for laboratory tests. Almost one third of individuals with mental retardation do not have readily identifiable reasons for their disabilities. However, in many cases, enough factors can be ruled out to allay the guilt and anxiety of families as to their responsibility in causing the disability.

### References

Behrman RE, Kliegman RM, Arvin AM (eds): Nelson Textbook of Pediatrics, 15th ed. Philadelphia, WB Saunders, 1996, Chapters 17, 40.
Palmer FB, Capute AJ: Mental retardation. Pediatr Rev 15(12):473, 1994.

## VISION IMPAIRMENT

Significant visual impairment is a problem in many children. *Partial vision* (defined as visual acuity between 20/70 and 20/200) occurs in 1 in 500 schoolchildren in the United States, with about 35,000 children having visual acuity between 20/200 and total blindness. "Legal blindness" is defined as distant visual acuity of 20/200 in the better eye or a visual field that subtends an angle not greater than 20 degrees. Although this definition allows for considerable residual vision, such impairment can be a major barrier to optimal educational development.

The most common *etiology* of severe visual impairment in children is retinopathy of premature infants (see Chapter 6). Congenital cataracts due to a variety of causes occur in 1:250 newborn infants and can result in significant amblyopia; cataracts are also associated with other ocular abnormalities and developmental disabilities. Optic atrophy, retinal degeneration (Leber congenital amaurosis and retinitis pigmentosa), retinoblastoma, and congenital glaucoma are other common causes of significant visual impairment in childhood.

The *diagnosis* is commonly made between 4 and 8 mo of life based on parental suspicions aroused by unusual behavior, such as lack of smiling in response to appropriate stimuli or motor delays in beginning to reach for objects. Fixation and visual tracking behavior can be seen in most children by 6 wk post-term and by many infants at birth. This behavior can be assessed by moving a brightly colored object or the examiner's face across the visual field of a quiet but alert infant at a distance of 1 ft. The eyes should be examined for red reflexes and pupillary reactions to light, although optical alignment should not be expected until the child is beyond the newborn period. Persistent nystagmus is abnormal at any age. If abnormalities are seen, referral to an ophthalmologist should be made.

The developmental implications of visual impairment are many. Perceptual development is abnormal in terms of body image, and imitative behavior, such as smiling, is delayed. Delays in mobility may occur in children who are visually impaired from birth, although their postural milestones usually are achieved appropriately. Social bonding with the parents also is limited. Stereotypic behaviors ("blindisms") occur in these children and may at times be self-injurious, requiring intensive behavioral interventions to reduce trauma to eyes, periorbital structures, or other body parts.

*Treatment* of children with vision impairments is aimed at maximizing available visual skills and developing compensatory methods for individualized education. Classroom settings may be augmented with resource room assistance to present material in a nonvisual format; some schools utilize consultations with an experienced teacher of the blind. Segregated programs sometimes are necessary in training for mobility and for individuals with multiple disabilities. Fine motor activity development, listening skills, and Braille reading and writing are intrinsic to successful educational intervention with the child with severe visual impairment.

### References

Behrman RE, Kliegman RM, Arvin AM (eds): Nelson Textbook of Pediatrics, 15th ed. Philadelphia, WB Saunders, 1996, Chapters 569–574.
Moller MA: Working with visually impaired children and their families. Pediatr Clin North Am 40(4):881, 1993.
Repka MX: Common pediatric neuro-ophthalmologic conditions. Pediatr Clin North Am 40(4):777, 1993.

## HEARING IMPAIRMENT

The clinical significance of hearing loss varies with its type (conductive versus sensorineural), its frequency distribution, and its severity, as measured in number of decibels (Table 1–26). The most common *cause* of mild to moderate hearing loss in children is a conduction abnormality due to acquired middle ear disease. This abnormality may have significant impact on the development of speech and other aspects of language, particularly if there is chronic fluctuating middle ear fluid. Sensorineural hearing loss is more common as an etiologic factor as hearing loss becomes more severe. The age of onset of the hearing loss may suggest the etiology as well. Other causes of deafness are congenital infection with rubella or cytomegalovi-

TABLE 1-26. Neurodevelopmental-Behavioral Complications of Hearing Loss

| Severity of Hearing Loss | Possible Etiologic Origins | Complications | | | | Types of Therapy |
|---|---|---|---|---|---|---|
| | | Speech-Language | Educational | Behavioral | | |
| *Slight* 15–25 dB (ASA) | Serous otitis media Perforation of tympanic membrane Sensorineural loss Tympanosclerosis | Difficulty with distant or faint speech | Possible auditory learning dysfunction May reveal a slight verbal deficit | Usually none | | May require favorable class setting, speech therapy, auditory training Possible value in hearing aid |
| *Mild* 25–40 dB (ASA) | Serous otitis media Perforation of tympanic membrane Sensorineural loss Tympanosclerosis | Difficulty with conversational speech over 3–5 ft May have limited vocabulary and speech disorders | May miss 50% of class discussions Auditory learning dysfunction | Psychologic problems May act inappropriately if directions are not heard well Acting-out behavior Poor self-concept | | Special education resource help Hearing aid Favorable class setting Lip reading instruction Speech therapy |
| *Moderate* 40–65 dB (ASA) | Chronic otitis media Middle ear anomaly Sensorineural loss | Conversation must be loud to be understood Defective speech Deficient language use and comprehension | Learning disability Difficulty with group learning or discussion Auditory processing dysfunction Limited vocabulary | Emotional and social problems Behavioral reactions of childhood Acting out Poor self-concept | | Special education resource or special class Special help in speech-language development Hearing aid and lip reading Speech therapy |
| *Severe* 65–95 dB (ASA) | Sensorineural loss Middle ear disease | Loud voices may be heard 2 ft from ear. Identification of environmental sounds Defective speech and language No spontaneous speech development if loss present before 1 yr | Marked educational retardation Marked learning disability Limited vocabulary | Emotional and social problems that are associated with handicap Poor self-concept | | Full-time special education for deaf children Hearing aid, lip reading, speech therapy Auditory training Counseling |
| *Profound* 95 dB or more (ASA) | Sensorineural or mixed loss | Relies on vision rather than hearing Defective speech and language Speech and language will not develop spontaneously if loss present before 1 yr | Marked learning disability owing to lack of understanding of speech | Congenital and prelingually deaf may show severe emotional underdevelopment | | As above Oral and manual communication Counseling |

From Gottleib MI: Otitis media. *In* Levine MD, Carey WB, Crocker AC, Gross RT (eds): Developmental-Behavioral Pediatrics. Philadelphia, WB Saunders, 1983, p 469.
dB = decibel; ASA, Acoustical Society of America.

rus, meningitis, birth asphyxia, perinatal complications such as kernicterus, ototoxic drugs such as aminoglycoside antibiotics, and tumors and their treatments. Genetic deafness may be either dominant or recessive in inheritance pattern; this is the main cause of hearing impairment in schools for the deaf. In Down syndrome, there is a predisposition to both conductive loss caused by middle ear infection and sensorineural loss caused by cochlear disease.

Screening of children who are at risk may allow for early appropriate intervention. Hearing can be screened by means of an office audiogram, but other techniques are needed (e.g., auditory evoked brain stem potential or otoacoustic emission testing) for the young, neurologically immature or impaired, behaviorally difficult, or severely cognitively impaired child. The typical audiologic *assessment* includes pure tone audiometry over a variety of sound frequencies (pitches), especially over the range of frequencies in which most speech takes place. The response to actual speech at various volumes (decibel levels) is also tested. **Tympanometry** is used in the assessment of middle ear function and the evaluation of tympanic membrane compliance for pathology in the middle ear, such as fluid, ossicular dysfunction, and eustachian tube dysfunction. For the young infant or less cooperative child who nevertheless can consistently turn his or her eyes to sound stimuli, pure tone and speech audiometry can be done in a sound field, with and without masking of one ear at a time. A list of indications for referral has been shown in Table 1–8.

*Treatment* of hearing impairment may be medical or surgical. The audiologist may believe that amplification is indicated, in which case hearing aids can be tuned to preferentially amplify the frequency ranges in which the patient has decreased acuity. Educational intervention typically includes speech-language therapy and manual communication. For some children with significant language impairments, manual communication may be used as an adjunct to aid in language concept formation (Total Communication), even in the absence of severe hearing impairment. Even with amplification, many hearing-impaired children demonstrate deficits in processing information presented through the auditory pathway, requiring special educational services to aid in reading and other academic skills. Cochlear implants may be of benefit to some children.

## SPEECH AND LANGUAGE IMPAIRMENT

Among the most common and difficult developmental problems is the child with speech delay.

The most common causes are MR, hearing impairment, social deprivation, autism, and oral-motor abnormalities. If a problem is suspected based on screening, such as the Denver Developmental Screening Test (Denver II) or the Early Language Milestone Scale, a referral to a specialized hearing and speech center should be arranged.

Language development may be characterized by progress in both receptive and expressive areas of auditory and visual functioning. Simply assessing speech quality, although important, does not suffice for identification of significant language impairments. A child with severe motor impairments may, for example, have speech delays but have normal auditory reception and understanding, whereas a deaf child may lack the capability of speech and be unresponsive to auditory stimuli but have excellent communication abilities via the visual pathway (Table 1–27).

### References

Behrman RE, Kliegman RM, Arvin AM (eds): Nelson Textbook of Pediatrics, 15th ed. Philadelphia, WB Saunders, 1996, Chapters 17, 29.1, 31, 586, 587.
Coplan J: Normal speech and language development: An overview. Pediatr Rev 16(3):91, 1995.
Rapin I: Hearing disorders. Pediatr Rev 14(2):43, 1993.

## CEREBRAL PALSY

The term "cerebral palsy" (CP) includes a variety of nondegenerating neurologic disabilities caused by abnormal CNS development or injuries in the prenatal and perinatal period that result in abnormalities of motor function. In many children, the etiology is unknown and occurs before birth. The incidence is about 7:1000 live births, and the prevalence is about 500 cases/100,000 population. Significant cognitive handicap is also present in 30–70% of children with CP.

The *causes* of CP are presented in Table 1–28.

The *clinical manifestations* are varied but several distinct patterns can be identified.

**Spastic diplegia** (10–33%) typically occurs in low-birth-weight infants; it is related to cerebral asphyxia, with or without intraventricular hemorrhage from the immature germinal matrix. The lower extremities are more involved than the upper, with increased muscle tone (spasticity), increased deep tendon reflexes, and a Babinski reflex. Seizures may be present along with other impairments such as learning disabilities and language problems. Severe mental retardation is less common than in other forms of CP. Hip, knee, and ankle contractures can interfere with subsequent ambulation.

TABLE 1–27.  Language Disorders, Evaluative Techniques, and Interventions

| Disorder | Etiology | Evaluation | Treatment |
| --- | --- | --- | --- |
| *Disorders of Resonance* | | | |
| Hypernasality | Increased air through nose due to incompetent velopharyngeal seal | Examine for clefts (open or submucous) | ENT, dental evaluation<br>Functional therapy |
| Hyponasality | Decreased air through nose due to mucosal or lymphoid obstruction of nasal passage | Look in nose for edema<br>Look for tonsillar or adenoidal hypertrophy | ENT evaluation<br>Speech therapy not indicated |
| *Disorders of Voice* | | | |
| Abnormality of voice quality, pitch, or loudness | Vocal nodules<br>Voice misuse<br>Prolonged endotracheal intubation<br>Neuropathy<br>Nonmalignant tumors<br>Laryngeal trauma<br>Anxiety | History and physical<br>Listen to and describe voice quality<br>Laryngoscopy, direct and indirect | Voice therapy<br>Surgical intervention, when needed<br>Antihistaminic medications for allergy |
| *Disorders of Fluency* | | | |
| Stuttering | Normal development<br>Response to anxiety<br>Neurogenic (aphasic disorders) | History from family<br>Speech observation<br>Speech pathology evaluation in presence of severe stutter, attempts to hide behavior, avoidance of speaking, muscle tension | Observation in mild cases<br>Speech therapy referral in moderate–severe cases<br>Psychologic evaluation if emotional stressors present<br>Decrease stress of speaking, slow pace of conversation |
| *Disorders of Receptive/ Expressive Language* | | | |
| Auditory attention<br>Auditory discrimination<br>Narrative organization<br>Syntax abnormalities<br>Vocabulary problems<br>Word-finding problems | Hearing loss<br>Neurogenic causes<br>Unknown (functional problem in isolation)<br>Social/cultural factors | General:<br>  History and physical<br>  Oral examination<br>  Speech pathology<br>    evaluation | Speech therapy |

ENT = ear, nose, and throat.

**Spastic quadriplegia** (9–43%) involves all four extremities. It is associated with low birth weight and severe asphyxial insults, MR, seizures, and feeding difficulties. Scoliosis and other orthopedic problems are much more common in this type of CP.

**Spastic hemiplegia** (25–40%) is associated with the situations just described but also may be due to cerebrovascular insults, such as embolic phenomena or vascular malformations. Seizures are common, but cognitive function may be spared because only one side of the brain is involved. Motor impairments and language processing difficulties can be significant.

**Extrapyramidal CP** (9–22%) is characterized by hypotonia, choreoathetosis, and dystonic movements occurring later in life. It has been closely associated with the development of kernicterus and has become less common with aggressive management of neonatal hyperbilirubinemia (see Chap-

ter 6). There are fewer seizures and more normal cognitive function than in other forms of CP, although hearing impairment is more common and motor speech disorders may mimic retardation.

**Atonic CP** is associated with marked hypotonia, brisk reflexes, and severe cognitive delays. It easily can be confused with other spastic forms of CP that also may include hypotonia early in their course. The presence of brisk reflexes helps differentiate atonic CP from hypotonic disorders not originating in the CNS, such as muscular dystrophy and Werdnig-Hoffmann disease.

**Mixed forms** (9–22%) of CP are due to combinations of insults to multiple cerebral areas and typically are associated with more complications, including sensory deficits, seizures, and cognitive/ perceptual impairments.

*Prognosis* in CP depends on the individual's spectrum of disability and on the type and intensity of habilitative intervention.

**TABLE 1–28.** Etiologic Classification of Cerebral Palsy

**Developmental Anomalies**
Disorders of neuronal migration (polymicrogyria)
*Spastic diplegia*
Schizencephalies (double porencephalies)
*Double or bilateral hemiplegia*

**Congenital Infection (TORCH, HIV)**

**Perinatal Trauma**
Intracerebral hemorrhage, cerebral infarction, or both
*Spastic states*

**Metabolic Disorders in Perinatal Period**
**Hypoxia-ischemia**
Premature infant
*Spastic diplegia*
Full-term infant
*Spastic states*
*Choreoathetosis*
*Ataxia*

**Hypoglycemia**
*Spastic states*

**Hyperbilirubinemia**
*Choreoathetosis*

**Thromboembolic**
*Spastic hemiplegia*

**Unknown**
*Spastic states*

Adapted from Eiben RM, Crocker AC: Cerebral palsy within the spectrum of developmental disabilities. *In* Thompson GH, Rubin IL, Bilenker RM (eds): Comprehensive Management of Cerebral Palsy. New York, Grune & Stratton, 1983, p 20.
TORCH = *t*oxoplasmosis, other (syphilis, hepatitis, zoster), *r*ubella, *c*ytomegalovirus, and *h*erpes simplex; HIV = human immunodeficiency virus.

*Treatment* depends on the pattern of dysfunction that is present. Physical and occupational therapies can facilitate optimal positioning and movement patterns, increasing function of the affected parts. Management of seizures, spasticity, orthopedic impairments, and sensory impairments all aid in providing optimal educational stimulation. Family support is essential to allow for emotional growth.

### References

Behrman RE, Kliegman RM, Arvin AM (eds): Nelson Textbook of Pediatrics, 15th ed. Philadelphia, WB Saunders, 1996, Chapters 40, 548.1.
Taft LT: Cerebral palsy. Pediatr Rev 16(11):411, 1995.

## SCHOOL DYSFUNCTION

The inability to function normally in school may be caused by a variety of problems (Table 1–29). This dysfunction may itself result in somatic complaints, such as headache, abdominal pains, sleep disorders, and other problems. Learning disabilities and the attention deficit disorders are particularly important causes of school dysfunction that are discussed here.

### Learning Disabilities

Learning disabilities occur in 5–15% of school-aged children. Parents may become aware of behavioral difficulties that may interfere with learning in the preschool years when a child demonstrates hyperactivity and inattention, but usually learning disabilities do not become evident until the child enters the primary grades. Teachers then may identify weaknesses in specific areas of school performance or behavior that interfere with learning. The physician may be asked to evaluate the child for evidence of neurologic impairment or other medical illness.

Vision and hearing should be screened, but they are usually normal. In an extended neurologic examination, markers of neurologic immaturity ("soft signs") and gross and fine motor incoordination may be observed. These findings are physical concomitants that suggest that many learning disabilities are neurologically based at some level; the findings should be used only in conjunction with other tests to describe the child's strengths and weaknesses. They are not predictive of learning disorders because they may occur in the absence of educational disability. An expanded neurodevelopmental examination can better describe skills, whereas specialized psychoeducational testing must be done to characterize particular learning disabilities.

**TABLE 1–29.** Causes of School Dysfunction

Systemic medical illness

Learning disability

Medication effects (e.g., chronic administration of bronchodilators, anticonvulsants, decongestants, drug abuse)

Anxiety due to social and emotional factors (e.g., child abuse/neglect, sexual abuse, parental divorce)

Sensory impairments

Classroom-student mismatch (e.g., language barriers, classwork too simple, classwork too hard)

Conduct disorder

Attention Deficit Hyperactivity Disorder

Occult seizure activity

Environmental toxins (e.g., lead poisoning)

Conduct disorder

## Attention-Deficit Hyperactivity Disorder

The diagnosis of Attention-Deficit Hyperactivity Disorder (ADHD) is based on the presence of a complex of behaviors that characterize the child as inattentive, easily distracted, overactive, and impulsive to such an extent that his or her behavior interferes with the ability to function socially and academically. Restlessness and fidgetiness (hyperactivity) are common but not essential concomitants of this syndrome. Current classifications include the predominantly Impulsive-Overactive Type (more common in boys), the predominantly Inattentive Type, and mixed combination forms. Specific learning disabilities also are commonly associated, and some children may display aggressive or oppositional behavior.

The *clinical manifestations* of ADHD usually are obvious to teachers. Inattentiveness is demonstrated by failure to complete tasks once begun, failure to grasp directions, and making errors through inattention rather than lack of understanding of the material presented. "Impulsivity" refers to the child's difficulty in controlling reactions and responses when he or she faces uncertainty or the need to attend carefully. Impulsive children commonly act without thinking, shifting quickly from one activity to another, and often exhibit the right behavior at the wrong time, such as calling out in class with an inappropriate answer. They often get into trouble with their peers because they seem "socially inept." Distractibility presents as a reaction to environmental noises or visual stimuli that others can ignore. Distractible children also may be distracted by their own bodies, clothing, or other objects (e.g., touching clothes or hair or running their hands over furniture or walls).

Overactivity, although the most noticeable feature of ADHD, is not uniformly present. Children with ADHD commonly can be observed swinging their legs, rocking their bodies, tapping fingers, or making odd noises. In more obvious cases, they may be in near-constant motion, darting around the room, often ignoring their own or others' safety. The male-to-female ratio is 4:1. Girls more typically present with inattention but without hyperactivity.

The physical examination findings typically are normal, although there may be a suggestion of neurologic immaturity. Cranial imaging and EEG are not of benefit in diagnosing or treating ADHD or other forms of school dysfunction. They should be performed only when seizures or focal neurologic findings are suggested by history and physical examination.

Some infants and preschool children who are later characterized as having ADHD are colicky, irritable, and occasionally more active than their peers, spending a shorter time than normal playing with a given toy and requiring more supervision than other children.

As the child with ADHD ages, neurologic maturation may result in symptomatic improvement. However, adolescents who had ADHD in their early school years often continue to demonstrate school dysfunction, low self-esteem, and social inappropriateness, and many benefit from ongoing medical treatment.

Primary *treatment* of the child with ADHD combines pharmacologic and environmental interventions. However, such management often is complicated by the presence of associated learning disabilities that require specific educational interventions. Moreover, many such children have developed emotional reactions to what may be years of social inappropriateness and school dysfunction, and both family behavior patterns and the child's psychologic reactions must be assessed to avoid continuation of undesirable stereotyping. The beneficial effects of medication are decreased significantly in the presence of unaddressed emotional or educational needs.

The drugs most commonly used in treating ADHD are presented in Table 1–30. They are presumed to have their neuropharmacologic effects on dopaminergic neurons in the brain stem reticular activating system. Such psychostimulants are most effective when used in conjunction with behavior modification techniques. Major side effects of these drugs are sleep and appetite impairment, elevation of pulse rate and blood pressure, rebound overactivity, irritability on withdrawal of the medication, and attentional overfocusing. Motor tics may be exacerbated by these drugs. The child should play an active role in decisions about medications in terms of administration and monitoring the effect of the drug, both to give the child a measure of control in managing his or her problem and to avoid non-compliance.

There are no significant beneficial effects of specific dietary interventions in children with ADHD or other forms of school dysfunction.

## References

Behrman RE, Kliegman RM, Arvin AM (eds): Nelson Textbook of Pediatrics, 15th ed. Philadelphia, WB Saunders, 1996, Chapters 27, 30.2, 31.

Biederman J, Faraone, Milberger S, et al: A prospective 4 year follow-up study of attention-deficit hyperactivity and related disorders. Arch Gen Psychiatry 53:437, 1991.

Committee on Children with Disabilities and Committee on Drugs: Medication for children with attentional disorders. Pediatrics 98:301, 1996.

TABLE 1–30.  Stimulant Medications Used for Treatment of Attention Deficits

| Generic Name | Brand Name | Preparations | Dosage Range (mg/kg/Dose) | Onset of Action | Duration of Action | Comments |
|---|---|---|---|---|---|---|
| Methylphenidate | Ritalin | Tablets: 5, 10, 20 mg; 20-mg sustained release | 0.3–1.0 | 30 min | 3–5 hr | Not recommended below 6 yr |
| Dextroamphetamine | Dexedrine | Tablets: 5 mg; sustained-release capsules: 5, 10, 15 mg | 0.15–0.5 | 30 min | 3–5 hr | Not recommended below 3 yr |

Adapted from Levine MD, Brooks R, Shonkoff JP: Pediatric Approach to Learning Disorders, New York, John Wiley, 1980, p. 184. Copyright © 1980, John Wiley. Reprinted with permission of John Wiley & Sons.

Diagnostic and Statistical Manual of Mental Disorders: DSM-IV, 4th ed. Washington, DC, American Psychiatric Association, 1994, pp 78–85.
Snowling M: Dyslexia: A hundred years on. BMJ 313: 1096, 1996.

## CHRONIC DISEASE

Chronic diseases may be characterized by long-term disability, a variable relapsing course, or a gradual declining course. Some examples of such disorders include arthritis, asthma, autism, traumatic brain injury, cerebral palsy, chronic renal failure, congenital heart disease, cystic fibrosis, diabetes mellitus, mental retardation, visual impairments, seizure disorders, sickle cell disease, leukemia, acquired immunodeficiency syndrome (AIDS), hearing impairment, neural tube defects, cleft palate/lip, hemophilia, and phenylketonuria. The goal in managing such patients is to maximize their potential for productive adult functioning and for a high quality of life by treating the primary disease and aiding the patient and family to deal with the stresses incurred because of the disease. The factors that influence responses to chronic diseases include disease-related factors (such as pain, treatment, and visibility of condition), age of onset, age and developmental level of the child, and family attitudes and stress.

Whenever a chronic disease is diagnosed, family members typically go through grieving processes similar to those seen at the time of death, including anger, denial, negotiation in an attempt to forestall the inevitable, and depression. However, because the child with the chronic disease is a constant reminder of the object of this grief, it may take family members a long time to accept the condition. Understanding and support on the part of the physician can facilitate this process by sharing both the known and the unknown and by allaying guilty feelings and fear. In order to minimize de-nial, it is helpful to confirm the family's observations about the child. Once the diagnosis has been presented, the family may not be able to absorb any additional information, so written material and the option for further discussion at a later date should be offered.

When children with chronic diseases are acutely ill, treatment becomes a common goal for all concerned. However, as stabilization takes place and the child is not "cured," it is important that the family not feel abandoned by staff who are involved in the case. There are predictable times in the course of a chronic illness when stress is greatest (Table 1–31).

A major goal of care for the family of the child with a chronic disease is that the family and child feel in control of the situation. Although in the acute health care setting the locus of control is with the medical management team, as the child moves into a more routine home-based life the control should shift to the family and the child. Treatment

TABLE 1–31.  Predictable Crises and Stress in the Medical Course of Chronic Disease

Onset and diagnosis

Disease-specific, emotionally distressing medical symptoms

Hospitalization(s)

Response to appearance of initial major complication

Confrontation with significant therapeutic choices

Failure(s) of an expected therapeutic response

Threat of imminent death

Unpredictable complications

From Hamburg BA: Chronic illness. In Levine MD, Carey WB, Crocker AC, Gross RT (eds): Developmental-Behavioral Pediatrics. Philadelphia, WB Saunders, 1983, p 456.

plans should be organized to allow for the greatest degree of normalization of the child's life.

Among chronic diseases, the most difficult with which to deal are those with major multiple system involvement, such as spina bifida, severe cerebral palsy, cystic fibrosis, sickle cell disease, inborn metabolic errors, and a variety of congenital anomaly syndromes. The combination of sensory, motor, and cognitive handicap and emotional/behavioral abnormality is a particularly difficult problem, requiring multiple medical and habilitative specialists. The primary physician may assume the role of coordinator of care.

## References

Behrman RE, Kliegman RM, Arvin AM (eds): Nelson Textbook of Pediatrics, 15th ed. Philadelphia, WB Saunders, 1996, Chapters 30, 40.
Desguin BW, Holt IJ, McCarthy SM: Comprehensive care of the child with a chronic condition: Part 1. Understanding chronic conditions in childhood. Curr Probl Pediatr 24(6):199, 1994.
Desguin BW, Holt IJ, McCarthy SM: Comprehensive care of the child with a chronic condition: Part 2. Primary care management. Curr Probl Pediatr 24(7):230, 1994.

## AUTISM AND PSYCHOSES IN CHILDHOOD

These disorders may have a distinctive early onset in infancy and preschool years or an adult-like presentation in older children.

**Autism spectrum** conditions are clinical disorders of a variety of causes and variable prognoses that usually are characterized by significant impairment of the child's ability to relate to people, including parents. They affect 0.7–4.5:10,000 children. *Clinical manifestations* typically indicate that, as an infant, the autistic child was noticeably "uncuddly," with delayed or absent smiling. Later the young child may spend hours in solitary play and be withdrawn in the presence of other children or adults and indifferent to attempts to communicate. Intense, absorbing interests, ritualistic behavior, and compulsive routines are characteristic, and their disruption may invoke tantrum or rage reactions. Eye contact is abnormal or absent. Head banging, teeth grinding, rocking, diminished responsiveness to pain and external stimuli, and even self-mutilation may be noted. Speech often is delayed and, when present, frequently is dominated by echolalia, pronoun reversal, nonsense rhyming, and other unusual language forms. The child's IQ is difficult to evaluate because of language and socialization deficits and often falls in the functional retarded range by conventional testing. Some children with autism spectrum disorders show remarkable isolated abilities ("savant skills"). Suspicion of this diagnosis requires referral to a specialist for further evaluation and treatment. Higher measured intelligence and the presence of meaningful language by age 5 yr are favorable prognostic indicators. Early intensive intervention may dramatically improve outcomes. A relationship between autism and schizophrenia has been suspected, but these children rarely go on to develop classic schizophrenic symptoms.

The onset of *affective psychosis* and *schizophrenia* in older children resembles that in adults. The same diagnostic criteria are applied but must be interpreted in terms of the developmental stage of the child. Long-term psychiatric care often is required for these chronic disorders.

## References

Bauer S: Autism and the pervasive developmental disorders: Parts 1 and 2. Pediatr Rev 16(4):130, 1995; 16(5):168, 1995.
Behrman RE, Kliegman RM, Arvin AM (eds): Nelson Textbook of Pediatrics, 15th ed. Philadelphia, WB Saunders, 1996, Chapters 17, 29, 30.2.
Brent DA, Puig-Antich J, Rabinovitch H: Major psychiatric disorders in childhood and adolescence. *In* Levine MD, Carey WB, Crocker AC (eds): Developmental-Behavioral Pediatrics, 2nd ed. Philadelphia, WB Saunders, 1992, pp 569–588.

# Chapter 2

# PEDIATRIC NUTRITION AND NUTRITIONAL DISORDERS

Andrew M. Tershakovec

Virginia A. Stallings

Proper nutrition is central in promoting the normal growth and development of children. Rapidly growing infants, children, and maturing adolescents have specific but not necessarily fixed requirements for macronutrients (protein, fat, carbohydrates, fluids) and micronutrients (vitamins, trace elements, minerals). Pathophysiologic mechanisms present during various disease states may adversely affect nutritional status, thus retarding growth and development even in the presence of normal recommended intakes of both macro- and micronutrients. Diseases associated with inflammation (infectious diseases, systemic lupus erythematosus, inflammatory bowel disease), trauma (fractures, burns), malignancy, malabsorption (cystic fibrosis, celiac disease, sprue), inborn errors of metabolism (galactosemia, maple syrup urine disease), and chronic cardiopulmonary insufficiency (heart failure, bronchopulmonary dysplasia) place additional stress on nutritional balance, may alter energy and nutrient needs, and thus may require nutrient supplementation or special diets (Fig. 2–1). These disease processes may limit the genetic potential and may even modify the eventual expression of growth.

Nutritional disorders are not confined to children living in areas of famine and starvation. Deficiencies and excesses of nutrient intake are common problems among infants and children in the United States, as evidenced by the continued existence of iron-deficiency anemia and the increasing rate of childhood obesity, respectively. Furthermore, specific nutritional deficiency syndromes are relatively common among low-birth-weight infants, children with malabsorption (cystic fibrosis, short bowel syndrome, cholestatic jaundice), breast-fed infants of strict vegetarian parents, and acutely or chronically ill hospitalized children with multiorgan system dysfunction requiring intensive care.

## BODY COMPOSITION AND GROWTH

Nutrition plays a central role in growth and the changing body composition. Growth and maturation begin at the moment of conception and cease with the end of puberty. Prenatal growth is part of a continuous developmental and genetic process modified by maternal variables; during postnatal growth this process is also dependent on familial, socioeconomic, and environmental factors. The normal growth patterns after birth are shown in Chapter 1, Figures 1–2 to 1–14. The velocity (rate of change) of body mass and length accretion is greater at 32 wk gestation (15 kg/yr and 65 cm/yr, respectively) than in any subsequent period, including puberty. Growth in length reflects the differential growth of the head, trunk, and long bones of the legs (see Fig. 1–15). Head size increases most rapidly after 28 wk of gestation and growth slows before 2–3 yr of age. The trunk increases during the same period but continues to lengthen at a slower rate from 2 yr through puberty. The legs grow fastest during the period covering the last 14 wk of gestation through the first 6 mo of life (18 cm/yr). This rate exceeds that of leg growth in male puberty (4 cm/yr). Linear growth and mass growth are differentially reduced by malnutrition but synchronously increased by obesity. (See Chapters 1 and 17 for measurement of growth.)

Height and weight measurements provide only a crude estimation of body composition. Organ weights increase with maturation; some organs assume a smaller proportion of body mass (brain),

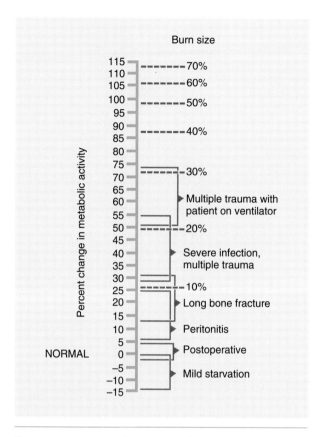

FIGURE 2–1. Increased energy needs with stress. (Adapted from Witmore D: The Metabolic Management of the Critically Ill. New York, Plenum Publishing, 1977; revised *in* Walker W, Watkins J [eds]: Nutrition in Pediatrics: Basic Science and Clinical Application. Boston, Little, Brown & Co, 1985, p 873.)

puberty. The effect of malnutrition on development depends on the stage of development. Because the brain develops early, it is relatively protected from malnutrition in later childhood; delayed puberty is seen in malnourished adolescents.

The embryo contains 95% water, which decreases to 80% at 28 wk gestation. During the 3rd trimester, as significant fat (which is anhydrous) is deposited, the proportion of body water decreases further to 72%. By 8 yr of age, it has reached the adult proportion of 60%. The extracellular fluid compartment is substantially greater than the intracellular fluid compartment during fetal life. Before 6 mo of age, intracellular fluid increases and extracellular fluid decreases so the components become equal. This trend continues so that, by adulthood, the intracellular fluid compartment has twice the volume of the extracellular compartment (Fig. 2–3). The relatively high extracellular fluid volume in the young infant results in a vulnerability to abnormal fluid losses during illness.

The chemical composition of lean body mass (LBM) changes with growth. The concentrations of nitrogen and potassium increase and the concentration of chloride decreases as the relationship between extracellular and intracellular water compartments changes. After the 7th mo of gestation, the fall in total extracellular sodium is counterbalanced by an increase in total sodium in bone. Calcium is confined primarily to bone, but phosphorus

while the percentage of body mass that is composed of muscle and adipose tissue increases as the child grows. Little adipose tissue is deposited during early fetal development, but a rapid deposition occurs during the last 3 mo of gestation. The term infant's body contains approximately 20–25% adipose tissue, 80% of which is subcutaneous and 20% visceral. After early infancy, the percentage of fat decreases to 15% and is fairly constant until the acceleration during pubertal growth. During puberty the proportion of fat increases to 20–30% in the average girl (Fig. 2–2). The largest tissue of the body is skeletal muscle, which makes up 25% of body mass during fetal life and increases to 45% in the adult. The rate of increase is greatest between birth and 5 yr, with an additional small increase in boys at puberty.

Different organ systems develop at different times and different rates. Seventy-five percent of brain growth is completed by 3 yr of age and 90% by 7 yr; the reproductive system grows little until

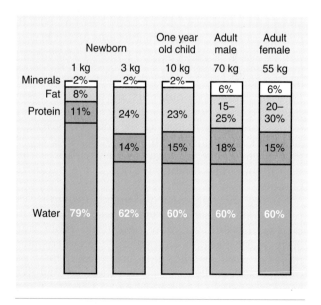

FIGURE 2–2. The changes in the proportions of body composition with growth. (Adapted from Pencharz P: Body composition and growth. *In* Walker W, Watkins J [eds]: Nutrition in Pediatrics: Basic Science and Clinical Application. Boston, Little, Brown & Co, 1985, p 81.)

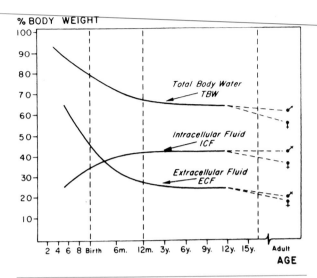

FIGURE 2–3.    Change with age in total body water (TBW) and its major subdivisions. (Data from Friis-Hansen: Body water compartments in children: Changes during growth and related changes in body composition. Pediatrics 28:169, 1961; revised *in* Winters RW [ed]: The Body Fluids in Pediatrics. Boston, Little, Brown & Co, 1973, p 100.)

is an equally important constituent of soft tissues. During the first 2 mo of gestation, the phosphorus concentration is greater than that of calcium. Skeletal calcification begins thereafter, and body calcium concentration increases more rapidly than that of phosphorus. At term, 98% of body calcium, 80% of phosphorus, and 60% of magnesium are in bones. During the adolescent growth period, a male accumulates 12 kg of protein, 1.2 kg of calcium, 0.7 kg of phosphorus, 26 g of magnesium, 4 g of iron, and 1.5 g of zinc. These nutrients are accumulated in specific tissues, which cease to grow when they reach a size proportional to the total body length and mass. The genetic coordination of tissue accretion is remarkable, but various dietary deficiencies may become rate limiting for any of these growth processes.

Energy and nutrient requirements generally are proportional to lean body mass; these requirements increase as children grow and attain more lean body mass. Because women have proportionally more fat mass and less lean body mass, their requirements usually are less than those of men. For some nutrients, women have equal (vitamin C) or greater (iron) needs than men. To meet the recommended dietary allowance (RDA), a woman needs to ingest a more nutrient-dense diet than a man. Thus, women are at risk for deficiencies of some of those specific nutrients.

## DIET OF THE NORMAL INFANT

In the first 4–6 mos of life, human milk or various infant formulas can provide complete nutrition to the growing infant. However, breast milk is the recommended source of nutrition for almost all children. Nonetheless, few infants are exclusively breast-fed beyond 2–3 mos of age. Every effort should be made to encourage and promote breast-feeding.

Although infant formulas simulate the composition of human milk, human milk has several subtle nutritional and non-nutritional advantages over infant formula. From a practical point of view, breast milk does not need to be warmed, is ready to serve, does not need a clean water supply, is generally free of microorganisms, and does not need a clean serving container. These issues are significant concerns in less developed areas of the world. Breast-feeding also encourages maternal-infant bonding. By limiting the exposure to potential antigens, human milk may reduce the incidence of cow's milk protein allergy and eczema. Breast milk also contains protective bacterial and viral antibodies (immunoglobulin A) and macrophages, which help limit infections. Although the iron content of human milk is relatively low, the iron is more biologically available than that in cow's milk. Human milk also contains lactoferrin, an iron-binding whey protein that inhibits the growth of *Escherichia coli*. In addition, there are other nutrients contained in breast milk that are not present in most formulas (e.g., cholesterol, taurine, omega-3 fatty acids, nucleotides), whose function or importance is not well understood. Breast-feeding is recommended for 6–12 mo.

The alternative to human milk is iron-fortified formula, which permits adequate growth of most infants. No supplements are needed with such formulas. Cow's milk should not be introduced until after the 1st year of life.

After 4–6 mo, solid foods (beikost) and juices are introduced (using these nutrient sources initiates *weaning*), progressively replacing some of the calories and nutrients provided by human milk or formula. Although the growth rate of the child is decreasing, energy needs for greater activity increase (Fig. 2–4). A relatively high-fat and calorically dense diet (milk) still is needed to deliver adequate calories. Nutritional supplements become an important source of some nutrients (iron) in the second 6 mo of life.

### References

Behrman RE, Kliegman RM, Arvin AM (eds): Nelson Textbook of Pediatrics, 15th ed. Philadelphia, WB Saunders, 1996, Chapters 8–16.

Makrides M, Neumann M, Simner K, et al: Are long-chain polyunsaturated fatty acids essential nutrients in infancy? Lancet 345:1463, 1995.

Windowson EM: Growth and body composition in childhood. *In* Brunser O, Carrazza FR, Gracey M, et al (eds): Clinical Nutrition of the Young Child. New York, Raven Press, 1984, pp 1–14.

## NUTRIENT NEEDS
### (Tables 2–1 and 2–2)

The *minimum daily requirement* (MDR) of a nutrient is set at a level of consumption below which signs of deficiency develop. The RDA is generally 2–6 times the MDR and takes into consideration modifications needed for weight, sex, age, pregnancy, and lactation. The RDA for nutrients usually is 2 standard deviations above the mean requirement for each food group, while it is at the mean for energy requirements. Some nutrients have no RDA and thus recommendations are based on quantities known to be safe within a given adequate range (see Table 2–2). Caloric needs are determined by resting energy expenditure plus energy needed for exercise, growth, and the thermic effect of food. More often caloric needs are estimated by the following rule of thumb: 100 kcal/kg for the first 10 kg, 50 kcal/kg for the next 10–20 kg, and 20 kcal/kg for weight above 20 kg (see Chapter 6); or by

**FIGURE 2–4.** Energy requirements of infants. (From Waterlow JC: Basic concepts in the determination of nutritional requirements of normal infants. *In* Tsang RC, Nichols BL [eds]: Nutrition During Infancy. Philadelphia, Hanley and Belfus, 1988, p 6.)

the use of World Health Organization (WHO) or other prediction equations and a factor adjusting for physical activity, stress, and so on.

## BREAST-FEEDING

Mothers should decide before delivery whether to breast-feed or bottle-feed their infants. When breast-feeding is chosen, mothers should be assisted to develop appropriate feeding skills and practices. The optimal goal is to produce sufficient milk to breast-feed an infant for 6–12 mo (see Chapter 6, Table 6–24 for composition of human milk). However, even short-term breast-feeding is probably beneficial.

### Beginning Breast-Feeding

The mother should be comfortable and the infant positioned so that nothing interferes with mouth-to-breast contact. The breast from which the infant nurses should be supported with the opposite hand, with the thumb and index fingers above the nipple to allow the infant easy access to the nipple. The *rooting reflex* should be explained to the parents to make initiation of breast-feeding easier. The nipple should be stroked against the infant's cheek nearest the nipple. The infant will turn toward the nipple (rooting reflex) and open the mouth, allowing the introduction of the nipple and areola. The entire nipple and most of the areola should be placed in the infant's mouth. The infant "latches on" by compressing the lips. The mechanics of normal suckling include: (1) suction of 4–6 cm of the areola, (2) compression of the nipple against the palate, (3) stimulation of milk ejection by initial rapid non-nutritive sucking, and (4) extraction of milk from the lactiferous sinuses by a slower suck-swallow rhythm of approximately 1/sec. One may remove the infant from the breast by placing a clean finger between the baby's gums and the areola to release suction. The mean feeding frequency during the first 2 wk is 8–12 times/day.

### Exclusive Breast-Feeding

Breast-feeding is the recommended method for feeding normal infants during the first 6 mo of life. If the mother can be made aware of possible nursing problems that may arise shortly after hospital discharge, many cases of lactation failure may be averted. *Colostrum*, a high-protein and low-fat and lactose product, is produced in small amounts during the first few postpartum days. It has some nutritional value but primarily has important im-

TABLE 2–1. Food and Nutrition Board, National Academy of Sciences–National Research Council Recommended Dietary Allowances (Revised 1989)*

| Category | Age (yr) or Condition | Weight† | | Height† | | Protein (g) | Fat-Soluble Vitamins | | | |
|---|---|---|---|---|---|---|---|---|---|---|
| | | kg | lb | cm | inch | | Vitamin A (µg RE)‡ | Vitamin D (µg)§ | Vitamin E (mg α-TE)‖ | Vitamin K (µg) |
| Infants | 0.0–0.5 | 6 | 13 | 60 | 24 | 13 | 375 | 7.5 | 3 | 5 |
| | 0.5–1.0 | 9 | 20 | 71 | 28 | 14 | 375 | 10 | 4 | 10 |
| Children | 1–3 | 13 | 29 | 90 | 35 | 16 | 400 | 10 | 6 | 15 |
| | 4–6 | 20 | 44 | 112 | 44 | 24 | 500 | 10 | 7 | 20 |
| | 7–10 | 28 | 62 | 132 | 52 | 28 | 700 | 10 | 7 | 30 |
| Males | 11–14 | 45 | 99 | 157 | 62 | 45 | 1000 | 10 | 10 | 45 |
| | 15–18 | 66 | 145 | 176 | 69 | 59 | 1000 | 10 | 10 | 65 |
| | 19–24 | 72 | 160 | 177 | 70 | 58 | 1000 | 10 | 10 | 70 |
| | 25–50 | 79 | 174 | 176 | 70 | 63 | 1000 | 5 | 10 | 80 |
| | 51+ | 77 | 170 | 173 | 68 | 63 | 1000 | 5 | 10 | 80 |
| Females | 11–14 | 46 | 101 | 157 | 62 | 46 | 800 | 10 | 8 | 45 |
| | 15–18 | 55 | 120 | 163 | 64 | 44 | 800 | 10 | 8 | 55 |
| | 19–24 | 58 | 128 | 164 | 65 | 46 | 800 | 10 | 8 | 60 |
| | 25–50 | 63 | 138 | 163 | 64 | 50 | 800 | 5 | 8 | 65 |
| | 51+ | 65 | 143 | 160 | 63 | 50 | 800 | 5 | 8 | 65 |
| Pregnant | | | | | | 60 | 800 | 10 | 10 | 65 |
| Lactating | 1st 6 mo | | | | | 65 | 1300 | 10 | 12 | 65 |
| | 2nd 6 mo | | | | | 62 | 1200 | 10 | 11 | 65 |

munologic and maturational properties. Primiparous women usually experience breast engorgement on the 3rd postpartum day; the breasts become hard and are painful, the nipples become nonprotractile, and the mother's temperature may increase slightly. Enhancement of milk flow is the best management. If severe engorgement occurs, areolar rigidity may prevent the infant from grasping the nipple and areola. Attention to proper latch-on and hand expression of milk assist drainage. The first appetite spurt of the infant is noted at 8–10 days of life by an increase in the demand for nursing, which serves to stimulate the production of a greater volume of milk. Hydration status is an index of the adequacy of intake. A well-hydrated infant voids 6–8 times/day. Each voiding should soak, not merely moisten, a diaper. Parents should be advised to contact the pediatrician if the infant voids less than 6 times/day. Telephone follow-up is valuable during the interim between discharge and the first pediatric visit in order to monitor the progress of lactation. Initial weight loss in the neonatal period is greater in the breast-fed than in the bottle-fed infant, but birth weight should be regained by 2 wk of age.

The duration of nursing varies widely. Longer nursing may be an adaptation to inadequate milk production or ineffective latch-on. Eighty percent of milk is consumed in the first 4 min of nursing at each breast. Milk volume increases rapidly during the first 2 wk after parturition. Women who breast-feed their infants exclusively produce approximately 750 mL/day. This level of production is maintained for at least 4–6 mo, but milk volume declines in response to decreased nursing after solid foods have been added to the infant's diet.

The characteristics of the stools of breast-fed infants often alarm mothers. Stools are unformed, yellow, brown, or green, and seedy in appearance. Stool frequencies are variable, though breast-fed babies tend to stool more frequently than formula-fed infants.

In the newborn period, elevated concentrations of bilirubin occur more often in breast-fed infants than in formula-fed infants. Feeding frequency during the first 3 days of life of breast-fed infants is related inversely to the serum level of bilirubin; frequent feedings stimulate meconium passage and excretion of bilirubin. The use of water supplements in breast-fed infants has no effect on serum bilirubin levels. If the concentration of serum bilirubin rises sufficiently to be of clinical concern, formula feedings should be temporarily substituted, which may prevent further increases in bilirubin levels. A temporary discontinuation of breast-feeding for 24–72 hours is of diagnostic value in identifying *breast milk jaundice* (see Chapter 6). Slight elevations in serum bilirubin com-

TABLE 2–1. Food and Nutrition Board, National Academy of Sciences–National Research Council Recommended Dietary Allowances (Revised 1989)* *Continued*

| Water-Soluble Vitamins | | | | | | | Minerals | | | | | | |
|---|---|---|---|---|---|---|---|---|---|---|---|---|---|
| Vitamin C (mg) | Thiamine (mg) | Riboflavin (mg) | Niacin (mg NE)¶ | Vitamin $B_6$ (mg) | Folate (µg) | Vitamin $B_{12}$ (µg) | Calcium (mg) | Phosphorus (mg) | Magnesium (mg) | Iron (mg) | Zinc (mg) | Iodine (µg) | Selenium (µg) |
| 30 | 0.3 | 0.4 | 5 | 0.3 | 25 | 0.3 | 400 | 300 | 40 | 6 | 5 | 40 | 10 |
| 35 | 0.4 | 0.5 | 6 | 0.6 | 35 | 0.5 | 600 | 500 | 60 | 10 | 5 | 50 | 15 |
| 40 | 0.7 | 0.8 | 9 | 1.0 | 50 | 0.7 | 800 | 800 | 80 | 10 | 10 | 70 | 20 |
| 45 | 0.9 | 1.1 | 12 | 1.1 | 75 | 1.0 | 800 | 800 | 120 | 10 | 10 | 90 | 20 |
| 45 | 1.0 | 1.2 | 13 | 1.4 | 100 | 1.4 | 800 | 800 | 170 | 10 | 10 | 120 | 30 |
| 50 | 1.3 | 1.5 | 17 | 1.7 | 150 | 2.0 | 1200 | 1200 | 270 | 12 | 15 | 150 | 40 |
| 60 | 1.5 | 1.8 | 20 | 2.0 | 200 | 2.0 | 1200 | 1200 | 400 | 12 | 15 | 150 | 50 |
| 60 | 1.5 | 1.7 | 19 | 2.0 | 200 | 2.0 | 1200 | 1200 | 350 | 10 | 15 | 150 | 70 |
| 60 | 1.5 | 1.7 | 19 | 2.0 | 200 | 2.0 | 800 | 800 | 350 | 10 | 15 | 150 | 70 |
| 60 | 1.2 | 1.4 | 15 | 2.0 | 200 | 2.0 | 800 | 800 | 350 | 10 | 15 | 150 | 70 |
| 50 | 1.1 | 1.3 | 15 | 1.4 | 150 | 2.0 | 1200 | 1200 | 280 | 15 | 12 | 150 | 45 |
| 60 | 1.1 | 1.3 | 15 | 1.5 | 180 | 2.0 | 1200 | 1200 | 300 | 15 | 12 | 150 | 50 |
| 60 | 1.1 | 1.3 | 15 | 1.6 | 180 | 2.0 | 1200 | 1200 | 280 | 15 | 12 | 150 | 55 |
| 60 | 1.1 | 1.3 | 15 | 1.6 | 180 | 2.0 | 800 | 800 | 280 | 15 | 12 | 150 | 55 |
| 60 | 1.0 | 1.2 | 13 | 1.6 | 180 | 2.0 | 800 | 800 | 280 | 10 | 12 | 150 | 55 |
| 70 | 1.5 | 1.6 | 17 | 2.2 | 400 | 2.2 | 1200 | 1200 | 320 | 30 | 15 | 175 | 65 |
| 95 | 1.6 | 1.8 | 20 | 2.1 | 280 | 2.6 | 1200 | 1200 | 355 | 15 | 19 | 200 | 75 |
| 90 | 1.6 | 1.7 | 20 | 2.1 | 260 | 2.6 | 1200 | 1200 | 340 | 15 | 16 | 200 | 75 |

From Recommended Dietary Allowances, 10th ed., National Academy Press, 1989, pp 15–17.

*The allowances, expressed as average daily intakes over time, are intended to provide for individual variations among most normal persons as they live in the United States under usual environmental stresses. Diets should be based on a variety of common foods in order to provide other nutrients for which human requirements have been less well defined.

†Weights and heights of Reference Adults are actual medians for the U.S. population of the designated age, as reported by National Health and Nutrition Examination Survey (NHANES II). The median weights and heights of those under 19 years of age were taken from Hamill et al. (1979). The use of these figures does not imply that the height-to-weight ratios are ideal.

‡Retinol equivalents. 1 retinol equivalent = 1 µg retinol or 6 µg β-carotene.

§As cholecalciferol. 10 µg cholecalciferol = 400 IU of vitamin D.

‖α-Tocopherol equivalents. 1 mg d-α-tocopherol = 1 α-TE.

¶1 NE (niacin equivalent) is equal to 1 mg of niacin or 60 mg of dietary tryptophan.

monly are observed when breast-feeding is resumed, and a less severe level of jaundice may persist for several weeks. Few detrimental effects of breast milk jaundice have been reported. If temporary formula feeding is introduced, the mother's milk production can be maintained by manual milk expression.

### Supplementation

Breast-fed term infants require supplementation with vitamin K (intramuscular ×1) at birth; they require vitamin D and, after 6 mo of age, fluoride. Iron or iron-fortified formula should be added at 4–6 mo of life. Vitamin $B_{12}$ should be included if the mother is a strict vegan (one who consumes no animal products). Formula and/or water supplements in addition to breast milk are usually not necessary for term breast-fed infants. Supplementary formula feedings in this period may increase the risk for feeding difficulties or lactation failure.

When nursing from an artificial nipple, the infant positions the tongue differently than when breast-feeding. If the infant has difficulty breast-feeding after nursing from a bottle, the mother should make certain that the infant's mouth is positioned well over the areola. Bottle feedings that are introduced before breast-feeding is well established may interfere with the continuation of breast-feeding.

Iron-fortified infant formula should be used as supplementary feedings, if such feedings are given to the infant younger than 12 mo of age. Alternatively, the working mother may express her milk and store it frozen for use by other caregivers.

After 4–6 mo of age, solid foods may be added to the diet. After 6 mo of age, the nutrients often found somewhat lacking in the diet of the exclusively. breast-fed infant are likely to be protein, iron, and zinc; total calories may be lacking as well. Thus, the most appropriate first food to add to the

TABLE 2-2. Estimated Safe and Adequate Daily Dietary Intakes of Selected Vitamins and Minerals*

| Category | Age (yr) | Vitamins | | Trace Elements† | | | | |
|---|---|---|---|---|---|---|---|---|
| | | Biotin (μg) | Pantothenic Acid (mg) | Copper (mg) | Manganese (mg) | Fluoride (mg) | Chromium (μg) | Molybdenum (μg) |
| Infants | 0–0.5 | 10 | 2 | 0.4–0.6 | 0.3–0.6 | 0.1–0.5 | 10–40 | 15–30 |
| | 0.5–1.0 | 15 | 3 | 0.6–0.7 | 0.6–1.0 | 0.2–1.0 | 20–60 | 20–40 |
| Children and adolescents | 1–3 | 20 | 3 | 0.7–1.0 | 1.0–1.5 | 0.5–1.5 | 20–80 | 25–50 |
| | 4–6 | 25 | 3–4 | 1.0–1.5 | 1.5–2.0 | 1.0–2.5 | 30–120 | 30–75 |
| | 7–10 | 30 | 4–5 | 1.0–2.0 | 2.0–3.0 | 1.5–2.5 | 50–200 | 50–150 |
| | 11+ | 30–100 | 4–7 | 1.5–2.5 | 2.0–5.0 | 1.5–2.5 | 50–200 | 75–250 |
| Adults | | 30–100 | 4–7 | 1.5–3.0 | 2.0–5.0 | 1.5–4.0 | 50–200 | 75–250 |

From Recommended Dietary Allowances, 10th ed, National Academy Press, 1989, p 284.
*Because there is less information on which to base allowances, these figures are not given in the main table of recommended daily allowance and are provided here in the form of ranges of recommended intakes.
†Because the toxic levels for many trace elements may be only several times usual intakes, the upper levels for the trace elements given in this table should not be habitually exceeded.

diet of exclusively breast-fed infants may be iron-fortified (rice) cereals.

### Common Breast-Feeding Problems

If a lactating woman reports fever, chills, and malaise, *mastitis* should be considered. Treatment includes frequent and complete emptying of the breast. Breast-feeding should not be stopped because the mother's mastitis has no adverse effects on the breast-fed infant. Antibiotic therapy, which is safe for the infant, is indicated. Untreated mastitis may progress to a *breast abscess*. If an abscess is diagnosed, breast-feeding should be discontinued from the affected breast until the condition is successfully treated. Milk expression from the affected breast should continue, but the milk should be discarded.

Maternal infections of active tuberculosis, syphilis, human immunodeficiency virus (HIV), typhoid, rubella, mumps, cytomegalovirus, or localized cutaneous herpesvirus are contraindications to breast-feeding. When the mother has active tuberculosis or syphilis, breast-feeding may be continued after initiating therapy.

The mother should be advised against the use of unprescribed drugs, including alcohol, nicotine, caffeine, or "street drugs." No medications (including over-the-counter drugs) should be taken without consulting a physician. Table 2–3 shows effects of selected maternal drugs on the breast-fed infant.

Lactation failure, resulting in malnutrition, failure to thrive, and hypernatremic dehydration is a serious problem that may be due, in part, to poor parent education and inadequate follow-up of an infant after discharge from the nursery.

### References

Behrman RE, Kliegman RM, Arvin AM (eds): Nelson Textbook of Pediatrics, 15th ed. Philadelphia, WB Saunders, 1996, Chapters 44.1.

Cooper W, Atherton H, Kahana M, et al.: Increased incidence of breastfeeding malnutrition and hypernatremia in a metropolitan area. Pediatr, 96:957, 1995.

Fomon SJ: Nutrition of Normal Infants. St. Louis, Mosby-Year Book, 1993, Chapter 26.

Freed G: Breast-feeding. JAMA 269:243, 1993.

## WEANING FOODS

Substitutes for and supplements to human milk are regarded as weaning foods in this section.

### Cow's Milk–Based Formulas

Cow's milk formulas (see Table 6-24) are composed of reconstituted, skimmed cow's milk or a mixture of skimmed cow's milk and electrolyte-depleted cow's milk whey or casein proteins. The fat used in infant formulas is a mixture of soy, palm, coconut, corn, oleo, or safflower oils; all contain lactose. Modern cow's milk–based formulas are generally equivalent to human milk in promoting growth during the first 6 mo of life. Complete cow's milk–based infant formulas are used as *substitutes* for breast milk for infants whose mothers choose not to or cannot breast-feed, as *supplements* for breast-fed infants whose mothers choose to omit occasional feedings, or as *complementary* feedings if breast-feeding alone does not result in normal growth or if other signs of malnutrition are present. Breast milk fortifiers (whey-casein protein, corn syrup, lactose, butterfat, minerals) also are available for use in special situations (as in the premature infant when breast milk is inadequate for growth).

### Soy Formula

Soy protein–based formulas are used if cow's milk–based formula intolerance occurs either from protein hypersensitivity or from lactose intolerance. These formulas are nutritionally sound and safe alternatives to cow's milk–based formulas (see Table 6–24). The soy protein is supplemented with l-methionine to improve its nutritional qualities. The carbohydrate in soy formulas is sucrose, glucose oligomers (smaller-molecular-weight corn starches), or a mixture of the two. The fat mixture is similar to that used in cow's milk formulas.

Soy protein formulas do not prevent the development of allergic disorders in later life, and clinical intolerances to soy milk proteins or cow's milk occur with equal frequency (see Chapter 11). Soy protein formulas can be recommended for use in vegetarian families choosing not to serve animal protein formulas and in the management of galactosemia and primary and secondary lactose intolerance. Although safe for the normal child, soy-based formula has been associated with protein-losing enteropathy in patients with cystic fibrosis and with neonatal rickets in premature infants. Too often soy and other "special" formulas are used indiscriminately to "treat" poorly evaluated patients with colic, formula intolerance, or more serious diseases.

### Premature Infant Formulas

See Chapter 6.

### Therapeutic Formulas

The composition of infant formulas has been further modified to meet specific therapeutic require-

TABLE 2–3.   Effect of Maternal Drugs on the Breast-Fed Infant

| Drug | Effect | Comment |
| --- | --- | --- |
| Amoxicillin | None | Safe |
| Antimetabolites | Carcinogenic | Contraindicated |
| Aspirin | Rare complication of bleeding | Usually safe |
| Atenolol | None | Probably safe |
| Bromocriptine | Suppresses lactation | Avoid |
| Carbamazepine | Unknown | Probably safe |
| Cascara | Colic, diarrhea | Avoid |
| Chloramphenicol | Gray baby syndrome | Contraindicated |
| Codeine | Lethargy | Usually safe |
| Diazepam | Lethargy, apnea | High doses contraindicated |
| Digoxin | None | Safe |
| Ergot | Gangrene, vasospasm | Contraindicated |
| Furosemide | None | Safe |
| Gold salts | Hepatonephrotoxicity | Contraindicated |
| Meperidine | Lethargy | Avoid |
| Methimazole | Hypothyroidism | Contraindicated |
| Metoprolol | None | Probably safe |
| Metronidazole | Carcinogenic? | Contraindicated |
| Phenindione | Hemorrhage | Contraindicated |
| Phenobarbital | Lethargy | Usually safe |
| Phenytoin | None | Safe |
| Prednisone | None | Probably safe |
| Propoxyphene | Lethargy | Usually safe |
| Propranolol | None | Probably safe |
| Propylthiouracil | Usually none; rare goiter | Probably safe |
| Radioactive material | Carcinogenic | Discontinue breast-feeding 1–2 wk |
| Tetracycline | Discolored teeth | Contraindicated |

ments (see Table 6-24). Therapeutic formulas designed to avoid digestive insufficiency or protein hypersensitivity contain hydrolyzed casein, whole casein, or soy protein as a source of amino acids. These formulas are also lactose free; some contain glucose oligomers and soluble starches, and some contain medium-chain triglycerides. Modular formulas allow stepwise introduction of specific carbohydrates and fats into the diet in a logical sequence for the purpose of therapeutic feeding trials. Modular formulas are nutritionally incomplete, are often hyperosmolar, and should be used only under close professional supervision.

## Whole Cow's Milk

Whole cow's milk should not be introduced into the diet before the age of 1 yr. The high solute load of cow's milk and its low iron content make it inappropriate to use earlier. Cow's milk ingested before 12 mo may cause gross or microscopic intestinal bleeding leading to iron deficiency anemia.

## Baby Foods

Commercially prepared or homemade foods fulfill the nutritional needs of the infant. Such foods are introduced at 4–6 mo. Because infant foods are calorically less dense than milk, they do not "fatten up" an infant. Furthermore, oropharyngeal coordination is immature before 3 mo. Vitamin- and mineral-enriched dry cereals are used as a source of calories (~375 calories/100 g), vitamins, and minerals (particularly iron) to supplement the diet of infants whose needs for these nutrients are not met by human milk, formula, or other milks. The manufacture of infant dry cereals involves the enzymatic hydrolysis of cereal flour and heat to precook and gelatinize the starches. Cereals are mixed with milk, water, or juice and later with fruits. To help identify possible allergies or food intolerances that may arise while adding new foods to the diet, single-grain cereals (rice, oatmeal, and barley) are recommended as starting cereals. Mixed cereal (oat, corn, wheat, soy) provides greater variety to older infants. High-protein cereal (soy, oat, wheat) offers the advantages of low cost and high protein in addition to variety.

Puréed fruits, vegetables, and meats are available in containers that provide an appropriate serving size. The caloric ranges are 40–80 calories/container for vegetables and 90–100 calories/container for fruit. Fruit and vegetable juices provide a maximum of only 4% of the total caloric intake of infants. The juices are strained, homogenized, and supplemented with vitamin C to achieve a uniform nutrient level that is equivalent to that of fresh orange juice. Excessive milk (>24 oz/day) or juice intake should be avoided in infants over 1 yr of age, because these products may reduce the intake of nutritionally important solid foods. Foods with high allergic potential that should be avoided during early infancy include fish, peanuts, egg whites, and various food additives. Hot dogs, grapes, and nuts also have a risk of aspiration and airway obstruction.

### References

Behrman RE, Kliegman RM, Arvin AM (eds): Nelson Textbook of Pediatrics, 15th ed. Philadelphia, WB Saunders, 1996, Chapters 44.2, 44.3.
Nichols BL: Infant feeding practices. *In* Tsang RC, Nichols BL (eds): Nutrition during Infancy. Philadelphia, Hanley and Belfus, 1988, pp 367–377.

## DIET OF THE NORMAL CHILD AND ADOLESCENT

Nutrient needs for children and adolescents are shown in Tables 2–1 and 2–2.

## OBESITY

*Pathology.* In infants and children of normal weight, increases in adipocyte size account for most of the increase in adipose mass during the first year of life. The total adipocyte number increases slowly between 6 mo and 2 yr of age and remains stable until 8–10 yr, when an increase in size and number occurs in association with puberty. Obese children have larger fat cells than normal-weight controls and have increased numbers of adipocytes.

In some circumstances in animals, obesity may be due to abnormalities in appetite suppression by a gene product of the **ob** gene in adipocytes. Normally, this protein (leptin) coded by the gene is secreted into the circulation and eventually suppresses the appetite center in the hypothalamus. Abnormalities of the leptin gene product or hypothalamic receptor may produce obesity in some patients.

*Epidemiology.* Although there are familial tendencies toward leanness or obesity, the critical issue is the extent to which such trends are due to similar genetic or environmental influences. In comparisons of adopted twin pairs, up to 80% of the variance in weight for height or skinfold thickness may be explained on the basis of genetics. A strong

relationship exists between the body mass index of adoptees and their biologic parents; a poorer relationship exists between adoptees and their adoptive parents.

Maternal obesity has been associated with increased adipose tissue in the newborn. Children from families in which either one or both parents are obese are susceptible to adult obesity (approximately 40% risk if one parent is obese; 80% if both are obese). There is a modest correlation between excessive weight gain or weight-gain velocity during the 1st yr of life and later obesity. However, overweight infants usually do not become obese children. Most obese infants and children do not become obese adults. The risk of obesity persisting to adulthood increases with a more advanced age of onset (adolescence versus infancy) and severity of obesity (100% adult obesity if the child weighs greater than 180% of his or her ideal body weight).

*Clinical Manifestations.* Complications of obesity often are noted during the preadolescent and teenage years (Table 2–4). During these periods, children develop increasing awareness of body types and generate negative stereotypic attitudes toward obesity. Medical complications usually are

TABLE 2–4. Complications of Obesity

| Complication | Effects |
|---|---|
| Psychosocial | Peer discrimination, teasing, reduced college acceptance, isolation, reduced job promotion* |
| Growth | Advanced bone age, increased height, early menarche |
| Central nervous system | Pseudotumor cerebri |
| Respiratory | Sleep apnea, pickwickian syndrome, infection |
| Cardiovascular | Hypertension, cardiac hypertrophy, ischemic heart disease,* sudden death* |
| Orthopedic | Slipped capital femoral epiphysis, Blount disease |
| Metabolic | Insulin resistance, type II diabetes mellitus, hypertriglyceridemia, hyperchloesterolemia, gout,* hepatic steatosis,* polycystic ovary disease, pancreatitis, cholelithiasis |
| Malignancy | Endometrial,* breast,* prostate,* colon* |

*Complications unusual until adulthood.

related directly to the degree of obesity and resolve with weight reduction.

The *diagnosis* of obesity is made by determining the percent deviation from the ideal body weight for height after adjusting for age. An actual weight greater than 120% of the ideal weight for age, gender, and height is considered obese. However, weight-for-height deviations may result in a muscular person incorrectly being identified as obese. Body mass index (weight/height$^2$) is commonly used in adults; however, because it is age-dependent in children, it is somewhat problematic to use in children. Therefore, caliper measurement of triceps skinfold thickness is a more accurate, readily available method for assessing adiposity; a measurement greater than the 85th percentile is considered overweight. In addition to obtaining anthropometric data, the pediatrician should direct the history and physical examination toward identifying the many potential complications noted among obese patients (see Table 2–4) in addition to specific diseases associated with obesity (Table 2–5).

*Treatment.* Obesity is difficult to treat, and management often includes a combination of education, behavior modification, exercise, drugs (in mature adolescents), and diet. A balanced diet consisting of an approximately 30% decrease in the previous caloric intake (total calories, 1000–1500) is an appropriate starting point for most obese patients. Dietary fat and thus total calories are reduced; portion size and meal patterns also are modified. More severe dietary restriction, such as the very-low-calorie diet or "protein modified fast," may be needed when a life-threatening complication, such as alveolar hypoventilation, sleep apnea, or significant hypertension, is present. Such restrictive diets require close supervision; supplementation with potassium, magnesium, calcium, and multiple vitamins; and the use of high-quality protein sources. Pharmacotherapy with appetite suppressant drugs is usually reserved for severely obese adolescent patients. Surgical therapy for morbid obesity includes gastric stapling or ileal bypass but is rarely indicated in children or adolescents.

*Prevention.* There is no recognized method of prevention, although increasing exercise and decreasing fat intake may be helpful. Despite constant energy intake/unit weight, there are large differences among normal children for rate of fat accumulation. Thus, an "appropriate" level of calories for a given child may be difficult to specify. Dietary recommendations, therefore, should be based on an acceptable rate of growth rather than on a fixed number of calories per kilogram of body weight.

### References

Behrman RE, Kliegman RM, Arvin AM (eds): Nelson Textbook of Pediatrics, 15th ed. Philadelphia, WB Saunders, 1996, Chapter 42.2.

Danforth E, Sims EAH: Obesity and efforts to loss weight. N Engl J Med 327:1947, 1992.

Lindpaintner K: Finding an obesity gene—a tale of mice and men. N Engl J Med 332:679, 1995.

Must A, Jacques PF, Dallal GE, et al: Long-term morbidity and mortality of overweight adolescents: A follow up of the

TABLE 2–5.   Diseases Associated with Childhood Obesity*

| Syndrome | Manifestations |
| --- | --- |
| Alström syndrome | Hypogonadism, retinal degeneration, deafness, diabetes mellitus |
| Carpenter syndrome | Polydactyly, syndactyly, cranial synostosis, mental retardation |
| Cushing syndrome | Adrenal hyperplasia or pituitary tumor |
| Fröhlich syndrome | Hypothalamic tumor |
| Hyperinsulinism | Nesidioblastosis, pancreatic adenoma, hypoglycemia, Mauriac syndrome (poor diabetic control) |
| Laurence-Moon-Bardet-Biedl syndrome | Retinal degeneration, syndactyly, polydactyly, hypogonadism, mental retardation; autosomal recessive |
| Muscular dystrophy | Late onset of obesity |
| Myelodysplasia | Spina bifida |
| Prader-Willi syndrome | Neonatal hypotonia, normal growth immediately after birth, small hands and feet, mental retardation, hypogonadism; some have partial deletion of chromosome 15 |
| Pseudohypoparathyroidism | Variable hypocalcemia, cutaneous calcifications |
| Turner syndrome | Ovarian dysgenesis, lymphedema, web neck; XO chromosome |

*These diseases represent fewer than 5% of cases of childhood obesity.

Harvard Growth Study of 1922 to 1935. N Engl J Med 327:1350, 1992.

# EATING DISORDERS

## ANOREXIA NERVOSA

The prevalence of anorexia nervosa has been estimated to be 1–5% in teenage girls. The female-to-male ratio is approximately 20:1 and shows a familial pattern. The cause of anorexia nervosa is unknown.

*Clinical Manifestations.* The clinical manifestations of weight loss usually begin with moderate efforts to lose weight, which accelerate into a fear of obesity and a preoccupation with becoming thin (Tables 2–6 and 2–7). Predisposing factors include perfectionist behavior, low self-esteem, and, in 40% of cases, a history of being mildly overweight. An almost invariable feature of anorexia nervosa is the patient's pleasure in the achievement of low weight for personal and emotional reasons. Any weight gain generates severe anxiety; weight loss reduces this anxiety. Vitamin and nutrient deficiency disorders are infrequently observed. Nonetheless, scalp hair loss is common; fine lanugo-like hair grows on the face and the trunk. The skin becomes rough, scaly, and petechial.

Two types of dieting prevail: (1) the fasting, abstaining, or restricting type, and (2) the so-called bulimic type. In the bulimic type of dieting, binge eating initially occurs in spurts but gradually becomes a habit. Binge eating ends with self-induced vomiting, either alone or in combination with laxative and/or diuretic abuse as a means to get rid of excess weight. Intense compulsive exercise is another weight-control method.

Additional features include bradycardia, osteopenia, delayed gastric emptying, lymphopenia,

low voltage on electrocardiogram, decreased 1-sec forced expiratory volume ($FEV_1$), hypothermia, myopathy, neuropathy, and, if severe, organic brain syndrome.

*Endocrine changes* are starvation-induced (see Tables 2–7 and 2–11). For most female patients, amenorrhea, which occurs when body weight drops below the normal range, is due to low plasma luteinizing hormone levels, which result in reduced ovarian stimulation, low estradiol levels, and nonmeasurable progesterone levels. The hypothalamic-pituitary-thyroid axis changes are identical to those in marasmic patients. The cortisol production rate is elevated. When dexamethasone is administered, plasma cortisol levels are not suppressed. Weight gain to the normal premorbid level reverses all the endocrine changes in patients with anorexia nervosa.

*Diagnosis.* The *differential diagnosis* includes Addison disease, hyperthyroidism, diabetes mellitus, inflammatory bowel disease, malignancy (including brain tumors), drug abuse, primary depression, schizophrenia, and obsessive-compulsive disorders.

*Treatment and Prognosis. Treatment* requires a multidisciplinary approach consisting of a feeding program and individual and family therapy. Therapy is difficult because the patients and families involved often deny the severity of the illness and may conceal symptoms. Goals of therapy are to restore normal function and body weight and to re-establish normal eating patterns. Adequate nutrition is of lifesaving importance in the acutely ill, severely underweight patient, but weight restoration and refeeding require the patient's cooperation if this therapy is to succeed.

When vital signs are stable, discussion and negotiation of a detailed treatment contract with the patient and the parents are essential before further treatment begins. The first step is to restore body weight; the patient's weight should be increased to more than 80% of normal levels for height and age. This is accomplished by voluntary intake of regular foods or of a nutritional formula ingested orally or by nasogastric tube. Occasionally parenteral nutrition is indicated to improve the nutritional status to a safe level. During the second step, the patient is given freedom to gain weight at a personal pace. Hospitalization is indicated when:

1. Weight loss exceeds 25% of ideal body weight.
2. Personal and family dynamics place the patient at excessive risk for suicide or abuse.
3. Metabolic disturbances (dehydration, hypokalemia, severe dysrhythmias, severe recur-

TABLE 2–6.    Diagnostic Criteria for Anorexia Nervosa

Refusal to maintain minimal normal body weight for age and height

Weight loss leading to body weight 15% below expected or failure to have expected weight gain during growth leading to weight 15% below expected

Disturbance of body image: feels fat despite emaciation

Intense fear of becoming obese, even with progressive weight loss

Absence of at least three consecutive menstrual cycles when expected to occur

No known physical illness to account for weight loss

TABLE 2-7. Comparative Characteristics of Anorexia Nervosa and Bulimia Nervosa

| Characteristics | Anorexia Nervosa | Bulimia Nervosa |
|---|---|---|
| Intense preoccupation with food | Yes | Yes |
| Weight loss | Severe | Fluctuates |
| Female | 90–95% | 90–95% |
| Family history | + for anorexia nervosa | + for depression |
| Methods of weight control | Severe food restrictions, emesis, exercise | Restriction and binges with self-induced vomiting and diuretic and/or laxative purging |
| Guilt/shame | None | Yes |
| Denial | Yes | None |
| Personality | Withdrawn/asexual | Outgoing/heterosexual |
| Onset (age) | Bimodal (13–14 yr and 17–18 yr) | 17–25 yr |
| Endocrinopathy/metabolism | Amenorrhea, increased growth hormone, osteoporosis, hypercarotenemia, hypothermia | Menstrual irregularities, hypokalemia |
| Cardiovascular complications | Bradycardia, hypotension, arrhythmias | Ipecac toxicity |
| Gastrointestinal | Constipation, elevated hepatic enzymes | Gastric dilation and rupture, Mallory-Weiss syndrome, esophagitis, parotid enlargement, dental enamel erosion |
| Psychiatric | Depression, suicide, obsessional fears | Impulsive behaviors, alcohol-drug addictions, depression, suicide |
| Renal | Calculi Edema | Hypokalemia secondary to diuretics |

rent induced vomiting or laxative abuse) are noted.

4. Outpatient therapy fails.

Antidepressant drug therapy may be indicated for depressed patients.

The *prognosis* includes a 3–5% mortality (suicide, malnutrition) rate, the development of bulimic symptoms (30%), and persistent problems (20%).

## BULIMIA NERVOSA

The diagnostic indicators in the behavior of a patient with bulimia nervosa are binge-eating episodes and the loss of control during overeating (Table 2–8). Although often considered a symptom of anorexia nervosa, the term "bulimia" also is applied to a distinct eating disorder. Previous dieting is usually a precondition for the development of bulimia. It occurs predominantly in young women of normal weight or in slightly overweight women. The prevalence may be as high as 5% of female college students; the female-to-male ratio is 10:1.

In the fully developed syndrome, binge eating is precipitated by a variety of conditions. During these episodes, patients tend to consume large volumes of "forbidden" foods that are high in carbohydrate and fat content; others may eat leftovers of unpalatable foods. The food is consumed rapidly and secretly without dwelling on the taste. Vomiting eventually becomes coupled to binge eating. Most patients overeat with the forethought of vomiting afterward. Most metabolic abnormalities are the result of excessive vomiting (see Table 2–7). The excessive use of laxatives or diuretics also increases the risks of metabolic disturbance, such as hypokalemia.

In contrast to patients with anorexia nervosa, patients with bulimia are more likely to present with personality disturbances, impulse control difficulties (stealing, drug abuse, sexual promiscuity), personal and family history of affective disorders, and a positive response to antidepressant therapy. These patients often feel embarrassed, guilty, and ashamed. Repetitive binge eating and vomiting can result in salivary gland enlargement, esophagitis, fluid and electrolyte imbalance, callus formation on knuckles due to abrasion from teeth while vomiting was induced, and erosion of dental enamel.

TABLE 2–8.  Diagnostic Criteria for Bulimia Nervosa

1. Recurrent episodes of binge eating (rapid consumption of large food quantities in short time periods); at least two episodes a week for 3 mo
2. Overconcern with body shape and weight
3. Three of the following:
   a. Consumption of high-caloric, easily ingested food during a binge
   b. Inconspicuous eating during a binge
   c. Termination of binge by abdominal pain, self-induced vomiting, sleep, or social interruption
   d. Repeated attempts to lose weight by restrictive diets, cathartics, diuretics, or self-induced vomiting
   e. Frequent weight fluctuations of more than 4.5 kg due to binges and fasts
4. Awareness of abnormal eating patterns and fear of being unable to stop eating voluntarily; lack of control during binges
5. Depression and self-deprecating thoughts after binge
6. Exclusion of anorexia nervosa or known physical causes of bulimic episodes

Ipecac abuse (to induce emesis) may cause cardiomyopathy.

A combination of nutritional, educational, and self-monitoring techniques is employed to increase awareness of the maladaptive behavior, after which efforts are made to change the eating behavior. Antidepressants have a place in the treatment of bulimia. Suicide occurs in up to 5% of patients, with many more patients attempting suicide.

References

Behrman RE, Kliegman RM, Arvin AM (eds): Nelson Textbook of Pediatrics, 15th ed. Philadelphia, WB Saunders, 1996, Chapter 107.

Fairburn CG: Bulimia nervosa. BMJ 300:485, 1990.
Patton G: The course of anorexia nervosa. BMJ 299:139, 1989.

## ARTERIOSCLEROSIS
(See Chapter 5)

Evidence suggests the utility of adult cardiovascular disease prevention beginning in children. Elevated low-density lipoprotein (LDL) cholesterol levels are associated with heart disease in adults; dietary modification reduces LDL cholesterol levels in adults and children. The childhood origin of atherosclerosis is suggested by finding vascular atherosclerotic lesions in young soldiers killed in wars and in autopsies of younger children. Childhood cholesterol levels are associated with subsequent cholesterol levels and heart disease in adulthood. Given the known influences (diet, exercise, smoking) on LDL cholesterol and the development of heart disease and the resistance of many adults to behavioral intervention, children should be encouraged to adopt healthier lifestyles to reduce the risk of atherosclerotic heart disease. The Prudent or Step-One Diet (Table 2–9) is proposed for all children over 2 yr of age, and especially those with elevated cholesterol levels, whereas the Step-Two Diet is reserved for those with more significant elevations in LDL cholesterol that have not responded to the original dietary intervention. Drug therapy is reserved for older children (generally >10 yr) with severe elevations in LDL cholesterol after failing 6–12 mo of dietary management. Drug therapy in children should be considered only after consultation with a pediatric lipid specialist.

Several questions have been raised about the safety and efficacy of dietary interventions in children. Some children fail to thrive when put on very-low-fat, low-calorie diets by well-meaning but misguided parents. Dietary intervention should be

TABLE 2–9.  Characteristics of Step-One and Step-Two Diets for Lowering Blood Cholesterol

| | Recommended Intake | |
|---|---|---|
| Nutrient | Step-One Diet | Step-Two Diet |
| Total fat | Average of no more than 30% of total calories | Same |
| Saturated fatty acids | Less than 10% of total calories | Less than 7% of total calories |
| Polyunsaturated fatty acids | Up to 10% of total calories | Same |
| Monounsaturated fatty acids | Remaining total fat calories | Same |
| Cholesterol | Less than 300 mg/day | Less than 200 mg/day |
| Carbohydrates | About 55% of total calories | Same |
| Protein | About 15–20% of total calories | Same |
| Calories | To promote normal growth and development and to reach or maintain desirable body weight | Same |

From National Cholesterol Education Program: Report of the Expert Panel on Blood Cholesterol Levels in Children and Adolescents. Pediatrics 89(Suppl):556, 1992.

undertaken with appropriate guidance (a registered dietitian with pediatric experience) to ensure that the diet has sufficient calories and nutrients for growth while fulfilling the guidelines of the Prudent Diet.

There is concern about the psychosocial consequences of labeling children as hypercholesterolemic (i.e., the development of the "sick child" role). For this to be avoided, intervention programs should focus on the positive changes the child and family can make to help limit their risk. Another concern is the mislabeling of children based on a single or inaccurate screening test as a result of inherent biologic and laboratory variability in cholesterol testing. Any measure of cholesterol should be completed with adequate quality assurance; repeated measurements are required to define a child's lipid status (Table 2–10).

The current National Cholesterol Education Program guidelines recommend screening children with a positive family history of early (before 55 yr of age) cardiovascular disease or hypercholesterolemia (>240 mg/dL). Those children with unknown histories or other cardiovascular risk factors may be screened at the physician's discretion. To prevent heart disease, it is also important to focus on lifestyle interventions to minimize other risk factors—smoking, hypertension, obesity, diabetes mellitus, and physical inactivity.

### References

Behrman RE, Kliegman RM, Arvin AM (eds): Nelson Textbook of Pediatrics, 15th ed. Philadelphia, WB Saunders, 1996, Chapter 72.4.
Committee on Nutrition: Statement on cholesterol. Pediatrics 90:469, 1992.
National Cholesterol Education Program: Report of the expert panel on blood cholesterol levels in children and adolescents. Pediatrics 89:525, 1992.
Writing Group for the DISC Collaborative Research Group: Efficacy and safety of lowering dietary intake of fat and cholesterol in children with elevated low-density lipoprotein cholesterol. JAMA 273:1429, 1995.

## PITFALLS IN CHILD AND ADOLESCENT NUTRITION

When dietary intakes are compared with recommendations (see Tables 2–1 and 2–2), the intake of preschool children in the United States is deficient in zinc. The deficiency is profound in the diets of children living in families of low socioeconomic status (70% in 1–3 yr olds and 79% in 4–5 yr olds). Calcium intake is inadequate (82%) in these children unless the families participate in federal food stamp programs. Latent calcium and zinc deficiencies are likely to be buffered by adaptive mechanisms; however, the presence of illness may precipitate clinical signs and symptoms of deficiency.

Iron intake tends to be inadequate (65%) in children between 1 and 3 yr of age in the United States. The incidence of iron-deficiency anemia is decreasing in the United States in part as a result of participation in the Women, Infants and Children (WIC) program, but is still significant. Dietary iron deficiency is the major nutritional risk for the 1- to 2-yr age group.

Osteoporosis (osteopenia) from poor dietary calcium intake or absorption of ingested calcium in children and adolescents is becoming more clinically recognized and treated. Poor calcium intake during adolescence may predispose females to osteoporotic hip fractures in later life.

In the United States, 20% of all children and 50% of all black and Hispanic children live in families of low socioeconomic status. Among those families who participate in federal assistance programs, 2–3 times the expected number of children have weight-for-height measurements below the 5th percentile. This problem is evident in infants from 3

TABLE 2–10.  Cutpoints of Total and Low-Density Lipoprotein (LDL) Cholesterol for Dietary Intervention in Children and Adolescents with a Family History of Hypercholesterolemia or Premature Cardiovascular Disease

| Category | Total Cholesterol (mg/dL) | LDL Cholesterol (mg/dL) | Dietary Intervention |
|---|---|---|---|
| Acceptable | <170 | <110 | Recommended population eating pattern |
| Borderline | 170–199 | 110–129 | Step-One Diet prescribed, other risk factor intervention |
| High | ≥200 | ≥130 | Step-One Diet prescribed, then Step-Two if necessary |

From National Cholesterol Education Program: Report of the Expert Panel on Blood Cholesterol Levels in Children and Adolescents. Pediatrics 89(Suppl):556, 1992.

mo through the 2nd yr of life. Surveillance of growth velocity is essential in this population, and evidence for macronutrient and micronutrient deficiencies should be sought in all children placed below the 5th percentile of weight-for-height measurements.

## References

Nationwide Food Consumption Survey: Continuing Survey of Food Intakes by Individuals. Women 19–50 Years and Their Children 1–5 Years, 1 Day. Washington, DC, U.S. Department of Agriculture, 1985, pp 40–41, 66–77.

Popkin B, Siega-Riz A, Haines P: A comparison of dietary trends among racial and socioeconomic groups in the United States. N Engl J Med 335:716, 1996.

# MACRONUTRIENT DEFICIENCIES

Worldwide, protein-energy malnutrition (PEM) is a leading cause of death among children younger than 5 yr of age. PEM is a spectrum of conditions due to varying proportions of protein and calorie deficiencies. Primary PEM is due to social or economic factors that result in lack of food. Secondary PEM occurs in children with various diseases associated with increased caloric requirements (infection, trauma, cancer), increased caloric loss (malabsorption, cystic fibrosis), reduced caloric intake (anorexia, cancer, oral intake restriction, social factors), or a combination of these three variables.

## MARASMUS

Marasmus is the most common form of primary PEM and is due to severe caloric depletion. Many secondary forms of marasmic PEM are associated with diseases such as cystic fibrosis, tuberculosis, cancer, acquired immunodeficiency syndrome (AIDS), or celiac disease.

The principal *clinical manifestation* in a child with severe malnutrition is emaciation with a body weight below 60% of that expected for age or below 70% of the ideal weight for height and depleted body fat stores. Although growth stunting may be observed with longer-term malnutrition, the ratio of observed to expected weight to height reveals a reduction in body mass exceeding that of any coexisting growth stunting. Visible loss of muscle mass and subcutaneous tissue is confirmed by inspection or palpation and quantified by anthropometric measurements. The head appears large but generally is proportional to the body length. Edema usually is absent. The skin is dry and thin, and the hair is thin and sparse and easily pulled out. Marasmic children are apathetic and

weak. Bradycardia and hypothermia signify severe and life-threatening malnutrition. Atrophy of the filiform papillae of the tongue is common, and monilial stomatitis is frequent. Recent weaning of the child or inappropriate weaning practices and chronic diarrhea are common findings in developing countries.

## ROLE OF CHRONIC DIARRHEA

Malnutrition often is associated with chronic diarrhea as a result of the effects of malnutrition on the gastrointestinal tract (mucosal atrophy, secondary malabsorption) and the increased susceptibility to viral, bacterial, protozoal, and parasitic infections related to a secondary T and B cell immunodeficiency state. Recurrent episodes of diarrhea treated with prolonged periods of fasting or oral electrolyte solutions reduce caloric intake and contribute to malnutrition. Diarrhea may worsen during rehabilitation (in 10–20% of children) as a result of excessive refeeding or formula intolerance (transient lactose or monosaccharide malabsorption or milk protein intolerance). Nonetheless, cow's milk formulas are used routinely to rehabilitate malnourished children with good results. In very severe cases of diarrhea, malabsorption, and malnutrition, intravenous refeeding may be necessary.

## KWASHIORKOR

Kwashiorkor, presenting with pitting edema that starts in the lower extremities and ascends with increasing severity, is due to inadequate protein intake in the presence of fair to good caloric intake. It is common in developing countries if children are weaned to low-protein foods, but it also may be a complication of critical illness (burns, cancer, acute and chronic infections, multiorgan system failure, inflammatory bowel disease, anorexia nervosa, and postoperative surgery) when inadequate amounts of protein are provided for a prolonged time.

The major *clinical manifestation* of kwashiorkor is that the body weight of the child ranges from 60–80% of the expected weight for age; weight may not represent the nutritional status because of the presence of edema. Physical examination reveals a relative maintenance of subcutaneous adipose tissue and a marked atrophy of muscle mass. Edema varies from a minor pitting of the dorsum of the foot to generalized edema accompanied by involvement of the eyelids and scrotum. The hair is sparse, easily pluckable, and appears dull brown, red, or yellow-white. Adequate protein intake restores hair color (flag sign). Skin changes are common and range from hyperpigmented hyperkeratosis to an erythematous macular rash on the trunk and extremities. In its most severe form, a superficial desquamation occurs over pressure surfaces. Angular cheilosis and the atrophy of the filiform papillae of the tongue are common. Monilial stomatitis is frequent. Examination of the abdomen may reveal a large, soft liver with an indefinite edge. Lymphatic tissue commonly is atrophic. Chest examination may reveal basilar rales. The abdomen is distended, and bowel sounds tend to be hypoactive.

## TREATMENT OF MALNUTRITION

The basal metabolic rate and immediate nutrient needs during malnutrition are decreased. When nutrients are provided, the metabolic rate increases, stimulating anabolism and thus increasing nutrient requirements. The malnourished child may have compensated for vitamin and mineral deficiencies with lower metabolic and growth rates; refeeding may unmask these deficiencies. Furthermore, the gastrointestinal tract may not tolerate a rapid increase in intake. Nutritional rehabilitation, therefore, should be initiated and advanced slowly to minimize these complications. Fluid and solute load must be monitored to avoid stressing the compromised myocardial function. The caloric intake should be kept stable until the edema begins to resolve.

Calories can be safely initiated at 20% above the child's recent intake. If no estimate of the caloric intake is available, 50–75% of the normal energy requirement is safe. Caloric intake can be increased 10–20%/day, with monitoring for electrolyte imbalances, poor cardiac function, edema, or feeding intolerance. If any of these occurs, further caloric increases are not made until the status stabilizes. Caloric intake is increased until appropriate regrowth is initiated. This may require 150% or more of the recommended calories for an age-matched, well-nourished child. Protein needs also are increased as anabolism begins and are provided in proportion (10–20%) to the caloric intake.

In most cases, cow's milk–based formulas are tolerated and provide an appropriate mix of nutrients. Other easily digested foods, appropriate for the age, also may be introduced slowly. If feeding intolerance occurs, lactose-free or, rarely, other regimens (parenteral nutrition) may be considered (see Marasmus earlier). During 2–3 wk of dietary rehabilitation and rapid growth, a hypermetabolic *"nutritional recovery syndrome"* may develop that is characterized by postprandial diaphoresis, hepatic glycogenesis, and eosinophilia.

Vitamin and mineral intake in excess of the RDA is provided to account for the increased requirements. Potassium, phosphorus, calcium, and magnesium status is carefully monitored. Potassium, as a major component of lean body tissue, is needed during growth and healing; serum levels may decrease dangerously in response to a glucose load, with subsequent insulin-induced transcellular shift of potassium. Phosphorus is needed for phosphorylated intermediates because it becomes "trapped" intracellularly by such phosphorylation in response to a glucose load, increased anabolism, and increased metabolic rate. Magnesium, a cofactor for adenosine triphosphatase, is needed when the metabolic and anabolic rates increase. Hypomagnesemia blunts the parathyroid response to hypocalcemia, which may be exacerbated by the vitamin D and calcium deficiencies associated with malnutrition (see Chapter 17). Electrolyte imbalances can further alter cardiac function, exacerbating heart failure. Overzealous refeeding has been documented to cause life-threatening abnormalities of these and other nutrients.

### References

Behrman RE, Kliegman RM, Arvin AM (eds): Nelson Textbook of Pediatrics, 15th ed. Philadelphia, WB Saunders, 1996, Chapter 45.1.

Torún B, Chew R: Protein-energy malnutrition. *In* Shils ME, Olson JA, Shike M (eds): Modern Nutrition in Health and Disease, 8th ed. Philadelphia, Lea & Febiger, 1994, pp 950–976.

## COMPLICATIONS OF MALNUTRITION

Malnourished children are more susceptible to infection, especially sepsis, pneumonia, and gastroenteritis. Hypoglycemia is common after periods of severe fasting but also may be a sign of sepsis. Apnea may be associated with hypoglycemia. Hypothermia may signify infection or, with bradycardia, may signify a decreased metabolic rate to conserve energy. Bradycardia and poor cardiac output predispose the malnourished child to heart failure, which is exacerbated by acute fluid or solute loads. Vitamin deficiencies also can complicate malnutrition. Vitamin A deficiency is common in the developing world and is an important cause of altered immune response and increased morbidity (infections, blindness) and mortality (especially from measles). Depending on the age of onset and the duration of the malnutrition, such children may suffer permanent growth stunting (malnutrition in utero, infancy, adolescence) and delayed development (malnutrition in infancy). Environmental (social) deprivation may interact with the effects of the malnutrition to further impair development and cognitive function.

### Pathophysiology of Macronutrient Deficiencies

Protein-energy malnutrition represents a complex interrelationship between reduced protein and calorie intake, inciting events such as weaning or gastrointestinal infection, some chronic illnesses, and the complications associated with PEM and infection. The child's adaptation to reduced protein and calorie intake is typical for that of starvation, and secondary immune dysfunction and continued exposure to infectious diseases increase the morbidity and mortality of PEM.

### Endocrine Adaptation

The hormonal responses to malnutrition are noted in Table 2–11. The net effects of nutrient deficiency and these hormonal events are to reduce (spare) tissue glucose utilization and to increase alternate fuel mobilization and use (proteolysis, lipolysis, ketogenesis). Initially, free fatty acids and ketones may spare proteolysis, but with profound deficiencies muscle breakdown continues and net protein synthesis is reduced.

### Metabolic Substrates

There are several stages of metabolic adaptation in PEM. The first is a reduction in voluntary energy expenditure used for spontaneous physical activity, the second is a reduction in the rate of gain of body mass and length, and the last is a reduction in resting energy expenditure. The marasmic form of malnutrition results in a more striking reduction in resting energy expenditure than the reduction produced by kwashiorkor.

Inadequate macronutrient intake, especially when amplified by concurrent infection, results in growth arrest. Normal nitrogen balance may be sustained if protein intake has not been exceeded by excessive nitrogen losses; in both healthy children and those with PEM, the efficiency of nitrogen balance is greater than 95%. Protein turnover is a measure of total endogenous protein synthesis and degradation. In normal adults, the rate of turnover is influenced only modestly by starvation; in children with kwashiorkor, however, the rate of turnover is strikingly reduced. In contrast, turnover rates in normal children are increased in response to the stress of an infection.

The turnover of individual proteins is reduced under modest dietary restrictions. In both well-nourished and malnourished children, a reduced protein intake results in a few days in reduced rates of albumin synthesis and, later, if the reduction continues, in decreased concentrations of serum transferrin, retinol-binding protein, and pre-albumin. However, because of differences in half-life, serum albumin concentrations do not decrease for 1–2 weeks, whereas pre-albumin levels, for example, decrease within a few days. The synthesis of hepatic acute-phase proteins, such as C-reactive protein, nonetheless is preserved under these conditions. In addition to the hepatic synthetic adaptations, there is increased degradation of muscle proteins. In the marasmic child, these mechanisms maintain the plasma levels of free amino acids and hepatic secretory proteins. In the child with kwashiorkor, the adaptation fails to maintain serum amino acids and hepatic protein synthesis, and the plasma levels of branched-chain amino acids decrease. In marasmus, the urea synthesis and concentration are normal, but in kwashiorkor, urea levels are below 7 mg/dL, reflecting a reduced amino acid pool. Hepatic steatosis occurs in patients with kwashiorkor owing to a failure to synthesize and secrete hepatic triglyceride-transporting proteins.

Macronutrient deficiency and specific infections (e.g., measles and rotavirus) also decrease the rate of synthesis of pancreatic enzymes and intestinal mucosa brush-border hydrolases, which can retard later dietary rehabilitation.

Body water content is increased in kwashiorkor as a result of reduced adipose tissue mass and fluid retention. Blood osmolality and serum sodium concentrations may be low, and serum concentrations of potassium and magnesium may be reduced. Total body magnesium and potassium are reduced in all malnourished children owing to loss of muscle mass. In kwashiorkor, there also are defects in the maintenance of the normal sodium-potassium membrane gradients in soft tissues. Calcium and phosphorus are uniformly low, but tetany is rare. Concentrations of serum zinc and copper are strikingly reduced in kwashiorkor but are normal in marasmus. If adequate micronutrient dietary supplements are not provided, serum zinc and copper concentrations fall rapidly during nutritional rehabilitation.

### References

Frenk S: Metabolic adaptation in protein-energy malnutrition. J Am Coll Nutr 5:371–381, 1986.
Waterlow JC: Metabolic adaptation to low intakes of energy and protein. Annu Rev Nutr 6:495–526, 1986.

TABLE 2-11. Summary of Selected Hormonal Changes and Their Main Metabolic Effects Usually Seen in Severe Protein-Energy Malnutrition (PEM)

| Hormone | Influenced in PEM by | Hormonal Activity in | | Metabolic Effects of Changes in PEM |
|---------|----------------------|----------------------|----------------------|-------------------------------------|
| | | *Energy Deficit* | *Protein Deficit* | |
| Insulin | Low food intake ($\downarrow$ glucose) ($\downarrow$ amino acids) | Decreased | Decreased | $\downarrow$ muscle protein synthesis <br> $\downarrow$ lipogenesis <br> $\downarrow$ growth |
| Growth hormone | Low protein intake ($\downarrow$ amino acids) Reduced somatomedin synthesis | Normal or moderately increased | Increased | $\uparrow$ visceral synthesis <br> $\downarrow$ urea synthesis <br> $\uparrow$ lipolysis |
| Somatomedins (IGF-I) | Low protein intake? | Variable | Decreased | $\downarrow$ muscle and cartilage protein synthesis <br> $\downarrow$ collagen synthesis <br> $\downarrow$ lipolysis <br> $\downarrow$ growth <br> $\uparrow$ production of growth hormone |
| Epinephrine | Stress of food deficiency, infections ($\downarrow$ glucose) | Normal but can increase | Normal but can increase | $\uparrow$ lipolysis <br> $\uparrow$ glycogenolysis inhibits insulin secretion |
| Glucocorticoids | Stress of hunger Fever ($\downarrow$ glucose) | Increased | Normal or moderately increased | $\uparrow$ muscle protein catabolism <br> $\uparrow$ visceral protein turnover <br> $\uparrow$ lipolysis <br> $\uparrow$ gluconeogenesis |
| Aldosterone | $\downarrow$ blood volume <br> $\uparrow$ extracellular K? <br> $\downarrow$ serum Na? | Normal | Increased | $\uparrow$ sodium retention and <br> $\uparrow$ water retention contribute to appearance of edema |
| Thyroid hormones | ? | $T_4$ normal or decreased; $T_3$ decreased | $T_4$ usually decreased; $T_3$ decreased | $\downarrow$ glucose oxidation <br> $\downarrow$ basal energy expenditure <br> $\uparrow$ reverse $T_3$ |
| Gonadotropins | Low protein intake? Low energy intake? | Decreased | Decreased | Delayed menarche |

From Shils M, Young V: Modern Nutrition in Health and Disease, 7th ed. Philadelphia, Lea & Febiger, 1988.
$\downarrow$ = low or reduced; $\uparrow$ = high or increased; IGF-I = insulin-like growth factor-I.

### Immune Function

Cell-mediated immunity is depressed in patients with PEM. Severely malnourished children fail to respond to tuberculin or *Candida albicans* skin tests, which reveals an inability of their system to demonstrate prior sensitization. They also do not react to dinitrofluorobenzene sensitization, indicating that noncommitted lymphocytes are unresponsive. Thymic, lymph node, tonsil, and splenic tissues are atrophic in malnourished children. Total circulating lymphocytes are reduced, indicating a reduction of the thymus-derived cells, or T lymphocytes; the T lymphocytes present have a poor response to in vitro mitogenic stimulation. Vitamin A deficiency produces a reduced CD4/CD8 ratio and total CD4 naive T cells. This immunocompromised status improves with dietary rehabilitation; functional recovery occurs within 2 wk, and the total lymphocyte count recovers within 4 wk.

The concentration of B lymphocytes in lymphoid tissues and in peripheral blood is normal.

Immunoglobulin (Ig) synthesis is increased, as reflected in elevated total circulating IgA, IgM, IgG, IgD, and IgE levels. The concentrations are greater in children with kwashiorkor than in those with marasmus. The quantitative antibody response to vaccines for yellow fever, influenza, and typhoid is reduced, although the response to cholera vaccine is not. The recovery of antigenic response is dependent on adequate protein intake. Malnourished children have reduced secretory IgA (sIgA) levels in nasal washings, duodenal fluids, and tears despite the elevated serum IgA. The reduction is reflected by the diminished response of sIgA to measles and polio vaccines. The loss of secretory immunity may contribute to an increase in respiratory and intestinal infections.

The response of polymorphonuclear (PMN) leukocytes to chemotactic stimulation is normal, but that of the macrophages is reduced in PEM. The PMN leukocytes are able to phagocytize bacteria but have reduced ability to kill *Staphylococcus aureus*, *E. coli*, and *C. albicans*.

Patients with kwashiorkor have reduced hemolytic complement (CH50) titers because of the presence of anticomplementary serum factors. Titers return to normal after a week of dietary rehabilitation. All subjects with PEM have depressed concentrations of specific complement factors (C1q, C1s, C3, C5, C6, C8, C9, and C3PA). The levels of C1q, C6, and C8 are more profoundly depressed in kwashiorkor but respond to dietary therapy within 4 wk. Levels of C9 may remain low for several months. Recovery of complement levels occurs more quickly in children who receive diets with adequate protein.

### Infection

A triangle of interactions exists among host defenses, infection, and macronutrient malnutrition. PEM may be initiated by primary dietary deficiencies or by illnesses that induce a secondary dietary deficiency. Infections induce anorexia and increase caloric requirements owing to hypermetabolism during the febrile response. Contributing infections may be bacterial (*E. coli* enteritis, pneumococcal pneumonia), viral (rotavirus, measles), protozoal (malaria, giardia), or a result of intestinal helminths (roundworms, flukes, tapeworms). The result is catabolism and a loss of body nutrient stores, leading to clinical malnutrition. The impaired host defenses associated with PEM are important factors in determining the frequency and severity of infection. Gastrointestinal infections also exacerbate intestinal malabsorption, mucosal atrophy, and micronutrient losses.

### References
Keusch GT, Farthing MJG: Nutrition and infection. Annu Rev Nutr 6:131–154, 1986.
Cunningham-Rundles S, Cervia J: Malnutrition and host defense. *In* Walker WA, Watkins JB (eds): Nutrition in Pediatrics, 2nd ed. Hamilton, Ontario, BC Decker, 1996, Chapter 19, pp 295–307.

## MICRONUTRIENT DEFICIENCIES

The causes of micronutrient deficiencies are diverse and relate to unusual diets; various malabsorption or maldigestion syndromes; drugs that alter nutrient absorption, metabolism, and excretion or that compete with vitamin action; and various genetic disorders associated with specific nutrient metabolic defects (Tables 2–12 and 2–13).

TABLE 2–12. Etiology of Vitamin and Nutrient Deficiency States

| Etiology | Deficiency |
|---|---|
| ***Diet*** | |
| Vegans (strict) | Protein, vitamins $B_{12}$, D, riboflavin |
| Breast-fed infant | Vitamins K, D |
| Cow's milk–fed infant | Iron |
| Bulimia, anorexia nervosa | Electrolytes, other deficiencies |
| Parenteral alimentation | Essential fatty acid, trace elements |
| Alcoholism | Calories, vitamin $B_1$, $B_6$, folate |
| ***Medical Problems*** | |
| Malabsorption syndromes | Vitamins A, D, E, K, zinc, essential fatty acids |
| Cholestasis | Vitamins E, D, K, A, zinc, essential fatty acids |
| ***Medications*** | |
| Sulfonamides | Folate |
| Phenytoin, phenobarbital | Vitamins D, K, folate |
| Mineral oil | Vitamins A, D, E, K |
| Antibiotics | Vitamin K |
| Isoniazid | Vitamin $B_6$ |
| Antacids | Iron, phosphate, calcium |
| Digitalis | Magnesium, calcium |
| Penicillamine | Vitamin $B_6$ |
| ***Specific Mechanisms*** | |
| Transcobalamine II or intrinsic factor deficiency | Vitamin $B_{12}$ |
| Other digestive enzyme deficiencies | Carbohydrate, fat, protein |
| Menkes kinky hair syndrome | Copper |
| Acrodermatitis enteropathica | Zinc |
| Reduced direct sunlight | Vitamin D |

TABLE 2–13.   Characteristics of Vitamin Deficiencies

| Vitamin | Purpose | Deficiency | Comments | Source |
|---|---|---|---|---|
| **Water Soluble** | | | | |
| Thiamine (B$_1$) | Coenzyme in ketoacid decarboxylation (e.g., pyruvate → acetyl-CoA transketolase reaction) | *Beri-beri:* polyneuropathy, calf tenderness, heart failure, edema, ophthalmoplegia | Inborn errors of lactate metabolism; boiling milk destroys B$_1$ | Liver, meat, milk, cereals, nuts, legumes |
| Riboflavin (B$_2$) | FAD coenzyme in oxidation-reduction reactions | Anorexia, mucositis, anemia, cheilosis, nasolabial seborrhea | Photosensitizer | Milk, cheese, liver, meat, eggs, whole grains, green leafy vegetables |
| Niacin (B$_3$) | NAD coenzyme in oxidation-reduction reactions | *Pellagra:* photosensitivity, dermatitis, dementia, diarrhea, death | Tryptophan is a precursor | Meat, fish, liver, whole grains, green leafy vegetables |
| Pyridoxine (B$_6$) | Cofactor in amino acid metabolism | Seizures, hyperacusis, microcytic anemia, nasolabial seborrhea, neuropathy | Dependency state; deficiency secondary to drugs | Meat, liver, whole grains, peanuts, soybeans, meat |
| Pantothenic acid | Coenzyme A in Krebs cycle | None reported | — | Meat, vegetables |
| Biotin | Cofactor in carboxylase reactions of amino acids | Alopecia, dermatitis, hypotonia, death | Bowel resection, inborn error of metabolism* and ingestion of raw eggs | Yeast, meats; made by intestinal flora |
| B$_{12}$ | Coenzyme for 5-methyl-tetrahydrofolate formation; DNA synthesis | Megaloblastic anemia, peripheral neuropathy, posterior lateral column disease, vitiligo | Vegans; fish tapeworm; transcobalamine or intrinsic factor deficiencies | Meat, fish, cheese, eggs |
| Folate | DNA synthesis | Megaloblastic anemia | Goat milk deficient; drug antagonists; heat inactivates | Liver, greens, vegetables, cereals, cheese |
| Ascorbic acid (C) | Reducing agent; collagen metabolism | *Scurvy:* irritability, purpura, bleeding gums, periosteal hemorrhage, aching bones | May improve tyrosine metabolism in preterm infants | Citrus fruits, green vegetables; cooking destroys it |
| **Fat Soluble** | | | | |
| A | Epithelial cell integrity; vision | Night blindness, xerophthalmia, Bitot spots, follicular hyperkeratosis | Common with protein–calorie malnutrition; malabsorption | Liver, milk, eggs, green and yellow vegetables, fruits |
| D | Maintain serum calcium, phosphorus levels | *Rickets:* reduced bone mineralization | Prohormone of 25- and 1,25-vitamin D | Fortified milk, cheese, liver |
| E | Antioxidant | Hemolysis in preterm infants; areflexia, ataxia, ophthalmoplegia | May benefit patients with G6PD deficiency | Seeds, vegetables, germ oils, green leafy vegetables |
| K | Post-translation carboxylation of clotting factors II, VII, IX, X and proteins C, S | Prolonged prothrombin time; hemorrhage; elevated PIVKA (protein induced in vitamin K absence) | Malabsorption; breast-fed infants | Liver, green vegetables; made by intestinal flora |

*Biotinidase deficiency.
FAD = flavin adenine dinucleotide; G6PD = glucose-6-phosphate dehydrogenase; NAD = nicotinamide adenine dinucleotide; DNA = deoxyribo-nucleic acid.

## WATER-SOLUBLE VITAMINS

### Ascorbic Acid

The first recognized micronutrient deficiency disease was that of ascorbic acid (vitamin C). The principal forms of vitamin C are L-ascorbic acid and the oxidized form dehydroascorbic acid. Ascorbic acid accelerates hydroxylation reactions in many biosynthetic reactions. The needs of full-term infants for ascorbic acid are calculated by estimating the availability of this vitamin in human milk. Commercially available cow's milk–based formulas are fortified to a comparable level of 5.5 mg/dL (8 mg/ 100 kcal).

A deficiency of ascorbic acid results in the clinical manifestations of **scurvy**. Infantile scurvy is manifested with irritability, bone tenderness with swelling, and pseudoparalysis of the legs; it may be seen if infants are fed unsupplemented cow's milk in the 1st yr of life. Subperiosteal hemorrhage, hyperkeratosis of hair follicles, and a succession of mental changes characterize the progression of the illness. Anemia, secondary to decreased iron absorption or to abnormal folate metabolism, also is seen in chronic scurvy.

*Treatment* is presented in Table 2–14.

### Thiamine

Vitamin B$_1$ functions as a coenzyme in biochemical reactions related to carbohydrate metabolism, to decarboxylation of alpha-keto acids and pyruvate, and to transketolase reactions of the pentose pathway. Thiamine also is involved in the decarboxylation of branched-chain amino acids. Loss of the vitamin occurs during milk pasteurization and sterilization. The thiamine content of commercial formulas for full-term and preterm infants is 59–156 $\mu$g/100 kcal and 100–250 $\mu$g/100 kcal, respectively.

**Infantile beriberi** occurs between 1 and 4 mo of life in breast-fed infants whose mothers have a thiamine deficiency, in infants with protein-calorie malnutrition, in infants receiving unsupplemented hyperalimentation fluid, or in infants receiving boiled milk. Acute cardiac symptoms and signs predominate. Anorexia, apathy, vomiting, restlessness, and pallor progress to dyspnea, cyanosis, and death from congestive heart failure. Infants with beriberi have a characteristic aphonic cry; they appear to be crying but no sound is uttered.

*Treatment* is noted in Table 2–14.

### Riboflavin

Vitamin B$_2$ is a constituent of two coenzymes, riboflavin-5′-phosphate and flavin-adenine dinucleotide, which are essential components of glutathione reductase and xanthine oxidase and which are involved in electron transport. A deficiency of riboflavin affects glucose, fatty acid, and amino acid metabolism. Riboflavin and its phosphate are decomposed by exposure to light and by strong alkaline solutions. The intake of riboflavin from standard infant formulations, which contain 147–156

TABLE 2–14.  Recommended Daily Dose Ranges for Treatment of Vitamin-Related Diseases

| Vitamin | Treatment of Vitamin Deficiency | Treatment of Deficiency in Patients with Malabsorption | Treatment of Dependency Syndrome |
|---|---|---|---|
| A (IU) | 5000–10,000 | 10,000–25,000 | — |
| D (IU) | 400–5000 | 4000–20,000 | 50,000–200,000 |
| Calcifediol ($\mu$g) | — | 20–100 | 50–100 |
| Calcitriol (1,25-(OH)$_2$-D) ($\mu$g) | — | 1–3 | 1–3 |
| E (IU) | — | 100–1000 | — |
| K (mg) | 1* | 5–10* | — |
| Ascorbic acid (C) (mg) | 250–500 | 500 | — |
| Thiamine (mg) | 5–25 | 5–25 | 25–500 |
| Riboflavin (mg) | 5–25 | 5–25 | — |
| Niacin (mg) | 25–50 | 25–50 | 50–250 |
| B$_6$ (mg) | 5–25 | 2–25 | 10–250 |
| Biotin (mg) | 0.15–0.3 | 0.3–1.0 | 10 |
| Folic acid (mg) | 1.0 | 1.0 | —† |
| B$_{12}$ ($\mu$g) | —* | —* | 1–40 |

From AMA Council on Scientific Affairs: Vitamin preparations as dietary supplements and as therapeutic agents. JAMA 257:1929–1936, 1987. Copyright 1987, American Medical Association.
*To be used parenterally as needed.
†To be used only in conjunction with multivitamin mixtures.

μg/100 kcal, is significantly greater than from human milk (uniform throughout lactation and averaging 49 μg/100 kcal). The processes of pasteurization, evaporation, and condensation of milk do not destroy riboflavin.

**Ariboflavinosis** is characterized by angular stomatitis, glossitis, cheilosis, seborrheic dermatitis around the nose and mouth, and eye changes that include reduced tearing, photophobia, corneal vascularization, and formation of cataracts. Subclinical riboflavin deficiencies have been found in diabetic subjects, children from low socioeconomic families, children with chronic cardiac disease, and infants undergoing prolonged phototherapy for hyperbilirubinemia.

*Treatment* is presented in Table 2–14.

### Niacin

Niacin consists of the compounds nicotinic acid and nicotinamide (niacinamide). Nicotinamide, the predominant form of the vitamin, functions as a component of the coenzymes nicotinamide adenine dinucleotide (NAD) and nicotinamide adenine dinucleotide phosphate (NADP). Niacin is involved in multiple metabolic processes, including fat synthesis, intracellular respiratory metabolism, and glycolysis.

When determining the needs for niacin, we must consider the content of tryptophan in the diet because tryptophan is converted to niacin. Niacin is stable in foods and can withstand heating and prolonged storage. The concentration of niacin in human milk remains stable throughout lactation and averages 0.29 mg/100 kcal. Approximately 70% of the total niacin equivalents in human milk are derived from tryptophan. Infants fed commercial formula receive 0.8–1.2 mg of preformed niacin/100 kcal. The deficiency disease **(pellagra)** is characterized by weakness, lassitude, dermatitis, inflammation of mucous membranes, diarrhea, vomiting, dysphagia, and, in severe cases, dementia.

*Treatment* is noted in Table 2–14.

### Vitamin B$_6$

Vitamin B$_6$ refers to three naturally occurring pyridines: pyridoxine (pyridoxol), pyridoxal, and pyridoxamine; the phosphates of the latter two pyridines are metabolically and functionally interrelated and are converted in the liver to the coenzyme form, pyridoxal-5-phosphate.

The metabolic functions of vitamin B$_6$ include interconversion reactions of amino acids, conversion of tryptophan to niacin and serotonin, metabolic reactions in the brain, carbohydrate metabolism, immune development, and the biosynthesis of heme and prostaglandins. The pyridoxal and pyridoxamine forms of the vitamin are destroyed by heat; heat treatment has been responsible for vitamin B$_6$ deficiency and seizures in infants fed improperly processed formulas. For this reason, heat-stable pyridoxine is presently used for the fortification of milk. The vitamin B$_6$ content in human milk reflects the mother's nutritional status. The concentration of vitamin B$_6$ in milk obtained from mothers whose intake exceeds the RDA is 18 μg/100 kcal. The range of vitamin B$_6$ concentrations in cow's milk–based formulas routinely used for full-term infants (59–62 μg/100 kcal) satisfies the recommended allowances. Goat's milk is deficient in vitamin B$_6$. Full-term infants become deficient in vitamin B$_6$ when fed human milk containing 9–12 μg/100 kcal.

*Dietary deprivation* or *malabsorption* of vitamin B$_6$ in children results in hypochromic microcytic anemia, vomiting, diarrhea, failure to thrive, listlessness, hyperirritability, and seizures. Children receiving isoniazid may require additional vitamin B$_6$ because the drug binds to the vitamin.

*Treatment* is noted in Table 2–14.

### Biotin

Biotin has coenzyme functions in the metabolism of fat and carbohydrate (e.g., it is a component of several carboxylase enzymes). Biotin is synthesized by intestinal bacteria, and thus a deficiency state is uncommon. The average biotin concentration in mature human milk is 0.9 μg/100 kcal. Biotin deficiencies have been reported when it was omitted from parenteral nutrition solutions. Deficiency of *biotinidase*, the enzyme needed for conservation of metabolically active biotin, produces biotin deficiency.

*Clinical manifestations* of biotin deficiency include anorexia, nausea, glossitis, pallor, mental changes, alopecia, and a fine maculosquamous dermatitis, which becomes exfoliative. Antibiotics may increase biotin requirements by decreasing enteric synthesis of the vitamin, and the protein avidin, in raw eggs, binds biotin.

*Treatment* is noted in Table 2–14.

### Vitamin B$_{12}$

For a discussion of vitamin B$_{12}$ deficiency, see Minerals, Nutritional Anemia.

References

Behrman RE, Kliegman RM, Arvin AM (eds): Nelson Textbook of Pediatrics, 15th ed. Philadelphia, WB Saunders, 1996, Chapter 45.3.
Guthrie HA: Water-soluble vitamins. *In* Introductory Nutrition. St. Louis, Times Mirror/Mosby College Publishing, 1989, pp 381–448.

## FAT-SOLUBLE VITAMINS

### Vitamin A

The basic constituent of the vitamin A group is retinol. Ingested plant carotene or animal-tissue retinol esters release retinol after hydrolysis by pancreatic and intestinal enzymes. Chylomicron-transported retinol esters are stored in the liver as retinol palmitate. Retinol is transported from the liver to target tissues by retinol-binding protein (RBP). After free retinol is delivered to the target tissues, the RBP is excreted by the kidney. Diseases of the kidney diminish excretion of RBP, whereas liver parenchymal disease or malnutrition lowers the synthesis of RBP. The uptake of retinol by target tissues is facilitated by specific cellular binding proteins. In the eye, retinol is metabolized to form rhodopsin; the action of light on rhodopsin is the first step of the visual process. Retinol also influences the growth and differentiation of epithelia and serves as a cofactor in glycoprotein synthesis. Retinoic acid can substitute for retinol in all functions except those for maintaining tissue growth and vision. The retinol content of human milk averages 50 μg/dL; the retinol content of formulas averages 100–200 μg/dL.

The *clinical manifestations* of vitamin A deficiency in humans appear in a group of ocular signs termed **xerophthalmia**. The earliest symptom is night blindness, which is followed by xerosis of the conjunctiva and cornea. Untreated, xerophthalmia can result in ulceration, necrosis, keratomalacia, and a permanent corneal scar. Clinical and subclinical vitamin A deficiencies are associated with immunodeficiency; increased risks of infection, especially measles; and increased risk of mortality, especially in developing nations.

*Treatment* is noted in Table 2–14. Hypervitaminosis A also has serious sequelae, including dry skin, alopecia, headaches, and hepatotoxicity. Death may occur (Table 2–15). Excessive vitamin A is also teratogenic.

### Vitamin E

There are eight naturally occurring compounds with vitamin E activity. The most active of these, α-tocopherol, accounts for 90% of the vitamin E present in human tissues and is commercially available as an acetate or succinate. The other compounds of importance are β- and γ-tocopherol, which possess 33% and 10%, respectively, of the activity of α-tocopherol.

In humans, vitamin E acts as a biologic antioxidant by inhibiting the peroxidation of polyunsaturated fatty acids (PUFAs) present in cell membranes. It scavenges free radicals generated by the reduction of molecular oxygen and by the action of oxidative enzymes. In the process, the α-tocopherol is oxidized to a quinone, which is excreted in the urine.

Human milk has a lower content of α-tocopherol and a lower ratio of vitamin E to PUFAs compared with currently utilized formulas. Nevertheless, term and preterm infants have higher serum α-tocopherol levels when fed human milk. The vitamin E requirement is increased in diets having high concentrations of PUFAs or iron, both of which facilitate membrane peroxidation and generation of free radicals.

Because colostrum contains high concentrations of vitamin E, the blood tocopherol of breast-fed term infants increases within a few days after birth and remains in the normal adult range of 1.46 ± 0.63 mg/dL until weaning. Term infants who are fed formulas low in vitamin E have low blood levels of α-tocopherol (<0.8 mg/dL) for many months. Complete formulas are fortified to contain a minimum of 0.3 IU of vitamin E/100 kcal and 0.7 IU of vitamin E/g of linoleic acid.

*Tocopherol deficiency* occurs in children with prolonged and profound fat malabsorption secondary to biliary atresia, cystic fibrosis, and abetalipoproteinemia; in these children, a syndrome of progressive sensory and motor neuropathy may develop late in the 1st decade of life. Deficient preterm infants at 1–2 mo of age have hemolytic anemia characterized by an elevated reticulocyte count, an increased sensitivity of the erythrocytes to hemolysis in hydrogen peroxide, peripheral edema, and thrombocytosis. All the abnormalities are corrected after oral vitamin E therapy (see Table 2–14). Toxicity due to excess vitamin E is noted in Table 2–15.

### Vitamin D

Cholecalciferol (D₃) is the mammalian form of vitamin D and is produced by ultraviolet irradiation of inactive precursors in the skin. Ergocalciferol (D₂) is derived from plants. Both vitamin D₂ and vitamin D₃ require further metabolism to become active and are of equivalent potency. Clothing, lack of sunlight exposure, and skin pigmentation de-

TABLE 2–15.   Toxic Effects of Vitamins and Other Nutrients

| Nutrient | Effects | Comments |
|---|---|---|
| **Fat-Soluble Vitamins** | | Toxicity noted at lower multiples of RDA than water-soluble vitamins |
| A | | |
| Acute | Lethargy, headache, papilledema, bulging fontanel | Megadoses used to prevent cancer,* treat acne |
| Chronic | Scaly dry skin, alopecia, sore tongue, hyperostoses, anorexia, increased intracranial pressure (pseudotumor cerebri); teratogenic | Consumption of polar bear liver; toxicity with chronic 20,000–50,000 IU/24 hr |
| D | | |
| Acute | Hypercalcemia, muscle weakness, anorexia, emesis, headache, polyuria | Hypercalcemia produces arrhythmias, hypertension, renal water wasting |
| Chronic | Nephrocalcinosis, bone pain, vascular calcification, renal insufficiency; idiopathic infantile hypercalcemia | Toxicity with chronic 3000–4000 IU/24 hr |
| E | Muscle weakness, diarrhea, antagonism of vitamin K, enhanced anticoagulant drug action | Megadoses used to improve libido*; toxicity with 300–800 IU/24 hr |
| K | Water-soluble analogues produce neonatal jaundice | Menadione induces neonatal hemolysis |
| **Water-Soluble Vitamins** | | |
| C | Uricosuria, oxalate stones, G6PD-deficient hemolysis, rebound scurvy in infants; false-positive test for glycosuria; false-negative test for hematochezia | Prevention of upper respiratory tract infections* |
| Niacin | Histamine release, ulcers, asthma, flushing, pruritus, gout, hepatotoxic | Orthomolecular treatment of schizophrenia*; toxicity with 200–1000 mg/24 hr |
| Pyridoxine (B$_6$) | Peripheral sensory neuropathy; fetal–neonatal dependency and seizures | Treat depression* and premenstrual syndrome*; toxicity with 2–6 g/24 hr |
| Tryptophan | Eosinophilia, myositis, fasciitis, scleroderma | Treat depression* and premenstrual syndrome*; possible toxic metabolite; toxicity with 0.5–4.0 g/24 hr |

*No established benefit.
G6PD = glucose-6-phosphate dehydrogenase; RDA = recommended daily allowance.

crease the generation of vitamin D in the epidermis and dermis.

Vitamin D (D$_2$ and D$_3$) is metabolized in the liver to calcidiol, or 25-(OH)-D; this metabolite, which has little intrinsic activity, is transported by a plasma-binding globulin to the kidney, where it is converted to the most active metabolite calcitriol, or 1,25-(OH)$_2$-D. The molecular action of 1,25-(OH)$_2$-D results in a decrease in the messenger ribonucleic acid (mRNA) for collagen in bone and an increase in the concentration of mRNA for vitamin D–dependent calcium-binding protein in the intestine (directly mediating increased intestinal calcium transport). Calcium transport is mediated by the specific local synthesis of the intestinal vitamin D–dependent calcium-binding protein. The antirachitic action of vitamin D probably is mediated by provision of appropriate concentrations of

calcium and phosphate in the extracellular space of bone and by enhanced intestinal absorption of these minerals. The direct effect of vitamin D on bone is probably similar to that of parathyroid hormone and results in bone resorption. Vitamin D also may have a direct anabolic effect on bone. 1,25-(OH)$_2$-D also has direct feedback to the parathyroid gland and inhibits secretion of parathyroid hormone.

The most prevalent form of vitamin D measured in plasma, 25-(OH)-D, ranges from 10 to 60 ng/mL. The values vary with dietary intake, sunlight (ultraviolet light) exposure, and body stores. The serum concentration of 1,25-(OH)$_2$-D ranges from 18 to 60 ng/mL.

*Vitamin D deficiency* appears as **rickets** in children and as osteomalacia in postpubertal adolescents. Inadequate direct sun exposure and vitamin

D intake are sufficient causes, but other factors (e.g., high cereal intake, a vegetarian diet, or various drugs [phenobarbital, phenytoin]) also may increase the risk of development of vitamin D–deficiency rickets.

The *pathophysiology* of rickets results from defective bone growth, especially marked at the epiphyseal cartilage matrix, which fails to mineralize. The uncalcified osteoid results in a wide, irregular zone of poorly supported tissue, the rachitic metaphysis. This soft, rather than hardened, zone produces many of the skeletal deformities through compression and lateral bulging or flaring of the ends of bones.

The *clinical manifestations* of rickets are most common during the first 2 yr of life and require several months of a vitamin D–deficient diet to become evident. Craniotabes is due to thinning of the outer table of the skull, which feels to the touch like a Ping-Pong ball when compressed. Enlargement of the costochondral junction (rachitic rosary) and thickening of the wrists and ankles may be palpated. The anterior fontanel is enlarged, and its closure may be delayed. In advanced rickets, there may be scoliosis and exaggerated lordosis. Bowlegs or knock-knees may be evident in older infants, and greenstick fractures may be observed in long bones.

The *diagnosis* of rickets is based on a dietary history of poor vitamin D intake and little exposure to direct ultraviolet sunlight. The serum calcium usually is normal but may be low, the serum phosphorus level always is reduced, and the serum alkaline phosphatase activity is elevated. When serum calcium levels decline below 7.5 mg/dL, tetany may occur. 24,25-$(OH)_2$-D levels are undetectable and serum 1,25-$(OH)_2$-D levels are commonly below 7 ng/mL, though 1,25-$(OH)_2$-D levels may also be normal. The best measure of vitamin D status is the level of 25-(OH)-D. Characteristic roentgenologic changes of the distal ulna and radius include widening, concave cupping, and frayed, poorly demarcated ends. The increased space between the distal ends of the radius and ulna and the metacarpal bones is the enlarged, nonossified metaphysis.

The *treatment* of vitamin D–deficiency rickets and osteomalacia is indicated in Table 2–14. Breast-fed infants born of mothers with adequate vitamin D stores usually maintain adequate serum vitamin D levels for the first 6 mo, but rickets may subsequently develop if these infants are not exposed to the sun or do not receive supplementary vitamin D. Toxic effects of vitamin D are noted in Table 2–15.

## Vitamin K

The plant form of vitamin K is phylloquinone or vitamin $K_1$. Another form, menaquinone or vitamin $K_2$, is one of a series of compounds with unsaturated side chains synthesized by the intestinal bacteria. Plasma factors II (prothrombin), VII, IX, and X in the cascade of blood coagulation factors depend on vitamin K for synthesis and for post-translational conversion of precursor proteins of these plasma factors. The post-translational conversion of glutamyl residues to γ-carboxyglutamic acid residues of a prothrombin molecule creates effective calcium-binding sites, making the protein active.

Other vitamin K–dependent proteins include proteins C, S, and Z in plasma and γ-carboxyglutamic acid (gla)–containing proteins in kidney, spleen, lung, uterus, placenta, pancreas, thyroid, thymus, testes, and bone. Bone contains a major vitamin K–dependent protein, osteocalcin, as well as lesser amounts of other glutamic acid–containing proteins.

Phylloquinone is absorbed from the intestine and transported by chylomicrons. The rarity of dietary vitamin K deficiency in humans with normal intestinal function suggests that the absorption of menaquinones is possible. Vitamin K deficiency has been observed in subjects with impaired fat absorption caused by obstructive jaundice, pancreatic insufficiency, and celiac disease; often these problems are combined with the use of antibiotics that change intestinal flora. Absorption of vitamin K also may be inhibited by mineral oil and high dietary intakes of vitamins A and E. The phylloquinone content of mature human milk averages 2.1 ng/mL, not different from that of colostrum samples. Average concentrations of phylloquinones are 11.5 ng/mL in supplemental soy-based formulas and 55–58 ng/mL in cow's milk formulas.

**Hemorrhagic disease of the newborn**, a disease more common among breast-fed infants, occurs at 2–10 days of life in those who do not receive prophylactic vitamin K on the first day of life. The recommended preventive dose is 0.5–1.0 mg intramuscularly. Hemorrhagic disease of the newborn usually is marked by generalized ecchymoses, gastrointestinal hemorrhage, or bleeding from a circumcision or umbilical stump; intracranial hemorrhage is uncommon (see Chapter 6).

## References

Behrman RE, Kliegman RM, Arvin AM (eds): Nelson Textbook of Pediatrics, 15th ed. Philadelphia, WB Saunders, 1996, Chapter 45.3.

Guthrie HA: Fat-soluble vitamins. *In* Introductory Nutrition.

St. Louis, Times Mirror/Mosby College Publishing, 1989, pp 339–378.

## MINERALS

### Calcium

Ninety-nine percent of calcium is in the skeleton; the remaining 1% is in extracellular fluids, intracellular compartments, and cell membranes. The 1% nonskeletal calcium serves a role in nerve conduction, muscle contraction, blood clotting, and membrane permeability. There are two distinct bone calcium phosphate pools, a large crystalline form and a smaller amorphous phase. Bone calcium constantly turns over, with concurrent bone resorption and formation. Bone mass peaks in the late teens and is influenced by prior and concurrent dietary calcium intake, exercise, and hormone status (testosterone, estrogen).

Dietary calcium intake depends on the consumption of dairy products. The calcium equivalent of 1 cup of milk is ¾ cup plain yogurt, 1½ oz cheddar cheese, 2 cups ice cream, ⅘ cup almonds, and 2½ oz sardines. Other sources of calcium include some leafy green vegetables (broccoli, kale, collards), lime-processed tortillas, and calcium-precipitated tofu ("bean curd" from soybeans).

There is no classical calcium deficiency syndrome, because blood and cell levels are closely regulated. The body can mobilize skeletal calcium and increase the absorptive efficiency of dietary calcium. *Osteoporosis* is characterized by diminished quantity of bone that is histologically normal. Osteoporosis occurs in childhood and is related to protein-calorie malnutrition, vitamin C deficiency, steroid therapy, endocrine disorders, immobilization and disuse, osteogenesis imperfecta, or calcium deficiency (premature infants)(see Chapter 6). The primary method of prevention of postmenopausal osteoporosis is to ensure maximum peak bone mass by providing optimal calcium intake during childhood and adolescence. Bone mineral status can be monitored by single-energy and dual-energy photon densitometry and dual-energy x-ray absorptiometry. The latter method is increasingly being used to diagnose osteoporosis or osteopenia in children and youths.

No adverse effects are observed in adults with dietary calcium intakes of up to 2.5 g/day. Nonetheless, there is concern that high intakes may increase the risk for urinary stone formation, constipation, and decreased renal function and inhibit intestinal absorption of other minerals (iron, zinc).

### References

Behrman RE, Kliegman RM, Arvin AM (eds): Nelson Textbook of Pediatrics, 15th ed. Philadelphia, WB Saunders, 1996, Chapter 50.
Guthrie HA: Macronutrient elements. *In* Introductory Nutrition. St. Louis, Times Mirror/Mosby College Publishing, 1989, pp 261–277.

## NUTRITIONAL ANEMIA
### (see Chapter 14)

The recognition of anemia in infancy requires knowledge of normal age-related and birth weight–related changes in hemoglobin concentration. Reference values are given in Table 14–2.

### Iron-Deficiency Anemia

In infancy, the major causes of iron-deficiency anemia are a decrease of body iron by rapid growth and an iron-poor diet. Blood loss results in more severe iron-deficiency anemia than is seen with the other two causes. Blood loss may be caused by conditions such as fetal-maternal transfusion, placenta previa, rupture of umbilical vessels, and twin-twin transfusion. Intestinal bleeding may be due to the ingestion of fresh cow's milk in early infancy or, rarely, pulmonary hemosiderosis, a bleeding Meckel diverticulum, esophagitis, or peptic ulcer. The removal of blood for laboratory studies in infants requiring intensive care also may result in iron-deficiency anemia.

Iron is used in the synthesis of hemoglobin, myoglobin, and enzyme iron. Iron-deficiency anemia occurs when a lack of iron is sufficient to restrict the production of hemoglobin and its concentration falls below the normal range. Body iron content is regulated primarily through modulation of iron absorption, which depends on the state of body iron stores, the form and amount of iron in foods, and the mixture of foods in the diet. Iron excretion occurs through the feces.

There are two categories of iron in food. The first is *heme iron*, present in hemoglobin and myoglobin; it is supplied by meat and rarely accounts for more than a quarter of the iron ingested by infants. The absorption of heme iron is relatively efficient and is not influenced by other constituents of the diet. The second category is *non-heme iron*, which represents the preponderance of iron intake consumed by infants and exists in the form of salts. The absorption of non-heme iron is determined by the composition of consumed foods. The fractional intestinal absorption of the small amount of iron in human milk is 50%, in contrast to 10% of iron absorbed from unfortified cow's milk formula and

4% absorbed from iron-fortified cow's milk formula. About 4% of the iron from iron-fortified infant dry cereals is absorbed. Enhancers of non-heme iron absorption are ascorbic acid, meat, fish, and poultry. Inhibitors are bran, polyphenols (including the tannates in tea), and phosphate. During pregnancy, iron is efficiently transported from the maternal circulation to the fetus, and transport is not impaired by maternal iron-deficiency anemia. In the *term infant*, there is little change in total body iron and little need for exogenous iron before 4 mo of age. Iron deficiency is rare among term infants during the first 4 mo unless there has been substantial blood loss.

After 4 mo of age, iron reserves become marginal for the remainder of infancy. From 4 to 12 mo, an average of 0.9 mg of iron/24 hr must be absorbed from the diet to provide 0.7 mg/24 hr for growth and 0.2 mg/24 hr to balance normal fecal losses. In term infants who receive unfortified cow's milk formula, depletion of storage iron occurs as early as 4 mo of age, as indicated by low serum ferritin concentrations (10 μg/liter). Breast-fed infants rarely deplete their iron stores until after 6 mo of age. In the absence of iron fortification or supplementation, iron stores eventually become inadequate in breast-fed infants at the age when solid foods are added to the diet. *Premature infants* have a lower amount of stored iron since significant amounts of iron are transferred from the mother in the third trimester. In addition, their postnatal iron needs are greater because of rapid rates of growth.

Term breast-fed infants need an alternative source of iron after 4–6 mo of age. Some pediatricians recommend ferrous sulfate supplementation, whereas others introduce iron-containing solid foods. Iron-fortified formula is the only alternative to breast milk in the child younger than 1 yr old.

Premature infants fed human milk may develop iron-deficiency anemia unless they receive iron supplements of 2 mg of iron/kg/24 hr. Formula-fed preterm infants should receive iron-fortified formula by approximately 1 or 2 mo of age.

In older children, iron deficiency is often the result of blood loss (menses, gastric ulceration). It is important to note that iron deficiency affects many tissues (muscle, central nervous system) in addition to producing anemia.

The *diagnosis* of iron-deficiency anemia is established by the presence of a microcytic hypochromic anemia, low serum ferritin levels, low serum iron levels, reduced transferrin saturation, normal to elevated red cell width distribution (RDW), and enhanced iron-binding capacity. The mean corpuscular volume (MCV) and red cell indices are reduced, and the reticulocyte count is between 0 and 1%. Iron deficiency may be present without anemia (see Chapter 14). *Clinical manifestations* are noted in Table 2–16.

*Treatment* of iron-deficiency anemia requires changes in the diet to provide adequate iron as well as the administration of 2–6 mg iron/kg/24 hr (as ferrous sulfate). Reticulocytosis is noted within 3–7 days of starting treatment, and the hemoglobin may rise as rapidly as 0.25–0.40 g/dL/24 hr; usually half-correction is achieved after 2 wk and two thirds correction after 4 wk. Oral treatment should be continued for 5 mo. Rarely, intramuscular or intravenous iron therapy is needed if oral iron cannot be given or if compliance is poor. Such parenteral therapy carries the risk of anaphylaxis.

### Megaloblastic Anemia

In infancy, these rare anemias are caused by folate deficiency, vitamin $B_{12}$ deficiency (see next), and inborn errors of metabolism. *Folate deficiency*, which may result from a low dietary intake, malabsorption, or vitamin-drug interactions, can develop within a few weeks of birth because infants require 10 times as much folate as adults per kilogram of body weight but have scant stores of folate in the newborn period. The recommended intake varies between 30 and 65 μg/day. **Heat-sterilizing** home-prepared formula can decrease the folate content by half. **Evaporated milk** has less than 20 μg of folate per reconstituted liter; **goat's milk** has less than 6 μg/L. Folate deficiency has been reported in healthy low-birth-weight infants who are fed formulas based on heated or boiled evaporated or pasteurized milk. In proprietary infant formulas, the presence of ascorbic acid decreases the loss of folic acid. Infants who are fed human milk or proprietary cow's milk formulas are not at risk for nutritional folate deficiency.

Very-low-birth-weight infants should be given supplemental folate to support their rapid growth, especially until their milk or formula volume intake provides adequate folate. Folate deficiency caused by malabsorption may occur with chronic diarrhea. The conjugated polyglutamate forms of folate in the diet may not be digested to the monoglutamate form that can be absorbed. Diarrhea also interferes with the normal enterohepatic circulation of folate. Patients with chronic hemolysis (sickle cell anemia, thalassemia) require extra folate to avoid deficiency caused by increased red blood cell production.

Folate deficiency should be suspected when hypersegmented neutrophils and/or elevation of

TABLE 2–16. Characteristics of Mineral Deficiencies

| Mineral | Function | Manifestations of Deficiency | Comments | Sources |
|---|---|---|---|---|
| Iron | Heme-containing macromolecules (e.g., hemoglobin, cytochrome, myoglobin) | Anemia, spoon nails, reduced muscle and mental performance | History of pica, cow's milk, gastrointestinal bleeding | Liver, eggs, grains |
| Copper | Redox reactions (e.g., cytochrome oxidase) | Hypochromic anemia, neutropenia, osteoporosis, hypotonia, hypoproteinemia | Inborn error, Menkes kinky hair syndrome | Liver, oysters, meat, nuts, grains, legumes, chocolate |
| Zinc | Metalloenzymes (e.g., alkaline phosphatase, carbonic anhydrase, DNA polymerase; wound healing | *Acrodermatitis enteropathica:* poor growth, acro-orificial rash, alopecia, delayed sexual development, hypogeusia, infection | Protein-calorie malnutrition; weaning; malabsorption syndromes | Meat, grains, cheese, nuts |
| Selenium | Antioxidant Glutathione peroxidase | Keshan cardiomyopathy in China | Endemic areas; long-term TPN | Meat, vegetables |
| Chromium | Insulin cofactor | Poor weight gain, glucose intolerance, neuropathy | Protein-calorie malnutrition, long-term TPN | Yeast, breads |
| Fluoride | Strengthening of dental enamel | Caries | Supplementation during tooth growth, narrow therapeutic range, fluorosis may cause staining of the teeth | Seafood, water |
| Iodine | Thyroxine, triiodothyronine production | Simple endemic goiter *Myxedematous cretinism:* congenital hypothyroidism *Neurologic cretinism:* mental retardation, deafness, spasticity, normal thyroxine level at birth | Endemic in New Guinea, the Congo; endemic in Great Lakes area prior to iodized salt | Seafood, iodized salt, most food in nonendemic areas |

TPN = total parenteral nutrition; DNA = deoxyribonucleic acid.

the MCV to about 100 fL is noted. The *diagnosis* is confirmed by the determination of both serum and red cell folate and serum vitamin $B_{12}$. A therapeutic dose of folate (0.5–1.0 mg of pteroylglutamic acid/ 24 hr, 10 or more times the daily allowance) is given when the diagnosis of folate deficiency is established (see Table 2–14).

*Treatment* is monitored by the reticulocyte response and by the rise in hemoglobin and hematocrit, responses similar to those noted during the iron treatment of iron-deficiency anemia. Folate supplementation during pregnancy reduces the risk of fetal neural tube defects and in adults may reduce the risk of coronary thrombosis. Folate therapy may mask the hematologic manifestations of vitamin $B_{12}$ deficiency.

## Vitamin $B_{12}$ Deficiency

Early diagnosis and treatment of this rare disorder in childhood are important because of the danger of irreversible neurologic damage. Most cases in childhood result from a specific defect in absorption (see Tables 2–12 and 2–13). Such defects include congenital pernicious anemia (absent intrinsic factor), juvenile pernicious anemia (autoimmune), and deficiency of transcobalamin II transport. Intestinal resection, small bowel bacterial overgrowth, or the fish tapeworm *Diphyllobothrium latum* also causes vitamin $B_{12}$ deficiency. An exclusively breast-fed infant ingests approximately 0.3 μg of vitamin $B_{12}$/24 hr unless the mother is a strict vegetarian. The absorption of vitamin $B_{12}$ depends on the formation of a complex between the vitamin and a mucoprotein, intrinsic factor. The complex is absorbed in the distal ileum. In the plasma, vitamin $B_{12}$ is bound to a specific serum transport protein, transcobalamin II. The vitamin is stored in the liver. These stores are large in the newborn and are rarely depleted before 1 yr of age.

Depression of serum vitamin $B_{12}$ below 100 pg/mL and the appearance of hypersegmented neutrophils are the earliest *clinical manifestations* of deficiency. Late findings of vitamin $B_{12}$ deficiency are similar to the findings of folate deficiency and include megaloblastic anemia, leukopenia, and thrombocytopenia. Neurologic manifestations include peripheral neuropathy, posterior column signs, dementia, and eventual coma; these signs do not occur in folate deficiency, but administration of folate in excess of 0.1 mg/24 hr to vitamin $B_{12}$–deficient individuals aggravates the neurologic manifestations.

The *diagnosis* is made by history and the presence of a macrocytosis accompanied by a megaloblastic bone marrow. Serum folate is normal, but red cell folate may be reduced with vitamin $B_{12}$ deficiency. Serum vitamin $B_{12}$ levels are reduced. Patients with vitamin $B_{12}$ deficiency also have increased urine levels of methylmalonic acid.

In nondietary deficiencies, a Schilling test must be performed to identify those patients with pernicious anemia and bacterial overgrowth. Vitamin $B_{12}$ (radiolabeled) is ingested, and 2 hr later a flushing intravenous dose of 1 mg of vitamin $B_{12}$ is given. If less than 7% of radiolabeled vitamin $B_{12}$ is excreted in urine, the test is repeated with the addition of oral intrinsic factor. Normal excretion following intrinsic factor confirms the diagnosis of pernicious anemia (absent endogenous intrinsic factor). If urinary excretion of labeled vitamin $B_{12}$ remains below 7% in 24 hr, an intestinal lesion such as bacterial overgrowth may be present; pretreatment with antibiotics and repetition of the test with subsequent normal results confirms the diagnosis.

Most cases of vitamin $B_{12}$ deficiency in infants and children are not of dietary origin and require *treatment* throughout life. An intramuscular dose of 50–100 $\mu$g is used to initiate therapy. Maintenance therapy consists of repeated monthly intramuscular injections.

## References

Behrman RE, Kliegman RM, Arvin AM (eds): Nelson Textbook of Pediatrics, 15th ed. Philadelphia, WB Saunders, 1996, Chapters 412, 413.
Dallmann PR: Nutritional anemia of infancy: Iron, folic acid and vitamin $B_{12}$. *In* Tsang RC, Nichols BL (eds): Nutrition During Infancy. Philadelphia, Hanley and Belfus, 1988, pp 216–235.

## Trace Elements

Trace element deficiencies are important clinical syndromes in persons with malabsorption and/or on parenteral nutrition. Many of these elements have a narrow therapeutic range and may cause toxicity.

**Copper.** Copper, as a constituent of many enzymes, is involved in energy production via oxidative phosphorylation, in the protection of cell membranes against oxidative damage, in the oxidation of iron released from storage, in erythropoietin synthesis, and in cerebral protein and myelin deposition. Some of the better known cuproenzymes are cytochrome oxidase, superoxide dismutase, ceruloplasmin, ferroxidase II, lysyl oxidase, tyrosinase, and dopamine $\beta$-hydroxylase.

Because copper is present in many foods (see Table 2–16), adequate intake levels are easily achieved. Large amounts of copper are deposited in the fetal liver during the 3rd trimester and gradually are depleted when ceruloplasmin synthesis and secretion begin. Transcuprein is the predominant vehicle of copper transport to the liver in the portal circulation. The liver of term infants contains a copper concentration 10–20 fold greater than that in the liver of adults. After its uptake from the portal circulation, copper is bound to hepatic metallothionein, from which it is released for enzyme synthesis in mitochondria and cytosol, transferred to the nuclei, and then incorporated into ceruloplasmin, which is released into the plasma compartment. Copper in plasma is found in four fractions: transcuprein and albumin, each 15%; ceruloplasmin, 60%; and various low-molecular-weight components, 10%. Synthesis and secretion in the liver occur with ceruloplasmin-bound copper, the preferred transport form to other tissues (e.g., brain, muscle, and bones). Copper breakdown products normally are sequestered in lysosomes and excreted in bile; copper overload may occur in patients with cholestasis. Urinary excretion of copper normally is minimal.

Serum levels of copper and ceruloplasmin are low at birth and remain low for several weeks in preterm infants. Levels rise, however, as ceruloplasmin synthesis begins between the 6th and 12th postnatal weeks, varying with the gestational age of the infant. Concentrations are not affected by the levels of oral copper intake.

*Copper deficiency* first was reported in infants recuperating from PEM whose diet was based on cow's milk. It also has been noted in infants and patients receiving total parenteral nutrition containing inadequate amounts of copper, with chronic antacid use, and after ingesting large amounts of zinc.

The *clinical manifestations* of copper deficiency may be traced to the specific cuproenzyme affected—depigmentation (hair, skin) and tyrosinase; hypothermia, hypotonia, and cytochrome C; altered elastin and collagen and lysyl oxidase deficiency; central nervous system degeneration (hypotonia, psychomotor retardation) and dopamine-β-hydroxylase. Other signs include apnea, scurvy-like hemorrhage, blood vessel rupture, failure to thrive, flaring of anterior ribs, fractures, osteoporosis, periosteal reaction, metaphyseal spurs, hypercholesterolemia, edema, diarrhea, altered glucose tolerance, anemia, and neutropenia.

**Wilson disease**, an autosomal-recessive disease (1:200,000 births) due to defective mobilization of copper from lysosomes, is characterized by increased copper deposition in brain, liver, kidney, and cornea and low serum copper and ceruloplasmin levels. Hepatic failure with cirrhosis, hepatitis, Fanconi renal syndrome, hemolytic anemia, Kayser-Fleischer corneal pigmented rings, and neurologic signs such as behavioral problems, tremor, spasticity, and poor fine motor control are noted after the age of 5 yr. Treatment is a low-copper diet and lifelong chelation therapy with D-penicillamine.

**Menkes kinky hair syndrome**, a lethal X-linked neurodegenerative condition due to a defect in copper absorption and transport across the intestines, is characterized by low serum copper and ceruloplasmin levels, and increased copper in fibroblasts and urine. Manifestations include hypotonia, myoclonic seizures, spasticity, failure to thrive, steely depigmented hair, osteoporosis, and arterial tortuosity. There is no specific therapy.

Excessive copper intake is associated with **Indian childhood cirrhosis**. Copper *toxicity* may produce nausea, hemolysis, and hepatic necrosis.

Unfortunately, no perfect measure of copper status exists. Thus, copper and ceruloplasmin levels and trends in these levels must be considered in the patient evaluation.

**Zinc.** Zinc is important in protein metabolism and synthesis, in nucleic acid metabolism, and in the stabilization of cell membranes. Zinc metalloenzymes include erythrocyte carbonic anhydrase, alcohol dehydrogenase, carboxypeptidases A and B, alkaline phosphatase, DNA and RNA polymerase, various dehydrogenases, and retinene reductase (see Table 2-16); many other enzymes use zinc as a cofactor.

Dietary zinc is absorbed (20–80%) in the duodenum and proximal small intestine. In zinc sufficiency, an increasing zinc pool triggers synthesis of intestinal mucosal metallothionein, which binds intracellular zinc. Protein-bound zinc and human milk zinc are the most readily absorbed forms of the mineral. Histidine and cysteine facilitate absorption, whereas phytase and fiber inhibit it. Excess dietary copper, iron, or cadmium decreases zinc absorption by competing for cellular uptake and metallothionein binding. After cellular uptake, the metal is secreted into the portal circulation, where it binds primarily to albumin. Zinc transported from the intestine is taken up rapidly by the liver, pancreas, kidneys, and spleen. Excretion occurs through fecal losses. Dietary requirements vary from 1.0 to 3.1 mg of zinc/day for 2 mo old infants. Zinc requirements for term infants receiving parenteral nutrition have been estimated at 100 μg/kg/day. In the presence of ongoing losses, such as chronic diarrhea, requirements can drastically increase.

The original account of *zinc deficiency dwarfism* syndrome was described in a group of children with low levels of zinc in their hair, poor appetite, diminished taste acuity, hypogonadism, and short stature.

*Acute acquired zinc deficiency* may occur in patients receiving total parenteral nutrition without zinc supplementation and in premature infants fed human milk. Transient zinc deficiency rarely has been reported in full-term, breast-fed infants. Mild clinical manifestations of zinc deficiency in infants include failure to thrive, and in children and adolescents include decreased growth velocity, anorexia, and hypogeusia. Moderately severe manifestations include delayed sexual maturation, rough skin, pica, and hepatosplenomegaly, and the severe signs include acral and periorificial skin lesions, failure to thrive, diarrhea, mood changes, alopecia, night blindness, and photophobia.

**Acrodermatitis enteropathica** is an autosomal recessive disorder that begins within 2–4 wk of weaning infants from breast milk. It is characterized by an acute perioral and perianal dermatitis, alopecia, and failure to thrive. The disease is due to severe zinc deficiency from an undefined but specific defect of intestinal zinc absorption. Plasma zinc levels are reduced, and serum alkaline phosphatase activity is low. Treatment is with oral zinc supplementation (1 mg/kg/24 hr).

Zinc *excess* produces nausea, emesis, abdominal pain, headache, vertigo, and seizures.

**Selenium.** The only well-defined function of selenium is as part of the enzyme glutathione peroxidase (GSHPx), one of the enzyme systems that, with catalase, superoxide dismutase, and vitamin

E, protect cells from oxidative damage by destroying cytosolic hydrogen peroxide (see Table 2-16). Selenium is well absorbed. The primary route of excretion is in the urine. An intake greater than 1.5 $\mu g/kg/24$ hr prevents a fall in blood selenium levels in young infants. Concentrations in human milk reflect selenium levels in the mother. The intake of selenium by exclusively breast-fed infants is approximately 10 $\mu g/24$ hr, compared with 7 $\mu g/24$ hr by formula-fed infants. Infants and children who receive total parental nutrition may have a rapid drop of blood selenium levels unless adequate amounts are provided in the solution ($\sim 1$ $\mu g/kg$ of body weight).

A *selenium deficiency syndrome* (Keshan disease) has been reported in rural China and is characterized by necrosis and fibrosis of the myocardium, which results in potentially fatal acute or chronic heart failure. Those most at risk include infants, young children, and women of childbearing age. Fatal cardiomyopathy has been reported in adults receiving long-term total parenteral nutrition and in a 2-yr-old child whose diet was very low in both selenium and animal protein. Blood selenium levels below 40 ng/mL in orally fed preterm infants also are associated with increased erythrocyte fragility. Muscle pain, myopathy, and nail bed changes may occur.

**Iodine.** Iodine is an integral part of the thyroid hormones (see Table 2-16). Circulating iodine is taken up avidly by the thyroid gland, where it is bound to thyroglobulin, an iodinated glycoprotein, from which the hormones thyroxine ($T_4$) and triiodothyronine ($T_3$) are formed. In iodine deficiency, the synthesis and release of thyroid hormones are decreased, low blood levels of $T_4$ and $T_3$ result, and the feedback mechanism involving the thyroid-hypothalamus-pituitary axis is stimulated. This sequence of events produces an increased output of thyroid-stimulating hormone (TSH) by the pituitary, which ultimately results in enlargement of the thyroid gland, or **goiter**.

Ingested iodine is readily absorbed; the main route of excretion is in the urine. Fifty percent of an adequate iodine intake is retained by healthy infants. A daily dietary intake of 40 $\mu g$ for infants from birth to 6 mo, increased to 50 $\mu g$ for infants from 6 to 12 mo, is recommended. The minimum intake by an exclusively breast-fed infant is 22 $\mu g/$ 24 hr, but this is well above the minimum estimated requirement of 1 $\mu g/kg/24$ hr. Infant formulas contain at least 5 $\mu g$ of iodine/100 kcal, and most formulas for both full-term and preterm infants supply 2–3 times this amount. For infants of iodine-sufficient mothers, additional iodine is not necessary during short-term intravenous feeding. Because of its potential for toxicity, all sources of iodine to the infant should be considered before supplementation is initiated.

Moderate *iodine deficiency* may produce a euthyroid state accompanied by hyperplasia and hypertrophy of the thyroid gland or goiter. Severe dietary iodine deficiency results in hypothyroidism. **Endemic cretinism** is seen in the same geographic areas as endemic goiter and may be characterized by ataxia, spasticity, deaf-mutism, and mental retardation with or without short stature, and little or no impairment of thyroid function. This variant affecting the nervous system is probably due to early fetal iodine deficiency. The **myxedematous type** of cretinism is characterized by retarded growth, delayed mental and sexual function, and the presence of myxedema in the absence of abnormal neurologic signs. This variant may be due to late fetal and postnatal iodine deficiency, which results in low thyroid hormone levels, elevated TSH concentration, and markedly delayed bone age. Both syndromes are prevented by iodine supplementation. *Excessive* iodine treatment may produce thyrotoxicosis or goiter.

**Fluoride.** Dental enamel is strengthened when fluoride is substituted for hydroxyl ions in the hydroxyapatite crystalline mineral matrix of the enamel. The resulting fluorapatite is more resistant to both chemical and physical damage. Fluoride is incorporated into the enamel during the mineralization stages of tooth formation and also by surface interaction after the tooth has erupted. Fluoride is similarly incorporated into bone mineral and may protect against osteoporosis later in life. Approximately 80% of fluoride in foods and fluids is absorbed; as much as 97% is absorbed from soluble supplements such as sodium fluoride. Fluoride is excreted mainly in the urine, with less than 10% of the intake appearing in the feces.

As a result of concern about the risk of fluorosis, infants should not receive fluoride supplements before 6 mo of age. In the formula-fed infant, the need for supplementation depends on the type of formula used. Commercial formulas now are made with defluorinated water and contain low amounts of fluoride. An infant older than 6 mo who receives only ready-to-feed formula should be given supplemental fluoride. The fluoride content of human milk is low, 5–15 ng/mL, and intakes by exclusively breast-fed infants are about 4–15 $\mu g/day$ in optimally fluoridated areas. Breast-fed infants older than 6 mo should receive fluoride supplements, especially if they are breast-fed longer than 6 mo. Fluoride levels of the water supply to which the child is exposed should be determined before fluoride supplements are prescribed. Fluorosis commonly stains the teeth.

## References

Behrman RE, Kliegman RM, Arvin AM (eds): Nelson Textbook of Pediatrics, 15th ed. Philadelphia, WB Saunders, 1996, Chapters 43.6, 522.

Casey CE, Walravens PA: Trace elements. *In* Tsang RC, Nichols BL (eds): Nutrition During Infancy. Philadelphia, Hanley and Belfus, 1988, pp 190–215.

# NUTRITIONAL MANAGEMENT DURING ILLNESS

## NUTRITIONAL ASSESSMENT

Pediatric nutritional assessment includes consideration of (1) medical and nutrition history, (2) dietary intake, (3) factors that alter nutrient utilization and absorption, (4) physical examination (including growth patterns and current anthropometry), and (5) laboratory assessment. The assessment is used to define nutritional status (Fig. 2–5) and nutrient needs in children.

Macronutrient depletion can be assessed by comparing height, weight, and head circumference measurements of the patient with normal standards. Recent weight loss or failure of normal growth is an important consideration. A low percentage of expected weight for height suggests recent macronutrient deficiency (usually calories), whereas low height for age suggests chronic deficiency. Loss of body fat is measured by determining triceps skinfold thicknesses, and loss of muscle mass is reflected in reduced arm circumference measurements corrected for skinfold thicknesses. Measurements of the triceps skinfold and the circumference of the upper arm are made midpoint in the distance between the palpated head of the humerus and the bony prominence of the elbow on the extensor (dorsal) surface when the elbow is flexed 90 degrees. Additional physical signs are noted in Table 2–17. Useful laboratory tests include measurement of hepatic secretory proteins in serum (Table 2–18). Albumin, retinol-binding protein, prealbumin, and transferrin are depleted during inadequate protein or calorie intake. Albumin is affected by non-nutritional influences; these other proteins have a shorter half-life and reflect recent macronutrient intake (days to weeks). Reduced total lymphocyte count and a failure of T-cell function are reflected in anergy in skin tests.

The nutritional management of the ill patient is accomplished by enteral or parenteral feeding. Priority should be given to oral feedings, followed by intragastric, duodenal, or jejunal tube delivery; peripheral intravenous infusions; and, finally, central intravenous infusions. The complexity and expense of nursing and dietary care increase exponentially with the progression through this management sequence. The immunologic and metabolic effects of malnutrition make the delayed introduction of adequate feeding a clinical risk that must be aggressively addressed.

FIGURE 2–5. Nutritional assessment form. Nutritional data for the patient are recorded and graphed on this form. Values falling in the area labeled "Depleted" are considered abnormal and those in the adjacent column borderline. (From Merritt RJ, Sinatra FR, Smith GA: Nutritional support of the hospitalized child. Adv Nutr Res 5:77–103, 1983.)

## References

Gibson RS: Principles of Nutritional Assessment. New York, Oxford University Press, 1990.

Hubbard VS, Hubbard LR: Clinical Assessment of Nutritional Status and Lo CW: Laboratory Assessment of Nutritional Status. *In* Walker WA, Watkins JB (eds): Nutrition in Pediatrics, 2nd ed. Hamilton, Ontario, BC Decker, 1996, pp 7–28, 29–43.

## ENTERAL NUTRITION

Contraindications to oral feeding include an obstructive ileus, gastric retention, intestinal perforation, anatomic obstruction, severe acute gastrointestinal hemorrhage, and severe diet-induced diarrhea. In all other conditions, feeding should

TABLE 2–17.  Physical Signs of Nutritional Deficiency Disorders

| System | Sign | Deficiency |
|---|---|---|
| General appearance | Reduced weight for height | Calories |
| Skin/hair | Pallor | Anemias (iron, $B_{12}$, vitamin E, folate, and copper) |
| | Edema | Protein, thiamine |
| | Nasolabial seborrhea | Calories, protein, vitamin $B_6$, niacin, riboflavin |
| | Dermatitis | Riboflavin, essential fatty acids, biotin |
| | Photosensitivity dermatitis | Niacin |
| | Acrodermatitis | Zinc |
| | Follicular hyperkeratosis (sandpaper-like) | Vitamin A |
| | Depigmented skin | Calories, protein |
| | Purpura | Vitamins C, K |
| | Scrotal, vulval dermatitis | Riboflavin |
| | Alopecia | Zinc, biotin, protein |
| | Depigmented, dull hair, easily pluckable | Protein, calories, copper |
| Subcutaneous tissue | Decreased | Calories |
| Eye (vision) | Adaptation to dark | Vitamins A, E, zinc |
| | Color discrimination | Vitamin A |
| | Bitot spots, xerophthalmia, keratomalacia | Vitamin A |
| | Conjunctival pallor | Nutritional anemias |
| | Fundal capillary microaneurysms | Vitamin C |
| Face, mouth, neck | Angular stomatitis | Riboflavin, iron |
| | Cheilosis | Vitamins $B_6$, niacin, riboflavin |
| | Bleeding gums | Vitamins C, K |
| | Atrophic papillae | Riboflavin, iron, niacin, folate, vitamin $B_{12}$ |
| | Smooth tongue | Iron |
| | Red tongue (glossitis) | Vitamins $B_6$, $B_{12}$, niacin, riboflavin, folate |
| | Parotid swelling | Protein |
| | Caries | Fluoride |
| | Anosmia | Vitamins A, $B_{12}$, zinc |
| | Hypogeusia | Vitamin A, zinc |
| | Goiter | Iodine |
| Cardiovascular | Heart failure | Thiamine, selenium, nutritional anemias |
| Genital | Hypogonadism | Zinc |
| Skeletal | Costochondral beading | Vitamins D, C |
| | Subperiosteal hemorrhage | Vitamin C, copper |
| | Cranial bossing | Vitamin D |
| | Wide fontanel | Vitamin D |
| | Epiphyseal enlargement | Vitamin D |
| | Craniotabes | Vitamin D, calcium |
| | Tender bones | Vitamin C |
| | Tender calves | Thiamine, selenium, vitamin C |
| | Spoon-shaped nails (koilonychia) | Iron |
| | Transverse nail lines | Protein |
| Neurologic | Sensory, motor neuropathy | Thiamine, vitamins E, $B_6$, $B_{12}$ |
| | Ataxia, areflexia | Vitamin E |
| | Ophthalmoplegia | Vitamin E, thiamine |
| | Tetany | Vitamin D, $Ca^{2+}$, $Mg^{2+}$ |
| | Retardation | Iodine, niacin |
| | Dementia, delirium | Vitamin E, niacin, thiamine |
| | Poor position sense, ataxia | Thiamine, vitamin $B_{12}$ |

TABLE 2–18.  Screening Tests for Nutritional
Deficiency Disorders*

| Test | Deficiency |
|------|------------|
| Hemoglobin + RBC indices | Iron, folate, vitamins $B_{12}$, $B_6$, copper |
| Lymphocyte count | Protein, calories |
| Delayed hypersensitivity skin tests | Protein, calories |
| Retinol-binding protein prealbumin, transferrin | Protein, calories |
| Albumin | Protein; affected by fluids, renal and hepatic dysfunction |
| Calcium, phosphate | Vitamin D |
| Prothrombin time | Vitamin K |
| Thyroxine | Iodine |
| Bone radiographs | Iodine, vitamins D and C, copper |
| Alkaline phosphate | Zinc |
| Ceruloplasmin | Copper |

*Specific assays are available for most vitamins. Macronutrients and trace elements are determined when indicated by the history and physical examination and screening tests.
RBC = red blood cell count.

begin with a diet appropriate for age given first in diluted form or in a limited amount. When tolerance is established, there should be as rapid a progression as reasonable toward full concentration and nutritional adequacy. The rate of this progression is governed by gastrointestinal tolerance as determined by emesis, abdominal distention, and diarrhea.

When intestinal digestion is abnormal or when protein hypersensitivity is suspected, an *oligomeric* or elemental enteral product can be utilized. In older children this commonly is administered by a continuous intragastric drip because of the objectionable taste. Some of these products have an increased osmolarity and may produce intestinal luminal water sequestration if delivered into the jejunum at rates adequate to meet nutrient requirements. The level of tolerance for oligomeric diets varies with each patient and the etiology of the gastrointestinal disease. Glucose polymers, medium-chain and long-chain triglycerides, and oligopeptides are available when needed for specific patients. Care must be taken to ensure the overall quality of the therapeutic diet. In moderately to severely affected patients, enteral feeding should be supplemented with peripheral intravenous nutrition until acceptable nutrient absorption and weight gain are established.

A number of complications can occur as a consequence of enteral feeding. Enteral catheter complications include erosion of the nasal septum, dis-

placement of the catheter tip into the esophagus, lung, or duodenum, and perforation of the gastric wall. Silastic catheters reduce irritation and the likelihood of perforation. A percutaneously placed gastrostomy feeding tube should be considered for long-term enteral feeding.

## PARENTERAL NUTRITION

Total parenteral nutrition (TPN) is indicated when enteral nutrients cannot meet the nutritional needs for nutritional rehabilitation or normal growth. Enteral nutrition is preferred, because it is more physiologic, less expensive, and associated with fewer complications. Often, the parenteral nutrition supplements the enteral intake until the latter route provides sufficient nutrients for growth. Indications for TPN include (1) congenital gastrointestinal anomalies, (2) necrotizing enterocolitis, (3) short bowel syndrome, and (4) intractable diarrhea unresponsive to enteral alimentation. TPN also is useful in patients with trauma, burns, malignant disease, multiple organ system failure, and severe inflammatory bowel disease.

Generally, TPN by peripheral venous access is instituted first, with central access established when peripheral access becomes unavailable. In patients who need long-term TPN, a central venous line is placed early in the course of care. With few exceptions (e.g., marked fluid limitations), adequate nutritional support can be provided by either central or peripheral line TPN. Intravenous nutrient solutions provide all of the protein, calorie, electrolyte, vitamin, mineral (except iron), trace element, and essential fatty acid requirements. Iron can be added or given separately in most situations. The nonprotein calories are provided by both carbohydrates (dextrose) and a 20% lipid emulsion.

### Peripheral Intravenous Nutrition

Peripheral TPN is based on a 10–12% dextrose solution with 2–3% amino acids solution to provide about 0.8–2.0 g protein/kg/24 hr for older children, 1.5–3.0 g/kg/24 hr for full-term and older infants, and 2.5–3.5 g/kg/24 hr for preterm infants. The caloric density of glucose and amino acid–based solutions is limited by the solution's osmolality (10% glucose = 550 mOsm). Solutions with greater than 600 mOsm/L cause phlebitis of peripheral veins. The high caloric density but low osmolar lipid emulsion usually provides additional calories in excess of the 3–5% of total calories needed to prevent essential fatty acid deficiency. The rate of lipid infusion is initiated at 0.5–1.0

g/kg/24 hr but is advanced to 2–4 g/kg/24 hr. Intravenous caloric requirement is approximately 10% less than the enteral requirement because of the omission of the caloric expenditure for the thermic effect of feeding (see Fig. 2–4).

### Central Venous Nutrition

Central TPN primarily differs from peripheral TPN in the dextrose concentration; usually 20% versus 10% with peripheral TPN. In situations with severe fluid limitations and/or lipid intolerance, up to 25–30% dextrose may be used centrally. For longer-term central access, a silicon-rubber cuffed catheter is surgically placed in a large vein tunneled subcutaneously to an exit site on the anterior chest wall, and threaded to the superior vena cava into the right atrium. The high blood flow in central veins reduces the risks of the hyperosmolar solutions. The lipid infusion ranges from the minimal 3–5% of calories to 2–4 g/kg/24 hr, as needed to meet the caloric requirements. The protein (amino acid), vitamin, and trace mineral intakes are individualized for the patient.

Careful monitoring of the venous line site and placement, fluid and electrolyte balance, growth, and metabolic response are essential to the safety and efficacy of TPN. *Laboratory evaluation* includes measurement of blood glucose, urea nitrogen, creatinine, calcium, phosphorus, magnesium, bilirubin, albumin, liver enzymes, and triglyceride. These are obtained prior to initiation of TPN and weekly during infusion. Serum triglycerides are monitored as the amount of lipids infused is increased from 1–2g/kg/24 hr to the level required for caloric needs (3–4 g/kg/24 hr).

Complications of TPN are categorized as metabolic, technical (catheter related), or infectious (Table 2–19). *Hepatobiliary dysfunction* is seen in some patients who require long-term (>2 wk) TPN. Cholestasis is associated with conjugated hyperbilirubinemia, modest elevation in the hepatocellular enzymes, and, rarely, irreversible hepatic failure. Although several factors (fasting, toxic amino acids) have been implicated in the pathogeneses of hepatobiliary dysfunction, no single causal factor has been identified. The diagnosis of TPN-induced cholestasis is one of exclusion; other causes of hyperbilirubinemia must be considered, such as sepsis, structural abnormalities, $\alpha_1$-antitrypsin defi-

---

TABLE 2–19.   Potential Complications of Total Parenteral Alimentation

**Catheter-Related**
Superior vena cava syndrome (thrombosis)
Pulmonary thromboembolism
Pulmonary hypertension
Pneumothorax
Pleural effusions (extravasated solution)
Cardiac arrhythmias
Pericardial effusion
Mural thrombosis (cardiac)
Intramyocardial infusion
Tricuspid valve injury
Hemorrhage
Flocculation precipitation of nutrients

**Infections**
Staphylococcal (*S. aureus, S. epidermidis*) sepsis
*Candida* sepsis
*Malassezia furfur* (intralipid)
Aspergillosis sepsis
Entry, exit site, tract infections
Contaminated solutions (rare organisms)

**Electrolyte (Minerals)**
Hyponatremia
Hypernatremia
Hypokalemia
Hypophosphatemia
Hypomagnesemia
Metabolic acidosis
Trace mineral deficiency (zinc, copper)
Aluminum toxicity

**Metabolic**
Hypoglycemia (infusion stopped)
Hyperglycemia (hyperosmolar state)
Hyperaminoacidemia (↑ protein intake)
Hyperammonemia (↑ protein intake)
Azotemia (↑ protein intake)
Hypoalbuminemia (↓ protein intake)
Essential fatty acid deficiency
Hypertriglyceridemia
Carnitine deficiency
Vitamin deficiencies (biotin)
Acanthocytosis (lipids)

**Systemic**
Cholestasis (hepatic dysfunction)
Cirrhosis
Fatty infiltration (liver, monocytes, lung; intralipid)
Altered myocardial function (phosphate, calcium depletion)
Intestinal mucosal atrophy
Platelet dysfunction (intralipid)
?Hemolysis (intralipid)
Osmotic diuresis (glucose)
Metabolic bone disease (osteopenia)
Isosmolar coma (protein, glucose)
Increased deposition of body fat
Increased extracellular fluid space
White blood cell dysfunction (phosphate depletion, lipids)
Poor sucking, swallowing (NPO)

---

NPO = nothing by mouth.

ciency, cystic fibrosis, viral hepatitis, and inborn errors of metabolism (galactosemia, tyrosinemia). The development of cholestasis increases the urgency to establish enteral support and discontinue TPN as soon as enteral intake is adequate. To avoid infection, trained personnel clean the catheter site with aseptic solutions; entry into the system is avoided and, if necessary, is performed with sterile technique.

Delays in behavioral development may result from the long-term administration of enteral nasogastric or parenteral feedings to young infants, in part because the development of oral feeding patterns is bypassed. The opportunity for non-nutritive sucking (i.e., the provision of a pacifier) may prevent this complication. When the infant has not learned to suck or swallow, a team approach is required to teach the infant these functions.

## References

Behrman RE, Kliegman RM, Arvin AM (eds): Nelson Textbook of Pediatrics, 15th ed. Philadelphia, WB Saunders, 1996, Chapters 44.2, 44.4, 54.

Heird W: Amino acid and energy needs of pediatric patients receiving parenteral nutrition. Pediatr Clin North Am 42:265, 1995.

Noel RA, Udall J: Parenteral nutrition. *In* Walker WA, Watkins JB (eds): Nutrition in Pediatrics, 2nd ed. Hamilton, Ontario, BC Decker, 1996, pp 734--746.

Stoker TW, Kleinman RE: Standard and specialized enteric feeding practices in nutrition. *In* Walker WA, Watkins JB (eds): Nutrition in Pediatrics, 2nd ed. Hamilton, Ontario, BC Decker, 1996, pp 727--733.

# Chapter 3

# THE ACUTELY ILL OR INJURED CHILD

Steven E. Krug

## RECOGNITION OF SHOCK AND RESPIRATORY FAILURE

The care of the acutely ill or injured child requires an evaluation and management approach that is quite different than that used to assess the well child or the child with a chronic or a minor illness. The assessment of the acutely ill child centers on the rapid identification of physiologic derangement in organ system function rather than the immediate development of a differential diagnosis. The goal of this efficient assessment is *triage*, or identifying children at risk for critical illness or injury. Because suspicion of critical illness warrants immediate resuscitation, such action may need to be based on very limited information.

Cardiopulmonary failure is rarely a spontaneous event in children. It is typically the end result of acute or chronic but progressive deteriorating respiratory and/or circulatory function. Unfortunately, once cardiopulmonary arrest has occurred, the outcome is generally poor, with 75–80% dying; and 75% of the survivors sustain permanent disability. The strategy for successful pediatric resuscitation relies on the recognition of a pre-arrest state, such as impending respiratory failure or shock. This recognition depends on one's ability to identify the symptoms or signs of those conditions or to identify those children who are at special risk for these life-threatening events.

The initial evaluation of the acutely ill child requires rapid cardiopulmonary assessment. This evaluation should take less than 60 sec to complete, follow the "ABC" (*a*irway, *b*reathing, *c*irculation) approach used in cardiopulmonary resuscitation (Table 3–1), and integrate pertinent physical findings and physiologic data into one of the following clinical impressions:

1. Stable.
2. Impending respiratory failure and/or shock.
3. Definite respiratory failure and/or shock.
4. Cardiopulmonary failure.
5. Cardiopulmonary arrest.

This assessment will then determine the priorities of patient management and their urgency. Initial treatment is directed toward the physiologic derangement (e.g. shock) rather than what might be the underlying cause (e.g., sepsis).

Objective data are then used both to assess the response to stabilization procedures and to make the ultimate diagnosis. Such data require ongoing

TABLE 3–1. Rapid Cardiopulmonary Assessment

| | |
|---|---|
| *Airway patency* | *Circulation* |
| Patent, able to be maintained independently | Heart rate |
| | Peripheral pulses |
| | Present/absent |
| Maintainable with positioning, suctioning | Volume/strength |
| | Skin perfusion |
| Unmaintainable, requires assistance | Capillary refill time |
| | Skin temperature |
| | Color |
| *Breathing* | Mottling |
| Rate | Blood pressure |
| Mechanics | Central pulse strength |
| Retractions | |
| Grunting | *CNS perfusion* |
| Use of accessory muscles | Responsiveness (AVPU) |
| Nasal flaring | Recognition of parents or caregivers |
| Air entry | Muscle tone |
| Chest expansion | Pupil size |
| Breath sounds | Posturing |
| Stridor | |
| Wheezing | |
| Paradoxical chest motion | |
| Color | |

AVPU = *a*lert, responds to *v*oice, responds to *p*ain, *u*nresponsive.

93

*monitoring of vital organ functions*, including brain, heart, kidney, bone marrow, lung, and liver. By using a combination of monitoring and therapeutic interventions, the physician is able to anticipate the further progression of the illness and can manage on-going physiologic derangements (Table 3–2).

*Respiratory failure* is the most common cause of cardiopulmonary arrest in children and is characterized by inadequate oxygenation or ventilation. It may be caused by intrinsic lung or airway disease, airway obstruction, or poor respiratory effort from central nervous system dysfunction. It is generally preceded by respiratory distress, a compensated state, characterized by signs of increased work of breathing (tachypnea, nasal flaring, intercostal muscle retraction, grunting, and accessory respiratory muscle use) (see Chapter 12).

*Shock* is defined as a physiologic state with insufficient delivery of oxygen and metabolic substrates to meet the metabolic needs of tissues. Shock is characterized by signs of inadequate tissue perfusion (pallor, cool skin, poor pulses, delayed capillary refill, oliguria, abnormal mentation) and may be further classified on the basis of the presence of a normal (compensated) or abnormal (uncompensated) blood pressure.

The clinical signs of respiratory failure and shock are caused by tissue hypoxia and the resulting metabolic or mixed (metabolic and respiratory) acidosis. Early in the course of acute illness, respiratory failure and shock may be clinically distinct entities. As both states progress, they deteriorate to a state of cardiopulmonary failure. Irregular respiration, bradycardia, and hypotension are ominous findings in acutely ill children, suggestive of impending cardiopulmonary arrest.

The goal of management of acutely ill patients is to recognize the early signs of impending respiratory failure or shock and to intervene before further deterioration develops. This requires careful observation and may be aided by the use of various clinical severity scoring systems (trauma, coma, acute injury scores). One system, PRISM (*pediatric risk of mortality*), combines physiologic (heart and respiratory rates, blood pressure, Glasgow Coma Scale, pupillary signs) and biochemical ($PaO_2/FiO_2$ or $FiO_2$ and arterial saturation $PaCO_2$, coagulation tests, bilirubin, potassium, ionized calcium, glucose, and bicarbonate) data to help predict the risk of progression.

Common causes of death among children over one mo of age include sudden infant death syndrome (SIDS), trauma (motor vehicle accidents, falls, child abuse, violence), burns, drowning, toxic ingestion, respiratory diseases (asthma), severe infections (meningitis, sepsis, human immunodeficiency virus [HIV], gastroenteritis), metabolic disorders (diabetes), and the consequences of treating congenital anomalies or malignancy.

## References

Behrman RE, Kliegman RM, Arvin AM, (eds): Nelson Textbook of Pediatrics, 15th ed. Philadelphia, WB Saunders, 1996, Chapter 60.

Chameides L, Hazinski MF (eds): Textbook of Pediatric Advanced Life Support. Dallas, American Heart Association, 1994, Chapter 2.

Joint Task Force on Advance Pediatric Life Support: APLS: The Pediatric Emergency Medicine Course, 2nd ed. Elk Grove Village, IL, American Academy of Pediatrics, 1993, Chapters 1, 3.

**TABLE 3–2.** Elements of Acute Care

**Examine**
 Initial assessment followed by complete and systematic evaluation
 Focus examination on areas of chief complaints; determine life-threatening and organ-threatening conditions
 Synthesize findings to plan further evaluation

**Monitor**
 Vital signs
 Physiologic parameters required to:
  1. make diagnosis, and/or
  2. ascertain response to therapy or progression of disease
 Prospectively determine allowable limits for changes in monitored parameters; generate and record objective data to guide therapy

**Intervene**
 Prior to initiating therapy, determine therapeutic goals and endpoints
 Prioritize life-threatening and organ-threatening conditions
 Initiate therapy based on recognized pathophysiologic derangements
 Adjust therapeutic strategies to individual patient needs
 Use objective data to guide alterations in therapy

**Anticipate**
 Requires understanding of the underlying pathophysiology
 Always plan for the "worst-case" scenario
 Use data obtained through examination and monitoring to update prognostic impressions continually

## EMERGENCY MEDICAL SERVICES FOR CHILDREN (EMS-C)

The outcome of the critically ill or injured child depends on the provision of timely and appropriate emergency care. This care begins with the early recognition of a life-threatening problem and continues through prehospital, in-hospital, and rehabilitative care. Because the occurrence of critical illness is much lower in children than in adults and the presenting signs of critical illness in children may be difficult to ascertain, existing components of emergency medical services (EMS) may not be prepared to meet the unique needs of children. The reductions realized in adult cardiac and trauma mortality and disability rates with the development of modern-day EMS and trauma systems have not been as dramatic in children. Efforts to integrate EMS-C and the special needs of children (via education and training, equipment, protocols) into existing EMS systems will improve the outcome of pediatric acute illness and injury.

## References

Behrman RE, Kliegman RM, Arvin AM (eds): Nelson Textbook of Pediatrics, 15th ed. Philadelphia, WB Saunders, 1996, Chapter 59.

Durch JS, Lohr KN: Emergency Medical Services for Children. Washington, DC, Institute of Medicine, National Academy Press, 1993.

Seidel J: Emergency medical services for children. Emerg Med Clin North Am 13:255, 1995.

# MAJOR TRAUMA

## EPIDEMIOLOGY

Injuries account for almost 50% of the deaths in children 1–14 yr of age. Almost 50% of these are due to motor vehicle accidents. A majority of the rest are due to falls (25–30%) and burns (10–15%). Gunshot wounds, assaults, and ingestions account for 5–10% of pediatric trauma. More than 50% of trauma fatalities occur at the scene of the accident rather than at a secondary site to which the victim may be transported, such as a hospital or the home. These deaths occur to patients who receive injuries to the brain stem, head, aorta, heart, and upper cervical spine. The next substantial group of deaths occurs within several hours of arrival in the emergency department; survival depends on the severity of shock at the time of presentation and the length of time the shock state was present. If the patient is taken to a center where definitive care can be provided and is stabilized within an hour of the time of the injury, the outcome is likely to be optimal. A final peak in mortality occurs days to weeks after the initial injury and results from severe, life-threatening complications because the injuries have not responded to medical and surgical management.

## EDUCATION FOR PREVENTING ACCIDENTAL TRAUMA

The recognition that much of the morbidity and mortality are determined at the scene of the acci-

dent has stimulated the development of prevention measures throughout the United States, including decreasing the speed limit, imposing more stringent automobile safety standards, mandating the use of child automobile restraining devices and bicycle helmets, promoting cardiopulmonary resuscitation (CPR) training, and the more frequent use of the Heimlich maneuver for the choking victim. The number of regional poison control centers also has grown throughout the United States, providing the lay public and medical professionals with information regarding toxic ingestions and exposures. Other primary prevention efforts have included fire safety programs, water safety and swimming programs, and legislative efforts to require the reporting of suspected child abuse and to control the temperature of hot water in order to prevent children from being scalded.

## PROVIDING PREHOSPITAL CARE

Trauma care begins at the scene of the injury. The prehospital phase of care is focused towards a rapid assessment of the "ABCs" (*a*irway, *b*reathing, *c*irculation), and initiation of basic or advanced life support interventions at the scene or en route to the hospital. The scope of care provided in the field is determined by the nature of the injured child's physiologic state and associated injuries, the anticipated transit time to the hospital, and the skill level or scope of practice of the prehospital care providers. The general goal of prehospital trauma care is rapid assessment, support of the ABCs, immobilization, and transportation.

Prehospital care providers, with the assistance of protocols and on-line medical direction, must also determine which injured children will require transport to a trauma center (Table 3–3). A number of trauma triage scoring tools have been developed to assist the evaluation of injury severity, trauma center triage decision making, and patient prognosis. The most appropriate objective scoring system for children is the Pediatric Trauma Score (Table 3–4).

## EVALUATING AND MANAGING THE TRAUMA PATIENT IN THE EMERGENCY DEPARTMENT

On the patient's arrival at the emergency department, an organized and synchronized response must be initiated by the responding team, based on the priorities and directives of the pediatric general surgeon. The initial assessment of the seriously injured child should employ a systematic

TABLE 3–3. Children Requiring Pediatric Trauma Center Care

Patients with serious injury to more than one system

Patients with one system injury who require critical care or monitoring in an intensive care unit

Patients with signs of shock who require more than one transfusion

Patients with fracture complicated by suspected neurovascular or compartment injury

Patients with fracture of axial skeleton

Patients with two or more long bone fractures

Patients with potential replantation of an extremity

Patients with suspected or actual spinal cord or column injuries

Patients with head injury with any one of the following:
    Orbital or facial bone fracture
    Cerebrospinal fluid leaks
    Altered state of consciousness
    Changing neural signs
    Open head injuries
    Depressed skull fracture
    Requiring intracranial pressure monitoring

Patients suspected of requiring ventilator support

approach which includes the following: (1) primary survey, (2) resuscitation, (3) secondary survey, (4) postresuscitation monitoring, and (5) definitive care.

The *primary survey* focuses on the *ABCDEs of emergency care,* as modified for trauma from the ABCs of cardiopulmonary resuscitation: "A" stands for *airway,* accompanied by *cervical spine control.* Effective care of the traumatized child should ensure immobilization. If there is a question regarding cervical spine stability, orotracheal intubation should be performed with the neck immobilized in the neutral position. Nasotracheal intuba-

tion may be contraindicated in facial trauma or basilar skull fracture, because the tube may enter the cranial vault. Needle cricothyrotomy also may be employed in instances of facial trauma or cervical spine fracture.

"B" stands for assessment of *breathing,* which is critical in the traumatized patient, even if an artificial airway is already in place. Ventilation can be assessed by observation, palpation, and auscultation. As a component of the primary survey, major thoracic injuries (Table 3–5) must be assessed and treated immediately to ensure a successful resuscitation.

"C" stands for *circulation and hemorrhage control.* Circulation can be assessed via observation (heart rate, skin color, mental status) and palpation (pulse quality, capillary refill, skin temperature). Control of bleeding is one of the primary responsibilities in the acute care of the traumatized child. Hemorrhage must be identified, then stopped, by the use of direct pressure or extremity tourniquets.

In trauma care, "D" stands for *disability,* which serves as a reminder to assess and monitor neurologic status, a condition that may be changing constantly. The rapid neurologic assessment in the primary survey has two components: (1) examination of pupil size and reactivity and (2) a brief mental status assessment (AVPU: *a*lert; responds to *v*oice; responds to *p*ain; *u*nresponsive). These changes may provide important diagnostic and prognostic information as well as therapeutic direction. Another common tool for assessing neurologic injury is the Glasgow Coma Scale (GCS). This scale is modified for use in preverbal children (Table 3–6). The GCS can direct decisions regarding the initiation of cerebral resuscitation (i.e. hyperventilation, osmolar therapy) in patients with suspected closed head injuries. Head injury is present in 80% of all multiple trauma patients, and in 60% of pediatric cases the head is the most severely affected part of

TABLE 3–4. Pediatric Trauma Score*

| Category Component | +2 | +1 | −1 |
|---|---|---|---|
| Size | >20 kg | 10–20 kg | <10 kg |
| Airway | Normal | Maintainable | Unmaintainable |
| Systolic BP† | >90 mm Hg | 50–90 mm Hg | <50 mm Hg |
| CNS | Awake | Obtunded/LOC | Coma/decerebrate |
| Skeletal | None | Closed fracture | Open/multiple fractures |
| Cutaneous/wounds | None | Minor | Major/penetrating |

Modified from Tepas J, Mollitt D, Talbert J, et al: The pediatric trauma score as a predictor of injury severity in the injured child. J Pediatr Surg 22:14, 1987.
*If score <8, refer to Pediatric Trauma Center.
†If proper size BP cuff is not available: +2 = palpable pulse at wrist; +1 = palpable pulse at groin; −1 = no palpable pulse.
BP = blood pressure; CNS = central nervous system; LOC = loss of consciousness.

**TABLE 3–5.** Life-Threatening Chest Injuries

**Tension Pneumothorax**
One-way valve leak from lung parenchyma
Complete collapse with mediastinal and tracheal shift to side opposite the leak
Compromises venous return and decreases ventilation of other lung
Clinically, becomes manifest by respiratory distress, unilateral absent breath sounds, tracheal deviation, distended neck veins, tympany to percussion of involved side, cyanosis
Relieve first with needle aspiration, then chest tube drainage

**Open Pneumothorax (Sucking Chest Wound)**
Effect on ventilation depends on size

**Major Flail Chest**
Usually due to blunt injury resulting in multiple rib fractures
Loss of bone stability of thoracic cage
Major disruption of synchronous chest wall motion
Mechanical ventilation and positive end-expiratory pressure required

**Massive Hemothorax**
Must be drained with large-bore tube
Initiate drainage only with concurrent vascular volume replacement

**Cardiac Tamponade**
Beck triad
  1. Decreased or muffled heart sounds
  2. Distended neck veins from increased venous pressure
  3. Hypotension with pulsus paradoxus (decreased pulse pressure during inspiration)
Must be drained

the body. The mortality rate in multiple trauma accompanied by head injury is 16% but only 6% in the absence of significant head injury.

"E", for *exposure*, has been added to the mnemonic as a reminder that for a full assessment of the patient, the child must be completely disrobed so that the entire body can be examined in detail. In doing so, the examiner should pay attention to maintaining a neutral thermal environment to prevent hypothermia.

On completion of the primary survey, a more detailed head-to-toe examination (the *secondary survey*) should ensue. The purpose of this careful reexamination is to identify life- and limb-threatening as well as less serious injuries. Coincident with the secondary survey, and dependent in part on the assessed physiologic status of the patient, certain procedures and resuscitative measures (i.e., large-bore vascular access, fluid therapy) are initiated. The prioritization of definitive care needs are determined by the injury findings collected from the primary and secondary surveys, the child's physiologic response to resuscitative care, and data from continuous monitoring.

## SPECIFIC ORGAN INJURIES

The initial physical examination in the emergency department, which is augmented by screening laboratory data (Table 3–7), should provide information and direction for further diagnostic evaluation. When one is subsequently focusing on various organ systems, evaluating and treating severe *head injury* is given a high priority. Major trauma to the *chest* and *mediastinal structures* usually requires immediate surgical intervention; except for pulmonary contusion, these injuries have a significant mortality. The *musculoskeletal system* also may require immediate attention. Fractures contribute most to the long-term morbidity associated with multiple trauma and, if inappropriately assessed, may lead to loss of limb or life. There is approximately a 12% failure rate in the diagnosis of significant fractures in and around the time of injury. Most fractures may be managed by closed techniques.

### Head Trauma

See Chapter 18.

### Abdominal Trauma

*Penetrating trauma* must be distinguished from blunt trauma. The former accounts for less than 10% of pediatric abdominal trauma but more than 50% of adult abdominal trauma. Pediatric patients experiencing penetrating trauma may be asymptomatic or in hypovolemic shock. Performing serial physical examinations is the primary method for obtaining information on which to base decisions regarding operative intervention. Abdominal computed tomography (CT) scanning is invaluable in assessing hemodynamically stable children with intra-abdominal trauma. Gunshot wounds to the abdomen, an important category of abdominal trauma, involve multiple organs in 80% of cases and have a mortality rate greater than 12%. Operative exploration may be indicated when peritoneal irritation, hypovolemia, free air on plain film, or positive results of paracentesis (Table 3–8) are present.

*Blunt abdominal trauma* occurs far more often in children than does penetrating abdominal trauma. The most frequently injured organs, in descending order, are the spleen, liver, genitourinary tract, stomach, intestine, colon, pancreas, pelvis, and major vessels. Optimal management in stable children with these injuries requires serial physical examinations with CT to confirm the presence and severity of organ injury. Operative intervention

TABLE 3–6.  Glasgow Coma Scales

| Glasgow Coma Scale | | | Modified Coma Scale for Infants | | |
|---|---|---|---|---|---|
| *Activity* | *Best Response* | *Score* | *Activity* | *Best Response* | *Score* |
| *Eye opening* | Spontaneous | 4 | *Eye opening* | Spontaneous | 4 |
| | To verbal stimuli | 3 | | To speech | 3 |
| | To pain | 2 | | To pain | 2 |
| | None | 1 | | None | 1 |
| *Verbal* | Oriented | 5 | *Verbal* | Coos, babbles | 5 |
| | Confused | 4 | | Irritable, cries | 4 |
| | Inappropriate words | 3 | | Cries to pain | 3 |
| | Nonspecific sounds | 2 | | Moans to pain | 2 |
| | None | 1 | | None | 1 |
| *Motor* | Follows commands | 6 | *Motor* | Spontaneous movements | 6 |
| | Localizes pain | 5 | | Withdraws to touch | 5 |
| | Withdraws to pain | 4 | | Withdraws to pain | 4 |
| | Flexion to pain | 3 | | Abnormal flexion | 3 |
| | Extension to pain | 2 | | Abnormal extension | 2 |
| | None | 1 | | None | 1 |

may be required in a patient whose vital signs are persistently unstable, even when there is no extravascular volume loss or no enlarging abdomen. The presence of peritoneal irritation or abdominal wall discoloration, together with signs of intravascular volume loss, indicates the need for

TABLE 3–7.  Initial Laboratory Evaluation of the Major Trauma Patient

**Hematology**
Complete blood count
Platelet count
Prothrombin time
Activated partial thromboplastin time
Fibrinogen
Type and cross-match

**Urinalysis**
Gross
Microscopic

**Clinical Chemistry**
Na, K, Cl, BUN, $CO_2$, glucose, calcium
Creatinine
Amylase
SGOT/SGPT

**Radiology**
Cervical spine films
AP chest roentgenogram
Roentgenograms of all apparent fractures
CT scans where indicated for head, chest, and abdominal trauma
IVP if urinalysis positive for blood

AP = anteroposterior; BUN = blood urea nitrogen; Cl = chloride; $CO_2$ = carbon dioxide; CT = computed tomography; IVP = intravenous pyelogram; K = potassium; Na = sodium; SGOT/SGPT = serum glutamic oxaloacetic transaminase/serum glutamic pyruvic transaminase.

laparotomy. Abdominal CT is an especially important adjunct in the patient who is unconscious as a result of a head injury. The use of high-fluid volumes to resuscitate this type of patient may exacerbate brain swelling; therefore, CT or, if it is unavailable, paracentesis and early surgery may be the judicious approach in some children.

### Injury to the Spleen

Splenic injuries often are signaled by pain at the tip of the shoulder or in the left chest, accompanied by respiratory distress, nausea, and vomiting. A positive *Kehr sign* (pressure on the left upper quadrant eliciting left shoulder pain) also is strongly suggestive of this diagnosis. No other consistent clinical or laboratory findings suggest a splenic injury.

Nonoperative management of serious splenic injuries is the treatment of choice. This treatment includes intensive care and serial observation by CT, radionuclide scan, or follow-up ultrasound ex-

TABLE 3–8.  Criteria for a Positive Paracentesis

Free aspiration ≥10 mL gross blood

Turbid or bloody fluid that prevents reading newsprint

Free egress through indwelling urinary catheter or chest tube

Presence of >500 WBC/mL or >100,000 RBC/mL

Amylase >175 U/mL

Presence of gross stool or food debris

RBC = red blood cells; WBC = white blood cells.

amination. Surgery is indicated for patients having an estimated blood loss greater than 40 mL/kg of transfused blood in 24–36 hr. The operative approach often involves repair of the lesion rather than removal of the spleen, but splenectomy is required if the organ is totally separated from its blood supply; if a severe head injury exists for which rapid, high-volume circulatory support might be hazardous; or if an increase in blood loss of unknown cause has occurred in the presence of fecal contamination of the peritoneal contents. If a splenectomy is performed, patients should remain on penicillin prophylaxis and receive pneumococcal and *Haemophilus influenzae* vaccines because there is an increased morbidity and mortality owing to overwhelming sepsis in asplenic patients.

### Renal Injury

The kidney commonly is injured by blunt abdominal trauma, and more than 40% of children with injured kidneys have other internal injuries. A young child's kidney is more vulnerable to trauma than an adult's because (1) it is positioned more anteriorly in the peritoneal cavity, (2) the child's rib cage is more compliant, and (3) the child's abdominal muscle development is immature. In the child in whom minor trauma has led to major renal injury, congenital renal anomalies also should be suspected. The diagnosis of renal injury is based on history and physical examination, coupled with a urinalysis showing blood and increased protein levels. An intravenous pyelogram (IVP) may be diagnostic; however, CT scans with renal contrast also are useful. In more than 80% of the children with positive IVPs, simple monitoring is all that is required; in the remaining patients, surgery usually is indicated for falling hemoglobin, refractory shock, or urinary obstruction caused by clots.

### Liver Trauma

Major trauma to the liver is a serious cause of morbidity and accounts for 40% of all deaths associated with blunt abdominal trauma in children. Almost 90% of these injuries involve the right lobe of the liver, and the diagnosis is usually made by the presence of pain in the right shoulder and right upper quadrant. Patients may have hypotension secondary to blood loss; hematobilia is rare. The site of the traumatic lesion may determine its severity. Subcapsular hematomas are less serious than capsular tears, which in turn are less serious than minor or deep lacerations. Burst injuries, with or without major vascular injury, are the most se-

vere of all traumatic injuries to the liver and almost invariably are fatal.

For most children experiencing liver trauma, conservative management is recommended. This management involves admission to an intensive care unit (ICU) and monitoring ongoing blood loss, hepatic function, and liver structure with serial CT scan or ultrasound examinations. Operative management should be reserved for life-threatening situations.

### Injuries of the Pancreas and Biliary Tree

Injuries of the pancreas and biliary tree are less common in children than in adults. Pancreatic injuries usually are present in association with injury to overlying structures, including the stomach, duodenum, extrahepatic biliary tree, and spleen. Pancreatic injury generally is identified by diffuse abdominal tenderness, pain, and vomiting. A midepigastric mass also is variably present. Hemodynamic instability, secondary to retroperitoneal hemorrhage, may be the presenting sign. Hyperamylasemia may not occur until 3–5 days after the injury. In managing these patients, nasogastric suction and parenteral nutrition are indicated. Surgical removal of part or all of the necrotic pancreas may be required in one third of the patients who have a pseudocyst or a persistent fistula. CT or ultrasonography may detect pancreatic injury, abscess formation, or pseudocyst.

Injury to the biliary tree is evident in children through the appearance of hematobilia after right upper quadrant trauma. The diagnosis usually is confirmed by the presence of bile in the peritoneal cavity or retroperitoneal space. When these children do not present with an acute injury, their chronic course is characterized by anorexia, weight loss, the development of bilious ascites, jaundice, and acholic stools. Biliary tree injury generally requires prompt surgical repair once it is identified.

### Intestinal Injury

In children, injury to the intestine usually is associated with other injuries requiring surgical treatment. The risk of intestinal injury varies with the amount of intestinal contents. A full bowel is likely to shear more easily than an empty bowel, and the shearing occurs at points of fixation (i.e., the ligament of Treitz, the ileocecal valve, and the ascending and descending peritoneal reflections). Perforation is more common in the jejunum and ileum than in the colon or stomach. Pneumoperitoneum that exists in association with intestinal perforation occurs in only 20% of patients. This diagnosis can be missed by CT and often is established by paracentesis that is positive for bowel contents. Prompt surgical intervention is required.

### References

Behrman RE, Kliegman RM, Arvin AM (eds): Nelson Textbook of Pediatrics, 15th ed. Philadelphia, WB Saunders, 1996, Chapter 58.

Galat JA, Grisoni ER, Gauderer MWL: Pediatric blunt liver injury: Establishment of criteria for appropriate management. J Pediatr Surg 25:1162, 1990.

Ghajar J, Hariri RJ: Management of pediatric head injury. Pediatr Clin North Am 39:1093, 1992.

Peclet MH, Newman KD, Eichelberger MR, et al: Thoracic trauma in children: An indicator of increased mortality. J Pediatr Surg 25:961, 1990.

Polhgeers A, Ruddy RM: An update on pediatric trauma. Emerg Med Clin North Am 13:267, 1995.

Yurt RW: Triage, initial assessment, and early treatment of the pediatric trauma patient. Pediatr Clin North Am 39:1083, 1992.

# BURNS

Burn injury results in 20,000 hospital admissions and 1400 deaths each year for children, making it the third leading mechanism of injury death. Overall, nearly 1% of all children sustain a burn injury each year. Burn risk is related to age, with a 2.5-fold increased risk for children under 5 yr of age. Mortality is primarily associated with burn severity (extent of body surface area and depth), although the presence of inhalation injury and young age are also predictors for mortality.

The upper extremities are the areas most frequently involved in burns (71%), followed by the head and neck (52%). Scalding injuries (75%) are most common and inhalation injuries are least common in pediatric patients.

The pathophysiology of burn injury is due to disruption of the three key functions of the skin: (1) regulation of heat loss, (2) preservation of body fluids, and (3) barrier to infection. Burn injury releases inflammatory and vasoactive mediators and promotes a number of hemodynamic changes, including increased capillary permeability, decreased plasma volume, and decreased cardiac output. Shock is common in children with burns that involve more than 10–12% of the total body surface area. For severe burns, admission to a qualified burn center is necessary.

## CLASSIFICATION

Burns usually are classified on the basis of four criteria:

1. Depth of injury.
2. Percent of body surface area involved.
3. Location of the burn.
4. Association with other injuries.

Most burn surgeons recommend that the depth of injury be assessed solely on clinical criteria of appearance.

*First-degree burns* are superficial (red, painful, dry) with damage limited to the epidermis. They are commonly seen with sun exposure or mild, hot, solid, or scald injuries. They heal in 3–6 days without scarring. They are not included in burn surface area calculations. *Second-degree* or partial-thickness burns may be superficial (red, painful, mottled, blistered, healing in 10–21 days with little or no scarring), or deep dermal (pale, painful, yellow), resulting from immersion (21–28 days to heal) or flames (≥3 wk to heal and potentially scarring). *Third-degree burns* are full thickness and require grafts (if >1 cm in diameter). They are avascular and are characterized by coagulation necrosis. *Fourth-degree* burns involve underlying fascia, muscle, or bone.

A *severe burn* is one that covers greater than 15% of the body surface area or involves the face or perineum. Second-degree and third-degree burns of the hands or feet as well as circumferential burns of the extremities also are classified as severe. Inhalation injuries resulting in bronchospasm and impaired pulmonary function also must be considered severe burns. A method for estimating the percentage of skin surface area involved in children of various ages is presented in Figure 3–1. The extent of skin involvement of older adolescent and adult patients is estimated as follows: each upper extremity, 9%; each lower extremity, 18%; anterior trunk, 18%; posterior trunk, 18%; the head, 9%; and the perineum, 1%.

The location of the burn is important in assessing the risk for disability. The risk is greatest when the face, eyes, ears, feet, perineum, or hands are involved. With partial-thickness burns, no disability generally results; however, full-thickness burns almost always result in permanent impairment. Inhalational injuries not only cause respiratory compromise but may result in difficulty in eating and drinking. Inhalational injuries also may be associated with burns of the face and neck.

## INITIAL EVALUATION

The triage decision for the physician caring for a burn patient is based on (1) the extent of the burn, (2) the body surface area involved, (3) the type of burn, (4) associated injuries, (5) any complicating medical or social problems, and (6) the availability

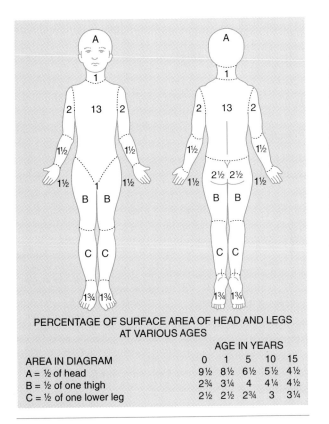

PERCENTAGE OF SURFACE AREA OF HEAD AND LEGS
AT VARIOUS AGES

| AREA IN DIAGRAM | AGE IN YEARS | | | | |
|---|---|---|---|---|---|
| | 0 | 1 | 5 | 10 | 15 |
| A = ½ of head | 9½ | 8½ | 6½ | 5½ | 4½ |
| B = ½ of one thigh | 2¾ | 3¼ | 4 | 4¼ | 4½ |
| C = ½ of one lower leg | 2½ | 2½ | 2¾ | 3 | 3¼ |

FIGURE 3–1. This chart of body areas, together with the table showing the percentage of surface area of head and legs at various ages, can be used to estimate the surface area burned in a child. (From Solomon JR: Pediatric burns. Crit Care Clin 1:159–174, 1985.)

of ambulatory management (Fig. 3–2). The initial treatment requires removing the patient from the site of injury, cleansing away any chemical or injurious contactants, and removing the clothing. The next priority is airway management; the upper airway is susceptible to burn injury, whereas the subglottic space appears protected. Few signs of injury may be present initially, although facial burns, singed nasal hairs or eyebrows, and acute inflammation of the oropharynx should suggest inhalation injury. Smoke inhalation may be associated with carbon monoxide toxicity; 100% humidified oxygen should be given if hypoxia or inhalation is suspected. A carboxyhemoglobin assessment should be performed for any suspected inhalation exposure (a house or closed-space fire or a burn victim who requires CPR. Hoarseness on vocalization also is consistent with a supraglottic injury. Some children with inhalation burns require endoscopy, an artificial airway, and mechanical ventilation.

## FLUID, ELECTROLYTE, AND NUTRITION MANAGEMENT

The initial fluid and electrolyte support of the burned child is critical. The first priority is to support the circulating blood volume, which requires the administration of intravenous fluids to provide both maintenance fluid and electrolyte requirements and to replace ongoing burn losses. Children with a significant burn should receive a rapid bolus of 20 cc/kg of lactated Ringer's solution. The resuscitation formula for fluid therapy in the first 24 hours is: 5000 mL/m²/% burned surface + 2000 mL/m² total body surface area (maintenance). This fluid is designed to cover "third space" losses associated with capillary leaking. Half the estimated burn requirement is administered during the first 8 hr after admission, and the remaining burn fluid requirement is divided over the subsequent 16 hr. This estimated fluid replacement should be titrated so that it results in ≥1 mL/kg/hr of urine output. During the second 24 hr, dextrose water in 0.25 normal saline is substituted for this regimen. Controversy exists over whether and when to administer colloid during fluid resuscitation. Colloid therapy may be needed only for burns ≥30%, and is given 8 to 24 hr from injury as 12.5 g of albumin in each liter of Ringer's lactated solution.

Because burn injury produces a hypermetabolic response, children with significant burns require immediate nutritional support. Although enteral feeding may be resumed on the 2nd or 3rd day of therapy, children with critical burn injury require parenteral nutritional support. The hypermetabolic state can be modulated to a degree through the effective management of anxiety and pain (sedation, analgesia) and the prevention of hypothermia by maintenance of a neutral thermal environment.

## INITIAL WOUND CARE

Wound care requires careful surgical management. The treatment is simple and noninvasive, and the involved areas should be covered with a sterile sheet. Wrapping with plastic, particularly for circumferential burns, may increase the child's comfort. Initial surgical attempts focus on relieving any pressure on the peripheral circulation by the developing eschar; then débridement is required for reclassifying the injury, a procedure that must occur prior to administering any topical therapy. After débridement, burns are generally covered with silver sulfadiazine (1%) applied to fine-mesh gauze or, if the burn is shallow, with polymyxin B/ bacitracin–neomycin (Neosporin) ointment. Silver nitrate (0.5%) and 11.1% mafenide acetate (painful,

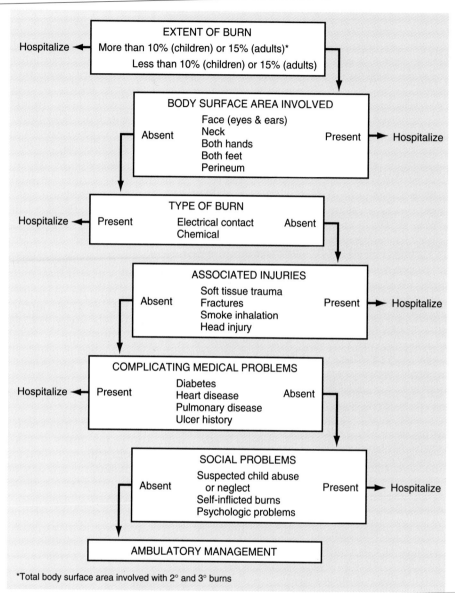

FIGURE 3–2. Triage of the burned patient. Additional considerations for hospitalization include involvement of major joints, third-degree burns of greater than 5%, and poor guardianship at home regarding wound care. (From Wachtel TL: Epidemiology, classification, initial care and administrative considerations for critically burned patients. Crit Care Clin 1:3–26, 1985.)

produces metabolic acidosis, penetrates eschar) are alternate antimicrobial agents. Such agents inhibit but do not prevent bacterial growth. Various grafts also have been used initially to cover wounds (cadaver allografts, porcine xenografts, artificial bilaminate [cross-linked chondroitin-6-sulfate, silicone] skin substitute, cultured patient's keratinocytes). For full-thickness burns, skin autografting and artificial skin substitutes are required for eventual closure. Burn management and rehabilitation are highly specialized skills and include recognizing many complications of burns (Table 3–9) and evaluating the wound and its cause for suspected child abuse or neglect. Tetanus toxoid and, if needed, immune globulin are indicated in the nonimmunized patient.

## PREVENTION

More than 600,000 children suffer burns each year; 94% occur in the home. Prevention is possible by using smoke and fire alarms, having identifiable escape routes and a fire extinguisher, and reducing hot water temperature to 120°F (49°C). Immersion full-thickness burns develop after 1 sec at 158°F (70°C), 5 sec at 140°F (60°C), 30 sec at 130°F (54.5°C), 60 sec at 127°F (53°C), 5 min at 122°F (50°C), and 10 min at 120°F (49°C).

TABLE 3–9.  Complications of Burns

| Problem | Treatment |
| --- | --- |
| Sepsis (*Staphylococcus aureus, Pseudomonas aeruginosa*) | Monitor for infection, avoid prophylactic antibiotics |
| Hypovolemia | Fluid replacement |
| Hypothermia | Adjust ambient temperature: dry blankets in field |
| Laryngeal edema | Endotracheal intubation, tracheostomy |
| Carbon monoxide poisoning | 100% $O_2$ |
| Cyanide poisoning | 100% $O_2$ plus amyl nitrate, sodium nitrate, and sodium thiosulfate |
| Cardiac dysfunction | Inotropic agents, diuretics |
| Curling gastric ulcers | $H_2$-receptor antagonist, antacids |
| Compartment syndrome | Escharotomy incision |
| Contractures | Physical therapy |
| Hypermetabolic state | Enteral and parenteral nutritional support |
| Renal failure | Supportive care, dialysis |
| Transient antidiuresis | Expectant management |
| Anemia | Transfusions as indicated |
| Psychologic trauma | Psychologic rehabilitation |
| Pulmonary infiltrates | |
| Burn injury | PEEP, ventilation, $O_2$ |
| Pulmonary edema | Avoid overhydration, give diuretics |
| Pneumonia | Antibiotics |
| Bronchospasm | Beta agonist aerosols |

PEEP = positive end-expiratory pressure.

### References

Behrman RE, Kliegman RM, Arvin AM (eds): Nelson Textbook of Pediatrics. 15th ed. Philadelphia, WB Saunders, 1996, Chapter 60.5.

Herdon DN, Rutan RL, Rutan TC: Management of the pediatric patient with burns. J Burn Care Rehab 14:3, 1993.

Monafo WW: Initial management of burns. N Engl J Med 335:1581, 1996.

Nguyen TT, Gilpin DA, Meyer NA, et al.: Current treatment of severely burned patients. Ann Surg 223:12, 1996.

# POISONING

## INGESTIONS

Accidental ingestions are most common in the 1–5 yr old age group, an incidence that reveals the young child's inquisitiveness and the adult's care-lessness in leaving drugs and household chemicals within reach. In older children, drug overdoses (poisonings) most often are associated with suicide attempts. Most ingestions are accidental (88%), occur in the home (92%), and produce no (82%) or minor (17%) toxicity; 0.01% are fatal. Common agents in young children include family members' medications, cleaning or polishing solutions, plants, and cosmetics. Fatal childhood poisonings are due to carbon monoxide, medications, hydrocarbons, and pesticides. The fatal medication poisonings are from salicylates, cyclic antidepressants, cardiovascular drugs, drugs of abuse, and pills containing iron.

### Clinical Assessment

Poisoning is usually a diagnosis of exclusion, but the history and physical examination often provide sufficient clues to distinguish between toxic ingestion and organic disease (Table 3–10). The comatose child should be considered to have ingested a poison until the facts prove otherwise. Because the comatose patient's history as well as physical examination may be unrevealing, using the toxicology laboratory to obtain information sometimes is helpful. Nonetheless, no toxicology screen can substitute for careful physical examination by someone who understands the signs and symptoms of various ingestions.

For a number of agents, the diagnosis can be established based on evaluating the level of consciousness; determining the pupillary size; and validating the presence of muscle fasciculations, cardiac arrhythmias, seizures, or hypothermia. Certain complexes of symptoms and signs are relatively specific to a given class of drugs (Table 3–11). Even in the absence of an obvious toxidrome, a careful and thorough examination is helpful in suggesting a diagnosis of poisoning. It also is important to determine whether the patient's vital signs are unstable, which warrants immediate supportive cardiopulmonary care.

The recognition of additional clinical manifestations is helpful in determining poisoning involving a particular agent (see Table 3–11). For example, an elevated body temperature may be related to sepsis or meningitis but also is typical of salicylate and anticholinergic overdose.

The patient's breath odors also may provide valuable clues to potential ingestions (see Table 3–10). A fruity smell may signify diabetic ketoacidosis, a silver polish smell is typical of cyanide, and a cleaning fluid–type odor is consistent with carbon tetrachloride ingestion. An evaluation of the lungs may reveal pulmonary edema, which can be due

TABLE 3–10.   Historic and Physical Findings in Poisoning

**Odor**
| | |
|---|---|
| Bitter almonds | Cyanide |
| Acetone | Isopropyl alcohol, methanol, salicylate |
| Alcohol | Ethanol |
| Wintergreen | Methyl salicylate |
| Garlic | Arsenic, thallium, organophosphates |
| Violets | Turpentine |

**Ocular Signs**
| | |
|---|---|
| Miosis | Narcotics (except meperidine), organophosphates, muscarinic mushrooms, clonidine, phenothiazines, chloral hydrate, barbiturates (late), PCP |
| Mydriasis | Atropine, alcohol, cocaine, amphetamines, antihistamines, cyclic antidepressants, cyanide, carbon monoxide |
| Nystagmus | Phenytoin, barbiturates, ethanol, carbon monoxide |
| Lacrimation | Organophosphates, irritant gas or vapors |
| Retinal hyperemia | Methanol |
| Poor vision | Methanol, botulism, carbon monoxide |

**Cutaneous Signs**
| | |
|---|---|
| Needle tracks | Heroin, PCP, amphetamine |
| Bullae | Carbon monoxide, barbiturates |
| Dry, hot skin | Anticholinergic agents, botulism |
| Diaphoresis | Organophosphates, nitrates, muscarinic mushrooms, aspirin, cocaine |
| Alopecia | Thallium, arsenic, lead, mercury |
| Erythema | Boric acid, mercury, cyanide, anticholinergics |

**Oral Signs**
| | |
|---|---|
| Salivation | Organophosphates, salicylate, corrosives, strychnine |
| Dry mouth | Amphetamine, anticholinergics, antihistamine |
| Burns | Corrosives, oxalate-containing plants |
| Gum lines | Lead, mercury, arsenic |
| Dysphagia | Corrosives, botulism |

**Intestinal Signs**
| | |
|---|---|
| Cramps | Arsenic, lead, thallium, organophosphates |
| Diarrhea | Arsenic, iron, boric acid |
| Constipation | Lead, narcotics, botulism |
| Hematemesis | Aminophylline, corrosives, iron, salicylates |

**Cardiac Signs**
| | |
|---|---|
| Tachycardia | Atropine, aspirin, amphetamine, cocaine, cyclic antidepressants, theophylline |
| Bradycardia | Digitalis, narcotics, mushrooms, clonidine, organophosphates, beta-blockers, calcium channel blockers |
| Hypertension | Amphetamine, LSD, cocaine, PCP |
| Hypotension | Phenothiazines, barbiturates, cyclic antidepressants, iron, beta-blockers, calcium channel blockers |

**Respiratory Signs**
| | |
|---|---|
| Depressed respiration | Alcohol, narcotics, barbiturates |
| Increased respiration | Amphetamines, aspirin, ethylene glycol, carbon monoxide, cyanide |
| Pulmonary edema | Hydrocarbons, heroin, organophosphates, aspirin |

**CNS Signs**
| | |
|---|---|
| Ataxia | Alcohol, antidepressants, barbiturates, anticholinergics, phenytoin, narcotics |
| Coma | Sedatives, narcotics, barbiturates, PCP, organophosphates, salicylate, cyanide, carbonmonoxide, cyclic antidepressants, lead |
| Hyperpyrexia | Anticholinergics, quinine, salicylates, LSD, phenothiazines, amphetamine, cocaine |
| Muscle fasciculation | Organophosphates, theophylline |
| Muscle rigidity | Cyclic antidepressants, PCP, phenothiazines, haloperidol |
| Paresthesia | Cocaine, camphor, PCP, MSG |
| Peripheral neuropathy | Lead, arsenic, mercury, organophosphates |
| Altered behavior | LSD, PCP, amphetamines, cocaine, alcohol, anticholinergics, camphor |

CNS = central nervous system; LSD = lysergic acid diethylamide; MSG = monosodium glutamate; PCP = phencyclidine.

TABLE 3–11.  Toxic Syndromes

| Agent | Manifestations |
|---|---|
| Acetaminophen | Nausea, vomiting, pallor, delayed jaundice–hepatic failure (72–96 hr) |
| Amphetamine, cocaine, and sympathomimetics | Tachycardia, hypertension, hyperthermia, psychosis/paranoia, seizures, mydriasis, diaphoresis, piloerection, aggressive behavior |
| Anticholinergics | Mania, delirium, fever, red dry skin, dry mouth, tachycardia, mydriasis, urinary retention |
| Carbon monoxide | Headache, dizziness, coma, skin bullae, other systems affected |
| Cyanide | Coma, convulsions, hyperpnea, bitter almond odor |
| Ethylene glycol (antifreeze) | Metabolic acidosis, hyperosmolarity, hypocalcemia, oxalate crystalluria |
| Iron | Vomiting (bloody), diarrhea, hypotension, hepatic failure, leukocytosis, hyperglycemia, radiopaque pills on KUB, late intestinal stricture, *Yersinia* sepsis |
| Narcotics | Coma, respiratory depression, hypotension, pinpoint pupils, hyporeflexia |
| Cholinergics (organophosphates, nicotine) | Miosis, salivation, urination, diaphoresis, lacrimation, bronchospasm (bronchorrhea), muscle weakness and fasciculations, emesis, defecation, coma, confusion, pulmonary edema, bradycardia, reduced erythrocyte and serum cholinesterase, late peripheral neuropathy |
| Phenothiazines | Tachycardia, hypotension, muscle rigidity, coma, ataxia, oculogyric crisis, miosis, radiopaque pills on KUB |
| Salicylates | Tachypnea, fever, lethargy, coma, vomiting, diaphoresis, alkalosis (early), acidosis (late) |
| Cyclic antidepressants | Coma, convulsions, mydriasis, hyperreflexia, arrhythmia (prolonged QT interval), cardiac arrest, shock |

KUB = kidney-ureter-bladder roentgenogram.

to cyclic antidepressants, organophosphates, or methaqualone.

## Major Patterns of Presentation

The poisoned child can present with any one of six basic clinical patterns: coma, toxicity, metabolic acidosis, heart rhythm aberrations, gastrointestinal symptoms, and seizures.

**Coma.** Coma is perhaps the most striking but leads to the greatest confusion because the comatose child is unarousable and unresponsive. Coma may be due to trauma, a cerebrovascular accident, a global asphyxial event, meningitis, or poisoning. A careful history and clinical examination are required to distinguish among these alternatives. The rapid loss of brain stem function usually suggests a supratentorial lesion, whereas the persistence of the pupillary light reflex in the presence of diminished respiratory effort and diminished level of consciousness often indicates a metabolic insult to the brain. The level of consciousness in the latter condition often is depressed out of proportion to other neurologic signs. Decorticate posturing strongly suggests structural or metabolic disorders rather than toxic ingestions. Pinpoint pupils suggest either a pontine lesion or the toxic ingestion of opiates, organophosphates, phenothiazines, or chloral hydrate. Dilated pupils often are associated with cyclic antidepressant overdoses (see Table 3–10). Structural lesions often may be accompanied by midpoint-fixed pupils or unilaterally dilated pupils and disturbances of ocular movement.

**Systemic and Pulmonary Toxicity.** *Hydrocarbon ingestion* may result in systemic and pulmonary (locally by aspiration) toxicity (Table 3–12). Halogenated hydrocarbons or those with toxic additives have the greatest systemic toxicities and should be removed by lavage. Hydrocarbons with low viscosity, low surface tension, and high volatility pose the greatest risk for producing aspiration pneumonia; once swallowed, however, they pose no risk unless emesis is induced. Emesis or lavage should *not* be initiated in the child who has ingested volatile hydrocarbons.

*Caustic ingestions* may cause dysphagia, epigastric pain, oral mucosal burns, and low-grade fever. Patients with esophageal lesions may have no oral burns or may have significant signs and symptoms. Treatment depends on the agent ingested and the

TABLE 3–12.   Acute Hydrocarbon Risk
            Assessments

**Systemic Toxicity Common***
  Trichloroethane (spot remover), trichlorethylene, carbon
   tetrachloride, methylene chloride, benzene, hydrocarbon
   additives (camphor, heavy metals, insecticides, aniline),
   toluene

**Local Toxicity by Aspiration Common,† Systemic Toxicity
Uncommon**
  Mineral seal oil, signal oil, furniture polish, turpentine,
   gasoline, kerosene, charcoal lighter fluid, toluene

**Nontoxic in 95% of Cases**
  Asphalt, tar, motor oil, mineral or liquid petroleum,
   lubricants, baby oil

*Chronic abuse of volatile hydrocarbons (e.g., sniffing) may cause
ataxia, tremor, seizures, coma, myopathy, peripheral neuropathy, and
renal tubular defects. Lead poisoning also is noted with abuse of lead-
containing gasoline.
†Hydrocarbons of low viscosity (30–60 standard Saybold universal
seconds [SSU]), low surface tension, and high volatility have the greatest
risk for inducing aspiration pneumonia.

presence or absence of esophageal injury. *Alkali agents* may be solid, granular, or liquid (Liquid Drano, 9.5% sodium hydroxide [NaOH]; Liquid Plumber, 8% potassium hydroxide [KOH]). Both of the latter agents are tasteless and produce full-thickness liquefaction necrosis of the esophagus or oropharynx. When the esophageal lesions heal, strictures form. There also is a long-term risk of esophageal carcinoma. Many do not recommend the routine use of diluents as a first aid measure because of the lack of proven efficacy and the potential risk of induced vomiting. Subsequent treatment includes antibiotics if there are signs of infection and dilation of late-forming (2–3 wk) strictures.

*Ingested button batteries* also may produce a caustic mucosal injury from NaOH, KOH, or mercuric oxide. If they pass to the stomach, no further therapy is needed because they are likely to be passed in the stool within a week. Those that do not pass through the esophagus may cause esophageal burns and erosion and should be removed with the endoscope.

*Acid agents*, such as Lysol Toilet Bowl Cleaner (8.5% hydrochloric acid [HCl]) or Vanish Toilet Bowl Cleaner (65% sodium acid sulfate), can injure the lungs (HCl fumes), oral mucosa, esophagus, and stomach. Because acids taste sour, children will immediately stop drinking the solution, thus limiting the injury. Acids produce a coagulation necrosis, which limits the chemical from penetrating into deeper layers of the mucosa and, therefore, damages tissue less severely than alkali. The signs and symptoms and initial therapeutic measures (dilution, no emesis or neutralization) are similar to those for alkali ingestion.

**Metabolic Acidosis.** The poisoned child also may present with metabolic acidosis (Table 3–13), which is assessed easily by measuring arterial blood gases, serum electrolytes, and urine pH. De-

TABLE 3–13.   Screening Laboratory Clues in Toxicologic Diagnosis

| Metabolic Acidosis (Mnemonic = MUDPIES) | | Radiopaque Substance on KUB (Mnemonic = CHIPPED) |
|---|---|---|
| Methanol,* carbon monoxide | Isoniazid, iron | Chloral hydrate, calcium carbonate |
| Uremia* | Ethanol,* ethylene glycol* | Heavy metals (lead, zinc, barium, arsenic, lithium, bismuth as in Pepto-Bismol) |
| Diabetes mellitus* | Salicylates, starvation, seizures | Iron |
| Paraldehyde,* phenformin | | Phenothiazines |
| **Hypoglycemia** | | Pla-Doh, potassium chloride |
| Ethanol | | Enteric-coated pills |
| Isoniazid | | Dental amalgam |
| Insulin | | |
| Propranolol | | |
| **Hyperglycemia** | | |
| Salicylates | | |
| Isoniazid | | |
| Iron | | |
| Phenothiazine | | |
| Sympathomimetics | | |
| **Hypocalcemia** | | |
| Oxalate | | |
| Ethylene glycol | | |
| Fluoride | | |

*Indicates hyperosmolar condition.
KUB = kidney-ureter-bladder roentgenogram.

termining serum sodium, potassium, chloride, glucose, urea nitrogen, and carbon dioxide ($CO_2$) levels permits the calculation of the serum anion gap (see Chapter 16) and osmolality

$$(Osm = 2 \times Na + (glucose/18) + (BUN/2.8)$$

which may be compared with measured osmolality. A difference of more than 10 between the measured and calculated osmolality, an **osmolal gap**, strongly suggests the presence of an unmeasured component, such as methanol or ethylene glycol. Because these ingestions require thorough assessment and prompt intervention, this approach allows a tentative diagnosis to be made pending access to the toxicology laboratory.

**Rhythm Abnormalities.** Rhythm abnormalities may be prominent signs of a variety of toxic ingestions, although ventricular arrhythmias are rare. Prolonged QT intervals may suggest phenothiazine or antihistamine ingestion, and widened QRS complexes are seen with cyclic antidepressants and quinidine. Because many drug and chemical overdoses may lead to sinus tachycardia, it is not a useful or discriminating sign; sinus bradycardia, however, should suggest digoxin, cyanide, or beta-blocker ingestion. A full 12-lead electrocardiogram should be part of the initial evaluation in all patients suspected of suffering from ingestions (Table 3–14).

**Gastrointestinal Symptoms.** Gastrointestinal symptoms of poisoning include emesis, nausea, abdominal cramps, and diarrhea. These may be due to direct toxic effects on the intestinal mucosa or to systemic toxicity following absorption.

**Seizures.** Seizures are the sixth major mode of presentation for children with toxic ingestions, but poisoning is an uncommon cause of afebrile seizures. When seizures do occur with intoxication, they may be life-threatening and require aggressive therapeutic intervention (see Table 3–14).

### Initial Therapy

**Supportive Care.** Prompt attention must be given to protecting and clearing the airway, establishing effective breathing, and supporting the circulation. This management sequence takes precedence over other diagnostic or therapeutic procedures. If there is a depressed level of consciousness and a toxic substance is suspected, glucose (1 g/kg IV), 100% oxygen, and naloxone should be administered. Laboratory studies helpful in the initial management include specific toxin-drug assays, arterial blood gases, electrolytes, blood glucose, electrocardiogram, and the calculation of the anion or osmolar gap. Urine screens for drugs of abuse or to confirm suspected ingestion of medications in the home may be revealing.

**Gastric Decontamination.** There is controversy about the most effective and safe means for gastric emptying and prevention of absorption of a toxic substance.

*Syrup of Ipecac.* Syrup of ipecac has been suggested as the drug of choice for ensuring rapid

TABLE 3–14. Drugs Associated with Major Modes of Presentation

| Common Toxic Causes of Cardiac Arrhythmia | Causes of Coma | Common Agents Causing Seizures (Mnemonic = CAPS) |
|---|---|---|
| Amphetamine | Alcohol | Camphor |
| Antiarrhythmics | Anticholinergics | Carbamazepine |
| Anticholinergics | Antihistamines | Carbon monoxide |
| Antihistamines | Barbiturates | Cocaine |
| Arsenic | Carbon monoxide | Cyanide |
| Carbon monoxide | Clonidine | |
| Chloral hydrate | Cyanide | Aminophylline |
| Cocaine | Cyclic antidepressants | Amphetamine |
| Cyanide | Hypoglycemic agents | Anticholinergics |
| Cyclic antidepressants | Lead | Antidepressants (cyclic) |
| Digitalis | Lithium | |
| Freon | Methemoglobinemia* | Pb (lead) (also lithium) |
| Phenothiazines | Methyldopa | Pesticide (organophosphate) |
| Physostigmine | Narcotics | Phencyclidine |
| Propranolol | Phencyclidine | Phenol |
| Quinine, quinidine | Phenothiazines | Phenothiazines |
| Theophylline | Salicylates | Proproxyphene |
| | | Salicylates |
| | | Strychnine |

*Causes of methemoglobinemia: amyl nitrite, aniline dyes, benzocaine, bismuth subnitrate, dapsone, primaquine, quinones, spinach, sulfonamides.

gastric emptying in patients of all ages with an acute ingestion. Ipecac works best if given immediately after the ingestion (e.g., at home), removes more gastric contents than lavage, and is more effective for substances (pills) too large to be removed by lavage and those toxins not absorbed by activated charcoal. Most toxicologists agree that ipecac has no role in the emergency department setting. The delayed and prolonged emesis may increase the risk of aspiration pneumonia and reduce the ability to administer the more effective activated charcoal. Doses of 15 mL (1 tablespoon) in children over the age of 1 yr and 30 mL (2 tablespoons) in adolescent and adult patients are effective in inducing emesis within 30 min of administration in 85–95% of patients. The response rate is improved to almost 100% if a second dose is given to those who have not responded to the first dose. In children under 1 yr of age, self-administered toxic ingestions are rare, but 1 mL/kg doses of syrup of ipecac have proved safe and effective.

It is recommended that syrup of ipecac be in the home of every family with children under the age of 12 yr, but it should be used only at the direction of a physician or the local poison control center. Syrup of ipecac is *contraindicated* in the comatose child, the child who has ingested a caustic agent, and the child younger than 6 mo of age, and in the presence of a foreign body, absent bowel sounds (ileus), shock, increased intracranial pressure, hypertension, pregnancy, drugs with rapid onset of central nervous system depression, and certain volatile petroleum distillates.

*Adverse reactions* to syrup of ipecac are rare when it is used as directed. These reactions include mild diarrhea, lethargy, irritability, and fever. Syrup of ipecac has been abused by young adolescent patients with anorexia nervosa and bulimia. This type of chronic overdose has been associated with cardiomyopathy and death.

*Gastric Lavage.* This procedure is an alternative to syrup of ipecac for patients who go to the hospital. Lavage does not interfere with activated charcoal and should be used in potentially lethal ingestions or with toxins not absorbed by activated charcoal. A large-diameter tube is placed into the stomach by either the nasal or oral route. Normal saline is recommended for lavage to prevent or minimize any electrolyte disturbances; cycles of 15 mL/kg are recommended, but large total volumes (5–20 L) are required for effectively removing toxins.

In children presenting in coma, gastric lavage should be undertaken only after intubation with a cuffed endotracheal tube. No intubation is required for children who are awake. In the responsive but obtunded child, endotracheal intubation may be necessary prior to gastric intubation, and this decision will require clinical judgment. Lavage is *contraindicated* in children who ingest caustic materials or hydrocarbons and in the presence of neurologic symptoms (coma, seizures) likely to impair normal mechanisms that are protective of the airway. Lavage is rarely indicated in patients who present more than one hour after ingestion.

*Complications* of gastric lavage include aspiration pneumonia, which appears secondary to vomiting during the lavage procedure, and laryngospasm, related to kinking of the lavage tube in the esophagus. Esophageal perforation also has been reported.

***Activated Charcoal.*** A binder, activated charcoal may be used as a primary gastric decontaminant with or without induced gastric emptying. Activated charcoal is prepared by pyrolyzing organic materials, such as wood pulp, and then activating them by exposing them to an oxidizing gas flow at a high temperature, which produces a fine network of pores.

Activated charcoal adsorbs a wide variety of organic materials from the gastrointestinal tract in a process that occurs within the first few minutes following administration. Because the surface area contained in the charcoal is large and because activated charcoal exhibits a relative affinity for certain compounds, it may prevent absorption of the toxin from the intestine. The charcoal also may serve as a reservoir for drugs removed from the blood that perfuses the intestine. Multiple doses of charcoal may enhance the elimination of numerous drugs that undergo enterohepatic recirculation, secretion across the gastric membranes into the bowel lumen, or continued prolonged absorption. Administering charcoal in divided doses over 72 hr is very effective in reducing the plasma half-life of phenobarbital, theophylline, digoxin, and methotrexate. An alternative to this intermittent dosing is administering the charcoal by continuous nasogastric infusion. Activated charcoal is ineffective against caustic or corrosive agents, hydrocarbons, alcohols, heavy metals (arsenic, lead, mercury, iron, lithium), glycols, and water-insoluble compounds. Charcoal may be given concomitantly with enteral *N*-acetylcysteine (NAC) therapy of acetaminophen ingestion; NAC is given in sufficiently high doses to overcome any clinical interference.

A dose of 15–30 g should be used for small children and a dose of 50–100 g for children older than 12 yr of age; alternatively; 1–2 g/kg can be given safely and effectively. The acceptance of oral charcoal as a slurry in water is variable, but its poor palatability may cause problems, and thus a variety of maneuvers have been attempted to increase its acceptance, including flavoring, cocoa powders, sweeteners, thickeners, and presentation in soft drink cans. If these fail, the charcoal may be given by nasogastric intubation.

One of the difficulties encountered with using multiple doses of charcoal relates to the effects when it is combined with cathartic agents, such as sorbitol. Several charcoal preparations are prepackaged in a slurry with 70% sorbitol. The sorbitol may result in significant diarrhea and fluid and electrolyte loss. In contrast, the use of activated charcoal alone in children may cause constipation. When multiple or continuous infusions of charcoal are used, the dose of sorbitol must be adjusted so that the amount being given is sufficient to prevent constipation, but not so much as to cause significant diarrhea. Hydration status must be rigorously monitored in these children. *Contraindications* include caustic or corrosive agents, an ileus, and poor control of the airway.

*Other Methods.* Catharsis alone (sorbitol, magnesium citrate) is an ineffective decontamination method. Whole-bowel irrigation (catharsis) removes coalesced pills (iron ingestion) and employs polyethylene glycol (GoLYTELY) as a nonabsorbable cathartic.

## Additional Therapy

After the initial resuscitation and gastric decontamination have been achieved, it is often difficult to determine whether or not further therapy is needed. There are basically three choices in the subsequent care of the child with a significant ingestion: (1) providing continued supportive care, (2) using specific antidotes where available, and (3) actively removing the toxin from the blood stream. In order to make a rational decision regarding these options, a judgment should be made as to whether or not the drug causes tissue damage (methyl alcohol, aspirin, acetaminophen, theophylline, iron, ethylene glycol). *Tissue damage* is defined as an irreversible or slowly reversible structural or functional change in an organ system as a direct result of ingestion of a poison; this definition precludes indirect effects such as respiratory depression or hypotension.

The decision should take into consideration (1) the amount taken; (2) the diagnostic assessment, including the condition of the patient at the time of presentation; and (3) the natural history of the suspected type of ingestion. All of these variables may be influenced by the child's prior clinical status or underlying medical problems. For example, in a patient with underlying severe hepatic or renal impairment, a more aggressive approach involving active removal might be selected, even though the ingestion ordinarily would require only the use of simple supportive care. Moreover, in the presence of a chronic ingestion, an acute overdose may require a lower dosage of the drug to cause significant clinical toxicity.

For most common ingestions, continued supportive care and treatment directed toward specific complications are appropriate for otherwise healthy individuals. Specific antidotes should be used according to prescribed guidelines (Table 3–15). Active removal (hemoperfusion, dialysis) should be undertaken only for those toxins that may cause tissue damage, those that have been ingested by a patient already exhibiting confounding medical problems, or to avoid very prolonged supportive care.

**Toxicology assays** are important for some agents, not only for identifying the specific drug but also for providing guidance for therapy and help in anticipating complications and estimating the prognosis. Serum iron levels below 300 μg/dL usually are safe following iron ingestion, but levels of free iron above 600 μg/dL usually are associated with significant toxicity. The timing of the physician's testing of the plasma level relative to the time of the patient's ingesting the drug also is useful in predicting the severity of illness for acetaminophen (Fig. 3–3) and salicylate (Fig. 3–4). Patients with drug levels (related to the time after ingestion) in the serious zone warrant immediate treatment.

## Preventing Ingestions

Most ingestions occur in the home, and the toxins involved are common household medications, household cleaning and work solutions, or vitamins. Accidental poisonings are more frequent in children under 5 yr of age, in boys, in families of low socioeconomic status, and during times of family disorganization; they occur most frequently in the kitchen, bathroom, or garage. Properly educating parents to use childproof medication containers, to store toxic substances in locked cabinets, and to label toxic chemicals properly is necessary for preventing ingestions. Kerosene and other toxic liquids should not be stored in soda pop bottles, and children should not come in contact with clothing exposed to pesticides. Old or unused medications should be discarded, and currently used medications should not be left on tabletops or in the mother's purse. If a child has ingested poison, the poison control center should be called. All households should have 30 mL of syrup of ipecac avail-

TABLE 3–15.    Emergency Antidotes

| Poison | Antidote | Dosage | Comments |
| --- | --- | --- | --- |
| Acetaminophen | N-Acetylcysteine | 140 mg/kg PO initial dose, then 70 mg/kg PO q4h × 17 doses | Most effective within 16 hr |
| Atropine | Physostigmine | Initial dose 0.01–0.1 mg/kg IV | Can produce convulsions, bradycardia |
| Benzodiazepine | Flumazenil | 0.1–0.3 mg IV adult dose | Possible seizures, arrhythmias |
| Beta-blocking agents | Atropine Isoproterenol | 0.01–0.10 mg/kg IV 0.05–5 μg/kg/min IV infusion | |
| | Glucagon | 1 mg IV | |
| Carbon monoxide | Oxygen | 100%; hyperbaric $O_2$ | Half-life of carboxyhemoglobin is 5 hr in room air but 1.5 hr in 100% $O_2$ |
| Coumarin | Vitamin K | 2.5–10 mg IV/IM | Monitor PT; fresh frozen plasma or plasma for acute bleeding; repeated vitamin K for super-warfarin |
| Cyanide | Amyl nitrite, then | 1–2 pearls every 2 min | Methemoglobin-cyanide complex |
| | Sodium nitrite | Initially 0.33 mL (10 mg 3% sol)/kg IV | Causes hypotension; dosage assumes normal hemoglobin |
| | Sodium thiosulfate | 25% solution; 1.65 mg/kg IV over 10 min | Forms harmless sodium thiocyanate |
| Cyclic antidepressants | Sodium bicarbonate | To produce pH 7.5–7.55 | — |
| Digoxin, digitoxin | Digoxin-specific Fab antibody fragments | Dose based on serum digoxin concentration and body weight; 1 vial (40 mg) neutralizes 0.6 mg digoxin | With acute life-threatening ingestion, dose and serum concentration are unknown; give contents of 20 vials |
| Iron | Deferoxamine | Initial dose 15 mg/kg/hr IV | Deferoxamine mesylate—forms excretable ferrioxamine complex; hypotension |
| Isoniazid | Pyridoxine | 1 mg/mg isoniazid | — |
| Lead | Edetate calcium (calcium disodium versenate [EDTA]) | 1500 mg/m²/day × 5 days; divided q6h or by continuous infusion | May lower to 1000 mg/m²/day if given with BAL; nephrotoxic |
| | BAL (British antiLewisite [dimercaprol]) | 500 mg/m²/day IM divided q4h × 3 days | May cause hypertension and sterile abscesses |
| | Penicillamine | 20 mg/kg/day PO divided q8h | Requires weekly monitoring for hepatic and bone marrow toxicity; should not be used in the presence of ongoing ingestion |
| | 2,3-dimercaptosuccinic acid (DMSA) | 30 mg/kg/day PO t.i.d. × 5 days then 20 mg/kg/day PO b.i.d. × 14 days | Few toxic effects, requires lead-free home plus compliant family |
| Mercury, arsenic, gold | BAL (British antiLewisite) | 5 mg/kg IM as soon as possible | Each mL BAL in oil has dimercaprol, 100 mg in 210 mL (21%) benzyl benzoate, and 680 mL peanut oil—forms stable nontoxic excretable cyclic compound |
| Methyl alcohol (ethylene glycol) | Ethyl alcohol in conjunction with dialysis | 1 mL/kg of 100% ethanol initially in glucose solution; maintain blood level of 100 mg/dL | Competes for alcohol dehydrogenase; prevents formation of formic acid and oxalates |
| Nitrites/Methemo-globinemia* | Methylene blue | 1–2 mg/kg, repeat in 1–4 hr if needed; treat for levels >30% | Exchange transfusion may be needed for severe methemoglobinemia; methylene blue overdose also causes methemoglobinemia |

TABLE 3–15.  Emergency Antidotes *Continued*

| Poison | Antidote | Dosage | Comments |
|---|---|---|---|
| Opiates, Darvon, Lomotil | Naloxone | 0.10 mg/kg IV, ET, SC, IM for children, up to 2 mg | Naloxone causes no respiratory depression (0.4 mg/1 mL ampule) |
| Organophosphates | Atropine | Initial dose 0.05–1.0 mg/kg IV | Physiologic: blocks acetylcholine; up to 5 mg IV every 15 min may be necessary in the critically ill adult patient |
| | Pralidoxime (2 PAM-chloride) (Protopam) | Initial dose 25–50 mg/kg IV | Specific: disrupts phosphate–cholinesterase bond; up to 500 mg/hr may be necessary in the critically ill adult patient |
| Sympathomimetic agents | Blocking agents: phentolamine; beta-blocking agents; other antihypertensives | | Must be used in a setting in which vital signs can be monitored effectively |

Data from Haddad LM, Winchester JF (eds): Clinical Management of Poisoning and Drug Overdose. Philadelphia, WB Saunders, 1983; Kulig K: Initial management of ingestions of toxic substances. N Engl J Med 326:1677, 1992; and Barkin R: Toxicologic emergencies. Pediatr Ann 19:629, 1990.
*See Table 3-14 for causes of methemoglobinemia.

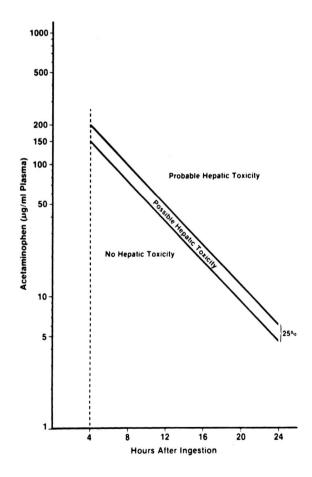

FIGURE 3–3. Semi-logarithmic plot of plasma acetaminophen levels versus time. Rumack-Matthew nomogram for acetaminophen poisoning. Cautions for use of this chart: (1) the time coordinates refer to time of ingestion; (2) serum levels drawn before 4 hr may not represent peak levels; (3) the graph should be used only in relation to a single, acute ingestion; and (4) the lower solid line, 25% below the standard nomogram, is included to allow for possible errors in acetaminophen plasma assays and estimated time from ingestion of an overdose. (Adapted from Rumack BH, Matthew H: Acetaminophen poisoning and toxicity. Pediatrics 55:871, 1975, with permission from the authors and the publisher.)

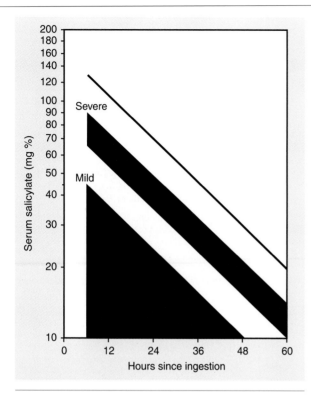

FIGURE 3–4. Nomogram relating serum salicylate concentration and expected severity of intoxication at various intervals following the ingestion of a single dose of salicylate. (From Done AK: Salicylate intoxication: Significance of measurements of salicylate in blood in cases of acute ingestion. Pediatrics 26:800, 1960.)

able and ready to administer as directed by the poison control center personnel or the physician.

### BITES, STINGS, AND ENVENOMATIONS

Toxic reactions to saliva or venom of living creatures or injuries caused by them are common and depend on exposure, provocation, and the species of specific indigenous insects or animals, or those encountered during travel. Most reactions produce local inflammation, with little progression or systemic manifestations. Some reactions may represent allergic responses to insect antigens (papular urticaria), whereas others may result in tissue necrosis, infection, paralysis, and death (Table 3–16).

### References

Behrman RE, Kliegman RM, Arvin AM (eds): Nelson Textbook of Pediatrics, 15th ed. Philadelphia, WB Saunders, 1996, Chapters 665–669.

Fine JS, Goldfrank LR: Update in medical toxicology. Pediatr Clin North Am 39:1031, 1992.

Goldfrank LR, et al (eds): Toxicologic Emergencies, 5th ed. Norwalk, CT, Appleton and Lange, 1994.

Kulig K: Initial management of ingestions of toxic substances. N Engl J Med 326:1677, 1992.

Litovitz T, Manoguerra A: Comparison of pediatric poisoning hazards: An analysis of 3.8 million exposure incidents. Pediatrics 89:999, 1992.

Vale JA, Proudfoot AT: How useful is activated charcoal? BMJ 306:78, 1993.

## SHOCK

Shock may result from a number of relatively common childhood disorders, including gastroenteritis, diabetes mellitus, trauma, infection, and accidental drug ingestion. The best opportunity to improve the clinical outcome of shock depends on early recognition and prompt, appropriate treatment.

Oxygen delivery is directly related to the arterial oxygen content (oxygen saturation, hemoglobin concentration) and cardiac output. Changes in metabolic needs are met primarily by adjustments in cardiac output, which are determined by the amount of blood ejected from the left ventricle (stroke volume) and by the heart rate (Fig. 3–5). Stroke volume is related to myocardial end-diastolic fiber length (preload), myocardial contractility (inotropy), and resistance of blood ejection from the ventricle (afterload) (see Chapter 13). In the young infant whose myocardium possesses relatively less contractile tissue, increased demand for cardiac output is met primarily by a neurally mediated increase in heart rate. In the older child and adult, cardiac output is most efficiently augmented by increasing stroke volume through neurohumorally mediated changes in vascular tone, resulting in increased venous return to the heart (increased preload), decreased arterial resistance (decreased afterload), and increased myocardial contractility.

### SHOCK SYNDROMES
(Table 3–17; Fig. 3–6)

#### Hypovolemic Shock

Acute hypovolemia is the most common cause of shock in pediatric patients and results from blood loss, from fluid and electrolyte depletion secondary to vomiting and diarrhea, from third space fluid losses due to capillary leak syndromes, and from pathologic renal fluid losses (Table 3–17). Hypovolemic shock is distinguished from other causes of shock by history and by the absence of signs of

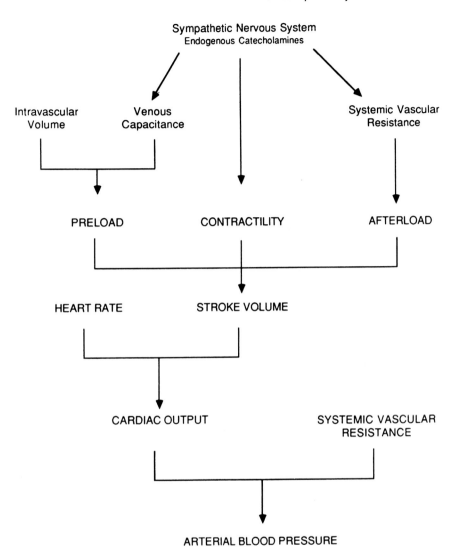

FIGURE 3–5. Determinants of cardiac output and arterial blood pressure. (From Witte MK, Hill JH, Blumer JL: Shock in the pediatric patient. Adv Pediatr 34:139–174, 1987.)

heart failure (such as hepatomegaly, rales, edema, jugular venous distention, or a gallop) or of sepsis (fever, leukocytosis, or focal infection). Reduced blood volume causes a decreased preload, stroke volume, and cardiac output. Recovery depends on the degree of hypovolemia, the patient's pre-existing status, and rapid diagnosis and treatment. The prognosis is good, with a low mortality (<10%) in uncomplicated cases.

Compensatory mechanisms include increased sympathoadrenal activity, which produces increased heart rate and myocardial contractility. Neurohumorally mediated constriction of the arterioles and capacitance vessels also maintains blood pressure, augments venous return to the heart to improve preload, and redistributes blood flow from nonvital to vital organs. Increased heart rate may impair coronary blood flow and ventricular

filling; elevated systemic vascular resistance increases myocardial oxygen consumption, resulting in poorer myocardial function. Intense systemic vaso-constriction and hypovolemia produce tissue ischemia, which impairs cell metabolism and releases potent vasoactive mediators from injured cells. The latter include arachidonic acid metabolites, cytokines, and other vasoactive peptides, which change myocardial contractility, vascular tone, and membrane permeability.

### Distributive Shock

Abnormalities in the distribution of blood flow may result in profound inadequacies in tissue perfusion, even in the presence of a normal or high cardiac output. These maldistributions of flow usually result from abnormalities in vascular tone.

TABLE 3–16.   Bites, Stings, and Envenomations

| Species | Characteristics | Agents or Venoms | Treatment |
|---|---|---|---|
| **Snakes** | | | |
| Pit vipers: rattlesnake, copperhead, cotton mouth; triangular head, elliptical pupils, heat-sensing pits | Strike on provocation; site: hand, leg, foot; only 75% of bites have venom release; pain, swelling, ecchymosis ± coagulopathy, rhabdomyolysis, shock, weakness, hemolysis; bites of head and neck are most severe | Phospholipases, proteases, hyaluronidase, thrombin, Mojave (paralytic) toxin | Keep extremity dependent, immobilized; avoid ice, aspirin; mechanically extract venom; gentle tourniquet; treat shock; antivenom (polyvalent) if severe*; tetanus check†; antibiotics‡ |
| Coral snake (cobra, mamba family) | Local pain and edema, hypesthesia, paresthesia, fasciculations, weakness, bulbar palsy, descending paralysis, respiratory paralysis | Paralytic toxin | Antivenom if severe* |
| Sea snake | Pinprick lesion, paralysis, myoglobinuria | Neurotoxin, phospholipase | Antivenom, antibiotics‡ |
| **Scorpions** | Usually benign; local pain, tingling, hypesthesia; paralysis, agitation, seizures rare; tachycardia, hypertension | Sympathetic and parasympathetic nervous system toxin | No treatment unless severe, then antitoxin; propranolol for tachyarrhythmia |
| **Hymenoptera** See Chapter 8 for allergy and anaphylaxis | | | |
| **Ticks** | Paralysis (spring, summer); tick located in scalp, groin | Paralytic toxin in saliva | Remove tick with forceps or gauze by constant, gentle, upward motion; prevention: DEET, permethrins |
| **Spiders** Black widow | Punctate lesions, local erythema, and immediate pain, muscle rigidity, spasms, abdominal pain, periorbital edema, hypertension, diaphoresis; spider has red hourglass marking on abdomen; lives in moist dark outdoor sites | Polypeptides producing spontaneous motor neuron depolarization | Analgesics, diazepam, intravenous calcium; antivenom if severe* |
| Brown recluse | Fiddle shape over cephalothorax; lives in dark, indoor dry areas; necrotic painful, pruritic skin lesion; vesiculation, hemorrhage, and eschar formation; hemolysis, DIC, headache, seizures | Sphingomyelinase, protease, esterase, hyaluronidase, hemolysin | Wound débridement; ice; Dapsone; steroids(?) |

TABLE 3–16.  Bites, Stings, and Envenomations *Continued*

| Species | Characteristics | Agents or Venoms | Treatment |
|---|---|---|---|
| Tarantula | Local pain, swelling, urticaria from hairs; usually benign | Polyamines, hyaluronidase | Analgesics, ice; remove hair with tape |
| *Marine Envenomation*<br>Stingray | Defensive attack; laceration, puncture plus venom; pain, edema, bleeding, limb paralysis | Serotonin, phosphodiesterase | Antivenom, hot water immersion, surgical wound exploration |
| Jellyfish, Portuguese man-of-war | Burning, painful urticaria, pain, lymphadenopathy, anaphylaxis, fever, chills, muscle spasm, paralysis, hypotension | Bradykinin, histamine, hyaluronidase, phosphodiesterase | Remove tentacles, avoid fresh water; topical vinegar, corticosteroids, papain, isopropyl alcohol; calcium IV |
| *Reptiles*<br>Gila monster | Local pain, edema, cyanosis, hypotension; animal jaws may clamp around the wound | Serotonin, phospholipase, protease, hyaluronidase | Analgesics, ice, immobilization; remove reptile |
| Toads | Salivation, cyanosis; seizures from placing toads in mouth | Bufotoxin | Supportive care |
| *Mammals*<br>Humans | Directly from a bite or indirectly from a fist fight; laceration, swelling, erythema, cellulitis | *Eikenella corrodens, Staphylococcus aureus,* streptococcal species | Débridement; tetanus check†; augmentin, nafcillin |
| Dogs | Swelling, erythema, cellulitis, lymphangitis; laceration, crush injury, tenosynovitis | *S. aureus,* streptococci; rabies | Débridement; tetanus check†; antibiotics per culture; rabies check |
| Cats | Laceration, swelling, cellulitis, osteomyelitis, tenosynovitis | *Pasteurella multocida, S. aureus,* streptococci; rabies | As for dogs; penicillin/ ampicillin for *P. multocida* |
| Rats | Local pain, inflammation (common); rat bite fever (rare) with chills, fever, leukocytosis, rash, arthritis, abscesses, endocarditis, may relapse (*Streptobacillus moniliformis*); *Spirillum minus* produces suppurative bite lesion | Skin, mouth flora; no rabies; *S. moniliformis; S. minus;* plague, leptospirosis | Penicillin for rat bite fever |
| Raccoons, skunks, foxes | Laceration, pain, swelling | Rabies, plus mouth and skin flora | Rabies vaccine and rabies immunoglobulin; tetanus check† |

Data from Banner W: Bites and stings in the pediatric patient. Curr Probl Pediatr 28:1, 1988;  Auerbach PS: Marine environments. N Engl J Med 325:486, 1991; and Gentile DA, Kennedy BC: Wilderness medicine for children. Pediatrics 88:967, 1991.
*Types of antivenom that are prepared in animals (horse, goat) as hyperimmune serum and as foreign proteins may cause anaphylaxis.
†Tetanus check for all animal bites includes evaluation for need of tetanus immune globulin and booster vaccine.
‡Antibiotics to treat human cutaneous and animal mouth flora.
DEET = diethyltoluamide; DIC = disseminated intravascular coagulation; ? = effect unproved.

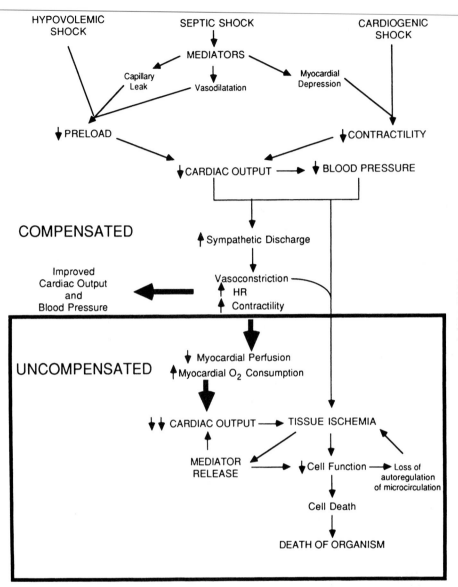

FIGURE 3–6. Sequence of pathophysiologic events in the clinical shock state. HR = heart rate. (From Witte MK, Hill JH, Blumer JL: Shock in the pediatric patient. Adv Pediatr 34:139–174, 1987.)

*Septic shock* is the most common type of distributive shock in children. It is commonly a complication of sepsis caused by gram-positive and gram-negative bacteria as well as infection due to rickettsiae and viruses (Table 3–18 and Fig. 3–7). Patients usually have fever, lethargy, petechiae or purpura, and an identified infectious focus. They often have tachycardia and poor peripheral perfusion, with cool, mottled extremities and poor capillary refill time. Hypotension, intense vasoconstriction, and a decreased cardiac index are present. Widespread cellular dysfunction, resulting from inadequate tissue perfusion in the early phases of shock, subsequently leads to diminishing organ function. In the early stages of shock, patients may be febrile and tachycardiac, with warm, flushed skin and poor urine output ("warm shock"). Systemic arterial blood pressure is normal, and cardiac output is normal or increased. The diagnosis of warm shock requires a high index of suspicion on the part of the physician and usually is made in the setting of a predisposing condition, such as a known infection or immunosuppression (see Chapter 10).

In the systemic inflammatory response syndrome (see Table 3–18 and Fig. 3–7), bacterial products stimulate the elaboration of a wide variety of vasoactive and inflammatory mediators. Endotoxins are bacterial cell wall lipopolysaccharides that activate macrophage production of tumor necrosis factor (TNF) and interleukin-1 (IL-1) in addition to

TABLE 3–17.  Classification of Shock and Common Underlying Causes

| Type | Primary Circulatory Derangement | Common Causes |
|---|---|---|
| Hypovolemic | Decreased circulating blood volume | Hemorrhage<br>Diarrhea<br>Diabetes insipidus<br>Diabetes mellitus<br>Burns<br>Adrenogenital syndrome<br>Capillary leak syndrome |
| Distributive | Vasodilation → venous pooling → decreased preload<br>Maldistribution of regional blood flow | Sepsis<br>Anaphylaxis<br>CNS/spinal injury<br>Drug intoxication |
| Cardiogenic | Decreased myocardial contractility | Congenital heart disease<br>Severe heart failure<br>Arrhythmia<br>Hypoxic/ischemic injuries<br>Cardiomyopathy<br>Metabolic derangements<br>Myocarditis<br>Drug intoxication<br>Kawasaki disease |
| Obstructive | Mechanical obstruction to ventricular outflow | Cardiac tamponade<br>Massive pulmonary embolus<br>Tension pneumothorax<br>Cardiac tumor |
| Dissociative | Oxygen not released from hemoglobin | Carbon monoxide poisoning<br>Methemoglobinemia |

CNS = central nervous system.

the complement, kinin, fibrinolytic, and coagulation pathways and result in the release of cellular histamine and prostaglandins. Additional inflammatory mediators include cytokines (IL-6), bioactive lipids (platelet-activating factor, leukotrienes), interferons, and the products of primary and secondary leukocyte granules. Direct injection of TNF produces cardiovascular, inflammatory, metabolic, hematologic, pulmonary, and renal abnormalities identical to those that occur in septic shock. The effect of TNF is blocked by neutralizing antibodies to TNF and only partially blocked by inhibition of prostaglandin synthesis. Most second mediators decrease vascular tone and increase vascular permeability, resulting in the maldistribution of blood flow. Arteriolar vasodilation (vasculopathy) results in reduced systemic vascular resistance, which serves to lower tissue perfusion pressure and impair coronary blood flow. The increased venous capacitance produced by venodilation results in venous stasis and decreased venous return to the heart. Mediator-induced changes in vascular permeability cause capillary leaks and loss of intravascular volume, which impair ventricular filling and thus cardiac output. Activated complement components and arachidonic acid metabolites promote leukocyte and platelet aggregation in capillary beds, producing obstruction to flow in the microcirculation. Vasculotoxins also directly depress cardiac output by decreasing intrinsic cardiac contractility or by inducing coronary vasospasm.

## Cardiogenic Shock

Cardiogenic shock is due to an abnormality in myocardial function and is expressed as depressed myocardial contractility and cardiac output with poor tissue perfusion. Primary cardiogenic shock occurs in children having congenital heart disease. Heart failure precedes cardiogenic shock in most patients who have congenital heart disease (except hypoplastic left heart syndrome) and in those who have circulatory obstruction (e.g., coarctation of the aorta, critical pulmonary stenosis; see Chapter 13).

In cardiogenic shock, compensatory mechanisms may contribute to the progression of shock by further depressing cardiac function. Neurohumoral vasoconstrictor responses increase afterload and add to the work of the failing ventricle. Tachycardia impairs coronary blood flow and decreases

TABLE 3–18. Definitions of Related Infectious and Shock States

**Infection:** Microbial phenomenon characterized by an inflammatory response to the presence of microorganisms or the invasion of normally sterile host tissue by those organisms

**Bacteremia:** The presence of viable bacteria in the blood

**Systemic Inflammatory Response Syndrome:** The systemic inflammatory response to a variety of severe clinical insults. The response is manifested by two or more of the following conditions:
    Temperature >38°C or <36°C
    Heart rate >90 beats/min*
    Respiratory rate >20 breaths/min* or PaCO$_2$ <32 torr
    WBC >12,000 cells/mm$^3$, <4000 cells/mm$^3$, or >10% immature (band) forms

**Sepsis:** The systemic response to infection. This systemic response is manifested by two or more of the following conditions as a result of infection:
    Temperature >38°C or <36°C
    Heart rate >90 beats/min*
    Respiratory rate >20 breaths/min* or PaCO$_2$ <32 torr
    WBC >12,000 cells/mm$^3$, <4000 cells/mm$^3$, or >10% immature (band) forms

**Severe Sepsis:** Sepsis associated with organ dysfunction, hypoperfusion, or hypotension. Hypoperfusion and perfusion abnormalities may include, but are not limited to, lactic acidosis, oliguria, or an acute alteration in mental status

**Septic Shock:** Sepsis with hypotension, despite adequate fluid resuscitation, along with the presence of perfusion abnormalities that may include, but are not limited to, lactic acidosis, oliguria, or an acute alteration in mental status. Patients who are on inotropic or vasopressor agents may not be hypotensive at the time that perfusion abnormalities are measured

**Hypotension:** A systolic BP of <90 mm Hg* or a reduction of >40 mm Hg from baseline in the absence of other causes for hypotension

**Multiple Organ Dysfunction Syndrome:** Presence of altered organ function in an acutely ill patient such that homeostasis cannot be maintained without intervention

From American College of Chest Physicians/Society of Critical Care Medicine Consensus Conference: Definitions for sepsis and organ failure and guidelines for the use of innovative therapies in sepsis. Crit Care Med 20:864, 1992.
    *Adults; must use age-appropriate norms.
    BP = blood pressure; WBC = white blood cell count.

myocardial oxygen delivery. Increased central blood volume caused by sodium and water retention and by incomplete emptying of the ventricles during systole results in elevated left ventricular volume and pressure, which impair subendocardial blood flow. Because of this self-perpetuating cycle, congestive heart failure progressing to death may be rapid. As compensatory mechanisms are overcome, the failing left ventricle produces increased ventricular end-diastolic volume and pressure, which leads to increased left atrial pressure, resulting in pulmonary edema. This sequence also contributes to right ventricular failure because of increased pulmonary artery pressure and increased right ventricular afterload. The liver usually enlarges, a gallop is present, and jugular venous distention may be noted. The spleen also may be enlarged. Because renal blood flow is poor, sodium and water are retained, contributing to the formation of peripheral edema.

Generally, *treatment* requires cardiotonic supportive drugs and diuretics to control pulmonary and tissue edema. In cardiogenic shock that develops in infants and children with underlying cardiovascular disease, the *prognosis* is poor.

Cardiogenic shock also may occur in previously healthy children secondary to viral myocarditis, dysrhythmias, toxic or metabolic derangement, or following a hypoxic-ischemic injury. In this circumstance, shock may be reversed by administering cardiotonic drugs.

### Obstructive Shock

Obstructive shock results from the patient's inability to produce adequate cardiac output, despite normal intravascular volume and normal myocardial contractility, because the ventricular outflow is mechanically obstructed; the major cause of the obstruction is pericardial tamponade. Clinically, tamponade should be suspected in the setting of trauma or previous heart surgery whenever a patient has a narrow pulse pressure, a muffled heart tone, an enlarged heart as determined by percussion or roentgenogram, or electromechanical dissociation. Echocardiography may be diagnostic, but attempts at needle pericardiocentesis should not await confirmation by diagnostic studies in symptomatic patients.

### Dissociative Shock

Dissociative shock refers to conditions in which tissue perfusion is normal but oxygen cannot be utilized by the cells because the hemoglobin has an abnormal affinity for oxygen, preventing its release to the tissues (see Table 3–17).

### THERAPY FOR SHOCK

### General Principles

The key to therapy is the *recognition of shock* in its early state, when many of the hemodynamic and metabolic alterations may be reversible. Therapy for shock is directed largely at treating the signs

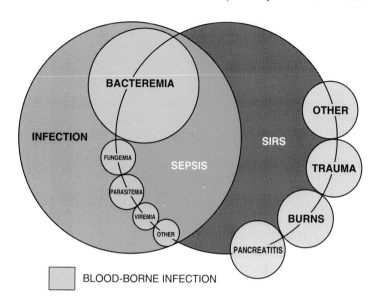

FIGURE 3–7. Interrelationship between various host responses to infections and other potential inflammatory injuries (burns, trauma). The systemic inflammatory response syndrome (SIRS) may be initiated by multiple inciting events; the inflammatory mediators released by these events initiate and perpetuate the SIRS. (American College of Chest Physicians/Society of Critical Care Medicine Consensus Conference: Definitions for sepsis and organ failure and guidelines for the use of innovative therapies in sepsis. Crit Care Med 20:864, 1992. Copyright Williams & Wilkins.)

and symptoms as they appear rather than directly addressing the primary cause or mechanisms involved.

Therapy should minimize cardiopulmonary work while ensuring cardiac output, blood pressure, and gas exchange. Intubation plus mechanical ventilation with 100% oxygen improves oxygenation and decreases or eliminates work of breathing but may impede venous return if distending airway pressures (positive end-expiratory pressure [PEEP], peak inspiratory pressure) (see Chapter 6) are excessive. Blood pressure support is critical because the vasodilation in sepsis may reduce perfusion despite supranormal cardiac output.

*Monitoring* a child in shock or in impending shock requires maintaining access to the central venous circulation to record pressure measurements, to perform blood sampling, and to measure systemic blood pressure continuously through an indwelling arterial catheter. These measurements facilitate the estimation of preload and afterload. When it is critical to know the patient's left atrial pressure, it can be measured through a left atrial catheter connected to a pressure monitor or estimated by measuring pulmonary capillary wedge pressure with a flow-directed balloon tip catheter. Directly measuring the cardiac index by thermodilution, injection of indocyanine green, or a Fick procedure also may be helpful. In addition, the management of shock requires monitoring arterial blood gases for oxygenation, ventilation ($CO_2$), and acidosis and frequently assessing serum electrolytes, calcium, magnesium, phosphorus, and blood urea nitrogen (BUN).

### Organ-Directed Therapeutics

**Cardiovascular Support.** In general, shock states are characterized by some form of primary or secondary impairment of myocardial function. Therefore, efforts to improve cardiac output are a basic component of shock therapy. Cardiovascular therapy should be targeted at fluid resuscitation and improvement of cardiac output, heart rate and rhythm, preload, afterload, and contractility.

**Fluid Resuscitation.** Alterations in preload dramatically affect cardiac output. In hypovolemic and distributive shock, decreased preload significantly impairs cardiac output. However, in cardiogenic shock, an elevated preload contributes to pulmonary edema. Table 3–19 lists fluids available for volume resuscitation. Plasma volume may be

TABLE 3–19.   Intravenous Fluids Available for Pediatric Volume Resuscitation

| Crystalloids | Colloids |
|---|---|
| 0.9% sodium chloride | 5% human serum albumin in 0.9% sodium chloride |
| Ringer's lactate | 25% human serum albumin in 0.9% sodium chloride |
| Hypertonic saline (3%) | 6% hydroxyethyl starch in 0.9% sodium chloride |
| | 10% dextran 40 in 5% dextrose in water |
| | Fresh frozen plasma |
| | Whole blood |

restored successfully with the use of crystalloid solutions, provided that sufficient volumes are employed, but edema fluid may accumulate (as a result of capillary leakage) if excessive amounts are infused. This accumulation may be unavoidable but nonetheless may be associated with a good outcome. Colloids contain larger molecules that theoretically may stay in the intravascular space longer than crystalloid solutions, and thus colloids exert oncotic pressure and draw fluid out of the tissues into the vascular compartment.

Selecting fluids for resuscitation and for ongoing use is dictated by the clinical circumstances. Crystalloid volume expanders are generally recommended as initial choices because they are effective and inexpensive. Most acutely ill children with signs of shock may safely receive, and usually benefit greatly from, a 20 cc/kg bolus of an isotonic crystalloid over 15 to 30 min. However, care must be exercised in treating cardiogenic shock with volume expansion because the ventricular filling pressures may rise without improvement of the cardiac performance. Carefully monitoring cardiac output or central venous pressure helps guide safe volume replacement. In patients with significant cerebral edema, the need to improve cardiac output by fluid replacement should be balanced by the requirement to reduce intracranial pressure with the need to maintain an acceptable cerebral perfusion pressure (mean blood pressure − intracranial pressure); intensive fluid resuscitation may increase intracranial pressure, exacerbating cerebral edema. However, the restoration of blood pressure and cardiac output have the highest priority in this situation.

**Cardiotonic and Vasodilator Therapy.** In an effort to improve cardiac output after volume resuscitation or when further volume replacement may be dangerous, a variety of cardiotonic and vasodilator drugs may be useful. Therapy is directed toward increasing myocardial contractility and decreasing left ventricular afterload, respectively.

Currently, five sympathomimetic agents are available (Table 3–20), but the hemodynamic status of the patient dictates the choice of the agent.

Therapy usually is initiated with dopamine or dobutamine. Combinations of these agents are highly effective. In children who fail to respond to several increases in either the dopamine or dobutamine infusion rate, a more potent cardiotonic agent, such as epinephrine or norepinephrine, may be indicated.

In addition to improving contractility, certain catecholamines may also cause an increase in systemic vascular resistance. The addition of a vasodilator drug may improve cardiac performance by decreasing the resistance against which the heart must pump (i.e., they may decrease afterload). The greatest clinical experience has been with nitroprusside and nitroglycerine. Afterload reduction also occurs with dobutamine, isoproterenol, amrinone, and angiotensin-converting enzyme (ACE) inhibitors. The use of these drugs may be particularly important in late shock, when vasoconstriction is prominent.

## Respiratory Support

The lung is a target organ for inflammatory mediators in shock and the systemic inflammatory response syndrome. Respiratory failure may develop rapidly and become progressive. Intervention requires endotracheal intubation and mechanical ventilation accompanied by the use of supplemental oxygen and PEEP. The *acute respiratory distress syndrome* (ARDS) may occur in children who are in shock (see Chapter 12). The mechanism underlying this syndrome is increased vascular permeability (noncardiogenic pulmonary edema) from the release of mediators. Vascular permeability, which results from direct damage to the alveolar-capillary endothelium, with leakage of proteinaceous fluid into the interstitium and alveoli, may interfere with surfactant action and is treated with diuretics,

TABLE 3–20.  Catecholamines Used for Cardiopulmonary Resuscitation

| | Positive Inotrope | Positive Chronotrope | Direct Pressor | Indirect Pressor | Vasodilator |
|---|---|---|---|---|---|
| Dopamine | + + | + | + / − | + + | + +* |
| Dobutamine | + + | + / − | − | − | + |
| Epinephrine | + + + | + + + | + + + | − | − |
| Isoproterenol | + + + | + + + | − | − | + + + |
| Norepinephrine | + + + | + + + | + + + | − | − |

*Primarily splanchnic and renal in low doses (3–5 μg/kg/min).

cardiotonics, combinations of a diuretic and a colloid, and PEEP to prevent atelectasis and pulmonary edema. Severe cardiopulmonary failure may be managed with inhaled nitric oxide and, if needed, extracorporeal membrane oxygenation (ECMO; see Chapter 6).

### Renal Salvage

Poor urine output during shock may be due to acute tubular necrosis (ATN) or to prerenal factors. Hypotension associated with shock may lead to acute renal failure. Prerenal azotemia may be due to poor cardiac output accompanied by decreased renal blood flow; however, severe hypotension may produce ATN. The former is corrected when blood volume deficits are replaced or myocardial contractility is improved, but ATN does not improve immediately once shock is corrected. Prerenal azotemia is associated with a serum blood urea nitrogen-creatinine ratio of greater than 10:1 and a urine sodium level below 20 mEq/L; ATN has a ratio of 10:1 and a urine sodium level of between 40 and 60 mEq/L (see Chapter 16). Aggressive fluid replacement often is necessary to improve oliguria associated with prerenal azotemia. Because the management of shock requires administering large volumes of fluid (often >50 mL/kg during resuscitation), maintaining urine output greatly facilitates patient management.

Preventing ATN and the subsequent complications associated with acute renal failure (e.g., hyperkalemia, acidosis, hypocalcemia, edema) or treating electrolyte imbalances or ATN with continuous arteriovenous hemofiltration or conventional peritoneal and hemodialysis are of paramount importance. Thus, using pharmacologic agents to augment urine output is indicated once the intravascular volume has been replaced. The use of loop diuretics, such as furosemide and bumetanide, mannitol, or combinations of a loop diuretic and a thiazide may enhance urine output. Infusing doses of dopamine, which produce renal artery vasodilation, also may improve urine output. Nevertheless, if hyperkalemia, refractory acidosis, hypervolemia, or the altered mental status associated with uremia occurs, dialysis or hemofiltration should be initiated. ATN is a self-limited condition that requires good supportive care to avoid potential complications until renal function improves, usually 3–7 days after the renal tubular injury.

### References

Behrman RE, Kliegman RM, Arvin AM (eds): Nelson Textbook of Pediatrics, 15th ed. Philadelphia, WB Saunders, 1996, Chapters 60.3, 60.7.

Bone R: Toward an epidemiology and natural history of SIRS (systemic inflammatory response syndrome). JAMA 268:3452, 1992.
Carcillo J, Davis A, Zaritsky A: Role of early fluid resuscitation in pediatric shock. JAMA 266:1242, 1991.
Gattinoni L, Brazzi L, Pelosi P, et al: A trial of goal-oriented hemodynamic therapy in critically ill patients. N Engl J Med 333:1025, 1995.
Huskisson L: Intravenous volume replacement: Which and why? Arch Dis Child 67:649, 1992.
LeGall J, Klan J, Lemeshow S, et al: The logistic organ dysfunction system. JAMA 276: 802, 1996.
Ognibene F, Cunnion R: Mechanisms of myocardial depression in sepsis. Crit Care Med 21:6, 1993.

## CARDIOPULMONARY RESUSCITATION

Cardiopulmonary resuscitation is rarely needed in pediatric practice. Most infants and children who do need CPR have had an isolated respiratory arrest. The outcome of cardiopulmonary arrest in children is poor; only 10–15% survive, and the majority of the survivors sustain permanent disability. Therefore, the ability to anticipate or recognize pre-arrest conditions and initiate prompt and appropriate therapy not only may save the child's life but also may preserve the quality of that sustained life.

Hypoxia plays a central role in most of the potential events leading to cardiopulmonary arrest in children. Furthermore, the presence of hypoxia leads to subsequent organ dysfunction or to ischemic damage, no matter what underlying illness affects the child. Hypoxia may be acute or chronic and may result from either an acquired or a congenital illness. In some children, abnormal pulmonary vasculature or congenital heart disease, leading to right-to-left shunting, contributes to tenuous oxygenation. Physicians should be acutely aware of the potential damage that hypoxia and the resulting ischemia may produce in susceptible organs (Table 3–21) so that their approach to an infant or a child experiencing cardiopulmonary arrest extends beyond CPR to include efforts to preserve vital organ function.

The goal in resuscitating the pediatric patient who has sustained a cardiopulmonary arrest should be to optimize cardiac output and tissue oxygen delivery, which may be accomplished by using artificial ventilation and chest compression, and the judicious administration of pharmacologic agents.

The natural history and mechanism of pediatric and adult cardiopulmonary arrest are different. Adult arrests tend to be sudden in onset and cardiac in origin, with ventricular dysrhythmias or asystole preceding respiratory arrest.. Children go through a series of physiologic changes prior to

TABLE 3–21.  Target Organs for
             Hypoxic-Ischemic Damage

| Organ | Effect |
|---|---|
| Brain | Seizures, cerebral edema, infarction, anoxic damage, SIADH, diabetes insipidus |
| Cardiovascular | Heart failure, myocardial infarct, tricuspid insufficiency, peripheral gangrene |
| Lung and pulmonary vasculature | Adult respiratory distress syndrome |
| Liver | Infarction, necrosis, cholestasis |
| Kidney | Acute tubular necrosis, acute cortical necrosis |
| GI tract | Gastric ulceration, mucosal damage |
| Hematologic | Disseminated intravascular coagulation |

GI = gastrointestinal; SIADH = syndrome of inappropriate secretion of antidiuretic hormone.

the onset of ventricular fibrillation or asystole, and most often respiration ceases before or concurrently with the cardiopulmonary arrest. Therefore, a child who is at risk may be identified prior to the occurrence of cardiopulmonary arrest (Table 3–22); respiratory arrest may be anticipated and interventions started before asystole occurs.

## AIRWAY

On recognizing that a clinical situation requiring resuscitation exists, the physician should first make sure that there is a patent airway. In children, airway patency often is compromised by a loss of muscle tone, allowing the mandibular block of tissue, including the tongue, the bony mandible, and the soft surrounding tissues, to rest against the posterior pharyngeal wall. In adult patients, such problems can be corrected by using manual head tilt maneuvers; in infants and young children, however, this correction may result in the excessive overextension of the neck and further narrowing of the tracheal airway.

Pediatric patients requiring resuscitation should be endotracheally intubated. Oral intubation is the preferred method in a resuscitation and is technically easier than nasal intubation in children. Prior to intubation, the patient should be ventilated with 100% oxygen using a bag and mask. Cricoid pressure should be employed to minimize inflation of the stomach. Certain patients may require the use of induction medications (paralytics, sedatives) to assist intubation. The correct size tube may be estimated according to the size of the mid-5th phalanx or the following formula:

$$\frac{\text{patient age in years} + 16}{4}$$

As a result of the presence of a narrow airway segment at the level of the cricoid ring, cuffed endotracheal tubes should not be used in children younger than 8 yr of age.

Once the endotracheal tube is in place, the child must be assessed again for breathing, which requires not only assessing respiratory movements but also performing auscultations of the trachea and chest to detect bilateral and symmetric breath sounds. If air exchange is not heard or cyanosis continues, the position of the tube must be re-evaluated.

## BREATHING

The major role of endotracheal intubation is to ensure the delivery of adequate oxygen to the patient. Because hypoxemia is the final common pathway in pediatric arrests, providing oxygen is more important than correcting the respiratory acidosis that also develops. Thus, 100% oxygen, at a rate of 20 breaths/min, should be delivered through the tube using a tidal volume necessary to produce adequate chest rise and relieve cyanosis. This usually requires a tidal volume equal to 10–15 mL/kg of body weight.

Once a patent airway is established and oxygenation and ventilation are maintained, many chil-

TABLE 3–22.  Warning Signs and Symptoms
             Suggesting the Potential Need for
             Resuscitative Intervention*

| CNS | Lethargy, irritability, obtundation, confusion |
|---|---|
| Respiratory | Apnea, grunting, nasal flaring, dyspnea retracting, tachypnea, poor air movement, stridor, wheezing |
| Cardiovascular | Arrhythmia, bradycardia, tachycardia, weak pulses, poor capillary refill, hypotension |
| Skin and mucous membranes | Mottling, pallor, cyanosis, diaphoresis, poor membrane turgor, dry mucous membranes |

*One would seldom act if only one or two of these signs and symptoms were present, but the occurrence of several in concert foreshadows grave consequences. Intervention should be directed at the primary disorder.
CNS = central nervous system.

dren will re-establish cardiac output. Thus, carefully reassessing the patient before proceeding with other mechanical and pharmacologic maneuvers is essential. This evaluation should include observing the color of the skin and mucous membranes and palpating both central and peripheral pulses. If cyanosis persists or the brachial or femoral pulses remain weak or absent, adequate circulation has not been re-established.

## CIRCULATION

Because some children may still have effective circulation early in the history of an acute respiratory arrest, circulation should be independently assessed. Chest compressions should be initiated if a pulse cannot be palpated or if the heart rate is less than 60 beats/min with signs of poor systemic perfusion. To achieve optimal compressions, the child should be supine on a hard, flat surface. In infants and children, the area for compression is the lower half of the sternum. Effective CPR in infants requires a compression depth between 0.5 and 1 inch. The child (ages 1 to 8 yr) requires a compression depth of 1 to 1.5 inches. In both, compression rate should be at least 100/minute, coordinated with assisted ventilation at a 1:5 ratio. The effectiveness of compressions should be assessed via palpation of the carotid, brachial, or femoral artery.

## DRUGS
### (Table 3–23)

When mechanical means fail to re-establish adequate circulation, pharmacologic intervention is essential. Drug therapy during CPR is directed toward improving cardiac output and the delivery of oxygen to tissues. The special requirements of drugs used during CPR limit the number of potential routes for their administration. Administration through a central venous line is preferred. The effectiveness of peripheral intravenous administration is limited by poor circulation. Alternative routes for administration of some drugs are through the endotracheal tube or by intraosseus (bone marrow) infusion.

Perhaps the most important agent employed during CPR in children is *oxygen*. Whenever possible, 100% oxygen should be administered through an endotracheal tube. Short exposures to high oxygen tensions cause little pulmonary toxicity, and high oxygen tensions may be required to reverse some of the reactive pulmonary vascular responses to poor cardiac output.

The use of buffers is the subject of considerable controversy. *Sodium bicarbonate* is the most commonly used buffer, but its risk may outweigh its potential benefits. One of the hallmarks of poor cardiac output is acidemia. In pediatric patients, however, this acidemia is often respiratory rather than metabolic. Judicious use of sodium bicarbonate to correct the metabolic component of the acidosis may be beneficial. However, the use of sodium bicarbonate in an attempt to correct what is primarily a respiratory problem can exacerbate respiratory acidosis by inducing the production of more $CO_2$. Sodium bicarbonate may produce hypernatremia, hyperosmolality, hypokalemia, metabolic alkalosis (shifting the oxyhemoglobin curve to the left and impairing tissue oxygen delivery), reduced ionized calcium level, and impaired cardiac function.

*Catecholamines* constitute the mainstay of therapy for CPR. They are administered both as boluses during the acute phases of resuscitation and by continuous infusions during the maintenance therapy involved in postresuscitative stabilization. Epinephrine is the primary agent employed. It is a catecholamine with mixed alpha- and beta-agonist properties. The alpha-adrenergic effects are most important during the acute phases, because of the alpha-induced increase in systemic vascular resistance that results in a greater pressure gradient across the coronary bed and an improved coronary blood flow.

Prompt electrical defibrillation is indicated when ventricular fibrillation is noted (Table 3–24). Bolus administration of lidocaine is recommended prior to defibrillation. Defibrillation should be distinguished from *cardioversion* of supraventricular tachycardias which also may compromise cardiac output. Cardioversion requires a lower starting dose and a synchronization of the discharge to the electrocardiogram to avoid discharging during a susceptible period, which may convert supraventricular tachycardia to ventricular tachycardia or fibrillation.

Pediatric CPR requires a careful integration of mechanical skills and pharmacotherapy (see Table 3–23). Intervention should commence in an anticipatory fashion, and the drug doses provided should serve as a guide rather than a limit to therapy. Resuscitative efforts should be directed toward preserving vital organ function and reversing ongoing tissue damage rather than simply starting the heart. This clinical strategy should continue into the postresuscitative period.

References

American Heart Association: Neonatal resuscitation. JAMA 268:2276, 1992.

TABLE 3–23.  Drug Doses for Cardiopulmonary Resuscitation

| Drug | Indication | Dose |
|---|---|---|
| Adenosine | Supraventricular tachycardia | 0.1–0.2 mg/kg (may repeat at 0.4 mg/kg); maximum 12 mg |
| Atropine | Supraventricular or junctional bradycardia<br>Asystole? | 0.02 mg/kg/dose (minimum dose 0.1 mg); up to 0.5 mg (child), 1.0 mg (adolescent); higher doses needed in anticholinesterase poisoning |
| Bicarbonate | Metabolic acidosis?<br>Hyperkalemia | 0.5–1 mEq/kg bolus, if metabolic acidosis present; ensure adequate ventilation; use 4.2% solution in neonates |
| Bretylium | Ventricular tachycardia | 5 mg/kg IV bolus (may repeat at 10 mg/kg); may cause hypotension |
| Calcium | Hypocalcemia<br>Hyperkalemia<br>Wide QRS pattern? | 25 mg/kg calcium chloride; stop if bradycardia occurs |
| Dobutamine | Inotropy | 2–30 μg/kg/min |
| Dopamine | Inotropy<br>Renal preservation | 0.5–2 μg/kg/min splanchnic, renal dilation; 2–7 μg/kg/min inotrope; 7–20 μg/kg/min inotrope + pressor |
| Epinephrine | Chronotropy<br>Inotropy<br>Hypotension | 0.01 mg/kg bolus; 0.1 mg/kg as subsequent doses if 0.01 mg/kg is ineffective; 0.05–2 μg/kg/min drip, inotrope + pressor; may cause subendocardial ischemia and arrhythmias |
| Fluid | Hypovolemia<br>Sepsis | Use colloid or crystalloid tailored to patient's physiologic needs |
| Glucose | Hypoglycemia | 2 mL/kg 10% dextrose; follow Dextrostix |
| Isoproterenol | Chronotropy<br>Inotropy | 0.05–1 μg/kg/min inotrope + vasodilator effects; chronotropic response may limit dose; may cause subendocardial ischemia and arrhythmias |
| Lidocaine | Ventricular tachycardia | 1 mg/kg/bolus followed by 20–50 μg/kg/min continuous infusion; monitor serum concentration and widening of QRS for toxicity |
| Nitroprusside | Reduce systemic vascular resistance<br>Hypertensive crisis | 0.05–10.0 μg/kg/min by continuous infusion |
| Oxygen | Hypoxia | 100%, humidified |
| Phenytoin | Ventricular tachycardia, digitalis-induced arrhythmias | 15–20 mg/kg slow loading dose; titrate maintenance therapy to serum concentrations of 15–30 μg/mL |

Data from Committee on Drugs, American Academy of Pediatrics: Emergency drug doses for infants and children. Pediatrics 81:462, 1988; and American Heart Association: Pediatric advanced life support. JAMA 268:2262, 1992.
? = Controversial, uncertain, or unproven efficacy.

American Heart Association: Pediatric advanced life support. JAMA 268: 2262, 1992.
American Heart Association: Pediatric basic life support. JAMA 268:2251, 1992.
Behrman RE, Kliegman RM, Arvin AM (eds): Nelson Textbook of Pediatrics, 15th ed. Philadelphia, WB Saunders, 1996, Chapter 253.
Goetting MG: Mastering pediatric cardiopulmonary resuscitation. Pediatr Clin North Am 412:1147, 1994.
Goetting MG: Progress in pediatric cardiopulmonary resuscitation. Emerg Med Clin North Am 13:291, 1995.

## DRUG THERAPY IN THE ACUTELY ILL CHILD

The goal of pharmacotherapy for the critically ill child is to achieve a specific effect. Such goals are limited to the augmentation, ablation, or modulation of normal physiologic processes because drugs cannot create physiologic responses that are not intrinsic to the patient.

Two important groups of factors determine the efficacy of drug therapy: (1) *pharmacokinetic* determinants (Table 3–25) relate to the absorption, distribution, metabolism, and excretion of the drug, and (2) *pharmacodynamic* determinants reflect the drug's mechanism of action and its safety profiles. Effective therapy can be achieved if the selected drug has favorable pharmacokinetic and pharmacodynamic properties.

Various developmental changes affect each phase of pharmacokinetics as well as drug-receptor interactions and drug safety profiles. Changes in

**TABLE 3–24.** Recommendations for Defibrillation and Cardioversion in Children

**Defibrillation**
  Pretreat with 0.01 mg/kg epinephrine (1:10,000) IV
  Place saline gauze or conduction jellied pad at apex and upper right sternal border
  Use 4.5-cm diameter paddles for infants and 8–10-cm diameter paddles for children
  Notify all participating personnel before discharging paddles so that no one is in contact with patient or bed
  Begin with 2 watts/sec/kg (2 joules/kg)
  If unsuccessful, double current (4 joules/kg) and repeat rapidly ×3

**Cardioversion**
  Determine mechanism of the predominant rhythm
  Consider pretreatment with lidocaine, 1 mg/kg IV, for risk of inducing ventricular tachycardia and valium for sedation
  For symptomatic supraventricular tachycardia* or ventricular tachycardia with a pulse, synchronize signal with electrocardiogram
  Choose paddles, position pads, and notify personnel as above
  Begin with 0.5–1 watts/sec/kg (joules/kg)
  If unsuccessful, double the current

*Consider adenosine first (see Table 3–23).

gastric acidity and gastrointestinal motility affect the rate and extent of oral drug *absorption*. Once absorbed, the *distribution* of drug into tissues is influenced by several factors. In the newborn period, it is influenced by the presence of fetal albumin, which has binding characteristics that differ from those of adult albumin. Also in neonates, endogenous substances such as bilirubin and elevated free fatty acids may displace drugs from their albumin-binding sites. Finally, drug distribution in neonates is affected profoundly by the changes in extracellular fluid volume that occur during normal maturation. At birth, water may account for up to 80% of the infant's total body weight, whereas in adults the extracellular fluid volume comprises only 60% of the total body weight. This may account, in part, for the higher dosages that infants and young children require for effects to be obtained, compared with doses required by adults, when assessed on a milligram-per-kilogram basis.

Drug *metabolism* accounts for the major differences in interindividual responses to drugs. In addition, marked changes in the drug-metabolizing enzymes in the liver occur during early infancy and then again at the time of adolescence, when sex differences in drug metabolism may be due to changes in steroid hormone levels. These changes in drug metabolism coincide with the changes in

drug *excretion* by the kidney, which relate to the maturation of both glomerular filtration and tubular secretion (see Chapter 16).

Changes in the pharmacodynamics of drugs may result from developmental changes in receptor number and affinity or in receptor-effector coupling, so that a certain dosage producing particular therapeutic as well as adverse effects will change as the newborn progresses from infancy through childhood to adolescence and adulthood. This continuum of changing pharmacokinetics and pharmacodynamics related to growth and development is complicated further by the impact of the various physiologic derangements during an acute illness (see Table 3–25).

Pharmacodynamic alterations in critically ill children may result from vascular volume and electrolyte derangements and from the effects of acute alterations in acid-base status. Moreover, acutely ill patients generate endogenous substances that alter drug responsiveness, and the long-term use of certain hormones and autacoids may result in the down-regulation of their various receptors. Finally, patients who already are seriously ill are less likely

**TABLE 3–25.** Pharmacokinetic Considerations in Critically Ill Children

**Absorption Phase**
  Altered gastric emptying
  Decreased gastrointestinal blood flow, ileus
  Altered gastric pH; exogenous buffers—antacids, $H_2$-receptor antagonists, maturity
  Time delay
  Altered biliary function

**Distribution Phase**
  Hemodynamic instability
  Inflammation
  Decreased protein synthesis/increased protein loss
  Synthesis of acute-phase reactants
  Extravascular fluid collections—ascites, pleural effusions
  Drug interactions
  Maturational changes of extracellular fluid space (see Chapter 2)

**Metabolism Phase**
  Hemodynamic instability
  Hypoxemia
  Substrate deficiencies
  Polypharmacy—drug interactions
  Use of hormones and autacoids as pharmacologic rather than physiologic agents
  Enzyme maturational changes in biotransformation

**Excretion Phase**
  Altered vascular volume
  Altered renal blood flow (illness, maturation)
  Hypoxemia
  Nephrotoxic agents
  Altered hepatic function (illness, maturation)

to tolerate the potential side effects of various drugs, so that the safety profile of the drugs employed in a critical care setting may be altered drastically.

The superposition of acute illness on a developmental program controlling drug biodisposition and response presents a challenge to the development of effective therapeutic strategies. One strategy, the *target-concentration strategy*, consists of an attempt to achieve specific plasma levels of a drug. Therapeutic principles include an awareness of drug pharmacokinetics and active metabolites, having predetermined expectations of the manifestations of drug efficacy and toxicity, awareness of appropriate sampling times for drug levels, treating the patient and *not* the drug level, and, if inconsistencies develop, re-evaluating and re-examining the patient. This strategy often is applied to drugs used chronically to treat illnesses having intermittent clinical manifestations. Examples of such problems include reversible reactive airway disease, seizure disorders, and cardiac arrhythmias. Implementing this strategy requires effective use of the drug analysis laboratory (Table 3–26). The targeted concentrations may relate either to drug efficacy or to toxicity and generally are based on data obtained from large populations rather than from individual patients.

The types of drugs that lend themselves to the target-concentration strategy are those manifesting a wide interindividual variation in drug absorption, distribution, or elimination (Table 3–27). Therapeutic monitoring for drug efficacy is possible for theophylline, anticonvulsants (phenytoin, phenobarbital, valproate, carbamazepine ethosuximide), and antiarrhythmic agents (procainamide and its metabolite NAPA, quinidine, lidocaine, amiodarone). This strategy also is useful for administering drugs having a narrow therapeutic index and for

those designed to attain relatively sustained and constant effects over a long period of time. Such a strategy can be considered only when the concentrations of drug in the plasma relate directly to clinical effects of the drug that can be monitored. Knowing the therapeutic range and toxic level for each drug and the average values for absorption, distribution, and elimination of the drug permits intelligent use of serum drug levels. The pathophysiologic conditions that alter these parameters and the extent of this alteration also must be appreciated.

The *target-effect strategy* is the second approach to the drug treatment of acutely ill children. Two principles are essential to its application: the first is the dose-response relationship (i.e., the concept that most drugs show increasing clinical or adverse effects with increasing doses); the second is that, prior to the initiation of therapy, there must be a

**Table 3–27.  Drugs Amenable to Therapeutic Monitoring for Drug Toxicity**

**Antibiotics**
  Aminoglycosides—gentamicin, tobramycin, amikacin
  Chloramphenicol
  Vancomycin

**Immunosuppression**
  Methotrexate
  Cyclosporine

**Antipyretics**
  Acetaminophen
  Salicylate

**Other**
  Digoxin
  Lithium
  Theophylline
  Anticonvulsant drugs

**Table 3–26.  Prerequisites for Therapeutic Drug Monitoring**

The analytic method must be specific, sensitive, accurate, and available in an appropriate time frame.

The active drug and important metabolites are measured.

Development of tolerance at receptor sites does not occur.

Concentration of drug in serum is proportional to the concentration of drug at receptor sites.

There must be reasonably good correlation between concentration and therapeutic effects.

The therapeutic range must be well defined.

Proper care is taken in interpretation of values.

**Table 3–28.  Drugs for Employing a Target-Effect Strategy in Critically Ill Children**

*Catecholamines*—dopamine, dobutamine, epinephrine, isoproterenol, norepinephrine, terbutaline

*Vasodilators*—nitroglycerine, nitroprusside, hydralazine, angiotensin-converting enzyme inhibitors

*Anticoagulants*—heparin, warfarin

*Beta-lactam antibiotics*—penicillins, cephalosporins, carbapenems, monobactams

*Anxiolytics, sedatives*—diazepam, lorazepam, midazolam, morphine, fentanyl, chloral hydrate, secobarbital

*Oxygen*

*Diuretics*—furosemide, bumetanide, chlorothiazide, metolazone well-defined clinical endpoint (e.g., the physician prescribing the drug must have a reasonable understanding of the drug's pharmacodynamic action, including its side effects). There must also be a reasonable understanding of the impact of both ontogeny and disease on these pharmacodynamic actions. Finally, before therapy begins, a system must be set in place to monitor both the efficacy and toxicity of the drug.

The target-effect strategy is particularly appro-priate to the intensive care setting (Table 3–28). For example, if oxygen is being used as a drug to attempt to increase a patient's oxygen saturation in the presence of respiratory failure, the approach is to choose a clinically acceptable oxygen saturation level (e.g., >90%) and to increase the inspired oxygen concentration serially until the patient is receiving the desired oxygen saturation or until the patient is inspiring 100% oxygen. The essence of drug dosing using the target-effect strategy is to

TABLE 3–29. Pharmacologic Management of Pain

| Agent | Comments |
| --- | --- |
| **Nonopioid Analgesia** | |
| *Nonsteroidal anti-inflammatory drugs (NSAIDs)* | Greater efficacy than acetaminophen, equal to or greater than oral opioids. Opioid and NSAID combination reduces opioid tolerance and enhances analgesia. *Chronic complications:* decreased glomerular filtration rate; fluid retention, gastrointestinal ulceration; bleeding; perforation. No abuse potential but has ceiling effect. |
| Ibuprofen | |
| Naprosyn | |
| Tolectin | |
| Ketorolac | |
| *Acetaminophen* | Potency equivalent to aspirin; less than NSAIDs. *Acute ingestion:* hepatic toxicity. |
| **Opioid Analgesia** | |
| *Pure agonists* | Have no ceiling effect (e.g., higher dose, greater analgesia) and greater *side effects* (respiratory depression, sedation, miosis, nausea, histamine release–pruritus, decreased gut motility, constipation, increased sphincter of Oddi tone, urinary retention, biliary spasm). Opioid abstinence syndrome if withdrawn quickly. High abuse potential. |
| Morphine | |
| Codeine | |
| Fentanyl, alfentanil, sufentanil | |
| *Partial agonists/agonist-antagonists* | May produce dysphoria, acute withdrawal symptoms if given with pure agonist opioids. Possible reduced biliary spasm. |
| Pentazocine | |
| Nalbuphine | |
| Butorphanol | |
| Buprenorphine | |
| Propoxyphene | |
| Methadone | |
| *Meperidine* | No histamine release, possibly decreased biliary spasm. Toxic, active metabolite—normeperidine—produces seizures. |
| **Sedative–Hypnotics** | |
| *Benzodiazepines* | Produce anxiolysis, sedation, muscle relaxation, amnesia; useful in combination with opioids for painful procedures or postoperative pain. Tolerance possible. *Acute complications:* apnea, decreased blood pressure, decreased myocardial function. |
| Diazepam | |
| Midazolam (short-acting) | |
| Lorazepam (long-acting) | |
| *Other agents* | |
| Ketamine | Produces dissociative anesthesia, analgesia, amnesia, increased heart rate, increased blood pressure, increased bronchial secretions (decreased with atropine), bronchodilation and emergent delirium, hallucinations, vivid dreams (reduced with benzodiazepines). Contraindicated with increased intracranial pressure. |
| Propofol | Rapid onset, lipophilic. May decrease cardiovascular function. |
| Chloral hydrate | Predominantly sedative, weak analgesia. *Toxicity* includes emesis, gastrointestinal bleeding, esophageal stricture, hepatic dysfunction, arrhythmias, decreased blood pressure, and possible carcinogenesis. |
| Cyclic antidepressants | Useful as adjuvant analgesia for chronic pain (e.g., cancer pain). |
| Carbamazepine | Useful as adjuvant for various chronic neuralgias. |

Data from Med Lett 35:1, 1993; Committee on Drugs, American Academy of Pediatrics: Guidelines for monitoring and management of pediatric patients during and after sedation for diagnostic and therapeutic procedures. Pediatrics 89:1110, 1992; Brill JE: Control of pain. Crit Care Clin 8:203, 1992; and Zetter LK, Anderson CT, Schechter NL: Pediatric pain: Current status and new directions. Curr Probl Pediatr 20:411, 1990.

increase the dosage until the desired therapeutic effect is achieved, but if sequential increases produce no increased effect and the therapeutic effect has not been achieved or if drug toxicity supervenes, changing the drug rather than adding different drugs to the regimen is the appropriate response.

### References

Behrman RE, Kliegman RM, Arvin AM (eds): Nelson Textbook of Pediatrics, 15th ed. Philadelphia, WB Saunders, 1996, Chapter 63.
Blumer J: Principles of drug disposition in the critically ill child. *In* Fuhrman B, Zimmerman J (eds): Pediatric Critical Care. St. Louis, CV Mosby, 1992, pp 1055–1072.
Reynolds DJM, Aronson JK: Making the most of plasma drug concentration measurements. BMJ 306:48, 1993.
Snodgrass WR: Selected aspects of pediatric intensive care unit clinical pharmacology. Curr Opin Pediatr 3:314, 1991.

## PAIN MANAGEMENT

The critically ill neonate, child, or adolescent may experience pain, discomfort, and anxiety resulting from injury, surgery, and invasive procedures (intubation, bone marrow aspiration, central venous line placement) or during life-sustaining mechanical ventilation. Pain may be manifested as verbal or visible discomfort, crying, agitation, tachycardia, hypertension, and tachypnea. The physician has a commitment to relieve discomfort and treat pain. Common pharmacologic agents employed to manage acute and chronic pain are noted in Table 3–29.

### References

Behrman RE, Kliegman RM, Arvin AM (eds): Nelson Textbook of Pediatrics, 15th ed. Philadelphia, WB Saunders, 1996, Chapter 62.
Brill JE: Control of pain. Crit Care Clin 8:203, 1992.
Committee on Drugs, American Academy of Pediatrics: Guidelines for the monitoring and management of pediatric patients during and after sedation for diagnostic and therapeutic procedures. Pediatrics 89:1110, 1992.
Lebovitz DJ, Blumer JL: Sedation and analgesic therapy for critically ill children. Curr Opin Pediatr 4:305, 1992.

# Chapter 4

# HUMAN GENETICS AND DYSMORPHOLOGY

R. Stephen S. Amato

Thousands of known inherited genetic conditions are found in humans. Genetic conditions are common causes of acute and chronic diseases that occur during fetal life, immediately at birth, or during childhood, adolescence and adulthood. Genetic abnormalities may produce congenital malformations (e.g., trisomies 13, 18, and 21 [Down syndrome]), metabolic disturbances (e.g., phenylketonuria [PKU], galactosemia), specific organ dysfunction (e.g., mental retardation, congenital heart disease), or abnormalities of sexual differentiation (e.g., Turner syndrome). Approximately 1% of newborn infants will manifest monogenic diseases (e.g., cystic fibrosis, sickle cell anemia), and 0.5% will have chromosomal disorders (e.g., Down syndrome); 1–3% of children have diseases that are multifactorial in pathogenesis (e.g., congenital heart disease, spina bifida). Approximately 40% of childhood deaths are due to genetic disorders and birth defects.

## GENE STRUCTURE AND FUNCTION

The human genome consists of approximately 100,000 genes. Each gene is a unique sequence of a deoxyribonucleic acid (DNA) macromolecule, which is arranged as a double-stranded chain of deoxyribose residues linked by complementary base pairs. The purine bases adenine and guanine are paired with hydrogen bonds to the pyrimidine bases thymine and cytosine, respectively. There are about 3 billion of these base pairs in the haploid human genome contained in the 23 chromosomes.

Double-stranded DNA must *replicate* to produce new copies of genetic material for daughter cells. *Transcription* is the process of initiating protein synthesis by reading the DNA and copying the future amino acid sequence encoded in the DNA onto a single strand of messenger ribonucleic acid (mRNA). Mature mRNA from the nucleus then affixes to cytoplasmic ribosomes, where the genetic message is *translated* into a polypeptide chain as amino acids are carried to the ribosome-mRNA complex by transfer RNAs (tRNA), small RNA molecules that are specific for each amino acid.

Genes or fragments of DNA from specific genes can be cloned in the laboratory. Specific DNA probes can be labeled to identify the gene's DNA. Specific probes or endonuclease-derived characteristic *restriction fragment length polymorphisms* (RFLPs) can be used to identify mutant or absent genes from patients with genetic disorders. A probe is a radioactively labeled single-stranded DNA fragment that selectively binds or hybridizes to complementary DNA of a specific gene, to part of the DNA sequence of a gene, or to parts of the DNA flanking the gene. The patient's DNA fragments are separated by gel electrophoresis. A single-stranded $^{32}$P-labeled DNA probe then is hybridized to the patient's DNA. An x-ray plate then is exposed to the gel, which produces an autoradiograph, demonstrating the sites of $^{32}$P-DNA binding.

Because each human chromosome has hundreds of thousands of base pairs, smaller workable units must be produced to identify genes. *Restriction endonucleases* are enzymes that recognize specific 4–8 base pair sequences and cleave DNA into smaller fragments at these specific sites. Each of the over 150 endonucleases will produce a reproducible and characteristic fragment pattern, which can be separated by size on an agarose gel. Mutations at the site of cleavage will change the fragmentation pattern, thus producing a restriction fragment length polymorphism. DNA from the agarose gel can be transferred to cellulose nitrate, where single-stranded DNA fragments can hybridize with probe DNA to identify the fragment containing the complementary DNA (cDNA). Hybridization of single-stranded DNA to DNA is called *Southern blotting*; hybridization of RNA to DNA is *Northern blotting*. The demonstration of antibody to protein bands is called *Western blotting*.

The combination of cDNA probes, restriction fragment length polymorphism, and Southern blotting has made it possible to diagnose genetic diseases, to clone genes, to add to our basic understanding of genetic diseases, to offer prenatal diagnoses, and, in the future, to treat certain genetic disorders by replacing the missing normal gene. Small quantities of genomic DNA can be amplified with the *polymerase chain reaction* (PCR). The PCR is a powerful tool for making many copies of a DNA or RNA segment, which simplifies subsequent analysis.

## INHERITED CONDITIONS

Three basic mechanisms of inheritance exist for single-gene conditions. The three methods of human inheritance are (1) dominant, (2) recessive, and (3) sex-linked or X-linked. Except for genes on the X and Y chromosomes in males, all genes are duplicated in a normal diploid individual. If a single copy of the gene (a single allele) has a detectable effect when present, the condition is said to be *dominant*. If the effect of the allele is inapparent when only one allele is present and is expressed if two functionally identical alleles are present, the condition is described as *recessive*. If an individual has two identical alleles, the person is said to be homozygous for the gene. If an individual has two different alleles, the person is heterozygous for the gene in question. The effects of recessive conditions are observed only in homozygous persons, whereas the effects of dominant conditions are observed in the heterozygous individual. A person who is heterozygous for a hidden recessive allele is described as a *carrier*.

*X-linked* inheritance is a variation of dominant and recessive inheritance modified by the fact that males have only one X chromosome. Normal XY males will express any genes present on their X chromosome; they are *hemizygous* for genes on the X chromosome. Males also possess a Y chromosome that is passed from father to son (holandric distribution). The Y chromosome is important in determining maleness but appears to do little else.

## MENDELIAN INHERITANCE AND CYTOGENETICS

### AUTOSOMAL DOMINANT INHERITANCE

The ability to explain gene inheritance during genetic counseling requires an understanding of how a pattern of inheritance occurs. In autosomal dominant conditions (Table 4–1), if one parent displays a dominant condition and is heterozygous for the gene, each child has a 50% chance of receiving the gene's single allele and also of manifesting the condition. Not all patients with the affected gene may be symptomatic. *Penetrance* is the percentage of patients with the gene who manifest symptoms or signs; *expressivity* reflects the spectrum of severity among patients having clinical manifestations.

The *major histocompatibility complex* (MHC) genes illustrate another important type of autosomal dominant inheritance (Fig. 4–1). These genes determine cell surface antigens (proteins) and are located in a cluster close to the middle of the short (p) arm of the number 6 chromosome. Three *human leukocyte antigen* (HLA) genes in the MHC are designated HLA-A, HLA-B, and HLA-C and code for class MHC proteins located on all nucleated cells and platelets. Each HLA gene has a large number of possible alleles; the alleles are designated by number. An unusual feature of the HLA system is that most of the individual alleles have an effect that can be detected on the leukocyte surface. When the effects of each different allele can be detected, the alleles are called "codominants." In this special case, the appearance of the condition produced by the genes (phenotype) corresponds to the allelic composition (genotype). HLA alleles (haplotypes) of gene A are A1, A2, A3, and so forth, continuing past A32; alleles of gene C are C1 to C8; and alleles of gene B are B1 to B49. The HLA genes A, B, and C are all codominant, so that an individual will have two alleles for each HLA gene site (A,C,B) and, thus, six detectable HLA alleles. (The actual sequence of the genes is A, C, B rather than alphabetical order.)

Myotonic dystrophy, an autosomal dominant disorder, is unusual because a severe congenital form occurs by transmission from the mother and not the father. In addition, the disease demonstrates *anticipation*, the severity of the disease increasing with each subsequent generation. Mutatable expansion of a GCT trinucleotide repeat in a 3' untranslated region of the myotonic protein kinase

TABLE 4–1.  Autosomal Dominant Diseases

|  | Frequency | Comments |
|---|---|---|
| Peutz-Jeghers disease | Rare | Mucocutaneous pigment, GI hamartoma |
| Huntington disease | 1:2500 | Chromosome 4 (short arm) |
| Adult polycystic kidney disease | 1:1200 | Chromosome 16 (short arm) |
| Neurofibromatosis | 1:3000 | Chromosome 17, 50% new mutations |
| Bilateral acoustic neuroma (neurofibromatosis II) | $1:1 \times 10^6$ | Chromosome 22 (long arm) |
| Protein C deficiency | 1:15,000 | Gene cloned; chromosome 2 (short arm) spontaneous thrombosis |
| Hereditary angioedema Type I (decreased protein) Type II (dysfunctional protein) | 1:10,000 | Deficiency of C1 esterase inhibitor, chromosome 11, idiomorphic variants |
| Hereditary hemorrhagic telangiectasia (Osler-Weber-Rendu disease) | 1–2:100,000 | Angiodysplasia |
| Myotonic dystrophy | 1:25,000 | Chromosome 19 (long arm) |
| Familial retinoblastoma | 1:20,000 | Multifocal tumor, chromosome 13, gene cloned |
| von Willebrand disease | 1:100 | Chromosome 12, male = female incidence |
| Tuberous sclerosis | 1:29,900 | Chromosome 19; adenoma sebaceum, seizures, retardation |
| Gilbert disease | ? | Indirect hyperbilirubinemia |
| Hereditary spherocytosis | 1:5000 | Spectrin deficiency, some variants autosomal recessive |
| Marfan syndrome | 1:20,000 | Variable penetrance |
| Achondroplasia | 0.5–1.5:10,000 | 90% new mutations |
| Alpha$_1$-antitrypsin deficiency | 1:3000 | Gene cloned: chromosome 14 cirrhosis, emphysema |
| Hyperlipidemia | 1:500 | Possible prevention of heart disease |

GI = gastrointestinal.

gene develops with each meiosis (especially maternal), thus explaining the genetic anticipation or increasing severity in the next generation. Other conditions result from unstable trinucleotide repeats, including Huntington disease and fragile X syndrome (see A Sex-Linked Condition with a Cytogenetic Marker).

## AUTOSOMAL RECESSIVE INHERITANCE

In autosomal recessive conditions, the phenotype is expressed when identical alleles are present. Consanguinity increases the risk of expressing an autosomal recessive disorder. For example, located on the distal segment of the q (long) arm of chromosome 12 is a gene for the enzyme phenylalanine hydroxylase. If an individual is homozygous for a gene that codes for an abnormal enzyme (or for a nonfunctional gene product) in this location, that person is not able to convert the essential amino acid phenylalanine to tyrosine. Under these cir-

cumstances, excess phenylalanine cannot be metabolized and will accumulate along with phenylalanine metabolic by-products to produce PKU. Elevated levels of phenylalanine can be neurotoxic and can lead to mental retardation (see Chapter 5). The risk of two carriers having a child with PKU is 1:4 (25%). To determine the gene frequency in a population, one uses the equation

$$p^2 + 2\,pq + q^2 = 1$$

where p = the frequency of one gene and q = the frequency of the other gene. For cystic fibrosis,

$$p^2 = 1:2500$$

Thus, the gene frequency is 1:25, or approximately 4% of the population has one abnormal cystic fibrosis gene. Other autosomal recessive conditions are shown in Table 4–2.

Homologous pair
paternal chromosomes 6

A1

At the completion of
meiosis the sperm will
have only one
6 chromosome

At the completion of
meiosis the ovum will
have only one
6 chromosome

The possibilities for HLA-A alleles in offspring
can be diagrammed using the Punnett square method

FIGURE 4–1. Chromosome 6 showing segregation of HLA-A alleles. HLA = human leukocyte antigen.

|  | Paternal contribution | |
|  | A1 | A2 |
| A3 | A1A3 | A2A3 |
| A10 | A1A10 | A2A3 |

Maternal contribution

TABLE 4–2.  Autosomal Recessive Diseases

|  | Frequency | Comments |
| --- | --- | --- |
| Congenital adrenal hyperplasia (21-hydroxylase) | 1:5000–15,000; 1:700 in Yupik Eskimo | Chromosome 6, linked to HLA groups |
| Phenylketonuria | 1:14,000 | Gene cloned; chromosome 12 |
| Sickle cell anemia | 1:625 in African Americans | Gene cloned; chromosome 11 |
| Cystic fibrosis | 1:2500 in whites | Gene cloned; chromosome 7 |
| Gaucher disease | 1:2500 in Ashkenazi Jews | Gene cloned; chromosome 1 (long arm) |
| Tay-Sachs disease | 1:3000 in Ashkenazi Jews | Gene cloned; chromosome 15 (long arm) |
| Galactosemia | 1:60,000 | Gene cloned; chromosome 9 (short arm) |
| Infantile polycystic renal failure | 1–2:14,000 | Renal and hepatic cysts |
| Wilson disease | 1:200,000 | Gene cloned; chromosome 13 (long arm) |
| Fanconi anemia | ? | Absent thumb, chromosomal breaks |

HLA = human leukocyte antigen.

## SEX-LINKED INHERITANCE

A sex-linked condition occurs when the gene locus appears on the X chromosome. There are many more sex-linked recessive conditions than sex-linked dominant conditions, and for this reason males are subject to a much larger number of inherited disorders than females (Table 4–3). Hemophilia A, a sex-linked recessive condition, exemplifies this mode of inheritance. The gene for clotting factor VIII is located on the distal q arm of the X chromosome. An absence of normal factor VIII leads to "classic" hemophilia. When the maternal parent is a carrier for hemophilia (factor VIII deficiency), 50% of the male offspring will have hemophilia, and 50% of the female offspring will be carriers like their mothers.

An inspection of the segregation of the sex chromosomes also leads to other important conclusions. The daughters of a man with a sex-linked recessive condition such as hemophilia will all be "obligate carriers" for the condition. Because a male cannot usually pass a sex-linked condition to his sons, male-to-male transmission establishes an autosomal pattern of inheritance.

Males with hemophilia can be identified because of an absence of factor VIII, but female carriers are extremely difficult to identify on the basis of factor VIII levels. Direct molecular analysis of the gene is possible using molecular techniques but is difficult. The hemophilia gene is very large; it includes 25 intervening sequences (introns) and 27,000 bases that code for mRNA. There is the potential for a great number of deletions and mutations in many areas of the single gene, all leading to the same disease. Carrier detection is facilitated by knowledge of the specific deletion in the affected male family member.

There is normally an inactivation of one X chromosome in females, a phenomenon called the *Lyon rule* (or *Lyon hypothesis*). According to the Lyon rule, early in embryogenesis, one of the two X chromosomes in each cell of a female embryo is randomly inactivated, leaving just one in the active state. All of the subsequent cells developing from this active ancestor have the same active X chromosome. For most of the genes on the X chromosome, females display a phenomenon called *mosaicism*, in which some cells have one X active and other cells have the alternative X active. Therefore, unless there is a test for the presence of the gene itself, tests for sex-linked gene products are very difficult to interpret. In many cells, the inactive X chromosome often can be seen as the Barr body (a clump of heterochromatin) adjacent to the nuclear membrane. There is ordinarily one Barr body for every X chromosome exceeding the active X (normal females who are 46,XX have one Barr body; a female who is 47,XXX would have two Barr bodies).

### A Sex-Linked Condition with a Cytogenetic Marker

A number of sex-linked conditions lead to mental retardation, and for many years it had been observed that there were many more males with mental retardation than comparably handicapped females. A chromosome marker called the "**fragile X**," so named for a breakage gap that can be induced on the distal q arm of the X chromosome, is present in many of these males. The condition is characterized by the following:

1. The fragile X marker (enhanced by special treatment of the cells in tissue culture).
2. Macro-orchidism in the postpubertal male.

TABLE 4–3.  X-Linked Recessive Diseases

| | Frequency | Comments |
|---|---|---|
| Lesch-Nyhan syndrome | 1:100,000 | Hypoxanthine-phosphoribosyl transferase |
| Ornithine transcarbamoylase deficiency | ? | Gene cloned—milder disease in females |
| Duchenne muscular dystrophy | 1:5000 | Gene cloned—high spontaneous mutation rate |
| Hemophilia A + B | 1:10,000 | Gene cloned; factor replacement needed |
| Fragile X syndrome | 1:2000 | 25% of mentally retarded males—macrocephaly, macro-orchidism, demonstrates anticipation |
| Bruton agammaglobulinemia | $1:1 \times 10^5$ | Recurrent infections |
| Chronic granulomatous disease | $1:1 \times 10^6$ | Recurrent infections, some variants autosomal recessive |
| Glucose-6-phosphate dehydrogenase deficiency | 10% of American blacks | Oxidant-induced hemolysis |
| Color blindness | $1:1 \times 10^5$ | |

3. Disproportionately severe delays in expressive language development.
4. Mild to moderate mental retardation.
5. In general, a normal appearance, except occasionally for some superficial findings such as prominent ears.

Fragile X is another example of *anticipation*, with mutatable expansion of a CGG trinucleotide repeat. This amplification occurs only during maternal meiosis, thus explaining transmission through carrier mothers and not through an unaffected "carrier" father. Amplification of CGG trinucleotide repeats creates the heritable unstable element of the X chromosome.

## GENES AND LINKAGE

Adjacent genes on the same chromosome are likely to be inherited together unless another genetic event separates the genes from each other. In *recombination*, a genetic event that takes place in meiosis, segments of DNA are exchanged (crossing over) in a reciprocal fashion between homologous chromosomes. The chance of this happening generally is proportional to the distance between the loci. The unit that is used to describe the distance between loci is the centimorgan (cM). A centimorgan does not represent a specific physical distance; rather, it is a number that reflects the chance that recombination will occur between two linked genes. If two loci are separated by 10 cM, recombination between the loci will occur about 10% of the time.

It is possible in a clinical situation to use the concept of linkage to determine genetic composition in a particular individual. If two genes are known to be linked in a given family and one of the genes is detectable by its normal effect but the other, mutated gene is undetectable, the individual demonstrating that he or she has the linked normal gene might be assumed to have the deleterious one also. The degree of certainty of this assumption depends on the chance that recombination has not occurred between the gene loci.

By employing appropriate methodology using restrictive endonucleases to digest DNA, we may presume a mutated gene to exist based on identification of the presence of a known closely linked DNA restrictive fragment polymorphism. The degree of certainty still is based on the chance for recombination occurring between the polymorphism and the mutated gene. The use of several closely linked polymorphic DNA fragments, especially those that flank the gene in question, can increase the certainty that recombination has not occurred and that the mutated gene is present.

When the actual abnormal DNA sequence responsible for the mutated allele is known (through a probe) and can be tested for directly, there is no uncertainty.

*Contiguous gene syndromes* occur when multiple neighboring or contiguous genes on a chromosome are deleted, often producing a cytogenetic alteration of chromosomal banding. DiGeorge (velocardiofacial) syndrome is an example and manifests abnormalities of the heart, thymus, parathyroid glands, and face.

## PEDIGREE ANALYSIS

Constructing a family pedigree is a quick way of surveying family history; the pedigree also helps to analyze the family visually for a specific pattern of inheritance. The conventional symbols used in pedigree construction are shown in Figure 4–2. *Autosomal dominant conditions* should occur in each generation and should not be passed on by individuals who do not manifest the condition (see Table 4–1). (An obvious exception would be an individual in whom there is no detectable expression of the gene, even though the gene is present.) Affected males should approximately equal affected females. An example is a pedigree of three generations affected with neurofibromatosis. Each child has a 50% chance of receiving the gene (i.e., 1:2 will be affected), and male-to-male transmission is present, excluding a sex-linked condition.

If a child is affected with a condition that is known to follow a dominant mode of inheritance

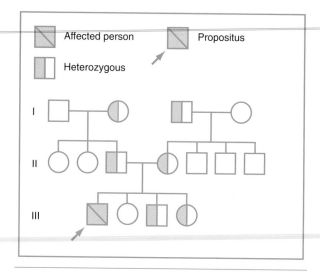

FIGURE 4–2. A pedigree showing an autosomal recessive pattern of inheritance.

but no family history can be constructed, several possibilities must be considered: (1) the child represents a new mutation; (2) a parent is affected but the expression cannot be detected or the parental mutation is limited to the germ cells; (3) the condition is genetically heterogeneic and in this family it follows another pattern of inheritance, such as an autosomal recessive pattern; (4) this condition is a *phenocopy* with another cause entirely; or (5) an identified parent is not the biologic parent.

*Autosomal recessive conditions* typically appear without an antecedent family history. Occasionally, the parents will be consanguineous (i.e., they have relatively close ancestors in common). Related persons have a greater chance of sharing the same hidden recessive genes than unrelated persons do. If a child is found to have a known autosomal recessive condition, the parents are carriers and the risk of recurrence for each subsequent child is 25%. Figure 4–2 shows a pedigree for autosomal recessive conditions (see Table 4–2).

An exception to the biparental carrier state in instances of autosomal recessive conditions has been discovered. This exception, called *uniparental disomy*, must be considered as an occasional mechanism for explaining the occurrence of recessive conditions. In uniparental disomy, two chromosomes of a pair are derived from one parent. If the pair of chromosomes are not just homologs but replicates of each other (a condition called *uniparental isodisomy*, which would happen if the chromosomes failed to separate at metaphase II of meiosis), then virtually all genes on the chromosomes would be identical (homozygous). If a mutation is present, a recessive disease will occur. If the nondisjunction (failure of the chromosomes to separate) occurs in metaphase I of meiosis, the two chromosomes are uniparental but not identical. Uniparental disomy can also result from a trisomy cell that loses one chromosome from the trisomy set in early embryogenesis. This event is called *trisomy rescue*. (See Chromosomal Imprinting.)

*Sex-linked recessive conditions* (see Table 4–3) are far more common than sex-linked dominant conditions. Males most often are affected, and transmission is through the mother, who often has affected male relatives (brothers or maternal uncles). Figure 4–3 shows a typical pedigree.

## MULTIFACTORIAL INHERITANCE: CONDITIONS WITH AN EMPIRIC RECURRENCE RISK

For genetic disease inherited by autosomal recessive and by dominant or sex-linkage patterns, the

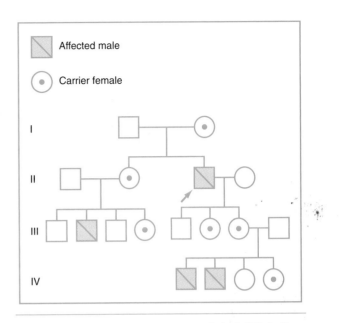

FIGURE 4–3. A pedigree showing a sex-linked (X-linked) recessive condition.

recurrence or inheritance risks are based on classic mendelian genetic laws. There is, however, no definitive genetic explanation for the inheritance of multifactorial genetic conditions. A large number of conditions occurring in children or adults seem to confer an increased risk of also occurring in parents, close relatives, and subsequent generations in the family. In this type of genetic disorder, it is postulated that a gene or a spectrum of genes confers a vulnerability for the condition in the individual and that some precipitating environmental factors interact to bring the condition about. By evaluating the reproductive outcomes of many families with similar conditions, we can calculate a pooled empiric recurrence risk. For most multifactorial disorders, the recurrence rate is 4–10%. Some have a sex predilection (e.g., pyloric stenosis in males and congenital dislocated hips in females), whereas others have a racial predilection (e.g., neural tube defects in whites or facial clefts in people of Asian ancestry).

The *inheritance of birth defects* often is multifactorial. It is likely that the causation of complex birth defects is heterogeneous and the defect may represent a final common pathway with many different causes. Congenital heart anomalies, neural tube defects, and cleft lip and cleft palate have empiric recurrence risks that exceed the general population risk, but the empiric recurrence risk is never as high as the recurrence risk for a classic specific gene disorder. Congenital heart anomalies affect about 5–10 infants per 1000 live births; the empiric recurrence is probably 5–10%. Neural tube defects, such as anencephaly and meningomyelocele, may affect as few as 1 infant per 1000 live births. There are significant differences in the prevalence of neural tube defects from area to area in the United States and from country to country; the incidence is higher in the United Kingdom and the Republic of Ireland than in the United States. The recurrence risk is 1–5%; however, recurrence risk can be lowered by preconception and early gestation maternal folic acid supplementation.

In evaluations of multifactorial genetic conditions, studies of twins may differentiate genetic from environmental factors. If twins have a disorder in common, they are said to be in *concordance* for their disorder; if they differ, they are described as *discordant* for the finding. With multifactorial genetic disorders, there is never 100% concordance, even in monozygotic twins (twins resulting from cleavage of a single egg). For example, concordance for all types of facial clefts is only about 33% in monozygotic twins and about 7% in dizygotic twins. Thus, other factors contribute to producing facial clefts.

Some multifactorial genetic diseases are associated with HLA types. Diabetes mellitus is associated with histocompatibility markers DR3 and DR4, whereas ankylosing spondylitis and post-venereal or enteric spondyloarthropathy are associated with HLA B27. Enteric spondyloarthropathy illustrates an interaction of environmental variables with a genetic predisposition to produce specific diseases.

## MITOCHONDRIAL INHERITANCE

Mitochondrial inheritance is another exception to mendelian or nuclear chromosomal inheritance. Many mitochondrial proteins and enzymes are determined by nuclear genes, but approximately 37 are dependent on the mitochondrial circular chromosome. Mitochondria are derived from the maternal parent exclusively, and mutations in the mitochondrial chromosome can be expected to follow a maternal pattern of inheritance. Therefore, both sexes are equally likely to inherit a mitochondrial mutation; expression may vary, depending on environmental and genetic factors. Leber optic neuropathy (sudden adult-onset blindness, cardiomyopathy, cardiac conduction defects; mitochondrial DNA [mtDNA] mutation of electron transport); myoclonic epilepsy and ragged red fiber–MERRF (myoclonus, seizures, optic atrophy, retinopathy, seizures, deafness, ataxia; mtDNA mutation of

tRNA genes); mitochondrial myopathy, encephalopathy, lactic acidosis; stroke-like episodes–MELAS (emesis, hemiplegia, cortical blindness, ataxia, dementia, seizures, diabetes; mtDNA mutation of transfer RNA gene); and Kearns-Sayre syndrome (ophthalmoplegia, ptosis, diabetes, ataxia, cardiomyopathy, retinal degeneration, ataxia; mtDNA deletion) are examples of maternal inheritance because of a mitochondrial chromosome mutation. Pearson marrow-pancreas syndrome (refractory sideroblastic anemia, pancreatic exocrine failure) is an atypical variant of Kearns-Sayre syndrome.

## CYTOGENETICS

Cytogenetics, the study of chromosome number and morphology, is an important part of the study of human inheritance.

It is possible to analyze the chromosomes of any cell capable of division. In a clinical setting, most cytogenetic analyses are performed using a mitosis-stimulating agent to cause division of peripheral blood lymphocytes placed in a tissue culture medium. Fibroblasts, bone marrow cells, amniocytes, and chorionic villi also can be used. Mitotic cells undergoing division are arrested in metaphase and ruptured, and the chromosomes spread out. Each pair of chromosomes has its own pattern of substructure that is expressed as a sequence of light and dark bands when the chromosomes are stained appropriately. The banding relates to the distribution of repetitive spacer DNA and nonrepetitive genomic DNA and a complex of DNA in association with acidic proteins and histones. These methods permit the identification of each pair of chromosomes and allow the chromosomes to be studied in detail; more than 1000 bands can be detected for the diagnosis of deletions and duplications of parts of chromosomes. Banding techniques vary: Q banding is detected with quinacrine, G banding with Giemsa, and C banding when the centromere region is stained.

A powerful cytogenetic tool involves in situ chromosome hybridization with a fluorescent tagged probe specific for a distinct locus on a chromosome. Deletions, translocations, and other small chromosomal changes can be detected even when conventional banding cannot detect any change. Probes for entire chromosomes are available, which makes it possible to karyotype an entire metaphase based on color analysis without banding. These techniques are called fluorescent in situ hybridization (FISH), chromosome painting, and spectral analysis.

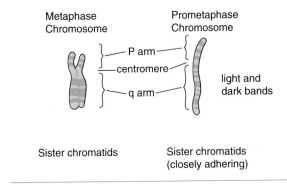

Metaphase Chromosome      Prometaphase Chromosome

P arm

centromere

q arm

light and dark bands

Sister chromatids      Sister chromatids (closely adhering)

FIGURE 4–4.  Chromosome morphology.

An understanding of cytogenetics and chromosomal abnormalities requires a special vocabulary and technology (Fig. 4–4).

## CHROMOSOMAL ABNORMALITIES

Chromosomal abnormalities may arise de novo during gametogenesis, so that an individual can be conceived with a chromosomal abnormality without any prior family history. Chromosomal abnormalities and chromosomal rearrangements also can be present in a parent and passed to an offspring. Sometimes this is associated with a family history of multiple spontaneous abortions or a higher-than-chance frequency of giving birth to children with chromosomal abnormalities. Chromosomal abnormalities or rearrangements also can occur in somatic cells at any time. If they arise early in embryogenesis, they can give rise to a clone that may have adverse consequences for the mosaic individual. Chromosomal alterations that occur later in life also may have adverse consequences on health; a high percentage of malignant neoplasms are associated with chromosomal abnormalities when the constitutional karyotype of the individual is normal.

Chromosomal abnormalities present at conception often lead to spontaneous abortion; about 50% of first trimester spontaneous abortions are chromosomally abnormal. Even the chromosomal abnormalities that are observed at term, such as trisomy 21 and Turner syndrome (45,X), represent only a fraction of the individuals conceived with these chromosomal problems. In general, abnormalities involving somatic chromosomes have a greater negative impact on the individual than do abnormalities of sex chromosomes.

Indications for obtaining chromosome studies include confirmation of a suspected chromosomal syndrome, multiple organ system malformations,

significant developmental delays or mental retardation not otherwise explained, short stature or very delayed menarche in girls, infertility or a history of several spontaneous abortions, ambiguous genitalia, and advanced maternal age (the fetus should be tested). The only way to establish that an individual has a normal karyotype is to perform a chromosome analysis. Higher-resolution banding studies have revealed subtle chromosomal alterations in a number of conditions.

FISH techniques have shown that there are a number of conditions, previously thought to be multifactorial and sporadic, that are due to chromosomal deletions. Williams syndrome (deletion 7) and DiGeorge-velocardiofacial syndrome (deletion 22q11.1-13) are examples.

## TRISOMY 21
### (Down Syndrome)

Trisomy 21 is the most common autosomal chromosomal abnormality in humans. A detailed review of this condition serves as a helpful model for understanding other chromosomal abnormalities.

Trisomy 21 occurs in all areas of the world and among all racial groups. The prevalence is 1:700 live births. The incidence of this and other chromosomal aneuploidy increases in frequency with increasing maternal age; the incidence is 1:2000 at 20 yr and 2–5% above 40 yr. Many trisomy 21 conceptuses result in spontaneous abortion. At 20 wk of gestation, a fetus with trisomy 21 has few phenotypic findings to suggest the diagnosis; however, at term, most infants have clinical manifestations suggesting the diagnosis.

### Cytogenetics

About 92% of children with Down syndrome have trisomy with an extra 21 chromosome present in all body cells, for a total chromosome count of 47. Chromosomal nondisjunction during *maternal meiosis* is responsible for 80–90% of cases of trisomy 21. About 5% of children have a translocation involving the 21 chromosome; the extra chromosome is attached to another chromosome, most often another acrocentric chromosome (chromosome numbers 13, 14, 15, 21, or 22), and the total chromosome count is 46. The majority of cases of trisomy due to translocation represent a new event. However, when a child is found to have trisomy owing to a translocation, parental karyotype analysis should be undertaken; it reveals a parent with a balanced translocation 20–40% of the time. If a parent has a balanced translocation, the other immediate family members should be studied to determine who may be at risk for having affected children. About 3% of the time mosaicism occurs; some cells display trisomy 21, but others have a normal karyotype.

## Clinical Manifestations

Infants born with trisomy 21 are the survivors of embryogenesis and fetal development. There is no clinical difference between children with transloca-tion trisomy and those with simple trisomy. In children with mosaicism, the clinical consequences of trisomy depend on the location and percentage of chromosomally normal cells. In many instances of mosaicism, the normal cells represent a minor clone that does not significantly alter the clinical manifestations. Cytogenetic analysis cannot predict the extent of organ malformation.

Children with trisomy 21 have almost a 40% chance of congenital heart disease. Virtually all children with Down syndrome are smaller than their siblings and smaller than peer age children. The intelligence is adversely affected, but the range of abilities is wide and approximates a bell-shaped curve shifted below the normal mean. Craniofacial manifestations include a small midface with up-turned nose, epicanthal folds, brachycephaly, flat occiput, speckled iris (Brushfield spots), and palpe-bral fissures that slant down to the midline. The Asian appearance of these infants led to the term "mongolism." Because of the small mandible and maxillae, the tongue may be prominent and the palate high and narrow. Eighty percent of infants with trisomy 21 are hypotonic at birth, but this feature often disappears with time. Additional neo-natal features include a poor Moro reflex (85%), joint hyperflexibility (80%), excess skin at the back of the neck (80%), and flat facies. Table 4–4 lists some of the clinical findings that may be present in trisomy 21.

## OTHER AUTOSOMAL TRISOMIES

Down syndrome accounts for the majority of chro-mosomal aneuploidy at birth. Trisomy 13 (1:5000) and trisomy 18 (1:8000) are other trisomies that can be differentiated by their spectra of clinical find-ings (Table 4–5). These trisomies carry a higher risk of spontaneous death in utero than Down syn-drome. Most children with these trisomies die in infancy; very few survive more than 1 yr. Definitive diagnosis is through chromosome analysis.

TABLE 4–4.  Clinical Findings That May Be Present with Trisomy 21*

Stature smaller than peer age group

Developmental delays

Congenital heart disease

Structural abnormalities of the bowel (tracheoesophageal atresia, duodenal atresia, annular pancreas, duodenal web, Hirschsprung disease)

Central hypotonia

Brachycephaly

Delayed closure of fontanels

Small midface, hypoplastic frontal sinuses, myopia, small (short) ears

Lax joints, including laxity of the atlantoaxial articulation (the latter predisposing the patient to C1–C2 dislocation)

Short, broad hands, feet, and digits; single palmar crease, clinodactyly

Exaggerated space between 1st and 2nd toe

Velvety, loosely adhering mottled skin (cutis marmorata) in infancy; coarse, dry skin in adolescence

Statistically increased risk for leukemia, Alzheimer disease, hypothyroidism

*An individual may show any combination of these findings. There is no correlation between the number of physical findings and eventual level of mental performance. The increased risk for leukemia is signifi-cant but probably no greater than 1.0% for any individual. Alzheimer disease is relatively common in persons with trisomy 21 who die in middle adult life, but the frequency in all adults with Down syndrome is not known.

## RECURRENCE RISK FOR AUTOSOMAL CHROMOSOMAL ABNORMALITIES

If a mother is younger than 35 yr of age, the recurrence risk for de novo chromosome abnormal-ities is about 1%. For couples in which the mother is over 35 yr, recurrence risk seems to approximate the empiric age risk.

## CHROMOSOMAL IMPRINTING

The sex of the parent contributing a specific chro-mosome may affect the expression of some of the genes on the chromosome. *Imprinting* is a strong parental (chromosomal) influence on the expres-sion of a particular gene. A small deletion of the q arm adjacent to the centromere of a number 15 chromosome (15 q11-q13) appears to give rise to *Prader-Willi syndrome* (PWS), if the deletion is in the paternal 15 chromosome. A normal gene on the paternal chromosome 15 prevents the syn-drome, but two maternal chromosomes 15 (mater-

TABLE 4–5. Findings That May Be Present in Trisomy 13 and Trisomy 18

|  | Trisomy 13 | Trisomy 18 |
|---|---|---|
| Head and face | Scalp defects (cutis aplasia)<br>Microphthalmia, corneal abnormalities<br>Cleft lip and palate (60–80%)<br>Microcephaly<br>Sloping forehead<br>Holoprosencephaly (arhinencephaly)<br>Capillary hemangiomas<br>Deafness | Small and premature appearance<br>Tight palpebral fissures<br>Narrow nose and hypoplastic nasal alae<br>Narrow bifrontal diameter<br>Prominent occiput<br>Micrognathia<br>Cleft lip and/or palate |
| Chest | Congenital heart disease (VSD, PDA, ASD) 80%<br>Thin posterior ribs (missing ribs) | Congenital heart disease (VSD, PDA, ASD)<br>Short sternum, small nipples |
| Extremities | Overlapping of fingers and toes (clinodactyly)<br>Polydactyly<br>Hypoplastic nails, hyperconvex nails | Limited hip abduction<br>Clinodactyly and overlapping fingers: index over 3rd,<br>  5th over 4th<br>Rocker-bottom feet<br>Hypoplastic nails |
| General | Severe developmental delays and prenatal and<br>  postnatal growth retardation<br>Renal abnormalities<br>Nuclear projections in neutrophils<br>Only 5% live >6 mo | Severe developmental delays and prenatal and postnatal<br>  growth retardation<br>Premature birth, polyhydramnios<br>Inguinal or abdominal hernias<br>Only 5% live >1 yr |

ASD = atrial septal defect; PDA = patent ductus arteriosus; VSD = ventricular septal defect.

nal uniparental disomy) produces Prader-Willi syndrome. Seventy percent of affected children demonstrate a cytogenetic visible deletion. Prader-Willi syndrome is characterized by transient neonatal hypotonia, obesity (onset 6 mo–6 yr), almond-shaped palpebral fissures, small hands and feet, and mild to moderate mental retardation. The incidence is 1:15,000. An entirely different condition, *Angelman syndrome*, seems to result if the deletion is in the maternal 15 chromosome.

## SEX CHROMOSOME ABNORMALITIES

The clinical consequences of sex chromosome abnormalities in term infants are much less severe than those associated with autosomal chromosomal abnormalities. However, Turner syndrome has a dramatic association with fetal death. Its frequency is about 1 affected individual per 10,000 female live term births, but the condition may be present in almost 1% of female fetuses.

### TURNER SYNDROME

Turner syndrome is associated with functional monosomy of the p arm of the X chromosome. The most common karyotype in Turner syndrome is 45,X with the second sex chromosome missing, but many affected females are mosaics. 45,X/46,XX is

the most common mosaic, but 45,X/47,XXX and 45,X/46,XY are also observed. Some females with Turner syndrome do have two X chromosomes, but in these instances one X has a missing p arm. The risk of Turner syndrome does not increase with advancing maternal age. These findings suggest an abnormality of embryonic cell division rather than fertilization by an abnormal gamete as the cause of Turner syndrome.

In utero mortality in Turner syndrome often is associated with severe and generalized edema and cystic hygroma. If swallowing is obstructed, polyhydramnios results. In many instances of severe fetal edema, pulmonary effusions impair lung development. However, live-born infants have an excellent prognosis. The gonads are present at birth and are appropriately infantile; during childhood, they often regress and may be absent at puberty.

The main *clinical manifestations* of Turner syndrome are short stature (adult height less than 150 cm in the untreated woman), sexual infantilism, and the consequences of congenital anomalies. Females with Turner syndrome have an increased incidence of bicuspid aortic valve and coarctation of the aorta. Furthermore, even in the absence of coarctation there is a higher frequency of hypertension later in life. In neonates there also may be carpal and/or pedal edema; this spontaneously resolves but may recur in adolescence when estrogen treatment is initiated. Additional features include a low hairline, webbed neck, widely spaced hypoplastic nipples, horseshoe kidney, and cubitus valgus of the elbow. Some children have problems with spatial relationships and geometric visual problem solving. As a consequence of having only one functional X chromosome, females with Turner syndrome display the same frequency of sex-linked conditions as do males with such conditions as hemophilia A or B.

*Treatment* of short stature has been successful using parenteral human growth hormone and oral anabolic steroids. Secondary sexual characteristics can be developed with estrogen or a combination of estrogen and progesterone (or their synthetic substitutes). A few girls will produce estrogen on their own, but most do not and have elevated gonadotropins, which reflects ovarian failure. Girls who are mosaic for cells containing a Y chromosome should have their gonads removed in adolescence to eliminate the risk for later gonadal neoplasm. A few women have become pregnant and have carried to term (presumably they had functioning ovaries). Several women with Turner syndrome have had in vitro fertilization with donor eggs and have carried to term.

### KLINEFELTER SYNDROME

Klinefelter syndrome occurs at a frequency of about 1:1000 live male infants, and the frequency at birth appears to increase with advancing maternal age. The typical karyotype is 47,XXY, but Klinefelter syndrome has occurred with multiple X chromosomes and one (or more) Y chromosomes. Infants and prepubertal boys are not identified owing to absence of recognizable clinical features. In the postpubertal male, there is infertility resulting from hypogonadism, with hypospermia or aspermia. Gonadotropin levels usually are elevated unless normal levels of testosterone are produced. Additional clinical manifestations may include mild mental retardation, long limbs, small penis, small and soft testes, and gynecomastia. Testosterone treatment may be indicated at adolescence.

### OTHER SEX CHROMOSOMAL ABNORMALITIES

Nature is extremely tolerant of variation in the sex chromosome composition. At least one normal X chromosome is essential for viability, but monosomy of the X chromosome, as in Turner syndrome, is compatible with normal but infertile life. Klinefelter syndrome and all its cytogenetic variants (47,XXY, 48,XXXY, 49,XXXXY, 48,XXYY, and others) are compatible with life, are not associated with elevated fetal loss, and also are associated with sterility. Klinefelter syndrome has been associated with personality disorders. Two other relatively frequent sex chromosomal abnormalities occur in humans—the karyotype 47,XXX (triple-X female) and the karyotype 47,XYY (the double-Y male). Each abnormality occurs with a frequency of about 0.1% and does not lead to sterility or to unique phenotypes. Because these karyotypes increase in frequency with maternal age, they are apt to be detected during prenatal diagnosis. The XYY male occasionally has been associated with antisocial behavior.

### GENETIC COUNSELING

For the family, inherited conditions and chromosomal abnormalities can create long-term and expensive health problems (mental retardation, major correctable or noncorrectable congenital anomalies, and multispecialized comprehensive care hospitalization). The success in the prevention of environmentally caused illness, especially infectious diseases, has led to an increased focus on genetic diseases and birth defects as causes of infant mortality and childhood morbidity. Only some birth defects are inherited, but the scope of clinical genetics includes all conditions with a familial recurrence risk that is higher than normal. Genetic evaluation should be followed by genetic counseling to estimate the recurrence risk for the family and relatives. Often, treatment for a genetic condition can be started before a definitive diagnosis is made, but appropriate genetic counseling requires a correct diagnosis.

Genetic counseling is a process of family education about inherited conditions or conditions that may affect future children. It is initiated as soon as a person begins to be evaluated, and it continues for as long as the physician is in contact with the family. This responsibility to communicate also may extend into the indefinite future if a new treatment is found or if new methods for screening or for prenatal diagnosis become available. Birth defects, whether genetic or not, and genetic conditions have the potential for significant emotional impact on the family, often because of the potential for parental feelings of guilt. Because these disorders frequently occur without prior history, the family may not understand the nature of the condition and may develop maladaptive coping mechanisms, which will adversely affect the long-term outcome for the child. Genetic counseling can help the family understand the condition, cope with hidden fears and superstitions, and proceed with the process of dealing constructively with the problem. Genetic counseling should include a discussion in understandable terms of the nature of the condition and the mode of inheritance; if the condition is not inherited, this should be explicitly stated. The estimated recurrence risk, the possibilities for prenatal diagnosis, the prognosis, and the treatment alternatives also should be included in the counseling.

## RECURRENCE RISK

Conditions inherited in mendelian fashion have a very precise recurrence risk that can be described and explained. An empiric risk for recurrence, if present, also should be explained to families. Couples should understand that no elevated recurrence risk is not the same as no risk.

## PRENATAL DIAGNOSIS

A significant number of inherited disorders and virtually all chromosomal abnormalities can be diagnosed prenatally. With the use of fetal ultrasonography, many dysmorphologic conditions with an empiric recurrence risk also can be diagnosed before birth.

## PROGNOSIS

Predictions for the outcome of a disease or the long-term development of a child are approximations at best. Specific predictions often are inappropriate, but the range and variation of a disease or condition can be described.

## TREATMENT ALTERNATIVES

Some treatments, of course, are dramatic and potentially lifesaving, such as the surgical correction of duodenal atresia. However, other less dramatic treatments include the recommendation for the avoidance of cigarette smoking in an individual with alpha$_1$-antitrypsin deficiency, or the dietary and medical management of a person with elevated cholesterol and an abnormal pattern of triglycerides and lipoproteins.

## EVALUATION OF THE PATIENT: PROBLEMS OF HUMAN SIMILARITIES AND VARIATIONS

Evaluating an individual whose condition potentially is genetic is a challenging diagnostic problem.

The pediatrician needs to consider a number of questions, such as:

Is this a "known" inherited condition?

Is it a chromosomal disorder?

Is it a "known" syndrome (a combination of nonrandom findings that seem to be associated in affected individuals)?

Is the condition due to a disruption of normal development?

Is the condition one that can arise because of exposure to an environmental agent (viral, bacterial, chemical, physical)?

Finally, is it a condition that may be inherited or that has an elevated recurrence risk, or is it one that is known to occur as a random event without elevated recurrence risk?

If there is a positive family history for the condition, the evaluation may be easier than if there is no history; however, many genetic conditions arise without a prior family history. Recessive conditions typically occur in a family without a prior history because most carriers are unaware of their status. New mutation dominant conditions also arise de novo, and even sex-linked conditions can occur as new mutations. In addition, minimal expressivity or nonpenetrance in other family members can result in a genetic condition without an apparent antecedent history. Genetic conditions or chromosomal disorders occur regardless of the general health of the mother or father.

In the evaluation of an individual child, several general points about heredity should be kept in mind. Children resemble their parents and other family members, although each individual will have a unique personal appearance. It is therefore a good idea to observe the appearance of parents and siblings.

There are also *group or racial similarities among individuals* that may need to be taken into account. Similarity of appearance in population groups may be explained at least partially by geographic and racial clustering of family members and ancestors. Groups originating from limited geographic areas must have had many ancestors in common. It is not surprising, therefore, that inbreeding and limited gene mixing are common among physically, socially, or religiously isolated populations (e.g., Amish, Ashkenazi Jews, and others).

There often is appreciable *variability among families with the same genetic disease.* The early discovery that sickle cell hemoglobin resulted from a point mutation leading to a single amino acid substitution in the beta chain of hemoglobin in every case of sickle cell disease encouraged geneticists to attribute specific gene disorders to identical changes in a single gene. Now we know that human genes are quite complex and that changes in different parts of the same gene can result in significant variation in the expression of the disease. It is probable that individuals homozygous for a recessive gene condition probably are actually heterozygous for specific alleles but that both alleles are abnormal. Data extracted from studies of families with hemophilia A (factor VIII deficiency) indicate that most families have gene alterations specific only to that family. It is probable that inherited conditions will display many kinds of gene changes. Some changes will be quite specific and common to many families (as with the sickle cell point mutation), but differences in disease expression may depend on the modulating effects from other components of the genome. Other gene changes may be variable because the gene is affected in different ways by a plethora of mutational mechanisms, duplications, deletions, and frame shifts. Mechanisms relating to expressivity always can be expected to operate to alter the clinical condition.

*Heterogeneity* refers to the fact that a condition may have separate causes. The condition, disease, or phenotype may represent the final common pathway in an abnormal process. For example, if a patient is found to have a hemolytic anemia, there are numerous causes, some acquired and some inherited. Even if we limit the cause of the hemolytic anemia to an inherited hemoglobinopathy, there still are numerous abnormalities of hemoglobin synthesis to consider. These include thalassemia, hemoglobin SS, hemoglobin SC, and others. The concept of heterogeneity must be kept in mind in the practice of medicine as well as in the practice of genetics. In genetic heterogeneity, separate genetic mechanisms may produce the same phenotype.

Another important concept is *expressivity*, which refers to the extent to which an individual is phenotypically affected by a gene or genes. For example, some patients with sickle cell anemia have a mild clinical course due in part to persistent production of fetal hemoglobin. *Penetrance* refers to the difference between the persons with a gene composition who show the effects of the gene and those with the same gene composition who do not show the effects. If a gene has a penetrance of 80%, 8:10 persons with the gene can be expected to show some effects of the gene. It does not mean that a person with the gene will be 80% affected; a gene is either penetrant or not penetrant in an individual.

*Pleiotropism* means that one gene or pair of genes can have many effects on the individual. When the mechanism of action of the gene or genes is not known, it may be difficult to explain why a single gene pair can have so many different effects on the

person. For example, without knowing the molecular and cellular pathology of sickle cell disease, the separate clinical manifestations of the condition would be difficult to explain on the basis of one homozygous gene pair because the effects seem so diverse. Persons with sickle cell disease would be described as having anemia, susceptibility to bacterial infections, renal disease, musculoskeletal pain, hand and foot swelling, and a predisposition to cerebral vascular accidents. When the molecular basis of the condition is understood, the multiple effects of the gene make more sense.

## EVALUATING AN INFANT WITH UNUSUAL PHYSICAL FINDINGS AND CLINICAL MALFORMATIONS (DYSMORPHOLOGY)

The challenge in physical diagnosis of an infant or child with unusual findings is describing as clearly as possible, in nonjudgmental terms, what is observed in the patient. Human variation is extensive but occurs on a continuum, with significant overlaps between what we call "normal" and what we term "abnormal." The subset of genetics that deals with the study of structural defects that alter appearance is called *dysmorphology*.

During the evaluation of an infant with unusual physical findings, a careful history is important even if it proves to be negative. Measurements of height, weight, and head circumference are essential, as are careful observations, documented in detail, for syndrome identification. Judicious laboratory tests can identify metabolic acidosis quickly, and chromosome analysis may be helpful. Sonography, computed tomography (CT), and magnetic resonance imaging (MRI) can identify internal abnormalities.

Congenital malformations (anomalies) usually occur early in gestation during tissue embryogenesis (Table 4–6) and may result from a variety of causes (Table 4–7). Malformations may be isolated and affect one organ system (spina bifida) or multiple, affecting unrelated tissues (trisomy 21). A *malformation sequence* is due to a single but localized abnormal tissue formation during development, which initiates a chain of subsequent defects. The prechordal mesoderm defect in the holoprosencephaly sequence produces deficits of midfacial development resulting in varying degrees of forebrain, ocular (hypotelorism to cyclopia), and nasal malformations. The *DiGeorge sequence* is due to a primary defect of the 4th branchial arch and derivatives of the 3rd and 4th pharyngeal pouches and results in varying degrees of thymus and parathy-

TABLE 4–6.  Relative Timing and Developmental Pathology of Certain Malformations

| Tissues | Malformation | Defect In | Causes Prior To | Comment |
|---|---|---|---|---|
| **Central nervous system** | Anencephaly | Closure of anterior neural tube | 26 days | Subsequent degeneration of forebrain |
| | Meningomyelocele | Closure in a portion of the posterior neural tube | 28 days | 80% lumbosacral |
| **Face** | Cleft lip | Closure of lip | 36 days | 42% associated with cleft palate |
| | Cleft maxillary palate | Fusion of maxillary palatal shelves | 10 wk | |
| | Branchial sinus and/or cyst | Resolution of branchial cleft | 8 wk | Preauricular and along the line anterior to sternocleidomastoid |
| **Gut** | Esophageal atresia plus tracheoesophageal fistula | Lateral septation of foregut into trachea and foregut | 30 days | |
| | Rectal atresia with fistula | Lateral septation of cloaca into rectum and urogenital sinus | 6 wk | |
| | Duodenal atresia | Recanalization of duodenum | 7 to 8 wk | |
| | Malrotation of gut | Rotation of intestinal loop so that cecum lies to the right | 10 wk | Associated incomplete or aberrant mesenteric attachments |
| | Omphalocele | Return of midgut from yolk sac to abdomen | 10 wk | |
| | Meckel diverticulum | Obliteration of vitelline duct | 10 wk | May contain gastric and/or pancreatic tissue |
| | Diaphragmatic hernia | Closure of pleuroperitoneal canal | 6 wk | |
| **Genitourinary system** | Exstrophy of bladder | Migration of infraumbilical mesenchyme | 30 days | Associated müllerian and wolffian duct defects |
| | Bicornuate uterus | Fusion of lower portion of müllerian ducts | 10 wk | |
| | Hypospadias | Fusion of urethral folds (labia minora) | 12 wk | |
| | Cryptorchidism | Descent of testicle into scrotum | 7 to 9 mo | |
| **Heart** | Transposition of great vessels | Directional development of bulbus cordis septum | 34 days | |
| | Ventricular septal defect | Closure of ventricular septum | 6 wk | |
| | Patent ductus arteriosus | Closure of ductus arteriosus | 9 to 10 mo | |
| **Limb** | Aplasia of radius | Genesis of radial bone | 38 days | Often accompanied by other defects of radial side of distal limb |
| | Syndactyly, severe | Separation of digital rays | 6 wk | |
| **Complex** | Cyclopia, holoprosencephaly | Prechordal mesoderm development | 23 days | Secondary defects of midface and forebrain |

Modified from Jones KL (ed): Smith's Recognizable Patterns of Human Malformation, 5th ed. Philadelphia, WB Saunders, 1997, p 704.

TABLE 4–7.  Causes of Congenital Malformations

| | | | |
|---|---|---|---|
| **Monogenic** | (7.5% of serious anomalies)<br>X-linked hydrocephalus<br>Achondroplasia<br>Ectodermal dysplasia<br>Apert disease<br>Treacher Collins syndrome | **Environmental agents** | (% unknown)<br>Polychlorinated biphenyls<br>Herbicides<br>Mercury<br>Alcohol |
| **Chromosomal** | (6% of serious anomalies)<br>Trisomies 21, 18, 13<br>XO, XXY<br>Deletions 4p–, 5p–, 7q–, 13q–, 18p–, 18q–,<br>    22q<br>Prader-Willi syndrome (50% have deletion<br>    of chromosome 15) | **Medications** | (% unknown)<br>Thalidomide<br>Diethylstilbestrol<br>Phenytoin<br>Warfarin<br>Cytotoxic drugs<br>Isotretinoin (vitamin A)<br>D-Penicillamine<br>Valproic acid |
| **Maternal infection** | (2% of serious anomalies)<br>Intrauterine infections (herpes simplex,<br>    varicella-zoster, rubella, toxoplasmosis) | **Unknown etiologies** | |
| **Maternal illness** | (3.5% of serious anomalies)<br>Diabetes mellitus<br>Phenylketonuria<br>Hyperthermia | *Polygenetic* | Anencephaly/spina bifida<br>Cleft lip/palate<br>Pyloric stenosis<br>Congenital heart disease |
| **Uterine environment** | (% unknown) | *Sporadic syndrome<br>complexes<br>(anomalads)* | CHARGE syndrome<br>VATER syndrome<br>Pierre Robin syndrome<br>Prune-belly syndrome |
| *Deformation* | Uterine pressure, oligohydramnios: clubfoot,<br>    torticollis, congenital hip dislocation,<br>    pulmonary hypoplasia, 7th nerve palsy | **Nutritional** | Low folic acid–neural tube<br>    defects |
| *Disruption* | Amniotic bands, congenital amputations,<br>    gastroschisis, porencephaly, intestinal<br>    atresia | | |
| *Twinning* | Conjoined twins, intestinal atresia,<br>    porencephaly | | |

CMV = cytomegalovirus; HIV = human immunodeficiency virus; CHARGE = *c*oloboma, *h*eart defects, *a*tresia choanae, *r*etarded growth, *g*enital anomalies, *e*ar anomalies (deafness); VATER, *v*ertebral defects, *a*nal atresia, *t*racheoesophageal fistula with *e*sophageal atresia, and *r*adial and renal anomalies.

roid gland hypoplasia, facial hypoplasia (micrognathia), and congenital heart disease (truncus arteriosus, interrupted aortic arch). Most patients with DiGeorge sequence have a partial monosomy of the proximal long arm of chromosome 22 or a microdeletion of 22q11.2. The recurrence rates for sequences are 1–5%.

A *malformation syndrome* is a nonsequential grouping of anomalies with multiple defects in more than one tissue and is often due to teratogens or chromosomal abnormalities. A *malformation association* is a nonrandom grouping of abnormalities with a specific pattern of affected tissues. The VATER syndrome includes varying rates of tissue involvement with *v*ertebral anomalies (70%), *a*nal atresia (80%), and *t*racheo*e*sophageal atresia (70%), *r*adial bone (65%), and kidneys (50%).

A *disruption sequence* often occurs later in gestation and manifests as amniotic bands with distal extremity amputations or constriction bands and pseudosyndactyly. Intrauterine infection or tissue infarction may also produce a disruption sequence.

A *dysplasia sequence* is due to poor tissue organization or migration of precursor cells. Abnormal neural crest cell migration is one example and may result in the neurocutaneous melanosis sequence. Abnormal cell metabolism, such as in *Hurler syndrome*, may also result in dysplasia in multiple tissues (cloudy cornea, mitral regurgitation, stiff joints, mental retardation, and coarse facies).

A *deformation sequence* is secondary to abnormal mechanical forces that influence tissue growth, position, and shape often after organogenesis is completed. Uterine compression due to oligohydramnios secondary to renal agenesis produces the *Potter syndrome* (pulmonary hypoplasia, breech position, club feet, flattened facies), while other causes of uterine constraint (bicornuate uterus, less severe degrees of oligohydramnios) may result in craniofacial (flat nose, crumpled ear, craniosynostosis, craniotabes) and limb deformations (metatarsus adductus, congenital dislocated hip).

A variety of specific terms are used to describe discrete features or structures. Word descriptions

TABLE 4–8.  A Glossary of Selected Terms Used in Dysmorphology

**Terms Pertaining to the Face and Head**

| | | | |
|---|---|---|---|
| Brachycephaly | A head shape that is shortened from front to back along the sagittal plane; the skull is rounder than normal | Scaphocephaly | A head elongated from front to back in the sagittal plane; most normal skulls are scaphocephalic |
| Canthus | The lateral or medial angle of the eye formed by the junction of the upper and lower lids | Synophrys | Eyebrows that meet in the midline |
| | | Telecanthus | A wide space between the medial canthi |
| Columella | The fleshy tissue of the nose that separates the nostrils | **Terms Pertaining to the Extremities** | |
| | | Brachydactyly | Short digits |
| Glabella | Bony midline prominence of the brows | Camptodactyly | A digit that is bent or fixed in the direction of flexion (a "trigger finger"–type appearance) |
| Nasal alae | The lateral flaring of the nostrils | | |
| Nasolabial fold | Groove that extends from the margin of the nasal alae to the lateral aspects of the lips | Clinodactyly | A crooked digit that curves toward or away from adjacent digits |
| | | Hypoplastic nail | The nail of a digit is unusually small |
| Ocular hypertelorism | Increased distance between the pupils of the two eyes | Melia | A suffix meaning limb (e.g., amelia—missing limb; brachymelia—short limb) |
| Palpebral fissure | The shape of the eyes based on the outline of the eyelids | | |
| | | Polydactyly | Six or more digits on an extremity |
| Philtrum | The vertical groove in the midline of the face between the nose and the upper lip | Syndactyly | Two or more digits are at least partially fused (can involve any degree of fusion, from webbing of skin to full bony fusion of adjacent digits) |
| Plagiocephaly | A head shape that is asymmetric in the sagittal or coronal planes; this can result from asymmetry in suture closure or from asymmetry of brain growth | | |

also can serve; for example, one can say that the eyebrows meet in the midline or, alternatively, that *synophrys* is present. Table 4–8 lists a glossary of some additional terms used in clinical morphology. Syndromes are identified from the detailed description of unusual findings. If an infant does not fit any specific condition, the child can be observed over time for growth, development, and physical changes that eventually may define the condition. In uncertain diagnostic situations, photographs can be helpful for discussion of the child with colleagues.

Throughout the physical examination, the taking of a family history, and each step of the evaluation, the physician should be compassionate, truthful, and respectful of patient, parents, and principles of the medical profession. Particularly, the physician should appreciate that diagnostic labels may produce untoward as well as beneficial effects on the family and, later, on the patient.

## PRENATAL DIAGNOSIS AND GENETICS

Prenatal diagnosis is a process for evaluating the health status of a fetus as early in gestation as possible. It includes analysis of cells from the developing chorion frondosum sampled at the 8th embryonic wk (chorionic villus sampling, [CVS]), maternal serum analysis for alpha-fetoprotein (MSAFP) or other substances of embryonic or fetal origin (chorionic gonadotropin and unconjugated estriol) after the 14th menstrual wk, ultrasound examination of the embryo/fetus during gestation, and analysis of amniotic fluid and/or amniotic cells removed by amniocentesis or fetal blood by cordocentesis during the middle trimester of gestation (Table 4–9).

Genetic indications for prenatal diagnosis include parental age and the risk of a detectable genetic condition based on the history or a known carrier state (X-linked or autosomal recessive). Maternal serum triple screen testing (maternal alpha-fetoprotein [AFP], unconjugated estriols, human chorionic gonadotropin [hCG]) is indicated for every pregnant woman. Chromosome analysis of amniotic fluid is virtually 100% accurate in detecting chromosomal abnormalities (see Table 4–9). The combination of ultrasound, amniotic fluid AFP analysis, and amniotic fluid acetylcholinesterase measurement is capable of detecting 95–98% of all neural tube defects. Hemoglobinopathies and a

TABLE 4–9.  Prenatal Diagnosis

| | |
|---|---|
| DNA analysis | Alpha$_1$-anitrypsin deficiency, thalassemia, sickle cell anemia, muscular dystrophy, hemophilia A, congenital adrenal hyperplasia, phenylketonuria, many others |
| Enzyme assay | Tay-Sachs disease, galactosemia, Hunter syndrome, maple syrup urine disease, Wolman syndrome, Lesch-Nyhan syndrome, Gaucher disease, I-cell disease, Menkes disease |
| Chromosome disorders | Trisomy 13, 18, 21; chromosome deletions; Turner syndrome; Klinefelter syndrome; fragile X |
| Alpha-fetoprotein | |
|   Elevated | Twins, neural tube defects, intestinal obstruction, congenital hepatitis, congenital nephrosis, impending fetal demise, omphalocele |
|   Decreased | Trisomy 21 and possibly other chromosomal disorders |
| Chorionic gonadotropin | |
|   Elevated | Trisomy 21, triploidy |
|   Decreased | Trisomy 13, trisomy 18 |
| Unconjugated estriol | |
|   Decreased | Trisomy 21 |
| Ultrasonography | Hydrops fetalis, hydronephrosis, neural tube defects, intestinal obstruction, congenital heart disease, diaphragmatic hernia, gastroschisis, omphalocele, limb reduction anomalies, assessment of growth |
| Cordocentesis | Fetal anemia, fetal acid-base and oxygenation disorders, fetal hypoalbuminemia, thrombocytopenia, thalassemia, cells for DNA |
| Fetal skin biopsy | Albinism, epidermolysis bullosa, xeroderma pigmentosum |

number of other gene disorders can be detected by DNA analysis or gene product (hemoglobin electrophoresis) assay (see Table 4–9). Many birth defects occur without a previous history in couples not at identifiable risk; therefore, it is unlikely that all major congenital malformations will be identified unless, as recommended by many obstetricians, all pregnant women receive antenatal ultrasonography.

## ENVIRONMENTAL AGENTS CAPABLE OF PRODUCING BIRTH DEFECTS

Many environmental agents have been alleged to produce birth defects, and it is best to consult the current literature and regional "hot lines" that are available for evaluating potential agents of embryo and fetal injury. If a structure has formed before the exposure, the agent cannot affect its formation. It is rare for an environmental agent to affect every exposed fetus, so most risks will be estimates of probable effects. Table 4–8 includes a list of some known environmental agents that present a risk to the developing fetus.

## References

Aase JM: Dysmorphologic diagnosis for the pediatric practitioner. Pediatr Clin North Am 39:135, 1992.

Austin KD, Hall JG: Nontraditional inheritance. Pediatr Clin North Am 39:335, 1992.

Behrman RE, Kliegman RM, Arvin AM (eds): Nelson Textbook of Pediatrics, 15th ed. Philadelphia, WB Saunders, 1996, Chapters 64–69, 86.

Jones K: Smith's Recognizable Patterns of Human Malformation, 5th ed. Philadelphia, WB Saunders, 1997.

Korf B: Molecular medicine. Parts I and II. N Engl J Med 332:1218, 1499, 1995.

Leppig KA, Werler MM, Cann CI, et al: Predictive value of minor anomalies: I. Association with major malformations. J Pediatr 110:531-536, 1987.

McKusick VA: Mendelian Inheritance in Man, 11th ed. Baltimore, Johns Hopkins University Press, 1996.

Seaver LH, Hoyme HE: Teratology in pediatric practice. Pediatr Clin North Am 39:111, 1992.

Shoffner JM: Maternal inheritance and the evaluation of oxidative phosphorylation diseases. Lancet 348:1283, 1996.

Tarleton J, Saul R: Molecular genetic advances in fragile X syndrome. J Pediatr 122:169, 1993.

Thornton JG, Hewison J, Lilford RJ, et al: A randomised trial of three methods of giving information about prenatal testing. BMJ 311:1127, 1995.

Yates JRW: Medical genetics. BMJ 312:1021, 1996.

# Chapter 5

# INBORN ERRORS OF METABOLISM

John F. Nicholson

The term "inborn errors of metabolism" was introduced by Garrod in 1908 to indicate recognizable abnormalities in human chemistry. We now recognize a great number of such abnormalities, many of which are best considered in the context of specific organ systems (e.g., sickle cell disease and congenital adrenal hyperplasia). Garrod's term now usually is applied to *intermediary* metabolism, loosely defined as the chemistry of dietary organic compounds and of the fuels derived from them, to which are added multisystem genetic diseases of biochemical origin.

Each of these diseases is caused by a deficiency of enzymatic catalysis or of an enzyme that facilitates the transport of biologic substances. In general, failure of enzymatic function leads to the accumulation of a reactant, which may or may not have toxic effects (Table 5–1). The product of the blocked reaction, if not available otherwise, becomes deficient. Defects in transport can impair intestinal absorption of dietary constituents, renal tubular reabsorption of filtered compounds, and the disposition of compounds within the body and even within the cell (Table 5–2).

The molecular nature of the many defects that have been described is diverse. In some instances, therapeutic strategies can be developed to deal with specific defects. For some disorders, the chemical problem can be defined as failure of interaction between an enzyme and a cofactor, usually a vitamin, in which case provision of a large excess of the vitamin can lead to chemical and clinical correction of the defect (e.g., cobalamin-responsive methylmalonic acidemia). Other therapeutic strategies deal with basic pathogenetic mechanisms—reducing the toxic reactant and providing the deficient product. In galactosemia, dietary elimination of galactose can be helpful. This can be done safely because galactose residues necessary for the formation of glycoproteins, polysaccharides, and complex lipids can be synthesized readily by humans. In contrast, treatment of phenylketonuria (PKU) requires reduction but not elimination of dietary phenylalanine, because phenylalanine cannot be synthesized by humans. In biotinidase deficiency, which impairs the recycling of biotin, supplementation of the diet with biotin is curative.

## GENERAL CONSIDERATIONS

### FAMILY HISTORY

Inherited metabolic disease frequently is discovered when the first affected child has distinct biochemical and clinical features or when the particular clinical disorder develops in the second child. Consanguinity is common in the family history of such patients. When parents are closely related (e.g., first cousins), the possibility of two rare inherited disorders in a single child becomes significant. For this reason, correlation of clinical findings with a single genetic defect is suspect when the correlation is based solely on the product of a consanguineous union.

### FAILURE TO THRIVE

Infants with inborn errors of metabolism frequently exhibit failure to thrive. Generally, metabolic defects severe enough to cause failure to thrive also produce readily recognizable chemical abnormalities. Additional clinical clues include recurrent emesis, lethargy, seizures, hypotonia, tachypnea, and unusual odors. Chemical clues to metabolic disease include hyperammonemia, hy-

TABLE 5–1.  Pathogenesis of Enzymatic Disorders

| Enzymatic Disorder | Reactant | | Product | | Clinical Disease |
| | Accumulated | Toxic? | Not Made | Deficient? | |
| --- | --- | --- | --- | --- | --- |
| Galactosemia | Galactose-1-phosphate | Yes | UDP-galactose | No | Yes |
| Biotinidase deficiency | Lysyl biotin | No | Biotin | Yes | Yes |
| Essential fructosuria | Fructose | No | Fructose-1-phosphate | No | No |

UDP = uridine diphosphate.

poglycemia, acidosis, ketonuria, abnormalities in hepatic transaminases, and hyperbilirubinemia.

## LABORATORY TESTS

*Plasma glucose*, as measured by the usual laboratory methods, averages 80 mg/dL in the fasting state, with a range of 60–100 mg/dL. During acute illness with temporary starvation, the blood glucose may fall to levels below 60 mg/dL in individuals who have no primary metabolic disorder. Therefore, it always is necessary to judge whether a given low value for blood glucose represents an appropriate physiologic adaptation or a true disorder. Autonomic manifestations (pallor, sweating, tremor, diplopia), seizures, and coma are clear manifestations of hypoglycemia as a disorder, whereas irritability and lethargy are defined as hypoglycemic in origin only when they respond dramatically to the administration of glucose. Hypoglycemia is an integral part of a number of metabolic diseases (see Chapter 17). In some of these diseases, acidosis or hyperammonemia may so dominate the clinical picture that the serious effects on glucose homeostasis are neglected. Hypoglycemia secondary to an inborn error may or may not be associated with ketonuria.

*Plasma ammonia* is present in very small concentrations (10–50 μmol/L) in normal fasting individuals. Blood samples should be collected on ice and analyzed within ½ hr because ammonia spontaneously rises rapidly. In general, elevations of less than twice the upper limit of normal in acutely ill patients do not indicate a significant disorder of nitrogen elimination.

In older infants and children, *ketonuria* is a normal response to starvation but not to a normal overnight fast. In the neonate, ketonuria is indicative of metabolic disease.

*Urine screening tests* for metabolic disease include the ferric chloride test (PKU, tyrosinosis, and others), the dinitrophenylhydrazine test (PKU, maple syrup urine disease), and the cyanide-nitroprusside test (homocystinuria, cystinuria). When the clinical manifestations suggest the diagnosis, these tests can be used as a basis for initiating therapy, but they should never be considered definitive. Abnormalities in the concentrations of metabolites (amino acids, organic acids) in body fluids and urine can provide diagnoses that are sufficient for long-term management and genetic counseling, but definitive diagnosis is made only by demonstration of a specific enzymatic or transport deficiency.

## DISORDERS OF METABOLISM FOR WHICH NEONATAL SCREENING IS PERFORMED

The purpose of neonatal screening is the detection and treatment of disorders during their preclinical

TABLE 5–2.  Pathogenesis of Disorders of Transport

| Disease | Transport System | Organs or Organelles Affected | Pathogenesis |
| --- | --- | --- | --- |
| Cystinuria | Cystine/arginine Lysine/ornithine | Kidney/intestine | Cystine stone formation |
| Hartnup disease | Monocarboxylic monoamino acids | Kidney/intestine | Tryptophan malabsorption |
| Glycogen storage disease Ib | Glucose-6-phosphate | Microsome | Hypoglycemia Excess glucose-6-phosphate |

phases. For PKU and homocystinuria, this strategy can be effectively carried out. Galactosemia and maple syrup urine disease (MSUD) usually do not remain subclinical for the time necessary to perform and report the tests.

## PHENYLKETONURIA

Phenylketonuria is an autosomal recessive disease that affects primarily the brain. It occurs in 1:10,000 persons. Classic PKU is the result of a defect in the hydroxylation of phenylalanine to form tyrosine (Fig. 5–1); the activity of phenylalanine hydroxylase in the liver is absent or greatly reduced. A small percentage of phenylketonuric infants have a variant disorder, **malignant** PKU, that results from a defect in the synthesis or metabolism of tetrahydrobiopterin, the cofactor for phenylalanine hydroxylase and for other enzymes involved in the intermediary metabolism of aromatic amino acids.

Affected infants are normal at birth, and the only constant *clinical manifestation* of PKU is the evolution of severe mental retardation (i.e., an intelligence quotient < 30). In addition, children may have blond hair, blue eyes, eczema, and mousy odor of the urine. In infants whose disease is caused by an error in the synthesis or metabolism of tetrahydrobiopterin (2% of PKU), a progressive, lethal central nervous system disease develops, reflecting abnormalities in other neural enzymatic reactions for which tetrahydrobiopterin is necessary.

In classic PKU, the *diagnosis* is made by demonstrating:

1. Hyperphenylalaninemia—1.2 mM (20 mg/dL) or higher (normal, ~0.06 mM, or 1 mg/dL) *and*
2. Normal or reduced plasma tyrosine (normal, ~0.06 mM, or 1 mg/dL).

The screening test for PKU measures whole blood phenylalanine; elevations should be confirmed by column chromatography of plasma amino acids. It is necessary to demonstrate normal (or lower) levels of tyrosine in blood because the pathway for phenylalanine metabolism develops late in gestation, with the result that a significant percentage of premature infants and a few full-term infants have transient elevations in both phenylalanine and tyrosine during the neonatal period. This condition, **transient tyrosinemia**, carries much less risk of permanent sequelae than classic PKU.

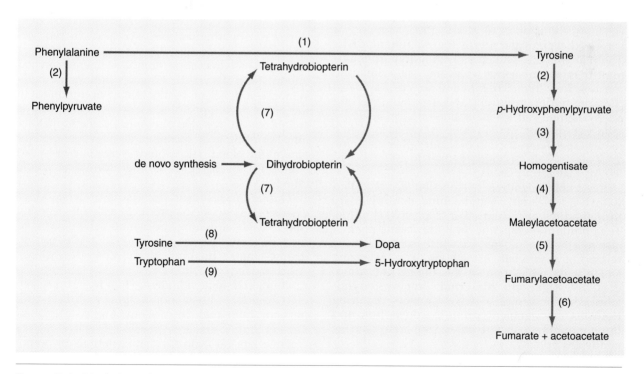

FIGURE 5–1. Metabolism of aromatic amino acids: (1) phenylalanine hydroxylase, (2) transaminase, (3) *p*-hydroxyphenylpyruvate oxidase, (4) homogentisate oxidase, (5) maleylacetoacetate isomerase, (6) fumaroylacetoacetate hydrolase, (7) dihydrobiopterin reductase, (8) tyrosine hydroxylase, (9) tryptophan hydroxylase.

Phenylpyruvic acid is present in the urine of phenylketonuric infants after the neonatal period and can be detected by adding a few drops of 10% ferric chloride to freshly voided urine. In the presence of phenylpyruvic acid, a deep green color develops immediately.

The diagnosis of malignant PKU is made by measuring dihydrobiopterin reductase in erythrocytes and analyzing biopterin metabolites in urine. Screening for malignant PKU is carried out in all hyperphenylalaninemic infants because there is no other way to differentiate the hyperphenylalaninemia caused by deficiency of phenylalanine hydroxylase from that caused by deficiency of tetrahydrobiopterin.

Achievement of normal intelligence is possible in most infants with classic PKU by *treatment* with a diet specifically restricted in phenylalanine begun within the first 3 wk of life. For infants with malignant PKU, restriction of dietary phenylalanine reduces plasma phenylalanine but does not ameliorate the clinical disease, which must be treated by replacement of the cofactor if biopterin synthesis is impaired and by neuropharmacologic agents if tetrahydrobiopterin reductase is deficient. Success in the management of malignant PKU is less predictable than with classic PKU.

In practice, a significant percentage of infants who are shown to be hyperphenylalaninemic by neonatal screening do not satisfy the chemical criteria for the diagnosis of classic PKU and do not satisfy the clinical criteria for malignant PKU. These infants are defined as having **hyperphenylalaninemia**. In some, plasma phenylalanine remains less than 0.6 mM (10 mg/dL) without therapeutic intervention, and in others, plasma phenylalanine can be maintained at that level by reducing dietary protein to 2 g/kg/day. A few require specific restriction of dietary phenylalanine to achieve "safe" (arguably, 0.4–0.6 mM or 7–10 mg/dL) levels in plasma.

Reversible cognitive dysfunction is associated with high plasma phenylalanine in previously treated adults and children with phenylketonuria. The optimum therapeutic level for plasma phenylalanine, the age (if any) at which control can be relaxed, and alternative methods for normalizing amino acids in the brain are the subjects of continuing investigation. **Maternal hyperphenylalaninemia** constitutes a major problem requiring rigorous management prior to conception and throughout pregnancy to avoid fetal brain damage and microcephaly.

### Related Disorders

Abnormalities in the catabolism of tyrosine can produce positive test findings for phenylketones in the urine but not elevations in blood phenylalanine. Although **tyrosinemia** can occur as a nonspecific consequence of severe liver disease, it is the most striking finding in fumaroylacetoacetate hydrolase deficiency (see Fig. 5–1), a rare disease in which metabolites that accumulate as a result of the impaired reaction produce severe liver disease (bleeding disorder, hypoglycemia, hypoalbuminemia, elevated transaminases, cirrhosis) and defects in renal tubular function. There are two clinical forms of the disease: *acute* highly lethal liver disease in the first months of life, and *chronic* liver disease, frequently associated with rickets, that manifests itself later in infancy or childhood. A high proportion of patients develop hepatic malignancies in later childhood.

*Treatment* includes a low-phenylalanine, low-tyrosine diet, NTBC (an inhibitor of the oxidation of para-hydroxyphenylpyruvic acid), and liver transplantation. There are more benign forms of hereditary tyrosinemia in which enzymes catalyzing tyrosine transamination and the oxidation of *para*-hydroxyphenylpyruvate are specifically deficient.

### HOMOCYSTINURIA

Homocystinuria, an autosomal recessive disease (1:200,000 live births) involving connective tissue, brain, and the vascular system, is caused by deficiency of cystathionine beta-synthase. In the normal metabolism of the sulfur amino acids, methionine gives rise to cystine; homocysteine is a pivotal intermediate (Fig. 5–2). When cystathionine beta-synthase is deficient, homocysteine accumulates in the blood and appears in the urine. There also is enhanced reconversion of homocysteine to methionine, resulting in an increase in the level of methionine in the blood. The neonatal screening test most commonly used measures methionine in whole blood.

Through mechanisms not clearly understood, an excess of homocysteine produces a slowly evolving *clinical syndrome* that includes in its fully developed form dislocated lenses, the habitus of Marfan syndrome, malar flushing, and livedo reticularis. Arachnodactyly, scoliosis, pectus excavatum or carinatum, and genu valgum are features of the skeletal disorder. Mental retardation, psychiatric illness, or both may be present. Major arterial or venous thromboses are a constant threat.

There are no neonatal manifestations of homocystinuria. Confirmation of the *diagnosis* requires demonstration of homocysteine in blood and urine.

*Treatment* of homocystinuria sometimes can be accomplished by giving, together with supplemen-

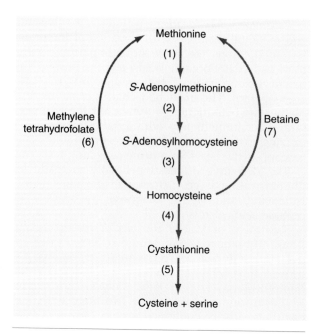

FIGURE 5–2. Metabolism of methionine and homocysteine: (1) methionine adenosyltransferase, (2) *S*-methyltransferase, (3) *S*-adenosylhomocysteine hydrolase, (4) cystathionine beta-synthase, (5) cystathionase, (6) homocysteine methyltransferase, (7) betaine-homocysteine methyltransferase.

tal folate, large doses of pyridoxine (100–1000 mg/day) to provide a great excess of the cofactor for cystathionine beta-synthase. If pyridoxine therapy fails, the accumulation of homocysteine can be controlled by a diet restricted in methionine and supplemented with cystine and folate. The use of supplemental betaine, to stimulate the alternative pathway for resynthesis of methionine from homocysteine, also appears to have a role in the management of pyridoxine-unresponsive patients. The prognosis is good for infants whose plasma homocysteine is controlled.

## GALACTOSEMIA

Galactosemia is an autosomal recessive disease (1:60,000 births) caused by an extreme deficiency of the enzyme galactose-1-phosphate uridyl transferase (Fig. 5–3). *Clinical manifestations* are most striking in the neonate, who, when fed milk, generally exhibits evidence of liver failure (bilirubinemia, disorders of coagulation, hypoglycemia), disordered renal tubular function (acidosis, glycosuria, aminoaciduria), and, frequently, cataracts. The neonatal screening test has limited usefulness for severely affected infants because they may die before the test result is available. When neonatal

manifestations are mild or nonexistent, failure to thrive may evolve. Major acute effects on liver and kidney function and the development of cataracts are limited to the first few years of life, but older children tend to have learning disorders. Ovarian failure is a late sequela.

*Laboratory manifestations* depend to a large extent on dietary galactose. When galactose is ingested (generally as lactose), plasma galactose and erythrocyte galactose-1-phosphate are elevated. Hepatocellular enzymes (alanine aminotransferase and aspartate aminotransferase) rapidly increase in plasma. Elevations of plasma conjugated and unconjugated bilirubin follow quickly, as do reductions in coagulation factors synthesized by the liver. Hypoglycemia is frequent, and albuminuria is always present in infants with clinical disease. Galactose frequently is present in the urine and can be detected by a positive reaction for reducing substances (Clinitest tablets) but no reaction with glucose oxidase on urine strip tests. Absence of urinary reducing substance cannot be relied on to exclude the diagnosis. Renal tubular dysfunction may be evidenced by hyperchloremic metabolic acidosis. The *diagnosis* is made by demonstrating extreme reduction in erythrocyte galactose-1-phosphate uridylyltransferase.

*Treatment* by the elimination of dietary galactose results in rapid correction of abnormalities, but infants who are extremely ill prior to treatment may die before therapy is effective. In addition, galactosemic infants are at increased risk for severe neonatal *Escherichia coli* infections.

Generally, it is possible to relax the dietary galactose restriction in later childhood. Congenital cataracts and mild brain damage have occurred even when galactosemic infants are treated from birth. For this reason, dietary galactose is elimi-

FIGURE 5–3. Pathway of galactose metabolism: (1) lactase (intestinal), (2) galactokinase, (3) galactose-1-phosphate uridyl transferase, (4) uridine diphosphoglucose 4-epimerase.

nated during pregnancy in mothers who have delivered galactosemic infants. Because the galactosemic fetus can synthesize galactose-1-phosphate, this therapeutic approach may have limited value.

### Related Disorders

**Galactokinase deficiency**, an autosomal recessive disorder (1:250,000), also leads to the accumulation of galactose in body fluids (see Fig. 5–3), which results in the formation of galactitol (dulcitol) through the action of aldose reductase. Galactitol, acting as an osmotic agent, can be responsible for cataract formation and, rarely, for increased intracranial pressure. These are the only clinical manifestations. Persons homozygous for galactokinase deficiency develop cataracts in the neonatal period, whereas heterozygous individuals are at risk for cataracts as adults. *Treatment* consists of lifelong elimination of galactose from the diet.

**Hereditary fructose intolerance** in many ways is analogous to galactosemia. When fructose is ingested, deficiency of fructose-1-phosphate aldolase leads to the intracellular accumulation of fructose-1-phosphate with resultant emesis, hypoglycemia, and severe liver and kidney disease. Elimination of fructose and sucrose from the diet cures the clinical disease.

*Fructosuria* is analogous to galactokinase deficiency in that it is caused by fructokinase deficiency, but the defect in fructosuria is entirely harmless.

### MAPLE SYRUP URINE DISEASE

This autosomal recessive disease, more properly named *branched-chain ketoaciduria*, is caused by deficiency of the decarboxylase that initiates the degradation of the ketoacid analogues of the three branched-chain amino acids—leucine, isoleucine, and valine (Fig. 5–4). MSUD is rare (1:250,000) in the general population but much more common in some population isolates (e.g., Pennsylvania Mennonites, 1:150). Neonatal screening programs commonly include MSUD.

Although intermittent and late-onset forms of the disease occur, clinical manifestations of the classic form typically begin within 1–4 wk of birth. Poor feeding, vomiting, and tachypnea commonly are noted, but the hallmark of the disease is profound depression of the central nervous system associated with alternating hypotonia and hypertonia (extensor spasms), opisthotonus, and seizures. The urine has the odor of maple syrup in most cases.

*Laboratory manifestations* include hypoglycemia and metabolic acidosis with elevation of the undetermined anions; the latter is due in part to plasma branched-chain organic acids and in part to the usual "ketone bodies," beta-hydroxybutyrate and acetoacetate. The branched-chain ketoacids, but neither the beta-hydroxybutyrate nor the acetoacetate, react immediately with 2,4-dinitrophenylhydrazine to form a copious white precipitate. This reaction is the basis for a urine screening test.

The definitive *diagnosis* generally is made by demonstrating large increases in plasma leucine, isoleucine, and valine. Diagnosis by analysis of organic acids also is possible.

Treatment of MSUD consists of restricting the intake of branched-chain amino acids (all three are essential amino acids) to the amounts required for growth in severely affected infants. Hemodialysis, hemofiltration, or peritoneal dialysis can be lifesaving during acidotic crises. Treatment with special diets must be continued for life. Ordinary catabolic stresses, such as moderate infections, can precipitate clinical crises. If left untreated, MSUD is rapidly fatal.

**Biotinidase deficiency** (see below) also is included in some programs for neonatal screening.

## INBORN ERRORS CAUSING CLINICAL DISEASE IN THE NEONATE

Virtually all of the diseases that cause metabolic acidosis, hyperammonemia, or hypoglycemia can produce clinical manifestations in the neonate. Because the fetus can be considered to undergo perpetual dialysis against an optimized nutrient solution, the infant with an inborn error of metabolism typically seems normal at birth. As the infant adapts to extrauterine life and the oral intake of nutrients, chemical abnormalities appear and symptoms follow at an interval that reflects both the type and the severity of the inborn error. Clinical recognition can occur as early as the 3rd day of life and generally is possible within the 1st wk. Poor feeding, vomiting, tachypnea, and seizures are manifestations common to neonates with inborn errors of metabolism, but these also are manifestations of a variety of other diseases, including neonatal septicemia. The most characteristic manifestation of metabolic disease is depression of the central nervous system exhibited by inattention to feedings, lethargy, and hypotonia, occurring in the absence of signs of disease of a specific organ or of neonatal septicemia. Laboratory evaluation of arterial blood gases, liver function, plasma glucose and ammonia, and routine urinalysis, including a

FIGURE 5–4. Metabolism of the branched-chain amino acids: (1) aminotransferases, (2) alpha-ketoacid dehydrogenase complex.

test for reducing substance, usually provides clues that lead to a diagnosis.

## NONKETOTIC HYPERGLYCINEMIA

Nonketotic hyperglycinemia, an autosomal recessive disease, is caused by a defect in the glycine cleavage system whereby glycine and serine are metabolically interconverted. As evidence that the fetus is affected by this disorder, malformations of the brain, most notably agenesis of the corpus callosum, are common.

*Clinically*, the disease produces profound deterioration in central nervous system function early in the neonatal period: alternating hypertonia and hypotonia, seizures, respiratory depression, inattentiveness, coma, and death within the first weeks of life. The $PCO_2$ may be increased as a result of respiratory depression and hyperglycinemia may be present, but the *diagnosis* rests on the demonstration of greatly increased glycine in cerebrospinal fluid and of an abnormal ratio of glycine in cerebrospinal fluid to glycine in plasma.

No effective *treatment* has been developed, but sodium benzoate, which lowers plasma glycine, has some efficacy, as do agents (diazepam, strychnine, ketamine, dextromethorphan) that antagonize glycine at receptors in the central nervous system. Although the genetic disease has a uniformly poor *prognosis*, there is a self-limited form of neonatal nonketotic hyperglycinemia that can mimic the genetic disease clinically and chemically but resolves spontaneously with no apparent residual effects.

## HYPERAMMONEMIA

Hyperammonemia can be considered to result from a failure of the liver to clear plasma ammonia. This failure can be caused mechanically by portal venous obstruction or chemically when an adequately perfused liver malfunctions, as occurs in hepatitis with cellular necrosis, in Reye syndrome with generalized hepatocellular dysfunction, and in a number of inborn errors of metabolism involving the synthesis of urea.

### Clinical Manifestations

Symptoms and signs depend on the underlying cause of the hyperammonemia, the age at which it develops, and its degree. Common constellations of findings in children are described next.

**Severe Neonatal Hyperammonemia.** Infants with complete genetic defects in urea synthesis, infants with *transient neonatal hyperammonemia* (see below), and, uncommonly, infants with interference in urea synthesis secondary to genetic disorders of organic acid metabolism can have levels of blood ammonia 100 times normal (>1000 μmol/L) in the first days of life. Poor feeding, hypotonia, apnea, hypothermia, and vomiting rapidly give way to coma and intractable seizures. Death occurs within days if the condition remains untreated.

**Moderate Neonatal Hyperammonemia.** Moderate neonatal hyperammonemia, in the range of 200–400 μmol/L, is associated with depression of the central nervous system, poor feeding, and vomiting, but seizures are not characteristic. This type of hyperammonemia may be caused by incomplete defects in urea synthesis and commonly is caused by disorders of organic acid metabolism that secondarily interfere with the elimination of nitrogen.

**Clinical Hyperammonemia in Later Infancy and Childhood.** Infants affected by defects in the urea cycle but who are not ill in the neonatal period may do well while receiving the low-protein intake of breast milk, but may later experience clinical hyperammonemia when dietary protein is increased or when catabolic stress occurs after the first few months of life. The clinical presentation is dominated by vomiting and lethargy, frequently progressing to coma. As protein intake is restricted by anorexia and vomiting, the sensorium clears and the infant recovers, only to develop symptoms again when the stimulus to hyperammonemia returns. Seizures are not typical of the disorder. During a crisis, the plasma ammonia level is usually 200–500 µmol/L, but when dietary protein is restricted, it becomes much lower and may even become normal. If the manifestations are not striking (i.e., if there is no coma), the condition may go unrecognized for years. When a crisis occurs during an epidemic of influenza, the child mistakenly may be thought to have Reye syndrome.

**Subclinical Hyperammonemia.** Infants and children with chronic elevations of plasma ammonia at the level of 100–200 µmol/L often do not have symptoms or signs of the derangement.

**Transient Neonatal Hyperammonemia.** Affected infants do not have a genetic disease, but striking hyperammonemia develops shortly after birth. Clinical manifestations may be extreme and include respiratory distress, apnea, and hypotonia. Exchange transfusion, hemofiltration, hemodialysis, or peritoneal dialysis may result in survival without neurologic sequelae. The etiology of this self-limited condition is unknown.

### Defects in the Urea Cycle

Inherited enzymatic deficiencies have been described for each of the steps of urea synthesis (Fig. 5–5). The following discussion considers, as examples, only two of these, ornithine carbamoyltransferase (OCT) deficiency and argininosuccinic aciduria (argininosuccinic acid lyase deficiency).

**Ornithine Carbamoyltransferase Deficiency.** This disease is unique among the defects in the urea cycle in that it is sex linked. Although the defective enzyme may have low-level activity, it generally is nonfunctional, resulting in absent OCT activity in the affected male, who will die in the neonatal period if untreated. Affected females are heterozygous, with one affected cell line and one unaffected cell line; the relative preponderance of each line is randomly determined according to the Lyon hypothesis (see Chapter 4). Because the liver is a mosaic of affected and unaffected nests of cells, it is not possible to define by needle biopsy the degree of enzymatic deficiency in clinically affected females, but it seems likely that overall activity of OCT must be reduced to roughly 20% of normal or lower in order to produce clinical disease. Thus, *clinical manifestations* range from lethal disease in the male to clinical normalcy in a high percentage of females. Manifestations in clinically affected females include recurrent emesis, lethargy, mental retardation, and psychiatric problems.

The *diagnosis* utilizes the fact that orotic acid, produced as a by-product of carbamoyl phosphate,

**FIGURE 5–5.** The urea cycle: (1) N-acetylglutamate synthase, (2) carbamoylphosphate synthetase, (3) ornithine carbamoyltransferase (OCT), (4) ornithine translocator, (5) argininosuccinic acid synthetase, (6) argininosuccinic acid lyase, (7) arginase.

is excreted in greatly increased quantities in the urine (see Fig. 5–5). The oroticaciduria, while much increased above normal, is not quantitatively significant for nitrogen excretion. Although some females heterozygous for the genetic defect excrete normal quantities of orotic acid, most affected females excrete excess orotic acid when given allopurinol.

**Argininosuccinic Aciduria.** Argininosuccinic acid lyase deficiency results in accumulation of argininosuccinic acid in tissues and blood; however, because the acid is cleared readily by the kidney, it is best identified in the urine, where it is found in gram quantities. Because the synthesis of argininosuccinic acid serves to fix ammonia nitrogen, hyperammonemia is not present at all times in all patients. However, the defect disrupts the urea cycle, and depletion of ornithine can lead to severe hyperammonemia. Death in the neonatal period has been reported, as has symptomatic hyperammonemia in later infancy and childhood. Failure to thrive, hepatomegaly, friable hair (trichorrhexis nodosa), slow motor and mental development, and seizures are characteristic features of the disease, whether or not there is clinical hyperammonemia. Argininosuccinic aciduria is an autosomal recessive disease.

### Treatment of Hyperammonemia

Reduction of dietary protein is the most important treatment for hyperammonemia. During episodes of extreme hyperammonemia, protein intake is eliminated and intravenous glucose is given in sufficient quantity to suppress catabolism of endogenous protein. Because 20% of total urea production is accounted for by detoxification of ammonia generated by bacterial urease in the intestine, sterilization of the intestine can provide brief benefit during acute episodes of hyperammonemia. Long-term benefit is possible with lactulose, a disaccharide not digestible by humans, which is fermented to lactic acid by intestinal bacteria. The resultant reduction in pH inhibits the transluminal absorption of ammonia.

Other important acute and chronic treatment modalities include sodium benzoate and phenylacetic acid (or its precursor, phenylbutyric acid), which are excreted in the urine as conjugates of glycine and glutamine, respectively. It must be noted as well that arginine is an essential amino acid when arginine synthesis via the urea cycle is grossly impaired. When hyperammonemia is extreme, direct removal of ammonia usually is carried out. For this purpose, hemodialysis or hemofiltration is more effective than exchange transfusion or peritoneal dialysis.

## ORGANIC ACIDOSES

**Metabolic acidosis** is a state in which acidification of urine is inadequate to maintain normal acid-base balance. **Renal tubular acidosis** frequently occurs in inborn errors of metabolism and is the result of disordered acidification of urine. Metabolic acidosis due to inborn errors of metabolism is the result of an overload of metabolic acids to be excreted. The latter condition is characterized by acidosis, acid urine, normal renal function, and an increase in circulating acids manifested by an abnormally large anion gap. In normal plasma, the **anion gap** as calculated by the formula $[Na - (Cl + HCO_3)]$ is 10–15 mEq/L. The metabolic acidosis results in values that are frequently 30 mEq/L or more as a result of the accumulation of organic acids. Both renal failure as a primary disorder and renal hypoperfusion associated with dehydration may increase the anion gap. Anion gaps exceeding 25 mEq/L usually do not occur in simple dehydration; however, for a given child, it may be neces-

sary to defer evaluation of the anion gap until rehydration has been accomplished.

### Starvation Ketosis and Ketotic Hypoglycemia

The most common circumstance in which acidosis is found in children is starvation associated with vomiting in the course of a viral illness. The *clinical manifestations* are those of the causative illness (see Chapters 2 and 11); the acidosis is mild, is associated with ketonuria, and promptly responds to the administration of carbohydrate. In this normal response to starvation, the blood glucose is relatively low (generally 50–70 mg/dL, but occasionally lower) and no symptoms referable to hypoglycemia appear (see Chapter 17).

In contrast, ketotic hypoglycemia is a common but abnormal condition in which tolerance for fasting is impaired to the extent that symptomatic hypoglycemia with seizures and/or coma occurs when the child encounters a ketotic stress. The stress may be significant (e.g., a viral infection with vomiting) or minor (e.g., a prolongation by several hours of the normal overnight fast). Ketotic hypoglycemia generally first appears in the 2nd yr of life. It occurs in otherwise healthy children and usually is treated by frequent snacks and the provision of glucose during periods of stress. *Clinical manifestations* typically are limited to the first 5–6 yr of life. Carbohydrate tolerance, gluconeogenesis, and hormone responses characteristically are normal.

### Lactic Acidosis

In most tissues, glucose is oxidized to carbon dioxide and water, with pyruvate as an intermediate (Fig. 5–6). Interference with mitochondrial oxidative processes results in an accumulation of pyruvate. Because lactate dehydrogenase is ubiquitous and because the equilibrium catalyzed by this enzyme greatly favors lactate over pyruvate, accumulation of pyruvate results in lactic acidosis. The most common interference with mitochondrial oxidation is oxygen deficiency owing to anoxia and/or poor perfusion. Hence, one expects lactic acidosis in the event of cardiac arrest, shock, severe cyanosis, and profound congestive heart failure. Poisons such as cyanide, sulfide, and carbon monoxide, which, like anoxia, block the terminal reaction of the mitochondrial respiratory chain, also produce lactic acidosis (see also Chapter 16).

Defects of the respiratory chain also can produce lactic acidosis. Given the complexity of the respiratory chain, it is not surprising that the defects

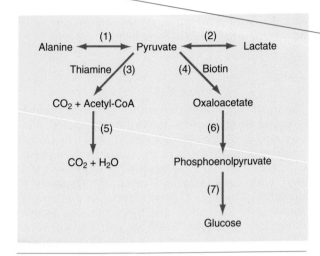

FIGURE 5–6. Metabolism of pyruvate and lactate: (1) alanine aminotransferase, (2) lactate dehydrogenase, (3) pyruvate dehydrogenase, (4) pyruvate carboxylase, (5) Krebs cycle, (6) phosphoenolpyruvate carboxykinase, (7) reverse glycolysis. CoA = coenzyme A.

described are varied in type and cause, some showing autosomal recessive inheritance, some showing mitochondrial (maternal) inheritance, and some showing no apparent inheritance pattern. Myopathy is very frequent, often showing ragged red fibers on muscle biopsy. Three striking entities are (1) **Kearns-Sayre syndrome** (ophthalmoplegia, retinal degeneration, and ragged red fibers), (2) **MERRF** (myoclonic epilepsy with ragged red fibers), and (3) **MELAS** (myopathy, encephalopathy, lactic acidosis, strokes). **Alpers syndrome** (degenerative disease of gray matter with seizures) and **Leigh disease** (subacute necrotizing encephalomyelopathy) are similar in molecular pathogenesis but clinically manifest primarily in the central nervous system.

Lactic acidosis also can occur when specific reactions of pyruvate are impaired. For practical purposes, pyruvate has three fates:

1. Transamination with glutamate to form alanine for gluconeogenesis and protein synthesis; the reaction is catalyzed by alanine aminotransferase.
2. Dehydrogenation and decarboxylation to form acetylcoenzyme A (CoA); the reaction is catalyzed by the pyruvate dehydrogenase complex (PDH).
3. Carboxylation to form oxaloacetate; the reaction is catalyzed by pyruvate carboxylase (PC).

Alanine, produced in muscle and other tissues, is an important precursor in hepatic gluconeogenesis.

The PDH reaction is the first step in pyruvate oxidation, and the PC reaction initiates gluconeogenesis. Inborn defects in both PDH and PC have been described. For *PDH deficiency*, the spectrum of reported clinical disease ranges from intractable, lethal acidosis in the first months of life to episodes of ataxia that improve with substitution of fat for carbohydrate in the diet. PDH deficiency also has been noted in some cases of Leigh disease. *PC deficiency* can produce a rapidly lethal neonatal disease that has as one of its elements hyperammonemia secondary to deficiency of aspartate, the product of transamination of oxaloacetate. Other infants with milder deficiencies show metabolic acidosis and mental retardation. In practice, the initial clinical manifestations associated with lactic acidosis due to inborn errors of metabolism frequently are nonspecific. The evaluation of the patient, therefore, must encompass a broad spectrum of both primary and secondary possibilities.

*Treatment* is limited for most mitochondrial defects. Disorders of gluconeogenesis may be treated with frequent carbohydrate feeding. Acidosis should be corrected (see Chapter 16).

### Disorders of the Propionate Pathway

Propionyl-CoA, a major catabolic metabolite of amino acids and lipids, is converted to succinyl-CoA in a series of reactions called the propionate pathway (Fig. 5–7). A key step in the sequence is the formation of succinyl-CoA from methylmalonyl-CoA, the cofactor for which is 5'-deoxyadenosyl cobalamin; this cofactor is the product of a series of reactions involving cobalamin (vitamin $B_{12}$). Defects in most steps of this pathway have been described, and all produce the **ketotic hyperglycinemia syndrome**. The specific entities are named for specific defects (e.g., propionic acidemia, methylmalonic acidemia, beta-ketothiolase deficiency).

The *clinical manifestations* of ketotic hyperglycinemia, which can begin in the neonatal period, consist of intermittent (1) ketoacidosis, (2) hyperglycinemia, (3) neutropenia, (4) thrombocytopenia, (5) hyperammonemia, and (6) hypoglycemia. After the first months of life, there is generally mild to moderate metabolic acidosis owing to the accumulation of the acid whose metabolism is impaired. Crises involving the intermittent elements of the syndrome occur during periods of catabolic stress but also may occur without an apparent precipitating event. During periods of neutropenia, the risk of serious bacterial infection is increased. Failure to thrive and impaired development are very com-

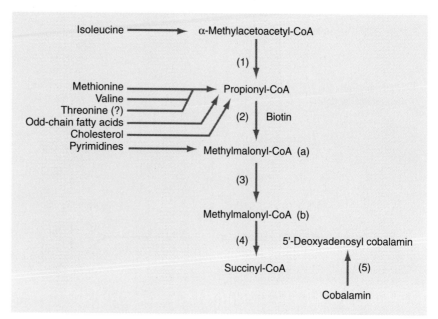

FIGURE 5–7. The propionate pathway: (1) β-ketothiolase, (2) propionyl-CoA carboxylase, (3) methylmalonyl-CoA isomerase, (4) methylmalonyl-CoA mutase, (5) cobalamin metabolic pathway. CoA = coenzyme A.

mon. The syndrome, caused by any of the reported defects, is inherited as an autosomal recessive trait.

*Treatment* with massive doses of vitamin $B_{12}$ is helpful in some cases of methylmalonic acidemia. For the remainder, management includes the restriction of dietary protein or of the specific amino acid precursors of propionyl-CoA (isoleucine, valine, methionine, threonine). Carnitine supplementation is indicated. Because intestinal bacteria produce a significant quantity of propionate, antibacterial treatment to reduce the population of bacteria in the gut has some beneficial effect in propionic acidemia and vitamin $B_{12}$–unresponsive methylmalonic acidemia.

### Isovalericacidemia

Isovalericacidemia is similar in its clinical manifestations to acidemias associated with defects in the propionate pathway; however, there are two significant differences:

1. Infants with isovalericacidemia have a "sweaty feet" odor.
2. Glycine therapy is beneficial through enhancement of the formation of isovalerylglycine, a relatively harmless conjugate of isovaleric acid (Fig. 5–8).

### Defects in Beta-Oxidation

The catabolism of fatty acids (Fig. 5–9) proceeds by the serial, oxidative removal of acetyl groups (each

as acetyl-CoA), the reactions catalyzed by a group of enzymes that exhibit specificities related to the chain length and other properties of the fatty acids, for example, very-long-chain acyl-CoA dehydrogenase (VLCAD), long-chain acyl-CoA dehydrogenase (LCAD), medium-chain acyl-CoA dehydrogenase (MCAD), short-chain acyl-CoA dehydrogenase (SCAD), and 3-hydroxyacyl-CoA dehydrogenases for at least two chain lengths of fatty acids. *MCAD deficiency* is the most common inborn error of beta-oxidation, prominently impairing hepatic adaptation to fasting. There is failure of normal fatty acid oxidation and of ketone body production and, thus, a failure to spare glucose utilization.

Hypoketotic hypoglycemia is a common mani-

FIGURE 5–8. Metabolism in isovalericacidemia: (1) leucine catabolic pathway (transamination and decarboxylation), (2) isovaleryl-CoA dehydrogenase, (3) glycine acyltransferase. CoA = coenzyme A.

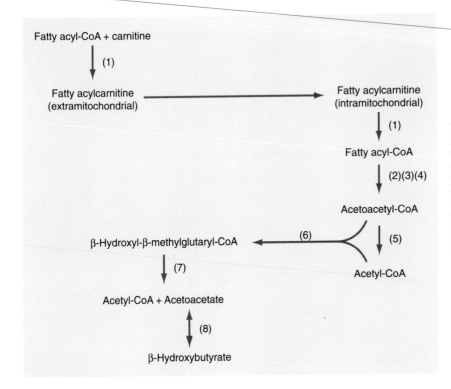

FIGURE 5–9. Scheme of fatty acid catabolism and ketone body formation: (1) carnitine acyl-CoA dehydrogenases, (2) long-chain fatty acyl-CoA dehydrogenase, (3) medium-chain fatty acyl-CoA dehydrogenase, (4) short-chain fatty acyl-CoA dehydrogenase, (5) β-ketothiolase, (6) β-hydroxy-β-methylglutaryl-CoA synthase, (7) β-hydroxy-β-methylglutaryl-CoA lyase, (8) β-hydroxybutyrate dehydrogenase.

festation, as is **Reye syndrome** (encephalopathy and fatty degeneration of the viscera with severe liver dysfunction). Reye syndrome–like illnesses may be recurrent in the patient or the family. Rarely, **sudden infant death syndrome** (SIDS) may occur in infants with MCAD deficiency. Most of the other, much rarer, disorders of fatty acid oxidation tend to involve skeletal and cardiac muscle more than does MCAD (see Glutaric Aciduria Type II). In all of the disorders of beta-oxidation, carnitine depletion can occur through excessive urinary excretion of carnitine and carnityl esters of incompletely oxidized fatty acids.

**Hydroxymethylglutaryl-CoA lyase deficiency**, although not a disorder of beta-oxidation, interferes profoundly with hepatic adaptation to fasting by impairing ketogenesis (see Fig. 5–9). The *clinical manifestations* are those of MCAD deficiency except that carnitine depletion is less prominent than in MCAD deficiency because hydroxymethylglutaric acid does not form an ester with carnitine.

The *diagnosis* of these disorders is suggested by the clinical picture and by hypoketotic hypoglycemia. The definitive diagnosis is made by analysis of urinary organic acids, acylcarnitine pattern, and enzyme characterization.

*Treatment* consists of a high-carbohydrate diet, carnitine supplements, avoidance of fasting, and aggressive administration of dextrose during intercurrent stresses.

## CARNITINE DEFICIENCY

Carnitine is a critically important cofactor in the transport of fatty acids across the mitochondrial inner membrane (see Fig. 5–9). It is synthesized from lysine by humans and also is present in dietary red meat and dairy products. Carnitine deficiency is either primary (i.e., due to failure of intake, synthesis, or transport to tissues of carnitine) or secondary (i.e., due to the excretion of excessive amounts of carnitine and carnitylesters in patients with inborn errors of metabolism). Primary carnitine deficiency has not been defined completely, but there are numerous examples of secondary carnitine deficiency among the organic acidurias, most prominently in disorders of the propionate pathway and in disorders of the beta-oxidation of long- and medium-chain fatty acids.

*Clinical manifestations* of carnitine deficiency include failure to produce acetoacetic and beta-hydroxybutyric acids, hypoglycemia, lethargy, lassitude, muscle weakness, and cardiomyopathy.

*Treatment* with carnitine has been dramatically effective in some cases and, in general, has facilitated the excretion of uncatabolizable organic acids and prevented carnitine depletion.

## BIOTINIDASE DEFICIENCY, BETA-METHYLCROTONYLGLYCINURIA, AND HOLOCARBOXYLASE DEFICIENCY

Biotin is a ubiquitous vitamin that is covalently linked to a number of carboxylases by holocarboxylase synthetase in a variety of tissues. Normal turnover of the carboxylases is accompanied by freeing of biotin for reutilization through the action of biotinidase. Inherited biotinidase deficiency greatly increases the dietary requirement for biotin, with the result that affected individuals can become biotin-deficient while consuming normal diets. Clinical disease can appear in the neonatal period or may be delayed until later infancy.

The *clinical manifestations* vary greatly—seizures, hypotonia, alopecia, skin rash, metabolic acidosis, and immune deficits—and undoubtedly are dependent on which enzymes in which tissues bear the brunt of the biotin depletion. Because carboxylation is a critical reaction in the metabolism of organic acids, most patients with biotinidase deficiency excrete abnormal amounts of several organic acids, prominent among which is beta-methylcrotonylglycine. In addition to biotinidase deficiency, an inherited deficiency of holocarboxylase synthetase gives rise to severe disease and to similar patterns of organic aciduria. Both conditions respond well to *treatment* with large (10–40 mg/day) doses of supplemental biotin.

## GLYCOGEN STORAGE DISEASES

The glycogen storage diseases enter into the differential diagnoses of hypoglycemia and of hepatomegaly (Table 5–3). Glycogen is the storage form of glucose and is found most abundantly in the liver, where it serves to modulate blood glucose, and in muscles, where it facilitates anaerobic work.

Glycogen is synthesized from uridine diphosphoglucose through the concerted action of glycogen synthetase and brancher enzyme (Fig. 5–10). Accumulation of glycogen is stimulated by insulin. Glycogenolysis occurs through a cascade phenomenon, initiated by epinephrine and/or glucagon and culminating in rapid phosphorolysis of glycogen to yield glucose-1-phosphate, accompanied by a lesser degree of hydrolysis of glucose residues from the branch points in glycogen molecules (see Fig. 5–10). In the liver and kidneys, glucose-1-phosphate can give rise to free glucose through the actions of phosphoglucomutase and glucose-6-phosphatase. The latter enzyme is not present in muscles.

Glycogen storage diseases fall into four categories:

1. Those that predominantly affect the liver and have direct influence on blood glucose (types I, VI, and VIII).
2. Those that predominantly involve muscles and affect the ability to do anaerobic work (types V and VII).
3. Those that can affect both the liver and muscles and directly influence both blood glucose and muscle metabolism (type III).

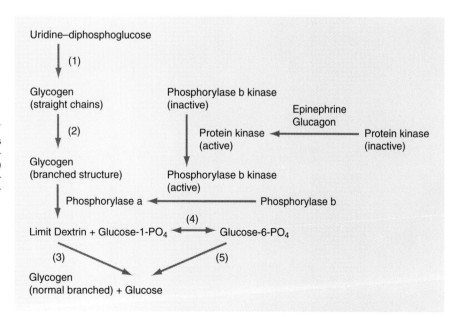

FIGURE 5–10. Glycogen synthesis and degradation: (1) glycogen synthetase, (2) brancher enzyme, (3) debrancher enzyme, (4) phosphoglucomutase, (5) glucose-6-phosphatase.

Table 5–3. Glycogen Storage Diseases*

| Disease | Affected Enzyme | Organs Affected | Clinical Syndrome | Neonatal Manifestations | Prognosis |
|---|---|---|---|---|---|
| Type I: von Gierke | Glucose-6-phosphatase | Liver, kidney, GI tract, platelets | Hypoglycemia, lactic acidosis, hepatomegaly, hypotonia, slow growth, diarrhea, bleeding disorder, gout, hypertriglyceridemia, xanthomas | Hypoglycemia, lactic acidemia, liver may not be enlarged | Early death from hypoglycemia, lactic acidosis; may do well with supportive management; hepatomas occur in late childhood |
| Type II: Pompe | Lysosomal α-glucosidase | All, notably striated muscle, nerve cells | Symmetric profound muscle weakness, cardiomegaly, heart failure, shortened PR interval | May have muscle weakness and/or cardiomegaly | Very poor; death in the 1st yr of life is usual; variants exist |
| Type III: Forbes | Debranching enzyme | Liver, muscles | Early in course hypoglycemia, ketonuria, hepatomegaly that resolves with age; may show muscle fatigue | Usually none | Very good for hepatic disorder; if myopathy present, it tends to be like that of type V |
| Type IV: Andersen | Branching enzyme | Liver, other tissues | Hepatic cirrhosis beginning at several months of age; early liver failure | Usually none | Very poor; death from hepatic failure before age 4 yr |
| Type V: McArdle | Muscle phosphorylase | Muscle | Muscle fatigue beginning in adolescence | None | Good, with sedentary lifestyle |
| Type VI: Hers | Liver phosphorylase | Liver | Mild hypoglycemia with hepatomegaly, ketonuria | Usually none | Probably good |
| Type VII: Tarui | Muscle phosphofructokinase | Muscle | Clinical findings similar to type V | None | Similar to that of type V |
| Type VIII | Phosphorylase kinase | Liver | Clinical findings similar to type III, without myopathy | None | Good |

*Except for hepatic phosphorylase kinase, which is X-linked, these disorders are autosomal recessive.
GI = gastrointestinal.

4. Those that affect various tissues but have no direct effect on blood glucose or on the ability to do anaerobic work (types II and IV).

In general, the *diagnosis* of hepatic glycogen storage disease can be made noninvasively by testing the response of blood glucose and lactate to glucagon (type I shows no rise in glucose, but a striking increase in lactate), by assaying enzymes (debrancher and brancher enzymes, phosphorylase, and phosphorylase kinase) in white blood cells, and by analyzing the structure of glycogen in erythrocytes. Type IV is best diagnosed by liver biopsy. Glycogen storage disease involving muscles can be assessed by electromyography (pathognomonic changes in type II), by measurement of the response of blood lactate to ischemic exercise (little change in type V in contrast to the normal brisk rise), and by muscle biopsy.

*Treatment* of hepatic glycogen storage is aimed at maintaining satisfactory blood glucose levels. This usually is not difficult, except in glucose-6-phosphatase deficiency (type I), the treatment for which requires nocturnal intragastric feedings of glucose during the 1st yr or two of life. Thereafter, snacks of uncooked cornstarch may be satisfactory. No specific treatment exists for the diseases of muscle that impair ischemic exercise. For both of the lethal glycogenoses (types II and IV), enzyme replacement has been attempted without success. Liver transplantation has been carried out successfully for severe hepatic glycogen storage disease.

## FAMILIAL HYPERLIPOPROTEINEMIA

### Type I Hyperlipoproteinemia

In type I hyperlipoproteinemia (familial hypertriglyceridemia), autosomal recessive deficiency of lipoprotein lipase or of its cofactor, apolipoprotein C-II, leads to the accumulation of chylomicrons in serum. Serum cholesterol may exceed 1000 mg/dL, but low-density lipoprotein (LDL) cholesterol is actually low; serum is grossly milky, with an easily visible layer of chylomicrons. This condition is rarer than type II disease.

*Clinical manifestations* of type I disease include eruptive xanthomata and periodic episodes of severe abdominal pain (pancreatitis), which may begin in infancy as colic. A diet very low in fat resolves the xanthomatosis and reduces the risk of the painful crises, which are sometimes fatal. Atherosclerotic disease does not occur.

### Type II Hyperlipoproteinemia

In type II hyperlipoproteinemia (familial hypercholesterolemia), hepatic clearance of LDL cholesterol is impaired because of genetic defects related to the LDL receptor. This results in large elevations in serum cholesterol (>500 mg/dL) in homozygous individuals and lesser elevations in heterozygotes.

The *clinical manifestations* include tendinous xanthomata and early atherosclerotic cardiovascular disease; angina pectoris and myocardial infarction may occur during late childhood and adolescence in homozygous individuals. The serum of affected subjects is clear.

## METABOLIC DISEASES ASSOCIATED WITH DYSMORPHIC SYNDROME

Most children who have inborn errors of metabolism are not dysmorphic; conversely, most dysmorphic children do not have currently recognized inborn errors of metabolism. Exceptions include homocystinuria, which can produce Marfan syndrome (see earlier), the glutaricacidurias, Zellweger syndrome, and the lysosomal storage diseases.

### Type I Glutaricaciduria

Type I glutaricaciduria is an autosomal recessive disease produced by deficiency of glutaryl-CoA dehydrogenase activity (Fig. 5–11). *Clinical manifestations* include macrocephaly, which may be present at birth; dystonia, which characteristically develops after 6 mo of age; and recurrent acute episodes of hepatic dysfunction, acidosis, hypoglycemia, and hyperammonemia (i.e., recurrent Reye syndrome). Intelligence is much less affected than motor function.

*Treatment* consisting of a low-protein diet, riboflavin, and agents (baclofen or valproic acid) that increase the concentration of gamma-amino butyric acid in the brain appears to be beneficial.

### Type II Glutaricaciduria

This clinical disease is produced by a defect in the transfer of electrons from flavine adenine nucleotides to the electron transport chain, caused by a deficiency of either electron transport flavoprotein or electron transfer flavoprotein-ubiquinone oxidoreductase (Fig. 5–11). When the enzyme essentially is nonfunctional, congenital anomalies are common—renal cysts, facial abnormalities, rocker-bottom feet, and hypospadias. Severely affected in-

TABLE 5–4. Lysosomal Storage Diseases

| Disease (Eponym) | Enzyme Deficiency | Clinical Onset | Dysostosis Multiplex | Cornea | Retina |
|---|---|---|---|---|---|
| *Mucopolysaccharidoses (MPS)* | | | | | |
| **MPS I (Hurler)*** | α-L-Iduronidase | ≈1 yr | Yes | Cloudy | — |
| MPS II (Hunter) | Iduronate-2-sulfatase | 1–2 yr | Yes | Clear | Retinitis, papilledema |
| **MPS III (Sanfilippo)** | One of several degrading heparan SO$_4$S | 2–6 yr | Mild | Clear | — |
| **MPS IV (Morquio)** | Galactose-6-sulfatase or β-galactosidase | 2 yr | No, dwarfism deformities | Faint clouding | — |
| MPS VI (Maroteaux-Lamy) | N-Acetylgalactosamine-4-sulfatase | 2 yr | Yes | Cloudy | — |
| MPS VII (Sly) | β-Glucuronidase | Variable neonatal | Yes | ± Cloudy | — |
| *Lipidoses* | | | | | |
| **Glucosylceramide lipidosis 1 (Gaucher 1)** | Glucocerebrosidase | Any age | No | Clear | Normal |
| Glucosylceramide lipidosis 2 (Gaucher 2) | Glucocerebrosidase | Fetal life to 2nd yr | No | Clear | Normal |
| Sphingomyelin lipidosis A (Niemann-Pick A) | Sphingomyelinase | 1st mo | No | Clear | Cherry-red spots (50%) |
| Sphingomyelin lipidosis B (Niemann-Pick B) | Sphingomyelinase | 1st mo or later | No | Clear | Normal |
| Niemann-Pick C | Unknown | Fetal life to adolescence | No | Clear | Normal |
| **GM$_2$ gangliosidosis (Tay-Sachs)** | Hexosaminidase A | 3–6 mo | No | Clear | Cherry-red spots |
| **Generalized gangliosidosis (Infantile GM$_1$)** | β-Galactosidase | Neonatal to 1st mo | Yes | Clear | Cherry-red spots (50%) |
| Metachromatic leukodystrophy | Arylsulfatase A | 1–2 yr | No | Clear | Normal |
| Fabry disease | α-Galactosidase A (cerebrosidase) | Childhood, adolescence | No | Cloudy by slit lamp | — |
| Galactosyl ceramide lipidosis (Krabbe) | Galactocerebroside β-galactosidase | Early months | No | Clear | Optic atrophy |
| Wolman disease | Acid lipase | Neonatal | No | Clear | Normal |
| Farber lipogranulomatosis | Acid ceramidase | 1st 4 mo | No | Usually clear | Cherry-red spots (12%) |

| Liver, Spleen | CNS Findings | Stored Material in Urine | WBC/Bone Marrow | Comment | Multiple Forms |
|---|---|---|---|---|---|
| Both enlarged | Profound loss of function | Acid mucopoly-saccharide | Alder-Reilly bodies (WBC) | Kyphosis | Yes—Schei and compounds |
| Both enlarged | Slow loss of function | Acid mucopolysac-charide | Alder-Reilly bodies (WBC) | X linked | Yes |
| Liver ± enlarged | Rapid loss of function | Acid mucopolysac-charide | Alder-Reilly bodies (WBC) | — | Several types biochemically |
| — | Normal | Acid mucopolysac-charide | Alder-Reilly bodies (WBC) | — | Yes |
| Normal in size | Normal | Acid mucopolysac-charide | Alder-Reilly bodies (WBC) | — | Yes |
| Both enlarged | ± Affected | Acid mucopolysac-charide | Alder-Reilly bodies (WBC) | Nonimmune hydrops | Yes |
| Both enlarged | Normal | No | Gaucher cells in marrow | Bone pain fractures | Variability is the rule |
| Both enlarged | Profound loss of function | No | Gaucher cells in marrow | — | Yes |
| Both enlarged | Profound loss of function | No | Foam cells in marrow | — | No |
| Both enlarged | Normal | No | Foam cells in marrow | — | Yes |
| Enlarged | Vertical ophthalmo-plegia, dystonia, cataplexy, seizures | No | Foam cells and sea-blue histiocytes in marrow | Pathogenesis not as for NP-A and NP-B | Lethal neonatal to adolescent onset |
| Normal | Profound loss of function | No | Normal | Sandhoff disease related | Yes |
| Both enlarged | Profound loss of function | No | Inclusions in WBC | — | Yes |
| Normal | Profound loss of function | No | Normal | — | Yes |
| Liver may be large | Normal | No | Normal | X linked | No |
| Normal | Profound loss of function | No | Normal | Storage not lysosomal | Yes |
| Both enlarged | Profound loss of function | No | Inclusions in WBC | — | Yes |
| May be enlarged | Normal or impaired | Usually not | — | Arthritis, nodules, hoarseness | Yes |

*Table continued on following page*

TABLE 5–4. Lysosomal Storage Diseases *Continued*

| Disease (Eponym) | Enzyme Deficiency | Clinical Onset | Dysostosis Multiplex | Cornea | Retina |
|---|---|---|---|---|---|
| *Mucolipidoses (ML) and clinically related diseases* | | | | | |
| Sialidosis II (formerly ML I) | Neuraminidase | Neonatal | Yes | Cloudy | Cherry-red spot |
| Sialidosis I (formerly ML I) | Neuraminidase | Usually second decade | No | Fine opacities | Cherry-red spot |
| Galactosialidosis | Neuraminidase and β-galactosidase | Usually second decade | Frequent | Clouding usually present | Cherry-red spot usually present |
| ML II (I-cell disease) | Mannosyl phosphotransferase | Neonatal | Yes | Clouding common | — |
| ML III (Pseudo-Hurler polydystrophy | Mannosyl phosphotransferase | 2–4 yr | Yes | Late clouding | Normal |
| Multiple sulfatase deficiency | Many sulfatases | 1–2 yr | Yes | Usually clear | Usually normal |
| Aspartylglycos-aminuria | Aspartylglucos-aminidase | 6 mo | Mild | Clear | Normal |
| Mannosidosis | α-Mannosidase | 1st mo | Yes | Cloudy | — |
| Fucosidosis | α-L-Fucosidase | 1st mo | Yes | Clear | May be pigmented |

*The more prominent storage diseases are in boldface type.
CNS = central nervous system; WBC = white blood cell.

fants experience hypoglycemia without ketosis, metabolic acidosis, and the odor of sweaty feet soon after birth, and may die within the neonatal period. Less severely affected infants may have a more episodic recurrent Reye-like illness. Skeletal and cardiac myopathy can be prominent in this complex, pansystemic disease, the manifestations of which may be delayed in some cases to adult life.

*Treatment* generally has not been effective in infants, but riboflavin in large doses (100–300 mg/day) has benefited some patients. Glutaricaciduria type II exhibits autosomal recessive inheritance.

### Zellweger Syndrome

Zellweger syndrome, an autosomal recessive disease (1:100,000 births), is also known as *cerebrohepatorenal syndrome*. Peroxisomes are virtually absent,

as are normal peroxisomal functions, which include the oxidation of very-long-chain fatty acids. Affected infants have high foreheads, flat orbital ridges, widely open fontanels, hepatomegaly, and hypotonia. Other anomalies are common. Failure to thrive, seizures, and nystagmus develop early, and death occurs within the 1st yr. The disease is not treatable. *Neonatal adrenoleukodystrophy, infantile Refsum syndrome,* and *rhizomelic chondrodysplasia punctata* are related peroxisomal disorders.

### Lysosomal Storage Diseases

At least a hundred diseases are now characterized as disorders of lysosomal function. Most of these diseases are associated with at least some degree of dysmorphism.

Lysosomes are ubiquitous cellular organelles that degrade various cellular constituents by hy-

| Liver, Spleen | CNS Findings | Stored Material in Urine | WBC/Bone Marrow | Comment | Multiple Forms |
|---|---|---|---|---|---|
| Both enlarged | Yes | Oligosaccharides | Vacuolated lymphocytes | — | Yes (also see galactosialidosis) |
| Normal | Myoclonus, seizures | Oligosaccharides | Usually none | Cherry-red spot/myoclonus syndrome | Severity varies |
| Occasionally enlarged | Myoclonus, seizures Mental retardation | Oligosaccharides | Foamy lymphocytes | Onset, from 1 yr to 40 yr | Congenital and infantile forms like sialidosis 2 |
| Liver often enlarged | Profound loss of function | Oligosaccharide | No | Gingival hyperplasia | No |
| Normal in size? | Modest loss of function | Oligosaccharide | No | — | No |
| Both enlarged | Profound loss of function | Acid mucopolysaccharide | Alder-Reilly bodies (WBC) | Icthyosis | Yes |
| Early, not late | Profound loss of function | Aspartylglucosamine | Inclusions in lymphocytes | Develop cataracts | No |
| Liver enlarged | Profound loss of function | Generally no | Inclusions in lymphocytes | Cataracts | Yes |
| Both enlarged commonly | Profound loss of function | Oligosaccharides | Inclusions in lymphocytes | — | Yes |

FIGURE 5–11. Scheme of flavoprotein metabolism with reference to glutaricaciduria types I and II: (1) glutaryl-CoA dehydrogenase (deficient in glutaricaciduria type I), (2) fatty acyl-CoA dehydrogenases, (3) other flavoprotein dehydrogenases, (4) electron transfer flavoprotein (ETF) (deficiency results in glutaricaciduria type II), (5) ETF-ubiquinone oxidoreductase (deficiency results in glutaricaciduria type II). CoA = coenzyme A.

drolysis, thus allowing the components of these cellular constituents to be utilized or reutilized. Absence of one or more hydrolytic activities leads to accumulation of nondegraded cellular material within the lysosome. Because tissues vary greatly in the rate of synthesis and degradation of specific constituents, the absence of a specific hydrolase affects one tissue more than another. If the stored material turns over (i.e., is degraded) rapidly under normal circumstances, the disease is likely to become manifest earlier than if the stored material turns over very slowly under normal circumstances.

Given the permutations of lysosomal hydrolases, cellular constituents, and tissues, it is not surprising that the known disease entities are large in number and increasing rapidly. Clinically, all of them are progressive, although some only slowly so. Defects of bones and joints with evolution of gargoylism or dysmorphic dwarfism (skeletal dysplasia), increasing hepatosplenomegaly, gingival hyperplasia, degenerative disease of the central nervous system, clouding of the corneae, and changes in retinal pigmentation are common manifestations in the group as a whole.

Some "rules of thumb" can help in the approach to a specific patient:

1. *Dysostosis multiplex* (gargoylism) is pathognomonic of mucopolysaccharide storage.
2. Macular cherry-red spots, seen on funduscopic examination, are pathognomonic of storage disease affecting the brain and specifically indicate lipid storage.
3. Rapid development of clinical manifestations over the first months of life often implies deficiency of more than one hydrolytic activity and frequently is associated with storage of both mucopolysaccharide and lipid.

Table 5–4 presents information regarding some of the known storage diseases. Unless otherwise indicated, the disorder is an autosomal recessive trait.

## References

Azen CG, Koch R, Friedman EG, et al: Intellectual development in 12-year-old children treated for phenylketonuria. Am J Dis Child 145:35, 1991.

Behrman RE, Kliegman RM, Arvin AM (eds): Nelson Textbook of Pediatrics, 15th ed. Philadelphia, WB Saunders, 1996, Part X.

Berry GT, Yudkoff M, Segal S: Isovaleric acidemia: Medical and neurodevelopmental effects of long-term therapy. J Pediatr 113:58, 1988.

Hudak ML, Jones MD Jr, Brusilow SW: Differentiation of transient hyperammonemia of the newborn and urea cycle enzyme defects by clinical presentation. J Pediatr 107:712, 1985.

Scriver CR, Beaudet AL, Sly WS, Valle D (eds): The Metabolic and Molecular Bases of Inherited Disease, 7th ed. New York, McGraw-Hill, 1995.

Tegtmeyer-Metzdorf H, Roth B, Günther M, et al: Ketamine and strychnine treatment of an infant with nonketotic hyperglycinemia. Eur J Pediatr 154:649, 1995.

Wagoner DD, Buist NR, Donnell GN: Long-term prognosis in galactosemia: Results of a survey of 350 cases. J Inherit Metab Dis 13:802, 1990.

Wraith J: The mucopolysaccharidoses: A clinical review and guide to management. Arch Dis Child 72:263, 1995.

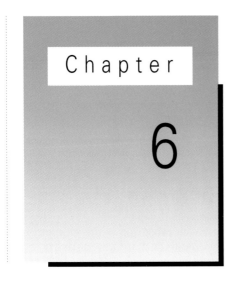

# Chapter 6

# FETAL AND NEONATAL MEDICINE

Robert M. Kliegman

The optimal care of both low-risk and high-risk newborn infants depends on knowledge of the family history, the history of prior and current pregnancies, and the events of labor and delivery. Thus, neonatal medicine, although focused on the care of the infant after birth, requires a continuum of understanding of the physiology of normal pregnancy; placental and fetal growth, function, and maturity; and any extrauterine or intrauterine pathologic events that affect the mother, placenta, or fetus. These latter adverse effects, which may result in an untoward neonatal outcome, often are interrelated and include such significant influences as poor maternal nutrition, poverty, physical or psychologic stresses, extremes of maternal age (<16 yr, >35 yr), black race, medical illness present prior to pregnancy, obstetric complications during the antepartum and intrapartum periods, and the inherent genetic predisposition of the fetus.

The late fetal and early neonatal period is the time of life exhibiting the highest mortality rate of any age interval. *Perinatal mortality* refers to fetal deaths occurring from the 20th wk of gestation until the 7th (or 28th) day after birth and is expressed as number of deaths per 1000 live births. Intrauterine fetal death represents 40–50% of the perinatal mortality rate. Such infants, defined as "stillborn," are born without a heart rate and are apneic, limp, pale, and cyanotic. Many have evidence of maceration, pale peeling skin, corneal opacification, and very soft cranial contents.

The *neonatal mortality rate* includes all infants dying during the period beginning after birth and continuing up to the first 28 days of life, and also is expressed as number of deaths per 1000 live births. Modern neonatal intensive care has delayed the mortality of many newborn infants who have life-threatening diseases, so that they survive the neonatal period, only to die of their original diseases or of complications of therapy sometime after the 28th day of life. This delayed mortality, as well as mortality due to acquired illnesses, occurs during the *postneonatal period,* which begins after 28 days of life and extends to the end of the 1st yr of life.

The *infant mortality rate* encompasses both the neonatal and the postneonatal periods and also is expressed as number of deaths per 1000 live births. The infant mortality rate in the United States declined in 1995 to 7.5:1000; the rate for black infants was approximately 14.9:1000.

The most common causes of perinatal and neonatal death are recorded in Table 6–1. Overall, congenital anomalies and diseases of the premature infant are the most significant etiologies of neonatal mortality.

*Low-birth-weight* (LBW) infants, defined as those having birth weights of less than 2500 g, represent a disproportionately large component of the neonatal and infant mortality rates. Although these low-weight births make up only about 7% of all births, they account for two thirds of all neonatal deaths.

*Very-low-birth-weight* (VLBW) infants, weighing less than 1500 g at birth, represent only about 1% of all births but account for 50% of neonatal deaths. In comparison with infants weighing 2500 g or more, LBW infants are 40 times more likely to die in the neonatal period, and VLBW infants have a 200-fold higher risk of neonatal death. In contrast to improvements in the infant mortality rate, there has been no recent improvement in the LBW rate. The LBW rate is one of the major reasons why the infant mortality of the United States is high compared with that of other large, modern, industrialized countries. If one calculates birth weight–specific mortality rates, the United States has one

**TABLE 6–1.** Major Causes of Perinatal and Neonatal Mortality

| Fetus | Preterm Infant | Full-term Infant |
|---|---|---|
| Placental insufficiency | Respiratory distress syndrome/ bronchopulmonary dysplasia | Congenital anomalies |
| Intrauterine infection | Severe immaturity | Birth asphyxia |
| Severe congenital malformations | Intraventricular hemorrhage | Infection |
| Umbilical cord accident | Congenital anomalies | Meconium aspiration pneumonia |
| Abruptio placentae | Infection | Persistent fetal circulation |
| Hydrops fetalis | Necrotizing enterocolitis | |

of the highest survival rates, but because of the large number of LBW infants, the total infant mortality remains relatively high.

Maternal factors associated with a LBW infant caused by premature birth or intrauterine growth retardation include a previous LBW birth, low socioeconomic status, low level of educational achievement, no antenatal care, maternal age younger than 16 yr or older than 35 yr, short time interval between pregnancies, cigarette smoking, alcohol and illicit drug abuse, physical (e.g., excessive standing or walking) or psychologic stresses (little social support), unmarried status, low prepregnancy weight (<45 kg or 100 lb) and poor weight gain during pregnancy (<10 lb), cervical infection, and black race. Race is especially significant because LBW and VLBW rates for black

women are twice those for white women. In addition, the neonatal and infant mortality rates are also 2-fold higher among black infants. These racial differences are explained only in part by poverty.

In addition to the sociodemographic variables associated with LBW, there are specific identifiable medical causes of preterm birth (Table 6–2). Factors such as uterine anomalies, hydrops fetalis, and most medical illnesses are not seen more frequently in blacks or in patients of lower socioeconomic status.

A comprehensive and multidisciplinary approach is required to identify and care for the high-risk pregnancy and to achieve the optimal neonatal outcome. Appropriate communication between the perinatal obstetrician and the pediatrician is essential. Additionally, the pediatrician must have a detailed up-to-date understanding of relevant perinatal obstetrics.

**TABLE 6–2.** Identifiable Causes of Preterm Birth

**Fetal**
Fetal distress
Multiple gestation
Erythroblastosis
Nonimmune hydrops fetalis
Congenital anomalies

**Placental**
Placenta previa
Abruptio placentae

**Uterine**
Bicornuate uterus
Incompetent cervix (premature dilation)
Short cervix

**Maternal**
Pre-eclampsia
Chronic medical illness (e.g., cyanotic heart disease)
Infection (e.g., group B streptococcal, herpes simplex, syphilis, bacterial vaginosis, genital mycoplasmal, chorioamnionitis)
Drug abuse (e.g., cocaine)

**Other**
Premature rupture of membranes
Hydramnios
Iatrogenic (e.g., cesarean section)
Trauma/surgery

### References

Barfield WD, Wise PH, Rust FP, et al: Racial disparities in outcomes of military and civilian births in California. Arch Pediatr Adolesc Med 150:1062, 1996.
Behrman RE, Kliegman RM, Arvin AM (eds): Nelson Textbook of Pediatrics, 15th ed. Philadelphia, WB Saunders 1996, Chapter 78.
Guyer B, Strobino D, Ventura S, et al: Annual summary of vital statistics 1995. Pediatrics 98:1007, 1996.
Meis P, Michielutte R, Peters T, et al: Factors associated with preterm birth in Cardiff, Wales: II. Indicated and spontaneous preterm birth. Am J Obstet Gynecol 173:597, 1995.
Sumits T, Bennett R, Gould J: Maternal risks for very low birth weight infant mortality. Pediatrics 98:236, 1996.

## PERINATAL OBSTETRICS

### RISK ASSESSMENT

Pregnancies associated with perinatal morbidity or mortality are considered high risk, and their identification is an essential component of obstetric care. These high-risk pregnancies may result in intrauterine fetal death, intrauterine growth retardation, congenital anomalies, excessive fetal growth, birth asphyxia and trauma, prematurity (birth before 38 wk) or postmaturity (birth at 42 wk or more), neonatal disease, or the long-term risks of cerebral palsy, mental retardation, and chronic sequelae of neonatal intensive care (Table 6–3). Between 10% and 20% of women can be considered to be at high risk at some time during their pregnancy. Although some obstetric complications are first seen during labor and delivery and cannot be predicted prior to parturition, many of these high-risk problems are present prior to labor and delivery. Overall, 50% of perinatal mortality and morbidity results from pregnancies identified as high risk prior to delivery. After identification, measures can be instituted to prevent complications, provide intensive fetal surveillance, and initiate appropriate treatments of the mother and fetus.

*Maternal factors* associated with high-risk status include the previously mentioned factors associated with LBW births. Additional maternal factors may be identified from past pregnancies. A history of premature birth, intrauterine fetal death, multiple gestation, intrauterine growth retardation, congenital malformation, explained or unexplained neonatal death, birth trauma, pre-eclampsia, gestational diabetes, grand multipara status (five or more pregnancies), or cesarean section is associated with additional risk for the subsequent pregnancy.

**Pregnancy complications** during the current gestation that increase risk include placenta previa, abruptio placentae, pre-eclampsia, diabetes, oligohydramnios or polyhydramnios, multiple gestation, blood group sensitization, abnormal levels of unconjugated estriols, chorionic gonadotropin, or alpha-fetoprotein, abnormal fetal ultrasonography, hydrops fetalis, trauma or surgery, abnormal fetal presentation (breech), exposure to prescribed or illicit drugs, prolonged labor, cephalopelvic disproportion, prolapsed cord, fetal distress, prolonged or premature rupture of membranes, cervical infections, and exposure to rubella, cytomegalovirus, herpes simplex, human immunodeficiency virus (HIV), toxoplasmosis, syphilis, and gonorrhea.

**Medical complications** associated with increased risk for maternal and fetal morbidity and mortality include maternal diabetes, chronic hypertension, congenital heart disease (especially with right-to-left shunting, Eisenmenger complex), glomerulonephritis, collagen vascular disease (especially systemic lupus erythematosus with or without antiphospholipid antibodies), lung disease such as cystic fibrosis, severe anemia such as sickle cell anemia, hyperthyroidism, myasthenia gravis, idiopathic thrombocytopenic purpura, inborn errors of metabolism such as maternal phenylketonuria, and malignancy. Furthermore, inheritance of maternal autosomal recessive genes, such as those for cystic fibrosis, galactosemia, and sickle cell anemia, places the newborn infant at increased risk for complications of these diseases that may become manifest in utero, in the newborn, or in the older infant.

## Obstetric Complications Associated with Fetal or Neonatal Risk

*Vaginal bleeding* in the 1st or early 2nd trimester may be due to a threatened or actual spontaneous abortion. If pregnancy continues, the fetus may be at increased risk for congenital malformations or chromosomal disorders. Vaginal bleeding that is painless, is not associated with labor, and occurs in the late 2nd or, more likely, the 3rd trimester often is due to placenta previa. Bleeding develops as the placental mass overlies the internal cervical os, which may produce maternal hemorrhagic

TABLE 6–3. Sequelae of Low-Birth-Weight Infants

| Immediate | Late |
| --- | --- |
| Hypoxia, ischemia | Mental retardation, spastic diplegia, microcephaly, seizures, poor school performance |
| Intraventricular hemorrhage | Mental retardation, spasticity, seizures, hydrocephalus |
| Sensorineural injury | Hearing, visual impairment, retinopathy of prematurity, strabismus, myopia |
| Respiratory failure | Bronchopulmonary dysplasia, cor pulmonale, bronchospasm, malnutrition, subglottic stenosis, iatrogenic cleft palate, recurrent pneumonia |
| Necrotizing enterocolitis | Short bowel syndrome, malabsorption, malnutrition, infectious diarrhea |
| Cholestatic liver disease | Cirrhosis, hepatic failure, carcinoma, malnutrition |
| Nutrient deficiency | Osteopenia, fractures, anemia, vitamin E deficiency, growth failure |
| Social stress | Child abuse or neglect, failure to thrive, divorce |
| Other | Sudden infant death syndrome, infections, inguinal hernia, cutaneous scars (chest tube, patent ductus arteriosus ligation, IV infiltration), gastroesophageal reflux, hypertension, craniosynostosis, cholelithiasis, urolithiasis, cutaneous hemangiomas |

Modified from Behrman RE, Kliegman RM, Arvin AM (eds): Nelson Textbook of Pediatrics, 15th ed. Philadelphia, WB Saunders, 1996, p 461.

shock, necessitating transfusions, and premature delivery. Painful vaginal bleeding is often the result of retroplacental hemorrhage and separation of an abruptio placentae. Associated findings may be hydramnios, twin gestation, and pre-eclampsia. Fetal asphyxia will ensue as the retroplacental hematoma causes placental separation that interferes with fetal oxygenation. Both types of bleeding are associated with fetal blood loss. Neonatal anemia may be more common with placenta previa.

*Abnormalities of the volume of amniotic fluid,* resulting in oligohydramnios or polyhydramnios, are associated with increased fetal and neonatal risk. **Oligohydramnios** is associated with intrauterine growth retardation and with major congenital anomalies, particularly of the fetal kidneys. Bilateral renal agenesis results in diminished production of amniotic fluid and a specific deformation syndrome (**Potter syndrome**) that is indicated by clubfeet, characteristic compressed facies, low-set ears, scaphoid abdomen, and diminished chest wall size accompanied by pulmonary hypoplasia and, often, pneumothorax. Uterine compression in the absence of amniotic fluid retards lung growth, and patients with this condition die of respiratory failure rather than of renal insufficiency. Twin-twin transfusion syndrome (donor) and complications from amniotic fluid leakage also are associated with oligohydramnios. Oligohydramnios (amniotic ultrasound fluid index ≤2 cm) increases the risk of fetal distress during labor (meconium-stained fluid, variable decelerations); the risk may be reduced by saline amnioinfusion during labor.

**Polyhydramnios** may be acute and may be associated with premature labor, maternal discomfort, and respiratory compromise. More often, polyhydramnios is chronic and is associated with diabetes, immune or nonimmune hydrops fetalis, multiple gestation, trisomy 18 or 21, and major congenital anomalies. Anencephaly, hydrocephaly, and meningomyelocele are neurologic problems associated with reduced fetal swallowing, whereas esophageal and duodenal atresia and cleft palate interfere with swallowing and gastrointestinal fluid dynamics. **Hydrops fetalis** may be due to Rh or other blood group incompatibilities with intrauterine hemolysis of fetal erythrocytes by maternal immunoglobulin G (IgG) sensitized antibodies crossing the placenta. Hydrops is characterized by fetal edema, ascites, hypoalbuminemia, and congestive heart failure. Causes of **nonimmune hydrops** include fetal supraventricular tachycardia, fetal anemia (resulting from bone marrow suppression, nonimmune hemolysis, twin-twin transfusion), severe congenital malformation, intrauterine infec-

tions, congenital neuroblastoma, inborn errors of metabolism (storage diseases), fetal hepatitis, nephrotic syndrome, and pulmonary lymphangiectasia. Twin-twin transfusion syndrome (recipient) also may be associated with polyhydramnios. Polyhydramnios is often due to unknown causes. If severe, polyhydramnios may be managed with bed rest, indomethacin, or amniocentesis.

*Premature rupture of the membranes,* which occurs in the absence of labor, and *prolonged rupture of the membranes* for greater than 24 hr are both associated with an increased risk of maternal or fetal infection (chorioamnionitis) and preterm birth. Typically, group B streptococcus, *Escherichia coli,* and *Listeria monocytogenes* are associated with fetal infection, although *Mycoplasma hominis, Ureaplasma urealyticum, Chlamydia trachomatis,* and anaerobic bacteria of the vaginal flora also have been implicated in infection of the amniotic fluid. The risk of serious fetal infection increases as the length of the time between rupture and labor (latent period) increases, especially if the period is greater than 24 hr.

*Multiple gestation* is associated with increased risk resulting from polyhydramnios, premature birth, intrauterine growth retardation, abnormal presentation (breech), congenital anomalies (such as intestinal atresia, porencephaly, and single umbilical artery), intrauterine fetal demise, birth asphyxia, and the **twin-twin transfusion syndrome.** The latter syndrome is associated with a high mortality and is seen only in monozygotic twins who share a common placenta and who demonstrate an arteriovenous connection between their circulations. The fetus on the arterial side of this shunt serves as the blood donor, which results in its fetal anemia, growth retardation, and oligohydramnios. The recipient, or venous-side twin, is larger or discordant in size, is plethoric and polycythemic, and may demonstrate polyhydramnios. Weight differences of 20% and hemoglobin differences of 5 g/dL confirm the diagnosis. Treatment includes amniocentesis and attempts to ablate the arteriovenous connection (laser). In addition to the twin-twin transfusion syndrome, the birth order of twins affects morbidity by increasing the risk of the second-born twin for breech position, birth asphyxia, birth trauma, and respiratory distress syndrome.

Overall, twinning is observed in 1:80 pregnancies, and 80% of all twin gestations are dizygotic twins. The diagnosis of the type of twins can be determined by placentation, sex, fetal membrane structure, and, if necessary, tissue and blood group typing.

*Toxemia of pregnancy,* or pre-eclampsia–

eclampsia, is a disorder of unknown but probably vascular etiology that may result in maternal hypertension, uteroplacental insufficiency, intrauterine growth retardation, intrauterine asphyxia, maternal seizures, and possible maternal death. Toxemia is more common in primiparous women and in women with twin gestation, chronic hypertension, or diabetes mellitus.

### Medical Problems During Pregnancy Associated with Fetal or Neonatal Risk

Medical diseases presenting during pregnancy can affect the fetus directly or indirectly (Table 6–4). Various immunologically mediated diseases affecting maternal tissues are due to autoantibodies; such antibodies also may cross the placenta. Because IgG immunoglobulins are transported actively across the placenta during the last half of the 3rd trimester, all IgG class antibodies will be present in the fetus. Pathologic antibodies can affect the same tissue in the fetus as in the mother. Other maternal illnesses, such as severe pulmonary disease (cystic fibrosis), cyanotic heart disease, and sickle cell anemia, may reduce oxygen availability to the fetus, whereas severe hypertensive or diabetic vasculopathy can result in uteroplacental insufficiency.

*Diabetes mellitus* that develops during pregnancy (gestational diabetes noted in about 5% of women),

TABLE 6–4.  Maternal Diseases Affecting the Fetus or Neonate

| Disorder | Effects | Mechanism |
|---|---|---|
| Cyanotic heart disease | Intrauterine growth retardation | Low fetal oxygen delivery |
| Diabetes mellitus | | |
| Mild | Large for gestational age, hypoglycemia | Fetal hyperglycemia—produces hyperinsulinemia; insulin promotes growth |
| Severe | Growth retardation | Vascular disease, placental insufficiency |
| Drug addiction | Intrauterine growth retardation, neonatal withdrawal | Direct drug effect, plus poor diet |
| Endemic goiter | Hypothyroidism | Iodine deficiency |
| Graves disease | Transient thyrotoxicosis | Placental immunoglobulin passage of thyrotropin receptor antibody |
| Hyperparathyroidism | Hypocalcemia | Maternal calcium crosses to fetus and suppresses fetal parathyroid gland |
| Hypertension | Intrauterine growth retardation, intrauterine fetal demise | Placental insufficiency, fetal hypoxia |
| Idiopathic thrombocytopenia | Thrombocytopenia | Nonspecific platelet antibodies cross placenta |
| Infection | See Table 6–28 | |
| Isoimmune neutropenia or thrombocytopenia | Neutropenia or thrombocytopenia | Specific antifetal neutrophil or platelet antibody crosses placenta following sensitization of mother |
| Malignant melanoma | Placental or fetal tumor | Metastasis |
| Myasthenia gravis | Transient neonatal myasthenia | Immunoglobulin to acetylcholine receptor crosses the placenta |
| Myotonic dystrophy | Neonatal myotonic dystrophy | Autosomal dominant with genetic anticipation |
| Phenylketonuria | Microcephaly, retardation | Elevated fetal phenylalanine levels |
| Rh or other blood group sensitization | Fetal anemia, hypoalbuminemia, hydrops, neonatal jaundice | Antibody crosses placenta directed at fetal cells with antigen |
| Systemic lupus erythematosus | Congenital heart block, rash, anemia, thrombocytopenia, neutropenia, stillbirth | Antibody directed at fetal heart, red and white blood cells, and platelets; lupus anticoagulant |

or diabetes that is present before pregnancy, adversely influences fetal and neonatal well-being. The effect on the fetus depends in part on the severity of the diabetic state in terms of age of onset of diabetes, duration of treatment with insulin, and the presence of arterial disease. Poorly controlled maternal diabetes results in maternal hyperglycemia, which in turn, because glucose levels in the fetus are slightly lower than but directly proportional to maternal glucose values, produces fetal hyperglycemia that stimulates the fetal pancreas, resulting in hyperplasia of the islets of Langerhans. Fetal hyperinsulinemia, which acts as a fetal growth hormone in the last trimester, results in increased fat and protein synthesis and fetal macrosomia, producing a fetus that is large for gestational age. After birth, hyperinsulinemia persists, resulting in fasting neonatal hypoglycemia. Strictly controlling maternal diabetes during pregnancy and avoiding hyperglycemia during labor and delivery prevent macrosomic fetal growth and neonatal hypoglycemia, respectively. Additional problems of the diabetic mother and her fetus and newborn are noted in Table 6–5.

In addition to the fetus' being directly affected by maternal illnesses, both the fetus and the newborn may be adversely affected by the medications used to treat those maternal illnesses. These effects may appear as teratogenesis (Table 6–6) or as an adverse metabolic, neurologic, or cardiopulmonary adaptation to extrauterine life (Table 6–7).

Acquired infectious diseases of the mother also may affect the fetus or newborn adversely (see Table 6–28).

**TABLE 6–6.** Common Teratogenic Drugs

| Drug | Results |
| --- | --- |
| Alcohol | Fetal alcohol syndrome, microcephaly, congenital heart disease |
| Aminopterin | Mesomelia, cranial dysplasia |
| Coumarin | Hypoplastic nasal bridge, chondrodysplasia punctata |
| Fluoxetine | Minor malformations, low birth weight, poor neonatal adaptation |
| Isotretinoin (Accutane) and vitamin A | Facial and ear anomalies, congenital heart disease |
| Lithium | Ebstein anomaly |
| Methyl mercury | Microcephaly, blindness, deafness, retardation |
| Penicillamine | Cutis laxa syndrome |
| Phenytoin (Dilantin) | Hypoplastic nails, intrauterine growth retardation, typical facies |
| Radioactive iodine | Fetal hypothyroidism |
| Stilbestrol (DES) | Vaginal adenocarcinoma during adolescence |
| Streptomycin | Deafness |
| Testosterone-like drugs | Virilization of female |
| Tetracycline | Enamel hypoplasia |
| Thalidomide | Phocomelia |
| Toluene (solvent abuse) | Fetal alcohol–like syndrome, preterm labor |
| Trimethadione | Congenital anomalies, typical facies |
| Valproate | Spina bifida |

**TABLE 6–5.** Problems of the Diabetic Pregnancy

**Maternal**
Ketoacidosis
Hypoglycemia
Pre-eclampsia
Polyhydramnios
Retinopathy

**Neonatal**
Prematurity
Macrosomia and birth trauma
Birth asphyxia
Respiratory distress syndrome
Transient tachypnea of newborn
Hypoglycemia
Hypocalcemia
Polycythemia
Unconjugated hyperbilirubinemia
Congenital malformations (heart, sacrum)
Cardiac septal hypertrophy
Small left colon syndrome
Renal vein thrombosis
Intrauterine fetal death

## ASSESSMENT OF FETAL WELL-BEING AND MATURITY

### Fetal Growth

Fetal growth can be assessed clinically by determining the fundal height of the uterus through bimanual examination of the gravid abdomen. In addition, ultrasonographic measurement of the fetal biparietal diameter, femur length, and abdominal circumference all have been employed to estimate fetal growth. A combination of these measurements will predict fetal weight accurately. Deviations from the normal fetal growth curve are associated with high-risk conditions.

*Intrauterine growth retardation* is present when fetal growth stops and, with time, falls below the 5th percentile of growth for gestational age or when growth proceeds slowly but the absolute size

TABLE 6–7.  Maternal Drugs Affecting Neonatal Status

| Drug | Effects |
| --- | --- |
| Anesthetics | Central nervous system depression |
| Angiotensin-converting enzyme inhibitors | Oligohydramnios, renal failure |
| Barbiturates | Central nervous system depression |
| Bromides | Rash |
| Cocaine | Preterm birth, growth retardation, behavioral disturbances |
| Coumarin derivatives | Bleeding |
| Indomethacin | PPHN? bleeding, reduced urination |
| Intravenous fluids | |
|   Salt-free | Hyponatremia |
|   High glucose loads | Hypoglycemia |
| Iodides | Goiter |
| Local anesthetic: "caines" | Bradycardia, neonatal seizures |
| Magnesium sulfate | Respiratory depression, meconium plug |
| Morphine (Demerol) | Central nervous system depression, apnea, hypotonia |
| Naphthalene and nitrofurantoin | Hemolytic anemia in glucose-6-phosphate dehydrogenase deficiency |
| Oxytocin | Hyponatremia, hyperbilirubinemia |
| Phenobarbital | Vitamin K deficiency |
| Phenytoin (Dilantin) | Bleeding, vitamin K deficiency |
| Propranolol | Hypoglycemia?, apnea? |
| Reserpine | Nasal stuffiness, drowsiness, poor temperature control |
| Sulfonamides | Bilirubin displaced from albumin binding, kernicterus |
| Tolbutamide | Hypoglycemia |
| Thiazides | Thrombocytopenia? |
| Vitamin K analogs (excessive amounts) | Jaundice |

PPHN = primary pulmonary hypertension of the neonate.

remains less than the 5th percentile (Fig. 6–1). Growth retardation may result from fetal causes producing reduced innate growth potential, such as fetal rubella infection, primordial dwarfing syndromes, chromosomal abnormalities, and congenital malformation syndromes. Reduced fetal production of insulin and insulin-like growth factor I (IGF-I) are associated with fetal growth retardation. Placental causes include villitis (congenital infections), placental tumors, chronic abruptio placentae, twin-twin transfusions, and placental insufficiency. Maternal causes of intrauterine growth retardation include severe peripheral vascular diseases that reduce uterine blood flow, such as chronic hypertension, diabetic vasculopathy, and pre-eclampsia–eclampsia. Additional maternal causes include reduced nutritional intake, alcohol or drug abuse, cigarette smoking, and uterine constraint noted predominantly in mothers of small stature with a low prepregnancy weight and reduced weight gain during pregnancy. The outcome of intrauterine growth retardation of the fetus or newborn depends on the cause of the reduced fetal growth and the associated complications after birth (Table 6–8). Fetuses subjected to chronic intrauterine hypoxia as a result of uteroplacental insufficiency are at an increased risk for birth asphyxia, polycythemia, and hypoglycemia. Fetuses with reduced tissue mass resulting from chromosomal or multiple congenital anomaly syndromes have poor outcomes based on the prognosis for the particular syndrome. Fetuses born to small mothers or fetuses with poor nutritional intake usually do well and may demonstrate catch-up growth after birth.

## Fetal Maturity

Fetal size can be accurately determined by means of ultrasonographic techniques. Unfortunately, fetal size does not always correlate with functional or structural maturity. The need to determine ma-

TABLE 6–8.  Problems of Intrauterine Growth Retardation (Small-for-Gestational Age)

| Problem* | Pathogenesis |
| --- | --- |
| Intrauterine fetal demise | Hypoxia, acidosis, infection, lethal anomaly |
| Perinatal asphyxia | ↓ Uteroplacental perfusion during labor ± chronic fetal hypoxia-acidosis; meconium aspiration syndrome |
| Hypoglycemia | ↓ Tissue glycogen stores, ↓ gluconeogenesis, hyperinsulinism, ↑ glucose needs of hypoxia, hypothermia, large brain |
| Polycythemia-hyperviscosity | Fetal hypoxia with ↑ erythropoietin production |
| Reduced oxygen consumption/hypothermia | Hypoxia, hypoglycemia, starvation effect, poor subcutaneous fat stores |
| Dysmorphology | Syndrome anomalads, chromosomal-genetic disorders, oligohydramnios-induced deformations, TORCH infection |

Modified from Behrman RE, Kliegman RM, Arvin AM (eds): Nelson Textbook of Pediatrics, 15th ed., Philadelphia, WB Saunders, 1996, p. 455.
*Other problems include pulmonary hemorrhage and those common to the gestational age–related risks of prematurity if born <37 wk.
TORCH = toxoplasmosis, other (syphilis, hepatitis, zoster), rubella, cytomegalovirus, and herpes simplex.

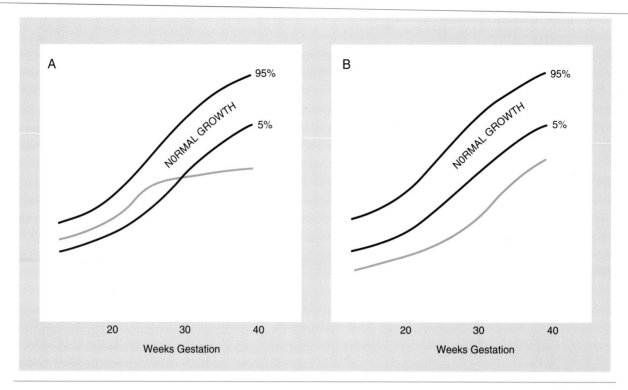

**FIGURE 6–1.** Hypothetical fetal growth curves depicting two patterns of intrauterine growth retardation. *A*, In this pattern, there is normal fetal growth during the 20th to 30th week of gestation. Thereafter, fetal growth stops and the fetal growth parameter (biparietal diameter, abdominal circumference, femur length) falls below 5%. In contrast to weight, head growth is usually spared and less severely affected. This "late flattening" pattern is noted in the donor twin involved in a twin-twin transfusion syndrome, in a fetus supplied by poor maternal nutrition, and in those growing within an environment of maternal pre-eclampsia. Catch-up growth is common after delivery from the adverse in utero environment. *B*, Fetal growth parameters are persistently below 5%. These fetuses demonstrate continued growth, albeit at a reduced rate. Fetuses with this "low-profile" pattern may have reduced growth potential, as noted in those with intrauterine viral infections, chromosome disorders, or malformation syndromes. Fetuses born to mothers who themselves were small for gestational age and who demonstrate reduced prepregnancy weight often have this characteristic growth profile. Some of these fetuses are normal in all other parameters except that they exhibit reduced intrauterine growth.

turity is critical when a decision has been made to deliver a fetus because of fetal distress or severe maternal pre-eclampsia. Fetal gestational age may be determined accurately on the basis of a correct estimate of the last menstrual period. Furthermore, clinically relevant landmark dates can be used to determine gestational age because the first audible heart tones by fetoscope are detected at 18–20 wk (12–14 wk by Doppler methods), and quickening of fetal movements is usually perceived at 18–20 wk. However, it is not always possible to determine fetal maturity by such dating, especially in a high-risk situation, such as preterm labor or a diabetic pregnancy.

**Fetal pulmonary maturity** may be determined through examination of the phospholipid profile present in the amniotic fluid. Surfactant, a combination of surface active phospholipids and proteins, is produced by the maturing fetal lung and eventually is secreted into the amniotic fluid. The amount of surfactant in amniotic fluid is a direct reflection of surface active material in the fetal lung and can be used to predict the presence or absence of pulmonary maturity. Because dipalmityl phosphatidylcholine, or lecithin, is a principal component of surfactant, the determination of lecithin in amniotic fluid is used to predict a mature fetus. Lecithin concentration increases with increasing gestational age, commencing at 32–34 wk (see Respiratory Distress Syndrome: Lung Development).

### Assessment of Fetal Well-Being

Methods employed to assess fetal well-being prior to the onset of labor attempt to identify the fetus at risk for asphyxia or the fetus currently experiencing hypoxia who is already compromised by uteroplacental insufficiency. The *oxytocin challenge test* simulates uterine contractions by an infusion of oxytocin sufficient to produce three contractions in a 10-min period. The development of periodic fetal bradycardia out of phase with uterine contractions (late deceleration) is a positive test and predicts the fetus at risk.

The *nonstress test* examines the heart rate response to fetal body movements: heart rate increments of greater than 15 beats/min, lasting 15 sec, are reassuring. If two such episodes occur in 30 min, the test is considered reactive (versus nonreactive) and the fetus is not at risk. Additional signs of fetal well-being include fetal breathing movements, gross body movements, fetal tone, and the presence of amniotic fluid pockets of greater than 2 cm as noted by ultrasound. The *biophysical profile* combines the nonstress test with these four parameters and offers the most accurate fetal assessment.

*Doppler examination* of the fetal aorta or umbilical arteries can permit identification of decreased or reversed diastolic blood flow, which is associated with increased peripheral vascular resistance, fetal hypoxia with acidosis and placental insufficiency. *Cordocentesis* (percutaneous umbilical blood sampling) can provide fetal blood for $PO_2$, pH, lactate, and hemoglobin. These values can be used to identify the hypoxic, acidotic, or anemic fetus who is at risk for intrauterine fetal demise or birth asphyxia. Cordocentesis also can be used to determine fetal blood type, platelet count, microbial culture, antibody titer, and rapid karyotype.

In the high-risk pregnancy, the fetal heart rate should be monitored continuously along with uterine contractions during labor. Fetal heart rate abnormalities may indicate (1) baseline tachycardia (>160 beats/min as a result of anemia, beta-sympathomimetic drugs, maternal fever, hyperthyroidism, arrhythmia, or fetal distress); (2) baseline bradycardia (<120 beats/min as a result of fetal distress, complete heart block, or local anesthetics); or (3) reduced beat-to-beat variability (flattened tracing resulting from fetal sleep, tachycardia, atropine, sedatives, prematurity, or fetal distress). In addition, periodic changes of the heart rate relative to the tracing of uterine pressure help determine the presence of hypoxia and acidosis caused by uteroplacental insufficiency or maternal hypotension (late or type II decelerations) or by umbilical cord compression (variable decelerations). In the presence of severe decelerations (any late or repeated prolonged variable), a fetal scalp blood gas level should be obtained to assess fetal acidosis. A scalp pH of less than 7.20 indicated fetal hypoxic compromise. A pH between 7.20 and 7.25 is in a borderline zone and warrants repeating the test.

**Fetal anomalies** may be detected by ultrasonography; emphasis should be placed on visualization of the genitourinary tract; the head, neck, and back (spina bifida); the skeleton; the gastrointestinal tract; and the heart. Four chamber and great artery views are required for detection of heart anomalies. *Chromosomal anomaly syndromes* may reveal choroid cysts, hypoplasia of the middle phalanx of the fifth digit, nuchal fluid, retrognathism, and low-set ears. In addition, chromosomal syndromes are often associated with an abnormal "triple test" (low estriols, low maternal serum alpha-fetoprotein, and elevated placental chorionic gonadotropin).

## DELIVERY ROOM CARE: RESUSCITATION

The approach to the birth of an infant, just as with the approach to any other medical situation, requires a detailed history (Table 6–9). Knowing the mother's risk factors (e.g., demographic risks and past and present medical illnesses, including a drug history, the prior pregnancy, and the problems of the current pregnancy) enables the delivery room team to anticipate problems that may occur after birth. Furthermore, the history of a woman's labor and delivery can reveal events that might lead to complications adversely affecting either the mother or neonate, even when the pregnancy was previously considered low risk. Anticipating the need to resuscitate a newborn as a result of its fetal distress increases the likelihood of successful resuscitation.

### Transition from Fetal to Neonatal Physiology

Oxygen transport across the human placenta results in a gradient between the maternal and the fetal $PaO_2$. Although fetal oxygenated blood has a low $PaO_2$ compared with that of adults and infants, the fetus is not anaerobic. Fetal oxygen uptake and oxygen consumption are similar to neonatal rates of oxygen utilization, even though the thermal environments and activity levels of fetuses and neonates differ significantly. Furthermore, the oxygen content of fetal blood is almost equal to that of older infants and children because fetal blood has a much higher concentration of hemoglobin.

Fetal hemoglobin (two alpha and two gamma chains) has a higher affinity for oxygen than adult hemoglobin does, thus facilitating oxygen transfer across the placenta. The fetal hemoglobin-oxygen dissociation curve thus is shifted to the left of the adult curve (Fig. 6–2); at the same $PaO_2$, fetal hemoglobin will be more saturated than adult hemoglobin. However, because fetal hemoglobin

TABLE 6–9.  Components of the Perinatal History

**Demographic Social Information**
Age
Race
Sexually transmitted diseases, hepatitis, AIDS
Illicit drugs, cigarettes, ethanol abuse
Immune status (syphilis, rubella, hepatitis B, blood group)
Occupational exposure

**Past Medical Diseases**
Chronic hypertension
Heart disease
Diabetes mellitus
Thyroid disorders
Hematologic/malignancy
Collagen vascular disease (SLE)
Genetic history—inborn errors of metabolism, bleeding, jaundice
Drug therapy

**Prior Pregnancy**
Abortion
Intrauterine fetal demise
Congenital malformation
Incompetent cervix
Birth weight
Prematurity
Twins
Blood group sensitization/neonatal jaundice
Hydrops
Infertility

**Present Pregnancy**
Current gestational age
Method of assessing gestational age
Fetal surveillance (OCT, NST, biophysical profile)
Ultrasonography (anomalies, hydrops)
Amniotic fluid analysis (L/S ratio)
Oligohydramnios-polyhydramnios
Vaginal bleeding
Preterm labor
Premature (prolonged) rupture of membranes (duration)
Pre-eclampsia
Urinary tract infection
Colonization status (herpes simplex, group B streptococcus)
Medications–drugs
Acute medical illness/exposure to infectious agents
Fetal therapy

**Labor and Delivery**
Duration of labor
Presentation—vertex, breech
Vaginal versus cesarean section
Spontaneous labor versus augmented or induced with oxytocin (Pitocin)
Forceps delivery
Presence of meconium-stained fluid
Maternal fever/amnionitis
Fetal heart rate patterns (distress)
Scalp pH
Maternal analgesia, anesthesia
Nuchal cord
Apgar score/methods of resuscitation
Gestational age assessment
Growth status (AGA, LGA, SGA)

AGA = average for gestational age; AIDS = acquired immunodeficiency syndrome; LGA = large for gestational age; L/S = lecithin/sphingomyelin ratio; NST = nonstress test; OCT = oxytocin challenge test; SGA = small for gestational age; SLE = systemic lupus erythematosus.

functions on the steep, lower end of the oxygen saturation curve ($PaO_2$ 20–30 mm Hg), oxygen unloading to the tissue is not deficient. In contrast, at the higher oxygen concentrations present in the placenta, oxygen loading is enhanced. In the last trimester, fetal hemoglobin production begins to decrease and adult hemoglobin production begins to increase, becoming the only hemoglobin available to the newborn by 3–6 mo of life. At this time, the fetal hemoglobin dissociation curve has shifted to the adult position (see Fig. 6–2).

A portion of the well-oxygenated umbilical venous blood returning to the heart from the placenta perfuses the liver; the remainder bypasses the liver through a shunt, the ductus venosus, and enters the interior vena cava. This oxygenated blood in the vena cava constitutes 65–70% of venous return to the right atrium. The crista dividens in the right atrium directs one third of this vena caval blood across the patent foramen ovale to the left atrium, where it is subsequently pumped to the coronary, cerebral, and upper extremity circulations by the left ventricle. Venous return from the upper body

combines with the remaining two thirds of the vena caval blood in the right atrium and then is directed to the right ventricle. This mixture of venous low-oxygenated blood from the upper and lower body enters the pulmonary artery, from which only 8–10% of it is pumped to the pulmonary circuit. The remaining 80–92% of the right ventricular output bypasses the lungs through a patent ductus arteriosus (PDA) and enters the descending aorta. The amount of blood (8–10%) flowing to the pulmonary system is low because vasoconstriction produced by medial muscle hypertrophy of the small pulmonary arterioles and fluid in the fetal lung increase vascular resistance to blood flow. Pulmonary artery tone also responds to hypoxia, hypercapnia, and acidosis by vasoconstriction, a response that may further increase pulmonary vascular resistance.

The ductus arteriosus remains patent in the fetus because of low $PaO_2$ levels and dilating prostaglandins (i.e., $PGE_2$). In utero, the right ventricle is the dominant ventricle, pumping 65% of the combined ventricular output, which is a very high volume

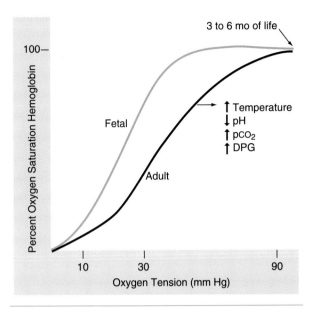

FIGURE 6-2. Hemoglobin-oxygen dissociation curves. The position of the adult curve depends on the binding of adult hemoglobin to 2,3-diphosphoglycerate (DPG), temperature, carbon dioxide tension ($pCO_2$), and hydrogen ion concentration (pH).

(450 mL/kg/min) compared with that pumped by the older infant's right ventricle (200 mL/kg/min).

The transition of the circulation occurring between the fetal and neonatal periods involves the phasing out of the low-resistance circulation of the placenta, the onset of air respiration and reduction of the pulmonary arterial resistance, and the closure of shunts that were used in utero. When the umbilical cord is clamped, the low-pressure system of the placenta is eliminated, increasing systemic blood pressure. Venous return from the placenta is reduced, thus also decreasing right atrial pressure. When the breathing process begins, air replaces lung fluid, maintaining the functional residual capacity. Fluid leaves the lung, in part, through the trachea and is either swallowed or squeezed out during vaginal delivery. The pulmonary lymphatic and venous systems reabsorb the remaining fluid.

Most normal infants require very little pressure to "open" the lungs after birth (5–10 cm $H_2O$); a few infants require greater opening pressures (20–30 cm $H_2O$). With the onset of breathing, pulmonary vascular resistance falls, in part a result of the mechanics of breathing and in part a result of the elevated arterial oxygen tensions. The increased blood flow to the lungs results in a greater quantity of pulmonary venous blood returning to the left atrium; left atrial pressure now exceeds right atrial pressure, and the foramen ovale closes. As the flow

through the pulmonary circulation increases and the arterial oxygen tensions become elevated, the ductus arteriosus begins to constrict. In the term infant, this constriction functionally closes the ductus arteriosus within 1 day after birth. A permanent closure requires thrombosis and fibrosis, a process that may take several weeks. In the premature infant, the ductus arteriosus is less sensitive to the effects of oxygen, and if circulating levels of vasodilating prostaglandins are elevated, the ductus arteriosus may remain patent. This patency is a common problem in the premature infant who is exhibiting the respiratory distress syndrome.

Ventilation, oxygenation, and normal pH and $PCO_2$ levels immediately reduce pulmonary artery vasoconstriction by causing smooth muscle relaxation. Remodeling of the medial muscle hypertrophy begins at birth and continues for the next 3 mo, resulting in a further reduction of pulmonary vascular resistance and a further increase of pulmonary blood flow. In infants with a ventricular septal defect (VSD), a significant left-to-right shunt and congestive heart failure usually do not develop until pulmonary vascular resistance declines. Thus, term infants with a VSD may become ill between 2 and 3 mo of age. Premature infants have not developed a full complement of pulmonary arteriole medial muscle and thus have a more rapid decline of the pulmonary vascular resistance. Because of a more rapid decline of pulmonary artery pressure, the preterm infant with a VSD experiences left-to-right shunting and symptoms sooner than the term infant does, often prior to discharge from the nursery. Persistence or aggravation of pulmonary vasoconstriction caused by acidosis, hypoxia, hypercapnia, hypothermia, polycythemia, asphyxia, shunting of blood from the lungs, or pulmonary parenchymal hypoplasia results in persistent pulmonary hypertension or a persistent fetal circulation (see Primary Pulmonary Hypertension of the Newborn [PPHN]). Failure to replace pulmonary alveolar fluid completely with air can result in respiratory distress (see Transient Tachypnea of the Newborn).

## Asphyxia: Resuscitation
### (See Hypoxic-Ischemic Encephalopathy)

Fetal or neonatal hypoxia, hypercapnia, poor cardiac output, and a metabolic acidosis can result from one or a number of many conditions affecting the fetus, the placenta, or the mother. Whether in utero or after birth, asphyxia-caused hypoxic-ischemic brain injury results from reduced gaseous exchange through the placenta or through the lungs, respectively. Asphyxia associated with severe bradycardia or cardiac insufficiency reduces or eliminates tissue blood flow, resulting in ischemia. The fetal and neonatal circulatory systems respond to reduced oxygen availability by shunting the blood preferentially to the brain, heart, and adrenal glands and away from the intestine, kidney, lung, and skin. When severe hypoxia and hypercapnia occur in utero, placental blood flow also is reduced.

The response to asphyxia also is characterized by:

1. Release of catecholamines (predominantly norepinephrine) from the adrenal glands.
2. Transient hypertension and tachycardia followed by bradycardia and shock, which are both mediated in part from the chemoreceptors and baroreceptors.
3. Production of a mixture of respiratory and metabolic acidosis.
4. Hypoxemia.

The metabolic acidosis is due to the combined effects of poor cardiac output secondary to hypoxic depression of myocardial function, systemic hypoxia, and tissue anaerobic metabolism. With severe or prolonged intrauterine or neonatal asphyxia, multiple vital organs will be affected (Table 6–10).

Many conditions that contribute to fetal or neonatal asphyxia are the same medical or obstetric problems associated with the high-risk pregnancy (Table 6–11). Maternal diseases that interfere with

**TABLE 6–11.** Etiology of Birth Asphyxia

| Type | Example |
| --- | --- |
| *Intrauterine* | |
| Hypoxia–ischemia | Uteroplacental insufficiency, abruptio placentae, prolapsed cord, maternal hypotension, unknown |
| Anemia–shock | Vasa previa, placenta previa, fetomaternal hemorrhage, erythroblastosis |
| *Intrapartum* | |
| Birth trauma | Cephalopelvic disproportion, shoulder dystocia, breech presentation, spinal cord transection |
| Hypoxia–ischemia | Umbilical cord compression |
| *Postpartum* | |
| Central nervous system | Maternal medication, trauma, previous episodes of fetal hypoxia–acidosis |
| Congenital neuromuscular disease | Congenital myasthenia gravis, myopathy |
| Infection | Consolidated pneumonia, shock |
| Airway disorder | Choanal atresia, severe obstructing goiter, laryngeal webs |
| Pulmonary disorder | Severe immaturity, pneumothorax, pleural effusion, diaphragmatic hernia, pulmonary hypoplasia |
| Renal disorder | Pulmonary hypoplasia/pneumothorax |

**TABLE 6–10.** Effects of Asphyxia

| System | Effect |
| --- | --- |
| Central nervous system | Hypoxic-ischemic encephalopathy, IVH, cerebral edema, seizures, hypotonia, hypertonia |
| Cardiovascular | Myocardial ischemia, poor contractility, tricuspid insufficiency, hypotension |
| Pulmonary | Persistent fetal circulation, respiratory distress syndrome |
| Renal | Acute tubular or cortical necrosis |
| Adrenal | Adrenal hemorrhage |
| Gastrointestinal | Perforation, ulceration, necrosis |
| Metabolic | Inappropriate ADH, hyponatremia, hypoglycemia, hypocalcemia, myoglobinuria |
| Integument | Subcutaneous fat necrosis |
| Hematology | Disseminated intravascular coagulation |

ADH = antidiuretic hormone; IVH = intraventricular hemorrhage.

uteroplacental perfusion, such as chronic hypertension, pre-eclampsia, and diabetes mellitus, place the fetus at risk for intrauterine asphyxia. Both maternal epidural anesthesia and the development of the vena caval compression syndrome may produce maternal hypotension, which decreases uterine perfusion. Maternal medications given to relieve pain during labor may cross the placenta and depress the infant's respiratory center, resulting in apnea at the time of birth.

Fetal conditions associated with asphyxia usually do not become manifest until delivery, when the infant must initiate and sustain ventilation, which requires an intact respiratory drive from the centers for respiration in the medulla. In addition, the upper and lower airways must be patent and unobstructed. The alveolus must be free from foreign material, such as meconium, amniotic fluid debris, and infectious exudate, which increase airway resistance, reduce lung compliance, and result in respiratory distress and hypoxia (see Table 6–11). Some very immature infants weighing less than 1000 g at birth may be unable to expand their lungs, even in the absence of pneumonia or other obvious signs of central nervous system dysfunction. Their compliant chest wall and surfactant deficiency may result in poor air exchange at birth, retractions, hypoxia, and apnea. Usually, more mature newborn infants do not manifest apnea in the delivery room as a sign of the respiratory distress syndrome.

Any condition resulting in hypoxia in the delivery room may cause apnea because the newborn infant, particularly the preterm infant, responds paradoxically to hypoxia by developing apnea rather than tachypnea, as occurs among adults. Episodes of intrauterine asphyxia also may depress the neonatal central nervous system. If recovery of the fetal heart rate occurs as a result of improved uteroplacental perfusion, fetal hypoxia and acidosis may resolve. Nonetheless, if the effect on the respiratory center is more severe, the newborn infant may not initiate an adequate ventilatory response at birth and thus will undergo another episode of asphyxia.

The *Apgar examination,* a rapid scoring system based on physiologic responses to the birth process, is a very good method for assessing the need to resuscitate a newborn infant (Table 6–12). At intervals of 1 min and 5 min after birth, each of the five physiologic parameters is observed or elicited by a qualified examiner. Full-term infants with a normal cardiopulmonary adaptation should score 8–9 at 1 and 5 min. Apgar scores of 4–7 warrant close attention to determine whether the infant's status will improve and to ascertain whether any pathologic condition resulting from labor or delivery or residing within the newborn is contributing to the low Apgar score.

By definition, an Apgar score of 0–3 represents either a cardiopulmonary arrest or a condition due to severe bradycardia, hypoventilation, and/or central nervous system depression. Most low

Apgar scores are due to difficulty in establishing adequate ventilation and not to primary cardiac pathology. Infants with the most severe types of complex congenital heart disease (such as lethal hypoplastic left heart syndrome) do not have low Apgar scores because of the cardiac lesion. In addition to an Apgar score of 0–3, most infants with asphyxia severe enough to cause neurologic injury also manifest fetal acidosis (pH < 7.00); seizures, coma, or hypotonia; and multiorgan dysfunction (see Table 6–10). Low Apgar scores may be due to fetal hypoxia or to other factors listed in Table 6–11. Most infants with low Apgar scores respond to assisted ventilation by face mask or by endotracheal intubation and usually do not need emergency medication.

*Resuscitation* of the newborn infant having a low Apgar score follows the same systematic sequence (see Cardiopulmonary Resuscitation in Chapter 3) as that for resuscitation of older patients, but in the newborn period this simplified "ABC" approach requires some qualification.

Although "A" stands for securing a patent airway by clearing amniotic fluid or meconium by suctioning, "A" should also remind us about "anticipation" and the need for knowing the events of pregnancy, labor, and delivery. This history also should include knowledge of fetal distress, fetal heart rate and acid-base status, abnormal position, vaginal bleeding, blood group sensitization, and ultrasonographic evidence of hydrops or congenital malformations because such knowledge may modify the approach to the airway. For example, evidence of a diaphragmatic hernia and a low Apgar score indicate that immediate endotracheal intubation is required. If a mask and bag are used, gas will enter both the lung and the stomach and the latter may act as an expanding mass in the chest that compromises respiration. Knowing the blood group sensitization and that fetal hydrops has occurred with pleural effusions may indicate the need for bilateral thoracentesis to evacuate the pleural effusions, so that adequate ventilation can be established.

"B" represents breathing. If the patient is apneic or hypoventilates and remains cyanotic, artificial ventilation should be initiated. It should be performed with a well-fitted mask that is attached to an anesthesia bag and a manometer to prevent very high pressures from being given to the newborn infant. One hundred percent oxygen should be given through the mask. If the infant does not revive, an endotracheal tube should be placed through the vocal cords and then attached to the anesthesia bag and manometer and 100% oxygen administered. The pressure generated should begin

TABLE 6–12.   Apgar Score

| Signs | Points | | |
|---|---|---|---|
| | *0* | *1* | *2* |
| Heart rate | 0 | <100/min | >100/min |
| Respiration | None | Weak cry | Vigorous cry |
| Muscle tone | None | Some extremity flexion | Arms, legs well flexed |
| Reflex irritability | None | Some motion | Cry, withdrawal |
| Color of body | Blue | Pink body, blue extremities | Pink all over |

at 20–25 cm $H_2O$, with a rate of 60 breaths/min. An adequate response to ventilation is indicated by good chest rise, return of breath sounds, well-oxygenated color, heart rate returning to the normal range (120–160 beats/min), and, later, by increased muscle activity and wakefulness. The usual recovery after a cardiac arrest is, first, a return to a normal heart rate. After that, cyanosis disappears and the infant will appear well perfused. An infant may remain limp and may be apneic for a prolonged time after return of cardiac output and correction of acidosis.

For the asphyxiated newborn infant, breathing should initially be briefly delayed if there is meconium-stained amniotic fluid. If the meconium is not cleared from the oropharyngeal and tracheal airways, it may be disseminated into the lungs, producing a severe **aspiration pneumonia.** If meconium is noted in the amniotic fluid, the oropharynx should be suctioned by the birth attendant once the head is delivered. After the birth of the infant, the oral cavity should be suctioned again; the vocal cords then should be visualized with a laryngoscope and the infant intubated with suction applied while the tube is below the vocal cords. If meconium is noted below the cords, intubation should be repeated quickly to clear the remaining meconium. During this time, the infant should not be stimulated to breathe and positive-pressure ventilation should not be applied.

"C" represents circulation and external cardiac massage. If artificial ventilation does not improve the bradycardia, if asystole is present, or if peripheral pulses cannot be palpated, external cardiac massage should be performed at a rate of 100–120 beats per minute. External cardiac massage usually is not needed, because most infants in the delivery room respond to ventilation.

"D" represents the administration of drugs. If bradycardia that is unresponsive to ventilation persists or if asystole is present, drugs should be added to the process of resuscitation. Intravenous epinephrine (1:10,000, 0.1–0.3 mL/kg) should be given through an umbilical venous line, or epinephrine may be injected into the endotracheal tube. If this dose is ineffective, 10 times the dose of epinephrine (1:1000) may be used. Additional medications for resuscitation may include 1–2 mEq/kg of sodium bicarbonate (0.5 mEq/mL) if acidosis is prolonged; calcium gluconate (2–4 mL/kg of 10% solution) if there is evidence of hypocalcemia; or a rapid infusion of fluids if poor perfusion suggests hypovolemia. Before medications are administered in the presence of electrical-mechanical dissociation, it is important to determine whether there is a pneumothorax because this is a common cause of electrical cardiac activity unaccompanied by palpable pulses or blood pressure. Transillumination of the thorax, involving the use of a bright light through each of the two sides of the thorax and over the sternum, may suggest pneumothorax if one side transmits more light than the other. Breath sounds are also decreased over a pneumothorax, and there is a shift of the heart tones away from the side of a tension pneumothorax.

If central nervous system depression in the infant is thought to be due to an analgesic medication, such as meperidine, that was given to the mother, naloxone (Narcan) can be given to the infant as a specific antidote. Before this drug is administered, however, the ABCs should be followed carefully, and naloxone should be given only after full resuscitation has been completed.

## OTHER NEONATAL EMERGENCIES IN THE DELIVERY ROOM

### Cyanosis

*Acrocyanosis* (blue color of the hands and feet with pink color of the rest of the body) is common in the delivery room and is usually normal. *Central cyanosis* of the trunk, mucosal membranes, and tongue can occur in the delivery room or at any time after birth and is always a manifestation of a serious underlying condition. Cyanosis is noted with 4–5 g/dL of deoxygenated hemoglobin. Central cyanosis can be due to problems in many different organ systems, although cardiopulmonary diseases are the most common (Table 6–13). Respiratory distress syndrome, sepsis, and cyanotic heart disease are the three most common causes of cyanosis among infants admitted to a neonatal intensive care unit (NICU). A systematic evaluation of these and other causes of cyanosis is required for every cyanotic infant after prompt administration of oxygen, with or without assisted ventilation as indicated.

### Life-Threatening Congenital Malformations
(Table 6–14)

Various congenital anomalies can interfere with vital organ function after birth. Some malformations, such as choanal atresia and other lesions obstructing the airway, may prevent ventilation. Intrathoracic lesions, such as cysts or bowel that has herniated into the chest, also interfere with respiration. Other malformations that obstruct the gastrointestinal system at the level of the esophagus, duode-

TABLE 6–13.  Differential Diagnosis of Neonatal Cyanosis

| System/Disease | Mechanism |
| --- | --- |
| *Pulmonary* | |
| Respiratory distress syndrome | Surfactant deficiency |
| Sepsis, pneumonia | Inflammation, pulmonary hypertension, ARDS |
| Meconium aspiration pneumonia | Mechanical obstruction, inflammation, pulmonary hypertension |
| Persistent fetal circulation | Pulmonary hypertension |
| Diaphragmatic hernia | Pulmonary hypoplasia, pulmonary hypertension |
| Transient tachypnea | Retained lung fluid |
| *Cardiovascular* | |
| Cyanotic heart disease with decreased pulmonary blood flow | Right-to-left shunt as in pulmonary atresia, tetralogy of Fallot |
| Cyanotic heart disease with increased pulmonary blood flow | Right-to-left shunt as in *d*-transposition, truncus arteriosus |
| Cyanotic heart disease with congestive heart failure | Right-to-left shunt with pulmonary edema and poor cardiac output as in hypoplastic left heart and coarctation of aorta |
| Heart failure alone | Pulmonary edema and poor cardiac contractility as in sepsis, myocarditis, supraventricular tachycardia, or complete heart block; high-output failure as in PDA or vein of Galen or other arteriovenous malformation |
| *Central Nervous System* | |
| Maternal sedative drugs | Hypoventilation, apnea |
| Asphyxia | CNS depression |
| Intracranial hemorrhage | CNS depression, seizure |
| Neuromuscular disease | Hypotonia, hypoventilation, pulmonary hypoplasia |
| *Hematologic* | |
| Acute blood loss | Shock |
| Chronic blood loss | Congestive heart failure |
| Polycythemia | Pulmonary hypertension |
| Methemoglobinemia | Low-affinity hemoglobin or red blood cell enzyme defect |
| *Metabolic* | |
| Hypoglycemia | CNS depression, congestive heart failure |
| Adrenogenital syndrome | Shock (salt-losing) |

ARDS = acute respiratory distress syndrome; CNS = central nervous system; PDA = patent ductus arteriosus.

num, ileum, or colon may result in aspiration pneumonia, intestinal perforation, or gangrene. Gastroschisis and omphalocele both are associated with intestinal necrosis and exposed bowel on the abdominal wall. Omphalocele also is associated with other malformations.

Many congenital malformations are obvious in the delivery room. By using fetal ultrasonography, the obstetrician is able to detect many serious congenital anomalies in utero. Immediate palliative medical or surgical treatment or corrective surgery must be planned for most infants with major congenital malformations. Prompt stabilization, as noted for the asphyxiated infant, is essential. In addition, specific attention must be given to the particular problems associated with the malformation.

### Shock

Shock in the delivery room is manifested by cyanosis, pallor, poor capillary refilling time, unpalpable pulses, hypotonia, and, eventually, cardiopulmonary arrest. Cyanosis in the presence of pallor, with or without purpuric ecchymosis, is very suggestive of shock. Blood loss prior to or during labor and delivery is a common cause of shock in the delivery room. Blood loss may be due to a fetal-maternal hemorrhage, placenta previa, vasa previa, a twin-twin transfusion, or displacement of blood from the fetus to the placenta as during asphyxia, hence the term *asphyxia pallida*. Hemorrhage into a viscus, such as the liver or spleen, may be noted in macrosomic infants, and hemorrhage into the cerebral ventricles may produce shock and apnea in preterm infants. Finally, anemia, hypoalbuminemia, hypovolemia, and shock at birth are common manifestations of Rh immune hydrops. Diseases causing nonimmune hydrops also can result in fetal anemia and hypovolemia.

Severe intrauterine bacterial sepsis may present with septicemic shock in the delivery room or im-

TABLE 6–14.    Common Congenital Anomalies

| Name | Manifestations |
| --- | --- |
| Choanal atresia | Respiratory distress in delivery room, apnea, unable to pass nasogastric tube through nares |
| Pierre Robin syndrome | Micrognathia, cleft palate, airway obstruction |
| Diaphragmatic hernia | Scaphoid abdomen, bowel sounds present in chest, respiratory distress |
| Tracheoesophageal fistula | Polyhydramnios, aspiration pneumonia, excessive salivation, unable to place nasogastric tube in stomach |
| Intestinal obstruction: volvulus, duodenal atresia, ileal atresia | Polyhydramnios, bile-stained emesis, abdominal distention |
| Gastroschisis/ omphalocele | Polyhydramnios; intestinal obstruction |
| Renal agenesis/Potter syndrome | Oligohydramnios, anuria, pulmonary hypoplasia, pneumothorax |
| Hydronephrosis | Abdominal masses |
| Neural tube defects: anencephalus, meningomyelocele | Polyhydramnios, elevated alpha-fetoprotein; decreased fetal activity |
| Down syndrome (trisomy 21) | Hypotonia, congenital heart disease, duodenal atresia |
| Ductal-dependent congenital heart disease | Cyanosis, murmur |

mediately after the infant is transferred to the nursery. Typically, these infants are mottled, hypotonic, and cyanotic and have diminished peripheral pulses. They have a normal hemoglobin concentration and usually manifest neutropenia, thrombocytopenia, and disseminated intravascular coagulation (DIC). Peripheral symmetric gangrene (purpuric rash) often is a sign of hypotensive shock among infants with severe congenital bacterial infections.

Congenital left ventricular cardiac obstruction (critical aortic stenosis, hypoplastic left heart syndrome) also produces shock, although not usually in the delivery room.

*Treatment* of newborn infants with shock should include the management approaches used for the sick infant (see Asphyxia: Resuscitation earlier). Problems may be anticipated through knowledge of the infant's immune status, evidence of hydrops, or suspicion of intrauterine infection or anomalies. Stabilization of the airway, institution of respira-

tory support, and external cardiac massage are essential. Hypovolemic shock should be managed with repeated boluses of 10–15 mL/kg of normal saline, lactated Ringer's solution, or albumin. If severe immune hemolysis is predicted, blood typed against the mother's blood should be available in the delivery room and should be given to the newborn infant if signs of anemia and shock are present. Thereafter, all blood should be cross-matched with both the infant's and the mother's blood prior to transfusion. Vasoactive drugs, such as dopamine, dobutamine, and epinephrine, may improve cardiac output and tissue perfusion.

### Birth Injury

Birth injury refers to both avoidable and unavoidable injury to the fetus during the birth process. Birth asphyxia has been discussed earlier in the chapter. Other traumatic injuries due to mechanical forces applied to the infant during parturition are discussed here.

*Caput succedaneum* is a diffuse, edematous, often dark swelling of the soft tissue of the scalp that extends across the midline and suture lines. In infants delivered from a face presentation, soft tissue edema of the eyelids and face is an equivalent phenomenon. Caput succedaneum may be seen after prolonged labor in both full-term and premature infants. Molding of the head often is associated with caput succedaneum and is the result of pressure induced from overriding the parietal and frontal bones against their respective sutures.

A *cephalhematoma* is a subperiosteal hemorrhage that does not cross the suture lines surrounding the respective bones. A linear skull fracture rarely may be seen underlying a cephalhematoma. With time, the cephalhematoma may organize, calcify, and form a central depression.

Infants with cephalhematoma and caput succedaneum require no specific treatment. Occasionally, a premature infant may develop a massive scalp hemorrhage. This *subgaleal bleeding* and the bleeding noted from a cephalhematoma may cause indirect hyperbilirubinemia that requires treatment with phototherapy.

*Retinal* and *subconjunctival hemorrhages* are common but usually are small and insignificant. No treatment is necessary.

*Spinal cord* or *spine injuries* may occur in the fetus, from the hyperextended "star gazing" posture, and in infants following excessive rotational (at C3-4) or longitudinal (at C7-T1) force transmitted to the neck during vertex or breech delivery. Fractures of vertebrae are rarer and may cause direct damage to the spinal cord that results in transection and permanent sequelae or hemorrhage, edema, and neurologic signs. Occasionally, a snapping sound indicative of cord transection rather than vertebral displacement is heard at the time of delivery. Neurologic dysfunction usually includes complete flaccid paralysis, absent deep tendon reflexes, and absence of responses to painful stimuli below the lesion. Painful stimuli may elicit reflex flexion of the legs. Infants with spinal cord injury often are flaccid, apneic, and asphyxiated, all of which may mask the underlying spinal cord transection. With time, these infants will experience bowel and bladder problems, spasticity, and hyperreflexia.

Injury to the nerves of the *brachial plexus* may result from excessive traction on the neck, producing paresis or complete paralysis, depending on the nerve roots involved. **Erb-Duchenne paralysis** involves the 5th and 6th cervical nerves. The infant cannot abduct the arm at the shoulder, externally rotate the arm, or supinate the forearm. The usual picture is one of painless adduction, internal rotation of the arm, and pronation of the forearm. There is an absent **Moro reflex** on the involved side; the hand grasp is intact. A **phrenic nerve palsy** (C3, 4, and 5) may result in diaphragmatic paralysis and respiratory distress. An elevated diaphragm caused by nerve injury must be differentiated from elevation resulting from eventration caused by congenital weakness or absence of diaphragm muscle. **Klumpke paralysis** is due to injury to the 7th and 8th cervical nerves and the 1st thoracic nerve, resulting in a paralyzed hand and, if the sympathetic nerves are injured, in ipsilateral *Horner syndrome* (ptosis, miosis). Complete arm and hand paralysis is noted with damage to C5, 6, 7, and 8 and T1. *Treatment* of brachial plexus injury is supportive and includes positioning to avoid contractures. Active and passive range-of-motion exercises also may be of benefit. If the deficit persists, nerve grafting may be beneficial.

*Facial nerve injury* may be due to compression of the 7th nerve between the facial bone and the mother's pelvic bones or the physician's forceps. This peripheral nerve injury is characterized by an asymmetric crying face whose normal side, including the forehead, moves in a regular manner. The affected side is flaccid, the eye does not close, the nasolabial fold is absent, and the side of the mouth droops at rest. When there is a central injury to the facial nerve, only the lower two thirds of the face (not the forehead) is involved. Complete agenesis of the facial nucleus results in a central facial paralysis; when this is bilateral, as in **Möbius syndrome,** the face appears expressionless.

*Fractures* of the cranium are rare, are usually linear, and require no treatment other than observation for very rare delayed (1–3 mo) complications (e.g., leptomeningeal cyst). Depressed **skull** fractures are unusual but may be seen with complicated forceps delivery. Fractures of the **clavicle** usually are unilateral and are noted in macrosomic infants following shoulder dystocia. Often a snap is heard following a difficult delivery, and the infant presents with an asymmetric Moro response and decreased movement of the affected side. The prognosis is excellent; many infants require no treatment or a simple figure-of-eight bandage to immobilize the bone.

**Extremity fractures** are less common than those of the clavicle and involve the humerus more often than the femur. *Treatment* requires immobilization and a triangular splint bandage for the humerus and traction suspension of the legs for femoral fractures. The *prognosis* is excellent.

Fractures of the **facial bones** are rare, but dislocation of the cartilaginous part of the nasal septum out of the vomeral groove and columella is common. *Clinical manifestations* include feeding difficulty, respiratory distress, asymmetric nares, and a flattened, laterally displaced nose. *Treatment* reduces the dislocation by elevating the cartilage back into the vomeral groove.

*Visceral trauma* to the liver, spleen, or adrenal gland is noted in macrosomic infants and in very premature infants, with or without breech or vaginal delivery. Rupture of the liver with subcapsular hematoma formation may result in anemia, hypovolemia, shock, hemoperitoneum, and disseminated intravascular coagulation. Infants with anemia and shock who are suspected of having an intraventricular hemorrhage but who have normal findings with head ultrasound examination should be evaluated for hepatic or splenic rupture. Adrenal hemorrhage may be asymptomatic, as noted by a high incidence of normal infants with calcified adrenal glands. Nonetheless, infants with severe adrenal hemorrhage may present with a flank mass, jaundice, and hematuria, with or without shock.

### Temperature Regulation

In utero thermoregulation of the fetus is performed by the placenta, which acts as an efficient heat exchanger. Fetal temperature is, nonetheless, higher than the mother's temperature. If maternal temperature becomes elevated during a febrile illness or on exposure to environmental heat, fetal temperature will increase further. Thus, the immediate temperature at birth of an infant born to a febrile mother with chorioamnionitis will be elevated regardless of the presence of infection in the infant unless the infant has cooled in the delivery room.

**Lowered Temperature.** After birth, the newborn infant begins life covered by amniotic fluid and situated in a cold environment (20–25°C). An infant's skin temperature may fall 0.3°C/min, and the core temperature may decline 0.1°C/min in the delivery room. In the absence of an external heat source, the infant must increase metabolism substantially to maintain body temperature.

Heat loss occurs by four basic mechanisms. In the cold delivery room, the wet infant loses heat predominantly by *evaporation* (cutaneous and respiratory loss when wet or in low humidity), *radiation* (loss to nearby cold solid surfaces), and *convection* (loss to air current). Once the infant is dry, radiation, convection, and *conduction* (loss to object in direct contact with infant) are important causes of heat loss. After birth, all high-risk infants should be dried immediately to eliminate evaporative heat losses (Table 6–15). Furthermore, a radiant or convective heat source should be provided for these high-risk infants. Normal term infants should be dried and wrapped in a blanket.

The ideal environmental temperature is the *neutral thermal environment*, the ambient temperature resulting in the lowest rate of heat produced by the infant while maintaining normal body temperature. The neutral thermal environmental temperature decreases with increasing gestational age and increasing postnatal age. Ambient temperatures be-

low the neutral thermal environment first result in increasing rates of oxygen consumption for heat production, which is designed to maintain normal body temperature. If the ambient temperature falls further or if oxygen consumption cannot increase sufficiently (as a result of hypoxia, hypoglycemia, or drugs), the core body temperature falls.

Heat production by the newborn infant is created predominantly by *nonshivering thermogenesis* from chemical reactions of adenosine triphosphate (ATP) hydrolysis in specialized areas of tissue containing brown adipose tissue. Brown fat is highly vascular, contains many mitochondria per cell, and is situated around large blood vessels, resulting in rapid heat transfer to the circulation. The vessels of the neck, thorax, and interscapular region are common locations of brown fat. These tissues also are innervated by the sympathetic nervous system, which serves as a primary stimulus for heat production by brown adipose cells. Shivering does not occur in newborn infants.

Severe *cold injury* in the infant is manifested by acidosis, hypoxia, hypoglycemia, apnea, bradycardia, pulmonary hemorrhage and a pink skin color. The color is due not to adequate oxygenation but, rather, to trapping of oxygenated hemoglobin in the cutaneous capillaries. Many of these infants appear dead, but most respond to treatment and recover. Milder degrees of cold injury in the delivery room may contribute to metabolic acidosis and hypoxia after birth. Conversely, hypoxia delays heat generation in cold-stressed infants.

*Treatment* of severe hypothermia should include resuscitation and rapid warming of both core (lung, stomach) and external surfaces. Fluid resuscitation also is needed to treat the hypovolemia seen in many of these infants. Reduced core temperature (32–35°C) in the immediate newborn period often requires only external warming with a radiant warmer or incubator, or both.

**Elevated Temperature.** Exposure to ambient temperatures above the neutral thermal environment results in *heat stress* and an elevated core temperature. Sweating is uncommon in newborn infants and may be noted only on the forehead. However, in response to moderate heat stress, infants may increase their respiratory rate in order to dissipate heat. Excessive environmental temperatures may result in heat stroke or in the hemorrhagic shock encephalopathy syndrome.

**TABLE 6–15.** General Management Strategies for Sick Newborns

| Procedure | Rationale |
| --- | --- |
| Warmth in a neutral thermal environment | Avoids cold stress, minimizes oxygen consumption |
| Humidification | Reduces insensible water losses |
| Intravenous fluids and glucose | Maintains fluid balance, avoids dehydration, hyperbilirubinemia, prevents prerenal azotemia, prevents hypoglycemia, provides supplemental calories to support oxygen consumption |
| Oxygen | Treats hypoxia, supports oxygen consumption, prevents cell injury and death |
| Monitor blood gases and arterial oxygen saturation | Avoids hyperoxic retinal injury and hypoxic brain injury, guides treatment with mechanical ventilation |

## ROUTINE DELIVERY ROOM CARE

Once the cardiopulmonary transition from fetal to newborn life has successfully occurred and no acute life-threatening conditions exist, routine delivery room or postpartum room care should be provided. Silver nitrate (1%) instilled into both eyes (without being washed out) is an indicated effective therapy for the prevention of neonatal gonococcal ophthalmia, which can result in severe panophthalmitis and subsequent blindness. Silver nitrate may produce a chemical conjunctivitis with a mucopurulent discharge and is not effective against *Chlamydia trachomatis.* Therefore, many hospitals use erythromycin drops to prevent neonatal gonococcal and chlamydial eye disease.

Bacterial colonization of the newborn may begin in utero when the fetal membranes have been ruptured before or during labor. Most infants undergo colonization after birth and acquire the bacteria present in the mother's genitourinary system, such as staphylococcus, *Escherichia coli,* and clostridial species. Colonization is common at the umbilicus, skin, nasopharynx, and intestine. Antiseptic skin or cord care is routine in most nurseries to prevent spread of pathologic bacteria from one infant to another and to prevent disease in the individual infant. Staphylococcal bullous impetigo, omphalitis, diarrhea, and systemic disease may result from colonization with virulent *Staphylococcus aureus.* For term infants, washing of the skin with 3% hexachlorophene is not routinely recommended but may avoid serious staphylococcal disease; preterm infants may absorb hexachlorophene, and neurotoxicity may develop. Triple dye or bacitracin may be applied to the umbilical cord to effectively reduce its colonization with gram-positive bacteria. Epidemics of *S. aureus* nursery infections are managed with strict infectious disease control measures (cohorting, hand washing, monitoring for colonization).

Vitamin K prophylaxis should be given to all infants to prevent hemorrhagic disease of the newborn.

Prior to discharge, infants should receive the hepatitis B vaccine.

References

Behrman RE, Kliegman RM, Arvin AM (eds): Nelson Textbook of Pediatrics, 15th ed. Philadelphia, WB Saunders, 1996, Chapters 79.3–85.
Carrero J, Torrents M, Mortera C, et al: Routine prenatal ultrasound screening for fetal abnormalities: 22 years experience. Ultrasound Obstet Gynecol 5:174, 1995.
Committee on Fetus and Newborn, American Academy of Pediatrics, and Committee on Obstetric Practice, American College of Obstetricians and Gynecologists: Use and abuse of Apgar score. Pediatrics 98:141, 1996.
Cusick W, Smulian J, Vintzileos A: Intrapartum use of fetal heart rate monitoring, contraction monitoring and amnioinfusion. Clin Perinatol 22:875, 1995.
Garner P: Type I diabetes mellitus and pregnancy. Lancet 346:157, 1995.
Hickok DE, Mills M, Western Collaborative Perinatal Group: Percutaneous umbilical blood sampling: Results from a multicenter collaborative registry. Am J Obstet Gynecol 166:1614, 1992.
Lopriore E, Frank PH, Vandenbussche A, et al: Twin-to-twin transfusion syndrome: New perspectives. J Pediatr 127:675, 1995.
Martin-Ancel A, Garcia-Alix A, Gaya F, et al: Multiple organ involvement in perinatal asphyxia. J Pediatr 127:786, 1995.
Perlman JM, Risser R: Cardiopulmonary resuscitation in the delivery room. Arch Pediatr Adolesc Med 149:20, 1995.
Steiner H, Staudach A, Spitzer D, et al: Growth deficient fetuses with absent or reversed umbilical artery end-diastolic flow are metabolically compromised. Early Hum Dev 41:1, 1995.

## PHYSICAL EXAMINATION AND GESTATIONAL AGE ASSESSMENT

The first physical examination of the newborn infant serves many important purposes. It may be a general physical examination of a well baby or an examination to determine the cause of various manifestations of neonatal diseases. Because the transition from fetal to neonatal life requires significant cardiopulmonary adjustments, problems in this transition may be detectable immediately in the delivery room or during the 1st day of life. Effects of the labor and delivery resulting from asphyxia, drugs, or birth trauma also may become evident by physical examination. Furthermore, the first newborn examination is an important way to detect congenital malformations or deformations (see Table 6–14). Congenital malformations are due to many different causes, for example, chromosomal trisomies, teratogens, or recognizable syndromes without identifiable causes. Significant congenital malformations may be present in as many as 1–3% of all births. Congenital deformations are due to compression of fetal parts by the uterus, usually in the absence of amniotic fluid. Thus, some cases of clubfoot are a result of compression of the fetal foot by the uterine wall (see Chapter 19).

### APPEARANCE

The general appearance of the infant should be evaluated first. Signs such as cyanosis, nasal flaring, intercostal retractions, and grunting suggest pulmonary disease. Meconium staining of the umbilical cord, nails, and skin suggests fetal distress and the possibility of aspiration pneumonia (see below). The level of spontaneous activity, passive muscle tone, quality of the cry, and apnea are useful screening signs to evaluate the state of the nervous system initially.

## VITAL SIGNS

The examination should then proceed with an assessment of vital signs, particularly heart rate (normal rate, 120–160 beats/min), respiratory rate (normal rate, 30–60 breaths/min), temperature (usually done initially per rectum and later as an axillary measurement), and blood pressure (often reserved for sick infants). In addition, length, weight, and head circumference should be measured and plotted on growth curves to determine whether growth is normal, accelerated, or retarded for the specific gestational age.

## GESTATIONAL AGE

Gestational age is determined by assessing various physical signs (Fig. 6–3) and neurologic characteristics (Fig. 6–4) that vary according to fetal age and maturity. Physical criteria that mature with advancing fetal age include increasing firmness of the pinna of the ear, increasing size of the breast tissue, decreasing fine, immature **lanugo hair** over the back, and decreasing opacity of the skin. Neurologic criteria that mature with gestational age include increasing flexion of the legs, hips, and arms; increasing tone of the flexor muscles of the neck; and decreasing laxity of the joints. These signs are determined during the 1st day of life and are assigned scores. The cumulative score is correlated with a gestational age, which is usually accurate to within 2 wk (Fig. 6–5).

Gestational age assessment permits the detection of abnormal fetal growth patterns, thus aiding in predicting the neonatal complications of large-

| EXTERNAL SIGN | SCORE | | | | |
|---|---|---|---|---|---|
| | 0 | 1 | 2 | 3 | 4 |
| Edema | Obvious edema of hands and feet; pitting over tibia | No obvious edema of hands and feet; pitting over tibia | No edema | | |
| Skin texture | Very thin, gelatinous | Thin and smooth | Smooth; medium thickness; rash or superficial peeling | Slight thickening, superficial cracking and peeling, especially on hands and feet | Thick and parchmentlike; superficial or deep cracking |
| Skin color (infant not crying) | Dark red | Uniformly pink | Pale pink; variable over body | Pale; only pink over ears, lips, palms, or soles | |
| Skin opacity (trunk) | Numerous veins and venules clearly seen, especially over abdomen | Veins and tributaries seen | A few large vessels clearly seen over abdomen | A few large vessels seen indistinctly over abdomen | No blood vessels seen |
| Lanugo (over back) | No lanugo | Abundant, long and thick over whole back | Hair thinning, especially over lower back | Small amount of lanugo and bald areas | At least half of back devoid of lanugo |
| Plantar creases | No skin creases | Faint red marks over anterior half of sole | Definite red marks over more than anterior half; indentations over less than anterior third | Indentations over more than anterior third | Definite deep indentations over more than anterior third |
| Nipple formation | Nipple barely visible; no areola | Nipple well defined; areola smooth and flat, diameter <0.75 cm | Areola stippled, edge not raised, diameter <0.75 cm | Areola stippled, edge raised, diameter >0.75 cm | |
| Breast size | No breast tissue palpable | Breast tissue on one or both sides <0.5 cm diameter | Breast tissue both sides; one or both 0.5 to 1.0 cm | Breast tissue both sides, one or both >1 cm | |
| Ear form | Pinna flat and shapeless, little or no incurving of edge | Incurving of part of edge of pinna | Partial incurving whole of upper pinna | Well-defined incurving whole of upper pinna | |
| Ear firmness | Pinna soft, easily folded, no recoil | Pinna soft, easily folded, slow recoil | Cartilage to edge of pinna, but soft in places, ready recoil | Pinna firm, cartilage to edge; instant recoil | |
| Genitalia Male | Neither testis in scrotum | At least one testis high in scrotum | At least one testis down in scrotum | | |
| Female (with hips half abducted) | Labia majora widely separated; labia minora protruding | Labia majora almost cover labia minora | Labia majora completely cover labia minora | | |

FIGURE 6–3. Physical criteria to estimate gestational age. (From Dubowitz L, Dubowitz V: Gestational Age of the Newborn. Reading, MA, Addison-Wesley, 1977.)

ness or smallness for gestational age. Infants born at a weight greater than the 90th percentile for their age are considered **large for gestational age** (LGA). Risks associated with being LGA include all the risks of the infant of a diabetic mother (see Table 6–5) and risks associated with postmaturity. Infants born at a weight less than the 10th percentile for their age (some growth curves use less than two standard deviations or the 5th percentile) are **small for gestational age** (SGA) and have intrauterine growth retardation. Problems associated with the SGA infant include congenital malformations in addition to those problems listed in Table 6–8.

FIGURE 6–4. Neurologic criteria to estimate gestational age to be used with physical findings. (From Dubowitz L, Dubowitz V: Gestational Age of the Newborn. Reading, MA, Addison-Wesley, 1977.)

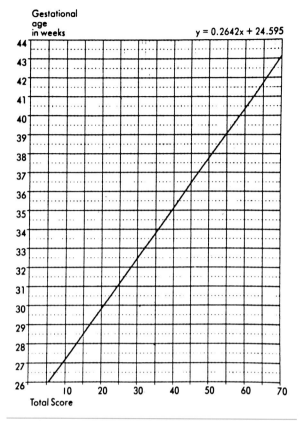

FIGURE 6–5. Score graph to determine gestational age. After adding the score from the physical criteria to that from the neurologic examination, the total score correlates with gestational age within ± 2 wk. (From Dubowitz L, Dubowitz V: Gestational Age of the Newborn. Reading, MA, Addison-Wesley, 1977.)

## SKIN

The skin should be evaluated for pallor, plethora, jaundice, cyanosis, meconium staining, petechiae, ecchymoses, congenital nevi, and neonatal rashes. Vasomotor instability with cutis marmorata, telangiectasia, phlebectasia (intermittent mottling with venous prominence), and acrocyanosis (feet and hands) is normal in the premature infant. Acrocyanosis also may be noted in the healthy term infant in the first days after birth. The **harlequin color change** is a striking transient but normal sign of vasomotor instability and divides the body from head to pubis through the midline into equal halves of pink and pale color.

The skin is covered with lanugo hair, which disappears by term gestation. **Hair tufts** over the lumbosacral spine suggest a spinal cord defect. **Vernix caseosa,** a soft, white, creamy layer covering the skin in preterm infants, disappears by term. Post-term infants often have peeling, parchment-like skin. **Mongolian spots** are transient dark blue to black pigmented macules seen over the lower back and buttock in 90% of black, Indian, and Asian infants. **Nevus simplex** (salmon patch), or pink macular hemangiomas, are common, usually transient, and noted on the back of the neck, eyelids, and forehead. **Nevus flammeus,** or the **port-wine stain,** commonly is seen on the face and should cause the examiner to consider the **Sturge-Weber syndrome** (trigeminal angiomatosis, convulsions, and ipsilateral intracranial "tram-line" calcifications).

Congenital melanocytic nevi are pigmented lesions of varying size noted in 1% of neonates. **Giant pigmented nevi** are uncommon but have malignant potential. **Capillary hemangiomas** are raised red lesions, whereas **cavernous hemangiomas** are deeper, blue-colored masses. Both increase in size after birth, only to resolve when the infant is 1–4 yr of age. When enlarged, these hemangiomas may produce high-output heart failure or platelet trapping and hemorrhage. **Erythema toxicum** is an erythematous, papular-vesicular rash common to neonates that develops after birth and has eosinophils in the vesicular fluid. **Pustular melanosis,** more common in black infants, may be seen at birth and consists of a small, dry vesicle on a pigmented brown macular base. Both erythema toxicum and pustular melanosis are benign lesions but may mimic more serious conditions such as the vesicular rash of disseminated herpes simplex or the bullous eruption of *Staphylococcus aureus* impetigo. Tzanck smear, Gram stain, Wright stain, direct fluorescent antibody stain, polymerase chain reaction (PCR) for herpes deoxyribonucleic acid (DNA), and appropriate cultures may be needed to distinguish these rashes. Other common characteristic rashes include **milia,** yellow-white epidermal cysts of the pilosebaceous follicles that are noted on the nose, and **miliaria** (prickly heat), which is caused by obstructed sweat glands. **Edema** may be present in preterm infants but should also suggest hydrops fetalis, sepsis, or lymphatic disorders.

## SKULL

The skull may be elongated and molded after a prolonged labor, but this resolves 2–3 days after birth. The sutures should be palpated to determine the width and the presence of premature fusion, or **cranial synostosis.** The anterior and posterior fontanel should be soft and nonbulging, with the anterior larger than the posterior. A **large fontanel** is associated with hydrocephalus, hypothyroidism, rickets, and other disorders. Soft areas away from the fontanel are **craniotabes**; these lesions have a Ping-Pong ball-like feeling and may be due to in utero compression. The skull should be examined carefully for signs of trauma or lacerations from internal fetal electrode sites or fetal scalp pH sampling; abscess formation may develop in these areas. (See Birth Injury for discussion of **caput succedaneum** and **subgaleal hemorrhage.**)

## FACE, EYES, MOUTH

The face should be inspected for dysmorphic features such as epicanthal folds, hypertelorism, preauricular tags or sinuses, low-set ears, long philtrum, and cleft lip or palate. Facial asymmetry may be due to 7th nerve palsy, and head tilt due to torticollis.

The eyes should open spontaneously, especially in an upright position. Under 28 weeks' gestational age, the eyelids may be fused. Coloboma, megalocornea, and microphthalmia should suggest other malformations or intrauterine infections. A cornea greater than 1 cm in diameter also may be seen in congenital glaucoma, uveal tract dysgenesis, and storage diseases. Conjunctival and retinal hemorrhages are common and usually of no significance. The pupillary response to light is present at 28 wk of gestation, and the **red reflex** of the retina is demonstrated easily. A white reflex, or **leukocoria,** is abnormal and may be due to cataracts, ocular tumor, severe chorioretinitis, persistent hyperplastic primary vitreous, or retinopathy of prematurity.

The mouth should be inspected for the presence of natal teeth, clefts of the soft and hard palate and uvula, and micrognathia. A bifid uvula suggests a submucosal cleft palate. White, shiny multiple transient epidermal inclusion cysts (Epstein pearls) on the hard palate are normal. Hard marble-sized masses in the buccal mucosa are usually transient idiopathic fat necrosis. The *tympanic membranes* are dull, gray, opaque, and immobile. These findings may persist for 1–4 wk and should not be confused with otitis media.

## NECK AND CHEST

The neck appears short and symmetric. Abnormalities include midline clefts or masses due to thyroglossal duct cysts or to goiter and lateral neck masses (or sinuses), which are, in turn, due to branchial clefts. Other masses include cystic hygromas and hemangiomas. Shortening of the sternocleidomastoid muscle with a fibrous "tumor" over the muscle produces head tilt and asymmetric facies (**neonatal torticollis**). The Arnold-Chiari malformation and cervical spine lesions also produce torticollis. Edema and webbing of the neck should suggest *Turner syndrome.* Both clavicles should be palpated for fractures.

Examination of the *chest* includes inspection of the chest wall to identify asymmetry resulting from absence of the pectoralis muscle and inspection of the breast tissue to determine gestational age and to detect a breast abscess. Both males and females may have breast engorgement and produce milk; milk expression should not be attempted. **Supernumerary nipples** may be bilateral and occasionally are associated with renal anomalies.

## LUNGS

Examination of the lungs includes observations of the rate, depth, and nature of intercostal or sternal retractions. Breath sounds should be equal on both sides of the chest, and rales should not be heard after the first 1–2 hr of life. Diminished or absent breath sounds on one side should suggest **pneumothorax,** collapsed lung, pleural effusion, or diaphragmatic hernia. Shift of the cardiac impulse away from a tension pneumothorax and diaphragmatic hernia and toward the collapsed lung is a helpful physical finding to differentiate these disorders. **Subcutaneous emphysema** of the neck or chest also suggests a pneumothorax, whereas bowel sounds auscultated in the chest in the presence of a scaphoid abdomen suggest a diaphragmatic hernia.

## HEART

The position of the heart in infants is more midline than in older children. The first heart sound is normal, whereas the second heart sound may not be split in the 1st day of life. Decreased splitting of the second heart sound is noted in primary pulmonary hypertension (PPHN) (also known as persistent fetal circulation [PFC]), transposition of the great vessels, and pulmonary atresia. **Heart murmurs** are common in the delivery room and during the 1st day of life. Most of these murmurs are transient and due to closure of the ductus arteriosus, peripheral pulmonary stenosis, or a small VSD. Pulses should be palpated in the upper and lower extremities, usually over the brachial and femoral arteries. Blood pressure in the upper and lower extremities should be measured in all patients with a murmur or heart failure. An upper-to-lower extremity gradient of more than 10–20 mm Hg suggests coarctation of the aorta.

## ABDOMEN

In the abdomen, the liver may be palpable 2 cm below the right costal margin, whereas the spleen tip may be felt less frequently. A left-sided liver suggests situs inversus and the asplenia syndrome. Both kidneys should be palpable in the 1st day of life with gentle deep palpation. The first urination occurs during the 1st day of life in over 95% of normal term infants.

**Abdominal masses** may represent hydronephrosis, dysplastic-multicystic kidney disease, ovarian cysts, intestinal duplication, neuroblastoma, or mesoblastic nephroma; masses should be evaluated immediately with ultrasound. Abdominal distention may be due to intestinal obstructions such as ileal atresia, meconium ileus, midgut volvulus, imperforate anus, or Hirschsprung disease. Meconium stool is passed normally within 48 hr of birth in 99% of term infants. The anus should be patent. An imperforate anus is not always visible; therefore, the first temperature should be taken carefully with a rectal thermometer. The abdominal wall musculature may be absent, as in prune-belly syndrome, or weak, resulting in diastasis recti. **Umbilical hernias** are common among black infants. The umbilical cord should be inspected to determine the presence of two arteries and one vein and the absence of a urachus or a herniation of abdominal contents, as occurs with an **omphalocele.** The latter is associated with extraintestinal problems such as genetic trisomies and hypoglycemia (*Beckwith-Wiedemann syndrome*). Bleeding from the cord should suggest a coagulation disorder, and a chronic discharge may be a granuloma of the umbilical stump or, less frequently, a draining omphalomesenteric cyst. Erythema around the umbilicus is **omphalitis** and may cause portal vein phlebitis and portal hypertension. The herniation of bowel through the abdominal wall 2–3 cm lateral to the umbilicus is a **gastroschisis.**

## GENITALIA

The appearance of the genitalia varies with gestational age. At term, the testes should be descended into a well-formed pigmented and rugated scrotum. The testes occasionally are in the inguinal canal; this is more common among preterm infants, as is **cryptorchidism.** Scrotal swelling may represent a hernia, transient hydrocele, in utero torsion of the testes, or, rarely, dissected meconium from meconium ileus and peritonitis. Hydroceles are clear and readily seen by transillumination, whereas testicular torsion in the newborn may present as a painless dark swelling. The urethral opening should be at the end of the penis. Epispadias or hypospadias alone should not raise concern about pseudohermaphroditism. However, if no testes are present in the scrotum and hypospadias is present, problems of sexual development should be suspected. Circumcision should be deferred with hypospadias, because the foreskin is needed for the repair. The prepuce is often too tight to retract in the neonatal period.

The female genitalia normally may reveal a milky white or blood-streaked vaginal discharge as a result of maternal hormone withdrawal. Mucosal tags of the labia majora are common. Distention of an **imperforate hymen** may produce **hydrometrocolpos** and a lower midline abdominal mass as a result of an enlarged uterus. Clitoral enlargement with fusion of the labial-scrotal folds (labia majora) suggests adrenogenital syndrome or exposure to masculinizing maternal hormones.

### EXTREMITIES

Examination of the *extremities* should include assessment of length, symmetry, and presence of hemihypertrophy, atrophy, polydactyly, syndactyly, simian creases, absent fingers, overlapping fingers, rocker-bottom feet, clubfoot, congenital bands, fractures, and amputations.

### SPINE

The spine should be examined for evidence of sacral hair tufts, a dermal sinus tract above the gluteal folds, congenital scoliosis (due to hemivertebra), and soft tissue masses such as a lipoma or meningomyelocele.

### HIPS

The hips should be examined for congenital dysplasia (dislocation). Gluteal fold asymmetry or leg length discrepancy is a suggestive sign of this condition, but the examiner should perform the **Barlow test** and the **Ortolani maneuver** to evaluate the stability of the hip joint. These tests determine whether the femoral head can be displaced from the acetabulum (Barlow test) and then replaced (Ortolani maneuver). The examiner's long finger is placed over the greater trochanter, and the thumb is placed medially just distal to the long finger. With the thighs held in midabduction, the femoral head is gently attempted to be pulled out of the acetabulum by lateral pressure of the thumb and by rocking the knee medially. The reverse maneuver is performed by pressing the long finger on the greater trochanter and rocking the knee laterally. A "clunking" sensation is palpated when the femoral head leaves and returns to the acetabulum.

### NEUROLOGIC ASSESSMENT

The neurologic examination should include assessment of active and passive tone, level of alertness, primary neonatal (primitive) reflexes, deep tendon reflexes, spontaneous motor activity, and cranial nerves (retinal examination, extraocular muscle movement, masseter power as in sucking, facial motility, hearing, and tongue function). Primary newborn reflexes include the **Moro reflex** (present at birth, gone between 3–6 mo), which is elicited by sudden slight dropping of the supported head from a slightly raised supine position. This slight drop should elicit opening of the hands and extension and abduction of the arms, followed by upper extremity flexion and a cry. The **palmar grasp** is present as early as 28 wk of age and gone by 4 mo of age. **Deep tendon reflexes** may be brisk in the normal newborn; 10–20 beats of ankle clonus are normal. The **Babinski sign** is extensor or upgoing. The sensory examination can be evaluated by withdrawal of an extremity, grimace, and cry in response to painful stimuli. The **rooting reflex,** or the turning of the head toward light tactile stimulation of the perioral area, is present as early as 32 wk of age.

References

Behrman RE, Kliegman RM, Arvin AM (eds): Nelson Textbook of Pediatrics, 15th ed. Philadelphia, WB Saunders, 1996, Chapter 79.2.
Illingworth R: The Normal Child, 10th ed. Edinburgh, Churchill Livingstone, 1991.
Leppig K, Werler M, Cann C, et al: Predictive value of minor anomalies: I. Association with major malformations. J Pediatr 110:530, 1987.

## RESPIRATORY DISORDERS

### APPROACH TO THE PATIENT

Respiratory distress that becomes manifest by tachypnea, intercostal retractions, reduced air exchange, cyanosis, grunting (a sound of distress), and flaring of the ala nasi is a nonspecific response

TABLE 6–16.  Etiology of Respiratory Distress

| Preterm Infant | Full-Term Infant | Preterm and Full-Term Infant |
|---|---|---|
| Respiratory distress syndrome<br>Erythroblastosis fetalis<br>Nonimmune hydrops<br>Pulmonary hemorrhage | Meconium aspiration pneumonia<br><br>Polycythemia<br>Amniotic fluid aspiration<br>Primary pulmonary<br>  hypertension of the neonate | Bacterial sepsis (GBS)<br>Transient tachypnea<br>Spontaneous pneumothorax<br>Congenital anomalies (e.g., congenital lobar<br>  emphysema, cystic adenomatoid<br>  malformation, diphragmatic hernia)<br>Congenital heart disease<br>Pulmonary hypoplasia<br>Viral infection (e.g., herpes simplex, CMV)<br>Inborn metabolic errors |

CMV = cytomegalovirus; GBS = group B streptococcus.

to serious illness. Not all of the disorders producing neonatal respiratory distress are primary diseases of the lungs. The differential diagnosis of respiratory distress includes pulmonary, cardiac, hematologic, infectious, anatomic, and metabolic disorders that may directly or indirectly involve the lungs (see Tables 6–13 and 6–16). Surfactant deficiency causes the *respiratory distress syndrome* (RSD), resulting in cyanosis and tachypnea; *infection* produces pneumonia demonstrated by interstitial or lobar infiltrates; *meconium aspiration* results in chemical pneumonitis with pulmonary hypertension; *hydrops fetalis* causes anemia and hypoalbuminemia with high-output heart failure and pulmonary edema; and congenital or acquired *pulmonary hypoplasia* causes pulmonary hypertension and pulmonary insufficiency. It also is useful to differentiate the common causes of respiratory distress according to gestational age (see Table 6–16).

In addition to the specific therapy of the individual disorder, the supportive care and evaluation of the infant with respiratory distress can be applied to all the problems mentioned earlier (see Tables 6–15 and 6–17). Blood gas monitoring and interpretation are key components of general respiratory care.

Treatment of hypoxemia requires knowledge of normal values. In term infants, the arterial $PaO_2$ is 55–60 mm Hg at 30 min of life, 75 mm Hg at 4 hr, and 90 mm Hg by 24 hr. Preterm infants have slightly lower values. $PaCO_2$ levels should be between 35 and 40 mm Hg, and the pH should be 7.35–7.40. It is imperative that arterial blood gas analysis be performed in all infants with significant respiratory distress, whether or not cyanosis is perceived. Cyanosis becomes evident when there are 5 g of unsaturated hemoglobin; thus, anemia may interfere with the perception of cyanosis. Jaundice also may interfere with the appearance of cyanosis.

Capillary blood gas determinations are useful in determining blood pH and $PCO_2$. Because of the nature of the heel-stick capillary blood gas technique, venous blood may mix with arterial blood, resulting in falsely low blood $PaO_2$ readings. Serial blood gases may be monitored by an indwelling

TABLE 6–17.  Initial Laboratory Evaluation of Respiratory Distress

| Test | Rationale |
|---|---|
| Chest roentgenogram | To determine reticular granular pattern of RDS; to determine presence of pneumothorax, cardiomegaly, life-threatening congenital anomalies |
| Arterial blood gas | To determine severity of respiratory compromise, hypoxemia, hypercapnia, and type of acidosis; the severity determines treatment strategy |
| Complete blood count | Hemoglobin/hematocrit to determine anemia and polycythemia; white blood cell count to determine neutropenia/sepsis; platelet count and smear to determine DIC |
| Blood culture | To recover potential pathogen |
| Blood glucose | To determine presence of hypoglycemia, which may produce or occur simultaneously with respiratory distress; to determine stress hyperglycemia |
| Echocardiogram, electrocardiogram | In the presence of a murmur, cardiomegaly, or refractory hypoxia; to determine structural heart disease or PPHN |

DIC = disseminated intravascular coagulation; PPHN = primary pulmonary hypertension of the neonate; RDS = respiratory distress syndrome.

arterial catheter placed through the umbilical artery to the aorta at the level of the T6-10 or the L4-5 vertebrae. This placement avoids catheter occlusion of the celiac (T12), superior mesenteric (T12-L1), renal (L1-2), and inferior mesenteric (L2-3) arteries. Another method for monitoring blood gases is to combine capillary blood gas techniques with noninvasive methods used to monitor oxygen (e.g., pulse oximetry or transcutaneous oxygen diffusion [TcPo$_2$]).

*Metabolic acidosis,* defined as a reduced pH (<7.25) and bicarbonate concentration (<18) accompanied by a normal or low Pco$_2$, may be due to hypoxia or to insufficient tissue perfusion; the origin of the disorder may be pulmonary, cardiac, infectious, renal, hematologic, nutritional, or iatrogenic. The initial approach to metabolic acidosis is to determine the cause and treat the pathophysiologic problem. This approach may include, as in the sequence of therapy for hypoxia, increasing the inspired oxygen concentration, applying continuous positive airway pressure nasally using oxygen as the gas, or initiating mechanical ventilation using positive end-expiratory pressure and oxygen. Patients with hypotension produced by hypovolemia require fluids and may need inotropic or vasoactive drug support. If metabolic acidosis persists despite specific therapy, sodium bicarbonate (1 mEq/kg/dose) may be given by slow intravenous infusion.

*Respiratory acidosis,* defined as an elevated Pco$_2$ and reduced pH without a reduction in the bicarbonate concentration, may be due to pulmonary insufficiency or central hypoventilation. Most disorders producing respiratory distress can result in hypercapnia. *Treatment* requires assisted ventilation but *not* sodium bicarbonate. If central nervous system depression of respirations is due to placental passage of narcotic analgesics, assisted ventilation is instituted first, and then the central nervous system depression is reversed by naloxone.

*Mixed metabolic/respiratory acidosis* is common and requires combined therapy. Other acid-base disturbances such as metabolic alkalosis and respiratory alkalosis are uncommon in the neonatal period, unless caused by chronic use of diuretics or by ventilator-induced hyperventilation, respectively.

## RESPIRATORY DISTRESS SYNDROME (HYALINE MEMBRANE DISEASE)

### Lung Development

An appreciation of lung development is basic to understanding the pathophysiology of RDS. The lining of the alveolus consists of 90% type I cells and 10% type II cells. After 20 wk of gestation, the type II cells contain vacuolated, osmophilic, lamellar inclusion bodies, which are packages of surface-active material (Fig. 6–6). This lipoprotein *surfactant* is 90% lipid and is composed predominantly of saturated phosphatidylcholine (dipalmityl phosphatidylcholine, or lecithin) but also contains phosphatidylglycerol, other phospholipids, and neutral lipids. The surfactant proteins SP-A, SP-B, SP-C, and SP-D are packaged into the lamellar body and contribute to surface-active properties and recycling of surfactant. Surfactant prevents at-

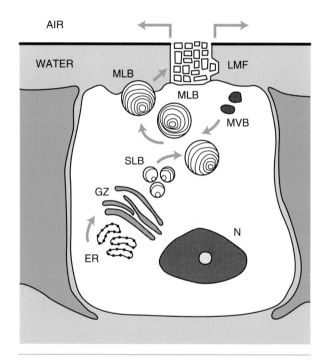

FIGURE 6–6. Proposed pathway of synthesis, transport, secretion, and reuptake of surfactant in the type II alveolar cell. Phospholipids are synthesized in the smooth endoplasmic reticulum (ER). The glucose/glycerol precursor may be derived from lung glycogen or circulating glucose. Phospholipids and surfactant proteins are packaged in the Golgi apparatus (GZ), emerge as small lamellar bodies (SLB), coalesce to mature lamellar bodies (MLB), migrate to the apical membrane, and are released by exocytosis into the liquid hypophase below the air-liquid interface. The tightly coiled lamellar body unravels to form the lattice (tubular) myelin figure (LMF), the immediate precursor to the phospholipid monolayer at the alveolar surface. Reuptake by endocytosis forms multivesicular bodies (MVB), which recycle surfactant. The enzymes, receptors, transporters, and surfactant proteins are controlled by regulatory processes at the transcriptional level in the nucleus (N). Corticosteroid and thyroid hormones are regulatory ligands that may accelerate surfactant synthesis. (From Hansen T, Corbet A: Lung Development and Function. *In* Taeusch HW, Ballard R, Avery ME [eds]: Diseases of the Newborn, 6th ed. Philadelphia, WB Saunders, 1991.)

electasis by reducing surface tension at low lung volumes when it is concentrated at end-expiration as the alveolar radius decreases; surfactant contributes to lung recoil by increasing surface tension at larger lung volumes when it is diluted during inspiration as the alveolar radius increases. Without surfactant, surface tension forces are not reduced and atelectasis develops during end-expiration as the alveolus collapses.

The timing of surfactant (lecithin) production in quantities sufficient to prevent atelectasis depends on an increase in fetal cortisol levels that begins between 32 and 34 wk of gestation. Between 34 and 36 wk, sufficient surface-active material is produced by the type II cells in the lung, is secreted into the alveolar lumen, and is excreted into the amniotic fluid. Thus, the concentration of lecithin in amniotic fluid indicates fetal pulmonary maturity. Because quantitation of lecithin is difficult to perform, the ratio of lecithin (which increases with maturity) to sphingomyelin (which remains constant during gestation) (L/S ratio) is determined. A ratio of 2:1 usually indicates pulmonary maturity. The presence of minor phospholipids such as phosphatidylglycerol also is indicative of fetal lung maturity and may be useful in situations in which the L/S ratio is borderline or possibly affected by maternal diabetes, which reduces lung maturity.

### Clinical Manifestations

Respiratory distress syndrome is due to a deficiency of pulmonary surfactant that results in atelectasis, a decreased functional residual capacity, arterial hypoxemia, and respiratory distress. In addition to the developmental deficiency, surfactant synthesis may be reduced as a result of hypovolemia, hypothermia, acidosis, and hypoxemia. These factors also produce pulmonary artery vasospasm, which may contribute to RDS in larger premature infants who have developed sufficient pulmonary arteriole smooth muscle to produce vasoconstriction. Surfactant deficiency–induced atelectasis causes alveoli to be perfused but not ventilated, which results in a pulmonary shunt and hypoxemia. As atelectasis increases, the lungs become increasingly difficult to expand and lung compliance decreases. Because the chest wall of the premature infant is very compliant, the infant attempts to overcome decreased lung compliance with increasing inspiratory pressures, resulting in retractions of the chest wall. The sequence of decreased lung compliance and chest wall retractions results in poor air exchange, an increased physiologic dead space, alveolar hypoventilation, and hy-

percapnia. A vicious circle of hypoxia, hypercapnia, and acidosis acts on type II cells to reduce surfactant synthesis and, in some infants, on the pulmonary arterioles to produce pulmonary hypertension.

Pathologic examination of the lung reveals atelectasis and acidophilic pink membranes (hyaline membranes) lining the air spaces. Hyaline membrane formation results from transudation of fluid through the capillary endothelium into the surfactant-deficient alveolus.

The infants at greatest risk for RDS are premature and have an immature L/S ratio. The incidence of RDS increases with decreasing gestational age. Nonetheless, RDS develops in only 30–60% of infants between 28 and 32 wk of gestation. Other risk factors include delivery of a previous preterm infant with RDS, being an infant of a diabetic mother, hypothermia, asphyxia, male sex, Caucasian race, being a second twin, and delivery by cesarean section without labor.

Signs of RDS may develop immediately in the delivery room in very immature infants at 26–30 wk of gestation. However, some more mature infants (34 wk of gestation) may not show signs of RDS until 3–4 hr after birth. Manifestations of RDS include cyanosis, tachypnea, nasal flaring, intercostal and sternal retractions, and a whining, crying, moaning sound called **grunting.** The latter sign is due to partial closure of the glottis during expiration, resulting in higher end-expiratory airway pressures that may ameliorate atelectasis. Atelectasis is well documented by the chest radiograph, which demonstrates a ground-glass haze in the lung surrounding air-filled bronchi (the air bronchogram) (Fig. 6–7). Severe RDS may demonstrate an airless lung field or a "whiteout" on roentgenogram, even obliterating the distinction between the atelectatic lungs and the heart.

During the first 72 hr, infants with RDS have increasing distress and hypoxemia. Infants with severe RDS develop edema, apnea, and respiratory failure necessitating mechanical ventilation. Thereafter, uncomplicated cases demonstrate a spontaneous improvement that often is heralded by diuresis and a marked resolution of edema. Complications include those noted in Table 6–18 plus the development of a PDA and bronchopulmonary dysplasia (BPD). The differential diagnosis of RDS includes diseases associated with cyanosis and respiratory distress (see Tables 6–13 and 6–16).

### Prevention and Treatment

Essential preventive measures for RDS include avoiding premature birth from either elective cesarean section or premature labor. In addition, pre-

FIGURE 6–7.   Respiratory distress syndrome. The infant is intubated, and the lungs show a dense reticulonodular pattern with air bronchograms *(A)*. Note how to evaluate rotation on the frontal chest: The lengths of the posterior ribs are compared from left to right *(arrows)*. Because the infant is supine, the side of the longer ribs indicates to which side the thorax is rotated. In this case, the left ribs are longer and this radiograph is thus a left posterior oblique view. Surfactant was administered, resulting in significant improvement in the density of the lung *(B)*. The right lung is slightly better aerated than the left. Uneven distribution of clearing is common. (From Hilton S, Edwards D: Practical Pediatric Radiology, 2nd ed. WB Saunders, Philadelphia, 1994, p 29.)

vention of cold stress, birth asphyxia, and hypovolemia reduces the risk of RDS and its severity. If premature delivery is unavoidable, the antenatal administration of corticosteroids to the mother (and thus to the fetus) stimulates fetal lung production of surfactant; this approach requires multiple doses for at least 48 hr.

After birth, RDS may be prevented or its severity reduced by the intratracheal administration of synthetic or natural surfactants to premature infants with immature amniotic L/S ratios. Synthetic

(lecithin, tyloxapol, hexadecanol) or natural (lecithin-fortified extract of cow lungs) surfactant also can be administered repeatedly during the course of RDS in patients receiving endotracheal intubation, mechanical ventilation, and oxygen therapy. Additional management includes the general supportive and ventilation care presented in Tables 6–15, 6–17, and 6–19.

The $PaO_2$ should be maintained between 60 and 70 mm Hg and pH kept above 7.25. An increased concentration of warm and humidified inspired oxygen administered by an oxygen hood may be all that is needed for larger premature infants. If hypoxemia ($PaO_2$ <50 mm Hg) is present and the needed inspired oxygen concentration is 70–100%, continuous positive airway pressure (nasal CPAP) should be added at a distending pressure of 8–10 cm $H_2O$. If respiratory failure ensues ($PcO_2$ >60 mm Hg, pH <7.20, and $PaO_2$ <50 on 100% $O_2$), mechanical ventilation using a respirator is indicated. Conventional rate (25–60 breaths/min), high-frequency jet (150–600 breaths/min), and oscillator (900–3000 breaths/min) ventilators each have been successful in managing respiratory failure due to severe RDS. Suggested starting settings on a conventional ventilator include: fraction of inspired oxygen ($FiO_2$), 60–100%; peak inspiratory pressure (PIP), 20–25 cm $H_2O$; positive end-expiratory pressure (PEEP), +5 cm $H_2O$; and a rate of 20–40 breaths/min. The inspiratory-to-expiratory time (I:E) ratio is 1:1.2 to 1:2.0.

In response to persistent hypercapnia, alveolar ventilation (tidal volume − dead space × rate) must be increased. This may be achieved by increasing the ventilator's rate or by increasing the tidal volume, which is the gradient between PIP and PEEP. In response to hypoxia, the inspired oxygen content may be increased. Alternately, the degree of oxygenation is dependent on the mean airway pressure ($\bar{P}aw$). $\bar{P}aw$ is directly related to PIP, PEEP, flow, and I:E ratio. Increased $\bar{P}aw$ may improve oxygenation by improving lung volume,

TABLE 6–18.   Acute Deterioration in Respiratory Distress Syndrome

Pneumothorax
Extubation
Endotracheal tube in right main stem bronchus
Mucous plug in endotracheal tube
Pulmonary hemorrhage
Intraventricular hemorrhage
Pneumopericardium
Sepsis
Intra-abdominal hemorrhage (liver, spleen, adrenal)
Acute pulmonary hypertension (shunting)

TABLE 6–19.  Ventilator Management of Respiratory Distress Syndrome

| Setting | Result | Rationale | Risks |
|---|---|---|---|
| ↑ $FiO_2$ | ↑ $Po_2$ | ↑ Alveolar $O_2$ | Oxygen toxicity |
| ↑ PIP | ↑ $Po_2$<br>↓ $Pco_2$ | ↑ $\overline{Paw}$<br>↑ Tidal volume | Pneumothorax, barotrauma, ↓ cardiac output? |
| ↑ PEEP | ↑ $Po_2$ | ↑ $\overline{Paw}$ | ↑ $Pco_2$ by ↓ tidal volume<br>↓ Cardiac output? |
| ↑ Rate | ↓ $Pco_2$ | ↑ Alveolar ventilation | ↓ Expiratory time causes gas trapping |
| ↑ I:E ratio | ↑ $Po_2$ | ↑ $\overline{Paw}$ | ↓ Expiratory time causes gas trapping |

$FiO_2$ = fraction of inspired oxygen; I:E = inspiratory to expiratory time ratio; $\overline{Paw}$ = mean airway pressure; PEEP = positive end-expiratory pressure; PIP = peak inspiratory pressure.

thus enhancing ventilation-perfusion matching (see Table 6–19).

Because of the difficulty in distinguishing sepsis and pneumonia from RDS, broad-spectrum parenteral antibiotics (ampicillin and gentamicin) are administered for 72 hr, pending the recovery of an organism from a previously obtained blood culture.

## Complications

**Patent Ductus Arteriosus.** The ductus arteriosus constricts after birth in normal term infants in response to an elevated $PaO_2$. The ductus arteriosus in the preterm infant is less responsive to vasoconstrictive stimuli, in part as a result of the persistent vasodilatory effect of $PGE_2$; this decreased vasoconstriction response, combined with hypoxemia during RDS, may result in a persistent PDA that may create a shunt between the pulmonary and systemic circulations.

During the acute phase of RDS, pulmonary arterial vasoconstriction and increased pressure are due to hypoxia, hypercapnia, and acidosis. Therefore, the pulmonary and systemic pressures may be equal, and flow through the ductus may be small or bidirectional. When RDS improves and pulmonary vascular resistance declines, flow through the ductus arteriosus increases in a left-to-right direction. Significant systemic-to-pulmonary shunting may result in heart failure and pulmonary edema. Excessive intravenous fluid administration may increase the incidence of a symptomatic PDA. The infant's respiratory status deteriorates owing to increased lung fluid, hypercapnia, and hypoxemia. In response to poor blood gases, the infant is subjected to higher inspired oxygen concentrations and higher peak inspiratory ventilator pressures, both of which damage the lung (see Bronchopulmonary Dysplasia).

*Clinical manifestations* of a PDA usually become apparent on the 3rd–5th day of life. Because the left-to-right shunt is to a low-pressure circulation from one of high pressure, the pulse pressure widens; a previously inactive precordium now demonstrates a very active precordial impulse, and the peripheral pulses become easily palpable and bounding. The murmur of a PDA may be continuous in systole and diastole, but usually only the systolic component is auscultated. Heart failure and pulmonary edema result in rales and hepatomegaly. A chest roentgenogram demonstrates cardiomegaly and pulmonary edema; a two-dimensional echocardiogram demonstrates patency, whereas Doppler studies demonstrate markedly increased left-to-right flow through the ductus.

*Treatment* of a PDA during RDS includes an initial period of fluid restriction and diuretic administration. If there is no improvement after 24–48 hr, indomethacin, a prostaglandin synthetase inhibitor, is administered (0.2 mg/kg) intravenously every 12 hr for three doses. Thereafter the drug is administered at 0.1–0.2 mg/kg every 24 hr for 5 days. This has been most successful in closing the PDA among premature infants in the first 2 wk of life, when prostaglandins may still be playing a significant role in maintaining ductal patency. Contraindications to using indomethacin include thrombocytopenia (<50,000), bleeding, serum creatinine measuring more than 1.8 mg/dL, and oliguria. Because 20–30% of infants do not respond initially to indomethacin and, of those who do, the PDA reopens in 10%, a repeated course of indomethacin or surgical ligation is required in a significant number of patients.

**Pulmonary Air Leaks.** High PIPs and PEEPs may cause overdistention of alveoli in localized areas of the lung. Rupture of the alveolar epithelial lining may produce **pulmonary interstitial emphysema** (PIE) as gas dissects along the interstitial space and the peribronchial lymphatics. Extravasation of gas into the parenchyma reduces lung compliance and worsens respiratory failure. Gas dissection into the mediastinal space produces a **pneumomediastinum,** occasionally with gas dissecting into the subcutaneous tissues around the neck, causing **subcutaneous emphysema.**

Alveolar rupture adjacent to the pleural space produces a **pneumothorax** (see Physical Examination and Gestational Age Assessment). If the gas is under tension, the pneumothorax shifts the mediastinum to the opposite side of the chest, producing hypotension, hypoxia, and hypercapnia. The diagnosis of a pneumothorax may be made by unequal transillumination of the chest and may be confirmed by chest roentgenogram (Fig. 6–8). *Treatment* of a symptomatic pneumothorax requires insertion of a pleural chest tube connected to negative pressure or to an underwater drain. Prophylactic or therapeutic use of exogenous surfactant has reduced the incidence of pulmonary air leaks.

Pneumothorax also is observed following vigorous resuscitation, meconium aspiration pneumonia, pulmonary hypoplasia, and diaphragmatic hernia. Spontaneous pneumothorax may be seen in fewer than 1% of deliveries and may be associated with renal malformations.

**Pneumopericardium** is a severe life-threatening

FIGURE 6–8. Pneumothorax. Right-sided hyperlucent pleural air is obvious. The findings of linear interstitial air and the resultant noncompliant but collapsed right lung are also noted. (From Heller R, Kirchner S: Advanced Exercises in Diagnostic Radiology: The Newborn. Philadelphia, WB Saunders, 1979, p 58.)

condition that may cause cardiac tamponade. Systemic gas embolism is another rare but lethal complication of mechanical ventilation.

**Bronchopulmonary Dysplasia.** Oxygen concentrations above 40% are toxic to the neonatal lung. Oxygen-mediated lung injury results from the generation of superoxides, hydrogen peroxide ($H_2O_2$), and oxygen-free radicals, which disrupt membrane lipids. Mechanical ventilation with high peak pressures produces barotrauma, compounding the damaging effects of high inspired oxygen levels. In most patients, BPD develops following ventilation for RDS that may have been complicated by PDA or PIE. Failure of RDS to improve after 2 wk, the need for prolonged mechanical ventilation, and oxygen therapy required at 36 wk postconception age are characteristic of patients with RDS who develop BPD. Infants weighing less than 1000 g who require mechanical ventilation for poor respiratory drive in the absence of RDS also may develop BPD.

The roentgenographic appearance of BPD may undergo phases characterized initially by lung opacification and, subsequently, by development of cysts accompanied by areas of overdistention and atelectasis, giving the lung a sponge-like appearance. The histopathology of BPD reveals interstitial edema, atelectasis, mucosal metaplasia, interstitial fibrosis, necrotizing obliterative bronchiolitis, and overdistended alveoli.

The *clinical manifestations* of BPD are oxygen dependence, hypercapnia, compensatory metabolic alkalosis, pulmonary hypertension, and the development of right-sided heart failure. Increased airway resistance with reactive airway bronchoconstriction also is noted, and is treated with bronchodilating agents. Severe chest retractions produce very negative interstitial pressure that draws fluid into the interstitial space. These chest retractions, together with cor pulmonale, cause fluid retention necessitating fluid restriction and administration of diuretics.

Patients with BPD may require *treatment* with mechanical ventilation for many months. To reduce the risk of subglottic stenosis, a tracheotomy may be indicated. To reduce oxygen toxicity and barotrauma, ventilator settings are reduced to maintain blood gases with slightly lower $PaO_2$ (50 mm Hg) and higher $PaCO_2$ (50–75 mm Hg) than for infants during the acute phase of RDS. Dexamethasone therapy may reduce inflammation, improve pulmonary function, and enhance weaning of patients from mechanical ventilation.

**Retinopathy of Prematurity (Retrolental Fibroplasia).** This disorder is caused by the acute and chronic effects of oxygen toxicity on the developing blood vessels of the premature infant's retina. The completely vascularized retina of the term infant is not susceptible to retinopathy of prematurity (ROP). ROP is a leading cause of blindness for VLBW infants (<1500 g). Excessive arterial oxygen tensions produce vasoconstriction of the immature retinal vasculature in the first stage of this disease, which is followed by vaso-obliteration if the duration and extent of hyperoxia are prolonged beyond the time when vasoconstriction is reversible. Hypercarbia and hypoxia may contribute to ROP. The subsequent proliferative stages are characterized by extraretinal fibrovascular proliferation, forming a ridge between the vascular and avascular portions of the retina, and by the development of neovascular tufts. In mild cases, vasoproliferation is noted at the periphery of the retina. Severe cases may exhibit neovascularization involving the entire retina, retinal detachment resulting from traction on vessels as they leave the optic disk, fibrous proliferation behind the lens producing leukocoria, and synechiae displacing the lens forward and resulting in glaucoma. Both eyes usually are involved, but severity may be asymmetric.

The incidence of ROP may be reduced by careful monitoring of arterial blood gases in all patients receiving oxygen. Although there is no absolutely safe $PaO_2$, it is wise to keep the arterial $O_2$ between 50 and 70 torr in premature infants. Cryotherapy may be used for vitreous hemorrhage or for severe progressive vasoproliferation. Surgery is indicated for retinal detachment. Less severe stages of ROP resolve spontaneously without visual impairment in the majority of patients.

## TRANSIENT TACHYPNEA OF THE NEWBORN

Transient tachypnea of the newborn (TTN) is a self-limited condition characterized by tachypnea, mild retractions, and occasional grunting, usually without signs of severe respiratory distress. Cyanosis, when present, usually requires no more than 30–40% $O_2$. TTN usually is noted in larger premature infants and in term infants born by cesarean section without prior labor. The infant of a diabetic mother or the infant with poor respiratory drive as a result of placental passage of analgesic drugs is also at risk. Chest roentgenograms show prominent central vascular markings, fluid in the lung fissures, overaeration, and occasionally, a small pleural effusion. Air bronchograms and a reticulogranular pattern are not seen in TTN, and their presence would suggest another pulmonary process such as RDS or pneumonia. TTN may be due to retained lung fluid and/or slow resorption of lung fluid.

## MECONIUM ASPIRATION SYNDROME

Meconium-stained amniotic fluid is seen in 10% of predominantly term, growth-retarded, and post-term deliveries. Although passage of meconium into amniotic fluid is very common among infants born in the breech presentation, meconium-stained fluid should be considered a sign of fetal distress for infants born in all presentations. Fetal scalp pH should be determined and biophysical evaluation should be done to assess the well-being of the fetus. The presence of meconium in the amniotic fluid suggests in utero asphyxia, hypoxia, and acidosis.

An additional risk is aspiration of amniotic fluid contaminated with particulate meconium. Aspiration may occur in utero in a distressed, gasping fetus, but more often meconium is aspirated into the lung immediately after delivery. More than 50% of infants born with meconium-stained fluid have meconium in the trachea at the time of birth. Half of these infants will have abnormal chest roentgenograms demonstrating a very high incidence of pneumonia and pneumothoraces.

*Meconium aspiration pneumonia* is characterized by tachypnea, hypoxia, hypercapnia, and small airway obstruction that results in a ball-valve effect, producing air trapping, overdistention, and extra-alveolar air leaks. Complete small airway obstruction produces atelectasis. Within 24–48 hr, a chemical pneumonia develops in addition to the mechanical effects of airway obstruction. The chest roentgenogram demonstrates patchy infiltrates, overdistention, flattening of the diaphragm, increased anteroposterior diameter, and a very high incidence of pneumomediastinum and pneumothoraces. Quite unexpectedly, many symptomatic infants with severe hypoxia demonstrate a completely normal-appearing chest film. The condition of these infants with severe pulmonary hypertension is very similar to that of infants with PPHN (PFC). Comorbid diseases include those associated with in utero asphyxia that initiated the passage of meconium (see Table 6–10).

*Treatment* of meconium aspiration includes general supportive care and mechanical ventilation. Infants with a PPHN-like presentation should be treated for PPHN. If severe hypoxia does not subside with conventional or high-frequency ventilation, inhaled nitric oxide (NO) or extracorporeal membrane oxygenation (ECMO) may be beneficial. Occasionally, surfactant is beneficial.

*Prevention* of meconium aspiration syndrome includes careful in utero monitoring to avoid asphyxia. When meconium-stained fluid is observed, the obstetrician should suction the oropharynx of the infant before delivering the rest of the infant's body. After birth the depressed or distressed infant's oropharynx should be suctioned, the vocal cords visualized, and the area below the vocal cords suctioned to remove meconium from the trachea. This procedure can be repeated two to three times as long as meconium is present, prior to either stimulating the infant to breathe or initiating artificial ventilation (see Asphyxia: Resuscitation). Saline intrauterine amnioinfusion during labor may reduce the incidence of aspiration and pneumonia.

## PRIMARY PULMONARY HYPERTENSION OF THE NEWBORN
### (Persistent Fetal Circulation)

PPHN is characterized by severe hypoxemia without evidence of parenchymal lung or structural heart disease that also may cause right-to-left shunting. The disorder is often seen in term or post-term infants who are asphyxiated or who have had meconium-stained fluid. The chest roentgenogram usually demonstrates normal lung fields rather than the expected infiltrates and hyperinflation that may accompany massive meconium aspiration pneumonia. Additional problems that may result in PPHN include congenital pneumonia, hyperviscosity–polycythemia, congenital diaphragmatic hernia, pulmonary hypoplasia, hypoglycemia, and hypothermia. Total anomalous venous return associated with obstruction of blood flow may produce a clinical picture that includes severe hypoxia and that is indistinguishable from PPHN; chest roentgenogram, however, reveals severe pulmonary venous engorgement and a small heart; echocardiography or rarely cardiac catheterization will confirm the diagnosis.

PPHN is characterized by significant right-to-left shunting through a patent foramen ovale, through a PDA, and through intrapulmonary channels. The pulmonary vasculature often demonstrates hypertrophied arterial wall smooth muscle, suggesting that the process of or predisposition to PPHN began in utero as a result of previous periods of fetal hypoxia. After birth, hypoxia, hypercapnia, and acidosis exacerbate pulmonary artery vasoconstriction, resulting in further hypoxia and acidosis. In addition to pulmonary hypertension, some infants with PPHN develop extrapulmonary manifestations as a result of asphyxia (see Table 6–10). Myocardial injuries include heart failure, transient mitral insufficiency, and papillary muscle or myocardial infarction. Thrombocytopenia, right atrial thrombi, and pulmonary embolism also may be noted.

The *diagnosis* may be confirmed by echocardiogram, which demonstrates elevated pulmonary artery pressures and sites of right-to-left shunting. Echocardiography also is helpful to rule out structural congenital heart disease and transient myocardial dysfunction.

*Treatment* includes general supportive care in addition to correction of hypotension, anemia, and acidosis and the management of complications associated with asphyxia. If myocardial dysfunction is present, dopamine or dobutamine will be needed. The most important therapy for PPHN is mechanical ventilation. Reversible mild pulmonary hypertension may respond to conventional ventilator settings (see Table 6–19). However, patients with severe PPHN do not always respond to conventional therapy and may require hyperventilation to reverse pulmonary vasoconstriction by reducing $PCO_2$ to 20 mm Hg and increasing pH to 7.5–7.6. Paralysis with pancuronium may be needed to assist such vigorous ventilation. If mechanical ventilation and supportive care are unsuccessful in improving oxygenation, inhaled nitric oxide, a selective pulmonary artery vasodilating agent, should be administered. If hypoxia persists, the patient may be a candidate for ECMO. Infants who require very high ventilator settings, marked by an alveolar-to-arterial oxygen gradient greater than 620 mm Hg, have a high mortality rate and may benefit from ECMO if they do not respond to nitric oxide.

## APNEA

Apnea is defined as the cessation of pulmonary airflow for a specific time interval, usually longer than 10–20 sec. Bradycardia often accompanies prolonged apnea. **Central apnea** refers to a complete cessation of airflow and respiratory efforts with no chest wall movement; **obstructive apnea** exhibits no airflow but the chest wall movements continue. A combination of these two events, **mixed apnea,** is the most frequent type. It usually begins as a brief episode of obstruction followed by a central apnea.

A careful *evaluation* to determine the cause should be performed immediately in any infant with apnea (Table 6–20). The incidence of apnea increases as gestational age decreases. Idiopathic apnea, a disease of premature infants, appears in the absence of any other identifiable disease states during the 1st week of life and resolves by 36 wk

TABLE 6–20.  Potential Causes of Neonatal Apnea

| CNS | IVH, drugs, seizures, hypoxic injury |
|---|---|
| Respiratory | Pneumonia, obstructive airway lesions, atelectasis, extreme prematurity (<1000 g), laryngeal reflex, phrenic nerve paralysis, severe RDS, pneumothorax |
| Infectious | Sepsis, necrotizing enterocolitis, meningitis (bacterial, fungal, viral) |
| Gastrointestinal | Oral feeding, bowel movement, gastroesophageal reflux, esophagitis, intestinal perforation |
| Metabolic | ↓ Glucose, ↓ calcium, ↓ $PO_2$, ↓↑ sodium, ↑ ammonia, ↑ organic acids, ↑ ambient temperature, hypothermia |
| Cardiovascular | Hypotension, hypertension, heart failure, anemia, hypovolemia, change in vagal tone |
| Idiopathic | Immaturity of respiratory center, sleep state, upper airway collapse |

CNS = central nervous system; IVH = intraventricular hemorrhage; RDS = respiratory distress syndrome.

of postconceptional age (gestational age at birth + postnatal age). The premature infant's process of regulating respiration is especially vulnerable to apnea. For example, preterm infants respond paradoxically to hypoxia by developing apnea rather than by increasing respirations, as mature infants do. Poor tone of the laryngeal muscles also may result in collapse of the upper airway, leading to obstruction. Isolated obstructive apnea, the least common type of apnea, also may occur as a result of flexion or extreme lateral positioning of the premature infant's head, obstructing the soft trachea.

*Treatment* of apnea of prematurity includes administration of oxygen to hypoxic infants, transfusion of anemic infants, and physical cutaneous stimulation for mild apnea. Persistent apnea with bradycardia can be treated with methylxanthines, caffeine, or theophylline. Theophylline decreases the incidence of apnea by acting as a central nervous system stimulant. Loading doses of 5 mg/kg followed by 1–2 mg/kg every 8–12 hr are sufficient. Elimination of theophylline is prolonged in preterm infants, and serum levels should be carefully monitored and maintained between 5 and 10 μg/mL. In the newborn infant, theophylline also is converted to caffeine, thus increasing its efficacy. Nasal CPAP of 3–5 cm $H_2O$ also is an effective method of treating obstructive or mixed apneas; it may work by splinting the upper airway.

## MISCELLANEOUS RESPIRATORY DISORDERS

**Pulmonary hypoplasia** becomes manifest as severe respiratory distress in the delivery room that progresses rapidly to pulmonary insufficiency. The lungs, which are very small, develop pneumothoraces with normal resuscitative efforts. A small chest size roentgenographically, joint contractures, and early onset of pneumothoraces, often bilateral, are early clues to the diagnosis. Pulmonary hypertension results from the decreased lung mass and hypertrophy of pulmonary arteriole muscle.

Pulmonary hypoplasia may be due to asphyxiating thoracic dystrophies (a small chest wall) or to decreased amniotic fluid volume that causes uterine compression of the developing chest wall, thus inhibiting lung growth. The latter failure of lung development may be associated with renal agenesis (Potter syndrome) or with a chronic leak of amniotic fluid from ruptured membranes. Isolated agenesis of one lung (usually the left lung) often is asymptomatic and familial. In contrast, serious pulmonary hypoplasia is noted in patients with a **diaphragmatic hernia.** Herniated bowel interferes with lung growth and also results in hypertrophy of the muscle layers of small pulmonary arteries, producing pulmonary hypertension. Pneumothoraces are common.

*Treatment* of a diaphragmatic hernia requires surgical evacuation of the chest and repair of the diaphragmatic defect. Respiratory care is similar to that for patients with PPHN.

Neuromuscular diseases that interfere with fetal breathing movements also may produce pulmonary hypoplasia (e.g., congenital anterior horn cell disease [**Werdnig-Hoffmann syndrome**]).

Another cause of bilateral pulmonary hypoplasia is **hydrops fetalis** (see Obstetric Complications Associated with Fetal or Neonatal Risks). Hydrops from any cause is characterized by anasarca, ascites, and pleural and pericardial effusions. Bilateral pleural effusions act as space-occupying masses that interfere with lung growth, resulting in pulmonary hypoplasia.

### References

Behrman RE, Kliegman RM, Arvin AM (eds): Nelson Textbook of Pediatrics, 15th ed. Philadelphia, WB Saunders, 1996, Chapters 87.1–87.10.

Cryotherapy for Retinopathy of Prematurity Cooperative Group: Multicenter trial of cryotherapy for retinopathy of prematurity. Arch Ophthalmol 114:417, 1996.

Davis P, Turner-Gomes S, Cunningham K, et al: Precision and accuracy of clinical and radiological signs in premature infants at risk of patent ductus arteriosus. Arch Pediatr Adolesc Med 149:1136, 1995.

Goldman AP, Tasker RC, Haworth SG, et al: Four patterns of response to inhaled nitric oxide for persistent pulmonary hypertension of the newborn. Pediatrics 98:706, 1996.

Le Souef PN: Persistent tachypnoea in neonates. BMJ 312:1113, 1996.

NIH Consensus Development Panel on the Effect of Corticosteroids for Fetal Maturation on Perinatal Outcomes: Effect of corticosteroids for fetal maturation on perinatal outcomes. JAMA 273:413, 1995.

Rojas MA, Gonzalez A, Bancalari E, et al: Changing trends in the epidemiology and pathogenesis of neonatal chronic lung disease. J Pediatr 126:605, 1995.

UK Collaborative ECMO Trial Group: UK collaborative randomised trial of neonatal extracorporeal membrane oxygenation. Lancet 348:75, 1996.

Upton CJ, Milner AD, Stokes GM: Upper airway patency during apnoea of prematurity. Arch Dis Child 67:419, 1992.

Wiswell TE, Henley MA: Intratracheal suctioning, systemic infection and the meconium aspiration syndrome. Pediatrics 89:203, 1992.

# HEMATOLOGIC DISORDERS

## ANEMIA

Embryonic hematopoiesis begins by the 20th day of gestation and is evidenced as blood islands in the yolk sac. In mid-gestation, erythropoiesis occurs in the liver and spleen; the bone marrow becomes the predominant site in the last trimester. Hemoglobin concentration increases from 8–10 g/dL at 12 wk to 16.5–18.0 g/dL at 40 wk. Fetal red blood cell production is responsive to erythropoietin, and the concentration of this hormone is increased with fetal hypoxia and anemia.

After birth, hemoglobin levels increase transiently at 6–12 hr and then decline to 11 g/dL at 3–6 mo. The prematurely born infant, who is less than 32 wk of gestational age, has lower hemoglobin concentration and a more rapid postnatal decline of hemoglobin level, which achieves a nadir 1–2 mo after birth. Fetal and neonatal red blood cells have a shorter life span (70–90 days) and a higher mean corpuscular volume (110–120 fL) than adult cells. Infants demonstrate a reticulocytosis of between 5% and 12% during the first days of life. Hemoglobin and hematocrit levels are higher in neonatal capillary samples obtained by skin pricks than they are in central venous or arterial samples.

In the fetus, *hemoglobin synthesis* in the last two trimesters of pregnancy produces fetal hemoglobin F, composed of two alpha chains and two gamma chains. Immediately prior to term, the infant begins to synthesize beta-hemoglobin chains; thus the term infant should have some adult hemoglobin (two alpha chains and two beta chains). Fetal hemoglobin represents 60–90% of hemoglobin at birth, and the levels decline to adult levels of less than 5% by 4 mo of age.

The time of presentation of hemoglobinopathy depends on the timing of chain synthesis. Thus, α-thalassemia caused by a four-gene defect produces no alpha chains and presents as severe anemia and hydrops (Bart hemoglobin, composed of four gamma chains). Hemoglobin H is due to a thalassemia three-gene defect resulting in four beta chains, and appears with hemolysis and anemia in the infant. In contrast, infants with beta chain abnormalities, such as Cooley anemia (β-thalassemia major) and sickle cell anemia, do not manifest anemia in the neonatal period.

The *blood volume* of the term infant is approximately 85 mL/kg. The placenta and umbilical vessels contain approximately 20–30 mL/kg of additional blood that, if clamping or milking ("stripping") of the umbilical cord is delayed at birth, can transiently increase neonatal blood volume and hemoglobin levels for the first 3 days of life. Delayed clamping increases the risk for polycythemia, increased pulmonary vascular resistance, hypoxia, and jaundice but improves glomerular filtration. Early clamping may result in anemia, a cardiac murmur, poor peripheral perfusion but lower pulmonary vascular pressures, and less tachypnea. To avoid both situations, one should clamp the cord at approximately 30 sec after birth. Hydrostatic pressure affects blood transfer between the placenta and the infant at birth, and an undesired fetal-to-placental transfusion will occur if the infant is situated above the level of the placenta.

The *physiologic anemia* noted at 2–3 mo of age in term infants and at 1–2 mo of age in preterm infants is associated with undetectable erythropoietin levels. Although hemoglobin levels decline during this period, an increase in tissue oxygen becomes available as a result of the production of hemoglobin A, which releases oxygen to the tissues (hemoglobin A becomes unsaturated) at a higher $Po_2$ than does hemoglobin F. (See the oxygen dissociation curve of hemoglobin A in Fig. 6–2 and also Transition from Fetal to Neonatal Physiology.)

### Etiology

Symptomatic anemia in the newborn period (Table 6–21) may be due to:

1. Blood loss.
2. Decreased red blood cell production.
3. Hemolysis.

**Blood Loss.** Anemia from blood loss at birth is manifested by two patterns of presentation, depending on the rapidity of blood loss. Acute blood

**TABLE 6–21.** Etiology of Neonatal Anemia

| | Blood Loss | Decreased Production | Hemolysis |
|---|---|---|---|
| *Common* | Fetal-maternal bleed<br>Placenta previa<br>Abruptio placentae<br>Twin-twin transfusion | Perinatal-congenital infections<br>Anemia of prematurity | Rh<br>ABO<br>Minor groups |
| *Rare* | Vasa previa<br>Rupture of umbilical cord<br>Hepatic hematoma<br>Splenic hematoma<br>Nuchal cord<br>Retroperitoneal hemorrhage | Parvovirus<br>Diamond-Blackfan syndrome<br>Osteopetrosis<br>Congenital leukemia<br>Congenital neuroblastoma<br>Sideroblastic anemia<br>Postintrauterine transfusions | RBC enzyme deficiency<br>Hemoglobinopathy<br>RBC membrane disorders<br>Disseminated intravascular coagulopathy<br>Maternal autoimmune disorder (SLE)<br>Perinatal-congenital infections |

RBC = red blood cell; SLE = systemic lupus erythematosus.

loss following fetomaternal hemorrhage, rupture of the umbilical cord, placenta previa, and internal hemorrhage is characterized by pallor, diminished peripheral pulses, and shock. There are no signs of extramedullary hematopoiesis and no hepatosplenomegaly. The hemoglobin content and serum iron levels initially are normal, but the hemoglobin levels decline during the subsequent 24 hr. Chronic blood loss due to chronic fetomaternal hemorrhage or a twin-twin transfusion presents with marked pallor, heart failure, hepatosplenomegaly with or without hydrops, a low hemoglobin level at birth, a hypochromic microcytic blood smear, and decreased serum iron stores. Fetomaternal bleeding occurs in more than 50% of all pregnancies, with fetal blood losses ranging between 1 and 50 mL.

The *diagnosis* of fetomaternal hemorrhage is confirmed by the acid elution test of Kleihauer and Betke; pink fetal red blood cells are observed and counted in the mother's peripheral blood smear because fetal hemoglobin is resistant to acid elution; adult hemoglobin is eluted, leaving discolored maternal cells.

**Decreased Red Blood Cell Production.** Anemia due to decreased production of red blood cells appears at birth with pallor, a low reticulocyte count, and absence of erythroid precursors in the bone marrow (see Table 6–21). There may be associated physical anomalies (see Chapter 14).

**Hemolysis.** Immunologically mediated hemolysis in utero may result in **erythroblastosis fetalis,** or the fetus may be spared and **hemolytic disease** may appear in the newborn infant. Hemolysis of fetal erythrocytes is due to blood group differences between the sensitized mother and fetus, resulting in the production of maternal IgG antibodies directed against an antigen on fetal cells. All mothers with type O blood have isohemagglutinins, which

are IgM antibodies. Because IgM does not cross the placenta, there is no risk of hemolysis.

**ABO blood group incompatibility** with neonatal hemolysis develops only if the mother has IgG antibodies from a previous exposure to A or B antigens. These IgG antibodies cross the placenta by active transport and affect the fetus or newborn. Sensitization of the mother to fetal antigens may have occurred by previous transfusions or by conditions of pregnancy that result in transfer of fetal erythrocytes into the maternal circulation, such as 1st trimester abortion, an ectopic pregnancy, amniocentesis, or even a normal pregnancy. The risk of fetomaternal transfusion is increased by manual extraction of the placenta and by version (external or internal) procedures.

ABO incompatibility with sensitization usually does not cause fetal disease other than very mild anemia. However, it may produce **hemolytic disease of the newborn** that is manifested as significant anemia and hyperbilirubinemia (see later). Because many mothers who are blood group O have IgG antibodies to A and B prior to pregnancy, the firstborn infant of A or B blood type may be affected. In contrast to Rh disease, ABO hemolytic disease does not become more severe with subsequent pregnancies. Hemolysis with ABO incompatibility is less severe than hemolysis in Rh-sensitized pregnancy because the anti-A or anti-B antibody may bind to nonerythrocytic cells that contain A or B antigen or because fetal erythrocytes have fewer A or B antigenic determinants than they have Rh sites. ABO incompatibility is the most common cause of isoimmune hemolysis of the newborn infant.

**Erythroblastosis fetalis** classically is due to Rh blood group incompatibility. Rh-negative women do not develop natural IgM antibodies, and most

Rh-negative women have no anti-Rh antibodies at the time of their first pregnancy. The Rh antigen system consists of five antigens, C, D, E, c, and e; the d type is not antigenic. In 90% of Rh-sensitized cases, the D antigen of the fetus sensitizes the Rh-negative (d) mother, resulting in IgG antibody production during the first pregnancy. A Du antigen is another Rh antigen that on initial assessment tests as Rh-negative. Mothers with Du are Rh-positive and thus are not at risk for sensitization.

Because most mothers are not sensitized to Rh antigens at the start of pregnancy, Rh erythroblastosis fetalis is usually a disease of the second and subsequent pregnancies. The first affected pregnancy results in an antibody response in the mother detected during antenatal screening with the Coombs test and determined to be anti-D antibody. The first affected newborn may demonstrate no serious fetal disease and may manifest hemolytic disease of the newborn only by the development of anemia and hyperbilirubinemia (see below). Subsequent pregnancies result in an increasing severity of response by having an earlier onset of hemolysis in utero. Fetal anemia, heart failure, and hypoalbuminemia result in **fetal hydrops,** which is characterized by ascites, pleural and pericardial effusions, and anasarca. There is a high risk of fetal death.

The *management* of the pregnancy complicated by Rh sensitization depends on the severity of hemolysis, its effects on the fetus, and the maturity of the fetus at the time it becomes affected. The severity of the hemolysis can be assessed by the quantity of bilirubin transferred from the fetus to the amniotic fluid, quantified by spectrophotometric analysis of the optical density (at 450 nm) of amniotic fluid. Bilirubin levels in normal pregnancies are higher at earlier gestational ages and decrease as the fetus matures.

Three zones of optical densities with decreasing slopes toward term gestation have been developed to predict the severity of the illness. The high-optical-density zone 3 is associated with severe hemolysis; fetuses in the lower zones probably are not affected. If a fetus's optical density measurement for bilirubin falls into zone 3 and the fetus has pulmonary maturity as determined by the L/ S ratio, it should be delivered and treated in the NICU. If the lungs are immature and the fetus is between 22 and 33 wk of gestational age, an intrauterine transfusion with O-negative blood, either into the peritoneal cavity or, more likely, into the umbilical vein, is indicated and may have to be repeated until pulmonary maturity is reached or fetal distress is detected. Indications for fetal intravascular transfusion in sensitized fetuses be-

tween 22 and 32 wk of gestational age include a fetal hematocrit of less than 25%, hemoglobin of less than 8 g/dL, fetal hydrops, and fetal distress too early in gestation for delivery and successful management with neonatal intensive care. Intravascular intrauterine transfusion corrects fetal anemia, improves the outcome of severe hydrops, and reduces the need for postnatal exchange transfusion but is associated with neonatal anemia as a result of continued hemolysis plus suppressed erythropoiesis.

*Prevention* of sensitization of the mother carrying an Rh-positive fetus is possible by treating her during gestation (after 28 wk) and within 72 hr after birth with anti-Rh-positive immune globulin (RhoGAM). The dose of RhoGAM (300 μg) is based on the ability of this amount of anti–Rh-positive antibody to bind all the possible fetal Rh-positive erythrocytes entering the maternal circulation during the fetal-to-maternal transfusion at birth (~30 mL). RhoGAM may bind Rh-positive fetal erythrocytes or interfere with maternal anti–Rh-positive antibody production by another unknown mechanism. RhoGAM is effective only in preventing sensitization to the D antigen. Other blood group antigens that can cause immune hydrops and erythroblastosis include Rh C, E, Kell, and Duffy.

Nonimmune causes of hemolysis in the newborn include *red cell enzyme deficiencies* of the Embden-Meyerhof pathway, such as pyruvate kinase or glucose-6-phosphate dehydrogenase deficiency. *Red cell membrane disorders* are another cause of nonimmune hemolysis. Hereditary spherocytosis is inherited as a severe autosomal recessive form or less severe autosomal dominant form and is due to a deficiency of the red blood cell membrane protein spectrin.

*Hemoglobinopathies* such as thalassemia are another cause of nonimmunologically mediated hemolysis (see Table 6–21).

### Diagnosis and Management

Hemolysis in utero due to any cause may produce a spectrum of *clinical manifestations* at birth. Severe hydrops with anasarca, heart failure, and pulmonary edema may prevent adequate ventilation at birth, resulting in asphyxia. Infants affected with hemolysis in utero have hepatosplenomegaly and pallor and become jaundiced within the first 24 hr after birth. Less severely affected infants manifest pallor and hepatosplenomegaly at birth and become jaundiced subsequently. Patients with ABO incompatibility often are asymptomatic and without physical signs at birth, and mild anemia with jaundice develops during the first 24–72 hr of life.

Because hydrops, anemia, or jaundice is secondary to many diverse causes of hemolysis, *a laboratory evaluation is needed in all patients with suspected hemolysis.* A complete blood count, blood smear, reticulocyte count, blood type, and direct Coombs test (to determine the presence of antibody-coated red blood cells) should be performed in the initial evaluation of all infants with hemolysis. Reduced hemoglobin levels, reticulocytosis, and a blood smear characterized by polychromasia and anisocytosis are expected with isoimmune hemolysis. Spherocytes are commonly observed with ABO incompatibility. The determination of the blood type and the Coombs test identify the responsible antigen and antibody in immunologically mediated hemolysis.

In the absence of a positive Coombs test and blood group differences between the mother and fetus, causes of nonimmune hemolysis must be considered. Red cell enzyme assays, hemoglobin electrophoresis, or red cell membrane tests (osmotic fragility; spectrin assay) should be performed. Internal hemorrhage also may be associated with anemia, reticulocytosis, and jaundice when the hemorrhage reabsorbs; ultrasonographic evaluation of the brain, liver, spleen, or adrenal gland may be indicated when nonimmune hemolysis is suspected. Shock is more typical in patients with internal hemorrhage, whereas heart failure may be seen with severe anemia from hemolytic diseases. Evaluation of a possible fetomaternal hemorrhage should include the Kleihauer-Betke test.

The *treatment* of *symptomatic* neonatal anemia is transfusion of cross-matched packed red blood cells. If immune hemolysis is present, the cells to be transfused must be cross-matched against both maternal and neonatal plasma. Acute volume loss may necessitate resuscitation with nonblood products such as saline or albumin if blood is not available; packed red blood cells can be given subsequently. Ten to 15 mL/kg of packed red blood cells should be sufficient to correct anemia and any remaining blood volume deficit. Cytomegalovirus (CMV)-seronegative blood should be given to CMV-seronegative infants, and all blood products should be screened for HIV, hepatitis B and C, and syphilis. Recombinant erythropoietin reduces the need for transfusions necessitated by anemia of prematurity. Supplementation with oral iron improves the response to erythropoietin.

## HYPERBILIRUBINEMIA

Hemolytic disease of the newborn is a common cause of neonatal jaundice. Nonetheless, because of the immaturity of the pathways of bilirubin metabolism, many newborn infants without evidence of hemolysis become jaundiced.

Bilirubin is produced by the catabolism of hemoglobin in the reticuloendothelial system. The tetrapyrrole ring of heme is cleaved by heme oxygenase to form equivalent quantities of biliverdin and carbon monoxide. Because no other biologic source of carbon monoxide exists, the excretion of this gas is stoichiometrically identical to the production of bilirubin. Biliverdin is converted to bilirubin by biliverdin reductase. One gram of hemoglobin produces 35 mg of bilirubin. Sources of bilirubin other than circulating hemoglobin represent 20% of bilirubin production; these sources include inefficient (shunt) hemoglobin production and lysis of precursor cells in bone marrow. Compared with adults, newborn infants have a two-fold to three-fold greater rate of bilirubin production (6–10 mg/kg/24 hr versus 3 mg/kg/24 hr). This is due, in part, to an increased red blood cell mass (higher hematocrit) and a shortened erythrocyte life span of 70–90 days, compared with the 120-day erythrocyte life span in adults.

Bilirubin produced following hemoglobin catabolism is lipid soluble, is unconjugated, and reacts as an indirect reagent in the van den Bergh test. Indirect-reacting, unconjugated bilirubin is toxic to the central nervous system and is insoluble in water, thus limiting its excretion. Unconjugated bilirubin binds to albumin on specific bilirubin binding sites; 1 g of albumin binds 8.5 mg of bilirubin in the newborn. If the binding sites become saturated or if a competitive compound binds at the site, displacing bound bilirubin, free bilirubin will be available to enter the central nervous system. Organic acids such as free fatty acids and drugs such as sulfisoxazole can displace bilirubin from its binding site on albumin.

Bilirubin dissociates from albumin at the hepatocyte and becomes bound to a cytoplasmic liver protein "Y" (ligandin). Hepatic conjugation results in the production of bilirubin diglucuronide, which is water soluble and capable of biliary and renal excretion. The enzyme UDP-glucuronyl transferase is the rate-limiting step of bilirubin conjugation. The concentrations of ligandin and glucuronyl transferase are lower in the newborn infant, particularly in the premature infant, than in the older child.

Conjugated bilirubin gives a direct reaction in the van den Bergh test. Most conjugated bilirubin is excreted through the bile into the small intestine and is eliminated in the stool. However, some bilirubin may undergo hydrolysis back to the unconjugated fraction by intestinal glucuronidase and then may be reabsorbed (enterohepatic recirculation). In addition, bacteria in the neonatal intestine do not convert bilirubin to urobilinogen or stercobilinogen, which is excreted in urine and stool respectively, and usually limits bilirubin reabsorption. Delayed passage of meconium, which contains bilirubin, also may contribute to the enterohepatic recirculation of bilirubin.

Bilirubin is produced in utero by the normal fetus and by the fetus affected by erythroblastosis fetalis. Indirect, unconjugated, lipid-soluble fetal bilirubin is transferred across the placenta and subsequently becomes conjugated by maternal hepatic enzymes. The placenta is impermeable to conjugated water-soluble bilirubin. Fetal bilirubin levels become only mildly elevated in the presence of severe hemolysis, but may increase when hemolysis produces fetal hepatic inspissated bile stasis and conjugated hyperbilirubinemia. Maternal indirect (but not direct) hyperbilirubinemia also may increase fetal bilirubin levels.

### Etiology of Indirect Unconjugated Hyperbilirubinemia
(Table 6–22)

*Physiologic jaundice* is a common cause of hyperbilirubinemia among newborn infants. It is a diagnosis of exclusion after careful evaluation has ruled out more serious causes of jaundice, such as hemolysis, infection, and metabolic diseases. Physiologic jaundice is due to many factors that are normal physiologic characteristics of the newborn infant: increased bilirubin production resulting from an increased red blood cell mass, shortened red blood cell life span, and hepatic immaturity of ligandin and glucuronyl transferase. Physiologic jaundice may be exaggerated among infants of Greek and Asian ancestry.

The clinical pattern of physiologic jaundice in term infants includes a peak indirect-reacting bilirubin level of no more than 12 mg/dL on the 3rd day of life. In premature infants, the peak is higher (15 mg/dL) and occurs later (5th day).

The peak level of indirect bilirubin during physiologic jaundice may be higher in breast milk-fed infants that in non-breast milk–fed infants (15–17 mg/dL versus 12 mg/dL). This may be due, in part, to the decreased fluid intake of the former. Jaundice is unphysiologic or pathologic if it is evident on the 1st day of life, if the bilirubin level increases more than 0.5 mg/dL/hr, if the peak bilirubin is greater than 13 mg/dL in term infants, if the direct bilirubin fraction is greater than 1.5 mg/dL, or if hepatosplenomegaly and anemia are present.

*Crigler-Najjar syndrome* is a serious, rare, permanent deficiency of glucuronyl transferase that results in severe indirect hyperbilirubinemia. The autosomal dominant variety responds to enzyme induction by phenobarbital, producing an increase in enzyme activity and a reduction of bilirubin levels. The autosomal recessive form does not respond to phenobarbital and manifests as persistent indirect hyperbilirubinemia, which often results in kernicterus (see later).

*Breast milk feeding* may be associated with unconjugated hyperbilirubinemia without evidence of hemolysis during the 1st to 2nd wk of life. Bilirubin levels rarely increase to above 20 mg/dL. Interruption of breast feeding for 1–2 days results in a rapid decline of bilirubin levels that do not increase significantly after breast-feeding is resumed. Breast milk may contain an inhibitor of bilirubin conjugation or increase the enterohepatic recirculation of bilirubin because of breast milk glucuronidase.

*Jaundice on the first day of life is always pathologic*, and immediate attention is needed to establish the cause. Early onset often is due to hemolysis, internal hemorrhage (cephalhematoma, hepatic or splenic hematoma), or infection (see Table 6–22). Infection also is often associated with direct-reacting bilirubin (see farther on) resulting from perinatal congenital infections or due to bacterial sepsis.

Physical evidence of jaundice is observable in infants when the bilirubin levels reach 5–10 mg/

TABLE 6–22.  Etiology of Unconjugated Hyperbilirubinemia

|  | Hemolysis Present | Hemolysis Absent |
|---|---|---|
| *Common* | *Blood group incompatibility:* ABO, Rh, Kell, Duffy<br>*Infection* | Physiologic jaundice, breast milk jaundice, internal hemorrhage, polycythemia, infant of diabetic mother |
| *Rare* | *Red cell enzyme defects:* glucose-6-phosphate dehydrogenase, pyruvate kinase<br>*Red cell membrane disorders:* spherocytosis, ovalocytosis<br>*Hemoglobinopathy:* thalassemia | Deficiency of glucuronyl transferase enzyme (Crigler-Najjar syndrome), pyloric stenosis, hypothyroidism, immune thrombocytopenia, Gilbert disease |

dL, versus only 2 mg/dL in adults. Once jaundice is observed, the laboratory evaluation for hyperbilirubinemia should include a total bilirubin measurement to determine the magnitude of hyperbilirubinemia. Bilirubin levels in excess of 5 mg/dL on the 1st day of life or in excess of 13 mg/dL thereafter in term infants should be evaluated further with indirect and direct bilirubin levels, blood typing, Coombs test, complete blood count, blood smear, and reticulocyte count. These tests must be done prior to the treatment of hyperbilirubinemia with phototherapy or exchange transfusion. In the absence of hemolysis or evidence for either the common or the rare causes of nonhemolytic indirect hyperbilirubinemia, the diagnosis is either physiologic or breast milk jaundice. Jaundice present after 2 wk of age is pathologic and suggests a direct reacting hyperbilirubinemia.

### Etiology of Direct Conjugated Hyperbilirubinemia

*Direct-reacting hyperbilirubinemia* should be evaluated according to the diagnostic categories noted in Table 6–23. Direct-reacting bilirubin (composed mostly of conjugated bilirubin) is not neurotoxic to the infant but signifies a serious underlying disorder involving cholestasis or hepatocellular injury. The diagnostic evaluation of patients with direct-reacting hyperbilirubinemia includes liver enzyme determinations (serum glutamic oxaloacetic transaminase, alkaline phosphatase, serum glutamic pyruvic transaminase, gamma-glutamyltranspepti-

**TABLE 6–23.** Etiology of Conjugated Hyperbilirubinemia

**Common**
Hyperalimentation cholestasis
CMV infection
Other perinatal congenital infections (TORCH)
Inspissated bile from prolonged hemolysis
Neonatal hepatitis
Sepsis

**Uncommon**
Hepatic infarction
Inborn errors of metabolism (galactosemia, tyrosinosis)
Cystic fibrosis
Biliary atresia
Choledochal cyst
Alpha$_1$-antitrypsin deficiency
Neonatal iron storage disease
Alagille syndrome (arteriohepatic dysplasia)
Byler disease

CMV = cytomegalovirus; TORCH = toxoplasmosis, other, rubella, cytomegalovirus, herpes simplex.

dase), bacterial and viral cultures, metabolic screening tests, hepatic ultrasonography, sweat chloride test, and, occasionally, liver biopsy. Additionally, the presence of dark urine and gray-white (acholic) stools with jaundice after the 2nd week of life strongly suggests biliary atresia.

The *treatment* of disorders manifested by direct bilirubinemia is specific for those diseases that are noted in Table 6–23. They do not respond to phototherapy or exchange transfusion.

### Kernicterus

Lipid-soluble, unconjugated, indirect bilirubin fraction is toxic to the developing central nervous system, especially when indirect bilirubin concentrations are high and exceed the binding capacity of albumin. Kernicterus results when indirect bilirubin is deposited in brain cells, disrupting neuronal metabolism and function, especially in the basal ganglia. Indirect bilirubin may cross the blood-brain barrier because of its lipid solubility; other theories propose that a disruption of the blood-brain barrier permits entry of a bilirubin-albumin or free bilirubin–fatty acid complex.

Kernicterus usually is noted at an excessively high bilirubin level for gestational age. Kernicterus does not usually develop in term infants when bilirubin levels are below 20–25 mg/dL. The incidence of kernicterus increases as serum bilirubin levels increase above 25 mg/dL. Kernicterus may be noted at bilirubin levels below 20 mg/dL in the presence of sepsis, meningitis, hemolysis, asphyxia, hypoxia, hypothermia, hypoglycemia, bilirubin displacing drugs, and prematurity. Other risks for kernicterus in term infants include hemolysis, jaundice noted within 24 hr of birth, and delayed diagnosis of hyperbilirubinemia. Very immature infants weighing less than 1000 g have developed kernicterus when bilirubin levels are less than 10 mg/dL.

The earliest *clinical manifestations* of kernicterus include lethargy, hypotonia irritability, poor Moro response, and poor feeding. A high-pitched cry and emesis also may be present. Early signs are noted after the 4th day of life. Later signs include bulging fontanel, opisthotonic posturing, pulmonary hemorrhage, fever, hypertonicity, paralysis of upward gaze, and seizures. Infants with severe cases of kernicterus die in the neonatal period. Spasticity resolves in surviving infants, who may later manifest nerve deafness, choreoathetoid cerebral palsy, mental retardation, enamel dysplasia, and discoloration of teeth as permanent sequelae. Kernicterus may be *prevented* by avoiding excessively high indirect bilirubin levels and by avoiding conditions or drugs that may displace bilirubin from albumin. Very early signs of kernicterus occasionally may be reversed by immediately instituting an exchange transfusion (see below).

### Therapy of Indirect Hyperbilirubinemia

*Phototherapy* is an effective and relatively safe method for reducing indirect bilirubin levels, particularly when initiated before serum bilirubin increases to levels associated with kernicterus. In term infants, phototherapy is begun when indirect bilirubin levels are between 16 and 18 mg/dL. Phototherapy is initiated in premature infants when bilirubin is at lower levels to avoid bilirubin reaching the high concentrations requiring exchange transfusion. Both blue lights and white lights are effective in reducing bilirubin levels.

Phototherapy acts by producing nontoxic photoisomers from the native bilirubin deposited in the skin. Unconjugated bilirubin (IX) is in the 4Z,15Z configuration (referring to the arrangement of atoms around the respective double bonds). Phototherapy causes a photochemical reaction producing the reversible, more water-soluble isomer 4Z,15E bilirubin IX. This configurational isomer is excreted readily in an unconjugated form in bile and is one of the mechanisms of the action of phototherapy. Another photochemical reaction results in the rapid production of lumirubin, a more water-soluble isomer than the aforementioned isomer, that does not spontaneously revert to unconjugated native bilirubin and also can be excreted in urine.

Complications of phototherapy include an increased insensible water loss, diarrhea, and dehydration. Additional problems include macular-papular red skin rash, lethargy, masking of cyanosis, nasal obstruction due to eye pads, and the potential for retinal damage. Skin bronzing may be noted in infants with direct-reacting hyperbilirubinemia. Infants with mild hemolytic disease of the newborn occasionally may be successfully managed with phototherapy for hyperbilirubinemia, but care must be taken to follow these infants for the late occurrence of anemia from continued hemolysis.

*Exchange transfusion* usually is reserved for infants with dangerously high indirect bilirubin levels who are at risk for kernicterus. As a rule of thumb, a level of 20 mg/dL indirect-reacting bilirubin is the "exchange number" for infants with hemolysis, weighing over 2000 g. Asymptomatic infants with physiologic or breast milk jaundice may not require exchange transfusion unless the indirect bilirubin level exceeds 25 mg/dL. The exchangeable level of indirect bilirubin for other infants may be estimated by calculating 10% of the birth weight in grams; thus the level in an infant weighing 1500 g would be 15 mg/dL. Infants weighing less than 1000 g usually do not warrant an exchange transfusion until the bilirubin exceeds 10 mg/dL.

Small infusions of whole blood cross-matched with that of the mother and infant are alternated with a withdrawal of an equivalent quantity of the infant's blood, which is discarded. Depending on the size of the infant, aliquots of 5–20 mL per cycle are withdrawn and infused, with the total procedure lasting 45–90 min. The total amount of blood exchanged is equal to twice the infant's blood volume, calculated as: weight (kg) $\times$ 85 mL/kg $\times$ 2. This volume should remove 85% of the infant's red blood cells (the source of bilirubin), maternal antibodies, and exchangeable tissue indirect bilirubin. The exchange transfusion usually is performed through an umbilical venous catheter placed in the inferior vena cava or, if free flow is obtained, at the confluence of the umbilical vein and the portal system. Serum bilirubin levels immediately after the exchange transfusion decline to levels that are about one half those prior to the exchange; levels rebound 6–8 hr later as a result of continued hemolysis and redistribution of bilirubin from tissue stores.

Complications of exchange transfusion include problems resulting from the blood (transfusion reaction, metabolic instability, infection), the catheter (vessel perforation, hemorrhage), or the procedure (hypotension, necrotizing enterocolitis). Unusual complications include thrombocytopenia and graft-versus-host disease. Continuation of phototherapy may alleviate the necessity for subsequent exchange transfusions.

*Heme oxygenase inhibitors* (zinc protoporphyrin, tin mesoporphyrin, or tin protoporphyrin) administered systemically may attenuate hyperbilirubinemia. The level of indirect bilirubin and the need for phototherapy are reduced.

### POLYCYTHEMIA
#### (Hyperviscosity Syndrome)

Polycythemia is an excessively high hematocrit (65% or more), resulting in hyperviscosity that produces symptoms related to vascular stasis, hypoperfusion, and ischemia. As the hematocrit increases from 40% to 60%, there is a very small increase of the blood viscosity. Once the central hematocrit increases above 65%, the blood viscosity begins to increase markedly and symptoms may appear. Neonatal erythrocytes are less filterable or deformable than adult erythrocytes, a fact that further contributes to hyperviscosity. A central venous hematocrit of 65% or more is noted in 3–5% of infants. Infants at special risk for polycythemia are term and post-term SGA infants, infants of diabetic mothers, infants with delayed cord clamping, and those having neonatal hyperthyroidism, adrenogenital syndrome, trisomy 21, twin-twin transfusion syndrome (recipient), and Beckwith-Wiedemann syndrome. In some infants, polycythemia may reflect a compensation for prolonged periods of fetal hypoxia from placental insufficiency; these infants have increased erythropoietin levels at birth.

Polycythemic patients appear plethoric or ruddy and may develop acrocyanosis. Symptoms are due to the increased red cell mass and to vascular compromise. Thus, seizures, lethargy, and irritability reflect abnormalities of microcirculation of the brain, whereas hyperbilirubinemia may be due to the poor hepatic circulation or to the increased amount of hemoglobin that is being broken down into bilirubin. Additional problems include respiratory distress and PPHN resulting, in part, from elevated pulmonary vascular resistance. The chest roentgenogram often demonstrates cardiomegaly, increased vascular markings, pleural effusions, and interstitial edema. Other problems include necrotizing enterocolitis, hypoglycemia, thrombocytopenia, priapism, and feeding intolerance. Many of these complications also are related to the primary condition associated with polycythemia (e.g., SGA infants are at risk for hypoglycemia and PPHN following periods of hypoxia in utero).

Long-term sequelae of neonatal polycythemia relate to neurodevelopmental abnormalities that may be prevented by treatment of symptomatic infants with partial exchange transfusion after birth. A partial exchange transfusion removes whole blood and replaces it with normal saline or albumin. The equation to calculate the volume exchanged is based on the central venous hematocrit (Hct), because peripheral hematocrits may be falsely elevated:

volume to exchange (mL) =

$$\frac{\text{blood volume (observed Hct} - \text{desired Hct)}}{\text{observed Hct}}$$

The desired hematocrit is 50%, and the blood volume 85 mL/kg.

## COAGULATION DISORDERS
(Also see Chapter 14)

Disorders of coagulation are very common in the neonatal period. Hemorrhage during this time may be due to trauma, inherited permanent deficiency of coagulation factors, transient deficiencies of vitamin K–dependent factors, disorders of platelets, and DIC seen in sick newborn patients with shock or hypoxia. Thrombosis is also a potential problem in the newborn because of developmentally lower circulating levels of antithrombin III, protein C (a vitamin K–dependent protein that inhibits factors VIII and V), and the fibrinolytic system.

There is no placental passage of coagulation factors, and newborn infants have relatively low levels of the vitamin K–dependent factors II, VII, IX, and X. Contact factors XI and XII, prekallikrein, and kininogen also are lower in newborn infants than in adults. Fibrinogen (factor I); plasma levels of factors V, VIII, and XIII; and platelet count are within the adult normal range.

Because of the transient, relative deficiencies of the contact and the vitamin K–dependent factors, the *partial thromboplastin time* (PTT), which is dependent on factors XII, IX, VIII, X, V, II, and I, is prolonged in the newborn period. Preterm infants have the most marked prolongation of the PTT (50–80 sec) compared with term (35–50 sec) and older, more mature (25–35 sec) infants. The administration of heparin and the presence of DIC, hemophilia, and severe vitamin K deficiency prolong the PTT.

The *prothrombin time* (PT), which is dependent on factors VII, X, V, II, and I, is a more sensitive test for vitamin K deficiency. The PT is only slightly prolonged in the term infant (13–20 sec) as compared with the preterm (13–21 sec) and the more mature patient (12–14 sec). Abnormal prolongations of the PT occur with vitamin K deficiency, hepatic injury, and DIC. Levels of *fibrinogen* and *fibrin degradation products* are similar in infants and adults. The *bleeding time*, which reflects platelet function and number, is normal during the newborn period in the absence of maternal salicylate therapy.

*Vitamin K* is a necessary cofactor for the carboxylation of glutamate on precursor proteins, converting them into the more active coagulation factors II, VII, IX, and X; gamma-carboxyglutamic acid binds calcium, which is required for the immediate activation of factors during hemorrhage. There is no congenital deficiency of hepatic synthesis of these precursor proteins, but, in the absence of vitamin K, their conversion to the active factor is not possible. PIVKA (protein induced by vitamin K absence) levels increase in vitamin K deficiency and are helpful diagnostic markers; vitamin K administration rapidly corrects the coagulation defects, reducing PIVKA to undetectable levels.

Although most newborn infants are born with

reduced levels of vitamin K–dependent factors, hemorrhagic complications develop only rarely. Those infants at risk for **hemorrhagic disease of the newborn** have the most profound deficiency of vitamin K–dependent factors, and these factors decline further after birth. Because breast milk is a poor source of vitamin K, infants fed breast milk are also at increased risk for hemorrhage that usually occurs between the 3rd and 5th days of life. Bleeding usually ensues from the umbilical cord, circumcision site, intestines, scalp, mucosa, and skin, but internal hemorrhage places the infant at risk for fatal complications, such as intracranial bleeding.

Hemorrhage on the 1st day of life resulting from a deficiency of the vitamin K–dependent factors often is associated with administration to the mother of drugs that affect vitamin K metabolism in the infant. This early pattern of hemorrhage has been seen with maternal warfarin therapy and in infants of mothers receiving phenobarbital and phenytoin. Bleeding also may occur as late as 1–3 mo after birth, particularly among breast-fed infants. Vitamin K deficiency in the latter group should also raise suspicion about the possibility of vitamin K malabsorption resulting from cystic fibrosis or antibiotic suppression of the colonic bacteria that produce vitamin K.

Bleeding due to vitamin K deficiency may be *prevented* by administration of vitamin K to all infants at birth. Prior to routine administration of vitamin K, 1–2% of all newborn infants had hemorrhagic disease of the newborn. One intramuscular dose (1 mg) of vitamin K prevents vitamin K–deficiency bleeding.

*Treatment* of bleeding resulting from vitamin K deficiency requires intravenous administration of 1 mg of vitamin K. If severe, life-threatening hemorrhage is present, fresh frozen plasma should also be given. Unusually high doses of vitamin K may be needed for hepatic disease and for maternal warfarin or anticonvulsant therapy.

### Clinical Manifestations and Differential Diagnoses of Bleeding Disorders

Bleeding disorders in the newborn may be associated with cutaneous bleeding such as cephalohematoma, subgaleal hemorrhage, ecchymosis, and petechiae. Facial petechiae are common in infants born by vertex presentation, with or without a nuchal cord, and usually are insignificant. Mucosal bleeding may appear as hematemesis, melena, or epistaxis. Internal hemorrhage results in organ-specific dysfunction such as seizures accompanied by intracranial hemorrhage. Bleeding from veni-puncture or heel stick sites, circumcision sites, or the umbilical cord also is common.

The *differential diagnosis* depends, in part, on the clinical circumstances associated with the hemorrhage. In the sick newborn, the differential diagnosis should include DIC, hepatic failure, and thrombocytopenia. Thrombocytopenia may be secondary to consumption by trapping of platelets in a hemangioma (**Kasabach-Merritt syndrome**) or may be associated with perinatal, congenital, or bacterial infections, necrotizing enterocolitis (NEC), thrombotic endocarditis, PPHN, organic acidemia, maternal pre-eclampsia, or asphyxia. Thrombocytopenia also may be due to peripheral washout of platelets following an exchange transfusion. *Treatment* of the sick infant with thrombocytopenia should be directed at the underlying disorder, supplemented by infusions of platelets and/or blood.

The etiology of DIC in the newborn infant includes hypoxia, hypotension, asphyxia, bacterial or viral sepsis, NEC, death of a twin while in utero, cavernous hemangioma, nonimmune hydrops, neonatal cold injury, neonatal neoplasm, and hepatic disease. The *treatment* of DIC should be focused primarily on the therapy of the initiating or underlying disorder. Supportive management of consumptive coagulopathy includes platelet transfusions and factor replacement with fresh frozen plasma. Heparin should be reserved for those infants with DIC who also demonstrate thrombosis.

Disorders of hemostasis in the well child are not associated with systemic disease in the newborn but reflect coagulation factor or platelet deficiency. *Hemophilia* initially is associated with cutaneous or mucosal bleeding and no systemic illness. If bleeding continues, hypovolemic shock may develop. Bleeding into the brain, liver, or spleen may result in organ-specific signs and shock.

In the well child, *thrombocytopenia* may be part of a syndrome such as Fanconi anemia (hypoplasia, aplasia of thumb), the radial aplasia–thrombocytopenia (TAR) syndrome (thumbs present), or Wiskott-Aldrich syndrome. Various maternal drugs also may reduce the neonatal platelet count without producing other adverse effects. These drugs include sulfonamides, quinidine, quinine, and thiazide diuretics.

The most common causes of thrombocytopenia in the well newborn infant are transient isoimmune thrombocytopenia and transient neonatal thrombocytopenia in well infants born to mothers with idiopathic thrombocytopenic purpura (ITP). **Isoimmune thrombocytopenia** is due to antiplatelet antibodies produced by the PLA1-negative mother after her sensitization to specific paternal platelet antigen (PLA1-positive) expressed on the fetal platelet. This response to maternal-sensitized antibodies that produce isoimmune thrombocytopenia is analogous to the response that produces erythroblastosis fetalis. The maternal antiplatelet antibody does not produce maternal thrombocytopenia, but after crossing the placenta, this IgG antibody binds to fetal platelets that are trapped by the reticuloendothelial tissue, resulting in thrombocytopenia. Infants with thrombocytopenia produced in this manner are at risk for development of petechiae, purpura, and intracranial hemorrhage after birth. Vaginal delivery may increase the risk for neonatal bleeding; thus cesarean section may be indicated.

Specific *treatment* for severe thrombocytopenia (<10,000 platelets/mm³) or significant bleeding is transfusion of maternal platelets. Because the antibody in isoimmune thrombocytopenia is directed against the fetal rather than the maternal platelet, plateletpheresis of the mother will yield sufficient platelets for carrying out a platelet transfusion to treat the affected infant. After one platelet transfusion, the infant's platelet count dramatically increases and usually remains in a safe range. Without treatment, thrombocytopenia resolves during the first month of life as the maternal antibody level declines. *Treatment* of the mother with intravenous immunoglobulin or the thrombocytopenic fetus with intravascular platelet transfusion (cordocentesis), is also effective.

**Neonatal thrombocytopenia in infants born to women with ITP** also is due to placental transfer of maternal IgG antibodies. In ITP, these autoantibodies are directed against all platelet antigens, and, therefore, both mother and newborn may have low platelet counts. The risks of hemorrhage in the infant born to the woman with ITP may be lessened by cesarean section and by treatment of the mother with corticosteroids.

*Treatment* of the affected infant born to the woman with ITP may include prednisone and intravenous immunoglobulin. In an emergency, random donor platelets may produce a transient rise in the infant's platelet count. Thrombocytopenia will resolve spontaneously during the 1st month of life as maternal-derived antibody levels decline. Elevated levels of platelet-associated antibodies also have been noted in thrombocytopenic infants with sepsis and thrombocytopenia of unknown cause, who were born to mothers without demonstrable platelet antibodies.

The *laboratory evaluation* of an infant (well or sick) with bleeding must include a platelet count, blood smear, PTT, and PT. Isolated thrombocytopenia in a well infant should suggest immune thrombocytopenia. Laboratory evidence of DIC should include a markedly prolonged PTT and PT

(minutes rather than seconds), thrombocytopenia, and a blood smear suggestive of a microangiopathic hemolytic anemia (burr or fragmented blood cells). Further evaluation reveals very low levels of fibrinogen (below 100 mg/dL) and elevated levels of fibrin degradation products. Vitamin K deficiency prolongs the PT more than the PTT, whereas hemophilia resulting from factors VIII and IX deficiency prolongs only the PTT. Specific factor levels confirm the *diagnosis* of hemophilia.

### References

Behrman RE, Kliegman RM, Arvin AM (eds): Nelson Textbook of Pediatrics, 15th ed. Philadelphia, WB Saunders 1996, Chapters 88.3–89.4.
Cohen DL, Baglin TP: Assessment and management of immune thrombocytopenia in pregnancy and in neonates. Arch Disease Child 72:F71, 1995.
Maisels MJ, Newman TB: Kernicterus in otherwise healthy, breast-fed term newborns. Pediatrics 96:730, 1995.
Ohls RK, Veerman MW, Christensen RD: Pharmacokinetics and effectiveness of recombinant erythropoietin administered to preterm infants by continuous infusion in total parenteral nutrition solution. J Pediatr 128:518, 1996.
Rubaltelli FF, Dario C, Zancan L: Congenital nonobstructive, nonhemolytic jaundice: Effect of tin-mesoporphyrin. Pediatrics 95:942, 1995.
Werner EJ: Neonatal polycythemia and hyperviscosity. Clin Perinatol 22:693, 1995.
Yao TC, Stevenson DK: Advances in the diagnosis and treatment of neonatal hyperbilirubinemia. Clin Perinatol 22:741, 1995.
Zipursky A: Vitamin K at birth. BMJ 313:179, 1996.

# NUTRITION AND GASTROINTESTINAL DISORDERS

## NUTRITION AND FEEDING

All newborn infants require water and a source of calories during the 1st day of life. In healthy, full-term infants, breast milk and/or formula is given on the 1st day of life as the source of fluid and nutrients during enteric alimentation; sick and very premature infants usually are managed with intravenous alimentation. Enteric alimentation of sick infants often is delayed until after the acute illnesses have resolved because of the risk of abdominal distention or ileus, either of which may lead to regurgitation and subsequent aspiration pneumonia, and because of the risk of the development of NEC. Delay in the onset of intravenous and enteric alimentation may be associated with fluid and electrolyte abnormalities such as hypernatremia, azotemia, dehydration, oliguria, fever, hypoglycemia, and hyperbilirubinemia.

Full-term infants usually are provided with breast-feeding or are fed formula by mouth during the first few hours after birth. Because premature infants before 32–34 wk of gestational age may not be able to coordinate the mechanisms for oral feeding, they usually are fed through a nasal or oral gastric tube. Such "gavage feedings" may be given continuously or intermittently by gravity drip every 1–3 hr. Subsequently, oral feedings are started when the infant can coordinate sucking, cheek and tongue movement, uvula closure of the nasopharynx, and epiglottal closure of the larynx; has acquired the esphageal motility to propel the milk feeding to the stomach; and has developed a gag reflex.

Problems of enteric alimentation are common in premature infants; these problems are due to immaturity of the gastrointestinal tract and to systemic disease states that alter gastrointestinal function. They include gastroesophageal reflux, gastric stasis and retention of formula, abdominal distention and ileus, failure to defecate, and a variety of abnormalities related to the composition of milk. Premature infants also may have bradycardia during enteral feedings, in part because of a reduced arterial oxygen content and gastric distention. Reflux of gastric contents may cause laryngospasm or aspiration pneumonia; both are associated with hypoxia, apnea, and bradycardia. Excessively large volumes of formula fed rapidly over a short time have been associated with the development of NEC. Problems associated with feeding tubes include erosive esophagitis, bowel perforation, fat malabsorption, and abnormal bacterial colonization of the upper intestine. There also may be a temporary loss of the ability to feed directly by mouth, if gavage or intravenous feeding is of long duration.

The composition of commonly used formulas and the indications for the initiation of *special infant formulas* are presented in Table 6–24. Breast milk is often the standard milk fed to newborn infants and serves as a nutritional reference point for comparison with other infant formulas.

The caloric requirements of the newborn infant include energy for growth, for regulation of body temperature, and for maintenance (replacement and turnover) of body macromolecules (Table 6–25). When fed 100–120 kcal/kg/24 hr, the infant should gain 10–30 g/24 hr. In term infants between 0 and 3 mo, weight gain is 25–35 g/24 hr; between 3 and 6 mo of life, it declines to 12–21 g/24 hr. The energy required for tissue synthesis is a small proportion, and that required for storage as macromolecules is a large proportion, of the energy required for growth. Energy partitioning for synthesis and storage depends on the composition of the new tissue; more calories are required for fat

synthesis than for protein synthesis. Net deposition of new tissue macromolecules (depositing 20–30% fat and 10–12% protein) requires 4–6 kcal/g tissue. Energy requirements may be spared for tissue synthesis if the infant is kept warm in a neutral thermal environment to avoid cold stress–induced energy utilization.

The *protein* requirement of the breast-fed, full-term infant may be as little as 1.5–2.0 g/kg/24 hr. Colostrum has a higher protein content than breast milk, which may contain as little as 0.9 g/dL. Standard formula for older premature infants and for full-term infants provides more protein than breast milk (see Table 6–24); growing infants consuming 150 mL/kg/24 hr will have a protein intake of 2.25 g/kg/24 hr. Preterm infants may have an increased requirement for protein to support growth but may develop an elevated blood urea nitrogen level, hyperaminoacidemia, hyperammonemia, and metabolic acidosis when fed casein-predominant (80%) formula or when fed greater than 4.5 g/kg/24 hr total proteins. The **late metabolic acidosis of prematurity** probably is due, in part, to increased endogenous acid production from casein-containing formula (high in sulfur and acidic amino acids). This disorder is characterized by metabolic acidosis and reduced weight gain in VLBW infants. *Treatment* includes substitution of a "humanized" whey-predominant formula and oral sodium bicarbonate.

All infants have an absolute requirement for the essential amino acids. Preterm infants also have an additional requirement for cystine and tyrosine because of immaturity of the enzymes required to convert cystathionine and phenylalanine to these amino acids. In addition, histidine and taurine also may be essential for the premature infant. Recommended protein intakes for the VLBW infant are 3.0–4.0 g/kg/24 hr of whey-predominant formula for the enteral route and 2.5–3.5 g/kg/24 hr of crystalline amino acids for intravenously alimented infants.

*Fat* absorption by the newborn infant may be reduced as a result of a small bile salt pool and a low pancreatic lipase activity. The latter may be compensated for by breast milk and lingual and gastric lipase activities. Reduced bile salt concentrations will be exacerbated by cholestatic jaundice. With the exception of human milk fat, animal fats are not well absorbed. Corn or soy oils are better tolerated, as are medium-chain triglycerides that do not require bile salts for absorption. Of the total calories, 3–5% should be in the form of essential fatty acids. Provision of linolenic and linoleic acids (unsaturated fatty acids) provide precursors for arachidonic acid, membrane phospholipids, and

Table 6–24. Composition of Breast Milk and Infant Formulas

| | Breast Milk (per dL) | Standard Formula (per dL) | Premature Formula (per dL) | Soy Formula (per dL) | Nutramigen (per dL) | Pregestimil (per dL) |
|---|---|---|---|---|---|---|
| *Calories (kcal)* | 67 | 67 | 67–81 | 67 | 67 | 67 |
| *Protein (g)* | 1.1 | 1.5 | 2.0–2.4 | 2.0 | 1.9 | 1.9 |
| (% calories) | (6%) | (9%) | (12%) | (12%) | (11%) | (11%) |
| Whey/casein protein ratio | 80/20 | 60/40, 18/82 | 60/40 | Soy protein, methionine | Casein hydrolysate, amino acid premix | Casein hydrolysate plus L-cystine, L-tyrosine, L-tryptophan |
| *Fat (g)* | 4.0 | 3.6 | 3.4–4.6 | 3.6 | 3.3 | 3.8 |
| (% calories) | (55%) | (50%) | (45%) | (48%) | (45%) | (48%) |
| MCT (%) | 0 | 0 | 40–50% | 0 | 0 | 55% |
| *Carbohydrate (g)* | 7.2 | 6.9–7.2 | 8.5–8.9 | 6.8 | 7.3 | 6.9 |
| (% calories) | (40%) | (41%) | (42%) | (40%) | (44%) | (41%) |
| Source | Lactose | Lactose | Lactose/glucose polymers, corn syrup | Corn syrup, sucrose | Sucrose, tapioca starch | Corn syrup solids, corn starch, dextrose |
| *Minerals (per L)* | | | | | | |
| Calcium (mg) | 290 | 420–550 | 750–1440 | 700 | 635 | 630 |
| Phosphorus (mg) | 140 | 280–390 | 400–720 | 500 | 420 | 420 |
| Sodium (mEq) | 8.0 | 6.5–8.3 | 6.5–15 | 13 | 14 | 12 |
| Vitamin D (IU) | Variable | 400 | 510–1200 | 400 | 400 | 400 |
| *Osmolality* (mOsm/L) | 273 | 300 | 250–310 | 240–260 | 320 | 320 |
| *Renal solute load* (mOsm/L) | 75 | 100–126 | 122–150 | 126 | 175 | 125 |
| *Comments* | Reference standard, deficient in vitamin K; may be deficient in Na+, Ca2+, protein, vitamin D for VLBW infants* | Risk of milk protein intolerance—gastrointestinal bleeding, anemia, wheezing, eczema | Specifically fortified with additional protein, Ca2+, P, Na+, vitamin D, and MCT oil | Useful for lactose and milk protein intolerance; may lead to soy protein intolerance; rickets develops in VLBW infants | Useful for lactose and milk protein intolerance (allergy) | Useful for malabsorption states, lactose and milk protein intolerance (allergy) |

*Can be supplemented with commercial fortifier (extra protein, energy, sodium, calcium, phosphorus, vitamins).
MCT = medium-chain triglyceride; VLBW = very-low-birth-weight.

TABLE 6–25.  Neonatal Caloric Requirements

| Source | kcal/kg/24 hr |
| --- | --- |
| Maintenance | 50 |
| Growth | 25–35 |
| Activity | 0–15 |
| Cold stress | 0–10 |
| Specific dynamic action (caloric cost of food) | 10 |
| Nutrient losses (stool) | 10–20 |
| TOTAL | 95–120 |

prostaglandin synthesis, thus avoiding **essential fatty acid deficiency.** The deficiency is characterized by growth failure, dermatitis, reduced pigmentation, and hypotonia. Poor intake of linolenic acid may impair visual function and neurodevelopment in VLBW infants. Excessive intake of polyunsaturated fatty acids may produce hemolysis by overcoming the antioxidant mechanisms of the erythrocyte. The provision of additional vitamin E may prevent this hemolysis.

Of milk calories, 40% are derived from *carbohydrates* (see Table 6–24). There is no absolute requirement for specific carbohydrates; however, both glucose and galactose can produce glycogen and prevent hypoglycemia. Lactose, a disaccharide of glucose and galactose, is the natural carbohydrate of human milk and of most formulas. Preterm infants have not developed normal full-term levels of the intestinal mucosal enzyme lactase, which is necessary to digest lactose. Malabsorption of lactose may result in watery, acidic stools from the production of organic acids by colonic bacteria. These organic acids may be absorbed and contribute to the development of late metabolic acidosis of prematurity. Newborn infants with gastrointestinal injury frequently become lactose-intolerant and require lactose-free formula. Because of the developmental immaturity of lactase activity, formulas for premature infants usually contain glucose polymers that will be digested by pancreatic amylase.

*Vitamin deficiency* is rare in the immediate newborn period; however, in breast-fed infants of strict vegan mothers vitamin $B_{12}$ deficiency may develop, and infants fed goat's milk may become folate-deficient. Vitamin D deficiency may be seen in infants of mothers with osteomalacia and in infants with cholestatic jaundice. Vitamin D deficiency may rarely occur in the breast-fed infant and may occasionally be a contributing factor to osteopenia of prematurity (see below). Preterm infants may need more vitamin C to improve tyrosine metabolism.

Vitamin E deficiency in the immediate newborn period may be due to an excess of oxidants, such as iron, and an abundance of oxidizable polyunsaturated fatty acids. Vitamin E deficiency of the premature infant may result in edema, anemia, reticulocytosis, and thrombocytosis.

Vitamin K deficiency is discussed under hemorrhagic disease of the newborn.

*Trace element deficiency* is unusual in formula-fed infants. It usually occurs during unsupplemented total parenteral alimentation. *Copper deficiency* was common before the addition of trace elements to intravenous alimentation solutions and manifests as anemia, neutropenia, and periosteal bone formation.

*Zinc deficiency* may be noted during total intravenous alimentation or among breast-fed infants whose mothers have low zinc levels in their milk. These infants have alopecia, growth failure, and dermatitis around the anus and on the hands and feet.

*Iron deficiency* rarely is manifested during the 1st mo of life. Prophylactic iron therapy should be started when preterm infants double their birth weight and in term infants after the 6th mo of life or at any age during treatment with erythropoietin; therapy for both should be in the form of iron-fortified formula and cereal or ferrous sulfate solution.

## FLUID REQUIREMENTS

Fluid balance in the normal, growing infant is always positive because of the high water content present during cellular growth. Oral feedings, intravenous solutions, or a combination of the two is the usual source of fluid intake. Water from oxidation is an additional internal source of small quantities of water (10 mL/kg/24 hr). Fluid intake is required because of continuous insensible, urine, and stool water losses (Table 6–26). Excessive fluid intake may predispose the premature infant to a PDA, congestive heart failure, BPD, NEC, hyponatremia, and edema. Too little fluid intake will result in dehydration, azotemia, hyperbilirubinemia, and hypernatremia.

The correct amount of fluid intake depends on the size of the infant, the postnatal age, and coexistent diseases affecting fluid balance. On the 1st day of life, most infants should receive 60–80 mL/kg/24 hr of fluid. On subsequent days, this amount should be increased to 100–140 mL/kg/24 hr. Fluid intake greater than 150–160 mL/kg/24 hr has been associated with PDA, BPD, and NEC and should be avoided unless there are excessive free water needs as a result of large insensible water losses. Hydration can be assessed by monitoring serum

TABLE 6–26. Components of Fluid Losses

| Source | Significance |
|---|---|
| Insensible water loss (IWL) | Varies with gestational and postnatal age; greatest in youngest, most immature (2–3 mL/kg/hr) versus term (0.5–0.8 mL/kg/hr); phototherapy, radiant warmer, low humidity increase IWL; ventilation, humidity, inner-plastic warmer shield decrease IWL |
| Urine output | Necessary to excrete obligate renal solute load; renal solute increases with fasting or a high-protein, high-electrolyte-containing formula; neonate has narrow range of urine concentration of diluting ability |
| Sweat | Uncommon in newborn; term infants sweat if overheated, with visible perspiration on forehead |
| Stool loss | Not a variable when on total parenteral alimentation; increased stool water loss with phototherapy and diarrhea |

blood urea nitrogen (BUN), Na+, urine output, and urine specific gravity (see below). Rising serum Na+, BUN, and urine specific gravity with weight loss suggest dehydration and a free water deficit.

Fluid balance in the newborn infant is tenuous because of very high rates of insensible water losses and immature renal function. Prior to 34 wk of gestation, the premature infant has a greatly reduced glomerular filtration rate (GFR). Although the GFR increases after 34 wk of age, the rate of filtration is still below adult values, even in full-term infants. Sodium reabsorption is reduced in the full-term infant and even more reduced in the preterm infant. Because of this, the fractional excretion of sodium is higher in the VLBW infant (up to 6–12%) than in the full-term infant or older child (< 2.0%). Thus, although the required sodium intake in the term infant is 1–3 mEq/kg/24 hr, the VLBW infant may require 3–5 mEq/kg/24 hr to prevent sodium wasting and hyponatremia. The newborn infant also has a limited ability to excrete a diluted or a concentrated urine. Maximum urinary concentrating ability of the newborn is 600–700 mOsm/L compared with 1200–1400 mOsm/L in the adult. Urine osmolality should be maintained between 50 and 300 mOsm/L, which corresponds to a urine specific gravity of 1.003–1.012; overhydration is a risk when urine osmolality is below 20–30 mOsm/L. The immature kidney also is limited in its capacity to excrete excessive solute, which may result in diminished excretion of sodium and other components of the renal solute load (also known as ash components of formula).

Additional signs of immaturity of renal function in the newborn include reduced sodium bicarbonate reabsorption, diminished capacity to acidify the urine, and reduced excretion of drugs such as the aminoglycosides.

## PARENTERAL ALIMENTATION

See Chapter 2.

## GASTROINTESTINAL DISEASES

For a discussion of obstruction and hemorrhage, see Chapter 11.

## GASTROINTESTINAL PERFORATION

Perforation of the small intestine associated with ileal atresia and cystic fibrosis results in sterile peritonitis in utero (*meconium peritonitis*). After birth, bacterial colonization of the intestines results in a combined bacterial and chemical peritonitis following a postnatal perforation. Neonatal intestinal perforation may be traumatic (iatrogenic), idiopathic (stomach), stress-related, drug-induced (dexamethasone, indomethacin), or associated with gastrointestinal obstruction.

**Necrotizing enterocolitis** is the most common cause of intestinal perforation during the neonatal period, but not all cases of NEC result in perforation. Patients with NEC are usually premature infants who are receiving oral feedings and have recovered from previous diseases of prematurity. The onset of symptoms is usually in the 1st wk of life but may be delayed 1–2 mo after birth.

The *clinical manifestations* include abdominal distention and tenderness, rectal bleeding, and a septic shock-like appearance. Abdominal roentgenograms reveal pneumatosis intestinalis and intrahepatic venous gas; pneumoperitoneum is noted with perforation.

Because epidemics of NEC are common and blood cultures are positive in 30% of patients, the *treatment* of NEC includes the initiation of broad-spectrum antibiotics as well as gastrointestinal decompression with a nasogastric tube and parenteral alimentation to put the bowel at rest. All newborn patients with evidence of intestinal perforation, such as pneumoperitoneum, require exploratory laparotomy.

References

Behrman RE, Kliegman RM, Arvin AM (eds): Nelson Textbook of Pediatrics, 15th ed. Philadelphia, WB Saunders, 1996, Chapters 44, 82.2.

Greer FR: Formulas for the healthy term infant. Pediatr Rev 16:107, 1995.

Lorenz JM, Kleinman LI, Ahmed G, et al: Phases of fluid and electrolyte homeostasis in extremely low birth weight infant. Pediatrics 96:484, 1995.

Makrides M, Neumann M, Simmer K, et al: Are long-chain polyunsaturated fatty acids essential nutrients in infancy? Lancet 345:1463, 1995.

Neu J: Necrotizing enterocolitis. Pediatr Clin North Am 43:409, 1996.

Wilson DC: Nutrition of the preterm baby. Br J Obstet Gynaecol 102:854, 1995.

## METABOLIC DISORDERS

### HYPOGLYCEMIA

Hypoglycemia is common during the neonatal period. Infants in many categories are at risk for neonatal hypoglycemia (Table 6–27). Serum glucose levels in healthy term infants are rarely less than 35 mg/dL between 1 and 3 hr of age, less than 40 mg/dL between 3 and 24 hr of age, and less than 45 mg/dL thereafter. Lower glucose levels among term or preterm infants suggest hypoglycemia. Alternately, symptoms compatible with hypoglycemia that respond to glucose infusions but with a higher glucose level are also considered to represent hypoglycemia.

Hypoglycemia in the **infant of a diabetic mother** is due to persistent hyperinsulinemia and a decreased ability to produce glucose (from glycogen) during neonatal fasting (see Medical Problems During Pregnancy Associated with Fetal or Neonatal Risk and Table 6–5). Poorly controlled maternal diabetes produces maternal and, hence, fetal hyperglycemia, which stimulates the fetal beta cells of the pancreas to produce large quantities of insulin. After birth, hyperinsulinemia persists, suppressing fasting hepatic glucose production (from glycogenolysis). Hyperinsulinemia also suppresses lipolysis and reduces levels of free fatty acids. Oxidation of fatty acids is an important source of energy after birth, as noted by a decline of the respiratory quotient from 1 at birth to 0.8 at 2–3 hr after birth. If free fatty acid mobilization is reduced, there is less alternate fuel available for oxidation. In normal infants, free fatty acid metabolism spares glucose utilization and helps prevent hypoglycemia.

In infants with **intrauterine growth retardation,** hypoglycemia occurs as a result of reduced tissue stores of glycogen and fat. Thus, glucose availability and fatty acid oxidation may be attenuated, resulting in a reduced total body energy production. The reduced level of oxygen consumption increases markedly with the provision of exogenous fuels during enteric feedings.

**TABLE 6–27.** Risk Factors for Neonatal Hypoglycemia

| Factors | Mechanism |
|---|---|
| *Common* | |
| Prematurity | Limited glycogen stores |
| Infant of a diabetic mother | Hyperinsulinism |
| Intrauterine growth retardation | Limited glycogen stores, hyperinsulinism |
| Asphyxia–perinatal stress | Depleted glycogen stores |
| Hypothermia | Increased glucose utilization |
| Starvation | Depleted glycogen stores |
| Large for gestational age | Possible hyperinsulinism |
| Maternal medications (tocolytics, propranolol, chlorpropamide, high-glucose infusion in labor) | Possible hyperinsulinism |
| *Uncommon* | |
| Erythroblastosis fetalis | Hyperinsulinism |
| Beckwith-Wiedemann syndrome | Hyperinsulinism |
| Islet cell adenoma | Hyperinsulinism |
| Nesidioblastosis | Hyperinsulinism |
| Familial hyperinsulinism | Hyperinsulinism |
| Polycythemia | Increased glucose utilization/decreased production |
| Sepsis | Increased glucose utilization |
| Inborn errors of metabolism | Decreased glycogenolysis, gluconeogenesis, or utilization of alternate fuels |
| Growth hormone deficiency | Increased glucose utilization, decreased gluconeogenesis |
| Adrenal insufficiency | Decreased glucose production (gluconeogenesis) |

The *clinical manifestations* of neonatal hypoglycemia usually are noted on the 1st or 2nd day of life and vary from asymptomatic patients to those with central nervous system and cardiopulmonary disturbances. Hypotonia, lethargy, apathy, poor feeding, jitteriness, and seizures are common. Congestive heart failure, tachycardia, cyanosis, pallor, diaphoresis, apnea, and hypothermia are additional manifestations. Because many of these symptoms and signs are not specific for hypoglycemia, systemic (congenital heart disease, sepsis, intraventricular hemorrhage) or other metabolic (hypocalcemia, hypomagnesemia, narcotic withdrawal) disorders must be considered. Hypoglycemia also may be seen in association with other diseases such as complex cyanotic heart disease and asphyxia.

The occurrence of hypoglycemia can be anticipated and may be *prevented* by identification of a high-risk population (see Table 6–27). Newborn infants who are at risk but who are asymptomatic and have no contraindications for oral feeding should be breast-fed or given formula within the 1st few hours of birth. When early feedings are not possible because of concomitant cardiopulmonary disease, 10% glucose should be given intravenously. All asymptomatic newborn infants who are at risk should be monitored with serial capillary blood glucose levels during the first day of life; a low glucose value on the Chemstrip should be confirmed by serum glucose determination.

*Treatment* of hypoglycemia requires an initial intravenous bolus infusion of 200–400 mg/kg (2–4 mL/kg) of 10% glucose solution that rapidly raises blood glucose to the physiologic range; it should be followed immediately by a continuous infusion of 8 mg/kg/min of glucose. If hypoglycemia recurs, the bolus is repeated and the glucose infusion rate is incrementally increased to maintain physiologic glucose concentrations.

The *prognosis* of symptomatic neonatal hypoglycemia with seizures is poor and is associated with abnormal neurointellectual development. The prognosis for other forms of hypoglycemia is better. Infants with nesidioblastosis often require surgical resection of most of the pancreas if medical management with diazoxide or somatostatin fails.

## HYPOCALCEMIA

Hypocalcemia is common among sick and premature newborn infants. Most infants are born with calcium levels that are higher in cord blood than in maternal blood because of active placental transfer of calcium to the fetus. Fetal calcium accretion in the third trimester approaches 150 mg/kg/24 hr, and fetal bone mineral content doubles between 30 and 40 wk of gestation. All infants show a slight decline of serum calcium levels after birth that reach trough levels at 24–48 hr, the point at which hypocalcemia usually occurs. Total serum calcium levels of less than 7 mg/dL and ionized calcium levels of less than 3.0–3.5 mg/dL are considered hypocalcemic.

The *etiology* of hypocalcemia varies with the time of onset and the associated illnesses of the child. **Early neonatal hypocalcemia** occurs in the first 3 days of life and is often asymptomatic. Transient hypoparathyroidism and a reduced parathyroid response to the usual postnatal decline of serum calcium levels may be responsible for hypocalcemia among premature infants and infants of diabetic mothers. Congenital absence of the parathyroid gland and DiGeorge syndrome also have been associated with hypocalcemia. *Hypomagnesemia* (<1.5 mg/dL) may be seen simultaneously with hypocalcemia, especially in infants of diabetic mothers. Treatment with calcium alone does not relieve symptoms or increase serum calcium levels unless the hypomagnesemia also is treated. Sodium bicarbonate therapy, phosphate release from cell necrosis, transient hypoparathyroidism, and hypercalcitoninemia may be responsible for early neonatal hypocalcemia associated with asphyxia. Early-onset hypocalcemia associated with asphyxia often occurs with seizures as a result of the hypoxic-ischemic encephalopathy and/or hypocalcemia. **Late neonatal hypocalcemia,** or **neonatal tetany,** often is due to ingestion of high-phosphate–containing milk or the inability to excrete the usual phosphorus in commercial infant formula. Hyperphosphatemia (>8 mg/dL) usually occurs in infants with hypocalcemia after the 1st week of life. Vitamin D deficiency states and malabsorption also have been associated with late onset hypocalcemia.

The *clinical manifestations* of hypocalcemia and hypomagnesemia include apnea, muscle twitching, seizures, laryngospasm, **Chvostek sign** (facial muscle spasm when the side of the face over the 7th nerve is tapped), and **Trousseau sign** (carpopedal spasm induced by partial inflation of a blood pressure cuff). The latter two signs are rare in the immediate newborn period. On occasion, congestive heart failure has been associated with hypocalcemia.

Neonatal hypocalcemia may be *prevented* by administering intravenous or oral calcium supplementation at a rate of 25–75 mg/kg/24 hr. Early asymptomatic hypocalcemia of preterm infants and infants of diabetic mothers often resolves spontaneously. Symptomatic hypocalcemia should be treated with 2–4 mL/kg of 10% calcium gluconate given intravenously slowly over 10–15 min; a continuous infusion of 75 mg/kg/24 hr of elemental calcium should then be administered. If hypomagnesemia is associated with hypocalcemia, 50% magnesium sulfate, 0.1 mL/kg, should be given by intramuscular injection and repeated every 8–12 hr.

The *treatment* of late hypocalcemia includes immediate management, as in early hypocalcemia, plus the initiation of low-phosphate-containing formula feedings. Subcutaneous infiltration of intravenous calcium salts can cause tissue necrosis; oral supplements are hypertonic and may irritate the intestinal mucosa.

## OSTEOPENIA OR METABOLIC BONE DISEASE OF PREMATURITY

The rate of fetal bone mineralization is not always maintained by the prematurely born infant fed breast milk or standard formula. Bone undermineralization or frank rickets may develop and result in pathologic fractures, altered growth, and respiratory insufficiency. Osteopenia predominantly is noted in infants weighing less than 1000 g and in infants with chronic diseases of prematurity, such as BPD, after the first 2–3 mo of life. Roentgenographic signs include bone demineralization and fractures. Serum alkaline phosphatase levels always are elevated, sometimes two to three times normal. The cause most probably is due to dietary deficiency of calcium and phosphate; vitamin D deficiency, copper deficiency, aluminum toxicity, diuretic-induced hypercalciuria, cholestatic jaundice–induced malabsorption of calcium, and altered metabolism of vitamin D are less likely causes or contributing factors.

*Prevention* may be possible with a formula containing higher concentrations of calcium, phosphate, and vitamin D (see Table 6–24). *Treatment* consists of dietary supplementation with calcium, phosphate, and vitamin D if indicated.

## NEONATAL DRUG ADDICTION AND WITHDRAWAL

Infants may become passively and physiologically addicted to medications or to drugs of abuse (heroin, methadone, barbiturates, tranquilizers, and amphetamines) taken by the mother during pregnancy and, subsequently, may have signs and symptoms of drug withdrawal. Many of these pregnancies are at high risk for other complications related to intravenous drug abuse, such as hepatitis, acquired immunodeficiency syndrome (AIDS) and syphilis. In addition, the LBW rate and the long-term risk for the sudden infant death syndrome (SIDS) are higher in the infants of these high-risk women.

### Heroin

Neonatal withdrawal signs and symptoms usually begin at 1–5 days of life with maternal heroin use and at 1–4 wk with maternal methadone addiction.

*Clinical manifestations* of withdrawal include sneezing, yawning, ravenous appetite, emesis, diarrhea, fever, diaphoresis, tachypnea, high-pitched cry, tremors, jitteriness, poor sleep, poor feeding, and seizures. The illness tends to be more severe during methadone withdrawal. The initial *treatment* includes swaddling in blankets in a quiet, dark room. When hyperactivity is constant and irritability interferes with sleeping and feeding or when diarrhea or seizures are present, pharmacologic treatment is indicated. Seizures usually are treated with phenobarbital. The other symptoms may be managed with replacement doses of a narcotic (usually tincture of opium) to calm the infant; weaning from narcotics may be prolonged over 1–2 mo.

### Cocaine

Cocaine use during pregnancy is associated with preterm labor, abruptio placentae, neonatal irritability, intraventricular hemorrhage, and decreased attentiveness. Usually no treatment is needed.

### References

Behrman RE, Kliegman RM, Arvin AM (eds): Nelson Textbook of Pediatrics, 15th ed. Philadelphia, WB Saunders, 1996, Chapters 92–93.

Burton BK: Inborn errors of metabolism: The critical diagnosis in early infancy. Pediatrics 79:359, 1987.

Jacobson SW, Jacobson JL, Sokol RJ, et al: New evidence for neurobehavioral effects of in utero cocaine exposure. J Pediatr 129:581, 1996.

Milner RDG: Nesidioblastosis unravelled. Arch Dis Child 74:369, 1996.

Rivers RPA: Neonatal opiate withdrawal. Arch Dis Child 61:1236, 1986.

Ryan S: Nutritional aspects of metabolic bone disease in the newborn. Arch Dis Child 74:F145, 1996.

## NEONATAL INFECTIOUS DISEASE
(see Chapter 10 and Appendix)

Systemic and local infections (lung, cutaneous, ocular, umbilical, kidney, bone-joint, and meningeal infections) are common in the newborn period. Infection may be acquired in utero through the transplacental or transcervical routes and during and after birth. Ascending infection through the cervix, with or without rupture of the amniotic fluid membranes, may result in amnionitis, funisitis (infection of the umbilical cord), congenital pneumonia, and sepsis. The bacteria responsible for ascending infection of the fetus are common bacterial organisms of the maternal genitourinary tract such as group B streptococcus, *E. coli*, *Haemophilus influenzae*, and *Klebsiella*. Herpes simplex virus (HSV) 2 also causes ascending infection that at times may be indistinguishable from bacterial sepsis. Syphilis and *Listeria monocytogenes* are acquired by transplacental infection.

Maternal humoral immunity may protect the fetus against some neonatal pathogens, such as group B streptococcus and herpes simplex type 2. Nonetheless, various deficiencies of the neonatal antimicrobial defense mechanism probably are more important than maternal immune status as a contributing factor for neonatal infection, especially in the LBW infant. The incidence of sepsis is approximately 1:1500 in full-term infants and 1:250 in preterm infants. The six-fold higher rate of sepsis among preterm infants compared with term infants relates both to the preterm infants' more immature immunologic system and to their prolonged period of hospitalization, which holds the added risk of nosocomially acquired infectious diseases.

Preterm infants prior to 32 wk of gestational age have not received the full complement of maternal antibodies (IgG), which cross the placenta by active transport predominantly in the latter half of the 3rd trimester. In addition, although LBW infants may generate IgM antibodies, their own IgG response to infection is reduced. These infants also have deficiencies of the alternate and, to a smaller degree, the classic complement activation pathways, which result in diminished complement-mediated opsonization. Newborn infants also demonstrate a deficit in phagocytic migration to the site of infection (e.g., to the lung) and in the bone marrow reserve pool of leukocytes. In addition, in the presence of suboptimal activation of complement, neonatal neutrophils ingest and kill bacteria less effectively than adult neutrophils do. Furthermore, neutrophils from sick infants seem to have an even greater deficit in bacterial killing capacity compared with phagocytic cells from normal neonates.

Defense mechanisms against viral pathogens also may be deficient in the newborn infant. Neonatal antibody-dependent cell-mediated immunity by the natural killer lymphocytes is deficient in the absence of maternal antibodies and in the presence of reduced interferon production; reduced antibody levels occur in premature infants and in infants born during a primary viral infection of the mother, such as with herpes simplex II or cytomegalovirus. In addition, antibody-independent cytotoxicity also may be reduced in lymphocytes of newborn infants.

## NEONATAL SEPSIS

Neonatal sepsis presents during three periods. **Early-onset sepsis** often begins in utero and usually is due to infection by the bacteria in the mother's genitourinary tract. These organisms include group B streptococcus, *E. coli, Klebsiella, L. monocytogenes,* and nontypable *H. influenzae.* Most infected infants are premature and show nonspecific cardiorespiratory signs such as grunting, tachypnea, and cyanosis at birth. Risk factors for early-onset sepsis include vaginal colonization with group B streptococcus, prolonged rupture of the membranes (>24 hr), amnionitis, maternal fever or leukocytosis, fetal tachycardia, and preterm birth. Black race and male sex are unexplained additional risk factors for neonatal sepsis.

Early-onset sepsis (birth to 7 days) is an overwhelming multiorgan system disease frequently manifested by respiratory failure, shock, meningitis (30%), DIC, acute tubular necrosis, and symmetric peripheral gangrene. Early manifestations—grunting, poor feeding, pallor, apnea, lethargy, hypothermia, or an abnormal cry—may be nonspecific. Profound neutropenia, hypoxia, and hypotension may be refractory to treatment with broad-spectrum antibiotics, mechanical ventilation, and vasopressors such as dopamine and dobutamine. In the initial stages of early-onset septicemia in the preterm infant, it is often very difficult to differentiate sepsis from RDS. Because of this difficulty, most premature infants with RDS receive-broad spectrum antibiotics.

Infants with early-onset sepsis should be *evaluated* by blood and cerebrospinal fluid (CSF) cultures; and by CSF Gram stain, cell count, protein, and glucose determinations. Buffy coat Gram stain or methylene blue stain also may help identify bacteria. Normal newborn infants generally have an elevated CSF protein content (100–150 mg/dL) and may have as many as 25 white blood cells (mean, $9/mm^3$), which are 75% lymphocytes in the absence of infection. Some infants with neonatal meningitis caused by group B steptococcus do not have an elevated CSF leukocyte count but demonstrate microorganisms on Gram stain of the spinal fluid. In addition to identification of the organism by culture, other methods to identify the pathogenic bacteria include the determination of bacterial antigen in samples of blood, urine, or spinal fluid by methods such as counterimmunoelectrophoresis or latex agglutination. Serial complete blood counts should be performed to identify neutropenia, an increased number of immature neutrophils (bands), and thrombocytopenia. C-reactive protein levels are often elevated in neonatal patients with bacterial sepsis.

A chest roentgenogram also should be obtained to determine the presence of pneumonia. In addition to the traditional neonatal pathogens, pneumonia in VLBW infants may be due to acquisition of maternal genital mycoplasmal agent (*U. urealyticum, M. hominis*). Arterial blood gases should be monitored to detect hypoxemia and metabolic acidosis that may be due to hypoxia, shock, or both. Blood pressure, urine output, and peripheral perfusion should be monitored to determine the need to treat septic shock with fluids and vasopressor agents.

A combination of ampicillin and gentamicin for 10–14 days is effective *treatment* against most organisms responsible for early-onset sepsis. If meningitis is present, the treatment is extended to 21 days, or 14 days after a negative CSF culture. Persistently positive CSF culture is common with neonatal meningitis caused by gram-negative organisms, even with appropriate antibiotic treatment, and may be present for 2–3 days after antibiotic therapy. If gram-negative meningitis is present, some authorities continue to treat with an effective penicillin derivative plus an aminoglycoside, whereas most change to a third-generation cephalosporin. High-dose penicillin (250,000 U/kg/24 hr) is appropriate for group B streptococcus meningitis. Inhaled nitric oxide and/or ECMO (in term infants) may improve the outcome of sepsis-related pulmonary hypertension.

**Late-onset sepsis** (8–28 days) usually occurs in the healthy full-term infant who was discharged in good health from the normal newborn nursery. *Clinical manifestations* may include lethargy, poor feeding, hypotonia, apathy, seizures, bulging fontanel, fever, and direct-reacting hyperbilirubinemia. In addition to bacteremia, hematogenous seeding may result in focal infections such as meningitis (75%), osteomyelitis (group B streptococcus, *Staphylococcus aureus*), arthritis (gonococcus, *S. aureus, Candida albicans,* gram-negative bacteria), and urinary tract infection (gram-negative bacteria).

The *evaluation* of infants with late-onset sepsis is similar to that for those with early-onset sepsis, with special attention given to a careful physical examination of the bones (infants with osteomyelitis may present with pseudoparalysis) and to the laboratory examination and culture of urine obtained by sterile suprapubic aspiration or urethral catheterization. Late-onset sepsis may be due to the same pathogens as early-onset sepsis, but those infants presenting late in the neonatal period also may have infections caused by the pathogens usually found in older infants (*H. influenzae, Streptococcus pneumoniae, Neisseria meningitidis*). In addition, viral agents (HSV, cytomegalovirus [CMV]) may present with a late-onset sepsis-like picture.

Because of the increased rate of resistance of *H. influenzae* to ampicillin, some centers begin treatment with ampicillin and a 3rd generation cephalosporin when sepsis occurs in the last week of the 1st mo of life. The treatment of late-onset neonatal sepsis and meningitis is the same as that for early-onset sepsis.

**Nosocomially acquired sepsis** (8 days to discharge) occurs predominantly among premature infants in the NICU; many of these infants have been colonized with the multidrug-resistant bacteria indigenous to the NICU. Frequent treatment with broad-spectrum antibiotics for sepsis and the presence of central venous indwelling catheters, endotracheal tubes, umbilical vessel catheters, and electronic monitoring devices increase the risk for such serious bacterial infection. Epidemics of bacterial or viral sepsis, bacterial or aseptic meningitis, staphylococcal bullous skin infections, cellulitis, pneumonia (bacterial, adenovirus, respiratory syncytial virus), omphalitis (*S. aureus*, gram-negative bacilli), and diarrhea (staphylococcal, enteroviral, rotavirus, and enteropathogenic *E. coli* and associated NEC) are not uncommon in the NICU or even in the nursery for well babies.

The initial *clinical manifestations* of nosocomial infection in the premature infant may be subtle and include apnea and bradycardia, temperature instability, abdominal distention, and poor feeding as early signs. In the later stages, there may be shock, DIC, worsening respiratory status, and local reactions such as omphalitis, eye discharge, diarrhea, and bullous impetigo.

The *treatment* of nosocomially acquired sepsis depends on the indigenous microbiologic flora of the particular hospital and their antibiotic sensitivities. Because *S. aureus* (occasionally methicillin-resistant), *Staphylococcus epidermidis* (usually methicillin-resistant), and gram-negative pathogens are common nosocomial bacterial agents in many nurseries, a combination of vancomycin or nafcillin with gentamicin is appropriate. The dose and interval for administering all aminoglycosides, such as gentamicin, vary with postnatal age and birth weight. In addition, treatment with aminoglycosides for more than 3 days requires monitoring of the serum peak and trough concentrations to optimize therapy and to avoid ototoxicity and nephrotoxicity. Persistent signs of infection despite antibacterial treatment should suggest candidal or viral sepsis.

## PERINATAL CONGENITAL (TORCH) INFECTIONS

The acronym "TORCH" represents a generic group of parasitic, bacterial, and viral pathogens that produce congenital or perinatally acquired infections:

*toxoplasmosis, other, rubella, cytomegalovirus,* and *herpes* simplex. The "other" is an increasing number of agents responsible for fetal infection, such as syphilis, varicella zoster, parvovirus, HIV, malaria, viruses, *Borrelia burgdorferi,* and hepatitis B, C or G.

Many of the *clinical manifestations* of TORCH infections are similar and include intrauterine growth retardation, nonimmune hydrops, anemia, thrombocytopenia, jaundice, hepatosplenomegaly, chorioretinitis, and congenital malformations. Some of the unique manifestations and epidemiologic characteristics of these infections are noted in Table 6–28.

*Evaluation* of patients thought to have TORCH infections should include attempts to isolate the organism by culture (rubella, CMV, HSV, gonorrhea, *Mycobacterium tuberculosis*); to identify the antigen of the pathogen (hepatitis B, *Chlamydia trachomatis*); to identify the pathogen's genome with the polymerase chain reaction; and to identify specific fetal production of antibodies (IgM or increasing titer of IgG for *Toxoplasma,* syphilis, parvovirus, HIV, *Borrelia*).

*Treatment* is not always available, specific, or effective. Nonetheless, some encouraging results have been reported for preventing the disease and for specifically treating the infant once the correct diagnosis is made (see Table 6–28).

### References

Behrman RE, Kliegman RM, Arvin AM (eds): Nelson Textbook of Pediatrics, 15th ed. Philadelphia, WB Saunders, 1996, Chapters 94–101.
Best J, Sutherland S: Diagnosis and prevention of congenital and perinatal infections: TORCH screening should be discouraged. BMJ 30:888, 1990.
Gaynes RP, Edwards JR, Jarvis WR, et al: Nosocomial infections among neonates in high-risk nurseries in the United States. Pediatrics 98:357, 1996.
Jakobi P, Goldstick O, Sujov P, et al: New CDC guidelines for prevention of perinatal group B streptococcal disease. Lancet 348:969, 1996.
Risser WL, Hwang L-Y: Problems in the current case definitions of congenital syphilis. J Pediatr 129:499, 1996.
Scott LL, Perinatal herpes: Current status and obstetric management strategies. Pediatr Infect Dis J 14:827, 1995.
Stoll BJ, Gordon T, Korones SB, et al: Early-onset sepsis in very low birth weight neonates: A report from the National Institute of Child Health and Human Development Neonatal Research Network. J Pediatr 129:72, 1996.
Stoll BJ, Gordon T, Korones SB, et al: Late-onset sepsis in very low birth weight neonates: A report from the National Institute of Child Health and Human Development Neonatal Research Network. J Pediatr 129:63, 1996.

## NEONATAL NEUROLOGY AND OUTCOME

The neonatal central nervous system is anatomically and functionally immature. Although division of cerebral cortical neuronal cells stops during the 2nd trimester of pregnancy, glial cell growth, dendritic arborization, myelination, and cerebellar neuronal cell number continue to increase beyond term gestation and into infancy. At birth, the human newborn spends more time asleep (predominantly rapid eye movement [REM] or active sleep) than in a wakeful state and is totally dependent on adults. Primitive reflexes, such as the Moro, grasp, stepping, rooting, sucking, and crossed extensor reflexes, are readily elicited and are normal for this age. In addition, the newborn infant has a wealth of cortical functions that are less easily demonstrated (e.g., the ability to extinguish repetitive or painful stimuli and to show visual preference for new or novel objects); the newborn also has the capacity for attentive eye fixation and differential responses to the mother's voice.

During the perinatal period, many pathophysiologic mechanisms can adversely and permanently affect the developing brain. These include prenatal events, such as hypoxia, ischemia, infections, malformations, maternal drugs, and coagulation disorders, and postnatal events, such as birth trauma, hypoxia-ischemia, inborn errors of metabolism, hypoglycemia, hypothyroidism, hyperthyroidism, polycythemia, hemorrhage, and meningitis.

### NEONATAL SEIZURES

Seizures during the neonatal period may be due to multiple causes with characteristic historic and clinical manifestations. Seizures due to **hypoxic-ischemic encephalopathy** (postasphyxial seizures), a common cause of seizures in the full-term infant, usually occur 12–24 hr after a history of birth asphyxia and often are refractory to conventional doses of anticonvulsant medications. Postasphyxial seizures also may be due to metabolic disorders associated with neonatal asphyxia, such as hypoglycemia and hypocalcemia. **Intraventricular hemorrhage** (IVH) is a common cause of seizures in premature infants and often occurs between 1 and 3 days of age. Seizures with IVH are associated with a bulging fontanel, hemorrhagic spinal fluid, anemia, lethargy, and coma. Seizures due to **hypoglycemia** often occur when blood glucose levels decline to the lowest postnatal value (e.g., 1–2 hr of age or after 24–48 hr of poor nutritional intake) (see Table 6–27). Seizures due to **hypocalcemia** and **hypomagnesemia** develop among high-risk infants and respond well to calcium and/or magnesium therapy.

Seizures noted in the delivery room often are due to (1) direct *injection of local anesthetic agents*

TABLE 6–28. Perinatal Congenital Infections (TORCH)

| Agent | Maternal Epidemiology | Neonatal Features |
|---|---|---|
| *Toxoplasma gondii* | Heterophil-negative mononucleosis<br>Exposure to cats or raw meat or immunosuppression<br>High-risk exposure at 10–24 wk gestation | Hydrocephalus, abnormal spinal fluid, intracranial calcifications, chorioretinitis, jaundice, hepatosplenomegaly, fever<br>Many infants asymptomatic at birth<br>*Treatment:* pyrimethamine plus sulfadiazine |
| Rubella virus | Unimmunized seronegative mother; fever ± rash<br>Detectable defects with infection:<br>   by 8 wk, 85%<br>   9–12 wk, 50%<br>   13–20 wk, 16%<br>Virus may be present in infant throat for 1 yr<br>*Prevention:* vaccine | Intrauterine growth retardation, microcephaly, microphthalmia, cataracts, glaucoma, "salt and pepper" chorioretinitis, hepatosplenomegaly, jaundice, PDA, deafness, blueberry muffin rash, anemia, thrombocytopenia, leukopenia, metaphyseal lucencies, B-cell and T-cell deficiency<br>Infant may be asymptomatic at birth |
| Cytomegalovirus | Sexually transmitted disease: primary genital infection may be asymptomatic<br>Heterophil-negative mononucleosis; infant may have viruria for 1–6 yr | Sepsis, intrauterine growth retardation, chorioretinitis, microcephaly, periventricular calcifications, blueberry muffin rash, anemia, thrombocytopenia, neutropenia, hepatosplenomegaly, jaundice, deafness, pneumonia<br>Many asymptomatic at birth<br>*Prevention:* CMV-negative blood products<br>*Possible treatment:* ganciclovir? |
| Herpes simplex type 2 virus | Sexually transmitted disease: primary genital infection may be asymptomatic; intrauterine infection rare, acquisition at time of birth more common | *Intrauterine infection:* chorioretinitis, skin lesions, microcephaly<br>*Postnatal:* encephalitis, localized or disseminated disease, skin vesicles, keratoconjunctivitis<br>*Treatment:* acyclovir |
| Varicella-zoster virus | Intrauterine infection with chickenpox during first trimester.<br>Infant develops severe neonatal varicella with maternal illness 5 days prior to or 2 days after delivery | Microphthalmia, cataracts, chorioretinitis, cutaneous and bony aplasia/hypoplasia/atrophy, cutaneous scars<br>Zoster as in older child<br>*Prevention of neonatal condition with VZIG*<br>*Treatment of ill neonate:* acyclovir |
| *Treponema pallidum* (syphilis) | Sexually transmitted disease<br>Maternal primary asymptomatic: painless "hidden" chancre<br>Penicillin, not erythromycin, prevents fetal infection | Presentation *at birth* as nonimmune hydrops, prematurity, anemia, neutropenia, thrombocytopenia, pneumonia, hepatosplenomegaly<br>*Late neonatal* as snuffles (rhinitis), rash, hepatosplenomegaly, condylomata lata, metaphysitis, cerebrospinal fluid pleocytosis, keratitis, periosteal new bone, lymphocytosis, hepatitis<br>*Late onset:* teeth, eye, bone, skin, CNS, ear<br>*Treatment:* penicillin |

*Table continued on opposite page*

into the fetal scalp (associated with transient bradycardia and fixed dilated pupils), (2) severe *anoxia*, or (3) *congenital brain malformation*. Seizures after the first 5 days of life may be due to (1) *infection* or (2) *drug withdrawal*. Seizures associated with lethargy, acidosis, and a family history of infant deaths may be due to an *inborn error of metabolism*. An infant whose parent has a history of a neonatal seizure also is at risk for *benign familial seizures*. In an infant who appears well, a sudden onset of seizures on days 1–3 that are of short duration and that do not recur may be due to a *subarachnoid hemorrhage*. Focal seizures often are due to local cerebral infarction.

Seizures may be difficult to differentiate from benign jitteriness or from tremulousness in infants of diabetic mothers, in infants with narcotic withdrawal syndrome, and in infants after an episode of asphyxia. In contrast to seizures, jitteriness and tremors are sensory dependent, elicited by stimuli,

TABLE 6–28.  Perinatal Congenital Infections (TORCH) *Continued*

| Agent | Maternal Epidemiology | Neonatal Features |
|---|---|---|
| Parvovirus | Etiology of fifth disease; fever, rash, arthralgia in adults | Nonimmune hydrops, fetal anemia<br>*Treatment:* in utero transfusion |
| Human immunodeficiency virus (HIV) | AIDS; most mothers are asymptomatic and HIV positive; high-risk history; prostitute, drug abuse, married to bisexual, or hemophiliac | AIDS symptoms develop between 3 and 6 mo of age in 25–40%; failure to thrive, recurrent infection, hepatosplenomegaly, neurologic abnormalities<br>*Management:* Intravenous immunoglobulin, trimethoprim/sulfamethoxazole, AZT<br>*Prevention:* Prenatal, intrapartum, postpartum AZT |
| Hepatitis B virus | Vertical transmission common; may result in cirrhosis, hepatocellular carcinoma | Acute neonatal hepatitis; many become asymptomatic carriers<br>*Prevention:* HBIG, vaccine |
| *Neisseria gonorrhoeae* | Sexually transmitted disease, infant acquires at birth<br>*Treatment:* cefotaxime, ceftriaxone | Gonococcal ophthalmia, sepsis, meningitis<br>*Prevention:* silver nitrate, erythromycin eye drops<br>*Treatment:* intravenous ceftriaxone |
| *Chlamydia trachomatis* | Sexually transmitted disease, infant acquires at birth<br>*Treatment:* oral erythromycin | Conjunctivitis, pneumonia<br>*Prevention:* erythromycin eye drops<br>*Treatment:* oral erythromycin |
| *Mycobacterium tuberculosis* | Positive PPD skin test, recent converter, positive chest roentgenogram, positive family member<br>*Treatment:* INH and rifampin ± ethambutol | Congenital rare septic pneumonia; acquired primary pulmonary TB; asymptomatic, follow PPD<br>*Prevention:* INH, BCG, separation<br>*Treatment:* INH, rifampin, pyrazinamide |
| *Trypanosoma cruzi* (Chagas disease) | Central South American native, immigrant, travel<br>Chronic disease in mother | Failure to thrive, heart failure, achalasia<br>*Treatment:* nifurtimox |

AIDS = acquired immunodeficiency syndrome; AZT = zidovudine (azidothymidine); BCG = bacille Calmette-Guérin; CMV = cytomegalovirus; CNS = central nervous system; HBIG = hepatitis B immune globulin; INH = isoniazid; PDA = patent ductus arteriosus; PPD = purified protein derivative; TB = tuberculosis; VZIG = varicella-zoster immune globulin.

and interrupted by holding the extremity. Seizure activity becomes manifest by coarse, fast and slow clonic activity, whereas jitteriness is characterized by fine, very rapid movement. Seizures may be associated with abnormal eye movements, such as tonic deviation to one side. The electroencephalogram (EEG) often demonstrates seizure activity when the clinical diagnosis is uncertain. It is often difficult to identify seizures in the newborn period because the infant, especially the LBW infant, usually does not demonstrate the tonic-clonic major motor activity typical of the older child (Table 6–29). Subtle seizures are a very common manifestation among newborn infants. The subtle signs of seizure activity include apnea, eye deviation, tongue thrusting, eye blinking, and staring. Continuous bedside EEG monitoring can help identify subtle seizures.

The *diagnostic evaluation* of infants with seizures should include an immediate determination of capillary blood glucose levels with a Chemstrip. In addition, determination of blood concentrations of sodium, calcium, glucose, and bilirubin should be obtained. When infection is suspected, appropriate specimens for culture should be obtained. After the seizure has stopped, a careful examination should be done to identify signs of increased intracranial pressure, congenital malformations, and systemic

TABLE 6–29.  Classification of Neonatal Seizures

| Type | Manifestations |
|---|---|
| Subtle | Eye deviation, blinking, mouth movements, apnea, fluctuation of vital signs |
| Focal clonic | Localized jerking movement |
| Multifocal clonic | Multiple random clonic movements |
| Tonic | Extensor posturing with tonic eye deviation |
| Myoclonic | Synchronized single or multifocal rapid jerks<br>Hypsarrhythmia on electroencephalogram |
| Tonic-clonic | Less common than in older children |

illness. In the absence of signs of elevated intracranial pressure, a lumbar puncture should be performed. If the diagnosis is not apparent at this point, further evaluation should include magnetic resonance imaging (MRI), computed tomography (CT), or cerebral ultrasonography and tests to determine the presence of an inborn error of metabolism. The latter determinations are especially important in infants with unexplained lethargy, coma, acidosis, ketonuria, or respiratory alkalosis.

The *treatment* of neonatal seizures may be specific, such as treatment of meningitis or the correction of hypoglycemia, hypocalcemia, hypomagnesemia, hyponatremia, and vitamin $B_6$ deficiency or dependency. In the absence of an identifiable cause, therapy should include an anticonvulsant agent, such as 20–30 mg/kg of phenobarbital, 10–20 mg/kg of phenytoin (Dilantin), or 0.1–0.3 mg/kg of diazepam (Valium), followed by one of the two longer-acting drugs. Treatment of status epilepticus requires repeated doses of phenobarbital and may also require a diazepam, midazolam, or paraldehyde drip titrated to clinical signs.

The long-term outcome for neonatal seizures usually is related to the underlying cause and to the primary pathology such as hypoxic-ischemic encephalopathy, meningitis, drug withdrawal, stroke, or hemorrhage.

## INTRACRANIAL HEMORRHAGE

Intracranial hemorrhage may be confined to one anatomic area of the brain, such as the subdural, subarachnoid, periventricular, intraventricular, intraparenchymal, or cerebellar region. **Subdural hemorrhages** are seen in association with birth trauma, cephalopelvic disproportion, forceps delivery, LGA infants, and postnatal head trauma. The subdural hematoma does not always cause symptoms immediately after birth, but with time the red blood cells undergo hemolysis and water is drawn into the hemorrhage because of the high oncotic pressure of protein, resulting in an expanding symptomatic lesion. Anemia, vomiting, seizures, and macrocephaly may occur in the 1–2 mo old infant with a subdural hematoma. *Child abuse* also must be suspected, and appropriate diagnostic evaluation undertaken to identify other possible signs of skeletal or soft tissue injury. Occasionally, a massive subdural hemorrhage in the neonatal period is due to rupture of the vein of Galen or to an inherited coagulation disorder, such as hemophilia. These infants present with shock, seizures, and coma. The *treatment* of all subdural hematomas is surgical evacuation.

**Subarachnoid hemorrhages** may be spontaneous, associated with hypoxia or due to bleeding from a cerebral arteriovenous malformation. Seizures are a common presenting manifestation, and the *prognosis* depends on the underlying injury. The *treatment* is directed at the seizure and the rare occurrence of posthemorrhagic hydrocephalus.

**Periventricular hemorrhage** and **intraventricular hemorrhage** are common among VLBW infants, and the risk decreases with increasing gestational age. Up to 50% of infants under 1500 g have evidence of intracranial bleeding. The *pathogenesis* for these hemorrhages is unknown (they usually are not due to coagulation disorders), but the initial site of bleeding may be the weak blood vessels in the periventricular germinal matrix. The vessels in this area have poor structural support and may rupture and hemorrhage because of passive changes in cerebral blood flow occurring with the variations of blood pressure that sick premature infants often exhibit (failure of autoregulation). In some sick infants, these blood pressure variations are the only identifiable etiologic factors. In others, the disorders that may cause the elevation or depression of blood pressure or that interfere with venous return from the head (venous stasis) increase the risk of IVH; these disorders include asphyxia, pneumothorax, mechanical ventilation, hypercapnia, hypoxemia, prolonged labor, breech delivery, PDA, heart failure, intravenous therapy with blood volume–expanding agents such as albumin, and therapy with hypertonic solutions such as sodium bicarbonate.

Most periventricular and intraventricular hemorrhages occur in the first 3 days of life. It is unusual for IVH to occur after the 5th day of life. The *clinical manifestations* include seizures, apnea, bradycardia, lethargy, coma, hypotension, metabolic acidosis, anemia not corrected by blood transfusion, bulging fontanel, and cutaneous mottling. Many infants with small hemorrhages (grade 1 or 2) are asymptomatic; those with larger hemorrhages (grade 4) often have a catastrophic event that rapidly progresses to shock and coma.

The *diagnosis* of IVH is confirmed and the severity graded by ultrasonographic examination through the anterior fontanel. Grade 1 IVH is confined to the germinal matrix; grade 2 is an extension of grade 1, with blood noted in the ventricle without ventricular enlargement; grade 3 is an extension of grade 2 with ventricular dilation; and grade 4 has blood in dilated ventricles and in the cerebral cortex, either contiguous with or distant from the ventricle. Grade 4 hemorrhage carries a poor prognosis, as does the development of periventricular small echolucent cystic lesions, with or without porencephalic cysts and posthemorrhagic hydrocephalus. Periventricular cysts often are noted after the resolution of echodense areas in the periventricular white matter and may correspond to the development of periventricular leukomalacia that may be a precursor to cerebral palsy. Extensive intraparenchymal echodensities represent hemorrhagic necrosis, are associated with a high mortality rate, and have a very poor neurodevelopmental prognosis for survivors.

*Treatment* of the acute hemorrhage involves standard supportive care, including ventilation for apnea and blood transfusion for shock. Posthemorrhagic hydrocephalus may be managed with serial daily lumbar punctures, external ventriculostomy tube, or permanent ventricular-peritoneal shunt. The latter often is delayed as a result of the very high protein content of the hemorrhagic ventricular fluid.

## HYPOXIC-ISCHEMIC ENCEPHALOPATHY
### (see also Asphyxia: Resuscitation)

Conditions known to reduce uteroplacental blood flow or to interfere with spontaneous respiration result in perinatal hypoxia, in lactic acidosis, and, if severe enough to reduce cardiac output or to cause cardiac arrest, in ischemia. The combination of the reduced availability of oxygen for the brain that occurs from hypoxia and the diminished or absent blood flow to the brain that occurs from ischemia results in reduced glucose for metabolism and in an accumulation of lactate that produces local tissue acidosis. After reperfusion, hypoxic-ischemic injury also may be complicated by cell necrosis and vascular endothelial edema, reducing blood flow distal to the involved vessel. Typically, hypoxic-ischemic encephalopathy in the term infant is characterized by cerebral edema, cortical necrosis, and involvement of the basal ganglia, whereas in the preterm infant it is characterized by periventricular leukomalacia. Both lesions may result in cortical atrophy, mental retardation, and spastic quadriplegia or diplegia.

The *clinical manifestations* and characteristic course of hypoxic-ischemic encephalopathy vary according to the severity of the injury (Table 6–30). Infants with severe stage 3 hypoxic-ischemic encephalopathy are usually hypotonic, although occasionally they appear hypertonic and hyperalert at birth. As cerebral edema develops, brain functions become affected in a descending order; cortical depression produces coma, whereas brain stem depression results in apnea. As cerebral edema progresses, refractory seizures begin between 12 and 24 hr after birth. At this time, the infant has no signs of spontaneous respirations, is hypotonic, and has diminished or absent deep tendon reflexes.

Survivors of stage 3 hypoxic-ischemic encephalopathy have a high incidence of seizures and serious neurodevelopmental handicaps. The prognosis of severe asphyxia also depends on other organ system injury (see Table 6–10). Another indicator of poor prognosis is time of onset of spontaneous respiration as estimated by Apgar score. Infants with Apgar scores of 0–3 at 10 min have a 20% mortality and a 5% incidence of cerebral palsy; if the score remains this low by 20 min, the mortality increases to 60% and the incidence of cerebral palsy rises to 57%.

TABLE 6–30. Hypoxic-Ischemic Encephalopathy in Term Infants

| Signs | Stage 1 | Stage 2 | Stage 3 |
|---|---|---|---|
| Level of consciousness | Hyperalert | Lethargic | Stuporous |
| Muscle tone | Normal | Hypotonic | Flaccid |
| Tendon reflexes/clonus | Hyperactive | Hyperactive | Absent |
| Moro reflex | Strong | Weak | Absent |
| Pupils | Mydriasis | Miosis | Unequal, poor light reflex |
| Seizures | None | Common | Decerebration |
| Electroencephalographic | Normal | Low voltage changing to seizure activity | Burst suppression to isoelectric |
| Duration | <24 hr if progresses, otherwise may remain normal | 24 hr to 14 days | Days to weeks |

Modified from Sarnat HB, Sarnat MS: Neonatal encephalopathy following fetal distress: A clinical and electroencephalographic study. Arch Neurol 33:696, 1976. Copyright, 1976, American Medical Association.

## NEONATAL HYPOTONIA

Decreased tone, floppiness, or hypotonia in the newborn infant may be transient and may resolve without future problems or may be due to serious permanent disease originating in the central nervous system, spinal cord, anterior horn cell, neuromuscular junction, or muscle. **Diseases of the brain** producing hypotonia may be due to hypoxic-ischemic encephalopathy, IVH, meningitis, metabolic toxins (organic acids, ammonia), or centrally acting drugs. The infant does not appear alert and has a weak cry, seizures, normal deep tendon reflexes, and an abnormal EEG.

**Spinal cord lesions** often are due to trauma or malformation and present in an alert-looking child with a strong cry, decreased deep tendon reflexes, reduced spontaneous movement below the cord lesions, and a normal EEG. *Anterior horn cell disease,* such as Werdnig-Hoffmann disease, is indicated by an alert-appearing infant with hypotonia, tongue fasciculations, absent deep tendon reflexes, reduced muscle mass, and a neurogenic electromyogram (EMG) and muscle biopsy.

**Neuromuscular junction disease,** such as neonatal transient myasthenia gravis (in a child born to a woman with myasthenia gravis), is indicated by an alert infant with a weak cry, ophthalmoplegia, ptosis, normal deep tendon reflexes, an abnormal EMG, and a positive physostigmine test.

**Muscle disease** may have onset prior to or immediately after birth and may be due to congenital muscular dystrophy, congenital myotonia, glycogen storage disease, mitochondrial defects, congenital lactic acidosis, or other myopathies. The infant with muscle disease is alert and has a good cry but also displays decreased muscle mass, contractures, myopathic EMG, characteristic muscle biopsy, and elevated serum creatine phosphokinase (CPK), with or without diminished deep tendon reflexes.

Respiratory difficulty is present in many of these conditions; the infants have difficulty swallowing secretions, which they may aspirate, or respiratory failure may occur as a result of weakness of the respiratory muscles. The evaluation of infants with hypotonia should include a family history of myasthenia gravis, myotonic dystrophy, muscular dystrophy, inheritable myopathies, and the existence of previous infants with metabolic diseases.

*Laboratory evaluation* depends on the history and physical examination and may include metabolic tests for organic acids and carnitine, muscle and head ultrasound, nerve conduction, EMG, serum CPK, physostigmine test, and muscle biopsy, with specific attention to electron microscopy. Chromosomal analysis also is helpful for diagnosing hypotonic infants with Prader-Willi syndrome, which has a deletion of the long arm of chromosome 15.

### References

Adamson S, Alessandi L, Badawi N, et al: Predictors of neonatal encephalopathy in full term infants. BMJ 311:598, 1995.

Bada HS, Korones SB, Perry EH, et al: Mean arterial blood pressure changes in premature infants and those at risk for intraventricular hemorrhage. J Pediatr 117:607, 1990.

Behrman RE, Kliegman RM, Arvin AM (eds): Nelson Textbook of Pediatrics. 15th ed. Philadelphia, WB Saunders, 1996, Chapters 84.7, 85, 543.5, 559, 563.

Sinha SK, D'Souza SW, Rivlin E, et al: Ischaemic brain lesions diagnosed at birth in preterm infants: Clinical events and developmental outcome. Arch Dis Child 65:1017, 1990.

Van Lieshout H, Jacobs J, Rotteveel J, et al: The prognostic value of the EEG in asphyxiated newborns. Acta Neurol Scand 91:203, 1995.

## OUTCOME AND FOLLOW-UP OF LOW-BIRTH-WEIGHT OR PREMATURE INFANTS

Most LBW infants survive neonatal illnesses without long-term sequelae. More than 90% of infants weighing more than 1500 g survive, whereas as many as 40% of infants weighing as little as 750 g survive. Between 10% and 25% of survivors have mild developmental problems, and 5–10% have severe developmental problems; the smallest at birth are at greatest risk. Long-term sequelae include retinopathy of prematurity with blindness, hearing loss, hydrocephalus, microcephaly, mental retardation, cerebral palsy (spastic diplegia), chronic pulmonary insufficiency (BPD), short bowel syndrome (post-NEC), and growth failure.

Many infants demonstrate transient neonatal hypotonia, which resolves by 8 mo "corrected age" and is not associated with future problems. However, it is difficult to diagnose cerebral palsy before this age, and all hypotonic infants should be considered at high risk until proven otherwise. Additionally, many VLBW infants have learning disabilities that may result in poor school performance or school failure. Although the intelligence quotient (IQ) often relates to adverse events affecting the central nervous system during the neonatal period, the intelligence of premature infants also is influenced directly by maternal socioeconomic status.

Most infants with cerebral palsy are not preterm infants or term infants with birth asphyxia. Perinatal causes account for fewer than 10% of older infants who have severe mental retardation. Furthermore, although 10–25% of VLBW infants demonstrate some handicap, the vast majority of these infants are functional and able to attend regular schools.

## PUBERTAL DEVELOPMENT IN SIZE OF FEMALE BREASTS

**Stage 1** The breasts are preadolescent. There is elevation of the papilla only.

**Stage 2** Breast bud stage. A small mound is formed by the elevation of the breast and papilla. The areolar diameter enlarges.

**Stage 3** There is further enlargement of breast and areola with no separation of their contours.

**Stage 4** There is a projection of the areola and papilla to form a secondary mound above the level of the breast.

**Stage 5** The breasts resemble those of a mature female as the areola has recessed to the general contour of the breast.

## PUBERTAL DEVELOPMENT OF FEMALE PUBIC HAIR
**Stage 1** There is no pubic hair.

**Stage 2** There is sparse growth of long, slightly pigmented, downy hair, straight or only slightly curled, primarily along the labia.

**Stage 3** The hair is considerably darker, coarser, and more curled. The hair spreads sparsely over the junction of the pubes.

**Stage 4** The hair, now adult in type, covers a smaller area than in the adult and does not extend onto the thighs.

**Stage 5** The hair is adult in quantity and type, with extension onto the thighs.

FIGURE 7–1. Typical progression of female pubertal development. (Adapted from Tanner JM: Growth at Adolescence, 2nd ed. Oxford, Blackwell Scientific Publications, 1962. Reprinted with permission of Ross Laboratories, Columbus, OH 43216, from Assessment of Pubertal Development, © 1986 Ross Laboratories.)

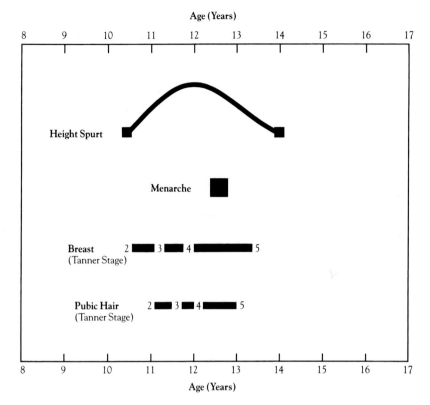

FIGURE 7–2. Sequence of pubertal events in the average American female. (Adapted from Brookman RR, Rauh JL, Morrison JA, et al: The Princeton Maturation Study, 1976, unpublished data for adolescents in Cincinnati, Ohio. Reprinted with permission of Ross Laboratories, Columbus, OH 43216, from Assessment of Pubertal Development, © 1986 Ross Laboratories.)

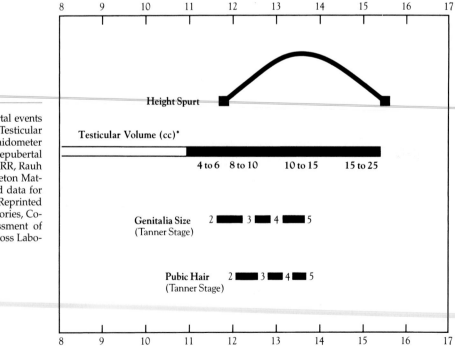

FIGURE 7–3. Sequence of pubertal events in the average American male. *Testicular volume less than 4 cc using orchidometer (Prader Beads) represents prepubertal stage. (Adapted from Brookman RR, Rauh JL, Morrison JA, et al: The Princeton Maturation Study, 1976, unpublished data for adolescents in Cincinnati, Ohio. Reprinted with permission of Ross Laboratories, Columbus, OH 43216, from Assessment of Pubertal Development, © 1986 Ross Laboratories.)

### PUBERTAL DEVELOPMENT IN SIZE OF MALE GENITALIA

**Stage 1** The penis, testes, and scrotum are of childhood size.

**Stage 2** There is enlargement of the scrotum and testes, but the penis usually does not enlarge. The scrotal skin reddens.

**Stage 3** There is further growth of the testes and scotum and enlargement of the penis, mainly in length.

**Stage 4** There is still further growth of the testes and scrotum and increased size of the penis, especially in breadth.

**Stage 5** The genitalia are adult in size and shape.

### PUBERTAL DEVELOPMENT OF MALE PUBIC HAIR
**Stage 1** There is no pubic hair.

**Stage 2** There is sparse growth of long, slightly pigmented, downy hair, straight or only slightly curled, primarily at the base of the penis.

**Stage 3** The hair is considerably darker, coarser, and more curled. The hair spreads sparsely over the junction of the pubes.

**Stage 4** The hair, now adult in type, covers a smaller area than in the adult and does not extend onto the thighs.

**Stage 5** The hair is adult in quantity and type, with extension onto the thighs.

FIGURE 7–4. Typical progression of male pubertal development. (Adapted from Tanner JM: Growth at Adolescence, 2nd ed. Oxford, Blackwell Scientific Publications, 1962. Reprinted with permission of Ross Laboratories, Columbus, OH 43216, from Assessment of Pubertal Development, © 1986 Ross Laboratories.)

ceded by the appearance of pubic hair at the base of the penis, followed by growth of axillary hair. Completion of testicular growth can occur any time between 13½ and 17 yr of age. Penile lengthening and widening begin normally between 10½ and 14½ yr of age; development of the penis reaches the SMR V stage between 12½ and 16½ yr of age. The growth spurt, as previously noted, is a relatively late event in males but normally is initiated from 10½ to 16 yr of age and is completed by 13½–17½ yr of age, depending on the individual. Growth does continue at a slower pace for several years after the spurt.

## Reproductive Endocrinology

Puberty is initiated following the release from inhibition of the gonadotropin-releasing hormone (GnRH) secreting medial-basal hypothalamic neurons. Decreased sensitivity to negative feedback by sex steroids results in pulsatile release of GnRH, which causes the pulsatile release of luteinizing hormone (LH) and follicle-stimulating hormone (FSH) from the pituitary gland. This occurs initially during sleep and, later in puberty, throughout wakefulness. Pituitary secretion of gonadotropins initiates gonadal growth and maturation. Ovarian estradiol and testicular testosterone affect breast and penis growth, respectively. Both hormones augment linear growth. Adrenarche (onset of pubic hair development) is mediated by adrenal androgens in females and testosterone in males.

## Precocious Puberty

See Chapter 17.

## Changes Associated with Physical Maturation

Sexual maturity rating is a marker of biologic maturity that can be related to both specific laboratory value changes and certain conditions (Tables 7–1 and 7–2). For example, higher hematocrit values in adolescent males than in adolescent females are due to greater androgenic stimulation of the bone marrow, not to loss through menstruation. Alkaline phosphatase levels in both males and females increase during puberty because there is rapid bone turnover, especially during the growth spurt. Wors-

TABLE 7–1.  Correlates of Female Pubertal Maturation

|  | Sexual Maturity Rating (Tanner Stage) | | | | |
|---|---|---|---|---|---|
|  | *1* | *2* | *3* | *4* | *5* |
| Hematocrit (%) | | | | | |
| White *mean* | 39.1 | 39.2 | 39.6 | 39.2 | 39.2 |
| *range* | 36.1–42.1 | 37.1–41.3 | 37.0–42.2 | 36.9–41.6 | 36.2–42.2 |
| Black *mean* | 37.3 | 38.9 | 39.0 | 38.4 | 38.7 |
| *range* | 34.6–39.9 | 35.7–42.1 | 35.2–42.6 | 34.9–42.8 | 35.9–41.5 |
| Alkaline phosphatase (IU/L) (serum) | | | | | |
| White *mean* | 70 | 89 | 76 | 33 | 38 |
| *range* | 51–90 | 49–134 | 36–108 | 16–60 | 23–76 |
| Black *mean* | 84 | 95 | 86 | 44 | 31 |
| *range* | 69–108 | 65–138 | 26–148 | 18–144 | 13–70 |
| Short female with growth potential | | + | | | |
| Short female with limited growth potential | | | | + | + + |
| Slipped capital femoral epiphysis | | + | + + | | |
| Acute worsening of scoliosis | | + | + + + | | |
| Osgood-Schlatter disease | | + | + | | |
| Oral contraceptive prescription | | | | + | + + |
| Diaphragm prescription | | | | | + |
| Acute worsening of straight back syndrome | | + | + + | + | |
| Acne vulgaris | | + | + + | + + | |
| Physiologic leukorrhea | | | + | | |
| Gonococcal vaginitis | + | | | | |
| Gonococcal cervicitis | | + | + | + | + |
| Regression of virginal breast hypertrophy | | | | | + |
| Timing of breast reduction or rhinoplasty | | | | | + |

Data from Copeland KC, Brookman RR, Rauh JL: Assessment of Pubertal Development. Columbus, Ross Laboratories, 1986; and Daniel WA: Growth at adolescence: Clinical correlates. Semin Adolesc Med 1:15–24, 1985.
+ = possible; + + = more likely than +; + + + = most likely.

TABLE 7–2.  Correlates of Male Pubertal Maturation

| | Sexual Maturity Rating (Tanner Stage) | | | | |
|---|---|---|---|---|---|
| | *1* | *2* | *3* | *4* | *5* |
| Hematocrit (%) | | | | | |
| White *mean* | 39.5 | 39.8 | 40.9 | 42.3 | 43.8 |
| *range* | 37.1–41.8 | 36.7–42.8 | 38.2–43.5 | 39.7–44.8 | 41.1–46.4 |
| Black *mean* | 37.7 | 38.4 | 39.7 | 41.1 | 42.7 |
| *range* | 35.2–40.2 | 36.0–40.9 | 37.3–42.0 | 38.3–43.8 | 39.6–45.9 |
| Alkaline phosphatase (IU/L) (serum) | | | | | |
| White *mean* | 72 | 77 | 101 | 75 | 58 |
| *range* | 54–110 | 42–106 | 53–141 | 41–158 | 21–120 |
| Black *mean* | 77 | 94 | 122 | 116 | 75 |
| *range* | 43–130 | 53–204 | 46–240 | 32–228 | 23–228 |
| Short male with growth potential | | + | | | |
| Short male with limited growth potential | | | | + | + + |
| Slipped capital femoral epiphysis | | + | + + | | |
| Acute worsening of scoliosis | | + | + + + | | |
| Osgood-Schlatter disease | | + | + | | |
| Acute worsening of straight back syndrome | | + | + + | + | |
| Gynecomastia | | + | + + | | |
| Acne vulgaris | | + | + + | + + | |
| Orchiopexy timing | + | | | | |
| Timing of rhinoplasty | | | | | + |

Data from Copeland KC, Brookman RR, Rauh JL: Assessment of Pubertal Development. Columbus, Ross Laboratories, 1986; and Daniel WA: Growth at adolescence: Clinical correlates. Semin Adolesc Med 1:15–24, 1985.
+ = possible; + + = more likely than +; + + + = most likely.

ening of scoliosis is especially common in adolescent females at the SMR II and III stages, during the growth spurt.

### Psychologic Growth and Development of Adolescents

See Table 7–3 and Chapter 1.

### References

Behrman RE, Kliegman RM, Arvin AM (eds): Nelson Textbook of Pediatrics, 15th ed. Philadelphia, WB Saunders, 1996, Chapter 16.
McAnarney ER, Kreipe RE, Orr DP, Comerci GD (eds): Textbook of Adolescent Medicine, Philadelphia, WB Saunders, 1992, Secs. 2 and 3.

## ADOLESCENT HEALTH CARE

### OVERVIEW

Adolescents present many challenges to health care providers because their physical symptoms often are related to psychosocial rather than biologic disorders. Nonetheless, adolescents frequently have chronic medical illnesses (Table 7–4), psychosocial problems, and causes of mortality specific for this age group (Table 7–5). Noncompliance with medical regimens is common. Limit testing, resistance to authority figures, and requests for confidentiality can complicate clinical care. Adolescents and their families usually respond well to health care that is based on respect, with attention to the adolescent's individual developmental needs (see Table 7–3).

Ideally, adolescent health care is provided in a setting where the self-conscious adolescent feels comfortable and welcome. Sufficient time and privacy should be allowed so that the adolescent and the clinician can adequately discuss sensitive topics, such as physical growth and development, medical and psychologic concerns, substance use, sexuality, and personal goals.

### The Interview

The successful interview of an adolescent resembles a conversation between two persons with a great many interests in common. Developmental principles are applied so that the interview of early adolescents is directed toward specific questions that concrete-thinking adolescents understand. The interview of older adolescents is directed toward open-ended questions that conceptually competent and rationalizing older adolescents understand (see Table 7–3, "Thinking").

TABLE 7–3.   Developmental Characteristics Related to Adolescent Health Care Needs

| Task | Characteristics | Health Care Needs |
|------|----------------|-------------------|
| **10–14 Year Olds** | | |
| Puberty | Wide variation in rapid physical changes; self-consciousness | Confidentiality; privacy |
| Independence | Ambivalence | Support for growing autonomy |
| Identity | Am I normal? peer group | Reassurance and positive attitude |
| Thinking | Concrete operational; egocentric; imaginary audience; focus on present | Emphasis on immediate consequences of actions |
| **15–17 Year Olds** | | |
| Puberty | Females ahead of males; chronic illness may delay puberty | Emotional support for adolescents who vary from "normal" |
| Independence | Limit testing; noncompliance; "experimental" behaviors; dating | Consistency; limit setting |
| Identity | Who am I?; introspection; global issues | Nonjudgmental acceptance; gentle reality testing |
| Thinking | Concrete → formal operational; personal fable; experiments with ideas | Problem solving; decision making; education |
| **18–21 Year Olds** | | |
| Puberty | Adult appearance; slow change | Minimal needs except in chronic illness |
| Independence | Ambivalence about real independence, separation/individuation from family | Support |
| Identity | Who am I with respect to others, sexuality, education, job? | Encouragement of identity allowing maximal growth |
| Thinking | Formal operational; contemplation of future; introspection; commitments | Approach as adult, but recognize that adolescent still changing |

## Confidentiality

There may be specific issues that adolescents prefer not to have discussed with their parents, but some issues cannot be kept confidential because of their serious adverse health consequences (e.g., suicidal ideation). Thus, it is important that clinicians caring for adolescents follow certain guidelines regarding confidentiality (Table 7–6) and discuss the issue of confidentiality at the outset.

Occasionally, an adolescent insists on absolute confidentiality. The clinician's decision whether or not to enter into this agreement depends on the reason for the request, the adolescent's developmental age, and whether this request is for one or several visits. Usually, one can see an adolescent once for exploration of a problem, but it is important to make it clear from the beginning, particularly for a younger adolescent who lives at home, that there may be a need to involve the parents.

## Legal Issues

Each adolescent health care provider should know the laws of the state and the policies of the institution in which the physician practices. The law confers certain rights on adolescents, allowing them to receive health services without parental permission (Table 7–7).

## Chaperons

It is often stated that a female chaperon should be present during the examination of a female by a male physician. In general, early adolescents may want a parent present, but middle adolescents and late adolescents usually prefer to be seen alone or with a chaperon of the same sex. A choice should be offered if one is available.

## WELL ADOLESCENT CARE

Guidelines for Adolescent Preventive Services (GAPS) and Bright Futures are recommendations for the organization and content of preventive services for individualized adolescent health supervision (Table 7–8). The focus of the visit is more on psychosocial evaluation than on physical examination.

TABLE 7–4.  Prevalence of Common Chronic Illnesses of Children and Adolescents

| Illness | Prevalence |
|---|---|
| *Pulmonary* | |
| Asthma | 3–5% |
| Cystic fibrosis | 1:2500 white, 1:17,000 black |
| *Neuromuscular* | |
| Cerebral palsy | 2:1000 |
| Mental retardation | 3% |
| Seizure disorder | 3:1000 |
| Auditory-visual defects | 10–30% |
| Traumatic paralysis | 2:1000 |
| Scoliosis | 5% males, 10% females |
| Migraine | 10% |
| *Endocrine–Nutrition* | |
| Diabetes mellitus | 2:1000 |
| Obesity | 10–25% |
| Anorexia nervosa | 0.5–1% |
| Bulimia | 1% (young adolescence), 5–10% 19–20 yr |
| Dysmenorrhea | 10% |
| Acne | 80% |

Modified from Gortmaker S, Sappenfield W: Chronic childhood disorders: Prevalence and impact. Pediatr Clin North Am 31:3, 1984.

### Early Adolescence (Ages 10–14 Yr)

Physical changes and behavior related to the physical changes of puberty are the major characteristics of this substage. The history focuses on an overall appraisal of the early adolescent's physical and psychosocial health.

### Middle Adolescence (Ages 15–17 Yr)

Independence and a global sense of identity are the major characteristics of this substage. The history focuses on the middle adolescent's interactions with family, school, and peers. High-risk behaviors as a result of experimentation are common.

### Late Adolescence (Ages 18–21 Yr)

Individuality and planning for the future are the major characteristics of this substage. The content

TABLE 7–5.  Leading Causes of Death in Adolescents

| Etiology | Comments |
|---|---|
| Accidents | Automobile, drug-related, guns, risk taking |
| Homicide | Drug-related, guns |
| Suicide | Males complete more often than females; guns, drugs |
| Cancer | Leukemia, lymphoma, Hodgkin disease, bone, central nervous system |

TABLE 7–6.  Guidelines for Confidentiality in Adolescent Health Care

Based on principles of adolescent growth and development (see Table 7–3)

Assumes a developing ability of the adolescent to take responsibility for his or her own health care that will culminate in full adult responsibility

Reflects mutual respect and trust between adolescent and health care provider

Extends to both the adolescent and the adolescent's parents (i.e., parental communication also is privileged)

Should be relative, with the scope determined by the individual situation

Should be discussed with patient and parents at the outset of adolescent health care

of the visit is similar to that of the visit with the middle adolescent, but greater emphasis is placed on the late adolescent's responsibility for his or her health. Transfer of health care to a physician who cares for adults and the details of that transfer may be discussed during this visit.

## PELVIC EXAMINATION

Comfort is maximized by using a padded examination table with stirrups, by keeping the examination room and instruments warm, and by performing the examination in an unhurried, but efficient manner. Control is afforded by allowing the patient to choose a supine or partially sitting position, by maintaining eye contact with the examiner, by being told the importance of the examination, by being informed of all maneuvers before they are performed, by being informed of normal

TABLE 7–7.  Legal Rights of Minors

Age of majority (≥18 yr of age in most states)

Exceptions in which health care services can be provided to a minor*:
  Emergency care (life-threatening condition, or condition in which a delay in treatment would significantly increase the likelihood of morbidity)
  Diagnosis and treatment of sexuality-related health care
  Diagnosis and treatment of drug-related health care
  Emancipated minors (physically and financially independent of family; Armed Forces; married; childbirth)
  Mature minors (able to comprehend the risks and benefits of evaluation and treatment)

All exceptions should be clearly documented in health record.

*Determined by individual state laws.

**TABLE 7–8.** Guidelines for Adolescent Health Supervision Visits

| Early Adolescent (10–14 Yr Old) | Middle Adolescent (15–17 Yr Old) | Late Adolescent (18–21 Yr Old) |
|---|---|---|
| *Health Guidance*<br>Parenting concerns<br>Normal development review<br>Discussing sexuality, drugs, etc.<br><br>Healthy lifestyle role-modeling<br>Positive qualities, strengths of adolescent | Parenting concerns<br>Normal development review<br>Discussing sexuality, drugs, and other topics<br>Healthy lifestyle role-modeling<br>Positive qualities, strengths of adolescent | Parents generally not interviewed unless specifically indicated |
| *Interview with Patient\**<br>Healthy lifestyles<br>Peer activities<br>High-risk behaviors (sexuality, drugs, smoking, violence, abuse)<br>Diet, fitness, exercise, body image<br>Safety (seat belt, helmet, guns)<br>Home and school<br>Self-esteem, positive qualities and personal strengths | Healthy lifestyles<br>Peer activities<br>High-risk behaviors (sexuality, drugs, smoking, violence, abuse)<br><br>Diet, fitness, exercise, body image<br><br>Safety (seat belt, helmet, guns)<br>Home and school<br>Self-esteem, positive qualities and personal strengths | Healthy lifestyles<br>Peer activities<br>High-risk behaviors (sexuality, drugs, smoking, violence, abuse)<br><br>Diet, fitness, exercise, body image<br><br>Safety (seat belt, helmet, guns)<br>Home and school<br>Self-esteem, positive qualities and personal strengths |
| *Physical examination†*<br>(patient alone, chaperon may be indicated for younger patients requiring pelvic examination):<br>Height/weight plotted on curve<br>Vision/hearing screening<br>Blood pressure<br>Tanner stage/external genital examination<br>Gynecomastia/breast asymmetry<br>Scoliosis screen<br>Skinfold thickness, acne<br>Self-examination of breast/testes, if mature<br>Pelvic examination if menstrual problem or sexually active | Height/weight plotted on curve<br>Vision/hearing screening<br>Blood pressure<br>Tanner stage/external genital examination<br>Gynecomastia<br>Scoliosis screen<br>Skinfold thickness, acne<br>Self-examination of breast/testes<br>Pelvic examination if menstrual problem or sexually active | Height/weight<br>Vision/hearing screening<br>Blood pressure<br>Tanner stage/external genital examination<br>Periodontal health<br>Skinfold thickness<br><br>Self-examination of breasts/testes<br>Pelvic examination |
| *Screening*<br>Hyperlipidemia (if family history)<br>Hypertension<br>Eating disorders, obesity<br>Tobacco, alcohol and drug use<br>Sexual behavior, if sexually active<br>STDs, including HIV if high-risk<br>Urine for WBCs (males)<br>Cervical cancer (Pap smear)<br>Abuse (physical sexual, emotional)<br>Depression/suicide<br>Learning problems<br>Tuberculin if indicated | Hypertension<br>Eating disorders, obesity<br>Tobacco, alcohol and drug use<br>Sexual behavior, if sexually active<br>STDs, including HIV if high-risk<br>Urine for WBCs (males)<br>Cervical cancer (Pap smear)<br>Abuse (physical, sexual, emotional)<br>Depression/suicide<br>Learning problems<br>Tuberculin if indicated | Hyperlipidemia (once in decade)<br>Hypertension<br>Eating disorders, obesity<br>Tobacco, alcohol and drug use<br>Sexual behavior; if sexually active<br>STDS, including HIV if high-risk<br>Urine for WBCs (males)<br>Cervical cancer (Pap smear)<br>Abuse (physical, sexual, emotional)<br>Depression/suicide<br>Learning problems<br>Tuberculin if indicated |
| *Immunizations*<br>Check immunization status<br><br><br>Mumps, measles vaccine if none previously<br>Rubella vaccine for nonimmune females if not pregnant<br>Hepatitis B vaccine, if not done previously | Check immunization status<br>Tetanus-diphtheria (Td) booster q 10 years<br>Mumps, measles vaccine if none previously<br>Rubella vaccine for nonimmune females if not pregnant<br>Hepatitis B vaccine, if not done previously | Check immunization status<br>Td booster q 10 years<br><br>Mumps, measles vaccine if none previously<br>Rubella vaccine for nonimmune females if not pregnant<br>Hepatitis B vaccine, if not done previously |

Adapted with permission from American Academy of Pediatrics: Guidelines for Health Supervision II. Elk Grove Village, IL, American Academy of Pediatrics, 1988.

Data from Green M (ed): Bright Futures: Guidelines for Health Supervision of Infants, Children and Adolescents. Arlington, VA, National Center for Education in Maternal and Child Health, 1994; and Elster AB, Kuznets NJ: AMA Guidelines for Adolescent Preventive Services: Recommendations and Rationale. Baltimore, Williams & Wilkins, 1994.

*Adolescents should be interviewed alone during talks about high-risk behaviors.

†Only three "routine" physical examinations are recommended during adolescence to allow time to address psychosocial issues.

HIV = human immunodeficiency virus; Pap = Papanicolaou; STD = sexually transmitted disease; WBC = white blood cell.

and abnormal findings, and by being encouraged to ask questions before, during, or after the examination.

Inspection of the genitalia includes evaluation of the pubic hair, labia majora and minora, clitoris, urethra, and hymenal ring. Bimanual palpation of the cervix, uterus, fallopian tubes, and ovaries should follow the speculum examination because the lubricant used interferes with samples obtained for microscopic and microbiologic evaluation. A Huffman or Pedersen speculum should be used with young virginal females; alternatively, a rectal examination can provide valuable information, since all of the midline internal genitalia are immediately anterior to the rectal wall. A nonvirginal introitus frequently admits a small to medium-sized adult speculum. Visualization of the vaginal walls and cervical os allows for the collection of appropriate specimens for Papanicolaou (Pap) smear, culture, Gram stain, and saline wet mount.

## References

American Academy of Pediatrics: Guidelines for Health Supervision: II. Elk Grove Village, IL, American Academy of Pediatrics, 1988.

Behrman RE, Kliegman RM, Arvin AM (eds): Nelson Textbook of Pediatrics, 15th ed. Philadelphia, WB Saunders, 1996, Chapter 15.

English A: Legal aspects of care. In McAnarney ER, Kreipe RE, Orr DP, Comerci GD (eds): Textbook of Adolescent Medicine. Philadelphia, WB Saunders, 1992, pp 164–171.

MacFarlane A, McPherson A: Primary health care and adolescence. BMJ 311:825, 1995.

# NORMAL VARIANTS OF PUBERTY

## BREAST ASYMMETRY

In normal females, one breast may develop before or more rapidly than the other, resulting in asymmetry. This can still be a source of concern for the early adolescent. The patient should be reassured that the asymmetry should become less noticeable as maturation progresses. The physical examination reveals no masses or discharge, although tenderness can occur in the breast-bud stage. A true breast mass is most commonly a benign fibroadenoma or cyst; cancer is exceedingly rare at this age (Table 7–9). For imaging, ultrasound is preferred to mammography because of the density of adolescent breast tissue.

## PHYSIOLOGIC LEUKORRHEA

Endogenous estrogen production stimulates glandular proliferation of the endometrium, often re-

**TABLE 7–9.** Etiology of Breast Masses in Adolescents

Classic or juvenile fibroadenoma (70%)
Abscess
Fibrocystic breast disease
Fat necrosis
Lipoma
Intraductal papilloma
Cystosarcoma phylloides (low-grade malignancy)
Carcinoma (very rare)

sulting in a vaginal discharge that usually occurs just prior to menarche, in SMR stage III. The discharge usually is scant, thin, mucoid, clear to milky, and neither pruritic nor foul-smelling. Characteristics other than these require further evaluation. Physiologic leukorrhea is associated with a few white blood cells and microscopic evidence of the maturational effect of estrogen on the vaginal epithelium. Pathogens are not present in cultures. Physical examination reveals only the changes of midpuberty, without evidence of introital trauma or inflammation. Rubbing due to self-consciousness or masturbation may result in mild erythema, but abrasions or tears should raise concern about sexual abuse. Unless specifically indicated, pelvic examination generally is not necessary.

## IRREGULAR MENSES

In the year following menarche, the menses often are irregular. Both the interval between periods and the duration of periods may vary as the hypothalamic-pituitary-ovarian system matures. On the average, it takes 18 mo to complete the first 12 menstrual periods. During most of that time, most females are infertile because of anovulation in more than half of the periods. Anovulatory periods often are irregular, with prolonged heavy bleeding but without midcycle or menstrual pain. However, some adolescents ovulate with their first cycle, as indicated by the fact that pregnancy can occur before menarche. The irregularity of early postmenarchal periods can be inconvenient, but treatment with birth control pills should be avoided. Reassurance, education about menstrual physiology, and awaiting more regular periods usually suffice.

## GYNECOMASTIA

Breast enlargement in the male, (gynecomastia), is usually a benign, self-limited condition, noted in

**TABLE 7–10.  Etiology of Gynecomastia**

Idiopathic
Hypogonadism (primary or secondary)
Liver disease
Renal disease
Hyperthyroidism
Neoplasms
   Adrenal
   Ectopic human chorionic gonadotropin (hCG) secreting
   Testicular
Drugs
   Antiandrogens
   Antibiotics (isoniazid, ketoconazole, metronidazole)
   Antacids ($H_2$ blockers)
   Cancer chemotherapy (especially alkylating agents)
   Cardiovascular drugs
   Drugs of abuse
      Alcohol
      Amphetamines
      Heroin
      Marijuana
   Hormones (female sex)
   Psychoactive agents (diazepam, phenothiazines, tricyclics)

50–60% of boys during early adolescence. Gynecomastia is often idiopathic but may be noted in various conditions (Table 7–10). Typical findings include the appearance of a 1–3 cm, round, freely mobile, often tender, firm mass immediately beneath the areola during SMR stage III. Large, hard or fixed enlargements and masses associated with any nipple discharge warrant further investigation. Reassurance that the condition is self-limited is usually the only treatment required. If the condition worsens and is associated with psychologic morbidity, pharmacologic treatment with bromocriptine may be used. Surgical treatment with reduction mammoplasty can be helpful with massive hypertrophy.

## SHORT STATURE (CONSTITUTIONALLY DELAYED PUBERTY)

See Chapter 17.

### References

Behrman RE, Kliegman RM, Arvin AM (eds): Nelson Textbook of Pediatrics, 15th ed. Philadelphia, WB Saunders, 1996, Chapters 516, 517.
Glass AR: Gynecomastia. Endocrinol Metab Clin North Am 23:825, 1994.
Kulin HE, Müller J: The biological aspects of puberty. Pediatr Rev 17:75, 1996.
Simmons PS: Diagnostic considerations in breast disorders of children and adolescents. Obstet Gynecol Clin North Am 19:91, 1992.

## PROBLEMS RELATED TO ADOLESCENT SEXUALITY

### MENSTRUAL DISORDERS

Lack of menstrual periods (*amenorrhea*) and irregularity of menstrual periods are among the most common complaints of early adolescents. As regular ovulatory cycles become established, painful menstruation (*dysmenorrhea*) becomes more frequent. *Dysfunctional uterine bleeding* is another common menstrual disorder.

#### Amenorrhea

*Primary amenorrhea* refers to a lack of menstruation by age 16 yr in the presence of breast development or by age 14 yr in the absence of breast development (most females have menarche within 2 yr of breast development). *Secondary amenorrhea* refers to the cessation of previously regular menstruation for more than 3 consecutive months any time after menarche. Within the first year after menarche, such irregularity of menses should be considered physiologic.

Amenorrhea may be due to functional or anatomic abnormalities of the hypothalamus, pituitary, ovary, or uterus, and it may result in inadequate hormonal stimulation of the endometrium, unresponsiveness of the endometrium to hormones, or obstruction to the flow of tissue and blood during endometrial shedding. The *differential diagnosis* of primary or secondary amenorrhea is broad (Tables 7–11 and 7–12). Physiologic immaturity, stress, exercise, and abnormal dietary patterns are usually the cause of amenorrhea. Secondary amenorrhea often is due to pregnancy.

The history and physical examination (Tables 7–13 and 7–14) provide the most valuable information and should guide the laboratory evaluation of any abnormality of vaginal bleeding, including amenorrhea. Thus, females with short stature and other stigmata of *Turner syndrome* (gonadal dysgenesis) should undergo chromosomal analysis, whereas those with signs of hypothyroidism, adrenogenital syndrome, or diabetes should be evaluated with specific tests for these diseases. If the patient with amenorrhea has normal secondary sex characteristics but no evidence of androgen excess (e.g., adrenogenital syndrome), pregnancy, or metabolic (e.g., thyroid disease) or uterine (imperforate hymen) pathology, the presence or absence of estrogen effect should be determined.

Superficial vaginal epithelial cells, representing greater than 10% of the cells on Pap smear obtained from the lateral vaginal wall, indicate the presence

TABLE 7–11. Differential Diagnosis of Primary Amenorrhea

| Etiology | History | Breast Development | Female Genitalia | Karyotype | Follicle-Stimulating Hormone | Prolactin | Thyroid |
|---|---|---|---|---|---|---|---|
| **Hypothalamic** | | | | | | | |
| Physiologic delay | Positive family history of delayed puberty | Delayed | Normal | Normal (46,XX) | Low/normal | Normal | Normal |
| Nutritional | History of dietary restriction, severe systemic diseases, or malabsorption | Delayed | Normal | Normal | Low/normal | Normal | Normal |
| Gonadotropin-releasing hormone (GnRH) deficiency | Anosmia (Kallmann syndrome); acquired or congenital anatomic lesions | Delayed | Normal | Normal | Low/normal | Normal | Normal |
| **Pituitary** | | | | | | | |
| Hypopituitarism | Other signs and symptoms of hypopituitarism | Variable | Normal | Normal | Low | Normal | Low/normal |
| **Gonadal** | | | | | | | |
| Chromosomally incompetent ovarian failure | Wide range of phenotypic expression of Turner syndrome | Delayed | Normal | 45,XO or mosaic | High | Normal | Normal |
| Chromosomally competent ovarian failure | May be congenital or acquired | Delayed | Small uterus | Normal | High | Normal | Normal |
| **Uterine** | | | | | | | |
| Congenital absence of uterus (Rokitansky syndrome) | May have associated renal anomalies | Normal | Absent uterus + varying degrees of vaginal dysgenesis | Normal | Normal | Normal | Normal |
| **Vaginal** | | | | | | | |
| Imperforate hymen | May have abdominal pain, pelvic, "mass" | Normal | Bulging hymen | Normal | Normal | Normal | Normal |
| **Biosynthetic/Hormone Defects** | | | | | | | |
| Hypothyroidism | May simulate pituitary tumor | Delayed | Normal | Normal | Low/normal | High | Low |
| Hyperprolactinemia | May not have galactorrhea | Normal | Normal | Normal | Low/normal | High | Normal |
| Hypercortisolism | Other signs and symptoms of Cushing syndrome | Normal | Normal | Normal | Low/normal | Normal | Normal |
| Androgen excess (polycystic ovarian disease) | Hirsutism, virilization | Minimal | Normal | Normal | LH high | Normal | Normal |
| Androgen resistance (testicular feminization) | Male pseudohermaphroditism | Normal | Absent uterus, shallow vagina, no pubic hair | 46,XY | Low/normal | Normal | Normal |

LH = luteinizing hormone.

**TABLE 7–12.** Differential Diagnosis of Secondary Amenorrhea

| Etiology | History | Physical Examination | Galactorrhea | Pelvic Examination | Prolactin | Thyroid | Response to Progesterone Challenge | Gonadotropins |
|---|---|---|---|---|---|---|---|---|
| **Hypothalamic** | | | | | | | | |
| Weight loss | Simple dieting; anorexia nervosa | Low weight, blood pressure, pulse, temperature | No | Normal | Normal | Normal | Bleeding | Low/normal |
| Weight gain | Overeating | Moderate to severe obesity | No | Normal | Normal | Normal | Bleeding | Low/normal |
| Exercise | Running >25 miles/wk, ballet | Physically healthy if weight normal | No | Normal | Normal | Normal | Bleeding | Low/normal |
| Stress | Family, school, peer problems | Normal | No | Normal | Normal | Normal | Bleeding | Low/normal |
| Chronic illness | Severe systemic illness | Signs of chronic illness | No | Normal | Normal | Normal | Bleeding | Low/normal |
| Idiopathic | Negative | Normal | No | Normal | Normal | Normal | Bleeding | Low/normal |
| Medication | Phenothiazines; oral contraceptive | No distinctive physical findings | Often | Normal | Normal/high | Normal | Bleeding | Low/normal |
| **Pituitary** | | | | | | | | |
| Destructive lesions | Symptoms of hypopituitarism | Signs of pituitary failure or tumor | No | Normal | Normal/high | Normal/low | No Bleeding | Low |
| **Gonadal** | | | | | | | | |
| Ovarian failure | Radiation, surgery | Signs of estrogen deficiency | No | Normal | Normal | Normal | No bleeding | High FSH |
| Polycystic ovarian disease | May have oligomenorrhea | Obesity, hirsutism and virilization | No | Enlarged ovaries | Normal | Normal | Bleeding | High LH |
| **Uterine** | | | | | | | | |
| Synechiae (Asherman syndrome) | Uterine curettage, endometritis | Normal | No | Normal | Normal | Normal | No bleeding | Normal |
| **Hormonal/Metabolic** | | | | | | | | |
| Pregnancy | Highly variable, may deny sexual intercourse | Breast engorgement, weight gain | No | Enlarged uterus; soft, cyanotic cervix | Normal | Normal | No bleeding | Low/normal |
| Hyperprolectinemia | Medications; may be negative | Usually normal physical examination | Often | Normal | High | High | Bleeding | Low/normal |
| Androgen excess | Concerns about virilization | Hirsutism, virilization | No | Clitoromegaly | Normal | Normal | Bleeding | Low/normal |
| Hypothyroidism | Symptoms of ↓ thyroid | May be normal | Often | Normal | Normal/high | Normal/high | Bleeding | Low/normal |
| Hypercortisolism | Symptoms of ↑ cortisol | Signs of Cushing syndrome | Often | Normal | Normal/high | Normal/high | Bleeding | Low/normal |

FSH = follicle-stimulating hormone; LH = luteinizing hormone.

TABLE 7–13.  History and Review of Systems in Abnormal Vaginal Bleeding

**History**

| | |
|---|---|
| Bleeding | How long; how much (number of pads or tampons per day); color (bright red or brown): presence of clots or tissue; cramping; bleeding from other sites (nose, gingiva, after tooth extraction or surgery); relationship to intercourse? |
| Menstrual | Age of menarche; frequency, duration, amount; last menstrual period (dates of last three episodes of bleeding); dysmenorrhea, spotting, mid-cycle pain? |
| Sexual | Sexual activity; sexual abuse; masturbation with foreign objects; sexually transmitted diseases; pelvic surgery; previous pregnancies, abortions (spontaneous or terminated pregnancies), dyspareunia; sharp pain during intercourse? |
| Contraceptive use | What kind, how often, any used since last period; missed contraceptive pills? |
| Medications | All prescription or over-the-counter medications, drug abuse |
| Illnesses | Recent, chronic, bleeding disorders, cancers? |
| Family | Bleeding disorders, diethylstilbestrol (DES) exposure, thyroid disease? |
| Diet | Anorexia, bulimia, crash diets, diet medications? |
| Exercise | Amount, frequency, competition, kind? |

**Review of Systems**

| | |
|---|---|
| General | Fatigue, weight loss, fever, chills, anorexia |
| Skin | Dry, ecchymosis, petechiae, acne |
| Hair | Dry, hair loss, brittle, hirsutism |
| Head/ENT | Visual changes, nosebleeds, gingival bleeding with flossing or brushing |
| Neck | Swelling or lumps, shoulder pain |
| Breasts | Soreness, enlargement, galactorrhea |
| Abdominal | Tenderness, swelling, waistband tight, pain |
| Genitourinary | Bleeding, dysuria, vaginal discharge, foreign body, trauma, abuse, hematuria, frequency, urgency |
| Gastrointestinal | Nausea, vomiting, diarrhea, rectal bleeding, mucus, cramps, tenesmus |
| CNS | Syncope or presyncope, headaches, fatigue |
| Endocrine | Weight change, nervousness, irritability, change in school performance, heat or cold intolerance |

From Anderson MM, Irwin CE, Snyder DL: Abnormal vaginal bleeding in adolescents. Pediatr Ann 15:697–707, 1986.
CNS = central nervous system; ENT = ear–nose–throat.

of estrogen, as does ferning of cervical mucus. Withdrawal bleeding 1–7 days after administration of medroxyprogesterone, 10 mg orally twice a day for 5 days, indicates estrogen priming of the endometrium and an intact hypothalamic-pituitary-ovarian axis (positive progesterone challenge). Withdrawal bleeding is reassuring and indicates that regular menses should begin soon. Absence of estrogen effect requires further evaluation and determination of LH/FSH levels. In the absence of estrogen effects, low levels of LH/FSH indicate hypothalamic-pituitary pathology, such as a prolactin-secreting tumor. High gonadotropin levels indicate primary ovarian failure, such as in Turner syndrome.

### Dysfunctional Uterine Bleeding

Normal periods are 28 ± 7 days apart, measured from the first day of one to the first day of the next period. Flow is usually not more than 7 days. Excessive flow may be quantified by the use of more than six pads or 10 tampons per day for more than 8 days; however, the frequency of pad change varies greatly among women. Excessive bleeding may cause iron-deficiency anemia and, rarely, hypovolemia.

Dysfunctional uterine bleeding, one of the few conditions in adolescent health care that is a diagnosis by exclusion, is any abnormal pattern of endometrial shedding not caused by an underlying pathologic process (Table 7–15). Anovulation occurs in 75% of cases. Without production of progesterone by the corpus luteum, unopposed estrogen production can result in two abnormal patterns of bleeding: mild breakthrough bleeding due to insufficient estrogen levels to support a proliferated endometrium, and heavy, prolonged, sometimes life-threatening menses resulting from lack of sufficient progesterone to stop menstrual flow by myometrial and vascular contractions. Once regular ovulatory cycles have continued for 1 yr, irregular bleeding usually indicates an organic abnormality.

Because the diagnosis of dysfunctional uterine bleeding can be made only after excluding underlying pathology (Table 7–16), one must be cautious in evaluating and treating this condition. A thor-

TABLE 7–14.  Physical Examination in the Evaluation of Abnormal Vaginal Bleeding

**General Physical Examination**

| | |
|---|---|
| Growth | Height, weight, obesity, overly thin |
| Vital signs | Heart rate and blood pressure changes with position, temperature |
| Skin | Ecchymosis, petechiae, pigmentation, pallor, sweating, capillary refill, striae, acne |
| Hair | Texture, amount, distribution, hirsutism, balding, low hair line |
| Eyes | Lid lag, proptosis, funduscopic examination (hemorrhages), visual fields |
| Nose/throat | Mucous membrane bleeding, petechiae, pallor |
| Neck | Enlarged thyroid, nodes, web neck |
| Breasts | Galactorrhea, Tanner stage |
| Cardiovascular | |
|   Heart | Heart rate, murmurs |
|   Pulses | Presence in extremities |
| Abdomen | Tenderness, masses, organomegaly, rebound |
| Rectal | Tone, blood, masses, fissures |
| Neurologic | Deep tendon reflexes, mental status, cranial nerves, visual fields |
| Nodes | Generalized lymphadenopathy |

**Pelvic Examination**

| | |
|---|---|
| External examination | Tanner stage; male vs. female hair pattern; clitoromegaly, discharge, condyloma, lacerations, erythema |
| Speculum examination | |
|   Vagina | Erythema, punctate hemorrhages, discharge; rotate speculum to look for lacerations, masses, condyloma |
|   Cervix | Color, discharge, punctate hemorrhages, tissue, erosion, friability, condyloma, polyps, abnormal shape |
| Bimanual examination | Palpate vaginal wall for masses or lacerations; cervical motion tenderness; softening of the cervix or uterocervical junction; adnexal tenderness or masses; size and shape of ovaries; uterine size, shape, and position; uterine tenderness |
| Laboratory evaluation | Cervical cultures for gonorrhea and *Chlamydia,* cervical smear for Gram stain, vaginal smears for potassium hydroxide (yeast, whiff test), saline (clue cells, *Trichomonas*), vaginal pH, cervical cytology (Papanicolaou [Pap] smear) |

From Anderson MM, Irwin CE, Snyder DL: Abnormal vaginal bleeding in adolescents. Pediatr Ann 15:697–707, 1986.

ough history and physical examination with pelvic examination should be combined with laboratory evaluation that minimally includes testing for pregnancy, genital infections, and thyroid and coagulation dysfunction and a complete blood count.

Approximately 20% of cases of adolescent menorrhagia are caused by coagulation disorders, with an additional 10% related to other types of pathology. If underlying pathology is discovered, treatment should be directed at the primary disorder as well as at the secondary menstrual dysfunction. Unpredictable, heavy, and prolonged menses may seriously impair an adolescent's ability to attend school and function socially. Thus, the health care provider also must attend to these psychosocial dysfunctions and provide appropriate treatment.

TABLE 7–15.  Abnormal Patterns of Menstrual Flow

| Pattern | Regularity of Cycles | Interval Between Cycles | Flow | | |
|---|---|---|---|---|---|
| | | | *Amount* | *Duration* | *Timing* |
| Amenorrhea | — | — | Absent >3 months | — | — |
| Hypomenorrhea | Regular | 28 ± 7 days | Decreased | Normal | Normal |
| Menorrhagia (hypermenorrhea) | Regular | 28 ± 7 days | Increased | Normal | Normal |
| Metrorrhagia (spotting) | Irregular | Normal | Decreased | Decreased | Intermenstrual as well as menstrual |
| Menometrorrhagia | Irregular | Decreased | Increased | Increased | Variable |
| Oligomenorrhea | Regular | >35 days | Decreased | Decreased | Variable |
| Polymenorrhea | Regular | <21 days | Decreased | Decreased | Variable |

TABLE 7–16.  Differential Diagnosis of Abnormal Uterine Bleeding

| Etiology | History | Pelvic Examination | Pregnancy Test | Coagulation Tests | Cervical Cultures |
|---|---|---|---|---|---|
| **Complications of Pregnancy** | | | | | |
| Threatened abortion | Abdominal cramps | Enlarged uterus | Positive | Normal | Negative |
| Ectopic pregnancy | Abdominal pain; syncope | Enlarged adnexa | Positive | Normal | Negative |
| **Systemic Conditions** | | | | | |
| Coagulation defects | | | | | |
| Secondary to liver disease | Chronic or severe acute liver disease | Normal | Negative | Abnormal | Negative |
| Secondary to blood dyscrasia | Leukemia | Normal | Negative | Thrombocytopenia | Negative |
| Primary coagulopathy | von Willebrand disease | Normal | Negative | Abnormal bleeding time | Negative |
| Hypothyroidism | Symptoms of ↓ thyroid; may be normal | Normal | Negative | Normal | Negative |
| Hypercortisolism or hypocortisolism | Symptoms of ↑ or ↓ cortisol | Normal | Negative | Normal | Negative |
| **Medications** | | | | | |
| Birth control pills | Low-dose estrogen; noncompliance | Normal | Negative | Normal | Negative |
| Aspirin | Aspirin ingestion | Normal | Negative | Abnormal bleeding time | Negative |
| **Pelvic Lesions** | | | | | |
| Ovarian cyst | Abdominal pain | Tender, enlarged ovary | Negative | Normal | Negative |
| Endometriosis | Dysmenorrhea | Tender uterus | Negative | Normal | May be + for STD |
| Foreign body (intrauterine device [IUD], retained tampon) | May have forgotton to remove tampon | Signs of foreign body | Negative | Abnormal if associated with toxic shock syndrome | May be + for *Staphylococcus aureus* |
| Cervicitis | Sexually transmitted disease (STD) contact | Severe inflammation | Negative | Normal | May be + for STD |
| Trauma | External genitalia may be normal | Signs of trauma | Negative | Normal | Negative |
| Diethylstilbestrol (DES) exposure | Maternal DES during pregnancy | Vaginal adenosis | Negative | Normal | Negative |
| Tumor | Often asymptomatic | Mass | Negative | Normal | Negative |
| **Hypothalamic** | | | | | |
| Anovulatory cycles | Symptoms related to anovulation | Normal | Negative | Normal | Negative |
| Stress | Family, school, peer problems; abnormal body image | Normal | Negative | Normal | Negative |

*Treatment* of dysfunctional uterine bleeding is essential if menstrual periods are heavy. The aim is to normalize the imbalance between estrogen and progesterone. Birth control pills are effective and have a rapid onset. In rare instances of uncontrollable bleeding, uterine curettage may be indicated. In the presence of a bleeding disorder (e.g., von Willebrand disease), estrogen may raise the level of factor VIII. Treatment with iron is also important for adolescents with continued excessive blood loss. Tranexamic acid, an antifibrinolytic agent, may be of value in patients with menorrhagia.

## Dysmenorrhea

Dysmenorrhea refers to cramping lower abdominal pains during the first 1–3 days of flow in a men-

TABLE 7–17.   Treatment of Primary Dysmenorrhea

| Severity | Characteristics | Treatment |
| --- | --- | --- |
| Mild | Mild cramps<br>Little interference with daily activities<br>No systemic symptoms | Ibuprofen, 400 mg PO q.i.d.<br>*or*<br>Naproxen sodium, 550 mg PO, then 275 mg q.i.d. treatment most effective if initiated at least 24 hr before menses begin |
| Moderate | Moderate cramps<br>Interference with daily activities<br>No systemic symptoms | Treatment of mild dysmenorrhea,<br>*and*<br>Cyclic combination oral contraceptive pills |
| Severe | Severe cramps<br>Restriction of activities for several days each mo<br>Systemic symptoms | Treatment for moderate dysmenorrhea<br>*and*<br>Re-evaluation for organic pathology, such as benign tumors, endometriosis, or anatomic abnormalities |

strual period. Painful uterine cramps are experienced by 65% of adolescent girls and are a leading cause of short-term school absenteeism among female students. **Secondary dysmenorrhea** is pain due to pelvic pathology (such as endometriosis, intrauterine device use, benign tumors, or anatomic abnormalities). **Primary dysmenorrhea** is more common and is not associated with a specific underlying structural problem. These two types of dysmenorrhea usually can be distinguished by history and physical examination (including pelvic examination) without the need for surgical or laboratory evaluation.

The *treatment* of secondary dysmenorrhea is directed at the underlying pathology. **Endometriosis**, which is becoming increasingly recognized as a common cause of secondary dysmenorrhea, requires management with birth control pills or danazol. Primary dysmenorrhea is associated with myometrial contractions related to local prostaglandin activity in the early phases of shedding of the endometrium. Because prostaglandin production is related to progesterone produced by the corpus luteum after ovulation, painful menstruation is associated with ovulatory cycles. Effective medical therapy is directed primarily at inhibiting the synthesis or action of prostaglandins (Table 7–17). Hormonal regulation with oral contraceptive pills can be tried if these approaches are not beneficial. Failure to respond to these regimens increases the likelihood of unrecognized pelvic pathology.

## References

Behrman RE, Kliegman RM, Arvin AM (eds): Nelson Textbook of Pediatrics, 15th ed. Philadelphia, WB Saunders, 1996, Chapter 111.

Hertweck SP: Dysfunctional uterine bleeding. Obstet Gynecol Clin North Am 19:129, 1992.
Emans SJH, Goldstein DP: Pediatrics and Adolescent Gynecology, 3rd ed. Boston, Little, Brown & Co, 1990.
Rosenfield RB, Barnes RB: Menstrual disorders in adolescence. Endocrinol Metab Clin North Am 22:491, 1993.

## PREGNANCY

Approximately 40% of 15 yr olds and 66% of 17-yr-olds in America have had sexual intercourse, resulting in 75 pregnancies per 1000 girls 15 to 17 yr old annually. Most adolescent pregnancies occur out of wedlock; about half end in abortion. Adolescent pregnancy is associated with premature birth, increased postneonatal mortality, child abuse, subsequent maternal unemployment, and poor maternal educational achievement. Most adolescents should not be considered high biologic risks, and in the presence of appropriate prenatal care, good nutrition, and social support and the absence of sexually transmitted diseases (STDs) the pregnant adolescent should have the same chance of delivering a healthy full-term infant compared with adult women of similar sociodemographic background.

### Diagnosis

Adolescent pregnancy most commonly is associated with secondary amenorrhea. Loss of menstrual periods in the adolescent should be presumed to be due to pregnancy until proven otherwise because adolescent pregnancy is prevalent and because frequently the pregnant adolescent delays seeking a diagnosis until several periods have been missed. However, serious consequences may result from a delayed diagnosis.

Pregnant girls in early adolescence often are seen with other symptoms, such as vomiting, vague pains, or deteriorating behavior. They may report normal periods. Pregnancy during early adolescence may result from rape or incest, and the patient is more likely to deny ever having had intercourse than older adolescents. Because of the varied presentations of adolescent pregnancy, a thorough menstrual history should be obtained in all menstruating females. Sensitive urine tests allow for diagnosis approximately 7–10 days after conception.

### Decision About Pregnancy

If pregnancy is confirmed, dating of the gestation should be done immediately. Most clinicians will not consider abortion after 20–24 wk of gestation. Pregnancy options include continuation of the pregnancy (the patient either keeps the infant or surrenders it for adoption) and termination of the pregnancy. During early adolescence, the clinician should urge the girl to involve the family in the decision because the adolescent may not be mature enough to make the decision alone.

**Continuation of the Pregnancy.** Adolescents who desire to carry their pregnancies to term require early, consistent, and comprehensive prenatal care by professionals. Although fewer than 5% of adolescents who deliver put their babies up for adoption, this is an option to discuss. Pregnancy is the most common cause of dropping out of school for females. Special attention should be given to keeping the adolescent in school, both during and after pregnancy.

**Termination.** If the pregnant adolescent chooses to terminate her pregnancy, she should be referred immediately to a setting in which abortion services are rendered. The choice of an abortion procedure depends on the gestational age of the fetus. The procedures include menstrual extraction, suction curettage, and intra-amniotic instillation of hypertonic saline or prostaglandin. "Chemical" termination with mifepristone (RU486) in combination with prostaglandin is under investigation in the United States as a safe and effective form of abortion. Psychosocial support should be available for adolescents who choose abortion.

### Prevention of Pregnancy

Sexual activity often is initiated without birth control. For those young people who initiate coitus, knowledge about and use of contraception is critical. Because unintended, unwanted pregnancy can be associated with significant psychosocial morbid-

ity for the adolescent mother, the adolescent father, and the child, prevention should be a primary goal. Reliable methods include the following, which are summarized in Table 7–18.

**Abstinence.** Abstaining from sexual intercourse remains the most commonly used and ideal adolescent birth control method. Unfortunately, a degree of self-control, self-assuredness, and self-esteem is necessary, but these qualities are not found in all adolescents. For those who choose to be sexually active, some form of birth control should be offered because there is a 70% chance that a regularly sexually active adolescent will become pregnant within a year without birth control.

**Birth Control Pills.** Birth control pills are extremely effective if taken regularly. The combined estrogen-progesterone pill prevents the LH surge, thus inhibiting ovulation. Contraindications are listed in Table 7–18. Following a detailed history and physical examination, birth control pills can be started on the first Sunday after the patient's next menstrual period. Condoms should be used both as a back-up method and to prevent STDs. Pills containing 30–35 $\mu$g of ethinyl estradiol (or the equivalent) and a progestin in packs of 28 pills are prescribed first.

Common side effects include nausea, breast tenderness, fluid retention, and breakthrough bleeding, especially if pills are missed. Some adolescents discontinue using the pill because they attribute normal weight gain to the contraceptive. If bleeding occurs in the early part of the cycle, it may be necessary to prescribe pills with increased estrogenic activity. If breakthrough bleeding occurs late in the cycle, a pill with more progestational activity can be prescribed. Before any change in pills, however, one should ask "How often do you forget to take your pills?" If the adolescent has forgotten to take the pill for 1 day, two pills may be taken on the subsequent day. If 2 days were missed, two pills may be taken on the 2 subsequent days. If 3 or more days are missed, the adolescent should use another form of birth control for the rest of this cycle and the next cycle while resuming regular pill use.

**Emergency (Postcoital) Contraception.** Emergency postcoital contraception may be effective (2–3% failure rate) if given within 72 hr of intercourse. *Treatment* consists of 100 $\mu$g ethinyl estradiol and 1 mg norgestrel (e.g., two Ovral tablets) administered twice, 12 hr apart (a total of four pills) or an equivalent contraceptive.

**Condoms and Foam.** When used with spermicidal foam in a conscientious manner, the effectiveness of the condom as a means of birth control can approach that of oral contraceptives. Advantages

TABLE 7–18. Birth Control Methods for Adolescents

| Method | Product | Contraindications | Pregnancy Rate | Side Effects/Problems | Advantages |
|---|---|---|---|---|---|
| **Birth Control Pills** | Combined birth control pills: 30–35 µg of ethinyl estradiol or its equivalent (50 µg of mestranol) and a progestin<br>Mini-pills: progestin only | *Absolute:*<br>Pregnancy<br>Active liver disease with abnormal liver function tests<br>Thrombophlebitis/ thrombotic disease<br>Undiagnosed uterine bleeding<br>Breast, uterine cancer<br>Congenital hyperlipidemia<br>*Relative:*<br>Hypertension<br>Migraine headache<br>Sickle cell disease<br>Active gallbladder disease or mononucleosis | ~1/100 women-years | *Common:*<br>Noncompliance<br>Nausea<br>Weight gain<br>Breast tenderness<br>Fluid retention<br>Break-through bleeding<br>Postpill amenorrhea<br>Acne<br>No protection against AIDS<br>*Uncommon, but serious and rare in adolescence:*<br>Thromboembolic phenomena<br>Cardiovascular sequelae (stroke, hypertension) | Used properly, optimum protection<br>↓ Dysmenorrhea<br>↓ Risk of fibrocystic breast disease, cystic ovarian disease<br>↓ Risk of pelvic inflammatory disease<br>↓ Risk of ovarian, endometrial cancer |
| ***Hormonal Injections/Implants*** | | | | | |
| Medroxyprogesterone (Depo-Provera) | 150 mg IM q 3 mo | Breast tumors? | ~0.2–0.6/100 women-years | Menstrual irregularity<br>Amenorrhea<br>IM injection | Compliance<br>Effective |
| Levonorgestrel (Norplant) | Subcutaneous implants | Obesity | ~0.4–0.6/100 women-years | Menstrual irregularity<br>Amenorrhea, weight gain<br>Minor surgery to place and to remove | Compliance<br>Effective |

# Barrier Methods

| Method | Advantages | Description | Contraindications | Effectiveness | Disadvantages |
|---|---|---|---|---|---|
| Condoms | Inexpensive, few side effects<br>No prescription needed<br>Male method<br>Protection against sexually transmitted diseases (STDs), including AIDS (especially latex condoms) | Condom (used with vaginal foam or with spermicidal lubricant) | Inability of adolescent to plan ahead and use method effectively | ~2–10/100 women-years | Interruption of coitus<br>Proper use<br>Motivation<br>Allergy to rubber (latex) in condom<br>Only water-based lubricants |
| Diaphragm | Safe and effective<br>Cream, jelly available without prescription<br>Protection against STDs<br>Use only when needed | Arcing, coil, flat spring diaphragm fitted by health professional—used with contraceptive cream or jelly | Inability of adolescent to plan ahead and use method properly | ~1.9–2.3/100 women-years | Preparation for coitus<br>Proper use and motivation<br>Toxic shock syndrome<br>"Messiness"<br>Recurrent cystitis |
| Intrauterine device (IUD) | Compliance not necessary<br>Effective | Progesterone- or copper-impregnated device placed by physician in uterine cavity | Multiple sexual partners<br>History of pelvic inflammatory disease or infection<br>Uterine abnormalities<br>Pregnancy | ~2/100 women-years | *High incidence of:*<br>Pelvic inflammatory disease among nulliparous women<br>Ectopic pregnancies<br>Extrusion<br>Heavy bleeding |

Data from Greydanus DE, McAnarney ER: Contraception in the adolescent: Current concepts for the pediatrician. Pediatrics 65:1–2, 1980; Med Lett 34:111, 1992; N Engl J Med 328: 1543, 1993; and Emans SJH, Goldstein DP: Pediatric and Adolescent Gynecology, 3rd ed. Boston, Little, Brown & Co, 1990.

AIDS = acquired immunodeficiency syndrome.

of this method include availability without a prescription and the prevention of STDs, particularly human immunodeficiency virus (HIV) infections, if latex condoms are used regularly.

**Diaphragm.** The diaphragm must be appropriately fitted to each adolescent, and spermicidal jelly or cream must be used with each act of intercourse. There are few side effects from the diaphragm, but adequate use requires comfort with manipulating one's own genitalia. For the more mature older adolescent who has sex infrequently, it is often the best method.

## HORMONAL INJECTIONS AND IMPLANTS

Intramuscular injection of 150 mg of medroxyprogesterone acetate (Depo-Provera) every 3 months is an effective form of birth control. Subdermal implantation of capsules containing levonorgestrel (Norplant) provides effective contraception for adolescents for up to 5 years or until removal. These forms of pregnancy prevention offer the advantage of not requiring use at each sexual encounter, minimizing problems of noncompliance. The main side effects are irregular menses, including amenorrhea (see Table 7-18).

**Coitus Interruptus.** Withdrawal is a common method of adolescent birth control used by sexually active adolescents, but it is ineffective because sperm often are released into the vagina prior to ejaculation or because withdrawal of the penis occurs after ejaculation.

**Rhythm Method (Periodic Coital Abstinence).** Few data support the use of the rhythm method in adolescents, whose irregular menses and whose common misunderstanding of the timing of ovulation may not allow its optimal use.

### References

Ammerman SD: The use of Norplant and DepoProvera in adolescents. J Adolesc Health 16:334, 1995.

Grimes D: A 17 year old mother seeking contraception, JAMA 276:1163, 1996.

Behrman RE, Kliegman RM, Arvin AM (eds): Nelson Textbook of Pediatrics, 15th ed. Philadelphia, WB Saunders, 1996, Chapters 108, 109.

Tafelski T, Boehm KE: Contraception in the adolescent patient. Prim Care 22:145,1995.

## SEXUALLY TRANSMITTED DISEASES

Adolescents have one of the highest rates of STDs. Compared with adults, sexually active adolescents are less likely to use any contraceptive method, are more likely to come into contact with an infected sexual partner, are less likely to receive health care when an STD develops, are more likely to believe that they cannot develop an STD, and are less compliant with treatment once an STD is discovered. In addition, there may be biologic factors that make adolescents more susceptible to certain STDs, such as *Chlamydia trachomatis*. STDs are associated with significant psychologic and biologic morbidity. Early diagnosis and treatment are important to prevent medical complications and infertility. Primary prevention of STDs should be a goal for all adolescent health care providers.

Infection with HIV is associated with behaviors in which other STDs are acquired, especially having multiple partners and exchanging sex for drugs or money. The presence of an STD increases the risk of acquiring HIV; HIV testing should be offered for any adolescent who has an STD.

### Differential Diagnosis

Numerous pathogens are capable of being transmitted venereally, often asymptomatically. However, there are a limited number of clinical presentations of STD (Tables 7–19 through 7–22). Genital ulcers occur with both syphilis and herpes simplex type 2. Genital warts or pubic lice cause nonulcerative external genital lesions or symptoms that are usually quite distressing to the adolescent. Candidal genital infection usually is not sexually transmitted but can cause severe external genital inflammation. Vaginal discharge can be noted in infection with *Candida albicans*, *Trichomonas vaginalis*, and *Gardnerella vaginalis*. Urethritis in the male and cervicitis or pelvic inflammatory disease in the female can result from infection with *Neisseria gonorrhoeae*, *C. trachomatis*, or both.

**Gonorrhea.** Gonorrhea is one of the most commonly reported STDs among adolescents; the most rapid rise in incidence is in the 15–19 yr old age group, especially females. The gram-negative diplococcus gains entry via the urethra, the periurethral Skene glands, the labial Bartholin glands, cervix, anus, pharynx, or conjunctiva. Purulent extension to the endometrium, fallopian tubes, and peritoneum is called **pelvic inflammatory disease** (PID), whereas perihepatitis with involvement of the liver capsule in females is termed the **Fitz-Hugh–Curtis syndrome**. In males, the prostate and epididymis also can be affected. Dissemination to the joints, skin, meninges, and endocardium can occur by the hematogenous route. Many patients may be asymptomatic or have only a mild symptom, such as vaginal or urethral discharge.

The *differential diagnosis* of PID includes simple

TABLE 7–19.  Features of Sexually Transmitted Diseases Characterized by Genital Ulcers in Adolescents

| | Chancroid | Genital Herpes | Syphilis | Granuloma Inguinale (Donovanosis) |
|---|---|---|---|---|
| *Agent* | *Haemophilus ducreyi* | Herpes simplex virus (HSV) 1, 2 | *Treponema pallidum* | *Calymmatobacterium granulomatis* |
| *Incubation (days)* | 3–10 | 4–14 | 10–90 | 8–80 |
| *Systemic Findings* | None | Headache, fever, malaise, myalgia in ⅓ of cases | Fever, rash, malaise, anorexia, arthralgia, adenopathy | Local spread only |
| *Inguinal Lymphadenopathy* | Early, rapid, tender, and unilateral Suppuration likely | Early, bilateral, tender, no suppuration | Late, bilateral, nontender, no suppuration | Lymphatic obstruction Pseudoadenopathy |
| *Primary Lesion* | Papule to pustule | Vesicle | Papule | Papule |
| *Ulcer Characteristics* | | | | |
| Number | <3 | Multiple | 1 or more | 1 or more, may coalesce |
| Edges | Ragged, undermined | Reddened, ragged | Distinct | Rolled, distinct |
| Depth | Deep | Shallow | Shallow | Raised |
| Base | Necrotic | Red, smooth | Red, smooth | Beefy red, clean |
| Secretion | Pus, blood | Serous | Serous | None |
| Induration | None | None | Firm | Firm |
| Pain | Often | Usual | None | None |
| *Diagnosis* | | | | |
| Serology | None | Complement fixation Ab rise only in 1° HSV; enzyme immunoassay | VDRL, ART, RPR, FTA-ABS, MHTP, TPI | None |
| Isolation | Aspirate of node, swab of ulcer on selective medium | Viral culture + in 48 hrs | No in vitro test; rabbit inoculation | None |
| Microscopic | Gram-negative pleomorphic rods | Pap smear; Tzanck smear; direct FA staining | Darkfield examination | Staining of ulcer biopsy material for "Donovan" bodies (Wright or Giemsa) |
| *Treatment (Treat Sexual Partners)* | Aspirate fluctuant nodes Incision and drainage of buboes > 5 cm Erythromycin 500 mg PO q.i.d. ×7 days *or* Ceftriaxone 250 mg IM ×1 dose *or* Azithromycin 1 g PO ×1 dose Ciprofloxacin* 500 mg PO b.i.d. ×3 days (alternative) | Soaks to keep lesions clean and dry; no occlusive ointments Avoid contacting lesions: use hand washing, gloves, condoms Acyclovir 400 mg PO t.i.d. ×7–10 days If proctitis, 800 mg PO t.i.d. ×7–10 days | *Early:* Benzathine penicillin G, 2.4 million U, IM ×1 *or* Doxycycline 100 mg PO b.i.d. ×14 days Repeat VDRL *Late:* (>1 yr duration) Benzathine penicillin G, 2.4 million U, IM q7d ×3 *or* Doxycycline 100 mg PO b.i.d. ×4 weeks Avoid contact with lesions | Doxycycline 100 mg PO b.i.d. ×1–3 weeks *or* TMP/SMX 1 DS PO b.i.d. ×14 days |

From Abramowicz M (ed): Drugs for sexually transmitted diseases. Med Lett 37:117, 1995; and Centers for Disease Control: 1993 STD treatment guidelines. MMWR 42 (RR-14):1–102, 1993.
*Contraindicated in pregnancy.
ART = automated reagin test; FA = fluorescent antibody; FTA-ABS = fluorescent treponemal antibody absorption; MHTP = microhemagglutination antibodies to *Treponema pallidum*; Pap = Papanicolaou; RPR = rapid plasma reagin; TMP/SMX = trimethoprim/sulfamethoxazole; TPI = *Treponema pallidum* immobilization test; VDRL = Venereal Disease Research Laboratory.

TABLE 7–20. Features of Sexually Transmitted Diseases Characterized by Nonulcerative External Genital Symptoms in Adolescents

| | Genital Warts | Vulvovaginal Candidiasis | Pediculosis Pubis (Crabs) |
|---|---|---|---|
| Agent | Human papillomavirus | *Candida albicans* | *Phthirus pubis* |
| Incubation (days) | 30–90 | Uncommon sexual transmission | 5–10 |
| Presenting complaints | Genital warts are seen or felt | Vulvar itching, discharge | Pubic itching, lice may be seen; sexual partner has "crabs" |
| Signs | Firm, gray to pink, single or multiple, fimbriated, painless excrescences on vulva, introitus, vagina cervix, perineum, anus | Inflammatory of vulva, with thick, white, "cottage cheese" discharge, pH <5<br>Friable mucosa that easily bleeds | Eggs (nits) at base of pubic hairs, lice may be visible<br>Excoriated, red skin, 2° infection |
| Clinical associations | Cervical neoplasia, dysplasia | Birth control pills, diabetes, antibiotics can lead to overgrowth | |
| Diagnosis | Clinical appearance; most infections asymptomatic; acetowhite changes on colposcopy<br>Enlarged cells with perinuclear halo and hyperchromatic nuclei | KOH (10%): pseudohyphae<br>Gram stain: gram (+) pseudohyphae<br>Nickerson or Sabouraud medium for culture | History and clinical appearance |
| Treatment (may need to treat sexual partner) | Cryotherapy with liquid nitrogen or cryoprobe<br>Podofilox or trichloracetic acid to external warts only repeated weekly up to ×4 (podophyllin not used during pregnancy)<br>Electrodesiccation; electrocauterization; laser; loop electrosurgical excision for internal, massive, or unresponsive warts<br>Intralesional alpha-interferon | Fluconazole 150 mg PO ×1 dose<br>*or*<br>Miconazole or clotrimazole cream intravaginally h.s. ×3–7 days<br>Lowest dose estrogen BCPs, glucose control, stop systemic antibiotics if possible | 5% permethrin or 1% pyrethrin<br>*or*<br>Pyrethrin/piperonyl shampoo, or lotion<br>May need to repeat |

Modified from Abramowicz M (ed): Drugs for sexually transmitted diseases. Med Lett 37:117, 1995; and Centers for Disease Control: 1993 STD treatment guidelines. MMWR 42 (RR-14):1–102, 1993.
BCP = birth control pill; KOH = potassium hydroxide; 2° = secondary.

cervicitis, pyelonephritis or cystitis, ectopic pregnancy, ovarian torsion, appendicitis, and mesenteric adenitis. Tubo-ovarian abscess may complicate PID. Pelvic ultrasonography is the imaging study of choice to determine the presence of these other diagnoses.

At least 30% of patients with gonococcal cervicitis, urethritis, proctitis, or epididymitis have a concomitant infection with *C. trachomatis*, which necessitates combined therapy for *C. trachomatis* in these syndromes (see Table 7–22). Doxycycline, which is effective against both these agents, is teratogenic and should not be given to pregnant females but often can be replaced by erythromycin. The compliance with outpatient treatment for PID is so poor that many authorities recommend treating all adolescent patients as inpatients.

**Chlamydial Infection.** This is the most frequently diagnosed bacterial STD in adolescents with a 5:1 female-to-male ratio (see Tables 7–19 and 7–22). *Chlamydia* may be a more important pathogen than *N. gonorrhoeae*, accounting for most cases of nongonococcal mucopurulent cervicitis and urethritis; it has an equal, if not a greater, capability to result in severe sequelae, such as female infertility, PID, and **Reiter syndrome** (conjunctivitis, uveitis, urethritis, buccal ulceration, peripheral arthritis, sacroiliitis, keratoderma blennorrhagia, and human leukocyte antigen [HLA]–B27). Serovar L1-3 produces lymphogranuloma ve-

TABLE 7–21.  Features of Syndromes with Vaginal Symptoms in Adolescents

| | Physiologic Leukorrhea (Normal) | Trichomoniasis | Nonspecific Bacterial Vaginosis (*Gardnerella vaginalis*-Associated Vaginitis) |
|---|---|---|---|
| *Agent* | Normal flora | *Trichomonas vaginalis* | *Gardnerella vaginalis* and anaerobes |
| *Incubation (days)* | — | 3–28 | Not necessarily sexually transmitted |
| *Predominant Symptoms* | | | |
| Itching | None | Mild to moderate | None to mild |
| Discharge | Minimal | Moderate to severe | Mild to moderate |
| Pain | None | Mild | Uncommon |
| *Discharge* | | | |
| Amount | Small | Profuse | Moderate |
| Color | Clear, milky | Yellow-green or gray | Gray |
| Consistency | Flocculent | Frothy | Homogeneous |
| Viscosity | Thin | Thin | Thin |
| Foul odor | None | None | Yes |
| Odor c̄/KOH | None | Possible | Characteristic fish odor (amine) |
| pH | <4.5 | >5.0 | >4.5 |
| *Vulvar* | | | |
| Inflammation | None | Common | Uncommon |
| *Vaginal* | | | |
| Infammation | None | Usual | None to mild |
| Discharge | Nonadherent | Nonadherent | Adherent, white to grey |
| Tenderness | None | Common | Minimal |
| *Cervical* | Normal | "Strawberry" hemorrhages | Normal |
| *Bimanual Exam* | Normal | Normal | Normal |
| *Microscopic Findings* | | | |
| Saline drop | Squamous and few white blood cells (WBCs) | Motile flagellates, slightly larger than WBCs, and WBCs | Squamous cells studded with bacteria ("clue cells") and WBCs |
| Gram stain | Gram-positive and -negative rods and cocci | *Trichomonas* killed | Predominance of gram-negative rods |
| *Culture* | Mixed flora with *Lactobacillus* predominant | Culture generally not indicated; antigen detection and antibody tests available | *Gardnerella vaginalis, Mobiluncus* anaerobes |
| *Treatment* | Reassurance | Metronidazole, 2 g PO × 1 dose, if not in first trimester<br>Avoid alcohol for 24 hr<br>Treat sexual partner<br>Clotrimazole, 100 mg intravaginal at night × 7 days if pregnant | *Intravaginal:* Metronidazole gel 0.75% b.i.d. ×5 days, *or* Clindamycin 2% cream h.s. ×7 days<br>*Oral:* Metronidazole 500 mg b.i.d. *or* Clindamycin 300 mg b.i.d. ×7 days<br>Treat sexual partner only if recurrent |

Modified from Abramowicz M (ed): Drugs for sexually transmitted diseases. Med Lett 37:117, 1995, and Centers for Disease Control: 1993 STD treatment guidelines. MMWR 42 (RR-14):1–102, 1993.

TABLE 7–22.  Features of Syndromes Characterized by Mucopurulent Cervicitis, Urethritis, or Pelvic Inflammatory Disease (PID)

| | Gonorrhea | Chlamydia |
|---|---|---|
| *Agent* | *Neisseria gonorrhoeae* | *Chlamydia trachomatis* |
| *Incubation (Days)* | 3–14 | 5–12 |
| *Possible Presentations* | The following possible presentations apply to both gonorrhea and chlamydiosis:<br><br>*Female*<br>  Asymptomatic<br>  Urethritis<br>  Skenitis/bartholinitis<br>  Pelvic inflammatory disease<br><br>  Anorectal/pharyngeal<br>  Disseminated (arthritis, dermatitis, endocarditis, meningitis) | *Male Partner*<br>  Asymptomatic<br>  Urethritis<br>  Epididymo-orchitis<br>  Proctitis<br>  Pharyngitis |
| *Typical Findings in Mucopurulent Cervicitis or Urethritis* | Cervical erythema, friability, ectopy, with thick, creamy discharge (penile discharge in males)<br>Mucopus >10 polymorphonuclear cells (PMNs) per high-power field (hpf)<br>Gram-negative intracellular diplococci<br>Mild cervical tenderness | Cervical erythema, friability, ectopy, with thick creamy discharge (penile discharge in males)<br><br>Mucopus >10 PMNs/hpf<br>May coexist with gonorrhea<br>Mild cervical tenderness |
| *Typical Findings in PID* | Onset day 3–10 of menstrual period<br>Lower abdominal pain (95%)<br>Adnexal tenderness, mass (95%)<br>Pain on cervical motion (95%)<br>Fever (35%)<br>Mucopurulent cervical discharge (variable)<br>Menstrual irregularities (variable)<br>Nausea, vomiting (variable)<br>Weakness, syncope, dizziness (variable)<br>Perihepatitis (5%) (may be seen without PID)<br>Laparoscopy: Definitive diagnosis = salpingitis<br>Pelvic ultrasound: Thickened adnexal structures<br>↑ Sedimentation rate (65%)<br>↑ WBC count (45%) | |
| *Important Differential Diagnoses for PID* | Ectopic pregnancy<br>Ovarian cyst (torsion, rupture)<br>Septic abortion<br>Urinary tract infection<br>Appendicitis<br>Mesenteric adenitis<br>Inflammatory bowel disease | |

nereum, whereas serovars B and D-K are associated with genital infections, such as mucopurulent cervicitis, urethritis, proctitis, epididymitis, salpingitis, endometritis, and perihepatitis. *Diagnosis* by culture, direct immunofluorescent antibody, or enzyme-linked immunoassay, radioimmunoassay, or newer methods based on deoxyribonucleic acid (DNA) technology are available.

*Treatment* of milder infections can be accomplished in an ambulatory setting. However, erythromycin frequently causes gastric upset, resulting in noncompliance, and doxycycline is teratogenic. A single oral dose of azithromycin (1 g) is also effective therapy for uncomplicated chlamydial genital infections; this can be combined with a single oral dose of cefixime (400 mg) to treat gonorrhea.

**Trichomoniasis.** Most cases of trichomonas infection are sexually transmitted (see Table 7–21). Females have vaginitis and are more likely to be

**TABLE 7–22.**  Features of Syndromes Characterized by Mucopurulent Cervicitis, Urethritis, or Pelvic Inflammatory Disease (PID) *Continued*

|  | Gonorrhea | Chlamydia |
|---|---|---|
| ***Laboratory Studies*** | Gram stain in cervicitis: 60% sensitivity, 95% specificity; diagnostic in males<br>Thayer-Martin selective medium<br>Antigen detection tests (LCR amplification) | Tissue culture<br>Antigen detection<br>(1) Fluorescent antibody<br>(2) Enzyme-linked immunoassay<br>(3) DNA probe<br>(4) Amplification with PCR or LCR |
| ***Treatment*** | | |
| Uncomplicated cervicitis, urethritis, pharyngitis, proctitis | Ceftriaxone 125 mg IM × 1 dose<br>*or*<br>Cefixime 400 mg PO × 1<br>*plus*<br>Doxycycline 100 mg PO b.i.d. × 7 days for *Chlamydia* | Doxycycline 100 mg PO b.i.d. × 7 days<br>*or*<br>Erythromycin 500 mg PO q.i.d. × 7 days<br>*or*<br>Azithromycin 1 g PO × 1 dose |
| PID | | |
| Outpatient | Ceftriaxone, 250 mg IM × 1 dose<br>*or*<br>Cefoxitin, 2 g IM × 1, with probenecid, 1 g PO<br>*plus*<br>Doxycycline, 100 mg PO b.i.d. × 14 days | |
| Inpatient | Cefoxitin, 2 g IV q6h<br>*or*<br>Cefotetan, 2 g IV q12h<br>*plus*<br>Doxycycline, 100 mg IV q12h until improved<br>*followed by*<br>Doxycycline, 100 mg PO b.i.d., to complete 14 days of treatment<br><br>Alternative (especially if anaerobic infection likely): clindamycin, 900 mg IV q8h<br>*plus*<br>Gentamicin, 2 mg/kg IV × 1 dose<br>*followed by*<br>Gentamicin, 1.5 mg/kg IV q8h until improved<br>*followed by*<br>Doxycycline, 100 mg PO b.i.d., to complete 14 days of treatment | |
| Disseminated gonococcal infection | Ceftriaxone, 1.0 g IV q24h until asymptomatic × 48 hr, then complete 1 wk of therapy with cefuroxime 0.5 g b.i.d. or amoxicillin 0.5 g t.i.d. with clavulanic acid<br><br>Cefoxitin, 1.0 g IV q8h<br><br>Cefotaxime, 1.0 g IV q8h | |

Modified from Abramowicz M (ed): Drugs for sexually transmitted diseases. Med Lett 37:117, 1995; and Centers for Disease Control: 1993 STD treatment guidelines. MMWR 42 (RR-14):1–102, 1993.

LCR = ligase chain polymerase; PCR = polymerase chain reaction; WBC = white blood cell.

symptomatic than males. A thin, frothy vaginal discharge and cervical "strawberry hemorrhages" are characteristic. *Diagnosis* is made by visualization of motile, flagellated protozoans in the urine or in a saline wet mount. Single-dose *treatment* of both sexual partners with 2 g of metronidazole is effective. Trichomoniasis often is associated with other STDs, such as gonorrhea and chlamydial infection.

**Nonspecific Bacterial Vaginosis.** In postpubertal females who have a thin, gray, foul-smelling vaginal discharge and mild vaginitis, *G. vaginalis* often is found on culture of the discharge (see Table 7–21). In addition to *G. vaginalis*, anaerobic bacteria such as *Bacteroides*, *Mobiluncus*, and *Peptostreptococcus* are important in the pathogenesis. The pH of the discharge is greater than 4.5, and on microscopic examination the squamous epithelial cells are studded with rod-shaped organisms (clue cells). With the addition of potassium hydroxide (KOH) to the discharge, there is a characteristic "fishy" odor because of the release of aromatic amines ("whiff" test). The clinical significance of this nonspecific bacterial vaginosis remains in doubt, but treatment with intravaginal or oral metronidazole or clindamycin is usually effective.

Vaginal discharge in prepubertal girls may be due to poor hygiene or irritants, such as bubble bath, deodorants, and detergents used to clean underwear. Nonabsorbent undergarments cause a moist environment to develop that may cause inflammation. Foreign bodies, pinworms, group A streptococcus, shigellosis, and sexual abuse also should be considered. *N. gonorrhoeae* also may cause vaginitis in the prepubertal female because of the thinner epithelial layer in this age group. When seen in prepubertal girls, gonorrhea almost invariably is due to sexual abuse.

**Candidiasis (Moniliasis).** See Table 7–20.

**Herpes Infection.** Primary genital *herpes simplex type* 2 (occasionally type 1) often is associated with headache, fever, malaise, myalgia, painful genital lesions, regional lymphadenopathy, discharge, and dysuria; some primary and many secondary lesions are asymptomatic (see Table 7–19). The multiple vesicles are red and painful. Secondary (recurrent or reactivation) eruptions are not as dramatic. Viral cultures are positive in 24 hr, but an immediate diagnosis can be made with a Tzanck test showing multinucleated giant cells. The Pap smear also demonstrates these cells. Latency develops as the virus becomes dormant in the sacral nerve ganglion. In primary herpes simplex infection, viral shedding lasts 10–14 days and ulcer healing occurs in 16–20 days; in recurrent disease, virus is present for less than 7 days and the time of healing is 8–10 days. Many patients experience five to eight recurrences per year.

Oral acyclovir is effective in reducing the severity and duration of symptoms in primary cases. Local hygiene and sitz baths may relieve some discomfort. Education of patients to use condoms and to avoid having sex with anyone who has genital ulcers can help prevent the spread of this disease.

**Genital Warts.** Warts can occur on the squamous epithelium or mucous membranes of the genital and perineal structures of both females and males (see Table 7–20). They are usually multiple, firm, gray to pink excrescences. They can become tender if macerated or secondarily infected. On cornified skin, cryotherapy with liquid nitrogen or cryoprobe is the recommended treatment, or topical podophyllin can be applied until the lesions regress. Warts on mucous membranes that are unresponsive to topical treatment or that occur during pregnancy can be treated with cryosurgery, laser ablation excision, or electrodesiccation, but they should not be treated with podophyllin; recurrences after treatment are common. Human papillomavirus infection most commonly is asymptomatic but has been associated with carcinoma of the cervix.

## References

Anonymous: Drugs for sexually transmitted diseases. Med Lett 37:117, 1995.
Behrman RE, Kliegman RM, Arvin AM (eds): Nelson Textbook of Pediatrics, 15th Philadelphia, WB Saunders 1996, Chapter 110.
Braverman PK, Strasburger VC: Sexually transmitted diseases. Clin Pediatr 33:26, 1994.
Centers for Disease Control: 1993 STD treatment guidelines. MMWR 42(RR-14):1–102, 1993.
Patel R, Cowan F, Barton S: Advising patients with genital herpes. BMJ 314:85, 1997.
Wald E: Pelvic inflammatory disease in adolescents. Curr Probl Pediatr 8:86, 1996.

## RAPE

Rape is a legal term for unlawful, nonconsensual intercourse; almost one half of victims are adolescents. The attacker is known in 50% of cases. Although gathering historic and physical evidence that may be used in later criminal investigation is important, the physician's primary responsibility to an alleged rape victim is to provide medical examination and treatment in a supportive, nonjudgmental manner. The acute trauma of rape can result in physical injury and untoward psychologic responses, ranging from a state of panic to extreme withdrawal. The history is important and should include details of the sexual assault, whether the victim cleaned herself, the last menstrual period, and previous sexual activity, if any.

Specimens from body surfaces, the mouth, vagina, and anus as well as any photographs taken to document the extent of injuries should maintain the "chain of evidence" that cannot be called into question in court. Specimens should be taken to identify sperm by microscopy, fluorescence in a Wood lamp, agglutination, and acid phosphatase content of posterior vaginal fornix and other locations. Attempts to identify *N. gonorrhoeae*, *Chlamydia* and *Trichomonas* also are helpful.

In addition to physical trauma, specific immediate medical issues include prevention of pregnancy and prophylaxis for STDs. Pregnancy may occur in 7–10% of victims and can be prevented reliably if treatment is instituted within 72 hr (see Emergency [Postcoital] Contraception). The risk of STDs is low, and the need for immediate treatment is controversial. One regimen includes ceftriaxone (250 mg IM) plus doxycycline (100 mg PO twice daily for 7 days) or azithromycin (1 g PO) plus metronidazole (2 g PO). Whether treatment is initiated or not, follow-up culture, Venereal Disease Research Laboratory (VDRL), and HIV studies are indicated. The regimen for STDs with the broadest coverage and highest compliance is doxycycline, 100 mg PO twice a day for 7 days. Long-term sequelae are common; patients should be offered immediate and ongoing psychologic support, such as that offered at local rape crisis services.

## SKIN CONDITIONS

### ACNE

Although acne usually is not a serious medical problem, at least 85% of adolescents have some form of this skin condition; it may have devastating effects on physical appearance, body image, and self-esteem. Effective treatment should be offered to any adolescent with acne, regardless of the extent of involvement, to avoid physical and psychologic scarring.

Many *pathogenic factors* cause acne. Androgenic stimulation of the sebaceous glands leads to an outpouring of lipid-rich sebum that lubricates the hair follicle. The epidermal cells lining the follicle canal obstruct the flow of sebum onto the surface of the skin. The retained material then acts as a medium for the growth of commensal bacteria, such as *Propionibacterium acnes* and coagulase-negative staphylococci. These bacteria produce lipases that hydrolyze the triglycerides contained in sebum, releasing free fatty acids. Inflammation occurs because neutrophils summoned by bacterial chemotactic factors produce hydrolases that disrupt the walls of the pilosebaceous unit. Because the adolescent may apply manual pressure to such lesions, the inflammatory products are released into the dermis rather than onto the surface of the skin. Open comedones are the earliest lesions and are due to dilation of the follicular canal from retained epidermal lining cells (blackheads). A whitehead, or closed comedo, is impaction of debris leading to inflammation and bacterial digestion of lipids, which results in the formation of papules, pustules, nodules, and cysts.

*Treatment* includes comedolytics (topical benzoyl peroxide, retinoic acid), topical bacteriostatics (benzoyl peroxide, erythromycin, clindamycin, tetracycline), oral bacteriostatics (tetracycline, erythromycin), oral contraceptives, and 13-*cis*-retinoic acid (Accutane). The latter drug causes congenital anomalies and should not be given to pregnant adolescents.

### CRAB LICE

Predominantly sexually transmitted, the pubic crab louse (*Phthirus pubis*) lives out its life cycle on pubic hair; therefore, the characteristic intense pruritus, erythematous papules, and egg cases (nits) of "crabs" are not seen before puberty (see Table 7–20). *Treatment* consists of education regarding personal and environmental hygiene and the application of an appropriate pediculicide, such as permethrin or pyrethrin.

### FUNGAL INFECTIONS (JOCK ITCH, ATHLETE'S FOOT)

See Chapter 10.

## EATING DISORDERS

See Chapters 1 and 2.

## BEHAVIORAL PROBLEMS

### PSYCHOSOCIAL CONDITIONS

#### Normal and Abnormal Behaviors

Normal adolescents may intermittently defy parents, provoke their teachers, and challenge physicians. They may refuse to participate in family events and argue incessantly with siblings. It is sometimes difficult to know whether these behaviors are a part of normal adolescent independence and individuality struggles or are pathologic. One can generally distinguish normal from abnormal behavior by taking into account the degree of interference that a particular behavior produces with regard to schoolwork, family life, activities with friends, or work.

#### Depression

Younger depressed adolescents, whose cognitive development usually is *concrete operational*, may not be able to acknowledge their affective state, but the condition may be indicated by boredom, restlessness, difficulty in concentrating or decreasing school performance, preoccupation with somatic complaints (fatigue, vague or localized pains), running away, fights with peers, flight to or from people, and other "acting-out" behaviors. Older adolescents who are *formal operational* in their thinking may be able to reflect on their feelings of depression and sadness. The mood disturbance in depression includes feeling sad or "blue" for more than 3 hr more than 3 times a week. Other symptoms include early morning awakening or hypersomnia, changes in appetite, loss of sexual interest, psychomotor retardation or fatigue, inability to concentrate, and feelings of excessive guilt, worthlessness, self-reproach, or hopelessness.

Biologic markers are not yet sufficiently specific to be used as diagnostic tests in adolescents. Antidepressant medication can be useful in adolescents who have a family history of depression or alcoholism (see discussion of suicide, under Violent Behaviors, next).

## Violent Behaviors

Violence is a major and increasing health problem among contemporary adolescents. Accidents are the leading cause, followed by suicide and homicide. Homicide is a particular problem among urban minority males.

Prevention of violent and destructive adolescent behavior is an important goal. Identifying high-risk antecedents of depression, Attention-Deficit/Hyperactivity Disorder, impulse control problems, risk-taking behavior, and substance abuse prior to accidents, homicides, or suicides is critical for prevention.

*Accidents,* particularly motor vehicle collisions, often result from risk-taking by adolescents; judgment impaired by alcohol or by drugs is frequently a contributing factor. Efforts have been made in several states to mandate seat belt use and to raise the drinking age to 21 yr. Data indicate a decrease in deaths from motor vehicle accidents following the use of such measures. Education programs do not appear to be as effective in changing behavior as legislation, but physicians should educate their young adolescent patients about the hazards of drinking, driving, or both.

*Homicide* is disturbingly common among young people of lower socioeconomic status living in crowded urban areas. A possible response to this situation may be to institute, at the local and national level, a combination of social programs providing perpetrators, potential perpetrators, and would-be victims with alternatives to violent behavior and destructive modes of thinking and relating to others. Gun control, improvements in education and economic opportunities, and training in conflict resolution may lower the number of disturbing and premature deaths.

*Suicide* is the second leading cause of death among adolescents 15–24 yr of age in the United States. Suicide and attempted suicide may result from despair over the breakup with a boyfriend or girlfriend, grief over the death of a loved one, or a chronic depression. Data suggest that adolescents are more likely to try to harm themselves after viewing programs depicting suicide or after friends or classmates commit suicide, resulting in so-called "cluster suicides." Other risk factors include poor impulse control, psychosis, family history of suicide, or risk-taking by the adolescent. Attempts outnumber completed suicides by a ratio of at least 100:1, with females accounting for more than 80% of attempts. Males outnumber females in completed suicide, however, because they are more likely to use a violent method, such as guns or hanging, rather than poisoning.

## References

American Academy of Pediatrics, Task Force on Adolescent Assault Victim Needs: Adolescent Assault Victim Needs: A review of issues and a model protocol. Pediatrics 98:991, 1996.

Behrman RE, Kliegman RM, Arvin AM (eds): Nelson Textbook of Pediatrics, 15th ed. Philadelphia, WB Saunders, 1996, Chapters 103, 104.

Fennig S, Carlson GA: Advances in the study of mood disorders in children and adolescents. Curr Opin Pediatr 7:401, 1995.

Weiner IB: Normality during adolescence. *In* McAnarney ER, Kreipe RE, Orr DP, Comerci GD (eds): Textbook of Adolescent Medicine. Philadelphia, WB Saunders, 1992, pp 86–90.

# SUBSTANCE ABUSE

Exploratory drug use may be seen as part of normal psychosocial development for the contemporary adolescent. Many adolescents abandon or lessen their drug use as they develop into adults. However, it is hazardous to adopt an "everybody's doing it" attitude, especially with the more vulnerable younger adolescent, for several reasons (Table 7–23). The use of drugs is often purposive, goal-directed, and psychologically adaptive. For example, drug use may allow the adolescent to attain independence from parental control and regulation; to express opposition to social norms; to cope with anxiety, frustration, and depression; or to gain admission to a peer group. The adolescent may fail to develop healthy ways of dealing with these problems if drugs are used as a ready solution.

Furthermore, the use of substances by young people is linked systematically to a larger constellation of problem behaviors that are also considered inappropriate by society, such as prostitution and stealing. Compared with nonusing peers, adolescents who abuse drugs have lower grades, higher truancy rates, and fewer plans to attend college; they work less, have less of a religious commitment, have more radical political views, spend less time at home, and spend more time dating.

Finally, the average age at which young people first use substances is declining, and younger age at first use is correlated with a higher likelihood of continued use and abuse. In this context, alcohol

TABLE 7–23.  Classification of Substance Use by Adolescents

| | |
|---|---|
| Nonuse | Abstinence from psychoactive or addictive substances for personal, family, or religious reasons |
| Experimental use | Infrequent, episodic use of various drugs during contact with peers that does not interfere with activities at home, in school, or at work |
| Recreational use | Episodic use of tobacco, alcohol, or marijuana during social encounters with peers, intended to make one feel accepted or at ease |
| Circumstantial use | Repeated substance use because of a learned association between its use and decreased anxiety or stress, with drugs serving as a coping tool; depending on stressors, such use can quickly lead to physical or psychologic dependency |
| Habitual use | Substance(s) use involves most, if not all, areas of life, with the adolescent being psychologically and socially addicted; because everything in the adolescent's life revolves around obtaining and using substance(s), drug use becomes its own reward |
| Compulsive use | Physiologic addiction to substance(s) so that the adolescent is unable to help himself or herself stop using the drug; because habituation underlies such use, it is best treated in a conscientiously prescribed program of abstinence, change of friends, change of school, and change of all other patterns that were associated with the substance(s) use |

From Obermeier G, Henry P: Inpatient treatment of adolescent alcohol and polydrug abuses. Semin Adolesc Med 1:293–301, 1985.

and tobacco are often "gateway drugs." When it provides a positive experience to a 7th grader, the experimental use of alcohol or tobacco can lead to experimentation with other psychoactive substances for which the risk of psychologic or physical addiction is great.

## Epidemiology

Approximately two thirds of teenagers in the United States try some form of illicit drug before finishing high school; almost all have tried alcohol, and 40% have used some illicit drug other than marijuana. About 5% of high school seniors smoke cigarettes daily, drink alcohol daily, or do both. Lifetime and current use of marijuana among 8th to 10th graders has increased substantially in the 1990s in the United States. The clinician must determine the epidemiology of substance use for the individual adolescent as part of routine health care or whenever the adolescent is seen for any problem.

## Clinical Manifestations

Important factors in the history include types, frequency, timing, setting, circumstances, and outcomes of substance use. Although alcohol use may be considered statistically normative, adolescent alcohol abuse is characterized by consumption of large amounts over a short time, often to the point of intoxication. Even though an adolescent may drink "only" with friends at weekend parties, he or she can still be the victim of a fatal motor vehicle accident while driving home intoxicated after a party.

Few physical findings are associated with most chronic adolescent substance use, except in cases of intoxication or overdose (Tables 7–24 and 7–25). However, this does not mean that the commonly used substances are harmless. In the late 1970s, cocaine snorting and smokeless tobacco dipping became popular "recreational" activities among some adolescents, behaviors often modeled after those of some sports and rock music heroes. Devastating reports of sudden death from the cocaine derivative "crack" and oral cancers from snuff are now being reported.

**Acute Overdose.** Many drugs (most commonly alcohol, amphetamine, opiates, and cocaine) can result in a toxicologic emergency, which occurs most often the first time an adolescent uses a substance, sometimes being unaware of its nature; such an initial reaction makes identification of the offending agent difficult. Initial management should be directed at appropriate supportive medical treatment, with follow-up counseling after the toxic effects have diminished (see Table 7–25).

**Acute Illness.** Heavy alcohol use can cause both acute gastritis and acute pancreatitis. Intravenous drug use can result in right-sided bacterial endocarditis, vertebral or sternoclavicular osteomyelitis, septic pulmonary embolism, hepatitis B infection, or acquired immunodeficiency syndrome (AIDS). Chronic marijuana or tobacco use is associated with bronchoconstriction and bronchitis.

**Chronic Use.** Compulsive drug or alcohol use results in the adolescent's being unable to help himself or herself out of drug dependency and the psychosocial sequelae that attend such habituation (stealing, prostitution, drug dealing, unemployment, school failure, and social isolation).

## Treatment

Specific management of substance use by adolescents depends on many individual patient factors.

TABLE 7–24. Effects, Duration of Action, Toxicity, Withdrawal Symptoms, and Treatment of Substance Abuse in Adolescents

| Substance | Immediate Effects | Duration of Action | Toxicity | Signs and Symptoms of Withdrawal | Treatment of Overdose |
|---|---|---|---|---|---|
| Alcohol | Respiratory depression, CNS depression, ataxia, slurred speech | Depends on amount ingested and adolescent's tolerance | Cirrhosis, gastrointestinal hemorrhage, thiamine and folate deficiency, CNS depression, impaired motor performance and mental function, stupor, deep anesthesia, death | Insomnia, restlesness, anxiety, tremulousness, hypertension, tachycardia, diaphoresis; auditory or visual hallucinations or both, seizures, delirium tremens are rare in adolescents | Supportive ventilation if needed |
| Amphetamine, other stimulants | ↑ blood pressure, activity, and alertness; tachycardia; insomnia, anorexia; ↓ fatigue, euphoria; excitation; aggression; hostility | 2–8 hr | Agitation; ↑ heart rate, blood pressure, and temperature; hallucinations; paranoia, psychosis; convulsions; death, arrhythmias, vasculitis | Apathy, hallucinations, irritability, excessive sleep, depression, psychosis, suicidal, sudden death | Paranoia with haloperidol; seizures with diazepam |
| Tobacco | ↑ blood pressure and heart rate; ↓ temperature, CNS stimulation, skeletal muscle relaxation | Minutes | CNS stimulation | Restlessness, anxiety, insomnia, agitation, nausea, headache, ↑ appetite, inability to concentrate | None |
| Cocaine, crack | ↑ alertness, exultation, euphoria, insomnia; ↓ appetite; ↑ blood pressure and heart rate, aphrodisiac, local anesthesia | 15–30 min | Agitation; ↑ temperature, pulse, and BP; tremors; convulsions, tachyarrhythmias; paranoia, psychosis; myocardial infarction; cerebral hemorrhage; death | Apathy, long periods of sleep, irritability, depression, suicidal, disorientation | Paranoia with haloperidol; seizures with diazepam; cooling for hyperthermia; nitroprusside, labetalol for hypertension |

| | Signs and symptoms of use | Duration of action | Signs and symptoms of overdose | Withdrawal syndrome | Treatment of overdose |
|---|---|---|---|---|---|
| Inhalants (solvents, gasoline) | Respiratory depression, CNS depression, ataxia, slurred speech, bradycardia | 5–30 min | Arrhythmias, ataxia, hallucinations, seizures, encephalopathy, renal tubular acidosis, peripheral neuropathy, lead poisoning, death | Rare: chills, hallucinations, headache, abdominal pain, muscle cramps, delirium tremens | See Chapter 3 |
| LSD, other hallucinogens | Dysphoria; hallucinations; anxiety; paranoia; psychosis; ↑ blood pressure, heart rate, and temperature; dilated pupils; incoordination; ↑ creativity | 2–12 hr; can produce exhaustion lasting for days | Long, intense "trips"; psychotic reactions not always reversible; flashbacks; suicide attempts; deaths with some drugs | None | Reassurance; haloperidol |
| Marijuana, hashish | Euphoria, ↓ reaction time, ↓ inhibitions, ↑ appetite | 2–4 hr | Dysphoria, acute anxiety attacks, acute psychosis, fatigue, paranoia, lack of motivation | Insomnia, hyperactivity, ↓ appetite | None |
| PCP and PCP analogs | Ataxia, nystagmus, ↑ blood pressure, slurred speech, dysphoria, hallucinations, paranoia, confusion | Hours to days | Psychosis; convulsions; paranoia; flashbacks; rhabdomyolysis; deaths have resulted from suicide, accidents | None | Haloperidol, diazepam |
| Opioids | Euphoria, ataxia, slurred speech, miosis, stupor | Hours | Respiratory depression, hypothermia, hypotension, pulmonary edema, apnea, coma, death | Increased sympathetic nervous system activity, hunger, antisocial behavior, gooseflesh, diaphoresis, rhinorrhea (flu), yawning; treatment with clonidine | Naloxone 2 mg IV, repeated up to 10 mg; ventilation |

Data from Jones RL: Substance abuse. *In* Shearin RB (ed): Handbook of Adolescent Medicine. Kalamazoo, MI, Upjohn Co, 1983, pp 133–152; and Abramowicz M (ed): Treatment of acute drug abuse reactions. Med Lett 38:43, 1996.

CNS = central nervous system; LSD = lysergic acid diethylamide; PCP = phencyclidine.

TABLE 7–25. Effects, Tolerance, Dependence, Adulteration, and Methods of Administration of Substances Abused by Adolescents

| Substance | Long-Term Effects | Tolerance | Dependence | | Adulteration or Substitution | Method of Administration |
|-----------|-------------------|-----------|------------|------------|------------------------------|--------------------------|
| | | | *Psychologic* | *Physical* | | |
| Alcohol | Blackouts; behavioral changes; ↑ accidents; homicide, suicide; gastritis; peptic ulcer; alcoholic hepatitis; fatty liver; pancreatitis | Yes | Yes | Yes | Methanol | Ingested |
| Amphetamine, other stimulants | Weight loss, insomnia, anxiety, paranoia, hallucinations; skin abscesses and amphetamine psychosis following injections | Yes | High | Yes | More than 90% of speed is adulterated with caffeine, asthma medications, PCP, LSD, strychnine, sugars | Ingested, injected |
| Tobacco | ↑ risk of chronic bronchitis, heart disease, and cancer (oral cancer with smokeless tobacco) | Yes | Yes | Yes | No | Smoke inhaled, snuff dipping, chewed |
| Cocaine, crack | Nasal perforation with snorting; weight loss, insomnia, anxiety, paranoia, hallucinations, soft tissue abscesses with injections | Yes | High | Yes, especially following smoking or injection | Local anesthetics, sugars, PCP | Snorted, smoked, ingested, injected |
| Inhalants (solvents, gasoline, "white out," etc) | Liver damage with toluene, trichloroethylene, gasoline; anemia with tetraethyl lead; leukemia with benzene; kidney damage with trichloroethylene | Yes, especially with toluene | Yes | Yes | None | Sniffing rags soaked with the compound, inhaling fumes through the mouth |

However, because of the highly addictive (physical or psychologic) nature of most substances, residential drug treatment facilities are becoming increasingly utilized, especially for younger adolescents.

## References

Behrman RE, Kliegman RM, Arvin AM (eds): Nelson Textbook of Pediatrics, 15th ed. Philadelphia, WB Saunders, 1996, Chapter 105.

Fuller PG, Kavanaugh RM: Basic assessment and screening for substance abuse in the pediatrician's office. Pediatr Clin North Am 42:295, 1995.

## FUNCTIONAL (PSYCHOSOMATIC) DISORDERS

Symptoms of pain or loss of function for which no physical cause is found are common during adolescence. Although the evidence for biologic disorders should be sought simultaneously with evidence for psychologic disorders, we must realize that our knowledge regarding the relationship between these two domains remains primitive. It is important that the adolescent not be led to believe that the physician, in finding no evidence of disease, judges the symptoms to be feigned or

TABLE 7–25. Effects, Tolerance, Dependence, Adulteration, and Methods of Administration of Substances Abused by Adolescents *Continued*

| Substance | Long-Term Effects | Tolerance | Dependence | | Adulteration or Substitution | Method of Administration |
| | | | *Psychologic* | *Physical* | | |
|---|---|---|---|---|---|---|
| LSD, other hallucinogens | Flashbacks, pronounced personality changes, ↑ risk of chronic psychosis | Yes, cross-tolerance with mescaline, DMT, and psilocybin | Degree unknown | No | Sold as tablets, in liquids, in microdots in many colors; often adulterated with or substituted for other drugs | Ingested, injected, sniffed |
| Marijuana, hashish | Great variety involving several body systems; ↓ motivation | Yes | Degree unknown | No | With PCP | Smoke inhaled, ingested |
| PCP and PCP analogs | Personality disorders, flashbacks, catatonia, neuropsychologic disturbances, increased risk of schizophrenia | Yes | High | Degree unknown | Often added to other drugs or advertised as other drugs | Ingested, injected, smoked |
| Opioids | ↓ motivation, antisocial behavior, crime to support habit, skin abscess, endocarditis, osteomyelitis, nephritis, hepatitis, HIV, amenorrhea | Yes | Yes | Yes | Quinine, sugar | Ingested, injected, subcutaneous (skin-popping), intravenous |

Modified from Jones RLK: Substance abuse. *In* Shearin RB (ed): Handbook of Adolescent Medicine. Kalamazoo, MI, Upjohn Co, 1983, pp 133–152. DMT = dimethyltryptamine; HIV = human immunodeficiency virus; LSD = lysergic acid diethylamide; PCP = phencyclidine.

imaginary ("all in your head"). In such a situation, psychologic factors may indeed play a role, but rarely does the physician have the adolescent's trust and confidence required for the treatment to be effective. Even if the physician and adolescent can agree that psychologic factors are operating, this does not guarantee that there is not some organic pathology underlying the symptoms. Thus, rather than labeling symptoms for which no organic cause can be determined "psychosomatic," it is preferable to categorize them as "functional" (Table 7–26), which avoids the connotation that the symptoms are psychologic (they are somatic) and allows the difficulty to be recast in terms of disordered bodily functioning (rather than in terms of the imagination), triggered by previously unappreciated stressors.

The *chronic fatigue syndrome* is another problem in adolescents. It is often a postviral phenomenon, but its etiology is undetermined.

## References

Behrman RE, Kliegman RM, Arvin AM (eds): Nelson Textbook of Pediatrics, 15th ed. Philadelphia, WB Saunders, 1996, Chapter 20.

Buchwald D, Smith MS: Chronic fatigue. *In* McAnarney ER, Kreipe RE, Orr DP, Comerci GD (eds): Textbook of Adolescent Medicine. Philadelphia, WB Saunders, 1992, pp 879–885.

Prazar G: Conversion reactions in adolescents. Pediatr Rev 8:279–286, 1987.

## SCHOOL PROBLEMS

School problems often indicate underlying psychologic or environmental difficulties. Common school problems include school phobia, truancy, and underachievement.

### School Phobia

Adolescents who avoid or refuse to go to school may have histories of separation anxiety and multi-

TABLE 7–26.  Features of Functional (Psychosomatic) Disorders of Adolescents

**Psychophysiologic Disorder**
  Presenting complaint is a physical symptom
  Physical symptom caused by a known physiologic mechanism
  Physical symptom is stress-induced
  Patient may recognize association between symptom and stress
  Symptom responds to medication, biofeedback, and stress reduction

**Conversion Reaction** (see also Chapter 1)
  Presenting complaint is physical (loss of function, pain, or both)
  Physical symptom not caused by a known physiologic mechanism
  Physical symptom related to unconscious idea, fantasy, or conflict
  Patient does not recognize association between symptom and the unconscious
  Symptom responds slowly to resolution of unconscious factors

**Somatization Disorder**
  Presenting complaint is >13 physical symptoms in females, >11 in males
  Physical symptoms not caused by known physiologic or pathologic mechanism
  Physical symptoms related to need to maintain the sick role
  Patient convinced that symptoms unrelated to psychologic factors
  Symptoms tend to either persist or change character despite treatment

**Hypochondriasis**
  Presenting complaint is a physical sign or symptom
  Physical sign or symptom is normal
  Physical symptom is interpreted by patient to indicate disease
  Conviction regarding illness may be related to depression or anxiety
  Symptom does not respond to reassurance; medication directed at underlying psychologic problems often helpful

**Malingering**
  Presenting complaint is a physical symptom
  Physical symptom is under voluntary control
  Physical symptom is used to gain reward (e.g., money, avoid military service)
  Patient consciously recognizes symptom as factitious
  Symptom may not lessen once reward is attained (need to retain reward)

**Factitious Disorder (e.g., Munchausen syndrome)**
  Presenting complaint is symptom complex mimicking known syndrome
  Symptom complex is under voluntary control
  Symptom complex is used to attain medical treatment (including surgery)
  Patient consciously recognizes symptom complex as factitious, but is often very psychologically disturbed so that unconscious
    factors also are operating
  Symptom complex often results in multiple diagnoses and multiple operations

ple vague somatic complaints, such as headaches, abdominal pain, and fatigue. They often have been seen by numerous specialists and undergo elaborate medical evaluations. Their absence from school often is mistaken as a consequence of their symptoms. In reality, the expression of their symptoms is a means of avoiding school and gaining the attention of a parent. These adolescents may have either a valid or an irrational concern about a parent and thus refuse to leave home, or they may have had an unpleasant experience in school. Rarely do they have a true phobia related to schoolwork. When challenged with the prospect of returning to school, these young people often become extremely anxious and incapacitated with escalating symptoms. School phobia that first becomes manifest during adolescence may be an expression of severe underlying psychopathology. If there is no medical contraindication for the young person to return to school and if he or she refuses to return, psychiatric consultation is indicated.

### Truancy

Truancy is absenteeism from school without permission. It is often peer-initiated. Truancy is more common in adolescents from lower socioeconomic status and low educational backgrounds. The truant adolescent leaves home ostensibly to attend school but either does not go to school or, once having arrived at school, leaves early. A review of the young person's curriculum for appropriateness and formal education testing is indicated because truancy is often a sign of borderline intellectual abilities or learning disability. Young people who are truant often drop out of school when they become 16 yr of age.

## Academic Failure

Academic difficulty is common during adolescence and often is a reflection of increasing demands of high school work and inability of adolescents to keep up with these demands for any number of reasons. Causes of academic failure should be sought. An initial history, physical examination, and laboratory evaluation by the pediatrician may define a physical cause, such as visual or hearing impairment or neurologic dysfunction, or previously undiagnosed chronic illness, such as anemia. A careful behavioral assessment may identify undiagnosed depression. School records should be sought to compare academic capability measured by intelligence quotient (IQ) tests, teacher observations of the student's ability, and the student's actual performance reflected in school grades. Formal educational and psychologic evaluation may be indicated if there is not sufficient information in the school records to identify the cause of academic failure. Intervention involves developing a concerted plan to remedy the situation. The adolescent, the parents, the pediatrician, and the school authorities should participate in this planning.

References

Behrman RE, Kliegman RM, Arvin AM (eds): Nelson Textbook of Pediatrics, 15th ed. Philadelphia, WB Saunders, 1996, Chapters 27, 31.
Koplewicz HS, Gallagher R: School-related anxiety and related conditions. In McAnarney ER, Kreipe RE, Orr DP, Comerci GD (eds): Textbook of Adolescent Medicine. Philadelphia, WB Saunders, 1992, pp 994–1002.
Sahler OJZ: The teenager with failing grades. Pediatr Rev 4:293–300, 1983.

## SERIOUS PSYCHIATRIC ILLNESS

Psychoses related to drug ingestion, schizophrenia, or manic-depressive illness or as isolated episodes of decompensation during emotional stress often first occur during adolescence. It is unusual for an adult with psychosis to have had an uneventful adolescence. If there is any question about the possibility of psychosis, or impending psychosis, early psychiatric evaluation is indicated.

*Schizophrenia* generally presents before adulthood. It is characterized by loosening of associative thought patterns, inappropriate affect, ambivalent emotional state, and gradual but marked withdrawal from family, school, and peers. Perceptual disturbances are frequent. Health care providers frequently see adolescents in the early stage of their schizophrenic decompensation because of behavioral or somatic symptoms.

*Manic-depressive (bipolar) disorder* often is misla-

beled as schizophrenia during adolescence. The distinct periods of elevated, expansive, or irritable moods associated with hyperactivity and distractibility may alternate rapidly with periods of severe depression lasting for several days or weeks. The family history usually is positive for mental illness.

*Acute confusional states* can be related to numerous panic inducers, including drugs. The hallucinogens (most notably lysergic acid diethylamide [LSD] and phencyclidine [PCP]), amphetamines, and marijuana all have been associated with an acute toxic psychosis marked by confusion, disorientation, anxiety, agitation, and disturbances of perception, judgment, or reason. Major tranquilizers and a quiet, safe, nonthreatening environment are helpful in such cases (see Table 7–24).

References

Behrman RE, Kliegman RM, Arvin AM (eds): Nelson Textbook of Pediatrics, 15th ed. Philadelphia, WB Saunders, 1996, Chapters 29, 30.
McAnarney ER, Kreipe RE, Orr DP, Comerci GD (eds): Textbook of Adolescent Medicine. Philadelphia, WB Saunders, 1992, Sec. 24.

## MISCELLANEOUS CONDITIONS

### RUNAWAY BEHAVIOR

Nearly 1 million young people run away from their families of origin during adolescence. Running away from home may indicate environmental stress, including abuse (more than two thirds of female runaways report sexual abuse), or it may indicate intrapsychic problems of the adolescent. Psychologic evaluation of the adolescent includes seeking evidence for depression, characterologic personality disturbance, or a combination of these conditions. Runaway youths are at particularly high risk of being used by adults for illicit activities, such as drug-related crimes or prostitution. Hotlines are available for runaway youths to seek help.

### ABUSE

Abuse of adolescents may be physical, verbal, or sexual. Adults often believe that adolescents are unlikely to be abused because they have developed the capacity to ask for outside help or to leave the family to seek care. However, adolescents may be reluctant to report the abusive situation because they may want to protect the abusing parent or may be too embarrassed to seek help. Evidence of physical trauma, including unexplained bruises and cuts, should be considered as evidence of abuse, as it would be in younger children. Sexual abuse or exploitation, either in incestuous relationships or for prostitution, may become evident when adolescents, particularly early adolescents, become pregnant. If a pregnant adolescent is unable to identify the father of the baby openly to the clinician, one should suspect either incest or prostitution.

## References

Behrman RE, Kliegman RM, Arvin AM (eds): Nelson Textbook of Pediatrics, 15th ed. Philadelphia, WB Saunders, 1996, Chapters 38, 42.

# Chapter 8

# IMMUNOLOGY AND ALLERGY

Dale T. Umetsu

## THE IMMUNE SYSTEM

The body resists infection by means of a number of integrated systems, including anatomic barriers as well as a complex interaction of serum proteins and bone marrow-derived cells collectively known as the immune system. When functioning effectively, host defenses rapidly eliminate pathogens and toxins. The hallmarks of immunodeficiency (frequent or unusually severe infections) appear when the immune system is ineffective or deficient. When the immune system develops inappropriate and deleterious responses, autoimmune or allergic disease results.

Children with *primary immunodeficiencies*, which are relatively rare diseases, present with infection; the pediatrician must be able to distinguish the rare child with true immunodeficiency from the immunologically normal child who has recurrent infections. The evaluation of children with recurrent infections, therefore, must be based on a comprehensive understanding of the immune system and the patient's age, the site, and the pathogens involved in those opportunistic infections (Table 8–1).

### MAJOR COMPONENTS OF THE HOST DEFENSE

The major components of host defense include the:

1. Anatomic/mucociliary barrier mechanism.
2. B-cell compartment (the major component of humoral immunity).
3. T-cell compartment (the major component of cell-mediated immunity).
4. Phagocytic compartment.
5. Complement system (a component of humoral immunity).

The phagocytic compartment and the complement system are responsible for *innate immunity*, which initiates an antigen-nonspecific first line of defense against pathogens, before the more versatile *adaptive immune* response begins, involving antigen-specific T cells and B cells (Fig. 8–1). Defects may occur in one or more of these compartments and lead to recurrent, opportunistic, or life-threatening infections. Anatomic integrity, at the interface between the body and its environment (skin, mucous membranes), is essential for protection against infection (Table 8–2). Such defects must not be overlooked as a potential source in children with recurrent infection.

### B-cell Compartment

*Humoral immunity* is the capacity of serum components to combat infection. The major components of humoral immunity are the immunoglobulins; other circulating components (complement proteins) are also involved in humoral defenses. Immunoglobulins attach specifically to antigens (glycoproteins, carbohydrates, toxins) and inactivate or agglutinate the antigen; or opsonize the antigen for phagocytosis; or allow the activation of complement causing pathogen cytolysis. Five major immunoglobulin (Ig) isotypes, IgG, IgM, IgA, IgD, IgE, are distinguished by antigenic and functional differences in their heavy chains (Fig. 8–2).

*IgG* is the major serum immunoglobulin (70–75% of all immunoglobulin), and it is the major immunoglobulin produced in secondary responses. IgG diffuses well into tissues, crosses the placenta, and has one of the longest half-lives of serum proteins (~21 days). IgG can be further subdivided into four subclasses—IgG1, IgG2, IgG3, IgG4—based on heavy-chain differences. In general, anti-

TABLE 8–1.   Clinical Characteristics of Primary Immunodeficiencies

**B-Cell Defects**
Recurrent pyogenic infections with extracellular encapsulated organisms, such as pneumococcus, *Haemophilus influenzae,* and streptococci
Otitis, sinusitis, recurrent pneumonia, bronchiectasis, conjunctivitis
Few problems with fungal or viral infections (except enterovirus encephalitis and poliomyelitis)
Decreased levels of immunoglobulins in serum and secretions
Diarrhea common, especially secondary to infection with *Giardia lamblia*
Growth retardation not striking
Compatible with survival to adulthood or for several years after onset unless complications occur

**T-Cell Defects**
Recurrent infections with less virulent or opportunistic organisms such as fungi, mycobacteria, viruses, and protozoa
Growth retardation, malabsorption, diarrhea, and failure to thrive are common
Anergy
Susceptible to graft-versus-host reactions if given unirradiated blood
Fatal reactions may occur from live virus or BCG vaccination
High incidence of malignancy
Poor survival beyond infancy or childhood

**Phagocytic Defects**
Recurrent dermatologic infections with bacteria and fungi, such as *Staphylococcus, Pseudomonas, Escherichia coli,* and *Aspergillus*
Subcutaneous, lymph node, lung, and liver abscesses
Pulmonary infections common, including abscess and pneumatocele formation, contributing to chronic disease
Bone and joint infection common

**Complement Defects**
Recurrent bacterial infections with extracellular pyogenic organisms, such as pneumococcus, *H. influenzae*
Unusual susceptibility to recurrent *gonococcal* and *meningococcal* infections
Increased incidence of autoimmune disease (SLE)
Severe or recurrent skin and respiratory tract infection

BCG = bacille Calmette-Guérin; SLE = systemic lupus erythematosus.

FIGURE 8–1.   Innate, adaptive, and anatomic mechanisms as major components of normal host defense.

globulin pool but is also the major protective antibody *(secretory IgA)* in saliva, lacrimal fluid, and colostrum. IgA is present in nasal, bronchial, and intestinal secretions, but because it does not activate complement, IgA is thought to function by clearing antigens from mucosal sites without evoking inflammatory responses. Secretory IgA (sIgA) is distinguished from serum IgA by the presence of a component (called secretory piece) and by a short polypeptide J chain.

TABLE 8–2.   Anatomic and Mucociliary Defects That Result in Recurrent or Opportunistic Infections

**Anatomic Defects in the Upper Airways**
Aspiration syndromes (gastroesophageal reflux, ineffective cough, foreign body or gastric aspiration)
Cleft palate, eustachian tube dysfunction
Adenoidal hypertrophy
Nasal polyps
Obstruction of paranasal sinus drainage (osteomeatal complex disease), encephaloceles
Post-traumatic or congenital sinus tracts (CSF rhinorrhea)

**Anatomic Defects in the Tracheobronchial Tree**
Tracheal esophageal fistula, bronchobiliary fistula
Pulmonary sequestration, bronchogenic cysts, vascular ring
Tumor, foreign body, or enlarged nodes

**Physiologic Defects in the Upper and Lower Airways**
Primary ciliary dyskinesia syndromes, Young syndrome
Cystic fibrosis, bronchopulmonary dysplasia, bronchiectasis
Allergic disease (allergic rhinitis, asthma)
Chronic cigarette smoke exposure

**Other Defects**
Burns
Chronic atopic dermatitis
Ureteral obstruction/vesicoureteral reflux
Intravenous drug use
Central venous lines, artificial heart valves, CSF shunts, peritoneal dialysis catheter, urinary catheter

CSF = cerebrospinal fluid.

body responses to polysaccharide antigens reside in the IgG2 subclass, whereas responses to protein antigens reside in the IgG1 and IgG3 subclasses.

*IgM* comprises 10% of all immunoglobulins and is confined to the intravascular pool. IgM circulates in the blood as a pentamer, joined by a J chain. IgM is secreted rapidly following primary antigenic stimulation, binds complement efficiently, and assists the reticuloendothelial system in clearing circulating bacteria by opsonization and agglutination.

*IgA* constitutes 15–20% of the serum immuno-

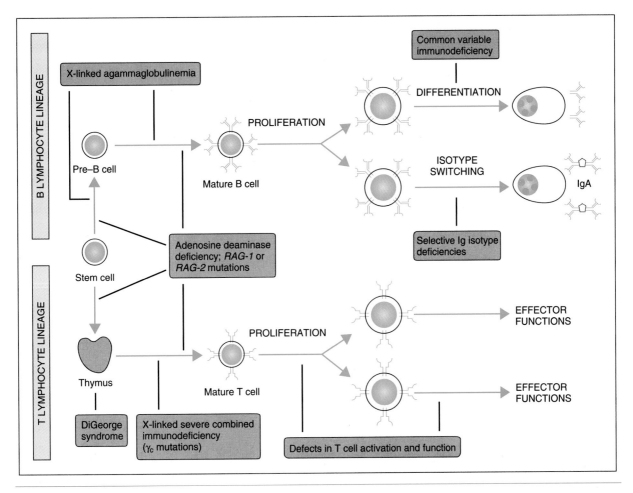

FIGURE 8–2. Sites of cellular abnormalities in congenital immunodeficiencies. In different congenital (primary) immunodeficiencies, the maturation or activation of B or T lymphocytes may be blocked at different stages. (From Abbas AK, Lichtman AH, Pober JS: Cellular and Molecular Immunology, 3rd ed. Philadelphia, WB Saunders, 1997, p 411.)

*IgD* accounts for less than 1% of total immunoglobulin and serves as an antigen receptor or receptor site on circulating B cells.

*IgE* is present in serum in very small amounts but is the principal mediator of immediate hypersensitivity reactions. IgE may play a role in immunity to metazoan parasites.

Immunoglobulin is produced by B lymphocytes, after they become activated and differentiate into plasma cells (see Fig. 8–2). B cells express cell surface receptors for the Fc region of IgG, receptors for complement, and receptors for major histocompatibility (MHC) class I and II molecules. They can be identified by staining for the CD19 and CD20 molecules.

## Complement

The complement system includes two parallel but independent pathways (classic and alternative or

properdin) that lead to the cascade-like sequential activation of factors; activated factors have various biologic activities which enhance phagocytosis and antibody-dependent and -independent cell lysis (Fig. 8–3). The complement system consists of 20 well-defined plasma complement components, five cell membrane regulatory proteins, and seven cell membrane receptors. The third component of complement, C3, is the most abundant, with a plasma concentration of 1 mg/mL. It is a pivotal factor, since the classical and alternative pathways converge at C3, after which the activation sequences are identical. The classical pathway is activated by antigen-antibody complexes and, nonimmunologically, by C-reactive protein and trypsin-like enzymes. The alternative pathway may be activated by C3b generated through classic complement activation and, nonimmunologically, by endotoxin or fungal antigens (zymogen). The complement com-

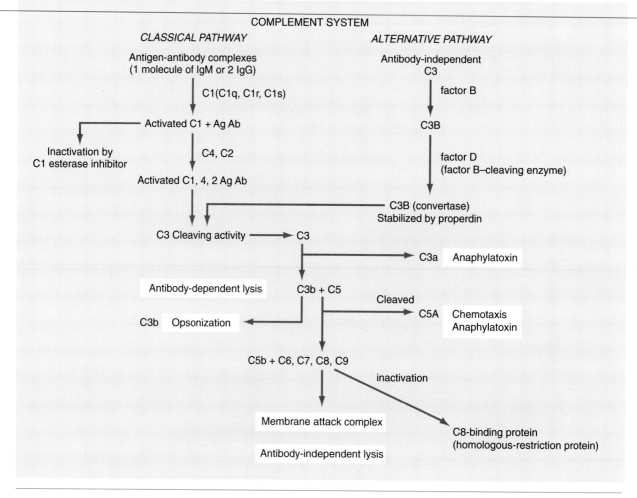

FIGURE 8–3.  Complement component cascade involving the classical and the alternate, or properdin, pathways. The initiating events for both pathways differ but result in production of C3 cleaving enzyme activity, which is the pivotal step as the two pathways converge to the terminal activation sequences. Ag Ab = antigen-antibody complex.

ponents amplify immunological stimuli in an antigen nonspecific manner, although complement can be activated in the classical pathway by aggregated antigen-specific antibody. When activated, complement components have potent opsonizing (C3b, iC3b), chemotactic (C5a), mast cell activating (C3a, C5a), and lytic (membrane attack complex, C5b–C9) activity; they can activate neutrophil respiratory burst activity (C3a, C5a).

## T-cell Compartment

T lymphocytes are lymphocytes that are responsible for the cytolysis of virus-infected cells, for inducing B cell activation and differentiation, and for recruiting, by means of their soluble products, macrophages, neutrophils, eosinophils, basophils,

and mast cells. T cells are greatly involved in immunity to intracellular organisms (viruses, *Mycobacterium, Toxoplasma, Legionella, Brucella*), fungal organisms (*Histoplasma, Candida*), and protozoa; in immune surveillance for cancer cells; and in causing graft-versus-host disease and transplant graft rejection. T cells can be divided into two major subsets: CD4+ and CD8+ T cells (see Fig. 8–2).

*CD4+ T cells*, the helper/inducer subset, help to regulate immune responses and produce a wide variety of cytokines, such as interleukin (IL)-2, IL-3, IL-4, IL-5, IL-10, and interferon-γ (IFN-γ) (Table 8–3). Th2 cells are CD4+ T cells that secrete cytokines such as IL-4, IL-5 and IL-10, and they are critical for the activation and differentiation of B cells (humoral immunity) and in downregulating immune responses. CD4+ T cells, which secrete cytokines

TABLE 8–3.  Interleukins and Their Functions

| Interleukin | Source | Function |
|---|---|---|
| IL-1 | Macrophages | Costimulatory effect on T cells enhance antigen presentation |
| IL-2 | T cells | T-cell growth factor, B-cell growth factor |
| IL-3 | T cells | Mast cell growth factor, multi–colony-stimulating factor |
| IL-4 | T cells | T-cell growth factor; enhances IgE synthesis, enhances B-cell differentiation, mast cell growth |
| IL-5 | T cells | Enhances immunoglobulin synthesis, enhances IgA synthesis, enhances eosinophil differentiation |
| IL-6 | T cells, macrophages, fibroblasts, endothelium | Enhances immunoglobulin synthesis, antiviral activity, hepatocyte-stimulating factor |
| IL-7 | Stromal cells | Enhances growth of pre–B cells and pre–T cells |
| IL-8 | T cells, macrophages, epithelium | Neutrophil-activating protein, T-lymphocyte chemotactic factor |
| IL-9 | T cells | Acts in synergy with IL-4 to induce IgE production, mast cell growth |
| IL-10 | T cells, macrophages | Cytokine synthesis inhibitory factor, suppresses macrophage function, enhances B-cell growth |
| IL-12 | Macrophages, neutrophils | Natural killer cell stimulatory factor, cytotoxic lymphocyte maturation factor, enhances IFN-$\gamma$ synthesis, inhibits IL-4 synthesis |
| IL-13 | T cells | Enhances IgE synthesis, enhances B-cell growth, inhibits macrophage activation |
| IL-18 | Macrophages | Enhances IFN-$\gamma$ synthesis |
| IFN-$\gamma$ | T cells | Macrophage activation, inhibits IgE synthesis; antiviral activity |
| RANTES | T cells, endothelium | Chemoattractant (chemokine) for monocytes, T cells, eosinophils |

IFN = interferon; Ig = immunoglobulin; RANTES = regulated upon activation, normal T expressed and secreted.

such as IFN-$\gamma$ and IL-2, are important in activating macrophages and in cell-mediated immunity. Development of Th1 cells expressing inappropriate cytokine profiles can exacerbate infection and cause allergy, autoimmune, and graft-versus-host disease.

CD8 + T cells (cytotoxic suppressor cells) kill virus-infected cells or tumor cells and suppress or limit immune responses. They kill target cells through several mechanisms, including pore formation by enzymes stored in the lytic granules of CD8+ cells, and induction of programmed cell death by triggering of Fas antigen (CD95) on target cells by the Fas ligand on the cytotoxic effector cells. Cytotoxicity is also mediated by natural killer (NK) cells, which express the CD16 and CD56 antigens but not T-cell receptors. NK cells express some form of antigen receptors; recognition by NK cells of MHC antigens on target cells inhibits lytic activity. NK cells secrete large quantities of IFN-$\gamma$ and tumor necrosis factor-$\alpha$ (TNF-$\alpha$), and they have cytolytic activity against virally infected and transformed target cells that express antigens to which they have not been previously sensitized. Therefore NK cells, as part of the innate immune system, are important early during immune responses, before immunologic memory (characteristics of adaptive immunity with T cells and B cells) becomes effective. The development of NK cell activity is enhanced by IL-12 and IL-2.

Tumor-infiltrating lymphocytes (TILs) are CD3 + T cells found in solid tumors that can be expanded in vitro when stimulated with IL-2. These cells are thought to be cytotoxic and tumor-specific, and when they are reinfused in the donor, they cause regression of the target tumor.

### Phagocytic Compartment

Phagocytic cells engulf and digest foreign antigens and microorganisms. The predominant phagocytic cell in blood is the polymorphonuclear neutrophil (PMN), which has a circulating half-life of 6–10 hr, is antigen-nonspecific, and does not divide; its major function is to ingest pyogenic bacteria and some fungi, in particular Aspergillus. Recruitment and chemotaxis of PMN to sites of inflammation are greatly aided by *adhesion molecules (selectins, integrins, and chemokines)*, which regulate specific interactions between PMNs and endothelial cells. Phagocytosis is initiated by the recognition of a foreign antigen; this is greatly facilitated by cell surface receptors for the Fc portion of immunoglobulin and three receptors for complement (CR1, CR2, CR3). These receptors allow antigen-specific immunoglobulin (with complement) to enhance recognition and phagocytosis of foreign material. Phagocytosis also triggers the cell's NADPH oxidase system that generates superoxide and hydrogen peroxide, which greatly aid in the killing of ingested organisms. Hydrolytic enzymes in granules, such as lysozyme and myeloperoxidase, also aid in the killing of microorganisms. Short peptides called *defensins* (29–42 amino acids), which constitute about 5% of the total cellular protein of neutrophils, have important antimicrobial and cytotoxic function against pathogens. The structure of defensins indicates that aggregation of defensins produce holes in the membranes of bacteria, mycobacteria, and fungi. Defensins are also secreted by tracheal cells and are important in resisting infection in the lungs.

The *macrophage*, another cell type in the phagocytic compartment, is a long-lived phagocytic cell that develops from circulating monocytes. It populates the lung, liver, kidneys, spleen, brain, and lymph nodes. Macrophages are effective in killing facultative intracellular organisms such as *Mycobacterium*, *Toxoplasma*, and *Legionella*. Macrophages are most effective when activated by IFN-γ and T cells. T cells can cross-link the CD40 molecule on macrophages, resulting in the expression of the inducible form of nitric oxide synthase and of B7-1 molecules (CD80) and B7-2 (CD86) in addition to the production of IL-12. The expression of B7 and the production of IL-12 enhance the capacity of macrophages to present antigens to T cells and to induce cell-mediated immunity (development of Th1 cells and cytotoxic T cells).

## ONTOGENY OF THE IMMUNE SYSTEM

T cells, B cells, neutrophils, and monocytes all derive from CD34+ stem cells in the bone marrow (see Fig. 8-2). T cells mature in the thymus through a complex process involving both negative and positive selection that determines the T-cell receptor repertoire. Approximately 90% of the developing T cells are eliminated by *negative selection*, eliminating autoreactive T cells, and by *positive selection*, eliminating T cells with receptors that do not recognize self-MHC antigens. T cells that leave the thymus then circulate and repopulate the lymphoid organs, including lymph nodes, spleen, and Peyer's patches.

B-cell development begins in the bone marrow and is dependent on the function of a gene called *Bruton's tyrosine kinase* (*Btk*), which is dysfunctional in patients with Bruton's X-linked agammaglobulinemia. In the bone marrow, B-cell differentiation involves deletional recombination of immunoglobulin genes and VDJ gene rearrangement. This process allows B cells to express cell surface IgM molecules and circulate and populate lymphoid follicles in the spleen, lymph nodes, tonsils and Peyer's patches.

Phagocytes, which also differentiate from stem cells, include circulating monocytes, from which tissue macrophages differentiate. Granulocytes, such as neutrophils, eosinophils, and basophils develop in the bone marrow before circulating in the blood. Mast cells develop from stem cells as a separate lineage, leave the bone marrow in an immature state, but complete their differentiation in the tissues.

## INITIATION OF IMMUNE RESPONSES

Immune responses are initiated by the presence of foreign materials or pathogens, which are taken up by antigen-presenting cells (APCs), such as dendritic cells, antigen-specific B cells, and macrophages. The initiation requires that the foreign material be accompanied by a "danger" signal, provided by endotoxin, other bacterial products, or tissue necrosis. These signals activate the APC, allowing for more efficient antigen presentation; in the absence of this "danger" signal, T-cell tolerance or anergy occurs. After uptake, the antigen is processed and antigen peptides associate with MHC class I or class II molecules. The antigen peptide-MHC complex is then expressed on the surface of the APC for recognition by T cells. T-cell activation occurs if the T-cell receptor is aggregated and if the APC also delivers costimulatory signals to the T cell through the expression of cell surface molecules, such as B7-1, B7-2, and intercellular adhesion molecule-1 (ICAM-1). T-cell activation results in the phosphorylation of multiple membrane and cytoplasmic proteins, hydrolyzation of membrane phosphatidylinositol bisphosphate, and an increase in intracellular free calcium; it is manifested by T-cell proliferation and production of cytokines, such as IL-2.

The activation of T cells sets off a number of events in the immune system, triggered by cell-cell interaction and by secreted cytokines. Activation of T cells induces the T cell to differentiate and produce other cytokines (such as IFN-γ) and, in some instances, IL-4, IL-5, and IL-10. Activation of the T cell also induces T-cell expression of other cell surface molecules, such as CD40 ligand, which is critical in activating dendritic cells and macrophages. Cross-linking of CD40 on the surface of dendritic cells and macrophages by CD40 ligand, in the presence of IFN-γ, activates the dendritic cells and macrophages to produce IL-12, which greatly enhances the production of IFN-γ from T cells and NK cells and the development of cytotoxic T cells. Activated macrophages can also produce nitric oxide, which effectively kills intracellular organisms such as *Mycobacterium*, *Listeria*, *Leishmania*, *Toxoplasma*, and other intracellular parasites. Cross-linking of CD40 on the surface of B cells, in the presence of IL-2, IL-4, and IL-5, induces B cell differentiation, isotype switch, and immunoglobulin production.

## PHYSIOLOGIC IMMUNODEFICIENCY IN THE NEONATE

Because immunity in young children, particularly neonates, is deficient compared to that in adults, children are more susceptible to infections than adults. The immune system in children is still developing and requires several years before reaching maturity. Infants produce only small amounts of immunoglobulin before 4–6 mo of age and by birth have received all of their immunoglobulins (IgG) transplacentally from the mother during the third trimester of gestation. Premature infants are frequently hypogammaglobulinemic because they receive only a fraction of the usual maternal antibody. The fetus can produce antibody but mostly of the IgM isotype. Neonates do respond to immunization, generally to potent proteins, but the ability to respond to bacterial antigens (carbohydrates) is not consistently acquired until after 2 yr of age. Normal levels of serum immunoglobulins reach a nadir at around 4–6 mo of age and increase slowly over several years. Acquisition of adult levels of IgM occurs by 1 yr of age, whereas adult levels of IgG are noted at 5–7 yr; adult levels of IgA are achieved at 10 to 14 yr of age.

T-cell function in young children is reduced, mainly because neonatal T cells are immature and have attenuated production of IFN-γ, IL-4, IL-5, and other cytokines. T-cell help for B cells is limited. Neonatal T cells express CD40L poorly; this expression is required for cognate interaction with B cells in the induction of antibody synthesis. Cyto-toxic responses are also reduced in the neonate, as is neutrophil function. Limited production of IFN-γ, which activates neutrophils, results in poor function of neutrophils. In neonates, there is also a reduced production of neutrophils and poor neutrophil chemotaxis. Complement levels particularly C8 and C9, are decreased; the neonate has less than 20% of the normal adult activity. Thus, multiple problems in the neonate contribute to the increased susceptibility to infection.

## IMMUNODEFICIENCY DISORDERS

The hallmark of immunodeficiency is increased susceptibility to infection; affected patients also have infections with increased severity or infections with opportunistic organisms. Infections primarily occur in the respiratory tract, the gastrointestinal tract (resulting in diarrhea or malabsorption), or the skin. Primary immunodeficiencies can be classified according to the location of the immune defect—in the B-cell, T-cell, phagocytic, or complement compartment. Deficiencies may also exist in one or more of these compartments; the deficiency may be congenital (X-linked [Bruton] agammaglobulinemia) or secondary (Table 8–4). There are more than 50 different primary immunodeficiencies. Although immunodeficiencies are rare, the overall frequency for severe primary immunodeficiency is about 1 in 10,000. Patients with B-cell defects constitute about 50% of primary immunodeficiencies, whereas about 30% of primary immunodeficiencies are due to T-cell defects. Phagocytic defects are even less common (~18% of all cases of primary immunodeficiency), but primary complement defects are the least common (~2% of all cases).

### B-CELL DEFECTS: ANTIBODY DEFICIENCY STATES

B-cell deficiencies are due to the absence of B cells, abnormal B-cell differentiation, or secondary to abnormal T-cell function (Table 8–5). Defects of antibody production may involve all antibody classes, selective antibody classes, selective deficiency of IgG subclasses, or an inability to respond to a specific antigen.

The *clinical manifestations* of abnormal B-cell function include recurrent sinopulmonary infections (otitis media, sinusitis, pneumonia), and bacteremia with encapsulated bacteria, such as *Streptococcus pneumoniae*, *Haemophilus influenzae*, and *Staphylococcus* (see Table 8–1). Antibody deficiency states do not become manifest until after 6 mo

TABLE 8–4.    Causes of Secondary
              Immunodeficiency

**Viral Infection**
  Measles (inhibits interleukin-12 production in macrophages)
  Roseola (human herpesvirus-6)
  Epstein-Barr virus (X-linked lymphoproliferative
    disease–Duncan syndrome)
  Cytomegalovirus
  Human immunodeficiency virus (destroys CD4+ T cells)

**Metabolic Disorders**
  Diabetes mellitus
  Malnutrition
  Uremia
  Sickle cell disease
  Zinc deficiency
  Multiple carboxylase deficiency
  Burns

**Protein-Losing States**
  Nephrotic syndrome
  Protein-losing enteropathy

**Other Causes**
  Prematurity
  Immunosuppressive agents (corticosteroids, radiation,
    antimetabolites)
  Malignancy (leukemia, Hodgkin disease, nonlymphoid
    cancer)
  Acquired asplenia
  Perodonitis
  Chronic (acute) blood transfusions
  Acquired neutropenia (autoimmune, viral, drug-induced)
  Bone marrow transplantation/graft-versus host disease
  Systemic lupus erythematosus
  Sarcoidosis

of age, when transplacentally acquired maternal antibody has been depleted. Deficiency of IgG synthesis can be observed in the 1st yr of life (X-linked agammaglobulinemia), or it may occur later in childhood or early adulthood (common variable agammaglobulinemia) (see Table 8–5). Isolated deficiency of IgA is associated with recurrent infection, but because many individuals with low IgA levels are asymptomatic, the precise mechanism that causes recurrent infection is unclear. Similarly, isolated IgG2 subclass deficiency is associated with a propensity for development of recurrent sinopulmonary infection, although asymptomatic individuals with low IgG2 levels have been identified.

### X-Linked Agammaglobulinemia

X-linked agammaglobulinemia is a congenital immunodeficiency in males characterized by a profound deficiency of B cells, resulting in severe hypogammaglobulinemia and absence of lymphoid tissue (see Fig. 8–2 and Table 8–5). The defect is limited to the B-cell lineage and is caused by muta-

tions of the B cell–specific tyrosine kinase, *Btk*, at chromosome Xq22. The major consequence is the arrest of B-cell development at the pre-B cell state. A similar phenotype has been described in females, with gene defects in the mu heavy-chain gene on chromosome 14. Patients with X-linked agammaglobulinemia present after the first few months of life; 20% of patients experience initial symptoms after 12 mo or as late as 3–5 yr. Infections with *S. pneumoniae*, *H. influenzae*, *Staphylococcus aureus*, and *Pseudomonas* species, organisms for which antibody is an important opsonin, develop. Gastrointestinal problems, except for enteroviral infection and giardiasis, are relatively rare in contrast to the frequency of gastrointestinal symptoms seen in **common variable immunodeficiency** (described farther on). Immunization with live poliomyelitis vaccine has resulted in poliomyelitis.

### Hyper-IgM Syndrome

Hyper-IgM syndrome is an X-linked immunodeficiency characterized by elevated serum levels of IgM but normal levels of IgG and IgA and by absent B-cell function (inability to produce antigen-specific antibody). Recurrent sinopulmonary infections, infection with *Pneumocystis carinii*, thrombocytopenia, hemolytic anemia, hypothyroidism, and neutropenia are common. The disease is caused by mutations in the gene coding for the CD40 ligand, an antigen expressed on the surface of T cells, making the T cells unable to interact with B cells and macrophages. B cells in such individuals, therefore, cannot undergo isotype switch, and macrophages cannot be activated. The result is an inability to generate normal antibody responses and a predisposition to infection with intracellular pathogens.

### Common Variable Immunodeficiency

Common variable immunodeficiency is a heterogeneous disorder characterized by initial normal immune function, followed by a severe reduction in serum IgG (generally <250 mg/dL), IgA, and IgM and by recurrent sinopulmonary infections. Antibody titers to protein antigens such as tetanus and diphtheria are absent, but T-cell function (proliferation to mitogens) is normal. B cells may be present. Patients often have normal-sized or enlarged tonsils and lymph nodes and may have splenomegaly. Initially, respiratory tract infections develop; as many as 50% of patients have gastrointestinal disease (malabsorption, chronic diarrhea) of unclear etiology as well as autoimmune diseases, such as hemolytic anemia, thrombocytopenia, and neutropenia. Malignancy is observed in 6–16%. These observations suggest that T-cell helper function may also be quantitatively abnormal. Common variable immunodeficiency is observed in families with IgA deficiency, or it may also occur as an idiosyncratic reaction to some drugs (e.g., phenytoin).

### Selective IgA Deficiency

Selective IgA deficiency is defined as serum IgA levels below 5–10 mg/dL accompanied by normal or increased levels of other immunoglobulins. It occurs in approximately 1 in 600 individuals; patients with selective IgA deficiency may be asymptomatic. IgA deficiency is also associated with recurrent sinopulmonary infections, IgG2 subclass deficiency, food allergy, autoimmune or rheumatologic disease, and celiac disease. IgA deficiency occurs in families, suggesting an autosomal inheritance. It also occurs in families with common variable immunodeficiency. The genes for IgA deficiency (and for some forms of common variable immunodeficiency) may reside in the MHC class III region on chromosome 6.

### Immunoglobulin G Subclass Deficiency

IgG subclass deficiency occurs when the level of antibodies in one or more of the four IgG subclasses is decreased. IgG2 subclass deficiency is the most common of these deficiencies and is often associated with IgA deficiency, ataxia telangiectasias, and a reduced capacity to produce antibody against carbohydrate antigens. In some patients, IgG2 subclass deficiency resolves spontaneously; in others, it progresses to common variable immunodeficiency.

### Transient Hypogammaglobulinemia of Infancy

Transient hypogammaglobulinemia of infancy is a temporary condition characterized by delayed immunoglobulin production of unknown cause coupled with the normal physiologic decline in immunoglobulin concentrations observed in the first 3–7 mo of life. The normal low point at 3–5 mo of age is accentuated, reaching levels of less than 200 mg/dL. B and T cells are present, and antibodies can be synthesized to protein antigens such as diphtheria and tetanus toxoids. Immunoglobulin levels remain diminished throughout the 1st yr of life but increase to normal age-appropriate levels, usually between 18 and 36 mo of age. The incidence of sinopulmonary infection is increased.

### Specific Therapies for B-cell Diseases

The *treatment* of X-linked agammaglobulinemia, common variable agammaglobulinemia, and hyper-IgM syndrome is replacement of IgG with intravenous human pooled immunoglobulin (IVIG), 400–500 mg/kg/dose, given every 4 wk. In spite of IVIG therapy, patients may continue to experience sinusitis and bronchitis, requiring aggressive antibiotic therapy as well as prophylactic antibiotics. Chronic bronchitis and bronchiectasis may develop, in which case chest physiotherapy and serial pulmonary function studies may be useful. Patients with other antibody deficiency states benefit from prophylactic antibiotics, but IVIG should be used in such patients only if prophylactic antibiotic therapy fails and when B-cell responsiveness on antigen challenge is impaired. In all patients, appropriate antibiotic therapy is indicated for specific infections as determined by culture and epidemiology (see Table 8–1).

### Complement Deficiencies

Complement deficiencies are rare diseases that occur when an individual is born without one of the 30 proteins that compose the complement system, or they may occur secondary to either increased consumption or decreased synthesis of any of the complement components. Deficiency may result in recurrent pyogenic infection, lupus-like disease, or vasculitis (Table 8–6). Acquired deficiency usually results from consumption of complement components from immune complex deposition (systemic lupus erythematosus, bacterial endocarditis, hepatitis) or protein loss. Sickle cell disease is associated with a defect in alternative pathway function that is needed for opsonization of pneumococci.

**C1 esterase inhibitor deficiency**, or **hereditary angioedema** (HANE), results in recurrent episodes of angioedema lasting 24–72 hr, which is nonpruritic and occurs after trauma, stress, or anxiety. Angioedema can occur in any tissue, but abdominal edema can cause acute abdominal pain, and edema of the upper airway can be life-threatening, requiring emergency tracheostomy. The *diagnosis* is suggested by family history (the disorder is transmitted as an autosomal dominant trait) and by chronically decreased C4 levels and decreased C2 levels during acute attacks. C1 inhibitor protein is markedly reduced or, if present, is not functional.

An antigen-nonspecific humoral factor of major importance in host defense is the *mannose-binding protein*. It binds and opsonizes high mannose-containing glycoproteins on the membranes of bacteria, mycobacteria, and yeast, and activates the

TABLE 8–5. Disorders of Lymphocyte Function

| Disorder | Genetics | Onset | Manifestations | Pathogenesis | Associated Features |
|---|---|---|---|---|---|
| Bruton agammaglobulinemia | X-linked (Xq21.3–q22) | Infancy (6–9 months) | Recurrent high-grade infections, sinusitis, pneumonia, meningitis | Arrest in B-cell differentiation (pre-B level); mutation in the Btk gene | Lymphoid hypoplasia |
| Common variable immunodeficiency | AR; AD | Second to third decade | Sinusitis, bronchitis, pneumonia, chronic diarrhea | Arrest in B-cell to plasma cell differentiation | Autoimmune disease, RA, SLE, Graves disease, ITP, malignancy |
| Transient hypogammaglobulinemia of infancy | | Infancy (3–7 months) | Recurrent viral and pyogenic infections | Delayed development of plasma cell maturation | Frequently in families with immunodeficiencies |
| IgA deficiency | X-linked, AR, ? 6p21.3 | Variable | Sinopulmonary infections Gastrointestinal infections; may be normal | Failure of IgA expressing B-cell differentiation | IgG subclass deficiency, common variable immunodeficiency, autoimmune diseases |
| IgG subclass deficiency | AR 2p11; 14q32.3 | Variable | Variable (normal to recurrent sinopulmonary infections and gastrointestinal infections) | Defect in isotype IgG production | IgA deficiency, ataxia–telangiectasia |
| IgM deficiency | AR | First year | Recurrent septicemia; pneumococcal, *Haemophilus influenzae* infections | Defective helper T-cell/B-cell interaction | Whipple disease, regional enteritis, lymphoid hyperplasia |
| Immunodeficiency with increased IgM | X-linked, AR, ? (Xq24–q26) | 2–3 years | Recurrent pyogenic infections (otitis media, sinusitis, tonsillitis, pneumonia) | Defect in IgG and IgA synthesis and of CD40 ligand | Hematologic autoimmune disease |
| DiGeorge anomaly | ? (22q11.2) | Early infancy | Variable | Hypoplasia of third and fourth pharyngeal pouch | Hypoparathyroidism, aortic arch anomalies, micrognathia, hypertelorism |

| Disease | Inheritance (locus) | Age of onset | Infections | Defect | Clinical features |
|---|---|---|---|---|---|
| Wiskott-Aldrich syndrome | X-linked (Xp11–p11.3) | Early infancy | Recurrent otitis media, pneumonia, meningitis with encapsulated organisms | 53-kD protein (WASP) defect | Recurrent infections, atopic dermatitis, platelet dysfunction, thrombocytopenia |
| Ataxia-telangiectasia | AR (11q22.3) | 2–5 years | Sinopulmonary infections | AT gene mutation | Neurologic and endocrine dysfunction, malignancy, telangiectasis; sensitive to radiation |
| Cartilage-hair hypoplasia (short-limbed dwarf) | AR | Birth | Variable | Unknown | Metaphyseal dysplasia, short extremities |
| Severe combined immunodeficiency | X-linked (Xq13.1–q21.1) AR | 1–3 months | Candidiasis, all types of infections (bacterial, viral, fungal, protozoal) | IL-2R γ depletion (severe T-cell depletion) ZAP-70 or Jak-3 kinase deficiency | Severe graft-versus-host disease from maternal fetal transfusions |
| Severe combined immunodeficiency (ADA deficiency) | AR (20q13-ter) | 1–3 months | Candidiasis, all types of infections (bacterial, viral, fungal, protozoal) | Enzyme deficiency results in dATP-induced lymphocyte toxicity | Multiple skeletal abnormalities, chondro-osseous dysplasia |
| Severe combined immunodeficiency (PNP deficiency) | AR 14q13.1 | 1–3 months | Candidiasis, all types of infections (bacterial, viral, fungal, protozoal) | Enzyme deficiency results in dGTP-induced T-cell toxicity | Neurologic disorders, severe graft-versus-host disease from transfusions |
| Severe combined immunodeficiency (reticular dysgenesis) | AR | 1–3 months | Candidiasis, all types of infections (bacterial, viral, fungal, protozoal) | Defective maturation of common stem cell affecting myeloid and lymphoid cells | Agammaglobulinemia, alymphocytosis, agranulocytosis |

Modified from Boxer L, Blackwood K: Recurrent infection. In Kliegman RM, Nieder ML, Super DM (eds): Practical Strategies in Pediatric Diagnostics and Therapy. Philadelphia, WB Saunders, 1996, p 866.

ADA = adenosine deaminase; AR = autosomal recessive; dATP = deoxy-adenosine triphosphate; dGTP = deoxy-guanosine triphosphate; Ig = immunoglobulin; IL = interleukin; IL-2R γ = interleukin-2 receptor gamma chain; ITP = idiopathic thrombocytopenic purpura; PNP = purine nucleoside phosphorylase; RA = rheumatoid arthritis.

TABLE 8–6.    Deficiency of Complement and
                        Associated Disease

| Deficient Protein | Associated Disease |
|---|---|
| C1q, C1r | SLE, glomerulonephritis; occasional pneumococcal infection |
| C2 | SLE, arthritis, JRA, recurrent infections in some patients, rare glomerulonephritis |
| C3 | Recurrent infections, rare glomerulonephritis, or SLE |
| C4 | SLE-like disease, pyogenic infection |
| C5 | Recurrent meningococcal or gonococcal infections, rare glomerulonephritis, or SLE |
| C6 | Recurrent meningococcal or gonococcal infections, rare glomerulonephritis, or SLE |
| C7 | Recurrent meningococcal or gonococcal infections, Raynaud phenomenon |
| C8 | Recurrent meningococcal or gonococcal infections |
| C9 | Occasional meningococcal infection, autoimmune disease in some patients |
| Properdin | Recurrent infections, meningococcemia (often fatal) |
| Factor H | Glomerulonephritis, meningococcal infection |
| Factor I | Recurrent infections |
| C4-binding protein | Collagen-vascular disease |
| C5a inhibitor | Familial Mediterranean fever |
| C3b receptor | SLE |
| C1 inhibitor | Hereditary angioedema |

JRA = juvenile rheumatoid arthritis; SLE = systemic lupus erythematosus.

classical complement pathway. Patients with mannose-binding protein defects experience skin infections, sepsis, chronic diarrhea, and failure to thrive.

Specific *treatment of complement deficiencies* with component replacement is not available; frequent and long courses of antibiotics constitute the therapy. Immunization of patients and close contacts with pneumococcal and meningococcal vaccine may be useful. Patients with C1 esterase inhibitor deficiency and frequent episodes of angioedema respond to prophylactic use of an oral attenuated androgen (stanozolol or danazol), which appears to increase serum concentrations of C1 esterase inhibitor. Use of androgens should be limited, however, because of side effects that include masculinization in females, growth arrest, and hepatitis. Prophylactic administration of fresh frozen plasma before surgery, for example, can prevent angioedema, but administration during an acute episode may exacerbate the episode. Angioedema of the airway can present as an acute emergency, requiring tracheostomy, since administration of epinephrine, antihistamines, or corticosteroids are ineffective in reversing this type of angioedema. Purified

C1 esterase inhibitor, if available, is for prophylactic and acute treatment of angioedema. Angiotensin-converting enzyme (ACE) inhibitors (captopril) should be avoided in patients with C1 esterase inhibitor deficiency, as they can precipitate episodes of angioedema by inhibiting degradation of kinins that mediate edema formation.

## DISORDERS OF T-CELL IMMUNITY

Because T cells have a wide range of functions, T-cell disorders have a broad range of *clinical manifestations* (see Fig. 8–2 and Table 8–5). Classically, patients with T-cell disorders have infections with fungi or pathogens that proliferate intracellularly in somatic cells and in macrophages (viruses, mycobacteria, toxoplasmosis, *Leishmania*). Cytotoxic CD8+ cells and CD4+ helper T cells that activate macrophages may be absent. In severe T-cell deficiency, B-cell function, which requires T-cell help, may also be impaired.

### DiGeorge Syndrome

DiGeorge syndrome is the classic example of T-cell deficiency that is the result of dysmorphogenesis of the third and fourth pharyngeal pouches, resulting in hypoplasia of the thymus through which T cells must mature (see Fig. 8–2 and Table 8–5). Genetically, the syndrome represents a subset of patients with a field defect on chromosome 22q11.2, the **velocardiofacial syndrome**, or **CATCH 22 syndrome** (*c*ardiac anomalies, *a*bnormal facies, *t*hymic hypoplasia, *c*left palate, and *h*ypocalcemia) (see Chapter 4). DiGeorge syndrome is classically characterized by hypocalcemic tetany, conotruncal and aortic arch anomalies (such as interrupted aortic arch type B, tetralogy of Fallot, and truncus arteriosus) and increased infections.

The *diagnosis* of CATCH 22 is made by fluorescent in situ hybridization (FISH) with a DNA probe to detect microdeletions in chromosome 22q11.2. Immunodeficiency in this syndrome varies markedly; indeed, immunologically significant defects are relatively rare. In severe cases, complete absence of T-cell function can occur, resulting in severe combined immunodeficiency (lack of both T-cell and B-cell function). In patients with partial thymic function, improvement in T-cell function is observed with time.

### Severe Combined Immunodeficiency

Severe combined immunodeficiency disease (SCID) is characterized by a profound lack of T-cell and

B-cell function (see Fig. 8–2 and Table 8–5). Many specific genetic mutations cause this syndrome, and consequently the clinical severity and manifestations of this disease are heterogeneous. In patients with the classic form of SCID, which is caused by mutations in the gene on the X chromosome coding for the gamma chain of the IL-2 receptor (this chain is also utilized by the receptors for IL-4, IL-7, IL-13, IL-9, and IL-15), no T cells, B cells, or NK cells are found in the peripheral blood. Symptoms of severe infection and failure to thrive occur within the 1st mo of life.

*Clinical manifestations* include severe bacterial infection, chronic candidiasis, infection with *P. carinii* and other opportunistic organisms, and intractable diarrhea. Patients often have skin disease similar to eczema, possibly related to graft-versus-host disease from maternal lymphocytes. **Omenn syndrome** is one variant form of SCID, but it is characterized by exfoliative erythroderma, lymphadenopathy, hepatosplenomegaly, marked eosinophilia, elevated serum IgE, and impaired T-cell function. Other forms of SCID are caused by genetic mutations in genes coding for enzymes or kinases such as *adenosine deaminase* (ADA).

ADA deficiency accounts for about 33% of all SCID patients and is caused by mutations in the ADA gene on chromosome 20, which affects purine metabolic pathways. T cells are particularly sensitive to the accumulation of toxic purine metabolites, especially deoxyadenosine triphosphate and deoxyadenosine. This results primarily in absent or markedly reduced T-cell function, often with absent or reduced B-cell function. Although many patients present early with severe infection, diagnosis in a number of patients with partial immune function has been made after the age of 5 yr. Patients with late onset are generally lymphopenic; they have B cells and normal total immunoglobulin levels but little functional antibody **(Nezelof syndrome)**. Immune function in these patients appears to wane with time.

Defects of various tyrosine kinases (Janus tyrosine kinase [Jak] or ZAP-70 kinase) that are important in T-cell activation also result in T-cell deficiency and SCID. In Jak deficiency, B cells can be present in normal numbers but are not functional; in ZAP-70 deficiency, normal numbers of nonfunctional CD4+ T cells are present. In **bare lymphocyte syndrome**, there is a deficiency of MHC class I or II or both. Lymphoid tissue as well as T and B cells may be present in normal amounts, but the cells are unable to respond to specific antigen.

### Partial Combined Defects

Several disorders feature a combination of T-cell and B-cell defects but are less severe than those of SCID. The **Wiskott-Aldrich syndrome** is an X-linked disorder characterized by thrombocytopenia, eczema, disorders in cell-mediated and humoral immunity, and a predisposition to lymphoproliferative disease. It is caused by mutations of the gene at chromosome Xp11 coding for the 53-kD Wiskott-Aldrich syndrome protein (WASP), expressed in lymphocytes, platelets, and monocytes. WASP deficiency results in elevated IgE and IgA levels, decreased IgM, poor responses to polysaccharide antigens, waning T-cell function, and profound thrombocytopenia. **Isolated X-linked thrombocytopenia** also results from mutations of the identical gene. One third of patients with Wiskott-Aldrich syndrome die from hemorrhage, while two thirds die from recurrent infection owing to bacteria, cytomegalovirus, *P. carinii*, or herpes simplex virus.

### Ataxia-Telangiectasia

Ataxia-telangiectasia (AT) is a syndrome caused by the ATM gene (AT, mutated) on chromosome 11, which codes for a phosphatidylinositol-3 kinase. Patients have cutaneous and conjunctival telangiectasias and progressive cerebellar ataxia with degeneration of Purkinje cells, IgA deficiency, IgG2 subclass deficiency of variable severity, along with low IgE levels, and variably depressed T-cell function. The gene's normal function is not clear, but it appears to be involved in detecting DNA damage blocking cell growth division until the damage is repaired, or both. AT cells are exquisitely sensitive to irradiation. Leukemias, lymphomas, and diabetes are also present, and sexual maturation is delayed. There is no uniformly effective therapy for this disease, but antimicrobial therapy and IVIG replacement therapy (with IgA-deficient preparations) may be helpful.

### Treatment of Severe T-cell Disorders

The therapy for severe T-cell disorders is bone marrow transplantation, preferably with bone marrow from an HLA-matched sibling. In patients with an accompanying humoral immunodeficiency, IVIG is also useful. Patients with the ADA deficiency form of SCID who lack histocompatible sibling donors can receive repeated intramuscular replacement doses of ADA, stabilized by coupling to polyethylene glycol (PEG-ADA). Gene therapy has been performed in several patients with ADA deficiency by transfer of a normal ADA gene into T cells and bone marrow stem cells.

Prenatal *diagnosis* is possible for ADA and PNP deficiencies in families with these disorders. Prenatal diagnosis of other immunodeficiency disorders (Wiskott-Aldrich syndrome, ZAP-70 deficiency, CD40L deficiency) can be made in specialized laboratories by restriction fragment length polymorphism (RFLP), when DNA or complementary DNA (cDNA) from the index case is available.

## DISORDERS OF THE PHAGOCYTIC COMPARTMENT

Disorders of the phagocytic compartment can be divided into those of deficient cell numbers (see Chapter 14) and those with insufficient function (Table 8–7). They are characterized by mucous membrane infections (gingivitis, abscesses in the skin and viscera), lymphadenitis, poor wound healing, delayed umbilical cord separation, and absence of pus (in disorders of cell numbers or of leukocyte migration). Microorganisms include *S. aureus*, certain fungi, and gram-negative bacteria.

### Chronic Granulomatous Disease

Chronic granulomatous disease (CGD) is a rare disorder of white blood cells that results from defective intracellular killing of bacteria and intracellular pathogens by neutrophils and macrophages.

CGD is inherited in an X-linked disorder (more severe form), caused by mutations in the gp91-*phox* gene on chromosome Xp21.1, or in an autosomal recessive fashion, resulting from mutations in several genes (p22-*phox*, p47-*phox*, or p67-*phox*), resulting in the failure of the cytochrome $b_{558}$ NADPH system to produce superoxide. Patients characteristically have lymphadenopathy, hypergammaglobulinemia, hepatosplenomegaly, dermatitis, failure to thrive, anemia, chronic diarrhea, and abscesses. Infections occur in the lungs resulting in chronic bronchitis as well as in the middle ear, gastrointestinal tract, skin, urinary tract, lymph nodes, liver, and bones. Granulomas may obstruct the pylorus or ureters. Common organisms include catalase-positive bacteria, such as *S. aureus*, enteric gram-negative bacteria (*Salmonella, Proteus, Klebsiella, E. coli, Serratia marcescens,* and *Burkholderia cepacia*), and fungi (*Aspergillus fumigatus, C. albicans,* and *Torulopsis glabrata*).

### Treatment of Neutrophil Disorders

Frequent courses of antibiotics (trimethoprim/sulfamethoxazole prophylaxis in the case of CGD) and surgical débridement of infections are required. Because *A. fumigatus* can cause serious infection in patients with CGD, avoidance of moldy hay, decomposing compost, and other nests of

TABLE 8–7. Phagocytic Disorders

| Name | Defect | Comment |
|---|---|---|
| Chronic granulomatous disease | Bactericidal | X-linked recessive (66%), autosomal recessive (33%); eczema, osteomyelitis, granulomas, abscesses caused by *Staphylococcus aureus, Burkholderia cepacia, Aspergillus fumigatus;* X-linked defect in cytochrome b produces negative nitroblue tetrazolium test |
| Chédiak-Higashi syndrome | Bactericidal plus chemotaxis, poor natural killer function | Autosomal recessive; oculocutaneous albinism, neuropathy, giant neutrophilic cytoplasmic inclusions; malignancy, neutropenia |
| Hyperimmunoglobulin E (Job syndrome) | Chemotaxis, opsonization | Eczema, staphylococcal abscesses, red hair; granulocyte and monocyte chemotaxis affected; antistaphylococcal IgE |
| Myeloperoxidase deficiency | Bactericidal, fungicidal | Reduced chemiluminescence; autosomal recessive (1:4000); persistent candidiasis in diabetics |
| Glucose-6-phosphate dehydrogenase deficiency | Bactericidal | Phenotypically similar to chronic granulomatous disease |
| Burns, malnutrition | Bactericidal plus chemotaxis | Reversible defects |
| Lazy leukocyte syndrome | Chemotaxis | Normal bone marrow cells but poor migration; granulocytopenia |
| Leukocyte adhesion deficiency; CD18 deficiency | Adherence, chemotaxis, phagocytosis; reduced lymphocyte cytotoxicity | Delayed separation or infection of umbilical cord; lethal bacterial infections without pus; autosomal recessive; neutrophilia; deficiency of LFA-1, Mac-1, CR3 |
| Schwachman syndrome | Chemotaxis, neutropenia | Pancreatic insufficiency, metaphyseal chondrodysplasia; autosomal recessive |

fungi is necessary. The frequency of infection in CGD is also decreased by treatment with recombinant IFN-$\gamma$, administered subcutaneously 3 times/wk. Recombinant granulocyte–colony-stimulating factor (G-CSF) and granulocyte monocyte–colony-stimulating factor (GM-CSF) also appear to be effective against some forms of neutropenia, and bone marrow transplantation may be needed in other cases.

## CLINICAL EVALUATION OF SUSPECTED IMMUNODEFICIENCY SYNDROMES
### (Fig. 8–4)

The frequency, type, location, and severity of the infections must be assessed. Separate episodes must be differentiated from relapse or recurrence of single episodes, which often occurs when episodes of otitis media or sinusitis are inadequately treated. Recurrent episodes of severe infection, such as meningitis or sepsis, are much more worrisome than recurrent otitis media, but antibody deficiency states initially present with common infections, such as otitis media and sinusitis. In patients having antibody deficiency states, ciliary dyskinesia, T-cell deficiencies, or neutrophil disorders, infections develop at multiple sites (ears, sinuses, lung, skin), whereas in individuals with anatomic problems (e.g., sequestered pulmonary lobe or ureteral reflux), infections are confined to a single anatomic site, such as a single pulmonary lobe or the urinary tract. The specific pathogens causing infections are helpful in the evaluation (see Tables 8–1, 8–5, and 8–7). Patients with primary immunodeficiency acquire infection with opportunistic organisms that do not ordinarily cause infection.

Recurrent infection in immunologically deficient children is associated with incomplete recovery at sites of infection, resulting in scarring of the tympanic membrane (TM) or of the skin, abnormal hearing, persistent perforation of the tympanic membrane, persistent ear drainage, chronic lung disease, persistent cough and sputum production, failure to thrive, digital clubbing, or anemia of chronic disease. The accrual of substantial morbidity from repeated infections (including minor infections) suggests the presence of significant immunologic disease. In addition, a history of persistent atypical rashes may suggest immunodeficiency. Atypical generalized rashes suggest graft-versus-host disease, whereas persistent eczema or petechiae suggest Wiskott-Aldrich syndrome, and telangiectasia suggests ataxia-telangiectasia. A history of neonatal tetany (DiGeorge), cardiac disease (DiGeorge), micrognathia (DiGeorge), delay in umbilical cord detachment (LFA-1 deficiency), or chronic atypical diarrhea and malabsorption (graft-versus-

host disease, chronic viral infection) are important facts that may suggest an immunologic diagnosis. The family history is also critical, since primary immunodeficiencies are genetic diseases. Family history of infants dying from infection or human immunodeficiency virus (HIV) risk factors (see Chapter 10) is important. Because primary immunodeficiency is rare, symptoms consistent with **anatomic disease** or **secondary immunodeficiency** should always be sought.

The height and weight percentiles, nutritional status, and presence of subcutaneous fat should be assessed. Evidence of persistent infection should be sought (thrush in the mouth, purulent nasal or otic discharge, chronic rales, scarring of the tympanic membranes or of the skin). Lymphoid tissue, such as the tonsils, and lymph nodes should be examined. Absence of tonsils suggests SCID or X-linked agammaglobulinemia, whereas increased size of lymphoid tissue suggests common variable agammaglobulinemia or HIV infection.

## LABORATORY EVALUATION OF SUSPECTED IMMUNODEFICIENCY

Screening tests can be employed initially for many patients (Table 8–8). More specific tests should be reserved for severe disease or when the history, physical examination, or screening tests suggest a specific immunologic diagnosis (see Fig. 8–4).

### B-cell Disease

Patients with B-cell disorders have decreased serum immunoglobulin levels. Normal values vary with age, with a physiologic nadir occurring at 6–8 mo of age. Low albumin with low immunoglobulin levels suggests low synthetic rates for all proteins or increased loss of proteins (nephrotic syndrome, protein-losing enteropathy). High levels of immunoglobulin levels suggest intact B-cell immunity (CGD, immotile cilia syndrome, cystic fibrosis). Very high levels suggest HIV infection.

In some patients with normal total immunoglobulin levels, it may be important to determine whether antibody function is present (see Table 8–8). If titers are low, the patient can be immunized with tetanus, diphtheria, or *H. influenzae* vaccines, or in patients older than 2 yr, with pneumococcal vaccine; titers are re-examined 2–4 wk later. Inadequate responses to bacterial polysaccharide antigens occur prior to age 2 yr, but they are also associated with IgG subclass deficiency. Patients with X-linked agammaglobulinemia have absent immunoglobulin and antibody titers, and they do not have circulating B cells, as assessed by fluorescent activated cell sorter (FACS) analysis.

**FIGURE 8–4.** Algorithm for the work-up of a patient with recurrent infections. AIDS = acquired immunodeficiency syndrome; CBC = complete blood count; Ig = immunoglobulin; G6PD = glucose-6-phosphate dehydrogenase; GSH = reduced glutathione; NBT = nitroblue tetrazolium; LAD = leukocyte adhesion deficiency syndrome. (From Boxer L, Blackwood R: *In* Kliegman RM, Nieder ML, Super DM [eds]: Practical Strategies in Pediatric Diagnosis and Therapy. Philadelphia, WB Saunders, 1996.)

## TABLE 8–8. Tests for Suspected Immune Deficiency*

**General**
*Complete blood count*, including hemoglobin, differential white blood cell count and morphology, and platelet count
*Roentgenograms* to document infection in chest, sinus, mastoids, long bones, if indicated by clinical history
Cultures, if appropriate
*Erythrocyte sedimentation rate*

**Antibody-Mediated Immunity**
*Quantitative immunoglobulin levels:* IgG, IgA, IgM, IgE
*Isohemagglutinin titers* (anti-A, anti-B): measures IgM function
Preexisting antibody levels: diphtheria, tetanus, polio, rubella, *Haemophilus influenzae, Streptococcus pneumoniae*

**Cell-Mediated Immunity**
*Lymphocyte count and morphology*
*Delayed hypersensitivity skin tests* (*Candida,* tetanus toxoid, tuberculin, mumps): measures T-cell and macrophage function
T- and B-cell subset enumeration by FACS analysis
T-lymphocyte function analyses

**Phagocytosis**
*Neutrophil cell count and morphology*
Nitroblue tetrazolium dye test
Staphylococcal killing, chemotaxis assay
Myeloperoxidase stain

**Complement**
Total hemolytic complement (CH50): measures complement activity
C3, C4 levels: measure important pathway components

*Initial screening tests for less severe disease are in bold italics.

### T-cell Disease

T-cell disorders demonstrate lymphopenia and absence of delayed type hypersensitivity (DTH) skin test reactions (tetanus, diphtheria, or *Candida*). Negative DTH reactions can be observed in 10–20% of normal individuals, but such individuals should receive boosters with tetanus or diphtheria toxoids and should be retested 2–4 wk later. T-cell (and B-cell) subsets can be assessed by FACS analysis to enumerate total numbers of CD4+ and CD8+ cells, NK cells, and monocytes and to evaluate expression of HLA antigens. In addition, functional T-cell studies, in vitro proliferation of T cells in response to mitogens (phytohemagglutinin, concanavalin A, or pokeweed mitogen) or antigens (tetanus toxoid or *Candida*) can also be performed. Tests for IL-2, IL-4, or IFN-γ production; expression of IL-2 receptor; and the presence of specific tyrosine kinases may be performed in specialized research laboratories. In patients thought to have DiGeorge Syndrome, FISH studies for microdeletions of chromosome 22 can be helpful; in patients suspected of having ataxia telangiectasia, chromosomal studies for multiple breakage of chromosomes 7 and 14 are useful.

### Complement Deficiency Diseases

The total hemolytic activity of serum (CH50) is a widely available test that is dependent on the presence of normal levels of the major components of complement. If the CH50 level is abnormal, individual components must be analyzed in specialized laboratories.

### Phagocytic Disease

Evaluation of neutrophil disorders begins with the complete blood count (CBC) and examination of neutrophil number and morphology. Further studies include the nitroblue tetrazolium test (NBT) for chronic granulomatous disease, and in vitro tests for neutrophil phagocytosis, chemotaxis, and bacterial killing. In addition, tests for expression of CD18 (LFA-1, Mac-1) cell antigens and for myeloperoxidase activity can be performed.

## GENERAL MANAGEMENT OF PATIENTS WITH RECURRENT INFECTIONS

Table 8–9 lists guidelines in the management of immunocompromised children. Immediate culture and aggressive antibiotic therapy should be instituted for fever or other manifestations of infection because infection may rapidly disseminate and become life-threatening. Continuous prophylaxis

### TABLE 8–9. General Management of Patients with Immunodeficiency

Avoid transfusions with blood products unless they are irradiated and cytomegalovirus-negative

Avoid live virus vaccines, especially in patients with severe T-cell deficiencies or severe agammaglobulinemia, and in household members

Follow pulmonary function in patients with recurrent pneumonia

Utilize chest physiotherapy, postural drainage in patients with recurrent pneumonia

Utilize prophylactic antibiotics, since minor infections can quickly disseminate

Examine diarrheal stools for *Giardia* and *Clostridium difficile*

Avoid unnecessary exposure to individuals with infection

Use intravenous immune globulin for severe antibody deficiency states at a dose of 400–500 mg/kg q 3–4 wk IV with antibacterial, antiviral, or antifungal agents may also be warranted if infection is difficult to control and likely to rapidly disseminate. Because children with immunodeficiency develop infections with uncommonly encountered organisms, poor response to commonly used antibiotics suggests the presence of a resistant or atypical pathogen, which must be specifically identified by culture or biopsy.

## References

Behrman RE, Kliegman RM, Arvin AM (eds): Nelson Textbook of Pediatrics, 15th ed. Philadelphia, WB Saunders, 1996, Chapters 116–131.

Flake A, Roncarolo M, Puck J, et al: Treatment of X-linked severe combined immunodeficiency by in utero transplantation of paternal bone marrow. N Engl J Med 335:1806, 1996.

Gelfand EW: SCID continues to point the way. N Engl J Med 322:1741, 1990.

Greenberg F: What defines DiGeorge anomaly? J Pediatr 115:412, 1989.

Ozsahin H, Le Deist F, Benkerrou M, et al: Bone marrow transplantation in 26 patients with Wiskott-Aldrich syndrome from a single center. J Pediatr 129:238, 1996.

Rosen F, Cooper M, Wedgwood R: The primary immunodeficiencies. N Engl J Med 333:431, 1995.

Stiehm ER: Immunologic Disorders in Infants and Children, 4th ed. Philadelphia, WB Saunders, 1996.

Yang K, Hill H: Assessment of neutrophil function disorders: Practical and preventative interventions. Pediatr Infect Dis J 13:906, 1994.

## HYPERSENSITIVITY REACTIONS

Hypersensitivity reactions are caused by an untoward, inappropriate immunologic response to a "foreign" substance involving antigen-specific antibody or antigen-specific memory lymphocytes. There are four major types of hypersensitivity reactions.

*Type I reactions* (IgE-mediated immediate hypersensitivity) are triggered by the binding of antigen to IgE molecules attached to IgE receptors (FcεRI) on the surface of mast cells (or basophils) (Fig. 8–5). This results in mast cell degranulation and release of preformed mediators, such as histamine and eosinophil chemotactic factors, causing urticaria, pruritus, mucus production, sneezing, wheezing, and hypotension within 20 min. The most severe life-threatening form of this reaction is *anaphylaxis*. The most common causes of anaphylaxis include penicillin (and other drugs), foods such as peanuts, pollen extracts, latex, and insect venom. Type I reactions cause allergic rhinitis and allergic asthma, initiated by the inhalation of allergens that deposit on the respiratory mucosa. Four to 12 hr after the initial response, a *late-phase reaction* may develop, characterized by local influx of basophils, eosinophils, monocytes, lymphocytes, and neutrophils causing persistent, more profound, and difficult-to-manage symptoms. Late-phase allergic inflammatory responses in the respiratory tract are associated with nasal or bronchial *hyperreactivity*. The infiltrating cells in the inflammatory response produce leukotrienes C4, D4, and E4; prostaglandins; IL-4, IL-5, and IL-13; and allergen-specific IgE, which amplify the response by enhancing the growth and differentiation of eosinophils, basophils, mast cells, and Th2 lymphocytes.

*Type II reactions* (antibody cytotoxicity) involve IgG (or IgM) antibodies binding to cell surface or tissue antigens with complement and a variety of Fc receptor-bearing effector cells that damage cells and surrounding tissues. The target antigens can be cell surface membrane antigens (such as red blood cell or platelet cell surface molecules leading to hemolysis or thrombocytopenia, respectively), basement membrane molecules in the kidney leading to Goodpasture syndrome, the α-chain of the acetylcholine receptor at the neuromuscular junction resulting in myasthenia gravis, and the thyroid-stimulating hormone (TSH) receptor on thyroid cells causing Graves disease. Other target antigens include drugs such as quinidine, which when bound to red cell membranes act as haptens, resulting in drug-induced hemolysis via complement activation.

*Type III reactions* involve the formation of soluble immune complexes of antigen and antibody (often IgG). Large immune complexes are removed by the reticuloendothelial system in the liver, spleen, and lungs; smaller complexes persist in the circulation and localize at the glomerular basement membrane or in the endothelium of other target organs (synovium, skin). Tissue deposition may be facilitated by the generation of C3a and C5a, which have anaphylactic and chemotactic properties, and occasionally by release of vasoactive amines from mast cells and basophils when antigen-specific IgE is present. Immune complex activation of complement attracts polymorphonuclear leukocytes, resulting in increased capillary permeability, release of proteases, and tissue damage. Local reactions caused by the injection of antigen into tissue are called **Arthus reactions**. Systemic administration of large amounts of foreign protein, some of which enters the circulation, causes **serum sickness**, with a clinical picture of fever, arthralgia, urticaria-like rash, lymphadenopathy, and proteinuria. Other type III-mediated diseases include farmer's lung, caused by inhalation of large quantities of mold spores, and some vasculitic syndromes (Kawasaki disease and Henoch-Schönlein purpura).

*Type IV reactions* (delayed hypersensitivity) are

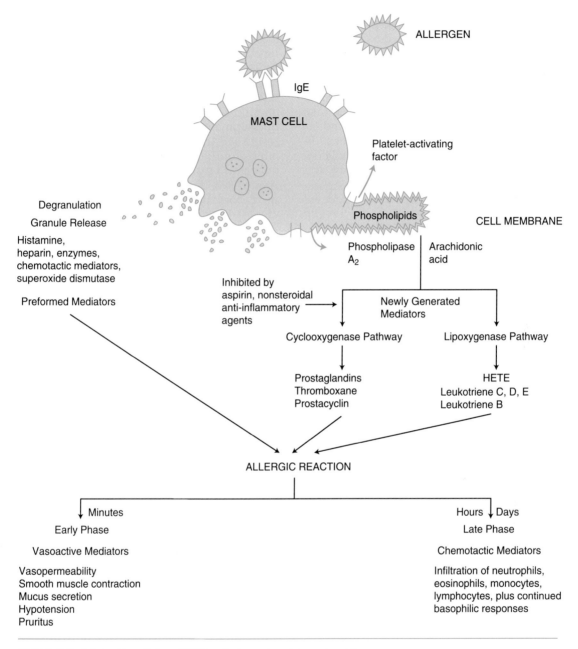

FIGURE 8–5. Mast cell mediators. HETE = hydroxyeicosatetraenoic acid.

mediated by antigen-specific T cells and macrophages and reach their peak 24–48 hr after antigen exposure. Memory T cells recognize antigen peptide/MHC class II complexes on APCs and release inflammatory cytokines (IFN-γ, TNF-β, GM-CSF) that activate macrophages. Type IV hypersensitivity includes contact hypersensitivity, for example, to pentadecacatechol (poison ivy) or nickel. Classically, tuberculin skin tests manifest the characteristics of type IV reactions. In addition, organ transplant rejection and graft-versus-host disease are type IV reactions.

## ATOPIC DISORDERS

Atopy is a condition in certain individuals that predisposes toward the development of IgE-mediated disorders, such as allergic rhinitis, asthma, and atopic dermatitis (eczema). There are genetic components to the atopic state; children of an atopic parent have a 30% risk for development of an atopic disorder. Expression also depends on environmental factors, such as allergen exposure. Breast-feeding may reduce the incidence of atopic diseases. Atopic individuals frequently have elevated levels of serum IgE (other diseases are also associated with elevated IgE) (Table 8–10) and eosinophilia (3–10% or > 250 eosinophils/mm³). Extreme eosinophilia should suggest a nonallergic disorder, such as a helminth parasite, a drug reaction, immunodeficiency, or an infiltrative lung disease (eosinophilic pneumonia). Asthma and elevated serum IgE levels have been linked to a region on chromosome 11q13, a gene for the β-chain of the high-affinity receptor for IgE, FcεR1, and to a cluster of cytokine genes at chromosome 5q31. Atopic disease is also thought to be caused by the overproduction of Th2 cell cytokines, such as IL-4, IL-5, and IL-10, in allergen-specific CD4+ T cells.

### Asthma

Asthma is defined as reversible obstruction of large and small airways due to hyperresponsiveness to various immunologic and nonimmunologic stimuli. The disease is intermittent and characterized by recurrent episodes of cough, chest tightness, dyspnea, and wheezing. Between 5% and 10% of all children are affected at some time with symptoms of asthma; 80–90% have the first episode by 4–5 yr of age. It is the most common chronic disease in children and is a leading cause of emergency room visits, hospital admissions, and school absenteeism. For reasons not entirely clear, the prevalence and mortality of asthma are increasing worldwide.

*Pathophysiology.* An allergic-type inflammatory response occurs in the airway mucosa of patients with asthma that results in bronchial hyperreactivity, the hallmark of asthma. Bronchial

hyperreactivity has been linked to a chromosomal loci (5q31) containing genes for a number of cytokines, including IL-3, IL-4, and GM-CSF. This is consistent with the idea that the airways inflammation in asthma is an allergic type, associated with the production of Th2 type cytokines (IL-4 and IL-5), and with the observation that the risk for development of asthma is associated with elevated serum IgE levels and hypersensitivity to perennial allergens. Viral respiratory infection (respiratory syncytial virus, parainfluenza virus, adenovirus, rhinovirus), bacterial infection in the large airways, or mycoplasmal respiratory infection can also increase airway inflammation and bronchial hyperreactivity.

Three major pathologic events contribute to airway obstruction: (1) mucosal edema, (2) smooth muscle contraction, and (3) production of mucus. Obstruction occurs during expiration as the airway approaches the closing volume and results in distal airway gas trapping; more severe asthma may have diminished air flow during inspiration. A number of anatomic and physiologic characteristics predispose infants and young children to an increased risk (smaller airway size, lower elastic recoil of the lung, decreased smooth muscle support of the small airways, relative mucous gland hyperplasia, and decreased collateral channels of ventilation [pores of Cohn] between alveoli).

In the setting of airway hyperreactivity (which is aggravated by infection or allergen exposure), a number of triggers can initiate asthmatic symptoms. These include (1) antigens (such as dust mites and roaches), (2) irritants (such as cold air, pollutants, or cigarette smoke), (3) air pollution (such as sulfur dioxide), and (4) solvents. Exercise, an important trigger, acts by increasing the exposure of the airways to cool (dry) air. In some individuals, particularly those with nasal polyps, aspirin and other nonsteroidal anti-inflammatory agents (NSAIDs) can trigger severe asthma symptoms, presumably by inhibiting prostaglandin and increasing leukotriene production. **Gastroesophageal reflux** (GER) has been associated with difficult-to-manage asthma, possibly by cholinergic mechanisms or as a direct result of aspiration. **Sinusitis**, a common problem in children, frequently aggravates asthma; allergic **bronchopulmonary aspergillosis** (ABPA) occurs in a small number of difficult-to-treat asthmatic individuals.

*Diagnosis.* Wheeze, cough, dyspnea, tachypnea, and chest pain are common during acute exacerbations but are late signs of asthma and may not always be present. A history of persistent cough (cough-variant asthma), night cough, exercise-induced cough, post-tussive emesis, and cough fol-

TABLE 8–10.    Disorders Associated with Elevated Serum Immunoglobulin E

Allergic disease
Atopic dermatitis (eczema)
Helminthic infections
Hyperimmunoglobulin E syndrome
Allergic bronchopulmonary aspergillosis
Wiskott-Aldrich syndrome
Bone marrow transplantation
Hodgkin disease
Bullous pemphigoid
Idiopathic nephrotic syndrome
Mononucleosis

lowing cold air exposure or with laughter are suggestive of asthma.

During acute episodes, the physical examination reveals a hyperinflated chest that is hyperresonant to percussion. Tachypnea, tachycardia, cough, inspiratory and more usually expiratory wheezing, a prolonged expiratory phase, and squeaky musical inspiratory rales are often present. As the attack progresses, the following signs develop: cyanosis, use of accessory muscles of respiration, decreased breath sounds (tight chest) and diminished wheezing, agitation, inability to speak, tripod sitting position, diaphoresis, and increased pulsus paradoxus.

*Differential Diagnosis.* Causes of wheezing are listed in Table 8–11. Wheezing before 3 mo of age should suggest another condition, such as infection, pulmonary malformations, cardiac and gastrointestinal abnormalities, or cystic fibrosis (especially in the presence of malabsorption or clubbing, which is not seen in asthma). In infants and toddlers, bronchiolitis caused by respiratory syncytial virus is a very common cause of wheezing. A foreign body in the airway or esophagus should be considered in patients above 1–2 yr of age who have sudden onset of wheezing (and/or coughing) and diminished breath sounds localized to one region.

TABLE 8–11.    Differential Diagnosis of Wheezing

**Respiratory**
*Common*
  Bronchial asthma
  Respiratory infection
  Foreign body
  Cystic fibrosis
  Vocal cord dysfunction
  Laryngotracheomalacia
*Uncommon*
  Bronchopulmonary dysplasia
  Alpha$_1$-antitrypsin deficiency
  Allergic bronchopulmonary aspergillosis
  Ciliary dyskinesia syndrome
  Hypersensitivity pneumonitis
  Bronchiectasis
  Pulmonary hemosiderosis

**Cardiovascular** (uncommon)
  Congenital heart disease
  Vascular rings and slings
  Cardiac failure

**Gastrointestinal**
  Gastroesophageal reflux
  H-type tracheoesophageal fistula
  Foreign body

**Miscellaneous**
  Immunodeficiency disorders
  Vasculitis, collagen vascular disease
  Psychogenic cough
  Mediastinal mass (tumor, lymphadenopathy)

ABPA results from immunologic reactions in the lung to antigens of the mold *A. fumigatus*. ABPA is not a result of fungal invasiveness. ABPA has been identified in corticosteroid-dependent asthma, in cystic fibrosis, and in bronchiectasis.

ABPA often is diagnosed initially as asthma with peripheral eosinophilia; irreversible lung damage may occur before the correct diagnosis is made. In addition, patients often demonstrate marked immediate skin reactivity to *A. fumigatus*. Acute exacerbations are characterized by anorexia, headache, fever, fatigue, and increased sputum production. Rales, wheezing, and bronchial breathing may be present, resembling an acute exacerbation of asthma.

Peripheral blood eosinophils in ABPA generally are greater than $1000/mm^3$. Large numbers of eosinophils and fungal mycelia may be present in the sputum. Specific IgE and/or IgG may be elevated. Prednisone is the drug of choice for ABPA because it reduces the clinical symptoms and sputum production, decreases the incidence of positive sputum cultures, and clears roentgenographic lesions. The total serum IgE level typically declines within 2 mo of initiating prednisone therapy in patients with ABPA. Adjunctive therapy with intraconazole may be beneficial.

*Laboratory Findings.* The evaluation of patients with suspected moderate to severe asthma includes a chest radiograph with both posteroanterior and lateral views to identify anatomic abnormalities, atelectasis, pneumomediastinum, pneumothorax, foreign bodies, or neoplasms. Such x-ray studies are particularly important in patients who respond poorly to bronchodilators. Peak expiratory flow rate (PEFR) monitoring is helpful in assessing the severity of disease and response to therapy in the acute phases of asthma. Spirometry, with measurement of forced expired volume in 1 second ($FEV_1$), forced vital capacity (FVC), and average flow between 25% and 75% FVC ($FEV_{25-75\%}$) is useful in assessing and monitoring large and small airways obstruction in less symptomatic children. Spirometry with bronchial provocation (exercise or methacholine) is particularly useful in evaluating airway hyperreactivity and in diagnosing asthma when the history is unclear. Such studies can be performed only in cooperative children, usually older than 5–6 yr. In the management of chronic asthma, skin testing and radioallergosorbent testing (RAST) are particularly useful in identification of environmental triggers. Skin testing is more sensitive and provides results within 30 min, but it cannot be performed in acutely ill children, patients with diffuse skin disease, or those who are receiving antihistamines.

In status asthmaticus, routine use of arterial blood gases is not needed if pulse oximetry is available; during severe episodes of wheezing, arterial blood gases are essential to evaluate respiratory ventilation. Because of V/Q mismatch (see Chapter 12), hypoxia develops in most, if not all, patients. As airway obstruction worsens and chest compliance diminishes, $CO_2$ retention develops. In the face of tachypnea, a "normal" $PCO_2$ (40 mm Hg) suggests moderate to severe disease, whereas hypercapnia, respiratory acidosis, and hypoxia-associated metabolic acidosis indicate severe disease and impending respiratory arrest.

**Treatment.** The goals of therapy are, first, to reverse asthmatic symptoms and, second, to prevent or diminish the frequency of recurrent symptoms, maintain normal or close to normal pulmonary function, and maintain normal activity levels, including exercise. Although treatment of asthma in inpatient and emergency department settings is common, the ultimate goal is to prevent serious exacerbations requiring hospital-based therapy. In the management of chronic asthma, there are four components to therapy:

1. Patient education.
2. Assessment and monitoring of asthma severity with objective measures of lung function.
3. Avoidance or control of asthma triggers.
4. Establishment of comprehensive plans of pharmacologic therapy, including plans for managing exacerbations.

Patient education provides information and training to enhance the effectiveness of and improve compliance with recommended therapy. Successful education involves improving patient skills in use of spacer devices for metered-dose inhalers (MDIs), in use of peak flow monitoring, and in uses of self-management and environmental control measures; it also includes information about medications and their side effects and when and how to respond to changes in symptoms.

The severity of asthma exacerbation is often underestimated by patients and physicians; therefore, objective assessment and monitoring of asthma severity and lung function are essential to prevent undertreatment and potentially fatal asthma. Measurement of respiratory function with home peak flow monitoring, which can be performed in children older than 5 yr, improves compliance by providing patients the capacity to self-manage their disease and allowing more appropriate use of asthma medications. Peak flow determinations between 50% and 80% of a patient's personal best efforts require changes in medical therapy, and repeated determinations below 50% of a patient's personal best efforts may require acute intervention.

Specific triggers for asthma (e.g., allergens and cigarette or wood-burning stove smoke exposure) should be identified and steps to avoid or reduce exposure should be instituted, particularly because avoidance of such triggers can decrease airway inflammation and hyperresponsiveness. In individuals allergic to dust mites, house dust mite control measures should be followed, including encasing mattresses and pillows in nonpermeable covers, removing carpets, and eliminating mites from stuffed toys. In patients allergic to animal dander, exposure to animals should be minimized, preferably by removal of the household pet. Aspirin and other NSAIDs as well as beta-blocker drugs should be avoided.

Pharmacologic treatment complements environmental avoidance measures and is based on disease severity and the frequency of symptoms. In patients with chronic asthma, pharmacologic intervention focuses on preventive, *anti-inflammatory therapies* (Fig. 8–6). Such agents include inhaled sodium cromoglycate such as cromolyn sodium (Intal) and nedocromil sodium (Tilade), available for metered-dose inhalers. Both drugs inhibit early and late-phase allergen-induced bronchospasm and acute bronchospasm after exercise or cold air; neither is a bronchodilator. Both are useful as prophylactic agents in children with mild to moderate asthma, particularly since they have virtually no known side effects.

Other anti-inflammatory agents include *inhaled corticosteroids*, such as beclomethasone (Vanceril, Beclovent) and triamcinolone (Azmacort), and *oral corticosteroids*. Inhaled corticosteroids are safe and extremely effective therapy for chronic asthma. Inhaled corticosteroids reduce airway hyperreactivity and reduce the need for rescue bronchodilator therapy. Long-term, high-dose regimens of inhaled corticosteroids in doses above 1 mg/day, although effective in severe asthma, may be associated with systemic effects. This is particularly true with newer, more potent, inhaled corticosteroids, such as fluticasone (Flovent) and budesonide (Pulmicort), with which growth retardation and adrenal suppression have been associated. These side effects are significantly less than that associated with chronic use of *oral* corticosteroids. Long-term oral use of corticosteroids should be reserved for chronic asthma only if other therapies fail; such use is preferable with an alternate-day schedule, which may reduce side effects (growth failure, diabetes, cataracts, immunosuppression). The side effects associated with short courses (<7 days) of oral corticosteroids are significantly less than those

**Step-up:**  Progression to the next higher step is indicated when control cannot be achieved at the current step and there is assurance that medication is used correctly. If PEFR ≤60% predicted or personal best, consider a burst of oral corticosteroids and then proceed.

**Step-down:**  Reduction in therapy is considered when the outcome for therapy has been achieved and sustained for several weeks or even months at the current step. Reduction in therapy is also needed to identify the minimum therapy required to maintain control.

**Outcome: Control of Asthma**
- Minimal (ideally no) chronic symptoms, including nocturnal symptoms
- Minimal (infrequent) episodes
- No emergency visits
- Minimal need for p.r.n. beta$_2$-agonist
- No limitations on activities, including exercise
- PEF circadian variation <20%
- (Near) normal PEF
- Minimal (or no) adverse effects from medicine

**Outcome: Best Possible Results**
- Least symptoms
- Least need for p.r.n. beta$_2$-agonist
- Least limitation of activity
- Least PEFR circadian variation
- Best PEFR
- Least adverse effects from medicine

**Therapy†**
- Short acting inhaled beta$_2$-agonist p.r.n., not more than 3 x a week
- Short acting inhaled beta$_2$-agonist or cromolyn before exercise or exposure to antigen

**Clinical Features Pretreatment***
- Intermittent, brief symptoms <1–2 x a week
- Nocturnal asthma symptoms <1–2 x a month
- Asymptomatic between exacerbations
- PEFR or FEV$_1$
  - >80% predicted
  - variability <20%

**STEP 1: MILD**

**Therapy†**
- Inhaled antiinflammatory daily
  - Initially: Inhaled corticosteroid 200–500 μg or cromolyn or nedocromil (Children begin with a trial of cromolyn)
  - If necessary: increase inhaled corticosteroid to 400–750 μg (Alternatively, particularly for nocturnal symptoms, proceed to Step 3 with additional long acting bronchodialator)
  and
- Short acting inhaled beta$_2$-agonist p.r.n., not to exceed 3–4 times a day

**Clinical Features Pretreatment***
- Exacerbations >1–2 x a week
- Exacerbations may affect activity and sleep
- Nocturnal asthma symptoms >2 x a month
- Chronic symptoms requiring short acting beta$_2$-agonist almost daily
- PEFR or FEV$_1$
  - 60–80% predicted
  - variability 20–30%

**STEP 2: MODERATE**

**Therapy†**
- Inhaled corticosteriods daily 800–1,000 μg (>1,000 μg under specialist's supervision) and
- Sustained release theophylline, oral beta$_2$-agonist, or long acting inhaled beta$_2$-agonist, especially for nocturnal symptoms; may consider inhaled anticholinergics and
- Short acting inhaled beta$_2$-agonist p.r.n., not to exceed 3–4 times a day

**Clinical Features Pretreatment***
(—)

**STEP 3: MODERATE**

**Therapy†**
- Inhaled corticosteroid daily 800–1,000 μg (>1,000 μg under specialist's supervision) and
- Sustained release theophylline, and/or oral beta$_2$-agonist, or long acting inhaled beta$_2$-agonist, especially for nocturnal symptoms with or without
- Short acting inhaled beta$_2$-agonist once a day; may consider inhaled anticholinergic and
- Oral corticosteroids (alternate day or single daily dose) and
- Short acting inhaled beta$_2$-agonist p.r.n., up to 3–4 times a day

**Clinical Features Pretreatment***
- Frequent exacerbations
- Continuous symptoms
- Frequent nocturnal asthma symptoms
- Physical activities limited by asthma
- PEFR or FEV$_1$
  - <60% predicted
  - variability >30%

**STEP 4: SEVERE**

**Step Down**
- Once control is reached at any step, and sustained, a step down—reduction in therapy—may be carefully considered and is needed to identify the minimum therapy required to maintain control.
- Advise patients of signs of worsening asthma and actions to control it.

*One or more features may be present to be assigned a grade of severity; an individual should usually be assigned to the most severe grade in which any feature occurs.

†All therapy must include patient education about prevention (including environmental control where appropriate) as well as control of symptoms.

FIGURE 8–6.  Management of asthma: a stepwise approach to asthma therapy. PEF = peak expiratory flow; PEFR = peak expiratory flow rate; FEV = forced expiratory volume. (Redrawn from International Consensus Report on the Diagnosis and Treatment of Asthma. National Heart, Lung, and Blood Institute. Bethesda, MD, National Institutes of Health Pub. No. 92-3091, 1992, p 34.)

associated with long-term use. Short courses of oral corticosteroids are beneficial in minimizing acute exacerbations in moderate to severe asthma.

Selective *beta₂-adrenergic agonists*, such as albuterol sulfate, are useful for the treatment of both acute and chronic asthma but alone do not give long-term control because they do not affect airway inflammation. Beta₂-adrenergic agonists relax airway smooth muscle, enhance mucociliary clearance, and may decrease mediator release from mast cells and basophils. They are available as metered-dose inhalers (more effective when used with spacer devices) and by nebulized aerosol, which is particularly useful in young children. Although beta₂-adrenergic agents are also available for oral administration, these cause more numerous and severe side effects (cardiovascular stimulation, tremor, and hypokalemia) than do inhaled agents. *Short-acting* inhaled beta₂-adrenergic agents are beneficial for *acute* exacerbations of asthma, for the pretreatment of exercise-induced asthma, and for rescue (quick-relief) therapy in the treatment of chronic asthma. If frequent or regularly scheduled use of short-acting inhaled beta₂-adrenergic agents is required for symptomatic control, inhaled anti-inflammatory agents should be added to control symptoms, since chronic use of inhaled beta₂-adrenergic agents alone has been associated with diminished control of asthma. *Long-acting* inhaled beta₂-adrenergic agents, such as salmeterol xinafoate (Serevent), have a duration of action more than 12 hr and are particularly useful for treating *chronic asthma* that is unresponsive to inhaled anti-inflammatory agents and for treating night-time cough. Long-acting agents must not be used for acute exacerbations.

Sustained-release preparations of *theophylline*, a bronchodilator with mild anti-inflammatory effects, are sometimes used for the treatment of asthma. Theophylline has the potential for significant adverse effects (gastrointestinal symptoms, nausea, vomiting, tachycardia, behavior problems, seizures); these can be reduced substantially by using low doses, aiming for serum levels between 3–12 μg/mL. Monitoring of serum levels is required when high doses are administered, when adverse side effects develop, or when liver metabolism is altered, as with febrile illness, pregnancy, liver disease, congestive heart failure, concomitant use of ciprofloxacin, cimetidine, or macrolide antibiotics, except azithromycin (Zithromax). Theophylline can be recommended when inhaled corticosteroids and inhaled beta₂-adrenergic agents fail to control symptoms, particularly for control of nocturnal symptoms, and if patient compliance is improved by once-daily or twice-daily oral (rather than inhaled) medication.

*Anticholinergic agents*, such as ipratropium bromide (Atrovent), are available in a metered-dose inhaler and as a nebulized solution. These drugs are potent bronchodilators that may also block reflex bronchoconstriction caused by inhaled irritants. They are less effective as bronchodilators than beta₂-adrenergic agents for the treatment of asthma but may be useful when nebulized together with a beta₂-adrenergic agent.

Other anti-inflammatory agents include *leukotriene antagonists* and *lipoxigenase inhibitors*. Zafirlukast (Accolate), an oral leukotriene D4 receptor antagonist, and zileuton, a lipoxygenase inhibitor, have been shown to significantly decrease asthma symptoms. These medications are not bronchodilators, and they may be used as adjunctive measures for the treatment of chronic asthma, particularly in patients with aspirin sensitivity.

Selection of specific medications or combinations is dependent on the asthma severity. Consideration is given to patient preference for oral versus inhaled medications and to the side effect profile in individual patients. Figure 8–6 illustrates a stepwise approach to therapy in which the number and frequency of medications are increased with increasing asthma severity. The goal is to achieve optimal symptom control with the least possible medication. If symptoms develop while a specific regimen is being prescribed, the next higher step in therapy is recommended. Plans for medical treatment of symptomatic exacerbation and for responding to changes in peak expiratory flow should be written out for every patient as part of the educational program for asthma self-management. Treatment of associated sinusitis or gastroesophageal reflux is essential.

***Emergency Treatment.*** In patients with significant airway hyperreactivity, asthma exacerbation can readily occur secondary to viral respiratory infection, acute sinusitis, bronchitis, or exposure to a major trigger (allergen). Exacerbation is characterized by significant respiratory distress, dyspnea, wheezing, cough, and major reduction in peak expiratory flow rates. Deterioration may progress over several days, or it may occur precipitously and may range in severity from mild to life-threatening. Evaluation should include assessment of the degree of cyanosis, breathlessness, mental status, respiratory rate, accessory muscle use, wheezing, pulsus paradoxus, PEFR, and oxygen saturation (in room air). In the emergency department, treatment should include repetitive administration of inhaled beta₂-agonists, oxygen, and early use of systemic corticosteroids. Epinephrine by subcutaneous or intramuscular injection is rarely indicated and is reserved for acute anaphylaxis or severe asthma unresponsive to continuous administration of inhaled beta$_2$-agonists. Arterial blood gases should be obtained if the PEFR is 30–50% of predicted value, if severe distress persists after initial treatment, or when oxygen saturation remains below 90% in room air. If the patient responds well to therapy (PEFR > 70% of predicted and oxygen saturation is greater than 95% in room air, marked reduction or elimination of symptoms) discharge is indicated, with a step-up in maintenance medication and plans for outpatient follow-up.

Hospital admission is indicated if:

1. Patient response is inadequate with persistence of symptoms.
2. PEFR is below (70%) of predicted value, particularly in patients at high risk for death (recent withdrawal from systemic corticosteroids, hospitalization or emergency care for asthma in the past year, previous intubation for asthma, psychiatric disease or psychosocial problems, or noncompliance with asthma medication plan).
3. Respiratory arrest is impending (signs of deterioration, confusion, $P_{O_2}$ < 60 mm Hg, and/or $P_{CO_2}$ > 45 mm Hg).

Inpatient therapy for asthma includes inhaled beta-agonists up to every 1–2 hr or by continuous nebulized aerosols and systemic corticosteroids (methylprednisolone, 2–4 mg/kg/day divided every 6 hr). Intravenous aminophylline (5 mg/kg loading dose, followed by 0.7–1.2 mg/kg/hr infusion) or intravenous terbutaline may be beneficial in patients who do not respond to aerosols and intravenous steroids; endotracheal intubation with mechanical ventilation may be required in the event of severe hypoxia and respiratory failure. Sedation is contraindicated unless the patient is intubated.

Discharge from the hospital is appropriate when:

1. Inhaled beta-agonists are being used no more than every 4 hr.
2. Clinical findings are normal or near-normal.
3. PEFR is above 70–80% of predicted value after short-acting inhaled beta$_2$-agonist.
4. PEF variability is below 20%.
5. Asthma education has been initiated (correct use of inhaler devices, development of an action plan, plans for discharge medication and outpatient follow-up understood, as appropriate, by patient and parent).

*Prognosis.* Although asthma can be a fatal disease, the long-term prognosis of childhood asthma is good. Most children with onset of asthma before age 5 yr are symptom-free by adolescence. Risk factors for persistence of asthma include severe asthma, concurrent allergic rhinitis, dust mite and cat allergy, a family history of asthma, lower respiratory infection in infancy, and maternal smoking. In patients who are dependent on corticosteroids, Cushing habitus, growth failure, acne, osteoporosis, cataracts, and opportunistic infections may develop.

### References

Adkinson NF, Eggleston PA, Eney D, et al: A controlled trial of immunotherapy for asthma in allergic children. N Engl J Med 336:324, 1997.

Behrman RE, Kliegman RM, Arvin AM (eds): Nelson Textbook of Pediatrics, 15th ed. Philadelphia, WB Saunders, 1996, Chapters 137, 230.

Burr M. Pollution: Does it *cause* asthma? Arch Dis Child 72:377, 1995.

Harding SM, Richter JE, Guzzo MR, et al: Asthma and gastroesophageal reflux: Acid suppressive therapy improves asthma outcome. Am J Med 100:335, 1996.

Kattan M: Management of acute asthma: A continuing challenge. J Pediatr 129:783, 1996.

Keeley D, Rees J: New guidelines on asthma management. BMJ 314:315, 1997.

McFadden ER, Hejal R: Asthma. Lancet 345:1215, 1995.

Nelson HS: β-adrenergic bronchodilators. N Engl J Med 333:499, 1995.

Postma DS, Bleecker ER, Amelung PJ, et al: Genetic susceptibility to asthma-bronchial hyperresponsiveness coinherited with a major gene for atopy. N Engl J Med 333:894, 1995.

Strachan D, Carey IM: Home environment and severe asthma in adolescence: A population based case-control study. BMJ 311:1053, 1995.

Suissa S, Dennis R, Ernest P, et al: Effectiveness of the leukotriene receptor antagonist zafirlukast for mild-to-moderate asthma. Ann Intern Med 126:177, 1997.

Szefler SJ, Bender BG, Jusko WJ, et al: Evolving role of theophylline for treatment of chronic childhood asthma. J Pediatr 127:176, 1995.

### Allergic Rhinitis

Allergic rhinitis (hay fever) affects 5–10% of children. Although not a life-threatening disorder, allergic rhinitis is a significant problem in terms of morbidity and health care costs, impeding education within the classroom, limiting outdoor or indoor activity, and predisposing to the development of sinusitis, otitis media, and asthma.

*Pathogenesis.* Allergic rhinitis is caused by a type I allergic response either to wind-borne pollens of grasses, trees, and weeds (classified as *seasonal allergic rhinitis*) or to house dust mite allergen, pet dander, or mold spores (classified as *perennial allergic rhinitis*). Both types of rhinitis may occur concomitantly.

*Clinical Manifestations.* Symptoms of allergic rhinitis include chronic recurrent sneezing, nasal congestion, clear rhinorrhea, and pruritus of the nose, eyes, soft palate, and ears. Patients frequently rub their nose with the palm of their hands (*allergic salute*) or rub the soft palate with their tongue, producing clucking sounds. Allergic symptoms, such as sneezing, classically occur immediately (within 20 min) following exposure to an offending allergen. Often, a more severe and persistent reaction, with nasal congestion, sneezing, and rhinorrhea, occurs 6–12 hr later. Seasonal symptoms caused by trees occur in late winter and early spring (in temperate climates), whereas symptoms due to grasses occur in the spring to early summer. In patients with perennial allergic rhinitis, chronic rather than intermittent exposure to allergen results in less acute symptoms than in seasonal rhinitis, which often obfuscates associations between exposure and onset of symptoms. Prominent symptoms in such patients include significant nasal congestion and snoring. Although seasonal allergic rhinitis rarely begins before the 2nd yr of life, perennial allergic rhinitis may occur occasionally before 2 yr if exposure to indoor allergens is great. Patients with allergic rhinitis often have a personal or family history of asthma or atopic dermatitis.

The *physical examination* demonstrates a clear nasal discharge and enlarged, often pale, turbinates. A transverse nasal crease may be present, secondary to the chronic practice of the allergic salute. The sclera may be injected, pruritic, and rarely edematous (chemosis); the lower eye lids may be darkened with **allergic shiners** from venous stasis, and creased with **Dennie's lines** from intermittent edema. In severe perennial rhinitis, an "allergic facies" with mouth breathing, high arched palate, and dental malocclusion or overbite is observed. Nasal polyps (gray, glistening membranous tissue, often with fine blood vessels) are uncommon and are seen mainly in older allergic children and adults. When **vernal conjunctivitis** is present, the palpebral conjunctiva is cobblestoned. A **geographic tongue** is common in atopic patients. The middle ear may contain fluid or may be infected; examination of the chest may reveal wheezing, rales, or rhonchi. Signs of asthma and atopic dermatitis may be present.

*Laboratory Findings.* The specific allergens to which the patient is allergic can be identified by (immediate) skin tests or by in vitro serum testing (RAST). For inhalant allergens, skin testing is sensitive, less costly, and gives results in minutes rather than weeks compared with RAST. Skin testing can provoke significant anxiety in young children. Identification of allergens is critical if specific environmental control measures are to be prescribed or if allergen immunotherapy is contemplated. Other relevant laboratory studies include nasal cytology which may show eosinophils (instead of neutrophils, as in sinusitis). An elevated serum IgE level suggests the presence of allergic disease. Because there is considerable overlap between the values of normal and allergic individuals, the total IgE test has low sensitivity and low specificity. IgE is also elevated in other conditions (see Table 8–10).

*Differential Diagnosis.* Problems that may be confused with allergic rhinitis are noted in Tables 8–12 and 8–13.

*Treatment.* The treatment of allergic rhinitis is based on (1) disease severity, (2) impact of the disease on the patient, and (3) the expected capacity of the patient to comply with recommendations. Treatment modalities include:

1. Environmental control and avoidance of allergens.
2. Pharmacologic therapy (systemic and topical).
3. Allergen immunotherapy.

Less severe disease can be treated solely with the first modality.

ENVIRONMENTAL CONTROL. Indoor allergens include many agents; specific control measures should be guided by symptom history and by skin testing to identify specific allergens. The house dust mite is a major indoor allergen, particularly in humid and warm conditions; dust mite control measures are focused on reducing mite content in

TABLE 8–12.    Differential Diagnosis of Nasal Symptoms in Childhood

| Congenital | Noninflammatory |
|---|---|
| Choanal atresia | Rhinitis medicamentosa |
| Posterior choanal stenosis | Vasomotor rhinitis |
| Encephalocele | Hypothyroidism, pregnancy, |
| Dermoid cyst | oral contraceptive agents |
| Glioma | Cerebrospinal fluid |
| Syphilis | rhinorrhea |
| | Encephalocele |
| **Anatomic** | |
| Septal anatomic deviation | **Neoplastic** |
| Adenoidal hypertrophy | Benign |
| Foreign body | Angiofibroma |
| | Papilloma |
| **Inflammatory** | Hemangioma |
| Eosinophilic | Malignant |
| Allergic | Lymphoma |
| Nonallergic (NARES) | Rhabdomyosarcoma |
| Neutrophilic (infection) | Neuroblastoma |
| Nasopharyngitis | |
| Sinusitis | |
| Nasal polyps | |
| Mastocytosis | |
| Granulomatous | |
| (Wegener) | |

NARES = nonallergic rhinitis with eosinophilia syndrome.

TABLE 8–13.   Differential Diagnosis of Rhinitis

| Diagnosis | Character of Nasal Discharge | Comments |
|---|---|---|
| Allergic rhinitis Seasonal rhinitis | Clear | Acute symptoms |
| Perennial rhinitis | Clear | Chronic nasal congestion and allergic shiners |
| Viral upper respiratory infection | Clear | Symptoms last 7–10 days; associated with sore throat, fever, poor appetite, exposure to others with upper respiratory infection |
| Sinusitis | Purulent or clear | Symptoms last >10 days, associated with cough, headache, halitosis, and abnormal sinus |
| NARES (nonallergic rhinitis with eosinophilia syndrome) | Clear | Negative skin tests; eosinophils on nasal smear |
| Vasomotor rhinitis | Clear | Profuse nasal discharge triggered by exercise or heat; associated with overuse of topical decongestants |
| Nasal polyps | Purulent or clear | Associated with cystic fibrosis or the aspirin triad (severe allergies, nasal polyps and sinusitis) or chronic rhinitis |

reservoirs, primarily mattresses, pillows, carpets, stuffed toys, blankets, and upholstered furniture. Environmental control measures (covering, cleaning, or eliminating mite reservoirs) are very effective and should be applied especially within the bedroom (dusting, vacuuming). Exposure to pet dander and to wind-borne pollens is somewhat more difficult to manage, but simple avoidance measures can be effective in reducing symptoms. These include avoidance of outdoor activity during high pollen count days, use of air conditioning, and washing hands and face and changing clothing after outdoor activity to remove pollen.

SYMPTOM THERAPY. *Antihistamines* (H$_1$ antagonists) are safe and effective medications for the treatment and prevention of allergic reactions and are particularly useful in controlling the symptoms of sneezing, nasal pruritus, and rhinorrhea. Although diphenhydramine (Benadryl) and hydroxyzine (Atarax) are effective in relieving acute allergic re-

actions, these should be avoided because they are especially sedating. Loratadine (Claritin), cetirizine (Zyrtec), and fexofenadine (Allegra) are nonsedating (but costly) antihistamines; the first two are available both as pills and liquids.

*Topical decongestants*, such as oxymetazoline hydrochloride (Afrin) and phenylephrine hydrochloride (NeoSynephrine) should not be used for the treatment of allergic rhinitis because after prolonged use they can cause severe rebound edema (*rhinitis medicamentosa*). Cromolyn sodium 4% nasal solution (Nasalcrom) is very effective and safe in preventing the symptoms of allergic rhinitis but must be used 2–6 times per day to be effective.

*Topical nasal steroids* (Flonase, Rhinocort, Vancenase, Beconase) are more effective than cromolyn in the treatment of allergic rhinitis; systemic effects rarely occur in children. Topical steroids should be used with some caution and only on a short-term basis in patients with significant symptoms. There is no indication for the use of systemic corticosteroids in the treatment of allergic rhinitis.

*Leukotriene antagonists* (Accolate and zileuton) may be effective therapy in allergic rhinitis. Ipratropium bromide (Atrovent nasal spray 0.03%, 0.06%) is used primarily for vasomotor rhinitis and rhinitis associated with viral upper respiratory infection, but it can also be used as adjunctive therapy for allergic rhinitis associated with profuse nonpurulent rhinorrhea.

IMMUNOTHERAPY. Allergen immunotherapy, which involves the subcutaneous administration of increasing doses of allergen, is highly effective in the patient with allergic rhinitis in whom specific allergens (inhalants and bee venom) are identified. It decreases the production of allergen-specific IgE and synthesis of allergen-induced IL-4, changing the underlying immunologic cause of allergy. Because of the high cost (time and pain), allergen immunotherapy should be reserved for older children with relatively severe allergic rhinitis. As a result of a small but real risk of anaphylaxis, allergen immunotherapy must be administered in a physician's office where treatment for systemic reactions is readily available.

## References

Behrman RE, Kliegman RM, Arvin AM (eds): Nelson Textbook of Pediatrics, 15th ed. Philadelphia, WB Saunders, 1996, Chapter 136.

Simons FER: Allergic rhinitis: Recent advances. Pediatr Clin North Am 35:1053, 1988.

## Atopic Dermatitis

Atopic dermatitis (AD) or eczema is a common childhood skin disorder of infancy and childhood affecting 3–5% of children before 5 yr of age. In approximately 60% of affected children, atopic dermatitis occurs in the 1st yr of life; in 90%, it occurs within the 1st 5 yr. Eczema has a genetic component, such that 70% of affected children have first-degree relatives exhibiting some form of allergic disease; 50–80% of children with eczema later develop allergic rhinitis or asthma.

*Pathogenesis.* Abnormalities within the skin and in lymphocytes of patients may contribute to the pathogenesis of AD. Patients have a reduced threshold for pruritus and a reduced threshold of irritant responsiveness. The skin reacts abnormally to light strokes (white dermographism) and demonstrates abnormal rates of cooling and warming, which suggest the existence of an abnormal balance between beta-adrenergic and cholinergic activity. Pruritus leads to skin trauma inflicted by scratching, which plays an important role in exacerbating the skin lesions.

Because AD is seen in immunodeficiency (Wiskott-Aldrich and Omenn syndromes) but is eliminated after bone marrow transplantation, bone marrow–derived cells also appear to be involved. Serum IgE levels are elevated in 80–85% of patients with AD; elevated levels of Th2 cytokines (IL-4, IL-5, and IL-10) are observed in the skin lesions of patients.

Although the role of food allergy in AD is controversial, food allergy can be demonstrated in a large number of patients with AD who may develop urticaria, pruritus, and lesions of AD after food challenge. Aeroallergen challenge (e.g., dust mites), either by inhalation and by direct contact, can exacerbate AD. Abnormal cutaneous immune responses also predispose to skin infections with viruses (herpes simplex, vaccinia, molluscum contagiosum, and papillomavirus), fungi (*Trichophyton rubrum, Pityrosporum ovale*), and bacteria (*S. aureus*).

*Diagnosis and Clinical Manifestations.* Because there is no specific feature or laboratory marker, the diagnosis (Table 8–14) is based on:

1. Skin lesions that are pruritic, dry, scaly, and often erythematous.
2. Lesions that have a typical distribution.
3. A chronic relapsing course.
4. A positive family history for atopic disease.

The most useful clue is the distribution of the lesions, which is very typical but varies with age. In the infantile form (2 mo to 5 yr), the face, extensor surface of arms, and chest are affected, with erythematous papules and vesicles. The diaper area is spared. In older children (4–12 yr), the lesions appear in the antecubital and popliteal fossa and on the wrists and hands. Typically, the lesions

**TABLE 8–14.** Criteria for the Diagnosis of Atopic Dermatitis in Children

A. **Major Features** (must have three)
  1. Pruritus
  2. Typical morphology and distribution
     a. Facial and extensor involvement during infancy and early childhood
     b. Flexural lichenification by adolescence
  3. Chronic or chronically relapsing dermatitis
  4. Personal or family history of atopy
B. **Minor or Less Specific Features**
  1. Xerosis
  2. Periauricular fissures
  3. Ichthyosis, hyperlinear palms, or keratosis pilaris
  4. IgE reactivity (increased serum IgE, RAST, or prick test positivity)
  5. Hand or foot dermatitis
  6. Cheilitis
  7. Scalp dermatitis (cradle cap)
  8. Susceptibility to cutaneous infections (especially *Staphylococcus aureus* and herpes simplex)
  9. Perifollicular accentuation (especially in pigmented races)

Modified from Hanifin JM: Atopic dermatitis in infants and children. Pediatr Clin North Am 38: 763–789, 1991.
IgE = immunoglobulin E; RAST = radioallergosorbent test.

are erythematous, dry, papular, excoriated or lichenified, and hyperpigmented. In the adult form, the dorsal surface of the hands and feet, eyelids, neck, flexor folds, and upper arms are affected. Associated findings include pityriasis alba (scaly, hypopigmented patches of skin, worse with sun exposure), keratosis pilaris (keratinified papules at the mouths of hair follicles, usually on the extensor surfaces of arms and thighs), and food allergies.

The *prognosis* in most patients with atopic dermatitis is extremely good, with a tendency for remission at 3–5 yr of age; approximately 75% of patients outgrow the problem by adolescence. Any "eczematoid" lesion can have the appearance of atopic dermatitis; these must be distinguished from atopic dermatitis (Table 8–15).

*Laboratory Findings.* Laboratory studies and skin biopsy, in rare circumstances, are performed to rule out other diseases that may mimic AD. Skin tests or RAST may be useful if food allergy is suspected but should be performed mainly when aggressive skin care fails.

*Therapy.* The goals of treatment are to assess the severity of the problem, which will vary with time, and to provide measures appropriate, for the disease severity, to control the symptoms. General measures include avoidance of soap, detergents, solvents, chemicals, and wool or acrylic clothing which dry or irritate the skin. The patient should wear loose-fitting clothing and should avoid becoming overheated. Because pruritus is a signifi-

TABLE 8–15.  Differential Diagnosis of Atopic Dermatitis

| Disease | Comment |
|---|---|
| Seborrheic dermatitis | Usually on scalp (cradle cap), sides of nose, with greasy, scaly lesions |
| Diaper dermatitis | Diaper area spared by atopic dermatitis |
| Contact dermatitis | Generally not chronic and recurring; distribution on exposed sites |
| Tinea dermatitis | Found in skin folds (neck, diaper area) rather than with distribution of atopic dermatitis |
| Langerhans cell histiocytosis (histiocytosis X) | Lesions generally hemorrhagic |
| Psoriasis | Lesions of raised plaques with sharply demarcated, irregular borders and silvery scales, occurring mainly on scalp, knees, elbows, and genitalia |
| Pyoderma | Lesions generally pustular |

Other

Immunodeficiency disorders (Wiskott-Aldrich syndrome, severe combined immunodeficiency disease, Omenn syndrome, hyper-IgE syndrome, Leiner disease [C5 deficiency], ataxia-telangiectasia, agammaglobulinemia)

Metabolic disorders (Hartnup syndrome, phenylketonuria, histidinemia, pellagra, acrodermatitis enteropathica [zinc deficiency], biotinidase deficiency)

Ectodermal dysplasia, ichthyosis

Scabies

cant feature of AD and because injury to the skin from scratching aggravates the disease, fingernails should be trimmed often and measures that reduce the pruritus should be provided. Skin hydration can significantly reduce pruritus and, therefore, is a major component of therapy. Although frequent baths with water can result in drying of the skin and has led some physicians to recommend limitations on bathing, improved skin hydration can be achieved by baths and showers one to four times per day, followed *immediately* by the application of lubricants to trap moisture in the skin. Depending on the severity of the problem, creams, mineral oil, or petroleum jelly (e.g., Vaseline) can be used, with the understanding that more severe disease requires greater occlusion, but that, occasionally, greater occlusion can result in folliculitis, particularly in hot weather. Conversely, increased occlusion (as well as humidification of the air) is required in winter months, when drying of the skin is worse because of the use of indoor heat.

Another major component of treatment is *topical steroids*, which are applied to affected skin, usually only on erythematous areas. These agents decrease pruritus, reduce inflammation, and cause vasoconstriction. Topical steroids are available in different strengths and in different vehicles. Compared with creams, ointments provide better penetration and, therefore, increased potency, whereas gels and lotions often dry the skin. Only low-potency steroids (1% hydrocortisone) should be used on the face to avoid skin atropy, and high-potency steroids (0.05% fluocinonide, 0.1% halcinonide) should be avoided except for limited periods of time and in limited areas, since systemic side effects can occur if large areas of the body are treated.

*Systemic steroids* are not necessary for the treatment of AD. Because fungal skin infections are likely to develop, it is critical that scaly, erythematous lesions without the usual distribution of AD and that are unresponsive to the usual therapy for eczema be examined for hyphae and treated with antifungal medications instead of topical steroids.

A third component in the treatment of AD consists of *antihistamines*, which are very effective in decreasing pruritus. Frequently used agents include hydroxyzine (Atarax, Vistaril); diphenhydramine (Benadryl); cetirizine (Zyrtec), a metabolite of hydroxyzine without the sedative effects of (hydroxyzine); and doxepin (Sinequan), a tricyclic compound with potent $H_1$ and $H_2$ receptor blocking action. Topical doxepin (Zonalon cream) may be used for short periods. Because pruritus and scratching are usually worse at night, night-time doses of oral antihistamines are important.

Most patients respond to treatment with good skin care, topical steroids, and antihistamines. In children who are resistant to such care, food allergies should be sought. As many as 30–50% of patients with severe AD, particularly younger children, have food allergies (see Food Allergy, which follows).

Disease severity in a given patient waxes and wanes. Acute exacerbations, caused by increased scratching, stress, heat, or infection, are characterized by increased pruritus and development of new skin lesions; these episodes should be treated with more aggressive skin care, including more frequent baths or cool soaks with Burow's solution, one to four times/day. When lesions become crusted, weepy, or vesicular, infection with *S. aureus* or herpes simplex (eczema herpeticum) should be suspected. Steroid medications and emollients should be discontinued at the involved sites. Staphylococcal infections should be treated with topical povidone and topical or systemic antibiotics if necessary, whereas herpes simplex infections can be treated with topical or systemic acyclovir.

## References

Behrman RE, Kliegman RM, Arvin AM (eds): Nelson Textbook of Pediatrics, 15th ed. Philadelphia, WB Saunders, 1996, Chapter 138.

Berhisel-Broadbent J, Sampson HA: Food hypersensitivity and atopic dermatitis. Pediatr Clin North Am 35:1115, 1988.

Hanifin JM: Atopic dermatitis. In Middleton E Jr, Reed CE, Ellis EF, et al (eds): Allergy Principles and Practice, 4th ed. St. Louis, Mosby-Year Book, 1993, p 1581.

Tan B, Weald D, Strickland I, et al: Double blind controlled trial of effect of house dust mites allergen avoidance on atopic dermatitis. Lancet 347:15, 1996.

## FOOD ALLERGY

Adverse reactions to foods are common. When severe reactions such as anaphylaxis occur immediately after ingestion, it may be easy to identify the offending food; however, if symptoms are more vague (as in headache, fatigue, increased irritability, behavior disorders, colic, diarrhea, vomiting) and do not occur immediately after ingestion of the food, identification of an offending food can be extremely difficult. Much of this difficulty is due to the fact that reactions to foods can occur via multiple mechanisms (Table 8–16), most of which are poorly understood. Food reactions are difficult to identify because reliable tests for *non*–IgE-mediated reactions are not available. To minimize the confusion regarding adverse reactions to food, the term "food allergy" will be used to define an abnormal response to a food that is triggered by an IgE-mediated immunologic reaction. IgE-mediated food reactions occur with higher frequency in families in which atopic diseases occur.

***Clinical Manifestations.*** Symptoms of food allergy include urticaria, exacerbation of atopic dermatitis, angioedema, nausea, vomiting, abdominal pain and diarrhea, wheezing, nasal congestion, sneezing, laryngeal edema, and anaphylaxis. In infants, food allergies may cause colic, vomiting, feeding problems, or growth failure. In young children, other reactions such as colitis, intestinal blood loss, and malabsorption may occur, in which case the mechanism may include T cells or immune complexes rather than IgE. Most food allergies in young children resolve with time, although IgE-mediated allergies to specific allergens (e.g., peanuts), which can be particularly severe, remain for life.

***Diagnosis and Laboratory Findings.*** The diagnosis is based on a careful history, with regard to the reproducibility of the reaction, timing of the reaction (reactions occurring soon after ingestion are more likely to be confirmed), and response to elimination of the food from the diet. Adverse reactions resulting from food poisoning, pharmacologic effects, and gastrointestinal disorders must be ruled out. A positive family history of food allergy or atopic dermatitis is common. IgA deficiency may be present. It is important to identify the specific problematic food so that specific dietary recommendations can be made.

Skin tests (or RAST) for foods can be performed to confirm IgE-mediated food allergies. The sensitivity of these tests is good, such that a negative result can eliminate the likelihood of IgE-mediated food allergy and can provide a guide for elimination diets and food challenge. Food skin testing has a relatively low specificity; results may be positive in patients not experiencing allergic reactions to the particular food.

Double-blind, placebo-controlled food challenge is a more definitive but more time-consuming test for food allergies and food intolerance; with this method, the patient is given increasing oral doses of the suspected food placed in gelatin capsules in a blinded fashion. The most common foods causing IgE-mediated reactions are cow's milk, eggs, legumes (peanuts and soy), shellfish, and wheat.

***Treatment.*** The treatment is dietary avoidance of the offending food or foods while the child continues to meet nutritional requirements. Some

TABLE 8–16.    Mechanisms for Development of Adverse Reactions to Food

| Mechanism | Example |
|---|---|
| IgE-mediated allergy | Anaphylaxis, urticaria, angioedema (peanuts, eggs) |
| Delayed allergic responses | Atopic dermatitis |
| Immune (non-IgE) mediated | Celiac disease, cow's milk protein enteropathy, eosinophilic gastroenteropathy |
| Food poisoning (toxins) | Botulism, *Staphylococcus aureus*, *Bacillus cereus*, *Escherichia coli* |
| Infection | Viral, *Salmonella*, *Shigella* |
| Pharmacologic effect | Caffeine, alcohol, tyramine, histamine |
| Gastrointestinal disorders | Peptic ulcer disease, lactase deficiency, cholelithiasis, inflammatory bowel disease |
| Reaction to additives | Sodium nitrate headaches, monosodium glutamate (headache, flushing), sorbitol (diarrhea) |
| Metabolic | Organic acidemias, hyperammonemias |
| Psychogenic | School phobia |

foods, such as celery, are easily avoided, though avoidance of other foods, such as milk and wheat, which are added to products such as bread, cakes, and cookies, warrants careful dietary planning. In infants, non–IgE-mediated cow's milk or soy allergy (frequency, ~2–4% of all infants) can be treated with hypoallergenic formulas, such as Pregestimil, Nutramigen, or Alimentum. The patient or parent must read food product labels carefully and communicate effectively with restaurants in order to avoid the offending foods. Overzealous dietary restriction may cause malnutrition and failure to thrive; substituted foods must be recommended. Because accidental ingestion of offending foods can occur despite precautions, antihistamines and bronchodilators for mild reactions and epinephrine for more severe reactions (anaphylaxis) should be available for administration. Patients with a history of food-induced anaphylaxis should be taught how to self-administer epinephrine using an EpiPen or Ana-Kit and should wear a Medic-Alert bracelet.

*Prevention.* In children with strong family histories of atopic disease, delayed exposure to food antigens may inhibit or postpone its development. Breast-feeding as the only source of nutrients for 6 mo is nutritionally sound and may prevent or delay the development of allergy. Because antigens from foods ingested by the mother are excreted into breast milk, breast-feeding decreases but does not eliminate exposure of the infant to food allergens. If breast-feeding is not possible, the infant at risk may be fed hydrolyzed milk-based formulas. Some recommend that eggs and fish be avoided by such infants until 12 mo of age.

## References

Behrman RE, Kliegman RM, Arvin AM (eds): Nelson Textbook of Pediatrics, 15th ed. Philadelphia, WB Saunders, 1996, Chapter 145.

Bock SA: Prospective appraisal of complaints of adverse reactions to foods in children during the first 3 years of life. Pediatrics 79:683, 1987.

Sampson HA, Mendelson L, Rosen JP: Fatal and near-fatal anaphylactic reactions to food in children and adolescents. N Engl J Med 327:380, 1992.

Yunginger JW: Lethal food allergy in children. N Engl J Med 327:421, 1992.

## ANAPHYLAXIS

Anaphylaxis is an acute, generalized allergic reaction in which signs and symptoms are mediated by an antigen-binding IgE on the surface of mast cells. An *anaphylactoid reaction* is clinically similar or identical to anaphylaxis, but it is not immunologically mediated; it occurs in the absence of an antigen-antibody interaction (e.g., with radiocontrast material or opioids).

*Etiology.* Antigen can be introduced by inhaled, oral, topical, and parenteral routes. Most cases of anaphylaxis are due to:

1. Hypersensitivity to drugs (antibiotics, blood products).
2. Food (peanuts, egg, seafood, milk).
3. Latex (particularly in patients with myelodysplasia).
4. Insect stings.

Penicillin causes anaphylaxis more frequently than any other drug. Occasionally, in recurrent idiopathic anaphylaxis or exercise-induced anaphylaxis, no etiologic agent is found.

*Pathophysiology.* Anaphylaxis is a type I hypersensitivity reaction mediated by IgE bound to mast cells, leading to release of granules containing histamine, tryptase, tumor necrosis factor (TNF), prostaglandin D2, leukotriene C4, platelet-activating factor (PAF); and IL-1, IL-4, IL-5, and IL-6. Histamine, TNF, and PAF all cause the production of nitric oxide, which results in vascular dilation and leakage. Agents that directly cause mast cell degranulation (opiates and complement components) do induce interleukin production but do not cause late-phase reactions.

*Clinical Manifestations and Diagnosis.* The symptoms of anaphylaxis include generalized urticaria, inspiratory stridor, laryngeal edema, difficulty swallowing, wheezing, nasal congestion, abdominal cramps, diarrhea, hypotension (decreased systemic vascular resistance, increased vascular permeability), and vascular collapse. Sneezing, pruritus (especially of hands and soles), a feeling of impending doom, or hoarseness in the throat and dysphonia may initiate the episode. Life-threatening manifestations usually involve respiratory symptoms (upper airway obstruction or bronchospasm) and/or cardiovascular involvement. The severity of the reaction is often proportional to the rapidity of onset and, in general, parallels the magnitude of the stimulus.

Anaphylaxis can be *protracted* or *biphasic*, presumably as a result of the development of late-phase responses. Concurrent illness, underlying asthma, or use of beta-blockers (Inderal) can also predispose to a more severe episode of anaphylaxis. Vasovagal reactions (bradycardia, nausea, weakness, sweating, and hypotension), hypoglycemic reactions to insulin, sepsis, and cardiac arrests can mimic and must be distinguished from anaphylaxis; these episodes are not associated with skin manifestations (except diaphoresis). Elevated histamine or tryptase levels can retrospectively help in diagnosis of the problem, as can cautious skin testing or RAST to specific antigens.

*Treatment.* Successful treatment of anaphylaxis requires prompt recognition and the immediate institution of appropriate therapy. The causative agent should be identified and exposure discontinued. Epinephrine, 0.01 mL/kg (up to 0.3–0.5 cc), subcutaneously or intramuscularly is indicated.

If anaphylaxis is due to an insect sting or allergy shot, another dose of epinephrine is indicated at the site of the sting or allergy shot and a tourniquet should be placed around the involved extremity. Supplemental oxygen should be administered and the patient's airway assessed and maintained. Intubation or tracheotomy may be required. If the blood pressure is reduced, IV fluids (normal saline, 10–20 cc/kg or more if needed) as well as an epinephrine drip should be administered. Diphenhydramine, 1–2 mg/kg IM, IV, or PO, should be administered in less severe cases. Cimetidine, an H₂ receptor antagonist, may also be helpful in a dose of 4 mg/kg. Corticosteroids, such as methylprednisolone (Solu-Medrol) IV, or prednisone, 1–2 mg/kg PO, when given early, may be helpful in limiting late-phase or prolonged responses.

Inhaled bronchodilator therapy (albuterol sulfate) or aminophylline may also benefit patients with wheezing. Patients having anaphylaxis who improve rapidly with treatment should be observed closely for late-phase reactions, which may occur 8–12 hr after the initial episode.

*Prevention.* Patients with a history of severe bee sting anaphylaxis benefit from immunotherapy with bee venom and from appropriate measures to avoid insects (including avoidance of perfumes, bright-colored clothes, and walking barefoot outdoors). Patients with a history of food, bee sting, or latex allergy and anaphylaxis should also be taught how to self-administer epinephrine using an EpiPen or Ana-Kit, should wear a Medic-Alert bracelet, and should have antihistamines available. Patients with a history of life-threatening bee sting anaphylaxis involving the respiratory or cardiovascular systems should be skin-tested to identify specific sensitivities (honeybee, wasp, yellow jacket, or hornet stings) and treated by immunotherapy with the appropriate venoms for 3–5 yr (see Insect Hypersensitivity).

Patients taking beta-blockers who are at risk for another anaphylaxis episode should be given a substitute for the beta-blocker if possible. Patients with radiocontrast allergy who require repeated imaging should be pretreated with oral steroids and antihistamines and given only low-ionic-strength contrast agents.

Patients with a history of egg anaphylaxis in rare instances may be at risk for anaphylaxis when given vaccines that contain egg protein (influenza and yellow fever vaccines). Skin testing with these vaccines prior to vaccine administration is prudent, and rapid desensitization can be performed in the event of a positive skin test result. Measles, mumps, rubella vaccine (MMR) (produced in chicken fibroblasts) does not contain sufficient egg antigens to cause anaphylaxis in allergic patients, although caution is advised when MMR vaccine is given to such patients.

### References

Behrman RE, Kliegman RM, Arvin AM (eds): Nelson Textbook of Pediatrics, 15th ed. Philadelphia, WB Saunders, 1996, Chapter 140.

Bochner B, Lichtenstein L: Anaphylaxis. N Engl J Med 324:1785, 1991.

Yunginger JW: Anaphylaxis. Curr Prob Pediatr 22:130, 1992.

## PENICILLIN HYPERSENSITIVITY

Penicillin is the most common cause of serious allergic drug reactions in children. Anaphylaxis has been reported to occur after parenteral, oral, topical, and inhalational administration, although parenteral treatment is the most likely route to produce anaphylaxis (~0.02% of treatments). Nonetheless, because of inappropriate diagnosis, as many as 85% of patients reported to have had some reaction to penicillin may be able to tolerate the drug on readministration.

*Pathophysiology.* Penicillin is a low-molecular-weight compound that is unable to elicit an immune response unless it combines with a carrier, such as a protein, polysaccharide, or cell membrane. When penicillin G (benzylpenicillin) is degraded, the beta-lactam ring opens and reacts with tissue proteins to form the benzylpenicilloyl (BPO) group, which is referred to as the "major determinant" because approximately 95% of benzylpenicillin reacts in this manner. The remaining available haptens, or "minor determinants," account for 5% of products responsible for immediate reactions.

Penicillin can elicit antibody responses of all major classes as well as produce delayed type hypersensitivity. Immediate reactions occurring within 1 hr after administration are mediated by IgE directed against the minor determinants and, on rare occasions, the major determinants. Accelerated reactions, occurring between 1 and 72 hr, and delayed reactions, occurring later than 72 hr after administration, are mediated by BPO-specific IgE, which may be modified by the presence of BPO-specific IgG acting as a "blocking antibody." BPO-specific IgG and IgM have been associated with hemolytic anemia, maculopapular eruptions, and urticaria. Delayed type hypersensitivity reactions have been associated with contact dermatitis.

*Clinical Manifestations.* Penicillin may produce a wide variety of hypersensitivity reactions. Reactions may be systemic (anaphylaxis, vasculitis), cutaneous (urticaria, angioedema, maculopapular eruptions), hematologic (Coombs-positive hemolytic anemia), and renal (interstitial nephritis). Occasionally, penicillin may be responsible for more severe cutaneous eruptions, such as Stevens-Johnson syndrome, exfoliative dermatitis, and toxic epidermal necrolysis.

A maculopapular, nonurticarial rash during *ampicillin* administration occurs in 5–10% of patients. This rash is non–IgE-mediated and does not correlate with a history of penicillin therapy. The incidence of the rash is higher in certain viral infections, such as mononucleosis and cytomegalovirus. The maculopapular eruption is not necessarily an indication to discontinue the drug, and the rash may resolve despite continued therapy. To avoid falsely labeling patients as penicillin-allergic, one should distinguish between penicillin hypersensitivity and the ampicillin rash.

*Diagnosis.* The diagnosis of penicillin hypersensitivity can be made by in vivo skin tests. Skin testing with both the major and minor determinants must be performed to detect the full spectrum of IgE activity. The major determinant is commercially available as a benzylpenicilloyl polylysine (Pre-Pen). The minor determinants are not commercially available but some persons sensitized to minor determinants can be identified by skin tests with diluted penicillin G. Skin testing is performed with a combination of prick testing and, if results are negative, intradermal testing with appropriate dilutions of the above antigens. Testing with both Pre-Pen and penicillin G identifies 95% of potential reactors. Skin tests are not predictive in non–IgE-mediated reactions.

*Treatment.* The treatment of a penicillin reaction is to discontinue the drug. If penicillin administration is mandatory in a penicillin-allergic patient, penicillin desensitization may be necessary. The desensitization procedure varies with the level of sensitivity and the route of drug administration. Desensitization has been successfully accomplished using the oral, subcutaneous, and intravenous routes. The desensitization process involves the administration of gradually increasing amounts of drug over a short time by personnel experienced in the procedure and capable of treating anaphylaxis. Once penicillin has been stopped for more than 48 hr following a desensitization procedure, the patient is no longer considered "desensitized" and future administration would require similar precautions.

### References

Behrman RE, Kliegman RM, Arvin AM (eds): Nelson Textbook of Pediatrics, 15th ed. Philadelphia, WB Saunders, 1996, Chapter 142.

Boguniewicz M, Leung D: Hypersensitivity reactions to antibiotics commonly used in children. Pediatr Infect Dis J 14:221, 1995.

## INSECT HYPERSENSITIVITY

### Stinging Insects

Allergic reactions to insect stings result in significant morbidity in children. Stinging female insects of the order Hymenoptera include honeybees, wasps, yellow jackets, hornets, and fire ants. Although most allergic reactions occur in individuals younger than 20 yr of age, children are at lower risk than adults for subsequent serious systemic reactions.

*Clinical Manifestations.* Reactions are classified as *immediate*, occurring within minutes to several hours after the sting, or *delayed*, occurring from several hours to weeks after the sting (Table 8–17). Anaphylaxis, the most serious reaction, follows a sting and occurs in 0.4–0.8% of the population. Symptoms of anaphylaxis may involve the skin

TABLE 8–17. Classification of Sting Reactions

| | |
|---|---|
| **Immediate** | |
| Normal | Localized swelling (<2 inches), transient pain, erythema, all lasting less than 24 hr |
| Toxic | Follows multiple stings, produced by exogenous vasoactive amines in venom |
| Large local | Swelling contiguous to sting lasting more than 24 hr |
| Systemic | Generalized symptoms involving signs or symptoms remote from sting site; may be non–life-threatening (distal urticaria, angioedema), or life-threatening (laryngeal edema, bronchospasm, hypotension) |
| **Delayed** | |
| Systemic | May take several clinical forms, including serum sickness–like reactions, myocarditis, transverse myelitis, nephrosis |

(generalized urticaria, flushing, angioedema), the cardiovascular system (circulatory collapse and hypotension), the respiratory tract (upper airway edema of the pharynx, epiglottis, and trachea; bronchospasm), and gastrointestinal tract (diarrhea, cramps).

*Pathophysiology.* Venom-specific IgE antibodies are produced following an initial exposure to insect venom and become bound to tissue mast cells and circulating basophils. Local reactions are due to venom-associated histamine, formic acid, hyaluronidase, and kinins. Following a sting, degranulation and release of mediators may result in local signs and symptoms or in anaphylaxis.

*Diagnosis.* A positive history of an immediate systemic reaction is necessary before venom testing and immunotherapy are to be considered. The honeybee has a barbed stinger that remains embedded after a sting. Even unprovoked, the more aggressive yellow jacket and hornet may sting repeatedly. Nonetheless, identifying the offending insect is usually difficult.

*Laboratory Findings.* Venom skin testing is the most sensitive means of detecting venom-specific IgE. Five purified venoms are available: honeybee, yellow jacket, wasp, white hornet, and yellow hornet. No good correlation exists between severity of the systemic reaction and degree of skin test positivity. Venom-specific IgE antibodies may also be measured by immunoassay.

*Treatment.* Avoiding brightly colored clothing and exterminating infested areas decrease the risk of accidental stings. Local reactions should be treated initially by removing the stinger if present, cleaning the site, applying cold compresses, and administering oral antihistamines and analgesics. In cases of severe, large local reactions, a short course of prednisone may be recommended.

Treatment of systemic reactions should be very aggressive. Epinephrine, 0.01 mL/kg of a 1:1000 solution (maximum, 0.3 mL), is the drug of choice instead of an antihistamine, although both drugs may be administered concurrently. Theophylline, pressor agents, and intravenous colloid solutions are necessary for more severe reactions. Glucocorticoids are not first-line drugs for the systemic reactions because of their delayed onset of action, but they should be administered to prevent recurrent or prolonged symptoms.

Patents who are at risk for systemic reactions should be instructed in the use of injectable epinephrine. Automatic injections, such as EpiPen (delivering 0.30 mg) and EpiPen Jr. (delivering 0.15 mg), are especially useful.

Patients with a history of normal, large local, toxic, or delayed systemic reactions are not candidates for *immunotherapy.* Venom immunotherapy is recommended for pediatric patients exhibiting a systemic reaction that involves the cardiovascular or respiratory tracts but not for patients having only cutaneous reactions. In childhood, cutaneous-systemic reactions carry a 10% risk that a subsequent systemic reaction will occur on re-sting. The therapy is effective, with almost a 98% nonreaction rate on subsequent stings.

## Biting Insects

In certain susceptible patients, unusually large local reactions to the salivary secretions of biting insects (mosquitos, flies, fleas) may develop. The reaction appears urticarial (papular urticaria) and probably results from vasoactive or irritant substances present in the insect secretions. The immune mechanism is unknown. *Treatment* consists of avoidance, antihistamines for pruritus, topical corticosteroids, and therapy for secondary infection, if present.

### References

Behrman RE, Kliegman RM, Arvin AM (eds): Nelson Textbook of Pediatrics, 15th ed. Philadelphia, WB Saunders, 1996, Chapter 143.

Valentine M, Schuberth K, Kagey-Sobotka A, et al: The value of immunotherapy with venom in children with allergy to insect stings. N Engl J Med 323:1601, 1990.

## SERUM SICKNESS

Serum sickness is a type III hypersensitivity reaction that results from an immunologic response to foreign proteins mediated by the deposition of immune complexes. It is frequently seen in response to heterologous (animal-derived) antisera (anti-lymphocyte, anti-snake venom, anti-botulism), in response to drugs (penicillin, cephalosporins), and, occasionally, with chronic viral infection.

*Pathogenesis.* Serum sickness follows the administration of large doses of antigen. Antigen must enter the circulation, where it forms soluble antigen-antibody complexes (in moderate antigen excess). These immune complexes deposit in small blood vessels; fix complement, producing C3a, C5a, and C567; and recruit polymorphonuclear leukocytes (PMNs). Capillary leak is triggered by vasoactive amines released either by antigen activation of IgE-coated mast cells or basophils or by complement activation with IgG and IgM, resulting in anaphylatoxin production. Proteolytic enzymes released from the lysosomal granules of the neutrophils mediate tissue damage and produce the vasculitis.

*Clinical Manifestations.* Serum sickness is characterized by pruritus, fever, polyarticular arthritis–arthralgia (particularly in the small joints of the hand and feet), lymphadenopathy, and urticaria–angioedema. It usually begins 7–14 days after antigen administration as antibody forms and begins to circulate. An accelerated reaction may develop with 2–4 days if prior sensitization has occurred. Symptoms generally improve in 1–2 wk as antigen is cleared. Skin eruptions occur in 90% of cases and may include urticaria, erythema multiforme, angioedema, and maculopapular and purpuric lesions (due to vasculitis). A characteristic serpiginous erythematous eruption on the sides of the hands and feet has been described. Generalized lymphadenopathy associated with splenomegaly, as well as gastrointestinal complaints (cramping, diarrhea, nausea), may occur. Cardiovascular (myocarditis, pericarditis), pulmonary (pleuritis, wheezing), and renal involvement is uncommon, although proteinuria is frequently seen. Involvement of the nervous system, including cranial nerve palsies, optic neuritis, transient hemiplegia, and Guillain-Barré syndrome, may occur rarely.

*Laboratory Findings.* Thrombocytopenia, leukopenia, or leukocytosis with or without associated eosinophilia is seen, as is an elevated erythrocyte sedimentation rate (ESR), proteinuria, microscopic hematuria, and hyaline casts. Serum C3 and C4 levels are variably depressed, and circulating immune complexes are occasionally observed. Circulating plasma cells are uncommon but are thought to be specific for serum sickness.

*Treatment.* Treatment involves discontinuing antigen administration, after which symptoms begin to improve slowly. Antihistamines may relieve the urticaria and, if given prophylactically at the time of antigen exposure, may potentially decrease immune complex deposition. Aspirin or another nonsteroidal agent is effective for fever and joint pain. If there is organ involvement, prednisone (1–2 mg/kg/24 hr) should be administered. Immediate skin testing with antigen does not predict the likelihood of serum sickness development.

### References

Behrman RE, Kliegman RM, Arvin AM (eds): Nelson Textbook of Pediatrics, 15th ed. Philadelphia, WB Saunders, 1996, Chapter 141.

Bielory L, Gascon P, Lawley TJ, et al: Human serum sickness: A prospective analysis of 35 patients treated with equine anti-thymocyte globulin for bone marrow failure. Medicine 67:40, 1988.

Heckbert S, Stryker W, Coltin K, et al: Serum sickness in children after antibiotic exposure: Estimates of occurrence and morbidity in a health maintenance organization population. Am J Epidemiol 132:336, 1990.

Lawley TJ, Frank MM: Immune complexes and allergic disease. *In* Middleton E Jr, Reed CE, Ellis EF, et al (eds): Allergy Principles and Practice, 4th ed. St. Louis, Mosby-Year Book, 1993, p 990.

## URTICARIA AND ANGIOEDEMA

Urticaria (hives) is characterized by raised, pruritic erythematous lesions that are evanescent and vary in size and pattern. Angioedema affects subcutaneous tissues and may accompany urticaria. When angioedema occurs alone, it is not pruritic. Urticaria can be "acute," present for less than 6 wk, or "chronic," occurring episodically for more than 6 wk.

*Etiology and Diagnosis.* Both acute and chronic urticaria may be produced by a number of factors (Table 8–18). Acute urticaria is more likely to be IgE-mediated; in younger patients, it is usually a benign condition. In contrast to chronic urticaria, the cause of acute urticaria is more likely to be identified. Allergy does not play a significant role in the pathogenesis of chronic urticaria; in most cases of chronic urticaria, no cause is found. A careful history regarding the specific appearance of the lesions, how and when they are provoked, often provides useful clues regarding the etiology

TABLE 8–18. Etiology of Urticaria

| Agent | Example |
|---|---|
| Drugs | Antibiotics (penicillin), aspirin, codeine, blood products |
| Foods and food additives | Eggs, peanuts, fish |
| Infectious diseases | Streptococcal pharyngitis, sinusitis, hepatitis, mononucleosis, viral infection, *Mycoplasma*, parasites |
| Insect stings | Bee stings, flea bites, mite bites |
| Collagen vascular diseases | Lupus erythematosus, vasculitis, polymyositis |
| Inhalant allergens | Cat, horse |
| Idiopathic | Unknown |
| Physical agents | Dermatographism, cold, heat, solar, cholinergic, pressure, water, vibration |
| Contact allergens | Cat scratches, moth scales, caterpillars, nettle plants |
| Neoplasms | Hodgkin disease, leukemia |
| Mastocytosis–urticaria pigmentosa | — |
| Endocrine disease | Hyperthyroidism, pregnancy, hypothyroidism |

of the urticaria. Factors that produce cutaneous vasodilation (exertion, heat, fever, hyperthyroidism) exacerbate urticaria.

*Treatment.* Skin testing or RAST may help identify the cause of acute urticaria; laboratory tests are not beneficial in evaluating chronic urticaria except to rule out collagen vascular diseases. Therefore, a CBC with differential, ESR, and urinalysis are more helpful for evaluation of chronic urticaria than skin testing or RAST.

The mainstay of treatment in acute and chronic urticaria is antihistamines ($H_1$ receptor antagonists). Hydroxyzine (Atarax) or diphenhydramine (Benadryl) is very effective, but each can be sedating. Nonsedating antihistamines, such as cetirizine (Zyrtec) and loratadine (Claritin), are also effective but more expensive. $H_2$ receptor antagonists can be added in refractory cases. If the offending agent can be identified, its avoidance will bring about rapid and dramatic improvement.

## ANGIOEDEMA

When angioedema occurs in the absence of urticaria, the diagnosis of C1 esterase inhibitor deficiency must be ruled out. Two forms exist: inherited form and acquired. The inherited form, or hereditary angioedema (HANE), has been discussed under Complement Deficiencies. Acquired C1-esterase inhibitor deficiency is associated with lymphoma or other syndromes with expanded B-cell populations or autoimmune deficiency with an autoantibody directed against the C1-esterase inhibitor. Patients with acquired C1-esterase inhibitor deficiency, in contrast to patients with HANE, have reduced levels of C1q.

*Treatment* is that of the underlying lymphoproliferative disease.

## References

Behrman RE, Kliegman RM, Arvin AM (eds): Nelson Textbook of Pediatrics, 15th ed. Philadelphia, WB Saunders, 1996, Chapter 139.
Huston DP, Bressler RB: Urticaria and angioedema. Med Clin North Am 76:804, 1992.
Kaplan AP: Urticaria and angioedema. *In* Middleton E Jr, Reed CE, Ellis EF, et al: (eds): Allergy, Principles and Practice, 4th ed. St. Louis, Mosby-Year Book, 1993, p 1553.

# Chapter 9

# RHEUMATIC DISEASES OF CHILDHOOD

Judyann C. Olson*

The rheumatic diseases of childhood (autoimmune, collagen vascular, or connective tissue diseases) are entities characterized by inflammatory changes that involve the connective tissues in the body. Common manifestations of rheumatic diseases include **synovitis** (arthritis), or inflammation of the joint synovium (Table 9–1); **enthesopathy**, or inflammation at the insertion of a ligament to a bone (sacroiliac joint arthritis, achilles tendinitis, plantar fasciitis); **serositis**, or inflammation of a serosal lining (Table 9–2); **myositis**, or muscle inflammation; **autoantibody** production (Table 9–3); and **vasculitis** (Table 9–4). Inflammation may be localized in one joint or tendon group or it may be generalized. Local inflammation is characterized by pain, swelling, erythema, limited range of motion, and warmth, whereas systemic inflammation is manifested by fever, malaise, anorexia, weight loss, and myalgias.

Currently, rheumatology is a descriptive subspecialty, and the pathophysiology of disorders included in this category is not precisely understood. Inflammation and tissue injury in rheumatic diseases are mediated by the immune response from the activation of monocytes, lymphocytes, polymorphonuclear leukocytes, complement, and antibodies. Specific autoantibodies may be produced, such as antiplatelet antibodies in **systemic lupus erythematosus** (SLE); or the injury may be mediated by deposition of non–tissue-specific antigen–antibody complexes in organs with large capillary beds, such as the glomerulus of the kidney. Furthermore, tissue damage may be mediated by local activation of macrophages and lymphocytes, as occurs in the synovium of patients with adult-type

rheumatoid arthritis. In the latter condition, local inflammatory cells accumulate, as a result of immune complexes, and activate complement, which attracts more inflammatory cells. Cytokines, phospholipids, kinins, and other mediators of inflammation are released into the tissue, and hydrolytic enzymes (e.g., proteases and collagenases) are released, producing local damage. Synovitis produces synovial hypertrophy (pannus), which migrates into the articular cartilage. This hypertrophy, together with hydrolytic enzymes, further destroys, demineralizes, and enhances mechanical

TABLE 9–1. Causes of Childhood Arthritis (Synovitis)

**Common**
 Juvenile rheumatoid arthritis
 Rheumatic fever
 Systemic lupus erythematosus
 Henoch-Schönlein purpura
 Pyogenic infection (septic or immune complex)
 Viral infection (parvovirus, rubella, mumps; possibly toxic synovitis)
 Lyme disease (*Borrelia burgdorferi*)
 Serum sickness
 Kawasaki disease

**Less Common**
 Hemophilia
 Endocarditis
 Leukemia
 Reiter syndrome (enteric, genital)
 Inflammatory bowel disease
 Dermatomyositis

**Rare**
 Acneiform arthritis
 Psoriatic
 Wegener granulomatosis
 Sarcoidosis
 Scleroderma

---

*This text is a revision of Dr. D. W. Kredich's chapter from the second edition.

TABLE 9–2.  Serositis

**Manifestations**
    Pericarditis
    Peritonitis
    Pleuritis

**Differential Diagnosis**
    Juvenile rheumatoid arthritis
    Systemic lupus erythematosus
    Tuberculosis
    Viral (coxsackievirus)
    Bacterial (pneumococcus, *Staphylococcus aureus*, group A
      streptococcus)
    Immune complex (meningococcus, gonococcus)
    Malignancy
    Spontaneous peritonitis (pneumococcus, *Escherichia coli*)

injury of the tissue. Although the description of each disorder is distinct, the individual patient often has overlapping signs and symptoms that may make a precise diagnosis difficult.

TABLE 9–3.  Manifestations of Autoantibodies

Coombs-positive hemolytic anemia
Immune neutropenia
Immune thrombocytopenia
Thrombosis (anticardiolipin, antiphospholipid, lupus
    anticoagulant)
Immune lymphopenia
Antimitochondrial (primary biliary cirrhosis, SLE)
Antimicrosomal (chronic active hepatitis, SLE)
Antithyroid (thyroiditis, SLE)
Antineutrophil cytoplasmic antibody (ANCA-cytoplasmic)
    (Wegener granulomatosis)
ANCA-perinuclear (microscopic polyangiitis)

**Antinuclear Antibodies to Specific Nuclear Antigens and
Associated Manifestations**
Single-stranded DNA* (nonspecific, indicates inflammation)
Double-stranded DNA* (SLE, renal disease)
DNA-histone (drug-induced SLE)
Sm (Smith) (SLE, renal, central nervous system)
RNP (ribonucleoprotein) (SLE; Sjögren syndrome,
    scleroderma, polymyositis, MCTD)
Ro (Robert: SSA) (SLE; neonatal lupus–congenital heart
    block: Sjögren syndrome)
La (Lane: SSB) (SLE, Sjögren syndrome)
Jo-1 (polymyositis, dermatomyositis)
Sc1-70 (scleroderma)
Centromere (CREST syndrome, variant scleroderma)
PM-Sc1 (scleroderma, UCTD)

Adapted from Condemi J: The autoimmune diseases. JAMA 268:2882, 1992. Copyright 1992, American Medical Association.

*Because antibodies to single-stranded DNA (ssDNA) are a nonspecific response to inflammatory diseases and because ssDNA may contaminate double-stranded DNA (dsDNA) preparations, the purer circular dsDNA of *Crithidia luciliae* (crithidia test) is preferred.

CREST syndrome = *c*alcinosis, *R*aynaud phenomenon, *e*sophageal dysfunction, *s*clerodactyly, *t*elangiectasia; DNA = deoxyribonucleic acid; MCTD = mixed connective tissue disease; SLE = systemic lupus erythematosus; SSA = Sjögren syndrome antigen A; SSB = Sjögren syndrome antigen B; UCTD = undifferentiated connective tissue disease.

# LABORATORY TESTS USED TO ASSESS RHEUMATIC DISEASES

## ACUTE-PHASE REACTANTS

The Westergren sedimentation rate (WSR), or erythrocyte sedimentation rate (ESR), is the most commonly used test to assess the activity of a rheumatic disease. It is nonspecifically increased in response to systemic inflammation (rheumatic disease, infection, malignancy). The sedimentation rate requires erythrocyte rouleaux formation and an interaction with fibrinogen or macroglobulins; afibrinogenemia, anemia, and sickle cell anemia may reduce the sedimentation rate. Other acute-phase reactants that are elevated in response to inflammation include (1) the C-reactive protein, which is rapidly synthesized by the liver; (2) platelet count; (3) ferritin; and (4) total hemolytic complement (CH50). Any of the acute-phase reactants may be helpful in following the disease course in a given patient, but some patients will have active inflammatory disease with normal values for one or more acute-phase reactants.

## RHEUMATOID FACTORS

Rheumatoid factors are antibodies directed against the Fc portion of immunoglobulin G (IgG). Most of the conventional tests for rheumatoid factor, such as the latex agglutination titer, detect rheumatoid factors that are IgM; IgG, IgA, and IgE rheumatoid factors can be measured by other techniques.

A positive rheumatoid factor is not diagnostic. Most children with **juvenile rheumatoid arthritis** (JRA) are negative for conventional rheumatoid factors, whereas children with SLE and Henoch-Schönlein purpura may have rheumatoid factors. Rheumatoid factors also are present in viral infections, such as hepatitis B, and in other conditions including bacterial endocarditis, sarcoidosis, tuberculosis, and congenital TORCH infections (*t*oxoplasmosis, *o*ther conditions, *r*ubella, *c*ytomegalovirus, and *h*erpes simplex).

## ANTINUCLEAR AND ANTICYTOPLASMIC ANTIBODIES

Autoantibodies against nuclear as well as cytoplasmic constituents often are found in the serum of patients with connective tissue diseases, but they also occur in individuals with nonrheumatic conditions (mononucleosis, endocarditis, chronic active

TABLE 9–4.  Vasculitis Syndrome

| Type | Comment | Type | Comment |
|---|---|---|---|
| *Polyarteritis Nodosa Group* | | *Wegener Granulomatosis* | Necrotizing granulomas; small and medium arteries; upper and lower respiratory tract, glomerulonephritis; positive antineutrophil cytoplasm antibodies |
| Polyarteritis nodosa | Multisystem—kidney, nerve, liver, skin; necrotizing vasculitis of small and medium muscular arteries | | |
| Churg-Strauss syndrome (allergic angiitis and granulomatosis) | Skin and pulmonary involvement; eosinophilia and asthma; granulomatous vasculitis of small and medium arteries | *Giant Cell Arteritis* | |
| | | Temporal/cranial | Medium-large arteries; retinal arteritis may cause blindness |
| Polyangiitis overlap | Overlap of more than one of any type vasculitis with skin, lung, kidney, nerve involvement | Takayasu | Young women, inflammation of aortic arch |
| | | *Others* | |
| *Hypersensitivity Syndromes* | | Behçet disease | Recurrent oral, gastrointestinal, and genital ulcers; uveitis; skin |
| Henoch-Schönlein purpura | Palpable purpura, kidney, joint, intestine; inflammation of arteriole, capillary, and venule; leukocytoclastic vasculitis, IgA immune complexes | Kawasaki disease | Arteritis, coronary artery aneurysm; immune complexes |
| Serum sickness (e.g., drug-related) | Antigen-antibody hypocomplementemic, skin, joint, kidney | Hypocomplementemic disease | Chronic urticaria |
| Vasculitis with infections | Meningococcemia, Rocky Mountain spotted fever, endocarditis, HIV, EBV, parvovirus B19, syphilis | | |
| Connective tissue vasculitis | SLE, JRA | | |

EBV = Epstein-Barr virus; HIV = human immunodeficiency virus; Ig = immunoglobulin; JRA = juvenile rheumatoid arthritis; SLE = systemic lupus erythematosus.

hepatitis, malaria, drug therapy such as hydralazine) (see Table 9–3). Antinuclear antibodies (ANAs) are determined by indirect immunofluorescence techniques in which the patient's serum is incubated with a source of nuclei and a fluorescent-labeled immunoglobulin; the greatest dilution of serum at which a positive immunofluorescent pattern is observed then is recorded. Procedures differ in many laboratories, but frequently a 1:40 titer is the lowest dilution considered positive. The pattern of staining also is reported. The four major patterns are as follows:

1. *Speckled*: nonspecific for SLE and occurs in many connective tissue diseases (antigens include Sm, RNP, Ro, La, Jo-1, Scl-70, centromere; see Table 9–3).
2. *Homogeneous*: also nonspecific and is the most common pattern seen in children with JRA in whom uveitis occurs.

3. *Rim (peripheral)*: usually diagnostic of SLE (double-stranded DNA; see Table 9–3) but is seen in a small proportion of patients with SLE.
4. *Nucleolar*: most commonly seen in patients with scleroderma-like illnesses (PM-Scl; see Table 9–3).

Between 60 and 70% of children with a positive ANA have autoimmune disease, which is often evident at the time of the positive ANA. JRA is the most common of these, followed by SLE, dermatomyositis, undifferentiated connective tissue disease, and uveitis. Patients with a positive ANA but no evidence of autoimmune disease may have nonspecific musculoskeletal complaints, hypermobility, dermatologic disease, or a viral syndrome.

## COMPLEMENT

The various complement components (see Chapter 8, Fig. 8–2) as well as the total hemolytic comple-

ment may be elevated, as are the acute-phase reactants in rheumatic diseases. Decreased complement levels are noted in active SLE, particularly in
SLE with nephritis; total hemolytic complement,
an important screening test, is depressed in SLE
and in various vasculitides. In addition, hereditary
complement component deficiencies have been associated with familial cases of SLE and vasculitis.

## HISTOCOMPATIBILITY ANTIGENS

Children with the human leukocyte antigen (HLA)
B27 locus are at increased risk for ankylosing spondylitis, Reiter syndrome, psoriatic arthritis, and arthritis associated with inflammatory bowel disease.
Seropositive polyarticular JRA is associated with
the HLA-DR4 locus.

### References

Behrman RE, Kliegman RM, Arvin AM (eds): Nelson Textbook
    of Pediatrics, 15th ed. Philadelphia, WB Saunders, 1996,
    Chapter 147.
Condemi J: The autoimmune diseases. JAMA 268:2882, 1992.
Deane P, Liard G, Siegel D, et al: The outcome of children
    referred to a pediatric rheumatology clinic with a positive
    antinuclear antibody test but without an autoimmune dis-
    ease. Pediatrics 95:892, 1995.

## JUVENILE RHEUMATOID ARTHRITIS

JRA is not a rare disease in childhood; it affects an
estimated 100,000–250,000 children in the United
States (incidence 1.4:10,000; prevalence 1:1000). The
age of onset shows peaks at 1–3 yr and in the early
teenage years.

### CLASSIFICATION

Chronic arthritis persisting for at least 6 wk in an
individual 16 yr of age or younger should suggest
JRA when there is no other reason for the arthritis.
JRA is divided into three broad onset types based
on the clinical manifestations in the first 6 mo of
illness. The most common type is **pauciarticular
disease**, which involves four or fewer joints. The
next most common is **polyarticular disease**, with
involvement of five or more joints. The least common is **systemic-onset disease**, which begins with
high spiking fevers to greater than 39.4°C (103°F).
The fever is frequently accompanied by a rheumatoid rash, which comes and goes with temperature
elevations. Joint involvement may occur either at
onset or later in the course of the disease.

## Pauciarticular Juvenile Rheumatoid Arthritis

About half of all children with JRA have this onset
type. There are two prominent subgroups of pauciarticular JRA: (1) a younger group of patients, primarily female, who often have chronic uveitis; and
(2) older children with later onset of disease, more
frequently male, who may develop features of a
spondyloarthropathy syndrome.

*Clinical Manifestations.* Pauciarticular arthritis
in the *younger* child has a peak age of onset at
about 2 yr. These children appear healthy with few
systemic signs of illness. The large joints are most
commonly involved. The knee is the most frequently involved joint, followed by ankles and elbows. Hip involvement is very rare. The child occasionally may have swelling in the small joints of
the hands or feet. Pain is uncommon in these children, and the diagnosis may be made after months
of asymptomatic swelling, leading to the slow development of contractures. The joint disease rarely
is destructive. Localized growth disturbance may
occur as a result of asymmetric joint disease. This
growth disturbance is particularly noticeable in the
knees, because it may lead to an overgrowth in the
length of the affected leg. Signs and symptoms of
uveitis are few (occasionally poor vision, red eye),
and the diagnosis usually is made at the time of a
regularly scheduled slit-lamp examination. Therefore, there is a risk of blindness secondary to late
diagnosis of eye disease. The differential diagnosis
includes Lyme disease (Table 9–5) because of the
pattern of few joints being involved.

Most *laboratory tests* are normal; these include
hemoglobin level, sedimentation rate, and white
blood cell count. Rheumatoid factor rarely is present, but many of the children have positive tests
for ANAs (>50%). The presence of ANAs in the
very young female patient with pauciarticular arthritis is closely associated with the development
of chronic iridocyclitis. The disease is associated
with HLA-DR5, HLA-DR6, and HLA-DR8.

*Treatment of uveitis* with local steroid eyedrops
and dilating agents usually is successful. A minority of patients may require systemic steroids for
severe eye disease. Severe arthritis occurs in 10% of
patients. Some patients progress to a polyarticular
course. If there is a *significant leg length discrepancy*
from overgrowth of a leg, the child may experience
a severe pelvic tilt, compensatory scoliosis, and a
gait abnormality that is easily corrected by placing
a lift on the shoe of the normal (shorter) leg. The
lift equalizes leg length and normalizes the gait.

Pauciarticular arthritis in *older* children usually
occurs after 8 yr of age and has a propensity to
involve the joints of the lower extremity in an

TABLE 9–5.  Differential Diagnosis of Pediatric Arthritis Syndromes

| Characteristic | Systemic Lupus Erythematosus | Juvenile Rheumatoid Arthritis | Rheumatic Fever | Lyme Disease | Leukemia | Gonococcemia | Kawasaki Disease |
|---|---|---|---|---|---|---|---|
| Sex | F > M | Type-dependent | M = F | M = F | M = F | F > M | M = F |
| Age | 10–20 yr | 2–16 yr | 5–15 yr | 2–20 yr | 2–10 yr | >12 yr | <4 yr |
| Arthralgia | Yes | Yes | Yes | Yes | Yes | Yes | Yes |
| Morning stiffness | Yes | Yes | No | No | No | No | No |
| Rash | Butterfly; discoid | Salmon-pink macules (systemic-onset) | Erythema marginatum | Erythema chronicum migrans | No | Palms/soles papulopustules | Diffuse maculopapular (nonspecific) |
| Monoarticular, pauciarticular | Yes | 50% | No | Yes | Yes | Yes | — |
| Polyarticular | Yes | Yes | Yes | Rare | Yes | No | Yes |
| Small joints | Yes | Yes | No | No | Yes | No | Yes |
| Temporomandibular joint | No | Rare | No | Rare | No | No | No |
| Eye disease | Uveitis/retinitis | Iridocyclitis (rare in systemic-onset) | No | Keratitis | No | No | Conjunctivitis, uveitis |
| Total WBC count | Decreased | Increased | Normal to increased | Normal | Increased or neutropenia ± blasts | Increased | Increased |
| ANA | Positive | Positive (50%) | Negative | Negative | Negative | Negative | Negative |
| Rheumatoid factor | Positive | Positive (10%) (poly-onset) | Negative | Negative | Negative | Negative | Negative |
| Other laboratory results | ↓ Complement | — | ↑ ASO | ↑ Cryoglobulin, ↑ immune complexes | + Bone marrow | + Culture for GC | Thrombocytosis, ↑ immune complexes |
| Erosive arthritis | No, rare | Yes | No, rare | Rare | No | Yes | No |
| Other clinical manifestations | Proteinuria, serositis | Fever, serositis (systemic-onset) | Carditis, nodules, chorea | Carditis, neuropathy | Thrombocytopenia | Sexual activity, menses | Fever, lymphadenopathy, swollen hands/feet, mouth lesions |
| Pathogenesis | Autoimmune | Autoimmune | Group A streptococcus | Borrelia burgdorferi | Acute lymphoblastic leukemia | Neisseria gonorrhoeae | Unknown |
| Treatment | NSAIDs, steroids, hydroxychloroquine, immunosuppressive agents | NSAIDs, methotrexate for resistant disease | Penicillin prophylaxis, aspirin, steroids | Penicillin, tetracycline, ceftriaxone | Steroids, chemotherapy | Ceftriaxone, cefoxitin | Aspirin, intravenous immunoglobulins |

ANA = antinuclear antibody; ASO = antistreptolysin-O titer; GC = gonococcus; NSAID = nonsteroidal anti-inflammatory drug; WBC = white blood cell.

303

asymmetric fashion; enthesopathy of the Achilles tendon, patellar tendon, or plantar fascia often occurs. Hips commonly are involved. The knee is the most commonly involved joint, and the ankle and the first metatarsophalangeal joint are the next. Some children have asymmetric upper extremity joint involvement. Many children have a positive family history of significant low back pain, psoriasis, inflammatory bowel disease, ankylosing spondylitis, or reactive (e.g., Reiter) arthritis.

The usual pattern is slowly diminishing motor performance and often attendant emotional depression. Commonly, the patient has a history of slowly decreasing exercise capacity, malaise, and nagging aches and pains. Occasionally, the child may have significant systemic signs accompanied by weight loss, fever, anorexia, and diffuse arthralgia/myalgia. In the first years of their illness, most children complain not of low back pain but rather of painful inflammation at points of insertion of tendons and ligaments (**entheses**). Joint swelling may develop later in the course. Uveitis, when it occurs, tends to be acute in nature (decreased visual acuity, erythema). This is in contrast to the younger children, who may have asymptomatic chronic uveitis. The differential diagnosis of seronegative spondyloarthropathy (inflammatory low back pain, enthesitis, asymmetric lower joint involvement) includes juvenile ankylosing spondylitis, Reiter disease, psoriatic arthritis, and arthropathies of inflammatory bowel disease. In each, there is a high incidence of HLA-B27.

*Laboratory Tests.* Older children with pauciarticular arthritis inevitably have normal findings on laboratory tests except, perhaps, children with constitutional symptoms, who may have markedly elevated sedimentation rates or depressed hemoglobin levels; these children frequently are positive for HLA-B27. Rheumatoid factor and ANA are negative.

### Polyarticular Juvenile Rheumatoid Arthritis

Children with the polyarticular onset (five or more joints involved in the first 6 mo) are further subcategorized into those who are seronegative (more common) and those who are seropositive for rheumatoid factor. Girls outnumber boys in both categories.

Invariably in *polyarticular disease* the small joints of the hands and, usually, the feet are involved. Large joint involvement also is common. The cervical spine, temporomandibular joint, sternoclavicular joint, and distal interphalangeal joints also may be affected. Systemic manifestations of disease are more frequently seen than in children with pauciarticular disease. Mild anemia of chronic disease, leukocytosis, fever, lymphadenopathy, and hepatosplenomegaly may be seen. Fatigue is common, and anorexia may occur.

Approximately one fourth of the *seronegative polyarticular JRA* patients have positive tests for ANAs; a few of these will have associated chronic uveitis. The onset of illness usually occurs when the child is 10 yr or younger. The course of the disease in this type of illness generally is favorable, with few extra-articular manifestations and 10–15% finally being categorized in functional class III or IV (Table 9–6). Seronegative JRA patients, in general, respond better to treatment with nonsteroidal antiinflammatory drugs (NSAIDs) than do seropositive patients. The *differential diagnosis* includes Lyme disease, rheumatic fever, and SLE (see Table 9–5).

Only about 5–8% of all children with chronic arthritis are *seropositive for rheumatoid factor.* The onset of illness usually occurs when the child is 9–16 yr of age. Most of these children have evidence of erosive, destructive arthritis on roentgenograms at the end of 1 yr of illness. Nodules over tendons (elbows, knees, scalp) are seen more frequently in seropositive than in seronegative polyarticular disease and are thought to indicate severe disease. Vasculitis (lung, skin) occurs uncommonly. Approximately half of these adolescents have severe unremitting disease with a functional outcome that puts them in class III or IV. Disease persists into adulthood, and the natural history is similar

**TABLE 9–6.** American College of Rheumatology Revised Criteria for Classification of Functional Status in Rheumatoid Arthritis*

| | |
|---|---|
| Class I | Completely able to perform usual activities of daily living (self-care, vocational, and avocational) |
| Class II | Able to perform usual self-care and vocational activities, but limited in avocational activities |
| Class III | Able to perform usual self-care activities, but limited in vocational and avocational activities |
| Class IV | Limited in ability to perform usual self-care, vocational, and avocational activities |

From Arthritis Rheum 35:498, 1992. © American College of Rheumatology.

*Usual self-care activities include dressing, feeding, bathing, grooming, and toileting. Avocational (recreational and/or leisure) and vocational (work, school, homemaking) activities are patient desired and age and sex specific.

to that of adult-onset rheumatoid arthritis. About 50% of patients have positive ANA tests, and there is an association with HLA antigens DW4 and DR4 (similar to adult rheumatoid arthritis).

## Systemic-Onset Juvenile Rheumatoid Arthritis

Systemic-onset JRA is the most dramatic and least common form of the illness. It is the only type of JRA that affects males as frequently as females.

*Clinical Manifestations.* The age of onset in children is usually 16 yr or younger, and the sexes are equally affected. These patients usually appear ill and often have high spiking fevers of at least 39.4°C (103°F) for many weeks. They usually have associated erythematous macular rash, splenomegaly, hepatomegaly, and lymphadenopathy. Irritability and arthralgia/myalgia are prominent features, particularly during fever spikes. The characteristic rash consists of small, salmon-colored macules located on the trunk and extremities that come and go with the fever spikes; rarely, the rash is pruritic. Arthritis often is absent during the first weeks or even 6–8 mo of illness. Later in the course, chronic polyarticular arthritis may occur; it may be severe. Therefore, JRA becomes a suspected diagnosis and one of exclusion. The *differential diagnosis* includes occult infection (Epstein-Barr virus), malignancy (leukemia or neuroblastoma), and acute rheumatic fever (see Table 9–5).

Other systemic features of the disease include pericarditis, pleuritis, and, uncommonly, abdominal serositis. Myocarditis occasionally is seen. Growth retardation is a prominent feature of this type of illness, particularly if long-term corticosteroid therapy has been required. Though uncommon, life-threatening abnormalities of coagulation have been seen. Bony fusion of the cervical spine can occur. Chronic uveitis is a rare manifestation of systemic JRA.

*Laboratory Findings.* There are no diagnostic laboratory features of systemic-onset JRA. The child typically has anemia that may be profound and is generally the normocytic/normochromic anemia of chronic disease. The white blood cell count frequently is markedly elevated and may show a shift to the left; often platelet counts are elevated, as are acute-phase reactants. Ferritin levels may be markedly elevated. Sedimentation rate usually is extremely high. The serum is uniformly negative for rheumatoid factors and ANAs.

*Prognosis.* Some children have intermittent episodes of febrile illness for years after onset; others (25%) progress to severe chronic, destructive polyarticular joint disease without recurrent fevers.

Death is uncommon in the course of JRA, but it is most likely to occur in the child with systemic onset disease. Death usually is due to myocarditis or infection, especially if the child has been immunosuppressed. The coagulopathy syndrome associated with JRA may also be life-threatening.

## GENERAL CHARACTERISTICS OF ARTHRITIS IN CHILDHOOD

**Morning stiffness** is characteristic of JRA. Children rarely complain specifically of stiffness as such; more often, they respond "yes" to questions regarding "slowness in the morning" or "needing time to loosen up." This morning stiffness may be ameliorated by setting an earlier time for arising, providing a warm morning bath, and using heating pads or electric blankets at night. Stretching exercises may also be beneficial. Stiffness also occurs after periods of immobility, and teachers need to be reminded that children with arthritis need extra freedom to move about the classroom throughout the day.

**Pain** is variable in JRA. Many children experience little or no pain, but later in life this lack of pain often may conceal the presence of a longstanding arthritis, possibly accompanied by significant flexion contractures, before the joint disease finally is appreciated. Contractures may occur as the child avoids the extremes of motion, the point at which pain may occur. Some children have significant pain or discomfort.

Generalized **growth retardation** may occur in the systemic form of the disease and in severe polyarticular disease and is accentuated if corticosteroids have been used. If the systemic illness remits, some catch-up growth occurs, but many children have such prolonged disease that their final height will be reduced.

**Localized overgrowth and undergrowth** occur in areas of asymmetric arthritis. In this case, there is generally marked overgrowth and acceleration of epiphyseal maturation in the affected joints so that, for example, the leg with the arthritic knee becomes much longer than the normal leg. If the cervical spine is involved, neck instability, stiffness, and torticollis may develop. Undergrowth of the mandible may result in a marked micrognathia and severe cosmetic and orthodontic deformity.

**Roentgenographic changes** in JRA usually are minimal. A child who has severe JRA for many years may have only osteopenia. Joint space narrowing may occur. Older children who are seropositive for rheumatoid factor may have evidence of erosive disease.

## PROGNOSIS OF JRA

One of the most difficult concepts for parents to accept is that it is not possible to predict accurately the ultimate outcome for any particular child. The outcome of most children is favorable. The prognosis is good in the young female with pauciarticular disease. It is most guarded in the child with seropositive polyarticular disease. However, a few children with pauciarticular JRA ultimately progress to a polyarticular involvement with severe destructive disease. Naturally, each time a child experiences a remission of disease, the family hopes that this is a permanent remission; relapse brings profound disappointment. The physician caring for the child should maintain a positive attitude, because meticulous medical management, physical therapy, splinting, and psychologic support can improve the quality of life for the child with JRA.

## TREATMENT

Most children respond to aspirin or NSAIDs (ibuprofen, naproxen, ketoprofen, meclofenamate, indomethacin, tolmetin) with a lessening of arthritis or systemic signs such as fever. Because aspirin is associated with Reye syndrome following influenza or varicella, NSAIDs are preferred by some rheumatologists. Influenza virus vaccine also may reduce this risk when aspirin is used. Splinting, physical therapy, and, rarely, joint replacement (e.g., total hip replacement) may be needed. Systemic corticosteroids are indicated for serious complications, such as pericarditis or when cricoarytenoid joint involvement obstructs the airway. Intra-articular corticosteroids may be used to control local joint involvement.

Second-line agents for patients not responding to NSAIDs include low-dose oral methotrexate (10 mg/m²). Sulfasalazine, hydroxychloroquine, and gold salts have been utilized in the treatment of JRA. Their role needs further clarification. Pulse methylprednisolone and cyclophosphamide in addition to methotrexate may benefit more refractory patients.

### References

Behrman RE, Kliegman RM, Arvin AM (eds): Nelson Textbook of Pediatrics, 15th ed. Philadelphia, WB Saunders, 1996, Chapter 148.

Giannini E, Cowkell G: Drug treatment in children with juvenile rheumatoid arthritis: Past, present, and future. Pediatr Clin North Am 42:1099, 1995.

Schneider R, Lang B, Reilly B, et al: Prognostic indicators of joint destruction in systemic-onset juvenile rheumatoid arthritis. J Pediatr 120:200, 1992.

# SYSTEMIC LUPUS ERYTHEMATOSUS

SLE is an autoimmune disease that may involve nearly every organ system in an inflammatory process. SLE occurs more frequently in females and has a higher incidence in the black population than in Caucasians. Peak ages of onset correlate roughly with menarche and menopause; the preponderance of females demonstrating onset of the disease during these ages and in the postpartum period is even more striking than that prior to puberty.

*Clinical Manifestations.* Arthritis or arthralgia, weight loss, fever, malaise, or rash are frequent symptoms at the onset of illness. The arthritis affects small more than large joints and is disproportionately painful relative to the physical findings. Many patients have a typical "butterfly" rash over the malar area of the face, sparing the nasolabial folds. Many other rashes are common with SLE and may vary from papular to bullous in character; some of these rashes exhibit photosensitivity. Any serosal surface also may be inflamed, resulting in pericarditis, pleuritis, or acute abdominal pain secondary to abdominal serositis. Vasculitis, myositis, pancreatitis, and the antiphospholipid antibody syndrome (with propensity for thrombosis) may be seen.

Renal disease is frequent in SLE, although in some patients it may be clinically inapparent. Renal biopsy demonstrates various lesions accompanied by deposition of complement and immunoglobulins within the glomerulus. At the onset of disease, some patients will have a diffuse proliferative nephritis with compromised renal function; others may have a mild mesangial involvement that may not be progressive.

Hematologic disorders are common and again reflect autoantibody formation. They include Coombs-positive hemolytic anemia, leukopenia secondary to antineutrophil antibodies, and thrombocytopenia associated with antiplatelet antibodies.

A broad spectrum of neurologic disorders may result from SLE, the most common being seizures or psychotic states. Mild cerebrospinal fluid (CSF) protein elevation and an abnormal magnetic resonance imaging study may occur. Neuropsychologic testing may be helpful. Other causes of central nervous system (CNS) symptoms, such as steroid psychosis, hypertension, uremia, infection (toxoplasmosis, cryptococcosis, *Nocardia*, *Listeria*), or stroke (from the antiphospholipid antibody syndrome) must be considered in the differential diagnosis. *Diagnostic criteria* for SLE and additional clinical manifestations are presented in Tables 9–7 and 9–8, respectively.

TABLE 9–7.   Clinical Diagnostic Criteria for Systemic Lupus Erythematosus*

**Physical Signs**

Butterfly rash (malar)
Discoid lupus
Photosensitivity
Oral and nasopharyngeal ulcers
Nonerosive arthritis (≥2 joints with effusion, tenderness)
Pleuritis *or* pericarditis (serositis)
Seizures *or* psychosis in absence of metabolic toxins or drugs

**Laboratory Data**

*Renal Disease (Nephritis)*
Proteinuria (greater than 500 mg/24 hr) *or*
Cellular casts (RBC, granular, tubular)

*Hematologic Disease*
Hemolytic anemia with reticulocytosis *or*
Leukopenia (<4000 on two occasions) *or*
Lymphopenia (<1500 on two occasions) *or*
Thrombocytopenia (<100,000)

*Serologic Data*
Positive anti-dsDNA *or*
Positive anti-Sm *or*
Positive LE prep *or*
False-positive VDRL for >6 mo
Positive ANA in absence of drugs known to induce lupus

*Table shows the 1982 revised criteria for diagnosing SLE. A patient must have four of the 11 criteria in order to establish the diagnosis of SLE. These criteria may be present at the same or at different times during the patient's illness. Additional, less diagnostic manifestations are noted in Table 9–8.
LE = lupus erythematosus; RBC = red blood cell.

*Laboratory Findings.* Nearly all patients have positive ANAs, although this is a screening test and is not diagnostic (see Table 9–3). Most patients with SLE have antibodies to double-stranded DNA and decreased levels of total hemolytic complement. With effective therapy, complement levels may return to normal, except in rare patients with familial complement deficiencies. Other less specific tests, such as a false-positive test for syphilis (VDRL) or the presence of a rheumatoid factor, may be seen. A usually reversible form of SLE also may be induced by various drugs (hydralazine, procainamide, isoniazid, chlorpromazine, phenytoin, carbamazepine, quinidine, propylthiouracil); in 95% of patients, this condition is associated with antihistone antibodies. When the drug is withdrawn, the lupus-like syndrome resolves.

*Treatment.* Treatment varies with the disease manifestation. Arthritis and less serious manifestations usually are managed with NSAIDs. The skin manifestations of lupus respond to sunscreens and sun avoidance. Hydroxychloroquine may be utilized for skin and/or joint involvement and may

have a steroid-sparing effect. Most patients have widespread organ system involvement that requires use of oral corticosteroids or, with very serious disease, intravenous pulses of steroids. Severe recalcitrant disease sometimes requires the use of cytotoxic agents (cyclophosphamide or azathioprine). Patients who have had a thrombotic event and evidence of the antiphospholipid antibody syndrome may require anticoagulation. Serologic parameters and complement levels may reflect disease activity, thus allowing the physician to use the lowest possible doses of medication for the shortest possible period of time.

Hypertension is a frequent complication of renal disease and steroid therapy and may require aggressive use of antihypertensive agents. End-stage renal disease may be managed with dialysis or transplantation. Children with CNS lupus and seizures require antiseizure medications in addition to the therapy for the lupus itself.

*Prognosis.* The outlook for long-term survival has improved in childhood lupus; most centers,

TABLE 9–8.   Additional Manifestations of Systemic Lupus Erythematosus

| | |
|---|---|
| **Systemic** | **Gastrointestinal** |
| Fever | Pancreatitis |
| Malaise | Mesenteric arteritis |
| Weight loss | Serositis |
| Fatigue | Hepatomegaly |
| | Hepatitis (chronic-lupoid) |
| **Musculoskeletal** | Splenomegaly |
| Myositis, myalgia | |
| Arthralgia | **Renal** |
| | Nephritis |
| **Cutaneous** | Nephrosis |
| Raynaud phenomenon | Uremia |
| Alopecia | Hypertension |
| Urticaria–angioedema | |
| Panniculitis | **Reproduction** |
| Livedo reticularis | Infertility |
| | Repeat abortions |
| **Neuropsychiatric** | Neonatal lupus |
| Personality disorders | Congenital heart block |
| Stroke | |
| Peripheral neuropathy | **Hematologic** |
| Chorea | Anticoagulants (factors |
| Transverse myelitis | VIII, IX, XII, others |
| Migraine headaches | causing hemorrhage) |
| Depression | Antiphospholipid |
| | antibodies (lupus |
| **Cardiopulmonary** | anticoagulant causing |
| Endocarditis | thrombosis) |
| Myocarditis | |
| Pneumonitis | **Endocrine** |
| | Hypothyroidism |
| **Ocular** | Hyperthyroidism |
| Episcleritis | |
| Sicca syndrome | **Treatment-Induced** |
| Retinal cytoid bodies | Steroid toxicity |
| | Immunosuppression |
| | Opportunistic infections |

using a variety of treatment regimens, report a better than 85% 5-yr survival rate. With earlier diagnosis and treatment, renal failure is less commonly a cause of death, but secondary infection with opportunistic organisms has become a leading cause of mortality. Cerebritis, vasculitis, and acute nephritis are less common causes of mortality.

As with any child with chronic disease, psychologic support is crucial to the long-term well-being of the patient with lupus.

### References

Behrman RE, Kliegman RM, Arvin AM (eds): Nelson Textbook of Pediatrics, 15th ed. Philadelphia, WB Saunders, 1996, Chapter 146.
Lehman T: A practical guide to systemic lupus erythematosus. Pediatr Clin North Am 42:1223, 1995.
McCurdy D, Lehman T, Bernstein B, et al: Lupus nephritis: Prognostic factors in children. Pediatrics 89:240, 1992.

## NEONATAL LUPUS SYNDROME

See Chapter 6.

## DERMATOMYOSITIS

Dermatomyositis is an inflammatory disease with characteristic skin changes and striated muscle involvement manifesting as proximal muscle weakness. Gastrointestinal involvement occurs in some patients, and there may be an underlying vasculopathy. The illness is more common in females and tends to peak in the 8–12 yr age range, although disease is seen from infancy to adulthood.

*Clinical Manifestations.* The clinical syndrome is associated with a characteristic rash, symmetric proximal muscle weakness, elevated muscle enzymes, an abnormal electromyogram, and a muscle biopsy that shows loss of muscle fibrils commensurate with damage to the blood supply of the affected muscle. The typical pattern of onset is insidious and, when the patient finally comes to medical attention, the history is one of very slowly diminishing capabilities, unnoticed by parents and teachers alike, until there is some major motor dysfunction (i.e., the child may no longer be able to climb stairs, step onto the school bus, comb his or her own hair, or get up out of a chair). In retrospect, the child may have had malaise or worsening endurance, but usually there have been no specific complaints. The fatigue and nonspecific complaints may have caused the parents to seek medical attention; it is usual for the child to have been seen by numerous physicians before a diagnosis is made.

The rash is said to be pathognomonic, but similar rashes occur in other disease entities. However, the rash is exceedingly characteristic and often overlooked. A "heliotrope" rash of purplish discoloration is present over the upper eyelids and is associated with periorbital edema and redness in the malar region. *Gottron papules* are areas of erythema, atrophy and/or hyperkeratosis over the metacarpophalangeal and proximal interphalangeal joints, without associated arthritis. Very commonly an associated nonspecific papular eruption covers the elbows and knees and, on occasion, occurs in the sun-exposed V-area of the neck as well. Telangiectasias of the nail fold capillaries may occur. A magnification aid, such as use of the ophthalmoscope, helps in visualization. Calcifications over pressure points (knee, elbow) or in soft tissue may occur later in the course of the illness. If the characteristic rash is present, only three of the other four criteria are necessary for diagnosis (Table 9–9).

Rarely, children may exhibit fulminant dermatomyositis/polymyositis with an acute course of proximal muscle weakness, often with dysphagia and/or respiratory muscle compromise. The rash may not be appreciated at onset and its course may be rapid enough to necessitate intensive care support. Cardiac involvement (conduction abnormalities, myopericarditis) may be present but is uncommon. A history of regurgitating liquids through the nose and laboratory evidence of markedly diminished vital capacity require that such a child be placed immediately in an intensive care facility. The status of palatal function and voluntary respiratory muscle function (spirometry) needs to be followed. Proximal muscle weakness also should be monitored and scored according to loss of function (Table 9–10). Hip, shoulder, neck flexor, and abdominal muscle weakness are common.

Involvement of the gastrointestinal tract with vasculopathy may result in massive gastrointestinal bleeding or intestinal perforation. Pulmonary involvement may be secondary to muscle weak-

**TABLE 9–9.** Dermatomyositis: Criteria for Diagnosis

Rash typical of dermatomyositis
Symmetric proximal muscle weakness
Elevated muscle enzymes (SGOT, SGPT, LDH, CPK, aldolase)
EMG abnormalities typical of dermatomyositis (fasciculations, needle insertion irritability, high frequency discharges)
Positive muscle biopsy with chronic inflammation

CPK = creatine phosphokinase; LDH = lactic dehydrogenase; EMG = electromyographic; SGOT = serum glutamic oxaloacetic transaminase; SGPT = serum glutamic pyruvic transaminase.

TABLE 9–10.  Scoring System for Muscle Weakness

| Score | Function |
|---|---|
| 0 | No movement or contraction |
| 1 | Contraction without extremity movement |
| 2 | No movement against gravity |
| 3 | Movement only against gravity |
| 4 | Movement against examiner resistance |
| 5 | Normal movement and strength |

ness, interstitial pneumonitis, or the development of fibrosing alveolitis.

The *differential diagnosis* includes relatively uncommon disorders, such as trichinosis, tropical pyomyositis, hypereosinophilic syndromes, steroid myopathy, metabolic myopathies, SLE, overlap syndrome, emetine abuse, azidothymidine, and hyperthyroidism or hypothyroidism. Chronic myositis also may be due to persistent coxsackievirus infection. Acute viral (enterovirus, influenza) myositis is common and associated with rhabdomyolysis, myoglobinuria, elevated creatine phosphokinase, and tender muscles.

*Treatment.* Most pediatric rheumatologists recommend 2 mg/kg of prednisone equivalent per day as initial therapy unless the child is so severely affected that intravenous pulse steroids are indicated. Usually, a child responds within weeks with improved muscle function and markedly decreased muscle enzymes; the steroid dose then can be tapered slowly over the course of months. Most children do not tolerate alternate-day steroids until they are well into their recovery. The natural history of the active disease spans approximately 2–3 yr, so most physicians plan a treatment regimen that involves at least alternate-day low-dose steroids for a total duration of 2 yr.

*Prognosis.* Before the advent of steroids, one third of children died in the acute phase of illness, one third were severely compromised by disease, and one third recovered. Currently, the mortality rate from dermatomyositis is significantly less than 10%. Most children totally recover after their disease has run its course. Some children have a remitting and exacerbating course, and a few unfortunate children have severe and unremitting disease, which may require them to receive immunosuppression with drugs such as methotrexate.

A complication of dermatomyositis is **calcinosis,** which occurs in patients with a prolonged disease course (at least 1 yr in duration) and, therefore, is not seen in patients during the acute onset of disease. The calcium deposition may be minimal, sporadic, and unimportant or may be severe enough to significantly retard movement in all joints, thus resulting in a major disability. No effective treatment exists for the calcinosis of dermatomyositis; it may remit spontaneously or progress unremittingly and produce severe debilitation.

### References

Behrman RE, Kliegman RM, Arvin AM (eds): Nelson Textbook of Pediatrics, 15th ed. Philadelphia, WB Saunders, 1996, Chapter 153.
Pachman LM: Juvenile dermatomyositis. Pediatr Clin North Am 42:1071, 1995.

## SCLERODERMA

In childhood, scleroderma (hardening of the skin) is a very rare condition that can be subdivided into localized and general disease entities. Girls are affected more than boys.

*Clinical Manifestations.* *Localized* scleroderma is the most frequent type of scleroderma in childhood and may appear as morphea or patch-like scleroderma on the trunk or as linear scleroderma that involves an extremity. The initial lesion may be inflammatory, exhibiting purplish discoloration and raised borders, some heat, and mild pain. Very rapidly progressing scleroderma lesions evolve into areas with hypopigmentation and atrophy. Even localized scleroderma can be a "full-thickness" entity in which not only skin and subcutaneous tissue but also muscle, supporting structures, and even bone are involved; in linear scleroderma this extensive involvement can lead to marked contractures and undergrowth of limbs, resulting in disability. When linear scleroderma involves the scalp, extension to underlying structures can produce seizures, hypoplasia of the face, and severe cosmetic problems. Skin softening may occur. The lesions of morphea are particularly likely to regress.

Localized scleroderma is differentiated from **progressive systemic sclerosis** (PSS), which involves organ systems that include the kidneys, resulting in severe hypertension and renal failure; the gastrointestinal tract, leading to esophageal and intestinal motility problems; the lungs, causing restrictive disease and pulmonary hypertension; and the joints, resulting in arthritis.

Progressive systemic sclerosis is extremely uncommon in childhood. **Raynaud phenomenon** is frequent and may be one of the first manifestations of the disease. The skin may initially be edematous and then becomes sclerotic; the hard, tightened skin is bound to subcutaneous structures. Digital involvement is common and may result in flexion contractures. Bone in the distal phalangeal tuft often disintegrates, resulting in tapering of the ends of the fingers, termed "sclerodactyly." Calcinosis is relatively common in patients with PSS. Skin involvement proximal to the metacarpophalangeal or metatarsophalangeal joints is an important feature of PSS. Antibodies to Sc1-70 may be seen.

The **CREST syndrome** represents a more benign pattern of illness that includes *c*alcinosis, *R*aynaud phenomenon, *e*sophageal hypomotility, *s*clerodactyly, and *t*elangiectasia. *Raynaud phenomenon,* which may precede scleroderma for as many as 10 yr, is characterized by intense pallor (vasoconstriction) followed by cyanosis (partial recirculation) and then by marked erythema (recirculation of blood) of the fingers in response to cold or stress. Anti-centromere antibodies may be seen.

*Scleroderma-like conditions* may occur secondary to drugs (bleomycin), toxins (polyvinyl chloride), and chronic graft-versus-host disease following bone marrow transplantation.

*Differential Diagnosis.* The differential diagnosis includes idiopathic Raynaud disease (rather than phenomenon), toxin exposure (toxic oil, vinyl chloride), carcinoid syndrome, hereditary telangiectasia, porphyria, lichen sclerosis et atrophicus, idiopathic pulmonary hypertension, and mixed connective tissue disease (MCTD). MCTD is an overlap syndrome with manifestations of arthritis, SLE, scleroderma, and myositis. Antibodies to extractable nuclear antigen and ribonucleoprotein are elevated in MCTD.

*Laboratory Findings.* There is no pathognomonic test for scleroderma, although the presence of ANAs, anti-centromere antibodies, and anti-Sc1-70 antibodies are common. Capillaroscopy may reveal nail fold capillary changes, such as enlarged capillary loops, disruption or loss of capillaries, tortuosity, and pseudoglomerular (bushy) capillaries. Vital capacity and carbon monoxide diffusion capacity are useful tests to evaluate pulmonary interstitial fibrosis and pulmonary endothelial damage, respectively.

*Treatment.* The treatment of localized scleroderma is not firmly established. Corticosteroids, D-penicillamine, and hydroxychloroquine have been utilized. Physical therapy is important if joint contractures have occurred.

The treatment of progressive systemic sclerosis or CREST syndrome is directed to the particular problems the patient is experiencing. Proton pump inhibitors have been useful for gastroesophageal reflux occurring in adults. Hypertension is treated with angiotensin-converting enzyme inhibitors.

Raynaud phenomenon is best treated by preventative measures, such as cold avoidance. Calcium channel blockers, such as nifedipine, may be of benefit. Biofeedback also may be of benefit.

## EOSINOPHILIC FASCIITIS

Eosinophilic fasciitis is a rare condition that resembles scleroderma. It may affect young adult and adolescent patients who may have engaged in strenuous physical activity and whose involved muscles subsequently have become swollen and edematous; these patients also exhibit marked skin changes characterized by an "orange peel" appearance without Raynaud phenomenon. Flexion contractures of the extremity are seen commonly and occur without active synovitis. Biopsy reveals evidence of eosinophilic infiltration into the fascia, peripheral eosinophilia, and an elevated ESR.

Therapeutic response to steroids usually is excellent, although the long-term outlook for children with eosinophilic fasciitis is unknown. Physical therapy may be used to avoid and treat contractures.

### References

Behrman RE, Kliegman RM, Arvin AM (eds): Nelson Textbook of Pediatrics, 15th ed. Philadelphia, WB Saunders, 1996, Chapter 154.
Uziel Y, Miller M, Laxer R: Sclerodermia in childhood. Pediatr Clin North Am 42:1171, 1995.

# VASCULITIS

## HENOCH-SCHÖNLEIN PURPURA

Henoch-Schönlein purpura is the most common vasculitis of childhood and is characterized by palpable nonthrombocytopenic purpura: periarticular, scrotal, and scalp swelling, edema, and inflammation; gastrointestinal bleeding (with or without intussusception); and nephritis (see Table 9–4). The cutaneous manifestations are striking, with circular purpuric lesions 2–3 cm in size typically occurring over the buttocks and the posterior surfaces of the arms and legs. Skin lesions and the renal glomeruli may contain IgA immune complexes.

*Clinical Manifestations.* The onset of the illness often follows a nonspecific upper respiratory tract infection in a 4–10 yr old child. The skin lesions are the hallmark of the disease, but cramping, intermittent abdominal pain, hematochezia, periarticular swelling, and tense scalp or scrotal edema may be present. Glomerulonephritis may occur within 1–2 months of onset and becomes manifest as asymptomatic hematuria, with or without proteinuria. Fewer than 5% of patients have acute renal insufficiency, and another 5% have a slow progression, with renal failure developing months to years later. Initial manifestations of nephritis, nephrotic syndrome, or nephritic nephrosis increase the long-term risks of hypertension, renal impairment, or pre-eclampsia. Encephalopathy and pulmonary hemorrhage are rare manifestations of Henoch-Schönlein purpura. Most patients recover without therapy, but a small percentage relapse and another small group has a much slower rate of recovery accompanied by the persistence of hematuria for 1–2 yr.

*Treatment.* Therapy is symptomatic because 90% of patients have a self-limited illness. Corticosteroids may relieve abdominal pain and joint, scalp, or scrotal edema, but this has not been proved in controlled studies. Steroids do not have a beneficial effect on established renal disease. Renal transplantation may be needed for the few patients with irreversible renal insufficiency; in some patients who have received a transplant, Henoch-Schönlein purpura has recurred in the transplanted kidney.

### References

Behrman RE, Kliegman RM, Arvin AM (eds): Nelson Textbook of Pediatrics, 15th ed. Philadelphia, WB Saunders, 1996, Chapter 152.1.

Goldstein A, White R, Akuse R, et al: Long-term follow-up of childhood Henoch-Schönlein nephritis. Lancet 339:280, 1992.

Mills J, Michel B, Bloch D, et al: The American College of Rheumatology 1990 criteria for the classification of Henoch-Schönlein purpura. Arthritis Rheum 33:1114, 1990.

### KAWASAKI DISEASE

Kawasaki disease, first described in Japan, now has been found throughout the world. There is a marked predilection for children of Japanese ancestry. It occurs in childhood, mostly in very young children, particularly under the age of 5 yr. The

**TABLE 9–11.** Kawasaki Disease: Criteria for Diagnosis

Fever persisting for 5 days or more

Changes of peripheral extremities
  Initial stage: reddening of palms and soles, indurative edema
  Convalescent stage: membranous desquamation from fingertips

Polymorphous exanthem

Bilateral conjunctival congestion

Changes of lips and oral cavity: reddening of lips, strawberry tongue, diffuse injection of oral and pharyngeal mucosa

Acute nonpurulent cervical lymphadenopathy (>1.5 cm in diameter)

**TABLE 9–12.** Complications of Kawasaki Disease

| | |
|---|---|
| Coronary artery aneurysms | Arthritis |
| Coronary artery thrombosis | Sterile pyuria (urethritis) |
| Myocardial infarction | Thombocytosis (late) |
| Myopericarditis | Peripheral artery aneurysm |
| Congestive heart failure | Diarrhea |
| Hydrops of gallbladder | Pancreatitis |
| Aseptic meningitis | Peripheral gangrene |
| Irritability | |

etiology is unknown, although many believe it is viral or toxin-mediated in origin.

*Clinical Manifestations.* This illness is primarily a multisystem vasculitis; a significant number of untreated children (20–25%) have coronary artery aneurysms as sequelae to the disease. Criteria for diagnosing Kawasaki disease are listed in Table 9–11; five of the six criteria are required to make a diagnosis, though incomplete forms of the disease are recognized. Other disease manifestations are noted in Table 9–12. In addition, other disease processes must be excluded (Table 9–13).

The disease can be subdivided into three stages. The *acute phase* lasts about 10 days, during which most of the diagnostic criteria are likely to be present. The children have high fever, conjunctivitis, changes in oral mucous membranes, extremity changes (puffiness of hands and feet and redness of palms and soles), and rash. A desquamating perineal rash may be present. Cervical lymphadenopathy is less frequent. Irritability is profound in children with Kawasaki disease, and aseptic meningitis frequently is found. Myocarditis and pericarditis may occur.

The *subacute phase* (from days 11 through 21) usually is associated with a decrease in fever. Arthritis occurs in many children at this time, although in a few children arthritis had already appeared in the acute phase of the disease. A

**TABLE 9–13.** Differential Diagnosis of Kawasaki Disease

Scarlet fever
Staphylococcal toxic shock syndrome
Stevens-Johnson syndrome (erythema multiforme)
Leptospirosis
Epstein-Barr virus
Juvenile rheumatoid arthritis (systemic-onset)
Measles
Acrodynia
Polyarteritis nodosa
Rocky Mountain spotted fever
Drug reaction
Scalded skin syndrome

dramatic skin desquamation occurs in virtually all children beginning on about day 14; usually this desquamation begins at the junction of the nail and the fingertip, is very thick in nature, and is not painful. It is most common on the hands and feet but may occur in other regions.

The third phase, the *convalescent phase*, begins about day 21. During this phase, coronary artery aneurysms are often detected by echocardiogram. Arthritis and thrombocytosis may persist, but generally the acute-phase reactants subside. Myocardial infarctions and rupture of aneurysms may occur in either the subacute or convalescent phases.

**Treatment.** High doses of aspirin generally are used in the acute phase (100 mg/kg/24 hr) and shorten the duration of fever; as the child improves, low doses of aspirin generally are employed for their effect in preventing platelet aggregation. Low-dose aspirin therapy (3–5 mg/kg/24 hr) generally is continued until both the thrombocytosis and the other acute-phase reactants have returned to normal (i.e., end of convalescent phase), provided coronary artery changes have not occurred, in which case it is continued. Intravenous immunoglobulin therapy (2 g/kg for 1 dose) during the acute phase reduces coronary aneurysm formation.

When Kawasaki disease was first described, the death rate was about 3%; this rate has dramatically decreased over the last 20 yr.

### References

Behrman RE, Kliegman RM, Arvin AM (eds): Nelson Textbook of Pediatrics, 15th ed. Philadelphia, WB Saunders, 1996, Chapter 152.2.
Burns J, Mason W, Glode M, et al: Clinical and epidemiologic characteristics of patients referred for evaluation of possible Kawasaki disease. J Pediatr 118:680, 1991.
Shulman ST, De Inocencio J, Hirsh R: Kawasaki disease. Pediatr Clin North Am 42:1205, 1995.

## POLYARTERITIS NODOSA

Polyarteritis nodosa (PAN) is an uncommon form of vasculitis characterized by inflammation of small and medium-sized arteries. Systemic features include weight loss, malaise, and anorexia. Multisystem organ involvement can occur and most commonly includes joint, muscle, kidney, peripheral nerve, and skin. Cutaneous nodules may be seen; a biopsy may help establish the *diagnosis*. Livedo reticularis and peripheral gangrene may occur. Other major organs may also be involved.

The etiology is not known; it may be associated with hepatitis B infection in adults and streptococcal infections in childhood. The outlook in the systemic form of the disease is guarded.

*Treatment* includes corticosteroids and cytotoxic agents. Patients with a more limited form, known as **cutaneous PAN**, may have a better outlook and require less aggressive treatment.

### References

Behrman RE, Kliegman RM, Arvin AM (eds): Nelson Textbook of Pediatrics, 15th ed. Philadelphia, WB Saunders, 1996, Chapter 152.3.
Sheth AP, Olson JC, Esterly NB: Cutaneous polyarteritis nodosa of childhood. J Am Acad Dermatol 31:561–566, 1994.

## WEGENER GRANULOMATOSIS

Wegener granulomatosis is an uncommon vasculitis in childhood (see Table 9–4). The disease may resemble Henoch-Schönlein purpura, exhibiting renal, skin, joint, and gastrointestinal involvement, or it may resemble an adult-type vasculitis, with lung, renal, sinus or nasopharynx, eye, and joint disease. Necrotizing midline upper respiratory tract granulomas (sinus, subglottic stenosis, nose, otitis) accompanied by renal vasculitis and pulmonary lesions (cavitary or nodular infiltrates) are typical in both age groups. Sinus disease is an early manifestation, demonstrating inflammation of the paranasal sinuses and, rarely, nasal septum perforation. Secondary infection may produce pyogenic sinusitis. Renal involvement may occur late and becomes manifest by hematuria, proteinuria, renal failure, and hypertension. Other manifestations include rash, arthralgia, peripheral neuropathy, and dacryocystitis.

Wegener granulomatosis can be differentiated from Henoch-Schönlein purpura by the presence of lung involvement, absence of IgA immune complexes in dermal capillaries, and presence of antineutrophil cytoplasmic antibodies and granulomas.

Without treatment, the prognosis is poor. Treatment with both cyclophosphamide and corticosteroids has resulted in improved prognosis.

### References

Behrman RE, Kliegman RM, Arvin AM (eds): Nelson Textbook of Pediatrics, 15th ed. Philadelphia, WB Saunders, 1996, Chapter 152.3.
Rottem M, Fauci A, Hallahan C, et al: Wegener granulomatosis in children and adolescents: Clinical presentation and outcome. J Pediatr 122:26, 1991.

## ACUTE RHEUMATIC FEVER

See Chapter 13.

## PAIN SYNDROMES IN CHILDHOOD

### RECURRENT LIMB PAIN

Many children, most frequently between ages 5 and 12 yr, complain of recurrent evening or night-time limb pains. These pains usually are intermittent and occur around and behind the knee, in the calves and thigh areas, and sometimes in the shins; occasionally upper extremity pain occurs. Typically, the pain occurs at the end of a day of strenuous activity and is resolved totally by the following morning. There is no associated limp, but the pain may interfere with normal sleep. Historically, these are likely to represent what people have called "growing pains."

Growth and development are normal, as is the physical examination. No associated effusions, limitations of joint motion, features of hypermobility syndrome, or "trigger points" are present. Systemic signs are absent and roentgenograms and laboratory studies are normal.

Treatment consists of reassurance and comfort measures, such as local heat and rubbing the limb. Stretching exercise for the Achilles tendons and hamstrings may be beneficial. Pain medication, such as acetaminophen, may be helpful. Recurrent limb pains may be episodic and may reappear over the course of months or years. Ultimately, the child outgrows the propensity for having these pains.

### FIBROMYALGIA

Fibromyalgia is a benign, intermittent, noninflammatory musculoskeletal pain syndrome seen in children as well as in adults; it is more common in females (5:1) and tends to occur much more often in adolescents than in younger children. There is arthralgia but no synovitis. A number of characteristically tender trigger points exist: those on the anterior chest (costochondral); on the inner aspect of the scapula medially (supraspinatus muscle); around the knee but beyond the joint margin; over the greater trochanters; and near the gluteus medius, low cervical spine (C5–C7), and low lumbar ligaments (L4–S1). Many patients relate their symptoms to changes in the weather, and some often experience an associated depression, morning stiffness, and a disturbance in sleep pattern. Many of these children miss an extraordinary amount of school. Some children may improve over time.

Associated nonrheumatic illnesses include headache, irritable bowel syndrome, major depression, and panic disorder.

The *treatment* of fibromyalgia includes education that it is not a crippling, deforming disease. NSAIDs may have an analgesic effect, but most controlled studies have not found them to be more effective than placebo. Amitriptyline and cyclobenzaprine have been more effective than placebo in adults. Controlled studies in adults have shown benefit from cardiovascular fitness training, electromyography–biofeedback, electroacupuncture, and hypnotherapy. Cognitive-behavioral interventions have been successful in some children.

### REFLEX SYMPATHETIC DYSTROPHY

Chronic, unilateral extremity pain may be due to reflex sympathetic dystrophy, which is character-

FIGURE 9–1. Features of hypermobility in children. *1*, Hyperextension of fingers. *2*, Apposition of thumbs. *3*, Hyperextension of elbows. *4*, Hyperextension of knees. *5*, Flexion of trunk. (From Gedalia A, Brewer EJ: Joint hypermobility in pediatric practice: A review. J Rheumatol 20:372, 1993.)

ized by local burning pain, hyperalgesia, allodynia (pain from usually nonpainful stimuli, such as light touch), cyanosis, sweating, mottling, coldness, excessive hair growth, swelling, and, if not treated, contractures, demineralization, and atrophy. A prior history of mild-moderate trauma may be present.

## BENIGN HYPERMOBILITY SYNDROME

Benign hypermobility syndrome is diagnosed in children with excessive joint mobility in the absence of a congenital disease of connective tissue, such as **Ehlers-Danlos syndrome** or **Marfan syndrome**. It likely represents a variation in normal joint range of motion. Children who meet three or more criteria (Fig. 9–1) are said to be hypermobile. Some children with joint hypermobility experience episodic arthralgia. It is generally thought that symptoms improve with maturation.

### References

Abu-Arafeh I, Russell G: Recurrent limb pain in schoolchildren. Arch Dis Child 74:336, 1996.

Behrman RE, Kliegman RM, Arvin AM (eds): Nelson Textbook of Pediatrics, 15th ed. Philadelphia, WB Saunders, 1996, Chapter 157.

Buskila D, Neumann L, Hershman E, et al: Fibromyalgia syndrome in children: An outcome study. J Rheumatol 22:525, 1995.

Gedalia A, Brewer EJ: Joint hypermobility in pediatric practice: A review. J Rheumatol 20:371, 1993.

Wilder R, Berde C, Wolohan M, et al: Reflex sympathetic dystrophy in children. J Bone Joint Surg 74A:910, 1992.

## SARCOIDOSIS

Sarcoidosis is a chronic disease of unknown cause. Multisystem ($\geq 5$) involvement is common. In pediatrics, the peak age is during adolescence, but it has occurred in children as young as 2 mo of age. The presentation varies by age, with children 4 yr or younger presenting with skin lesions, arthritis, and uveitis. This presentation may mimic JRA. Older children experience a disease presentation similar to that in adults with lung, lymph node, and eye involvement. Sarcoidosis is more common in blacks.

The *clinical manifestations* include weight loss, cough, fatigue, bone or joint pain, lymphadenopathy, dyspnea, parotid enlargement, fever, uveitis, nodules, maculopapular rash or erythema nodosum, and hepatosplenomegaly. Hilar adenopathy with pulmonary nodules or interstitial infiltrates also is common.

*Laboratory findings* are not specific, but hypercalcemia, polyclonal gammopathy, and elevated angiotensin-converting enzyme are common. Slit-lamp examination reveals granulomatous anterior uveitis, and tissue biopsy demonstrates noncaseating granulomas. Pulmonary function tests may show a restrictive pattern, and gallium scanning demonstrates increased pulmonary uptake. Renal disease becomes manifest as hematuria and proteinuria. Cutaneous anergy is common.

*Treatment* includes corticosteroids. The *prognosis* is fair to good; only 40–50% of patients remain symptomatic for 5 yr after therapy.

### References

Behrman RE, Kliegman RM, Arvin AM (eds): Nelson Textbook of Pediatrics, 15th ed. Philadelphia, WB Saunders, 1996, Chapter 658.

Hafner R, Vogel P: Sarcoidosis of early onset: A challenge for the pediatric rheumatologist. Clin Exp Rheumatol 11:685–691, 1993.

# Chapter 10

# INFECTIOUS DISEASES

Alice Prince

## BASIC PRINCIPLES OF PEDIATRIC INFECTIOUS DISEASES

### EPIDEMIOLOGY

The ability to diagnose and appropriately treat specific childhood infections depends on an understanding of the epidemiology and risk factors associated with each infectious agent as well as the population at risk for certain pathogens. Susceptibility to specific infectious agents is a direct consequence of the maturity of the immune system, exposure to potential infectious agents, and the presence of underlying diseases. The host response varies with age. Thus, neonates prior to the development of their own immunologic repertoire are at risk for different types of infections than school-aged children or adolescents. Clinical consequences of an excessive immune response may be more deleterious than the damage directly attributed to the pathogen. To approach the diverse types of infections seen in pediatrics, the clinician must consider the following questions:

1. Who gets a specific disease?
2. Does this occur in a normal host, an immunocompromised patient, or a child with a specific immunologic defect?
3. What organisms are involved?
4. Is the presentation one of a benign viral illness or more suggestive of bacterial infection?
5. How can the etiologic agent be identified?
6. What antimicrobial agents are available for treatment?
7. What can be done to prevent this disease?
8. What is the nature of the host immune response?

The likelihood of many infections can be esti-

mated by historic factors and host evaluation. Sociologic factors are important; for infants the adequacy of prenatal care, gestational age, maternal risk-taking behavior, and appropriate screening tests for congenital infection are helpful clues. The immunization history and living conditions, including exposure to infected adults or to other infants in a closed setting such as day care or an informal baby-sitting arrangement, may be factors in the transmission of common infections. Other environmental factors, such as travel, exposure to air conditioners, the season, construction sites, insects, and animals or exotic pets may help the clinician assess the possibility of specific etiologic agents.

A careful and complete physical examination is critical to the diagnosis of many infectious diseases. Although initial complaints, particularly in infants, may be nonspecific (irritability, poor feeding, or lethargy), certain physical findings, such as specific rashes, may be diagnostic. Particular care should be given to identifying the sites of infection (Table 10–1). Knowledge of these common sites permits identification of the infecting organism and guides appropriate treatment. Rashes are a common manifestation of infections; appropriate classification of the rash morphology can be diagnostic for many infections (Table 10–2).

### PREVENTION

The prevention of many previously fatal childhood diseases has been a triumph of pediatrics and has been accomplished through the use of routine vaccination (Fig. 10–1 and Table 10–3). Vaccines may be live attenuated viruses (measles, mumps, rubella, varicella, polio) or may consist of inactivated

TABLE 10–1.   Localizing Manifestations of Infection

| Site | Symptoms | Signs |
| --- | --- | --- |
| Upper respiratory | Rhinorrhea, sneezing, cough, sore throat, drooling, stridor, trismus, sinus pain, fever, ear pain or drainage, tooth pain | Nasal congestion; pharyngeal erythema; enlarged tonsils with exudate; swollen, red epiglottis; red, bulging tympanic membrane; regional lymphadenopathy |
| Lower respiratory | Cough, fever, chest pain, dyspnea; sputum production | Rales, wheezing, localized diminished breath sounds, intercostal retractions, tachypnea |
| Gastrointestinal | Vomiting, diarrhea, abdominal pain, anorexia, fever | Hyperactive bowel sounds, abdominal tenderness, hematochezia |
| Hepatic | Anorexia, vomiting; dark urine, light stools | Jaundice, hepatomegaly, hepatic tenderness, hemorrhage, coma |
| Genitourinary | Dysuria, frequency, urgency, fever, flank or suprapubic pain, vaginal discharge | Costovertebral angle or suprapubic tenderness, cervical motion and adnexal tenderness |
| Skeletal | Limp, bone pain, fever, pseudoparalysis | Local swelling, erythema, warmth, limited range of motion, tenderness |
| Central nervous system | Fever, lethargy, irritability, headache, neck stiffness, seizures | Kernig or Brudzinski sign, bulging fontanel, focal neurologic deficits |
| Cardiovascular | Dyspnea, palpitations, exercise intolerance, chest pain, fever, shock | Tachycardia, hypotension, cardiomegaly, hepatomegaly, splenomegaly, rales, petechiae, Osler nodes, Janeway lesions, new murmur, distended neck veins, pericardial friction rub, muffled heart tones |

immunogenic components of either viruses or bacteria (polio, hepatitis B, pertussis, influenza, diphtheria, tetanus, *Haemophilus influenzae* type b, pneumococcus). Vaccine efficacy is dependent on the age of the child, the immune status, appropriate administration, and booster immunizations.

In addition to those vaccines recommended for all children, various high-risk situations (e.g., repeated exposure to a pathogen, altered cardiopulmonary status, or increased susceptibility to various bacteria) warrant additional vaccinations (Table 10–4). When there are no specific effective vaccines and the patient is at increased risk for the infectious disease owing to repeated exposure or to increased host susceptibility, antimicrobial prophylaxis is administered for as long as the patient remains at risk (Table 10–5).

## CLINICAL USE OF THE MICROBIOLOGY LABORATORY

Laboratory diagnosis of infection involves a variety of techniques, ranging from the simple microscopic examination of bacterial morphology using the Gram stain to the more technical molecular microbiologic methods, such as the polymerase chain reaction (PCR). Current practices include:

1. Routine culture methods for isolation of specific pathogens from infected sites.

2. Antigen detection utilizing either latex agglutination or fluorescent antibody.
3. Detection of genomic deoxyribonucleic acid (DNA) or ribonucleic acid (RNA) sequences of pathogens using complementary probes and PCR.
4. Demonstration of an antibody response to an infection by serologic testing and/or Western hybridization technique.
5. Tissue culture to identify viruses and intracellular pathogens.

The laboratory also can provide critical information to optimize therapy and avoid toxicity, such as antimicrobial susceptibility testing, mean inhibitory (MIC) or bactericidal (MBC) concentrations of antimicrobial agents, or peak and trough drug levels.

## FEVER

Healthy individuals maintain their core body temperatures within 1 to 1.5°C (37°–38°C). Normal body temperature is considered to be 98.6°F (37°C, range from 97° to 99.6°F). Most individuals have a diurnal variation, with maximal levels achieved in the late afternoon. The normal body temperature is maintained by the anterior hypothalamus utilizing a complex regulatory system. Rectal temperatures greater than 38°C (100.4°F) generally are considered abnormal.

TABLE 10–2.  Differential Diagnosis of Fever and Rash

| Lesion | Pathogen or Associated Factor |
| --- | --- |
| *Maculopapular or Macular Rash* | *Viruses*<br>    Measles, rubella, roseola (human herpesvirus-6 or -7), fifth disease (parvovirus), Epstein-Barr virus, enteroviruses, hepatitis B virus (papular acrodermatitis or Gianotti-Crosti syndrome), human immunodeficiency virus<br>*Bacteria*<br>    Rheumatic fever (group A streptococcus), scarlet fever, erysipelas, *Arcanobacterium haemolyticum*, secondary syphilis, leptospirosis, *Pseudomonas,* meningococcal infection (early), *Salmonella,* Lyme disease<br>*Rickettsia*<br>    Early Rocky Mountain spotted fever, typhus (scrub, endemic), ehrlichiosis<br>*Other*<br>    Kawasaki disease, rheumatoid arthritis, drug reaction |
| *Diffuse Erythroderma* | *Bacteria*<br>    Scarlet fever (group A streptococcus), toxic shock syndrome (*Staphylococcus aureus*)<br>*Fungi*<br>    *Candida albicans* |
| *Urticarial Rash* | *Viruses*<br>    Epstein-Barr virus, hepatitis B, human immunodeficiency virus<br>*Bacteria*<br>    *Mycoplasma pneumoniae,* group A streptococci<br>*Other*<br>    Drug reaction |
| *Vesicular, Bullous, Pustular* | *Viruses*<br>    Herpes simplex, varicella-zoster, coxsackievirus<br>*Bacteria*<br>    Staphylococcal scalded skin syndrome, staphylococcal bullous impetigo, group A streptococcal crusted impetigo<br>*Other*<br>    Toxic epidermal necrolysis, erythema multiforme (Stevens-Johnson syndrome), rickettsialpox |
| *Petechial-Purpuric* | *Viruses*<br>    Atypical measles, congenital rubella, cytomegalovirus, enterovirus, human immunodeficiency virus, hemorrhagic fever viruses<br>*Bacteria*<br>    Sepsis (meningococcal, gonococcal, pneumococcal, *Haemophilus influenzae*), endocarditis<br>*Rickettsiae*<br>    Rocky Mountain spotted fever, epidemic typhus, ehrlichiosis<br>*Other*<br>    Vasculitis, thrombocytopenia, Henoch-Schönlein purpura, malaria |
| *Erythema Nodosum* | *Viruses*<br>    Epstein-Barr, hepatitis B<br>*Bacteria*<br>    Group A streptococcus, tuberculosis, *Yersinia,* cat-scratch disease<br>*Fungi*<br>    Coccidioidomycosis, histoplasmosis<br>*Other*<br>    Sarcoidosis, inflammatory bowel disease, estrogen-containing oral contraceptives, systemic lupus erythematosus, Behçet disease |
| *Distinctive Rashes* |  |
|   Ecthyma gangrenosum | *Pseudomonas aeruginosa* |
|   Erythema chronicum migrans | Lyme disease |
|   Necrotic eschar | Aspergillosis, mucormycosis |
|   Erysipelas | Group A streptococcus |
|   Koplik spots | Measles |
|   Erythema marginatum | Rheumatic fever |

| Age ►<br>Vaccine ▼ | Birth | 1 mo | 2 mos | 4 mos | 6 mos | 12 mos | 15 mos | 18 mos | 4-6 yrs | 11-12 yrs | 14-16 yrs |
|---|---|---|---|---|---|---|---|---|---|---|---|
| Hepatitis B[2,3] | Hep B-1 | Hep B-2 | | | Hep B-3 | | | | | Hep B[3] | |
| Diphtheria, Tetanus | | | DTaP or DTP | DTaP or DTP | DTaP or DTP | | DTaP or DTP[4] | | DTaP or DTP | Td | |
| H. influenzae type b[5] | | | Hib | Hib | Hib[5] | Hib[6] | | | | | |
| Polio[6] | | | Polio[6] | Polio | | Polio[6] | | | Polio | | |
| Measles, Mumps, Rubella[7] | | | | | | MMR | | | MMR[7] | MMR[7] | |
| Varicella[8] | | | | | | Var | | | | Var[8] | |

Vaccines[1] are listed under the routinely recommended ages. Bars indicate range of acceptable ages for vaccination. Bars with heavy borders indicate catch-up vaccination: at 11–12 years of age, Hepatitis B vaccine should be administered to children not previously vaccinated, and Varicella virus vaccine should be administered to unvaccinated children who lack a reliable history of chickenpox.

[1]This schedule indicates the recommended age for routine administration of currently licensed childhood vaccines. Some combination vaccines are available and may be used whenever administration of all components of the vaccine is indicated. Providers should consult the manufacturers' package inserts for detailed recommendations.

[2]*Infants born to HBsAg-negative mothers* should receive 2.5 μg of Merck vaccine (Recombivax HB®) or 10 μg of SmithKline Beecham (SB) vaccine (Engerix-B®). The 2nd dose should be administered ≥1 mo after the 1st dose.

*Infants born to HBsAg-positive mothers* should receive 0.5 mL hepatitis B immune globulin (HBIG) within 12 hrs of birth, and either 5 μg of Merck vaccine (Recombivax HB®) or 10 μg of SB vaccine (Engerix-B®) at a separate site. The 2nd dose is recommended at 1–2 mos of age and the 3rd dose at 6 mos of age.

*Infants born to mothers whose HBsAg status is unknown* should receive either 5 μg of Merck vaccine (Recombivax HB®) or 10 μg of SB vaccine (Engerix-B®) within 12 hrs of birth. The 2nd dose of vaccine is recommended at 1 mo of age and the 3rd dose at 6 mos of age. Blood should be drawn at the time of delivery to determine the mother's HBsAg status; if it is positive, the infant should receive HBIG as soon as possible (no later than 1 wk of age). The dosage and timing of subsequent vaccine doses should be based upon the mother's HBsAg status.

[3]Children and adolescents who have not been vaccinated against hepatitis B in infancy may begin the series during any childhood visit. Those who have not previously received three doses of hepatitis B vaccine should initiate or complete the series during the 11–12 year-old visit. The 2nd dose should be administered at least 1 mo after the 1st dose, and the 3rd dose should be administered at least 4 mos after the 1st dose, and at least 2 mos after the 2nd dose.

[4]DTaP (diphtheria and tetanus toxoids and acellular pertussis vaccine) is the preferred vaccine for all doses in the vaccination series, including completion of the series in children who have received ≥1 of whole-cell DTP vaccine. Whole-cell DTP is an acceptable alternative to DTaP. The 4th dose of DTaP may be administered as early as 12 mos of age, provided 6 mos have elapsed since the 3rd dose, and if the child is considered unlikely to return at 15–18 mos of age. Td (tetanus and diphtheria toxoids, absorbed, for adult use) is recommended at 11–12 yrs of age if at least 5 yrs have elapsed since the last dose of DTP, DTaP, or DT. Subsequent routine Td boosters are recommended every 10 yrs.

[5]Three H. infuenazae type b (Hib) conjugate vaccines are licensed for infant use. If PRP-OMP (PedvaxHIB® [Merck]) is administered at 2 and 4 mo of age, a dose at 6 mo is not required. After completing the primary series, any Hib conjugate vaccine may be used as a booster.

[6]Two polio virus vaccines are currently licensed in the US: inactivated polio virus vaccine (IPV) and oral polio virus vaccine (OPV). The following schedules are all acceptable by the ACIP, the AAP, and the AAFP, and parents and providers may choose among them:
  1. IPV at 2 and 4 mos; OPV at 12–18 mos and 4–6 yr
  2. IPV at 2, 4, 12–18 mo, and 4–6 yr
  3. OPV at 2, 4, 6–18 mo, and 4–6 yr
The ACIP routinely recommends schedule 1. IPV is the only polio virus vaccine recommended for immunocompromised persons and their household contacts.

[7]The 2nd dose of MMR is routinely recommended at 4–6 yr of age or at 11–12 yr of age, but may be administered during any visit, provided at least 1 mo has elapsed since receipt of the 1st dose, and that both doses are administered at or after 12 mo of age.

[8]Susceptible children may receive Varicella vaccine (Var) during any visit after the 1st birthday, and unvaccinated persons who lack a reliable history of chickenpox should be vaccinated during the 11–12 year-old visit. Susceptible persons ≥13 yr of age should receive 2 doses, at least 1 mo apart.

Approved by the Advisory Committee on Immunization Practices (ACIP), American Academy of Pediatrics (AAP), and American Academy of Family Physicians (AAFP).

FIGURE 10–1. Recommended childhood immunization schedule, United States, January–December 1997. (Modified from Centers for Disease Control and Prevention, JAMA 227:203, 1997; Pediatrics 99:136, 1997; and MMWR 46:35, 1997.)

TABLE 10–3. Recommended Schedule of Vaccinations for Adolescents Ages 11–12 Years

| Immunobiologic | Indications | Name | Dose | Frequency | Route |
|---|---|---|---|---|---|
| Hepatitis A vaccine (inactivated virus) | Adolescents who are at increased risk of hepatitis A infection or its complications | HAVRIX®* | 720 EL.U.†/0.5 mL§ | A total of two doses at 0,¶ 6–12 mo | IM** |
| | | VAQTA®* | 25 U/0.5 mL | A total of two doses at 0, 6–18 mo | IM |
| Hepatitis B vaccine (recombinant antigen) | Adolescents not vaccinated previously for hepatitis B | Recombivax HB®* | 5 μg/0.5 mL | A total of three doses at 0, 1–2, 4–6 mo | IM |
| | | Engerix-B®* | 10 μg/0.5 mL | A total of three doses at 0, 1–2, 4–6 mo | IM |
| Influenza vaccine (inactivated virus) | Adolescents who are at increased risk for complications caused by influenza or who have contact with persons at increased risk for these complications‖ | Influenza virus vaccine†† | 0.5 mL | Annually (September–December) | IM |
| Measles, mumps, and rubella vaccine (MMR) (live virus) | Adolescents not vaccinated previously with two doses of measles vaccine at ≥12 mo of age | MMR II®* | 0.5 mL | One dose | SC§§ |
| Pneumococcal polysaccharide vaccine | Adolescents who are at increased risk for pneumococcal disease or its complications# | Pneumococcal vaccine polyvalent†† | 0.5 mL | One dose | IM or SC |
| Tetanus and diphtheria toxoids (Td) | Adolescents not vaccinated within the previous 5 yr | Tetanus and diphtheria toxoids, adsorbed (for adult use)†† | 0.5 mL | Every 10 yr | IM |
| Varicella virus vaccine (live virus) | Adolescents not vaccinated previously and who have no reliable history of chickenpox | VARIVAX®* | 0.5 mL | One dose¶¶ | SC |

Modified from Centers for Disease Control and Prevention, MMWR 46:35, 1997.
*Manufacturer's product name.
†Enzyme-linked immunosorbent assay (ELISA) unit.
§Alternative dosage and schedule of 360 EL.U./0.5 mL and a total of three doses administered at 0, 1, and 6–12 mo.
¶0 months represents timing of the initial dose, and subsequent numbers represent months after the initial dose.
‖At risk includes patients with chronic cardiorespiration diseases (cystic fibrosis, bronchopulmonary dysplasia); patients with sickle cell anemia, those receiving chronic salicylate therapy, or those with chronic immunosuppressed conditions.
#At risk includes patients with chronic pulmonary disease, sickle cell anemia, functional or anatomic asplenia, nephrotic syndrome, and cirrhosis.
**Intramuscular injection.
††Generic name.
§§Subcutaneous injection.
¶¶Adolescents ≥13 yr of age should be administered a total of two doses (0.5 mL/dose) subcutaneously at 0 and 4–8 wk.

TABLE 10–4.  Additional Special Vaccines

| Vaccine | Indication |
|---|---|
| Meningococcal (polysaccharide A/C/Y/W135) | Functional or anatomic asplenia, travel to an endemic area, patients with terminal complement deficiency; type B meningococcus not covered |
| Bacille Calmette-Guérin (BCG) (live attenuated *M. bovis* vaccine) | Tuberculin-negative infant in household with active disease; high tuberculosis incidence areas |
| Typhoid (live attenuated bacteria) | Oral vaccine for travel to or living in endemic areas. Exposure to *S. typhi* chronic carrier. Recommended for children >6 yr of age. |
| Rabies (human diploid cell vaccine) Pre-exposure | High-risk groups (e.g., veterinarians, animal handlers, and laboratory workers) |
| Postexposure | Must include human rabies immune globulin passive immunization, plus vaccine on days 1, 3, 7, 14, and 28, following high-risk animal bites: dog, raccoon, skunk, fox, cat, coyote, and bat |

TOPV = trivalent oral polio vaccine.

## PATHOGENESIS OF FEVER

All infections can produce fever, which begins with the release of endogenous pyrogens into the circulation after an infectious or immunologically mediated event. The endogenous pyrogens reach the anterior hypothalamus via the arterial blood supply, liberating arachidonic acid, which is metabolized to prostaglandin E$_2$ (PGE$_2$), resulting in an elevation of the hypothalamic thermostat. Antipyretics work by altering the synthesis of prostaglandins, reducing production of PGE$_2$. Endogenous pyrogens are cytokines (interleukin [IL]-1, IL-6, tumor necrosis factor [TNF], and the interferons), which are released by monocytes, macrophages, mesangial cells, glial cells, epithelial cells, and B lymphocytes.

Intense muscle contraction (cocaine overdose) or muscle metabolism altered by drugs (neuroleptic agents) or anesthetics produces **malignant hyperthermia** (see Chapter 18). Heat stroke, a potentially fatal febrile illness, is due to excessively high environmental temperatures and failure of physiologic body heat-losing mechanisms.

The *pattern* of fever in children may vary, depending on the age of the child and the nature of the illness. Neonates may not have a febrile response or may be hypothermic despite a significant infection, whereas older infants and children younger than 5 yr may have an exaggerated febrile response with temperatures as high as 105°F in response to either a serious bacterial infection or a benign viral process. Fevers to this latter degree are unusual in older children and adolescents and suggest a significant pathologic process. Except in unusual circumstances, the fever pattern does not distinguish fever caused by bacterial, viral, fungal, or parasitic organisms from that resulting from malignancy, autoimmune diseases, or drugs.

Most febrile illness in children may be categorized as:

1. Fever of short duration accompanied by localizing signs and symptoms in which a diagnosis can be established by clinical history and physical examination.
2. Fever without localizing signs, usually occurring in a child under the age of 3 yr, in which a history and physical examination fail to establish a cause but a diagnosis may be suggested by laboratory studies.
3. Fever of unknown origin (FUO), fever present for more than 14 days (*in a child*) that does not have an etiology despite history, physical examination, and routine laboratory tests. In older children and adolescents, an FUO usually is defined as a fever over 38°F for more than 2 wk that remains undiagnosed despite detailed comprehensive evaluation for 7 days.

## FEVER WITHOUT A SOURCE: OCCULT BACTEREMIA

A common clinical pediatric problem is the evaluation of the febrile but well-appearing child with no localizing signs of infection. Although most of these children have self-limited viral infections, some (usually under the age of 3 yr) will have bacteremia, and a few will experience severe and potentially life-threatening illnesses, such as bacterial meningitis. Particularly in the early stages of such illness, it is difficult, even for experienced clinicians, to differentiate patients with bacteremia from those with benign illness (Table 10–6).

### Fever in Children between 3 Months and 2 Years of Age

*Etiology.* Children between 3 mo and 2 yr of age are at risk for infection resulting from organisms with polysaccharide capsules, such as *Strepto-*

TABLE 10–5.  Antimicrobial Prophylaxis

| | Pathogen | Preventive Therapy |
|---|---|---|
| Pertussis | *Bordetella pertussis* | Erythromycin, azithromycin |
| Diphtheria | *Corynebacterium diphtheriae* | Penicillin, erythromycin |
| Meningitis | *Haemophilus influenzae* type b | Rifampin |
| | *Neisseria meningitidis* | Rifampin |
| Tuberculosis | *Mycobacterium tuberculosis* | Isoniazid |
| Sepsis/asplenia* | *Streptococcus pneumoniae* | Penicillin |
| | *Haemophilus influenzae* type b | Amoxicillin |
| Rheumatic fever | Group A streptococci | Penicillin |
| Interstitial pneumonia | *Pneumocystis carinii* | Trimethoprim–sulfamethoxazole, pentamidine |
| Influenza | Influenza A virus | Amantadine |
| Hepatitis A | HAV | Immune serum globulin |
| Hepatitis B | HBV | Hepatitis B immune globulin (HBIG) |
| Chickenpox | Varicella-zoster virus | Varicella-zoster immune globulin (VZIG) |
| RSV | RSV | RSV-immune globulin |
| AIDS | HIV | Maternal prepartum and intrapartum plus neonatal postpartum therapy with AZT |
| Neonatal sepsis | Group B streptoccocus | Intrapartum ampicillin for at-risk mothers |
| Neonatal conjunctivitis | *Chlamydia trachomatis* | 0.5% erythromycin topically |
| | *Neisseria gonorrhoeae* | 1% silver nitrate or 0.5% erythromycin topically |
| Bacterial endocarditis | | |
| Dental procedure | Streptococci | Amoxicillin (PO), ampicillin and gentamicin (IV) |
| Genitourinary/gastrointestinal procedure | Enterococcus | Amoxicillin (PO), ampicillin and gentamicin (IV) (see Chapter 13) |

*Including sickle cell disease.

AIDS = acquired immunodeficiency syndrome; AZT = zidovudine (azidothymidine); HAV = hepatitis A virus; HBV = hepatitis B virus; HIV = human immunodeficiency virus; RSV = respiratory syncytial virus.

*coccus pneumonia, H. influenzae* type b, meningococci, and salmonella. Effective phagocytosis of these organisms requires opsonic antibody. Although neonates receive maternal immunoglobulin

G (IgG), transplacentally, this protection is gradually lost (3–6 mo), leaving the infant at risk for infection caused by encapsulated organisms until their own IgM and IgG are produced.

TABLE 10–6.  Differentiating Viral from Bacterial Infections

| Variable | Viral | Bacterial |
|---|---|---|
| Petechiae | Present | Present |
| Leukocytosis | Uncommon* | Common |
| Shift to left (↑ bands) | Uncommon | Common |
| Neutropenia | Possible | Suggests overwhelming infection |
| ↑ ESR | Unusual* | Common |
| ↑ CRP | Unusual | Common |
| ↑ TNF, IL-1, PAF | Uncommon | Common |
| Meningitis (pleocytosis) | Lymphocytic‡ | Neutrophilic |
| Meningeal signs positive† | Present | Present |

*Adenovirus and herpes simplex may cause leukocytosis and increased ESR; Epstein-Barr virus may cause petechiae and increased ESR.

†Nuchal rigidity, bulging fontanel, Kernig or Brudzinski sign.

‡Early viral (enterovirus, arbovirus) meningitis may initially have a neutrophilic pleocytosis.

CRP = C-reactive protein; ESR = erythrocyte sedimentation rate; IL = interleukin; PAF = platelet activating factor; TNF = tumor necrosis factor.

*Clinical Manifestations and Diagnosis.* In children between 3 mo and 2 yr of age, most febrile episodes demonstrate an obvious source of infection as elicited by history or physical examination (e.g., pharyngitis, otitis media, bronchitis, or upper respiratory tract infection). The evaluation of infants who are febrile, well-appearing, but without a focus of infection depends on the clinical assessment, which may include a complete blood count (CBC) with white blood cell (WBC) differential, erythrocyte sedimentation rate (ESR), blood culture, urinalysis with urine culture, and a chest radiograph (if respiratory symptoms are present) to attempt to find an infectious focus. In occult bacteremia, positive blood specimens for culture more often are obtained from children with fever higher than 104°F.

The WBC count does not always predict accurately whether a child is bacteremic. Nonetheless, it can be helpful in dividing the population into high-risk and low-risk (<15,000/μL) groups. This division may be helpful in selecting patients for further investigation or therapy. The ESR is no more useful than the WBC in predicting bacteremia in ambulatory febrile patients. Elevated C-reactive protein (CRP) and TNF levels have been correlated with bacterial disease. Other hematologic findings that have been considered suggestive of bacteremia but are too inconsistent and nonspecific include thrombocytopenia, Dohle inclusion bodies, neutrophil toxic granulations, and vacuolization of neutrophils. With or without thrombocytopenia, the finding of petechiae in a febrile child is suggestive of bacteremia. All patients should have a urinalysis to measure urine nitrites and leukocyte esterase, the presence of which suggests a urinary tract infection (see Chapter 16). Patients with diarrhea should have a stool checked for leukocytes. Variables that may help in differentiating viral from bacterial disease are noted in Table 10–6.

Occult bacteremia due to pneumococcus in otherwise healthy children between 3 and 24 mo may be transient, with serious infections developing in a small but important percentage of infants. In contrast, bacteremias caused by *H. influenzae* type b and *Neisseria meningitidis* are less benign, and serious localizing infections such as meningitis, septic arthritis, and pericarditis are possible sequelae.

Children with **sickle cell anemia** have deficiencies of splenic function and properdin-dependent opsonization, placing them at high risk for bacteremia, especially during the first 5 yr of life (see Chapter 14). Pneumococcal sepsis that is accompanied by meningitis, and, less commonly, bacteremia and meningitis that are due to *H. influenzae* type b are potentially serious and fulminant infections in patients with sickle cell disease. *Salmonella* bacteremia may result in osteomyelitis.

***Treatment.*** Because of the low incidence of occult bacteremia (4–5%) and because most episodes of occult bacteremia are due to pneumococci and may be transient in healthy immunocompetent children, most physicians do not administer antibiotics to febrile infants whose infection has no focus or to those patients who do not appear to be septic. After obtaining blood and urine specimens for culture, some physicians administer ceftriaxone (IM) and discharge the well-appearing infant with follow-up within 24 hr.

Any ill-appearing infant should be considered seriously infected, admitted to the hospital, and treated with antibiotics. A well-appearing febrile infant between 3 and 24 mo of age should be carefully evaluated, a blood specimen from the infant obtained, and the child sent home with follow-up in 24 hr. If the blood culture becomes positive for pneumococci and the child is afebrile, appears well, and has no localizing signs, the child does not need not be treated; a subsequent blood specimen should be obtained. If the initial blood culture is positive for pneumococcus and the child remains febrile or has localizing signs suggestive of pneumonia or meningitis, the child should be treated with appropriate antibiotics in the hospital.

If the bacteremia is due to *H. influenzae* type b or *N. meningitidis*, the child should be immediately re-evaluated, a lumbar puncture performed, and parenteral antibiotics administered. Prior to the administration of antibiotics, another blood specimen should be obtained in all children to determine the persistence of the bacteremia. (Antibiotic dosages are noted in Appendix I.)

### Fever in Infants Younger Than 3 Months of Age

Fever in infants under 3 mo may be associated with a higher risk of serious bacterial infections than fever in older infants. These younger infants may not demonstrate localizing signs, and bacteremia, meningitis, urinary tract infection, and pneumonia may be present in the infant exhibiting nonspecific signs, such as poor feeding. Often fever is the only manifestation of serious bacterial infection in very young infants. Urinary tract infection (*Escherichia coli*), bacteremia (*Salmonella*, group B streptococci, pneumococcus, *H. influenzae*, meningococcus), pneumonia (*Staphylococcus aureus*, pneumococcus), meningitis (viral or group B streptococci, meningococcus, pneumococcus, *H. influenzae* type b), and osteomyelitis (*S. aureus*, group B streptococci) are common types of infection. Nonetheless, most febrile diseases in this age group are due to common viral pathogens.

Differentiation between viral and bacterial infections often is difficult (see Table 10–6). Therefore, infants younger than 3 mo of age who appear sick and all infants younger than 1 mo of age (especially with uncertain follow-up) usually are admitted to the hospital.

After blood, urine, and cerebrospinal fluid (CSF) specimens are obtained for culture, broad-spectrum antibiotics are administered to many of these infants. The choice of antibiotics depends on the possible pathogens involved and any localizing findings, such as pneumonia, septic arthritis/osteomyelitis, or meningitis. Well-appearing febrile infants without an infectious focus (otitis media, skin, soft tissue, bone, or joint) who are older than 1 mo of age, with good follow-up, no history of prematurity or prior antimicrobial therapy, and a WBC count between 5000 and 15,000, less than 1500 bands, less than 10 WBC/high-power field (hpf) on examination of centrifuged urine (or negative leukocyte esterase), and fewer than 5 WBCs/

hpf on examination of stool in infants with diarrhea, may be discharged home without therapy. Some physicians administer ceftriaxone (IM) to these infants after obtaining a blood specimen for culture. In either case, careful outpatient management requires close phone contact for 48 hr and a return visit within 24 hr.

## References

Baraff LJ, Bass J, Fleisher G, et al: Practice guidelines for management of infants and children 0 to 36 months of age with fever without source. Pediatrics 92:1, 1993.

Behrman RE, Kliegman RM, Arvin AM (eds): Nelson Textbook of Pediatrics, 15th ed. Philadelphia, WB Saunders, 1996, Chapters 165–167.

Chiu C, Lin T, Bullard M: Identification of febrile neonates unlikely to have bacterial infections. Pediatr Infect Dis J 16:59, 1997.

Jones RG, Bass JW: Febrile children with no focus of infection: A survey of their management by primary care physicians. Pediatr Infect Dis J 12:179, 1993.

Rothrock S, Harper M, Green S, et al: Do oral antibiotics prevent meningitis and serious bacterial infections in children with *Streptococcus pneumonia* occult bacteremia? A meta-analysis. Pediatrics 99:438, 1997.

## FEVER OF UNKNOWN ORIGIN

FUO (fever >100.4°F lasting for more than 14 days with no obvious cause despite a complete history, physical examination, and routine laboratory evaluation) historically was a difficult problem because most patients remained undiagnosed despite in-hospital evaluation for 1 wk. The differential diagnosis between occult infections and neoplasms may require invasive procedures. With the improved capability of diagnostic imaging techniques (combined with imaging-guided needle biopsy), including ultrasound, computed tomography (CT), magnetic resonance imaging (MRI), and radionuclide scanning with gallium or technetium, the number of undiagnosed patients in this category has decreased substantially.

*Etiology.* In addition to carefully documenting several instances of an elevated temperature, a thorough *history* should be undertaken, including (1) the impact the fever has had on the child's health; (2) weight loss; (3) presence of an associated disease, such as diabetes mellitus or malignancy; (4) involvement of vital organs such as liver, heart, or brain; (5) use of drugs, medications, or immunosuppressive therapy; (6) exposure to industrial or hobby-related chemicals; (7) blood transfusions; (8) domestic or foreign travel to endemic areas (malaria, histoplasmosis, coccidioidomycosis, *Cryptococcus neoformans,* Colorado tick fever); (9) genetic background; (10) recent surgical procedure or den-

tal work; and (11) sexual activity. Specific attention should be paid to the social history and exposure to pathogens (malaria, tuberculosis, day care) or animals (birds, livestock, bats, reptiles, pets) and insects (tick, mosquito).

Because the etiology of most occult infections is an unusual presentation of a common disease, an evaluation for diseases typical to a geographic locale should pursued. Thus, an adolescent from an urban area with a FUO requires a careful evaluation for bacterial diseases, including tuberculosis, salmonellae, and spirochetes as well as viral entities, including Epstein-Barr virus (EBV), cytomegalovirus (CMV), human immunodeficiency virus (HIV), and hepatitis A, B, and C viruses. Inhabitants of or travelers to rural areas should be evaluated for zoonosis and insect or water-borne pathogens.

In the absence of localizing signs (heart murmur, abdominal pain, abnormal liver function), it may be difficult to focus the evaluation. Furthermore, entities such as sinusitis, endocarditis, intra-abdominal abscesses (perinephric, intrahepatic, subdiaphragmatic), and central nervous system (CNS) lesions (tuberculoma, cysticercosis, abscess, toxoplasmosis) may be relatively asymptomatic. A FUO also may be the presentation of an immunodeficiency disease.

*Differential Diagnosis* (Table 10–7). The three most common categories of FUO in children are (1) infectious diseases, (2) connective tissue or inflammatory diseases, and (3) neoplasms. A diagnosis is not established in 10–20% of children with FUO.

The bacterial diseases most commonly implicated in children can be grouped into two categories: *generalized* infections caused by specific organisms, and *localized* infections caused by a variety of organisms. In the United States, organisms and conditions most frequently associated with FUO in children that produce a generalized infection include oral streptococcal (endocarditis), *Bartonella* (cat-scratch disease), ehrlichiosis, *Salmonella,* mycobacteria, brucellosis, tularemia, spirochetes (leptospirosis, Lyme disease, rat-bite fever, syphilis), HIV, CMV, hepatitis viruses, and EBV. Localized infections include endocarditis, intra-abdominal or liver abscess, sinusitis, mastoiditis, osteomyelitis, pneumonia, and pyelonephritis or perinephric abscess.

The connective tissue (inflammatory) diseases that most commonly manifest as FUO are juvenile rheumatoid arthritis (JRA), systemic lupus erythematosus (SLE), polyarteritis nodosa, rheumatic fever, inflammatory bowel disease, and undefined vasculitis (see Chapter 9).

TABLE 10–7. Causes of Fever of Unknown Origin in Children

**Infections**

*Bacterial Diseases*

Specific organism causing systemic disease

    Bartonellosis

    Brucellosis

    *Campylobacter*

    Cat-scratch disease

    Gonococcemia (chronic)

    Meningococcemia (chronic)

    Salmonellosis

    *Streptobacillus moniliformis*

    Tuberculosis

    Tularemia

Localized infections

    Abscesses: abdominal, dental, hepatic, pelvic, perinephric, rectal, subphrenic, splenic, periappendiceal

    Cholangitis

    Endocarditis

    Mastoiditis

    Osteomyelitis

    Pneumonia

    Pyelonephritis

    Sinusitis

*Spirochete*

    *Borrelia* (borreliosis: *B. recurrentis, B. burgdorferi*)

    Leptospirosis

    Lyme disease

    *Spirillum minus*

    Syphilis

*Viral Diseases*

    Cytomegalovirus

    Hepatitis

    Human immunodeficiency virus (and its opportunistic-associated infections)

    Infectious mononucleosis (Epstein-Barr virus)

    Unidentified presumed virus

*Chlamydial Diseases*

    Lymphogranuloma venereum

    Psittacosis

*Rickettsial Diseases*

    *Ehrlichia canis*

    Q fever

    Rocky Mountain spotted fever

*Fungal Diseases*

    Blastomycosis (nonpulmonary)

    Coccidioidomycosis (disseminated)

    Histoplasmosis (disseminated)

*Parasitic Diseases*

    Extraintestinal amebiasis

    Babesiosis

    Giardiasis

    Malaria

    Toxoplasmosis

    Trypanosomiasis

    Visceral larva migrans

**Autoimmune Hypersensitivity Diseases**

    Drug fever

    Hypersensitivity pneumonitis

    Juvenile rheumatoid arthritis (systemic onset, Still disease)

    Polyarteritis nodosa

    Rheumatic fever

    Serum sickness

    Systemic lupus erythematosus

    Undefined vasculitis

**Neoplasms**

    Atrial myxoma

    Ewing sarcoma

    Hepatoma

    Hodgkin disease

    Leukemia

    Lymphoma

    Neuroblastoma

**Granulomatous Diseases**

    Granulomatous hepatitis

    Sarcoidosis

    Crohn disease

**Familial-Hereditary Diseases**

    Anhidrotic ectodermal dysplasia

    Cyclic neutropenia

    Deafness, urticaria, amyloidosis syndrome

    Fabry disease

    Familial dysautonomia

    Familial Mediterranean fever

    Hypertriglyceridemia

    Ichthyosis

**Miscellaneous**

    Behçet syndrome

    Chronic active hepatitis

    Diabetes insipidus (central and nephrogenic)

    Factitious fever

    Hemophagocytic syndromes

    Histiocytosis syndromes

    Hypothalamic-central fever

    Infantile cortical hyperostosis

    Inflammatory bowel disease

    Kawasaki disease

    Pancreatitis

    Periodic fever

    Postoperative (pericardiotomy, craniectomy)

    Pulmonary embolism

    Spinal cord injury–crisis

    Thyrotoxicosis

    Central fever

**Undiagnosed Fever**

    Persistent

    Recurrent

    Resolved

Modified from Behrman RE, Kliegman RM, Arvin AM (eds). Nelson Textbook of Pediatrics, 14th ed. Philadelphia, WB Saunders, 1996, p 701.

Malignancies are a less common cause of FUO in children than in adults, accounting for about 10% of all episodes. Malignancies that may be associated with FUO include Hodgkin and non-Hodgkin lymphoma, leukemia, Ewing sarcoma, and neuroblastoma.

*Factitious fever* is another important consideration, particularly if family members are health care providers. Fever should be documented in the hospital by a reliable individual who remains with the patient when the temperature is taken. Psychiatric disorders frequently are masked by the family's denial and desire to find an organic cause for their child's problems. Continuously observing the patient over a long period of time and repetitive evaluation are indicated.

**Clinical Manifestations.** By definition, *physical findings* are minimal in children with FUO but several important areas often are overlooked. Accurate weight measurements help document the impact of the FUO process on the nutritional status of the patient. Sweating should be noted; its absence suggests dehydration resulting from vomiting and diarrhea, central or nephrogenic diabetes insipidus, anhidrotic ectodermal dysplasia, familial dysautonomia, or exposure to atropine.

Red, weeping eyes may be a sign of systemic disease, particularly polyarteritis nodosa, sarcoidosis, inflammatory bowel disease, Kawasaki disease, or JRA. Palpebral conjunctivitis may be a clue to measles, coxsackievirus, tuberculosis, infectious mononucleosis, lymphogranuloma venereum, cat-scratch disease, or Newcastle disease. In contrast, bulbar conjunctivitis in a child with FUO suggests leptospirosis, Kawasaki disease, or rheumatologic disorders.

FUO may be caused by hypothalamic dysfunction. A clue to this disorder is the failure of the pupils to constrict because of the absence of the sphincter constrictor muscle of the eye. This muscle develops embryologically when hypothalamic structure and function also are undergoing differentiation. Lack of tears, insensitivity to pain, a smooth tongue displaying an absence of fungiform papillae, an absent corneal reflex, failure to thrive and gastroesophageal reflux may suggest fever from **familial dysautonomia.**

Tenderness to tapping over the sinuses and teeth should be sought, and the sinuses should be transilluminated. Oral candidiasis may be a clue to various disorders of the immune system, especially **acquired immunodeficiency syndrome** (AIDS). Fever blisters are common findings in patients with pneumococcal, streptococcal, malarial, or rickettsial infection. Hyperemia of the pharynx, with or without exudate, may suggest infectious mononucleosis or CMV.

Repetitive chills and temperature spikes are common in children with septicemia, regardless of cause, particularly when associated with renal, liver, or biliary tract disease; endocarditis; malaria; brucellosis; rat-bite fever; or loculated collections of pus. Careful ophthalmologic evaluation is helpful in establishing collagen vascular and granulomatous diseases, CMV, endocarditis, fungal infection, leukemia, sarcoidosis, syphilis, toxoplasmosis, and tuberculosis.

The muscles and bones should be palpated carefully. Point tenderness over a bone suggests osteomyelitis or neoplastic bone marrow invasion. Tenderness over the trapezius muscle may be a clue to a subdiaphragmatic abscess. Generalized muscle tenderness suggests dermatomyositis, trichinosis, polyarteritis, or mycoplasma, influenza, or arboviral infection.

Rectal or pelvic examination may reveal tenderness and suggest a deep pelvic abscess, iliac or mesenteric adenitis, or pelvic osteomyelitis. A guaiac test on stool should be performed because occult blood loss suggests inflammatory bowel disease. Hyperactive deep tendon reflexes suggest thyrotoxicosis.

**Diagnosis.** Children with unexplained fever should be evaluated in a logical sequence beginning with a meticulous history, comprehensive physical examination, and compilation of screening laboratory data. An organ system approach is helpful. The urgency of further testing will depend on the clinical status of the patient and the tempo of the disease processes. Not all patients with unexplained fever need to be evaluated for all of the conditions associated with FUO. Young infants with unexplained fever frequently have undefined viral illnesses, such as EBV infections. Other causes of FUO in infants include pyogenic bacterial infections, JRA and Kawasaki disease. A more aggressive approach would be required to evaluate an infant with daily fever spikes to 105°F and significant toxicity.

The *immunologic competency* of the host may need to be evaluated, by monitoring T-cell function by skin testing with an anergy panel as well as an intermediate-strength purified protein derivative, doing T-cell subsets, checking for lymphocytosis or leukocytosis with a WBC and differential count, evaluating B-cell function by immunoglobulin levels, and measuring complement. Additional tests for the evaluation of an FUO are listed in Figure 10–2. These additional tests should be used judiciously and should focus on areas suggested by the screening tests, physical findings, or historic data.

*CENTRAL NERVOUS SYSTEM.* The child with head-

FUO

Detailed chronologic history

Detailed general exam
+
Specific exam based on history

Repeat history and exam based on lab plus continued observation

Unstable vital signs
Organ/life-threatening signs
Signs of specific disease

Screening Lab tests*

Stable patient

Immediately obtain diagnostic tests and initiate empiric or specific therapy

Specific labs (special culture, PCR, serology titers, biopsy, aspiration, stains) or imaging (ultrasound, CT, MR, scans - bone, renal, gallium) studies based on history, exam, screening labs, continued observations

No diagnosis

Specific diagnosis

Repeat history, exam
Continued observation

Specific treatment

Consider antipyretics

*Screening laboratory tests include CBC with differential; ESR; CRP; urinalysis; liver enzymes; direct and indirect bilirubin; CPK; blood, urine, and stool culture (including ova and parasites); serology, VDRL, ANA, monospot-EBV titers; and radiologic studies such as chest x-ray.

FIGURE 10–2. Approach to the evaluation of fever of unknown origin (FUO) in children. ANA, antinuclear antibody; CBC = complete blood count; CRP = C-reactive protein; CPK = creatine phosphokinase; CT = computed tomography; EBV = Epstein-Barr virus; ESR = erythrocyte sedimentation rate; MR = magnetic resonance (imaging); PCR = polymerase chain reaction; VDRL = Venereal Disease Research Laboratory (see text for syphilis). (Modified from Corder WT, Aranoff SC: Fever of unknown origin. *In* Kliegman RM, Nieder ML, Super DM [eds]: Practical Strategies in Pediatric Diagnosis and Therapy. Philadelphia, WB Saunders, 1996, p 922.)

ache, possible sinusitis, or other signs suggestive of CNS involvement should first have a CT scan. Although acute bacterial meningitis is not a cause of FUO, a lumbar puncture and analysis of CSF may be informative and lead to a diagnosis such as SLE, Lyme disease, or syphilis. A parameningeal focus may be suggested by CSF findings that might then be identified by CT scan with contrast or MRI. Silent CNS lesions, such as small brain abscesses, tuberculomas, toxoplasmosis, and cysticercosis, may be identified.

*CARDIOVASCULAR DISEASE.* Bacterial endocarditis is

an important cause of FUO but may be difficult to diagnose because patients frequently are given oral antibiotics that sterilize blood cultures but are inadequate to sterilize intracardiac vegetations (see Chapter 13). A thorough cardiac evaluation is indicated to look for predisposing conditions (mitral valve prolapse, bicuspid aortic valve, patients with congenital heart disease). The evaluation of myocarditis, endocarditis, or pericarditis includes echocardiography and both transthoracic and transesophageal echocardiography.

*PULMONARY DISEASE.* Even in the absence of respiratory manifestations, pulmonary disease may be a cause of FUO. Patients with significant parenchymal disease, pleural disease, mediastinal widening, or hilar adenopathy may be asymptomatic. The determination of arterial blood gases may be helpful to define alveolar disease. CT scan or MRI may assist in the assessment of the extent of disease and suggest a diagnosis. Hilar adenopathy may suggest lymphoma, sarcoidosis, histoplasmosis, or tuberculosis. The diagnosis of sarcoidosis requires a tissue biopsy via fiberoptic or rigid bronchoscopy, or thorascopy. Interstitial infiltrates may be associated with histiocytosis, CMV, *Pneumocystis carinii* with or without HIV infection. Bronchoalveolar lavage and examination of fluid are indicated in such patients.

*GASTROINTESTINAL DISEASE.* Many causes of FUO originate from the gastrointestinal tract, either as walled-off occult abscesses from clinically inapparent appendiceal perforations or hepatic, pelvic, and splenic abscesses, or as inflammatory bowel disease. CT with contrast or MRI may be helpful following screening ultrasonography. These tests are useful in ruling out mass lesions and evaluating the integrity of the gastrointestional tract and bowel wall. When inflammatory bowel disease is suspected in children, contrast studies and endoscopy with mucosal biopsy may be required.

Weight loss and diarrhea may indicate parasitic infection, which may occur in a normal or immunodeficient child. In addition to the screening tests (above), careful evaluation for parasites also may include a total eosinophil count and a string test for *Giardia*. In HIV-infected patients, usually innocuous organisms such as *Blastocystis hominis*, cryptosporidium, or cyclospora may be associated with significant symptoms.

*GENITOURINARY DISEASE.* The genitourinary tract may be the source of several causes of FUO, including tuberculosis (heralded by sterile pyuria), perinephric abscess, and neuroblastoma. Ultrasound followed by CT or renal scan is utilized in the evaluation of possible renal pathology, pelvic abscess, pelvic inflammatory disease (PID), or other occult genitourinary infections.

*MUSCULOSKELETAL DISEASE.* The usual presentation of osteomyelitis or septic arthritis is that of an acute localized infection. However, vertebral or pelvic osteomyelitis that is not apparent may cause FUO. Similarly, a psoas abscess may present as vague back pain without localizing signs. Technetium pyrophosphate radionuclide imaging, which is highly sensitive for osteoclast and osteoblast activity, is extremely useful in detecting bony involvement. Similarly, a gallium scan, which indicates collections of polymorphonuclear leukocytes, may be

useful to screen for abscesses. CT scan or MRI is helpful in demonstrating the presence of Ewing sarcoma, which often presents as bone pain with FUO.

The presence or history of arthritis, even if evanescent or migratory, may be very important in establishing the diagnosis of Lyme disease, autoimmune processes (see Chapter 9), or one of the postinfectious arthritides, such as Reiter syndrome. Appropriate screening serologic tests may be helpful (see Fig. 10–2). Myositis frequently is suggested by myalgias, muscle tenderness, and a high serum creatine phosphokinase (CPK) level.

*HEMATOLOGIC DISEASE.* Children with FUO, chronic infection, or both are frequently anemic. Examination of a peripheral blood smear may indicate findings suggestive of the "anemia of chronic disease" or the toxic granulations suggestive of bacterial infection. An examination of the bone marrow may be indicated to exclude hematologic malignancy or storage cells. Bone marrow aspirates should be examined and cultured for fungi (histoplasmosis) and mycobacteria (*Mycobacterium tuberculosis* and *M. avium-intracellulare*) as well as for other bacteria (*Brucella*).

**Treatment.** By definition, a FUO is a chronic process. Every effort should be made to arrive at a specific diagnosis before initiating therapy, particularly with those modalities that may mask significant underlying diseases.

### References

Behrman RE, Kliegman RM, Arvin AM (eds): Nelson Textbook of Pediatrics, 15th ed. Philadelphia, WB Saunders, 1996, Chapter 167.

Knockaert DC, Vanneste LJ, Vanneste SB, et al: Fever of unknown origin in the 1980s: An update of the diagnostic spectrum. Arch Intern Med 152:51, 1992.

Miller L, Sisson B, Tucker L, et al: Prolonged fevers of unknown origin in children: Patterns of presentation and outcome. J Pediatr 129:419, 1996.

Steele RW, Jones SM, Lowe BA, et al: Usefulness of scanning procedures for diagnosis of fever of unknown origin in children. J Pediatr 119:526, 1991.

### FEVER IN THE IMMUNOCOMPROMISED HOST

The evaluation of fever in immunologically impaired patients is quite different than in normal hosts. Although a FUO may be the initial presentation of an immune deficiency, it is more common to be faced with a febrile patient with a known immunodeficiency. The types of infections and their management can be predicted by which parts of the immune system are abnormal.

## Fever and Neutropenia

Infection is the major cause of death in patients with hematologic malignancy or after transplantation. The use of antineoplastic agents that cause neutropenia (myelosuppression) as well as the regimens used for bone marrow transplantation deplete bone marrow granulocyte precursor cells, resulting in a high frequency of bacterial sepsis. As the peripheral WBC count decreases below 500, patients are at risk for bacterial sepsis caused by their own endogenous flora (gastrointestinal aerobic gram-negative rods or cutaneous staphylococci). Techniques to decrease the incidence of infection, such as the prophylactic use of fluoroquinolone antibiotics, fluconazole, or ganciclovir to prevent infection due to gram-negative bacteria, *Candida* species, and CMV, respectively, may also predispose these patients to infection as a result of highly drug-resistant organisms.

Febrile episodes in neutropenic patients routinely are treated with combinations of broad-spectrum antimicrobial agents (e.g., vancomycin or nafcillin–ceftazidime or antipseudomonal penicillin–aminogycoside) until the WBC count improves; some patients are prescribed prophylactic antimicrobial agents to prevent sepsis. The use of recombinant granulocyte colony-stimulating factor or granulocyte-macrophage colony-stimulating factor stimulates neutrophil production by the bone marrow, reduces the duration and severity of neutropenia, and decreases the risk of infection.

Fungal infection (*Candida,* aspergillosis) also becomes a problem in persistently neutropenic patients. A febrile neutropenic patient who remains febrile despite broad-spectrum antibacterial agents may require administration of amphotericin B. Fungal infections may produce fungemia, sinusitis, pneumonia, endophthalmitis and soft tissue, hepatic, splenic, or renal abscesses. Neutropenic patients may receive prophylactic antifungal agents (fluconazole).

In the absence of neutrophils to localize an infection, it often is difficult to determine the source of infection by physical examination. For example, chest examination findings may be negative despite significant infection, but abnormalities may be revealed by chest roentgenogram and arterial blood gases. Bronchoalveolar lavage is recommended to identify pulmonary pathogens. Many patients have indwelling central venous catheters to facilitate chemotherapy and blood drawing. Coagulase-negative staphylococci frequently colonize these catheters and are a source of infection in the absence of signs. Sinus infection (bacteria, *Aspergillus,* Zygomycetes) is common in neutropenic hosts and may be appreciated only by CT scan. Perirectal abscess is another focus of infection in neutropenic hosts; tenderness and erythema may be the only clues to a significant local infection. In addition to antibiotics effective against gram-negative and staphylococcal bacteria, metronidazole is indicated to treat anaerobic bacteria in perirectal abscesses.

## Fever in the Transplant Patient

The management of fever after an organ transplant is somewhat different than during leukemic or bone marrow transplantation. The use of cyclosporine and steroids decreases T-cell function. The transplant patient is more likely to develop infection with CMV, herpes simplex, varicella zoster, *P. carinii,* or toxoplasmosis. The transplanted organ itself may be the source of CMV or toxoplasmosis. Most transplant protocols use prophylactic antimicrobial agents, such as trimethoprim/sulfamethoxazole, acyclovir and/or ganciclovir, and fluconazole.

### References

Behrman RE, Kliegman RM, Arvin AM (eds): Nelson Textbook of Pediatrics, 15th ed. Philadelphia, WB Saunders, 1996, Chapter 173.
Pizzo PA, Rubin M, Freifeld A, et al: The child with cancer and infection: I. Empiric therapy for fever and neutropenia, and preventive strategies. J Pediatr 119:679, 1991.
Sable CA, Donowitz GR: Infections in bone marrow transplant recipients. Clin Infect Dis 19:273, 1994.

## BACTEREMIA AND SEPTICEMIA

Bacteremia is blood stream infection documented by positive blood cultures. This is distinguished from *sepsis,* which is the systemic response to infection and includes tachypnea, tachycardia, hyperthermia, hypothermia, and neutropenia or leukocytosis. The **sepsis syndrome,** also called the systemic inflammatory response syndrome (SIRS), includes the clinical diagnosis of sepsis with evidence of altered organ perfusion, including hypoxemia, oliguria, or elevated blood lactate levels. In approximately 10% of patients with a sepsis syndrome, the blood culture is negative. **Septic shock** includes the clinical diagnosis of the sepsis syndrome plus hypotension despite fluid resuscitation. See Chapter 3 and Table 3–18 for discussion of shock.

*Etiology and Epidemiology.* The age and immunization status of the child are important factors in determining which organisms must be considered (Table 10–8). In neonatal sepsis, the important microorganisms are group B streptococci, *E. coli,* other

**TABLE 10–8.** Risk Factors for Bacterial Sepsis

**Age**
  Premature > full term > infant under 2 yr old

**Immunodeficiency**
  Severe combined immunodeficiency syndrome
  B-cell defects (agammaglobulinemia)
  Neutropenia and immunosuppression (malignancy)
  Complement deficiency
  Sickle cell anemia *plus* other asplenic conditions
  Acquired immunodeficiency syndrome
  Neutrophil chemotactic defects
  Malnutrition

**Associated Disease States**
  Malignancy
  Nephrotic syndrome
  Galactosemia
  Intravenous drug abuse
  Paraplegia
  Gonococcal genitourinary infection
  Contact with *Neisseria meningitidis* or *Haemophilus influenzae*
    (e.g., day care)

**Medical Instrumentation/Procedures**
  Indwelling intravascular catheters
  Indwelling urinary catheter
  Endotracheal intubation
  Ventriculoatrial shunts
  Continuous peritoneal dialysis
  Surgery
  Prosthetic heart valves

streptococci, *S. aureus, Staphylococcus epidermidis* (coagulase-negative staphylococci) and *Listeria monocytogenes.* In preterm infants, infection due to coagulase-negative staphylococci is common; *Candida* species must also be considered. In the immunocompetent older febrile child with no localizing findings, the most common pathogens are *S. pneumoniae, N. meningitidis, Salmonella, S. aureus,* and group A streptococci. *H. influenzae* is now rarely seen, except in infants who have not been immunized. Infants with galactosemia and children with pyelonephritis often have gram-negative bacteremia (e.g., *E. coli*).

Immunocompromised children (those with asplenia, sickle cell disease, neutropenia, malignancy, AIDS, or indwelling foreign bodies) are infected by a broader spectrum of organisms and are more susceptible to development of septicemia. Illness may be due to common organisms or may be associated with a wide variety of bacteria or fungi.

In some patients, bacteremia or septicemia may be associated with focal infections (e.g., pyelonephritis, pneumonia, cellulitis, osteomyelitis, endocarditis, meningitis). In such cases, when bacteremia or septicemia is strongly suspected, specimens should be obtained for culture and intravenous broad-spectrum antibiotics administered.

*Pathophysiology of Septic Shock.* The pathophysiology of septic shock is based, in large part, on the body's response to microbial products: peptidoglysan fragments from gram-positive bacteria and lipopolysaccharide from gram-negative organisms. Lipid A (endotoxin) of gram-negative bacteria triggers a cascade of events, probably mediated by the resultant activation or production of inflammatory mediators (complement, prostaglandins, leukotrienes, kinins) and cytokines. Endotoxin stimulates the production of several cytokines from macrophages, including IL-1 and TNF, that produce fever, increased vascular permeability, and hypotension; increase the numbers of circulating neutrophils from the bone marrow; mobilize amino acids from skeletal muscle (catabolism); and amplify the immune response (see Chapter 3). Reactions in the lung lead to the development of the often fatal adult respiratory distress syndrome (ARDS) (see Chapter 12) and multiorgan system failure (see Chapter 3).

Certain bacteria, particularly *S. aureus* and *S. pyogenes,* may be associated with an unusually severe systemic inflammatory response syndrome, such as staphylococcal toxic shock syndrome. TSST-1 is a *superantigen,* a bacterial antigen that can interact with a superficial component of the T-cell receptor, without the usual requirement for presentation of a bacterial antigen within the context of major histocompatibility complex (MHC) and the antigen-binding groove. Superantigens can activate entire classes of T cells, which trigger cytokine production and initiate a cascade of biologic responses leading to shock. The clinical picture is that of shock, accompanied by multisystem dysfunction, such as a sunburn-type rash, renal failure, disseminated intravascular coagulation (DIC), hepatic abnormalities, and hypotension.

*Clinical Manifestations.* A clinical diagnosis of presumptive septicemia should be made when the child's fever and toxic appearance (tachycardia, hyperventilation, agitation, lethargy, poor perfusion) suggest serious illness. The history and physical examination may indicate the site of origin. The early features of septicemia are similar to those of many infections. The child usually is febrile; however, hypothermia may be an important sign of sepsis in the neonate, the neutropenic immunosuppressed patient, or the burn patient. Chills, hyperventilation, tachycardia, hypotension, and peripheral vasodilation are early signs. There may be petechiae and purpura. Apprehension, confusion, and agitation also are often early signs of septic shock, which often progresses to lethargy and coma. Profound hypotension with cold, clammy, mottled skin, cyanosis, poor capillary refill, a weak pulse, lethargy, and coma are observed later in the progression of shock.

Cutaneous lesions, such as purpura and petechiae, classically are seen in meningococcemia but may occur in infection with other organisms. *Pseudomonas aeruginosa* causes a characteristic skin lesion called **ecthyma gangrenosum.** These lesions are single round or oval lesions that look like a bull's eye, with a necrotic ulcer in the center surrounded by a rim of redness and induration. DIC is common and becomes manifest as purpura and bleeding from puncture sites. Hypotension may result in peripheral gangrene, anuric renal failure, and lactic acidosis.

***Diagnosis and Differential Diagnosis.*** In all patients, especially those immunocompromised by an underlying disease or by cancer therapy, the outcome of sepsis depends on early diagnosis and treatment. Several blood specimens should be obtained for culture to identify the specific organism. All suspected sites of infection should be examined by culture and Gram stain for evidence of bacterial infection; these sites include CSF, sputum, skin lesions, urine, and the buffy coat. The latter is the leukocyte-rich fraction of a centrifuged sample of blood and is located between the serum and erythrocyte interface. Gram stain, methylene blue, or acridine orange stained leukocytes demonstrate bacteria in some patients with bacteremia. Bacterial detection methods may be helpful to identify certain bacteria, including *H. influenzae* type b, *S. pneumonia, N. meningitidis,* and group B streptococci in less than 2 hr. These tests are particularly helpful when previous antibiotics were given before obtaining specimens. A chest roentgenogram is indicated to identify pneumonia, pleural effusions, or ARDS.

Neutropenia is an important early laboratory finding caused by infection-mediated neutrophil storage pool depletion and margination of cells. Thrombocytopenia and reduced factor VIII concentration reflect DIC, whereas fibrin split products are the result of fibrinolysis. Thrombocytopenia also may be due to platelet antibodies produced during sepsis. Clotting factor abnormalities also may be a result of liver failure. Lactic acidosis is due to tissue hypoxia from shock or pulmonary insufficiency.

Many infectious and noninfectious diseases are associated with systemic symptoms similar to those of bacteremia or septicemia. Infectious diseases include rickettsial disease, such as Rocky Mountain spotted fever, staphylococcal toxic shock syndrome, leptospirosis, plague, Lyme disease, tuberculosis, tularemia, viral sepsis (herpes simplex, enterovirus, hemorrhagic fever), malaria, and fun-gal diseases (candidiasis). Noninfectious diseases include anaphylactic shock, toxic ingestions, hemorrhagic shock, midgut volvulus, vasculitis, and Kawasaki disease.

***Treatment.*** The initial treatment of shock includes supportive therapy to maintain blood pressure, perfusion, and oxygenation as well as antimicrobial therapy. Broad-spectrum antibiotics that are bactericidal against both gram-negative and gram-positive bacteria should be initiated before the causative bacteria are identified. Therapy of suspected gram-negative sepsis includes an aminoglycoside plus an antipseudomonas penicillin (ticarcillin or piperacillin) or a broad-spectrum third-generation cephalosporin (such as ceftazidime) (see Appendix I for dosages). Treatment of nosocomial infections may be aided by knowledge of the susceptibility patterns of bacteria prevalent in the hospital setting. When methicillin-resistant *S. aureus* or coagulase-negative staphylococci are suspected, vancomycin should be added. Anaerobic bacteremia frequently complicates infections of the mouth, abdomen, rectum, or pelvis and requires therapy with either clindamycin or metronidazole in addition to antibiotics active against gram-negative enteric pathogens. Identifying the specific bacteria and performing antimicrobial susceptibility tests form the basis for administering antibiotics having a narrow spectrum, which avoids superinfection by yeast or resistant bacteria and reduces antibiotic toxicity.

Supportive care for shock is best performed in a pediatric intensive care unit where continuous monitoring of vital signs is possible (see Chapter 3). Venodilation, transcapillary fluid losses, and hemorrhage require the expansion of the circulating blood volume (with colloid or crystalloid solutions) to maintain the perfusion of vital organs. In addition to volume replacement, septic shock must be treated with sympathomimetic drugs, such as dopamine, dobutamine, and epinephrine. These drugs improve cardiac output and renal and systemic perfusion and may increase vascular tone. The mortality rate for patients with septic shock is 40–70%. When multiple organ systems fail (e.g., in ARDS or renal or hepatic failure), the mortality rate approaches 90–100%.

## References

Behrman RE, Kliegman RM, Arvin AM (eds): Nelson Textbook of Pediatrics, 15th ed. Philadelphia, WB Saunders, 1996, Chapter 168.
Bone RC, Balk RA, Cerra FB, et al: Definitions for sepsis and organ failure and guidelines for the use of innovative therapies in sepsis. Chest 101:644, 1992.
Martin MA, Silverman HJ: Gram-negative sepsis and the adult respiratory distress syndrome. Clin Infect Dis 14:1213, 1992.

Wenzel RP, Pinsky MR, Ulevitch RJ, et al: Current understanding of sepsis. Clin Infect Dis 22:407, 1996.

# OSTEOMYELITIS AND SEPTIC ARTHRITIS

Infections of bones (osteomyelitis) and joints (septic arthritis) usually are due to bacterial pathogens and must be differentiated from cellulitis, trauma, inflammatory reactions, and malignancy.

## OSTEOMYELITIS

Osteomyelitis may occur at any age but is most common in children between ages 3 and 12 yr and affects boys twice as frequently as girls.

*Pathogenesis.* Infections of the bone may result from hematogenous dissemination or by direct spread from a contiguous focus of infection. Osteomyelitis in children is most often the consequence of bacteremia and involves rapidly growing bone, particularly the metaphyses of long bones (distal femur, proximal tibia, distal humerus, distal radius). Bacteria lodge in sharp loops of nutrient arteries supplying the growth plates of these bones. Blood in the large sinusoidal veins flows slowly and there are no phagocytic cells in this area. Obstruction to flow by bacterial microemboli produce small areas of avascular necrosis with a resultant metaphyseal abscess. Trauma often is noted prior to the onset of osteomyelitis and may result in local

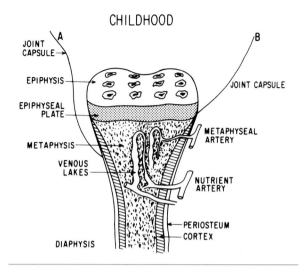

**FIGURE 10–4.** Major structures of the bone of a child. Joint capsule A inserts below the epiphyseal growth plate, as in the hip, elbow, ankle, and shoulder. Rupture of a metaphyseal abscess in these bones is likely to produce pyarthrosis. Joint capsule B inserts at the epiphyseal growth plate, as in other tubular bones. Rupture of a metaphyseal abscess in these bones is likely to lead to a subperiosteal abscess but seldom to an associated pyarthrosis. (From Gutman LT: Acute, subacute, and chronic osteomyelitis in children. Curr Probl Pediatr 15:7, 1985.)

areas of bone injury that predispose to infection. This may mislead the clinician to think the bone symptoms are due to trauma. In infants younger than 1 yr of age, the capillaries perforate the epiphyseal growth plate, permitting spread across the epiphysis, causing a septic arthritis (Fig. 10–3). In older children, the infection is contained in the metaphyseal sinusoidal veins because the vessels no longer cross the epiphyseal plate (Fig. 10–4). Osteoarthritis also may be seen in joints where the capsule inserts on the metaphysis proximal to the epiphyseal plate. Pyarthritis is common in these joints (hip, elbow, shoulder, knee) (see Fig. 10–4). Infection spreads through the haversian system and Volkmann canals; as infection spreads laterally, the periosteum is lifted. In chronic osteomyelitis, the infected periosteum may calcify into a shell of new bone around the infected portion of the shaft and is called an *involucrum.* The host defense mechanisms may wall off a metaphyseal abscess, producing a chronic infection with a sclerotic rim called a *Brodie abscess.* Dead bone within this space is called *sequestrum.*

*Contiguous osteomyelitis* is less common in children and usually occurs following spread of cellulitis as a result of an infected wound, such as a decubitus or sinus or periodontal disease, or after a surgical procedure. Osteomyelitis also may result

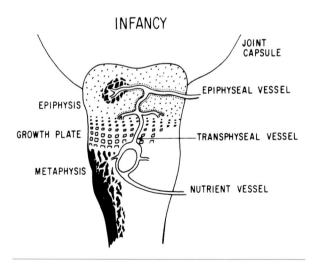

**FIGURE 10–3.** Major structures of the bone of an infant prior to maturation of the epiphyseal growth plate. Note the transphyseal vessel, which connects the vascular supply of the epiphysis and metaphysis, facilitating spread of infection between these two areas. (From Gutman LT: Acute, subacute, and chronic osteomyelitis and pyogenic arthritis in children. Curr Probl Pediatr 15:6, 1985.)

from direct inoculation from a penetrating wound, heel punctures, paronychia, open fracture, orthopedic surgery, and human or animal bites.

*Etiology.* *S. aureus* is responsible for most infections. Group B (in neonates) or other streptococci, anaerobic microorganisms, gram-negative enteric bacteria, and *M. tuberculosis* also cause osteomyelitis. Other factors that predispose the patient to osteomyelitis include furunculosis, infected lesions of varicella, infected burns, prolonged intravenous or central parenteral alimentation, intravenous drug abuse, and trauma. Sickle cell anemia and other hemoglobinopathies predispose the patient to osteomyelitis caused by *Salmonella* or *Staphylococcus* species or, less commonly, *S. pneumoniae*. Osteomyelitis secondary to dog or cat bites may be caused by *Pasteurella multocida*. *Pseudomonas* osteomyelitis commonly follows puncture wounds of the foot (in sneaker wearers) or intravenous drug abuse. Infection due to *H. influenzae*, type b is rarely seen in an immunized population.

*Clinical Manifestations.* Hematogenous osteomyelitis in children usually involves a single bone (after infancy) and occurs either as an acute illness with fever, focal bone pain, and sepsis or as a subacute illness with mild systemic signs but with local complaints at the site of involved bone. These complaints include severe pain, exquisite tenderness, warmth, erythema, and swelling. Weight bearing and spontaneous or requested motion are refused, which mimics paralysis (pseudoparalysis). Muscle spasm may make the extremity difficult to examine. Hematogenous osteomyelitis involving the vertebrae is notable for an insidious onset, vague symptomatology, backache, occasional spinal cord compression, and usually little associated fever or systemic toxicity. With osteomyelitis of the pelvis, presenting signs may include limp; abdominal, hip, groin, or thigh pain; and fever. Table 10–9 presents features of acute hematogenous osteomyelitis.

*Diagnosis.* Marked tenderness over the involved site identifies the infected bone. Leukocytosis may be present. The ESR usually is elevated and is of great help in monitoring the response to treatment. Blood specimens (positive in 60%), cultures of an aspirate of cellulitis, and a diagnostic aspirate of the periosteal space (or, if negative, of the bone itself) should be obtained before antibiotic therapy is begun. The evaluation of patients with chronic disease includes a tuberculin test and a chest roentgenogram. The tuberculin test may be especially helpful in establishing a diagnosis in vertebral osteomyelitis.

Roentgenograms of the affected areas should be obtained to allow observation of soft tissue swelling, periosteal elevation and calcification, and bone destruction and to consider a possible alternative diagnosis, such as bone tumors, bone cysts, leukemia, or histiocytosis. Plain films of the bone generally are normal during the early phase (10–14 days); the radionuclide technetium 99 bone scan may be valuable if plain films are normal. MRI is particularly useful for delineating the extent of infection in complex cases or when infection is a complication of trauma, surgery, or sickle cell anemia.

*Treatment.* Initial intravenous antibiotic therapy should be based on results of Gram stain of bone aspirate, blood culture reports, age, and associated diseases. Initial therapy should cover the staphylococci, all of which must be assumed to be penicillinase-producing (oxacillin, nafcillin, methicillin, clindamycin) (see Appendix I for dosages); the possibility of methicillin-resistant staphylococci should be considered. In patients with sickle cell anemia, *Salmonella* and *S. aureus* must both be covered (cefotaxime, ceftriaxone). Gram-negative organisms may be present if wound contamination or a history of intravenous drug abuse is discovered. *Candida*, *Aspergillus*, and *Rhizopus* are potential pathogens in immunocompromised patients or those

TABLE 10–9. Clinical Manifestations of Acute Hematogenous Osteomyelitis by Age Groups

| Age | Usual Site of Involvement | Symptoms and Signs | Expected Organism |
| --- | --- | --- | --- |
| Neonate | Varied; 40% may have multiple sites | Usually few systemic signs; local edema; reduced limb motion; joint effusion (60–70%) | Group B streptococci, *Escherichia coli*, *Staphylococcus aureus* or *Candida* |
| 1–24 mo | Long bones; may involve joints | Pseudoparalysis, fever, limp | *S. aureus*, group B streptococci |
| 2–20 yr | Metaphysis of long bones; rarely, vertebral bodies or pelvis | Focal pain with fever (90%) for days to weeks; focal tenderness (70%); focal swelling (70%) or joint effusion (20%) | *S. aureus* (60–90%), streptococci (10%), *Salmonella*; rarely, gram-negative bacilli, anaerobes, or fungi |

receiving long-term parenteral hyperalimentation and require appropriate antifungal therapy (amphotericin B).

The response to appropriate intravenous antibiotics usually occurs within 48 hr, and lack of improvement in fever and pain after this time indicates that surgical drainage may be necessary or that an unusual pathogen (*M. tuberculosis*) may be present. Surgical drainage may be appropriate at an earlier time if a sequestrum is present, if the disease is chronic or atypical, if the hip joint is involved, or if the disease occurs in the presence of spinal cord compression.

Standard therapy consists of administering antibiotics for 4–6 wk or longer. Oral antibiotics are effective after a good response to intravenous therapy (see Septic Arthritis). It is essential to ensure that patients are compliant with oral regimens, which may entail the assistance of social support services. In addition, there must be a good response to parenteral therapy (usually given for 7 days) and absorption, which is sufficient to produce serum bactericidal levels of 1:8–1:16 against the recovered organisms.

Inadequate or delayed antibiotic therapy of osteomyelitis often leads to chronic abscess formation, draining sinus tracts, pathologic fractures, orthopedic deformity, and amyloidosis.

## SEPTIC ARTHRITIS

Septic or suppurative arthritis is a serious infection of the joint space occurring most commonly during the first 2 yr of life and during adolescence.

*Pathogenesis.* Septic arthritis results from (1) hematogenous dissemination of bacteria, (2) contiguous spread from surrounding soft tissues, and (3) spread of osteomyelitis through the epiphysis into the joint space in young children (see Figs. 10–3 and 10–4). Septic arthritis must be differentiated from postinfectious joint effusions, which are sterile and often due to antigen-antibody complex deposition. Joint effusions developing after 7 days of a bacterial illness (bacteremia, meningitis, diarrhea, urethritis) more often are immunologically mediated, whereas those presenting in the first 3 days more often represent hematogenous spread of bacteria.

*Etiology.* S. aureus is the most common agent, followed by streptococci, pneumococci, and meningococci. Joint effusions may develop in patients with meningococcal sepsis and meningitis (see Pathogenesis). Meningococcal arthritis may occur in the absence of sepsis or meningitis. Gonococcal arthritis associated with disseminated gonococcal infection is the most common cause of polyarthritis or monoarticular arthritis in adolescents. In endemic areas, Lyme arthritis also must be considered. *H. influenzae* type b was the most common etiologic factor in children ages 3 mo to 4 yr but is now rarely seen in an immunized population.

*Clinical Manifestations.* The presentation has the typical features of infection: erythema, warmth, swelling, and tenderness over the affected joint, with a palpable effusion and decreased range of movement. The onset may be sudden, resulting in an ill-appearing child with fever and chills, or insidious, with symptoms only noted when the joint is moved, such as during a diaper change, or if parents become aware of decreased voluntary movement (pseudoparalysis) of a joint or limb. Toddlers may present with a limp. It is often difficult to assess septic arthritis of the hip, which may cause referred pain to the knee. The limb may be positioned in external rotation and flexion to minimize pain from pressure on the hip's joint capsule. Similarly, the knee and elbow joints usually are held in flexion. An acute septic arthritis most often involves a single joint (knee, hip, ankle, shoulder, elbow, wrist), with multiple joints affected in fewer than 10% of cases.

*Diagnosis and Differential Diagnosis.* Leukocytosis and an elevated ESR are common. Arthrocentesis is the test of choice for rapid diagnosis of suppurative arthritis (Table 10–10). During arthrocentesis, it is important to avoid crossing an overlying area of cellulitis to prevent the inoculation of bacteria and the conversion of a deep cellulitis into septic arthritis. Blood and/or joint cultures are positive in up to 85% of patients infected with *H. influenzae*. Joint fluid that exhibits the characteristics of pyogenic infection may not reveal bacterial pathogens in up to 30% of patients who have never received antibiotic therapy, because synovial fluid exerts a bacteriostatic effect. Gram stain, potassium hydroxide (KOH) preparation for fungi (neonates, immunosuppressed patients), and acid-fast stain are helpful if no bacteria are recovered. In chronic arthritis, synovial biopsy may distinguish between an infectious and a noninfectious process. Because septic arthritis may be present with osteomyelitis, roentgenograms or bone scans of the adjacent bone usually are indicated. Adolescents with acute septic arthritis should have urethral, cervical, rectal and pharyngeal culture examination for *N. gonorrhoea*.

The *differential diagnosis* of suppurative arthritis includes infections, postinfectious (Reiter syndrome rheumatic fever), and noninfectious (rheumatoid arthritis, SLE, and other collagen vascular diseases, serum sickness, and inflammatory bowel

TABLE 10–10. Synovial Fluid Findings in Various Joint Diseases

| Condition | Appearance | White Blood Cell Count (/µL) | Polymorphonuclear Cells (%) | Mucin Clot | Synovial Fluid–to–Blood Glucose Difference (mg/dL) | Comment |
|---|---|---|---|---|---|---|
| Normal | Clear, yellow | 0–200 (200)* | <10 | Good | No difference | — |
| Trauma | Clear, turbid, or hemorrhagic | 50–4000 (600) | <30 | Good | No difference | Common in hemophilia |
| Systemic lupus erythematosus | Clear or slightly turbid | 0–9000 (3000) | <20 | Good to fair | No difference | LE cell positive, complement decreased |
| Rheumatoid arthritis reactive arthritis (Reiter syndrome, inflammatory bowel disease) | Turbid | 250–80,000 (19,000) | >70 | Poor | 30 | Decreased complement |
| Infectious Pyogenic infection | Turbid | 10,000–250,000 (80,000) | >90 | Poor | 50–90 | Positive culture, positive Gram stain |
| Tuberculosis | Turbid | 2500–100,000 (20,000) | >60 | Poor | 40–70 | Positive culture, PPD, and acid-fast stain |
| Lyme arthritis | Turbid | 500–100,000 (20,000) | >60 | Poor | 70 | History of tick bite or erythema chronicum migrans |

*Average in parentheses.
LE = lupus erythematosus; PPD = purified protein derivative of tuberculin.

disease) diseases. Other entities that should be considered include Henoch-Schönlein purpura, leukemia, metabolic diseases involving joints, foreign bodies, and traumatic arthritis. Viral infections may cause arthritis (rubella, rubella vaccine, parvovirus, hepatitis B).

**Toxic tenosynovitis** of the hip is presumed to be viral in etiology and is a common condition of children ages 3–6 yr (see Chapter 19). This self-limited disorder is far more common than septic arthritis. Other bacterial infections causing arthritis including tuberculosis, syphilis, and Lyme disease. These must be considered in the child or adolescent with the signs of an acutely inflamed joint or joints but without typical findings of pyogenic infection.

*Treatment.* The therapy of septic arthritis is based on knowledge of the likely organism, the Gram stain of joint fluid, and the host's immunologic status. Parenteral antimicrobial agents are the mainstay of therapy, with surgical intervention reserved for specific situations. Pyogenic arthritis of the hip or shoulder caused by *S. aureus* usually requires prompt surgical drainage to prevent joint destruction and long-term sequelae. However, staphylococcal infection of the knee may be treated with repeated arthrocenteses to remove infected fluid and with continuation of appropriate parenteral antibiotics. Irrigation of the joints with antimicrobial agents is rarely, if ever, indicated. Infections caused by gonococci or meningococci rarely require surgical intervention in a normal host.

A number of antimicrobial agents are available that provide adequate antibiotic levels in joint spaces to eradicate the typical bacterial infections. For empiric therapy in the neonate, a cephalosporin with activity against staphylococci, group B streptococci, and aerobic gram-negative rods (cefotaxime or ticarcillin/clavulanate may be used, depending on the results of the joint fluid Gram stain. Infants aged 3 mo to 4 yr should receive antibiotics active against *S. aureus* and *H. influenzae* type b until culture results are known. These would include cefotaxime or ampicillin/sulbactam. Intravenous methicillin (nafcillin, oxacillin) is the treatment of choice for *S. aureus*; methicillin-resistant organisms are treated with vancomycin. The length of therapy depends on clinical resolution (afebrile, less pain) and reduction of the ESR. Infection with organisms such as *S. aureus* usually necessitates more lengthy treatment (14–21 days or more), whereas gonococcal or meningococcal arthritis responds to 7 days of penicillin. Ceftriaxone is preferred for gonococcal arthritis because of the large number of penicillin-resistant isolates. Treatment may be changed to oral antibiotics (see earlier, Osteomyelitis) for staphylococcal and other infec-

tions if compliance can be ensured. Oral agents with excellent activity against *S. aureus* include augmentin, cloxacillin, dicloxacillin, cephalexin, clindamycin, and ciprofloxacin (in older children); these are often used to complete therapy.

### References

Behrman RE, Kliegman RM, Arvin AM (eds): Nelson Textbook of Pediatrics, 15th ed. Philadelphia, WB Saunders, 1996, Chapter 172.
Lew D, Waldvogel F: Osteomyelitis. N Engl J Med 336:999, 1997.
Rodriguez AF, Kaplan SL: Outpatient management of skeletal infections in children. Semin Pediatr Infect Dis 1:365, 1990.

# CENTRAL NERVOUS SYSTEM INFECTIONS

## ACUTE BACTERIAL MENINGITIS BEYOND THE NEONATAL PERIOD

Meningitis is an inflammation of the leptomeninges. Although this may be caused by bacteria, viruses, or rarely fungi, bacterial meningitis is a common complication of septicemia in children and must be treated as an emergency. A limited number of bacteria are associated with meningitis in normal hosts; thus the principles of supportive management and the initial choice of antibiotics can be generalized. Meningitis during the neonatal period is discussed in Chapter 6.

*Etiology.* Bacterial meningitis in children 2 mo to 12 yr of age usually is due to *S. pneumoniae*, or *N. meningitidis*. *H. influenzae* type b was the most common cause of meningitis in children younger than 4 yr of age; the incidence of *H. influenzae* disease has decreased dramatically after the introduction of conjugated vaccine against the organism. Meningitis associated with ventricular-peritoneal shunts generally is due to coagulase-negative staphylococci or corynebacteria; meningitis in patients with an open neural tube defect may be due to *S. aureus* or enteric bacteria. Immunosuppressed patients with T-cell defects are susceptible to cryptococcal and *L. monocytogenes* meningitis. In patients with CSF leaks due to sinus fractures, pneumococcal meningitis is common, whereas in patients with penetrating head trauma or neurosurgical procedures, staphylococcal disease often develops.

*Epidemiology.* Bacterial meningitis occurs more frequently in the winter and spring, in more males than females, and most often between 2 mo and 2 yr of age. Close contact with a nasopharyngeal carrier (day care) or a patient ill with meningococcal infection has been associated with an increased risk of meningitis. Meningococcal disease often follows viral upper respiratory tract infections.

*Pathogenesis.* Bacterial meningitis is usually the result of hematogenous dissemination of microorganisms from a distant site of infection; bacteremia precedes the condition or occurs at the same time. Acquisition is by aerosol or droplet and leads to nasopharyngeal colonization, replication, invasion, and bacteremia. The hosts at risk for meningitis due to encapsulated organisms (*S. pneumoniae, H. meningitides, H. influenzae* type b) lack preformed anticapsular antibody. High-grade bacteremia is followed by meningeal seeding. Meningitis rarely may be due to bacterial spread from a contiguous focus of infection, such as sinusitis, otitis media, or mastoiditis. More often, brain, epidural, or subdural abscesses follow contiguous infections. Bacterial meningitis in children with otitis media generally follows bacteremia. Hematogenous spread to the meninges may occur with infective endocarditis, pneumonia, or thrombophlebitis. Because there is a direct communication between the skin and meninges, the meninges may be invaded from a dermoid sinus tract or meningomyelocele. Fracture of the cribriform plate and CSF rhinorrhea predispose to pneumoccal meningitis. Osteomyelitis of the skull or vertebral column also may produce meningitis.

Children with sickle cell anemia or asplenia have an increased incidence of meningitis caused by *S. pneumoniae.* Without antimicrobial prophylaxis, approximately 1 in 24 patients with sickle cell anemia develops pneumococcal meningitis prior to 4 yr of age. Terminal complement deficiency predisposes some children to *Neisseria* sepsis and meningitis.

The clinical manifestations of bacterial meningitis are due to the local immune response to unopposed bacterial replication, specifically to the immunogenic fragments of bacterial peptidoglycan. Endothelial cells and macrophages are activated, and local production of cytokines (IL-1β, TNF-α) is stimulated.

Neutrophil migration from capillaries is triggered, and the release of toxic neutrophil products further increases local damage. The ensuing inflammatory response increases the blood-brain barrier permeability, producing cerebral edema and increased intracranial pressure and activation of the coagulation system, producing local thrombosis and infarction. Increased CSF protein is due to this inflammatory response, whereas the reduced CSF glucose is due to alterations of the blood-brain barrier and increased CNS glucose utilization.

*Clinical Manifestations.* Manifestations of bacterial meningitis may be preceded by several days of upper respiratory tract symptoms. Rapid onset (<1 day) is common with *S. pneumoniae* or *N. meningitides,* whereas the course may be subacute (2–3 days) with *H. influenzae.* In young infants, signs of meningeal inflammation may be minimal; only irritability, restlessness, and poor feeding may be noted. Fever usually is present. Inflammation of the meninges is associated with headache, irritability, nausea, vomiting, anorexia, nuchal rigidity, lethargy, and, occasionally, photophobia. The older child may be confused, may complain of back pain, and usually demonstrates the Kernig and Brudzinski signs. Seizures and coma may occur.

Increased intracranial pressure is common and may be reflected in complaints of headache and diplopia. There may be a bulging fontanel. Ptosis, sixth nerve palsy, anisocoria, bradycardia with hypertension, and apnea are common signs of increased intracranial pressure and brain herniation, whereas a bulging fontanel usually is not associated with herniation. Papilledema is uncommon unless there are occlusions of the venous sinus, subdural empyema, or a brain abscess. Focal neurologic signs, arthralgia, myalgia, transient arthritis, anemia, petechial or purpuric lesions, and signs of DIC are additional manifestations.

*Diagnosis and Differential Diagnosis.* Lumbar puncture should be performed in every child when bacterial meningitis is suspected, except when signs (other than a bulging fontanel) of increased intracranial pressure are present. Infection at the lumbar puncture site, suspicion of a mass lesion, and extreme patient instability are other reasons to defer a spinal tap. CSF examination should include a WBC count, differential, protein and glucose levels, and Gram stain (Table 10–11). Specimens for culture should be obtained to look for bacteria and, when appropriate, for fungi, viruses, and mycobacteria. The Gram stain is helpful in 90% of patients with bacterial meningitis. Antigen detection methods may help with the diagnosis of bacterial meningitis due to *H. influenzae* type b, *S. pneumoniae,* and *N. meningitidis* groups A, C, D, X, Y, Z, and W 135 even if the patient was pretreated with antibiotics. Additional diagnostic tests include blood cultures (positive in 50–90% of patients), complete blood count, and sickle cell screening test.

Tuberculous meningitis, fungal meningitis, aseptic meningitis, spirochete infection (syphilis, Lyme disease), brain abscess, encephalitis, Rocky Mountain spotted fever, intracranial or spinal epidural abscesses, bacterial endocarditis with embolism, subdural empyema (with or without thrombophlebitis), subarachnoid hemorrhage, and brain tumors may mimic bacterial meningitis. The differentiation of these disorders depends on careful ex-

TABLE 10–11. Cerebrospinal Fluid (CSF) Findings in Various Central Nervous System Disorders

| Condition | Pressure | Leukocytes (/μL) | Protein (mg/dL) | Glucose (mg/dL) | Comments |
|---|---|---|---|---|---|
| Normal | 50–180 mm H$_2$O | <4; 60–70% lymphocytes, 30–40% monocytes, 1–3% neutrophils | 20–45 | >50 or 75% blood glucose | |
| Acute bacterial meningitis | Usually elevated | 100–60,000+; usually a few thousand; PMNs predominate | 100–500 | Depressed compared with blood glucose; usually <40 | Organism may be seen on Gram stain and recovered by culture |
| Partially treated bacterial meningitis | Normal or elevated | 1–10,000; PMNs usual but mononuclear cells may predominate if pretreated for extended period | 100+ | Depressed or normal | Organisms may be seen; pretreatment may render CSF sterile in pneumococcal and meningococcal disease, but antigen may be detected |
| Tuberculous meningitis | Usually elevated; may be low because of block in advanced stages | 10–500; PMNs early but lymphocytes predominate later | 100–500; may be higher in presence of block | <50 usual; decreases with time if treatment not provided | Acid-fast organisms may be seen on smear; organism can be recovered in culture or by PCR; PPD, chest x-ray positive |
| Fungal | Usually elevated | 25–500; PMNs early; mononuclear cells predominate later | 20–500 | <50, decreases with time if treatment not provided | Budding yeast may be seen; organism may be recovered in culture; India ink preparation or antigen may be positive in cryptococcal disease |
| Viral meningitis or meningoencephalitis | Normal or slightly elevated | PMNs early; mononuclear cells predominate later; rarely more than 1000 cells except in eastern equine | 20–100 | Generally normal; may be depressed to 40 in some viral diseases (15–20% of mumps) | Enteroviruses may be recovered from CSF by appropriate viral cultures |
| Abscess (parameningeal infection) | Normal or elevated | 0–100 PMNs unless rupture into CSF | 20–200 | Normal | Profile may be completely normal |

DNA = deoxyribonucleic acid; PMN = polymorphonuclear leukocyte; PPD = purified protein derivative of tuberculin.

amination of CSF and additional laboratory tests and roentgenographic studies (see Table 10–11).

*Treatment.* Treatment of bacterial meningitis focuses on decreasing the CNS damage caused by the inflammatory response, sterilization of the CSF by the use of appropriate antimicrobial agents that achieve cidal levels, and the maintenance of adequate CNS and systemic perfusion. As bacterial cell wall components elicit the damaging inflammatory response, the administration of dexamethasone (0.6 mg/kg every 6 hr for 2–4 days) beginning *prior to* the first dose of antibiotics is recommended for patients suspected of having *H. influenzae* meningitis and, possibly, for those having pneumococcal meningitis. Since the lysis of organisms, which occurs immediately after antimicrobial agents reach the CSF, triggers a huge cytokine response, the greatest benefit of steroids is in preventing this inflammatory response. The selection of empiric antimicrobial agents is also problematic. To cover *S. pneumoniae*, many of which are relatively resistant to penicillin (MIC 0.1–1.0 μg/ml), cefotaxime (200–300 mg/kg/24 hr) or ceftriaxone (100 mg/kg/24 hr) should be used *plus* vancomycin (60 mg/kg/24 hr) until antibiotic susceptibility testing is available. These higher doses are necessary to achieve adequate CSF levels in the presence of dexamethasone, which decreases penetration of these drugs across the blood-brain barrier. Alternatively, rifampin (20 mg/kg/24 hr) may be added to the β-lactam drug. A third-generation cephalosporin (cefotaxime or ceftriaxone) is also adequate to cover *N. meningitidis* or *H. influenzae* type b. For sensitive meningococci or pneumococci penicillin G (300,000 units/kg/24 hr) is recommended. For infants under age 2 mo, ampicillin (200 mg/kg every 6 hr) is added to cover the possibility of *L. monocytogenes.* Treatment for 7 days (meningococcus) or 10 days (*S. pneumoniae, H. influenzae*) is adequate because less antibiotic will cross the blood-brain barrier as the inflammation decreases.

*Supportive therapy* includes the treatment of shock, DIC, inappropriate antidiuretic hormone secretion, seizures, increased intracranial pressure, apnea, arrhythmias, and coma. Supportive therapy also includes the maintenance of adequate CNS perfusion in the presence of cerebral edema. Hypotension and hypoperfusion are much more common clinically than inappropriate antidiuretic hormone secretion, which may occur in severely ill patients. Subdural effusions (detected by CT scan) are common in infection with *H. influenzae* type b. Most subdural effusions are asymptomatic and do not require drainage unless associated with increased intracranial pressure or focal neurologic signs. Persistent fever is common with *H. influenzae*

type b infection but also may suggest a subdural effusion, pericardial or joint effusions, drug fever, thrombophlebitis, or nosocomial infection. Another lumbar puncture is not indicated for fever in the absence of other signs of persistent CNS infection.

*Prevention.* Chemoprophylaxis with rifampin for family contacts of individuals with *H. influenzae* type b and *N. meningitis* infections is recommended. Vaccines or prophylactic antibiotics against *N. meningitidis* are recommended for at-risk individuals, and routine immunization against *H. influenzae* is recommended for all infants (see Table 10–3 and 10–5).

*Prognosis.* Even with appropriate antibiotic therapy, the mortality rate for bacterial meningitis in children is significant (8%, *H. influenzae*; 15%, meningococcal; 25%, pneumococcal). As many as 35% of the survivors (particularly following pneumococcal infection) have some sequelae resulting from their disease, including, in order of frequency, deafness, seizures, learning disabilities, blindness, paresis, ataxia, or hydrocephalus. All patients with meningitis should have a hearing evaluation prior to discharge.

Poor prognosis is associated with (1) young age, (2) long duration of illness prior to effective antibiotic therapy, (3) late-onset seizures, (4) coma at presentation, (5) shock, (6) low or absent CSF WBC count in the presence of visible bacteria on Gram stain of the CSF, and (7) immunocompromised status.

*Relapse* may occur 3–14 days after treatment and is due to the same pathogen, possibly from parameningeal foci; *recrudescence* occurs during inappropriate therapy; and *recurrence* takes place later and may be due to the same or another pathogen, which suggests an underlying immunologic or anatomic defect that predisposes the patient to infection of the CNS.

## References

Behrman RE, Kliegman RM, Arvin AM (eds): Nelson Textbook of Pediatrics, 15th ed. Philadelphia, WB Saunders, 1996, Chapter 169.

Bonadio WA, Smith DS, Goddard S, et al: Distinguishing cerebrospinal fluid abnormalities in children with bacterial meningitis and traumatic lumbar puncture. J Infect Dis 162:251, 1990.

Pomeroy SL, Holmes SJ, Dodge PR, et al: Seizures and other neurologic sequelae of bacterial meningitis in children. N Engl J Med 323:1651, 1990.

Quagliarello V, Scheld W: Treatment of bacterial meningitis. N Engl J Med 336:708, 1997.

Spanos A, Harrell FE, Durack DT: Differential diagnosis of acute meningitis: An analysis of the predictive value of initial observations. JAMA 262:2700, 1989.

Tunkel AR, Scheld WM: Pathogenesis and pathophysiology of bacterial meningitis. Annu Rev Med 44:103, 1993.

Tuomanen EI, Austrian R, Masure HR: Pathogenesis of pneumococcal infection. N Engl J Med 332:1280, 1995.

## ACUTE ASEPTIC MENINGITIS

Aseptic meningitis, an acute inflammation of the meninges, is a common illness with many causes. CSF usually is characterized by lymphocytic pleocytosis, normal glucose, normal or slightly elevated protein levels, and absence of bacterial microorganisms on Gram stain or culture.

*Etiology.* Although an etiologic agent is not always identified, viruses are usually the responsible agents. Enteroviruses cause approximately 85% of all cases of aseptic meningitis; coxsackievirus B5 and echoviruses 4, 6, 9, and 11 are the most common types. St. Louis and California encephalitis viruses are the most commonly implicated arboviruses in the United States, accounting for 5–7% of all cases of aseptic meningitis. Other etiologic viral agents include human herpes virus 6 and 7, HIV, varicella, EBV, lymphocytic choriomeningitis, natural or vaccine-associated measles, mumps, rubella, or polio, rabies, influenza, and parainfluenza. A primary genital herpes simplex virus infection (type 2) in the adolescent can also be associated with a self-limited aseptic meningitis. Acute aseptic meningitis also may be caused by *Mycoplasma, Chlamydia,* various fungi and protozoa and other parasites as well as by postinfectious reactions to various viruses.

The most common cause of **nonviral aseptic meningitis** is partially or inappropriately treated bacterial disease; tuberculosis, parameningeal infections, toxoplasmosis, and Kawasaki disease should be considered. Less common causes include leptospirosis, syphilis, cryptococcosis, Lyme disease, Rocky Mountain spotted fever, malignancy, intracranial hemorrhage, and reactions to nonsteroidal anti-inflammatory drugs (NSAIDs), intravenous immunoglobulins, or trimethoprim/sulfamethoxazole.

*Epidemiology.* Because 85% of cases are a result of enteroviral infections, the epidemiologic pattern is typical of these agents. In temperate climates, most cases occur in the summer and fall. The epidemiology of aseptic meningitis due to other agents also depends on season, geography, climatic conditions, exposures to animals or insects, and other factors related to the specific pathogens.

*Clinical Manifestations.* The onset usually is acute, although it may be insidious or preceded by a nonspecific febrile illness. In older children, the initial manifestation is severe headache; in infants, it is irritability. Fever, nausea, and other neurologic complaints, such as vomiting, a stiff neck, photophobia, and retrobulbar pain, are frequent, but convulsions are uncommon. Examination often reveals nuchal rigidity without significant localizing neurologic signs. Exanthems that precede or accompany the infection may occur, especially in infections with echoviruses and coxsackieviruses. Parotitis or orchitis is noted with mumps, lymphadenopathy and hepatosplenomegaly with CMV, HIV, or EBV infections, and petechiae with Rocky Mountain spotted fever. The child with aseptic viral meningitis usually appears less ill than the child with bacterial meningitis; however, the two may be indistinguishable (see Table 10–6).

The disease may become manifest in a meningeal or an encephalitic pattern, but the children exhibiting the latter pattern have a great incidence of headache, confusion, altered consciousness, and seizures.

*Diagnosis.* The CSF contains a few to several thousand cells per microliter. Early in the disease, the cells may be polymorphonuclear; later, lymphocytes or mononuclear cells predominate (see Table 10–11). No organisms are seen on laboratory stain, and the protein level is normal to slightly elevated. The CSF glucose concentration is normal in most viral infections; glucose may be decreased with medulloblastoma, leukemia infiltration, *Mycoplasma pneumoniae* infection, inadequately treated bacterial meningitis, tuberculosis, and, rarely certain viral infections. Specimens for viral culture include CSF, throat swabs, and stool. Antigenic or genomic (PCR) methods also help determine the etiology. A serum specimen should be obtained early in the illness and again in 2–3 wk for serologic identification of the virus.

*Treatment.* Aseptic viral meningitis is usually a benign, self-limited disease. Hospitalization usually is necessary in young infants or more acutely ill children because of the possibility of bacterial disease. Treatment is supportive for viral meningitis except for aseptic meningitis caused by herpes simplex. Meningoencephalitis resulting from herpes simplex or complicated herpes zoster should be treated with acyclovir. Lyme disease should be treated with high-dose parenteral ceftriaxone. Headache, which may be severe in all cases of aseptic meningitis, should be treated with NSAIDs or mild narcotics, such as codeine.

## References

Behrman RE, Kliegman RM, Arvin AM (eds): Nelson Textbook of Pediatrics, 15th ed. Philadelphia, WB Saunders, 1996, Chapter 169.

Lyall E, Hons B, Hons C: Human herpes virus 6: Primary infection and the central nervous system. Pediatr Infect Dis J 15:693, 1996.

Walsh-Kelly C, Nelson D, Smith D, et al: Clinical predictors of bacterial versus aseptic meningitis in childhood. Ann Emerg Med 21:910, 1992.

Wildin S, Chonmaitree T: Importance of laboratory in the diagnosis and management of viral meningitis. Am J Dis Child 141:454, 1987.

## ENCEPHALITIS

Encephalitis is an inflammatory process of the brain parenchyma that is usually an acute process but may be a postinfectious encephalomyelitis, a chronic degenerative disease, or a slow virus infection. The diagnosis is established with absolute certainty by brain biopsy, but it usually is made in the presence of neurologic signs, epidemiologic data, and laboratory (CSF, electroencephalography [EEG], and brain imaging techniques) evidence of infection. Encephalitis may be diffuse or localized (e.g., cerebellar ataxia, brain stem encephalitis, a meningoencephalitis, meningoencephalomyeloradiculitis). There is considerable overlap between viral aseptic meningitis and meningoencephalitis. Neurologic manifestations suggestive of encephalitis but occurring in the absence of inflammation (intoxication, Reye syndrome, anoxia, inborn errors of metabolism) indicate **encephalopathy.**

*Etiology.* Encephalitis usually is caused by direct viral infection of the brain via a hematogenous or neuronal (peripheral or cranial) route. During epidemic seasons (summer or fall), arboviruses and enteroviruses are common pathogens. Other causes of encephalitis include varicella, mumps, measles, EBV, rubella, lymphocytic choriomeningitis, influenza, parainfluenza, adenovirus, and respiratory syncytial virus. Herpes simplex, the most common cause of sporadic encephalitis (herpes simplex virus [HSV] type I), is also a common encephalitis seen in neonates (HSV type II > type I). Cerebellar ataxia commonly is due to varicella virus. Postinfectious, allergic demyelinating encephalitis may follow either vaccination or a viral infection and is an autoimmune process. HIV is an increasingly common cause of encephalitis in children and may present as an acute febrile illness, but more commonly it is insidious in onset (see Human Immunodeficiency Virus Infection later in the chapter). Opportunistic CNS infections or lymphoma may also complicate HIV infection.

*Epidemiology.* St. Louis encephalitis virus, which is spread from the bird reservoir, is the most common arboviral (arthropod-borne) agent and is present throughout the United States. California encephalitis virus, common in the Midwest, is carried by rodents and spread by mosquitoes. The eastern equine encephalitis virus is limited to the East coast (mosquitoes, birds), whereas the western equine encephalitis virus is present throughout the Midwest and West (mosquitoes, birds). The spread of disease depends on the geographic area, season, arthropod vector, and animal reservoir. Epizootics in horses often precede human cases of eastern equine encephalitis, but the horse is not a direct source of disease to humans.

HSV infections account for approximately 10% of non-neonatal cases. Sporadic encephalitis caused by HSV occurs in newborn infants born to mothers with an active primary infection, or in adults as a primary infection or reactivation of latent virus (see Herpes Simplex Virus Infection).

Rabies is a rare but important cause of encephalitis in developing countries and is endemic in parts of the United States. In the northeast, raccoons may be infected; in the southeast, foxes and bats are potential sources. Management after exposure to potentially infected animals involves the aggressive postexposure use of vaccine plus hyperimmune globulin to prevent infection.

**Slow viral diseases** present months to years after infection with dementia, poor cognition, and personality changes; agents include HIV, natural or vaccine-related measles (subacute sclerosing panencephalitis), rubella, HSV (Mollaret meningitis), and papovavirus (progressive multifocal leukoencephalopathy). Slow CNS infection may be due to small proteinaceous particles (*prions*); illness includes Kuru or Creutzfeldt-Jakob disease. Slow viral or prion diseases are progressive and fatal; treatment is available only for HIV encephalopathy.

*Clinical Manifestations.* Signs and symptoms are similar to those in aseptic meningitis; in encephalitis, however, more abnormalities of mental function are noted. Headache and fever are associated with confusion, delirium, irritability, hallucinations, memory loss, combativeness, coma, seizures (sometimes focal), ataxia, and signs of increased intracranial pressure.

*Diagnosis and Differential Diagnosis.* A patient's history should take into account possible exposures to persons and animals with illnesses, to mosquitoes, and to ticks; the history also should note any extent of travel. Encephalopathy due to toxins, hypoglycemia, hypervitaminosis A, Reye syndrome, inborn errors of metabolism, or trauma should be considered. A patient with concurrent or recent mumps, measles, or varicella is at risk for infectious or postinfectious encephalitis; neurologic involvement may precede the development of other manifestations of these diseases.

Bacterial diseases to be considered include mycoplasmal infection, tuberculosis, syphilis, leptospirosis, rickettsia, Lyme disease, cat-scratch disease, and borreliosis. Parasites associated with encephalitis include *Toxoplasma gondii*, trypanosomiasis, cysticercosis, and malaria. Cryptococcal disease presents as an encephalitis and is common in older children with HIV infection. Noninfectious causes of an encephalitic disease include malignancy, sarcoidosis, Kawasaki disease, and primary CNS or systemic vasculitis.

Examination of the CSF in viral encephalitis usually reveals abnormalities. The findings may resemble those in aseptic meningitis, with elevated protein and lymphocytosis. Increased erythrocytes may be seen with HSV, whereas extreme elevations of protein and reductions of glucose should suggest tuberculosis or cryptococcal infection. The diagnosis of cryptococcal disease can be made by India ink smear and determination of CSF cryptococcal antigen. The EEG, CT scan, and MRI may be nonspecific, but in HSV infection they often reveal a temporal lobe focus. There are many causes of temporal lobe disease, and when HSV is suspected on clinical grounds, biopsy confirms the diagnosis in only 40–50% of cases. Viral cultures of the nasopharynx, rectum, and CSF for HSV occasionally are helpful. PCR has been most valuable in rapid diagnosis of HSV encephalitis. In many cases of viral encephalitis, paired serology of plasma is needed to determine a rise of specific antibodies. Brain biopsy may be necessary for definitive diagnosis, especially in patients with focal neurologic findings or at risk for CNS lymphoma or toxoplasmosis (both treatable).

*Treatment.* For HSV infections, acyclovir is the treatment of choice (see Appendix I). HIV infections may be treated with zidovudine and other antiretroviral agents. *M. pneumoniae* infections may be treated with doxycycline, erythromycin, azithromycin, or clarithromycin. Supportive care is extremely important to decrease elevated intracranial pressure and maintain cardiopulmonary function.

*Prognosis.* Most children with encephalitis recover without major sequelae. Disease caused by HSV, rabies, or *M. pneumoniae* is associated with a poorer prognosis. Encephalitis may be severe in young children (<1 yr) and those presenting with coma. Although most patients with epidemic forms of encephalitis (St. Louis, California, and enteroviral infections) do well, eastern equine encephalitis has a poorer outcome.

## References

Behrman RE, Kliegman RM, Arvin AM (eds): Nelson Textbook of Pediatrics, 15th ed. Philadelphia, WB Saunders, 1996, Chapter 169.

Cinque P, Cleator G, Weber T, et al: The role of laboratory investigation in the diagnosis and management of patients with suspected herpes simplex encephalitis: A consensus report. J Neurol Neurosurg Psychiatry 61:339, 1996.

Jeffery K, Read S, Peto T, et al: Diagnosis of viral infections of the central nervous system: Clinical interpretation of PCR results. Lancet 349:313, 1997.

Rautonen J, Koskiniemi M, Vaheri A: Prognostic factors in childhood acute encephalitis. Pediatr Infect Dis J 10:441, 1991.

# RESPIRATORY TRACT INFECTIONS

## UPPER RESPIRATORY TRACT INFECTIONS

### Ear Infections

**Otitis Externa ("Swimmers' Ear").** This is an acute infection of the external auditory canal. Trauma or prolonged exposure to moisture predisposes to infection. *P. aeruginosa* is the leading cause, followed by *S. aureus* and other skin flora. The child has severe unilateral pain localized to the ear. There is exquisite tenderness on manipulation of the pinna or tragus, a finding not observed in patients with otitis media. In otitis externa, the tympanic membrane is normal, whereas the canal is erythematous. **Malignant otitis externa** is noted in patients with diabetes and presents as a severe cellulitis due to *P. aeruginosa.* Rarely, herpes zoster may produce otitis externa.

The *differential diagnosis* includes the presence of a foreign body, such as small toys or insects, trauma, and referred pain. *Treatment* of uncomplicated otitis externa includes irrigation and topical antibiotics. For abscess formation, incision and drainage are required; for severe cellulitis, parenteral antistaphylococcal and antipseudomonas antibiotics are necessary.

**Otitis Media.** This is a suppurative infection of the middle ear cavity and is most common in healthy children between 6 mo and 2 yr of age; in certain high-risk populations, such as children with HIV, cleft palate, and Down syndrome; and in Eskimos and Native Americans. Otitis media is also more common in boys, in patients of lower socioeconomic status, in formula-fed infants, and in the winter months.

*Pathogenesis.* Bacteria gain access to the middle ear when the normal patency of the eustachian tube is blocked by local infection, pharyngitis, or hypertrophied adenoids. Air trapped in the middle ear is reabsorbed, creating negative pressure in this cavity, which permits reflux of bacteria. This bacterial reflux, plus obstruction of the flow of secretions from the middle ear to the pharynx, results in a middle ear effusion that becomes infected by nasopharyngeal bacteria. The common bacterial pathogens include the pneumococci, nontypable *H. influenzae, Moraxella catarrhalis,* and, less frequently, group A streptococci. Relatively resistant (penicillin, MIC 0.1–1.0 μg/mL) and highly resistant *S. pneumoniae* (penicillin, MIC >2 μg/mL) are being isolated with increasing frequency from young children, particularly those who attend day care. Bacteria recovered from the nasopharynx do not correlate with those isolated by tympanocentesis. Viruses (respiratory syncytial virus [RSV], CMV, rhinovirus) have been recovered as copathogens or alone in 20–25% of patients.

*Clinical Manifestations.* Patients with otitis media are febrile and irritable and may pull at their ears. The disease usually occurs 1–7 days following a nasopharyngitis. Vomiting, diarrhea, a bulging fontanel, vertigo, tinnitus, and a draining ear (with tympanic membrane perforation) also may be seen. The normal eardrum moves freely when negative or positive pressure is generated by the otoscope; it appears pink and translucent, and a cone of reflected light usually is noted radiating from the center to the anteroinferior margin. The otoscope examination in otitis media reveals a bulging, immobile, erythematous tympanic membrane, with loss of identifiable landmarks such as the short process and handle of the malleus. Perforation of the tympanic membrane also may occur and usually is associated with acute relief of pain. Otitis media may be associated with an ipsilateral conjunctivitis; both usually are due to nontypable *H. influenzae.*

*Treatment.* Oral antibiotics frequently used to treat otitis media include amoxicillin, amoxicillin-clavulanate, trimethoprim/sulfamethoxazole, and erythromycin/sulfisoxazole. Oral cephalosporins (cefaclor, cefuroxime, cefixime, cefpodoxime, cefprozil, loracarbef) have also been approved for the treatment of otitis media caused by β-lactamase–producing organisms and have convenient once-a-day or twice-a-day dosing schedules, although they are expensive. *S. pneumoniae* remains the most common significant pathogen causing acute otitis media; relatively and highly resistant pneumococci that are not susceptible to the above agents are increasingly frequent causes of infection. Higher doses of amoxicillin/clavulanate or clindamycin or a single dose of parenteral ceftriaxone may be efficacious, but there are no generally agreed on regimens for therapy of otitis media caused by highly resistant pneumococci. Tympanocentesis may be needed in difficult to treat patients or those who do not respond to therapy (see Appendix I).

Decongestants or antihistamines are not effective alone or when combined with antibiotics. *Complications* of otitis media include hearing loss, chronic effusion, cholesteatoma formation (mass-like keratinized epithelial growth), petrositis, and mastoiditis.

**Acute mastoiditis** is a suppurative complication of otitis media, with inflammation and potential destruction of the mastoid air spaces. The disease progresses from a periostitis to an osteitis with abscess formation and draining tracts (e.g., through the tympanic membrane or into the neck). Posterior auricular tenderness and swelling and erythema, in addition to the signs of otitis media, are present. The pinna is displaced downward and outward. Roentgenograms or CT of the mastoid reveals clouding of the air cells, demineralization, or bone destruction. Bacteria that cause acute otitis media are also those responsible for acute mastoiditis. *S. aureus, P. aeruginosa,* and anaerobic bacteria may be recovered in chronic cases. Culturing swabs of the external ear is not as specific as obtaining fluid by tympanocentesis, aspiration of posterior auricular cellulitis or the mastoid at surgery, or, rarely, a blood culture.

*Treatment* includes systemic antibiotics and incision and drainage if the disease has progressed to abscess formation.

## Nasopharyngitis

**Rhinorrhea (Nasal Discharge).** This is a common manifestation of infectious, allergic, or mechanical conditions. Infectious rhinitis is associated with a mucopurulent discharge that contains polymorphonuclear leukocytes and is due to rhinovirus and other respiratory viruses, such as RSV. Low-grade fever, nasal stuffiness, and sneezing may be present. Hypersensitivity to allergens is another common cause of rhinitis and is characterized by eosinophils in the discharge and by other allergic manifestations, such as allergic shiners; nasal polyps; a pale, edematous, nasal turbinate mucosa; and a transverse crease on the nasal bridge (see Chapter 8). Other less common causes of rhinorrhea include foreign body, choanal atresia, vasomotor rhinitis, CSF fistula, diphtheria, tumor, congenital syphilis, and Wegener granulomatosis. Persistent rhinorrhea following a cold should suggest sinusitis.

The *treatment* of viral rhinorrhea is usually supportive, with normal saline nose drops, steam, and, occasionally, decongestants.

**Sinusitis.** This is a suppurative infection of the paranasal sinuses and often complicates the common cold and allergic rhinitis. Patients with cyanotic heart disease, cystic fibrosis, immunoglobulin deficiency (total or subclass), HIV infection, nasotracheal intubation, immotile cilia syndrome, and dental infection have an increased incidence of sinusitis. It is also a frequent problem in immunocompromised children following organ transplantation. The maxillary, ethmoid, and sphenoid sinuses are present at birth, whereas the frontal sinus develops at 1 yr of life. Pneumatization of the sinuses is delayed relative to sinus formation; the frontal sinuses may not appear as air-filled spaces until 10 yr of age.

*Etiology.* Obstruction to mucociliary flow (preceding viral rhinitis) predisposes to bacterial proliferation. The bacteria producing acute sinusitis include pneumococci, nontypable *H. influenzae, M. catarrhalis*, anaerobic bacteria, and, rarely, streptococci and staphylococci. Nosocomial sinusitis occurs in children with indwelling nasogastric tubes and may be due to gram-negative bacteria (*Klebsiella, Pseudomonas, Enterobacter*); antibiotic-resistant organisms are often selected out by prior systemic antibiotic therapy. Neutropenic immunosuppressed patients may develop sinusitis as a result of infection by *Aspergillus* species or Zygomycetes. Culture of the nasal mucosa is not helpful in identifying the responsible bacteria. If necessary, antral puncture (for maxillary sinusitis) is the diagnostic procedure of choice.

*Clinical Manifestations.* These include persistent mucopurulent rhinorrhea; cough (especially at night); nasal stuffiness; nasal quality to voice; facial swelling, tenderness, and pain; and headache. Transillumination of the sinuses and sinus roentgenograms or CT reveals clouding or an air-fluid level. Sinus aspiration usually is not needed in patients with uncomplicated sinusitis.

*Treatment.* Amoxicillin or amoxicillin/clavulanate is usually effective in the treatment of uncomplicated sinusitis (see Appendix I). *Complications* should be treated with drainage and, if indicated, broad-spectrum parenteral antibiotics; these complications include orbital cellulitis, epidural or subdural empyema, brain abscess, dural sinus thrombosis, osteomyelitis of the outer or inner table of the frontal sinus (Pott's puffy tumor), and meningitis. Sinusitis also may exacerbate bronchoconstriction in asthmatic patients.

**Orbital Cellulitis.** This is a complication of sinusitis following spread of bacteria into the orbit through the wall of the infected sinus. Typically, ethmoid sinusitis spreads through the lamina papyracea, a thin bony plate that separates the orbit and the ethmoid sinus. Infection of the extraocular structures of the orbit progresses in stages from (1) an inflammatory edema to (2) orbital cellulitis (edema plus chemosis; mild proptosis; limited extraocular muscle motion, with or without reduced

visual acuity), to (3) a subperiosteal abscess (down-and-out position of globe in proptosis, resulting from abscess formation in periosteum), to (4) an orbital abscess (involvement of the orbital fat, muscle, and posterior cone of the orbit; severe ophthalmoplegia; vision loss; proptosis), to (5) cavernous sinus thrombosis (headache; nuchal rigidity; involvement of cranial nerves III, IV, V, and VI). The patient often has a high fever, orbital pain, limited extraocular motion (ophthalmoplegia), decreased vision, and proptosis. Infection of the orbit must be differentiated from that of the preseptal space (anterior to palpebral fascia, separating the eyelids and the orbit) or periorbital space. **Periorbital cellulitis** (preseptal) usually occurs in young children (<2 yr of age) who may, like those with orbital cellulitis, have fever, lid swelling, and appear toxic but do not have ophthalmoplegia or proptosis. These infections may be due to hematogenous infection (*S. pneumoniae; H. influenzae* type b is rarely seen in immunized children). Periorbital (preseptal) cellulitis may be a complication of sinusitis caused by the bacteria typically associated with sinusitis (*S. pneumoniae*, nontypable *H. influenzae, M. catarrhalis*) and the anaerobic organisms found in the upper respiratory tract. Periorbital cellulitis due to trauma is more often due to *S. aureus* or *S. pyogenes*.

*Diagnosis.* Orbital cellulitis is confirmed by a CT scan of the orbit. This essential examination determines the extent of orbital infection and the need for surgical drainage. Additional laboratory studies include blood culture, ESR, and CBC. Disorders to be considered in the differential diagnosis include mucormycosis, orbital aspergillosis, rhabdomyosarcoma, neuroblastoma, Wegener granulomatosis, inflammatory pseudotumor of the orbit, and trichinosis.

*Treatment.* Therapy for orbital cellulitis includes broad-spectrum parenteral antibiotics, such as oxacillin and ceftriaxone (see Appendix I). Draining the infected sinus or orbital abscess also is indicated in complicated cases.

**Pharyngitis (Pharyngotonsillitis).** Patients present with cough, sore throat, dysphagia, and fever. Pharyngitis is one of the most common pediatric infections. Inflammation confined to the pharynx is unusual, but if involvement of the tonsils is prominent, the term *tonsillitis* is used.

*Etiology.* Pharyngitis in children younger than 2 yr of age is often viral; group A streptococci are more common in children over age 5 yr, and *Mycoplasma*, gonococcus, and *Arcanobacterium haemolyticum* are more common among adolescents. Viral pathogens include rhinovirus, coronavirus, adenovirus, enteroviruses, EBV, CMV, and

HSV; the bacterial agent is predominantly group A streptococcus, which may be recovered from only 10–20% of patients. Less common causes include group C or G streptococcus, *Corynebacterium diphtheriae,* tularemia, toxoplasmosis, and gonorrhea.

*Clinical Manifestations.* Examination of the throat reveals erythema, exudate, palatine petechiae, enlarged tonsils, and, occasionally, anterior cervical lymphadenopathy. This appearance does not differentiate bacterial pathogens from viral pathogens. Nonetheless, vesiculation and ulceration suggest HSV and coxsackieviruses (herpangina); concomitant conjunctivitis suggests adenovirus; a gray-white fibrinous pseudomembrane with marked cervical swelling (bull neck), with or without carditis or neuropathy, suggests diphtheria; and a macular rash suggests group A beta-hemolytic streptococci (scarlet fever) or, less frequently, *A. haemolyticum.*

Rare *complications* of pharyngitis are anaerobic sepsis, usually due to *Fusobacteria,* extension to oropharyngeal or retropharyngeal spaces, peritonsillar abscess, and septic thrombophlebitis of the internal jugular vein (**Lemierre syndrome**). These latter patients present with painful adenopathy in the neck and often have evidence of metastatic foci of infection such as pneumonia.

*Diagnosis.* The diagnosis of streptococcal pharyngitis is made by throat culture or by rapid streptococcal antigen detection kits. It is important to identify streptococcal pharyngitis in all children because treatment (1) reduces symptoms; (2) prevents the poststreptococcal sequela of acute rheumatic fever; (3) prevents local suppurative complications; and (4) identifies the possibility of, but does not prevent the development of, the poststreptococcal sequela of acute glomerulonephritis. A CBC and heterophil testing may be used in the diagnosis of infectious mononucleosis, whereas cold agglutinins may be useful for mycoplasmal infection. Streptococcal pharyngitis may be present in 25% of patients with mononucleosis.

The *differential diagnosis* of infectious pharyngitis includes other local infections of the oral cavity, retropharyngeal abscesses (*S. aureus,* streptococci, anaerobes), peritonsillar abscess (quinsy sore throat; unilateral tonsil swelling; infections caused by streptococci, anaerobes, or, rarely, *S. aureus*), Ludwig angina (anaerobic bacterial cellulitis of the floor of the mouth, which may be due to an odontogenic source), and epiglottitis (see Chapter 12). In addition, neutropenic mucositis (leukemia, aplastic anemia), thrush (candidiasis secondary to T cell immune deficiency), autoimmune ulceration (SLE, Behçet disease), and Kawasaki disease may cause pharyngitis. Signs suggesting that the disease is not a simple pharyngitis include persistent clinical manifestations for more than 1 wk, stridor, trismus, poor clearance of secretions, difficulty in swallowing, pain in the absence of erythema, presence of a mass, and blood in the pharynx.

*Treatment.* The treatment of choice for group A streptococcal pharyngitis is penicillin. These organisms have remained highly penicillin-susceptible. Erythromycin (clarithromycin, azithromycin) is an acceptable alternative and is also active against *Mycoplasma* and *A. haemolyticum.* Failure to eradicate pharyngeal carriage of group A streptococci may be due to colonization with β-lactamase producing anaerobes, which destroy penicillin locally. Administration of clindamycin or amoxicillin/clavulanate usually eradicates the group A streptococci in these instances. Peritonsillar abscesses may be treated initially with high-dose penicillin and aspiration; following resolution of these abscesses, tonsillectomy may be indicated. Retropharyngeal abscesses frequently warrant drainage and the addition of antistaphylococcal antibiotics. Ludwig angina and other odontogenic infections may be treated with high-dose penicillin.

**Epiglottitis.** See Chapter 12.

## References

Alvarez A, Schreiber JR: Lemierre's syndrome in adolescent children: Anaerobic sepsis with internal jugular vein thrombophlebitis following pharyngitis. Pediatrics 96:354, 1995.

Behrman RE, Kliegman RM, Arvin AM (eds): Nelson Textbook of Pediatrics, 15th ed. Philadelphia, WB Saunders, 1996, Chapters 327, 332, 589, 596.

de Marie S, Tjon A, Tham RTO, van der Mey AGL, et al: Clinical infections and nonsurgical treatment of parapharyngeal space infections complicating throat infection. Rev Infect Dis 11:975, 1989.

Giebink GS, Canafax DM, Kempthorne J: Antimicrobial treatment of acute otitis media. J Pediatr 119:495, 1991.

Israele V, Nelson J: Periorbital and orbital cellulitis. Pediatr Infect Dis 6:404, 1987.

Komaroff AL, Aronson MD, Pass TM, et al: Serlogic evidence of chlamydial and mycoplasmal pharyngitis in adults. Science 222:927, 1993.

Ogle J, Laver B: Acute mastoiditis. Am J Dis Child 140:1178, 1986.

Shoemaker M, Lampe R, Weir M: Peritonsillitis: Abscess or cellulitis? Pediatr Infect Dis 5:435, 1986.

Shulman ST, Gerber MA, Tanz RR, et al: Streptococcal pharyngitis: The case for penicillin therapy. Pediatr Infect Dis J 13:1, 1994.

Waagner DC: *Arcanobacterium haemolyticum.* Biology of the organism and diseases in man. Pediatr Infect Dis J 10:933, 1991.

Wald ER: Sinusitis in children. N Engl J Med 326:319, 1992.

# LOWER RESPIRATORY TRACT INFECTIONS

## Bronchiolitis

See Chapter 12.

Pneumonia

See Chapter 12.

## URINARY TRACT INFECTIONS

See Chapter 16.

## BACTERIAL INFECTIONS

### ANTIBIOTIC THERAPY

#### Dosages

See Appendix I.

#### Principles

The chemotherapy of bacterial infections depends on the isolation of the offending agent, characterization of the agent's antibiotic susceptibility, and delivering the appropriate antibiotic to the site of infection in sufficient quantities to either kill the bacteria (bactericidal) or alter it to permit the body's immune response to eventually kill it. The two major strategies are as follows:

1. To use broad-spectrum, empiric antibiotics in high-risk situations, such as neonatal sepsis or bacteremia in an immunocompromised host.
2. To tailor antibiotic treatment to the specific pathogen in lower risk, immunocompetent patients. This second principle minimizes drug toxicity, the development of resistant microorganisms, superinfection by fungi and previously resistant bacteria, and cost to the family.

Antibiotic efficacy may be affected by several host factors. Antimicrobial agents are an adjunct to the host immune response. Infections of a foreign body, such as an intravascular catheter or a prosthetic device, are difficult to eradicate because polymorphonuclear leucocytes and macrophages do not readily engulf organisms on plastic surfaces. Similarly, in endocarditis it is difficult for phagocytic cells to eradicate bacteria amid vegetations of fibrin and platelets on infected heart valves. For these types of infections to be sterilized, prolonged therapy with bactericidal antibiotics is required and does not always result in a satisfactory outcome. Chronic osteomyelitis, with organisms sequestered from the circulation in abscesses or poorly perfused bone, is similarly difficult to cure

without surgical débridement of the infected tissue and re-establishment of a good vascular supply. Antimicrobial therapy alone may not cure infections in closed spaces with limited perfusion.

Optimal antimicrobial therapy requires an understanding of the pharmacokinetic properties of the drugs being administered to specific patient populations. Dosing schedules in the premature neonate take into account immaturity of renal function by increasing dosing intervals. In patients with cystic fibrosis, who often have larger volume of distribution of the hydrophilic antibiotics as well as increased renal clearance, larger doses are required to achieve therapeutic levels. Obese children may receive significant antibiotic overdoses if they are given dosage regimens on a per-kilogram basis that exceed the maximal adult doses recommended. These patients may have a significantly smaller volume of distribution for hydrophillic drugs and do not necessarily require as large doses as a leaner child of equivalent weight.

Another variable affecting antimicrobial therapy is the oral absorption of drugs. The bioavailability of orally administered antibiotics is highly variable, depending on the acid stability of the antimicrobial agent, the amount of gastric acidity, and whether the drug is taken with food, antacids, $H_2$ blockers, or other medications.

The site of infection is another important consideration. Aminoglycosides, which are only active against aerobic organisms, have significantly reduced activity in abscesses and milieus with low pH and oxygen tension. Infections of the CNS or the eye require treatment with antimicrobial agents that are able to penetrate and achieve levels in these sites.

Drug interactions must be considered when multiple antimicrobial agents are used to treat infection. For the empiric treatment of life-threatening infection, the use of two or more antimicrobial agents may be justified when broad-spectrum activity is needed prior to the identification of the organism. A few indications remain for the continuation of two drugs to treat infection, such as the use of a cell wall active agent (β-lactam or vancomycin) plus an aminoglycoside to effectively treat infections due to the highly resistant enterococci. Similarly, two drugs with different mechanisms of action are used against serious *P. aeruginosa* infections. Several drugs are dispensed together (trimethoprim–sulfamethoxazole, amoxicillin/clavulanate, ampicillin/sulbactam, ticarcillin/clavulanate) since the activity of the antibiotics in combination is significantly greater than when used alone. The addition of clavulanic acid (a β-lactamase inhibitor with modest antibacterial activity) to amoxicillin broadens the spectrum of the penicillin, allowing it to be used against gram-negative β-lactamase producers, such as *H. influenzae,* gram-positive organisms, such as *S. aureus,* and anaerobes. The use of a bacteriostatic drug, such as a tetracycline along with a β-lactam agent (which is only effective against growing organisms), may result in antibiotic *antagonism,* that is, less bacterial killing in the presence of both drugs than if either were used alone.

### Selection of Antibiotics

The choice of antibiotics depends on the epidemiology of the condition, site of infection, localizing manifestations (see Table 10–1), host factors, the need for antibiotic prophylaxis (see Table 10–5), and the spectrum of bacterial pathogens susceptible to the antibiotic (Table 10–12). The treatment of specific bacterial infections is covered in the following text.

## ANAEROBIC INFECTIONS OTHER THAN CLOSTRIDIAL

*Etiology.* Anaerobic bacteria are ubiquitous and are usually harmless commensal members of the normal human flora of the oropharynx, gastrointestinal tract, vagina, and skin. The fecal flora contains as many as 500 different species of anaerobes. Obligate anaerobes require special culture media to grow. Gram-negative nonsporulating rods include *Bacteroides* and *Fusobacterium* species; gram-positive nonsporulating rods include *Eubacterium* and *Propionibacterium*; cocci include *Peptostreptococcus, Peptococcus,* and *Veillonella.*

*Epidemiology.* Blood, peritoneum, oropharynx, lungs, and soft tissues are the main sites of anaerobic infection. Infection follows disruption of mucous membrane barriers. Several anaerobes, or both anaerobes and aerobes, may be recovered concomitantly from infected tissue. The major clinical settings for anaerobic infection are:

1. In the neonate following prolonged rupture of the membranes, amnionitis, or obstetric difficulty.
2. Peritonitis or septicemia associated with intestinal obstruction or perforation (appendicitis).
3. Aspiration pneumonia with lung abscess.
4. Salpingitis and tubo-ovarian abscess.
5. Orofacial infections.
6. Brain abscess.

*Clinical Manifestations.* Anaerobic infections of the *upper respiratory tract* have many different clinical manifestations. Periodontal infection ("trench mouth") often is due to poor dental hygiene. Periapical abscesses or anaerobic osteomyelitis of the mandible or maxilla may be present. Anaerobic microorganisms may be present in chronic sinusitis, chronic otitis media, mastoiditis, peritonsillar and retropharyngeal abscesses, and cervical lymphadenitis. Fusobacteria are important in the development of **Vincent stomatitis,** an infection characterized by ulcers covered by a brown or gray, foul-smelling exudate. Extensive tissue destruction can result in perforation of the carotid artery. **Ludwig angina** is an acute cellulitis of the sublingual and submandibular spaces that tends to spread rapidly without lymph node involvement or abscess formation. Edema of the tongue and airway may cause respiratory obstruction and require tracheotomy.

Anaerobic infection of the *lower respiratory tract* produces necrotizing pneumonia, putrid empyema, or lung abscess. A history of aspiration may be elicited. Aspiration pneumonia is a common problem in neurologically impaired children who may have repeated episodes of inapparent aspiration and less well-defined areas of pneumonia.

Anaerobic infection of the *CNS* produces brain abscess, subdural empyema, or septic thrombophlebitis of cortical veins and venous sinuses. These lesions originate by direct spread from a contiguous infection or by hematogenous spread. Purulent meningitis rarely is caused by anaerobes; identification of anaerobes from the CSF indicates another focus, such as a brain abscess or subdural empyema.

Peritoneal spillage of gastrointestinal contents, especially that of the colon, is associated with a high incidence of anaerobic *intra-abdominal infection.* Peritonitis and abscess formation (subdiaphragmatic, pelvic) are common after intestinal perforation. In sexually active adolescents, anaerobes are an important component of pelvic inflammatory disease in addition to the typical sexually transmitted pathogens, *N. gonorrhoeae* and *C. trachomatis,* and contribute to the formation of tubo-ovarian abscesses.

Anaerobic *bacteremia* is clinically indistinguishable from aerobic bacteremia. Anaerobic bacteremia frequently is associated with disease of the gastrointestinal and genitourinary systems.

*Diagnosis.* The diagnosis of anaerobic infection requires an awareness of anaerobe-associated infections and appropriate collection of specimens for cultures, with the use of special media and techniques. Factors that should increase the suspicion of an anaerobic infection include:

TABLE 10–12.  Commonly Used Antibiotics for Bacterial Infection

| Antibiotic | Mechanism of Action/Activity | Sensitive Bacteria/Indications | Comments |
|---|---|---|---|
| *Penicillins* | Bind to penicillin-binding proteins; inhibit transpeptidation reaction of cell wall, causing eventual cell lysis | | No activity for *Staphylococcus epidermidis, Mycoplasma, Chlamydia* |
| Penicillin | | Pneumococcus, meningococcus, gonococcus, streptococci, anaerobic bacteria (*Bacteroides melaninogenicus*), *Pasteurella multocida, Actinomyces* sp. | Penicillinase-producing *Gonococcus; Pneumococcus,* and some anaerobes are resistant |
| Ampicillin/ amoxicillin | Extended spectrum; beta-lactamase susceptible | *Haemophilus influenzae, Listeria monocytogenes, Escherichia coli, Salmonella, Shigella, Proteus mirabilis, Enterococcus* | Many of these organisms produce beta-lactamases and are resistant |
| Ticarcillin | Antipseudomonas | *E. coli, Pseudomonas aeruginosa, Proteus* sp. | Ureidopenicillins not beta-lactamase stable |
| Piperacillin/ tazobactam | Antipseudomonas | *P. aeruginosa, Klebsiella, Citrobacter, Acinetobacter, S. aureus,* anaerobes | Ureidopenicillins, tazobactam stable to penicillinases |
| Oxacillin/methicillin or nafcillin | Antistaphylococcus | *Staphylococcus aureus,* pneumococcus, *Streptococcus* | Penicillinase-resistant penicillins; *S. epidermidis* is usually resistant |
| Amoxicillin/ clavulanic acid | Extended spectrum | As for ampicillin, plus *S. aureus, Enterococcus, Bacteroides fragilis, Moraxella catarrhalis* | Clavulanic acid inhibits beta-lactamases; PO prep |
| Ampicillin/sulbactam | Extended spectrum | As for amoxicillin/clavulanic acid, plus anaerobes | Sulbactam inhibits β-lactamase; IV prep |
| Ticarcillin/clavulanic acid | Extended spectrum | As above, plus broader gram-negative coverage | IV prep |
| *Cephalosporins* | Bind to penicillin-binding proteins; inhibit cell wall cross-linking; produce cell lysis | | No activity against *Listeria* or *Enterococcus* |
| *1st generation* Cefazolin or cephalothin | | *S. aureus, E. coli, Klebsiella* | Good for *S. aureus,* other gram-positive organisms; *H. influenzae* type b is resistant |
| *2nd generation* Cefuroxime | Beta-lactamase stable | *H. influenzae* type b, *S. aureus, Klebsiella, E. coli* | |
| *Cephamycins* Cefoxitin, cefotetan | Anaerobic coverage | *B. melaninogenicus, Bacteroides fragilis, E. coli,* gonococcus | Abdominal and genital tract infections |
| *3rd generation* Cefotaxime or ceftriaxone | Extended spectrum | *E. coli, Klebsiella,* gonococcus, *H. influenzae,* pneumococcus, meningococcus, *S. aureus* | Better gram-negative enteric coverage, good CSF penetration |
| Ceftazidime, cefoperazone | Broad spectrum | Same as above, gram-negative plus *Pseudomonas;* not uniformly active against *B. cepacia* | Resistance may be induced during therapy |

*Table continued on following page*

TABLE 10–12.   Commonly Used Antibiotics for Bacterial Infection (*Continued*)

| Antibiotic | Mechanism of Action/Activity | Sensitive Bacteria/Indications | Comments |
|---|---|---|---|
| *Aminoglycosides* | Inhibition of bacterial protein synthesis at ribosomes | | Ototoxicity and nephrotoxicity, must monitor peak and trough serum concentrations |
| Gentamicin, tobramycin, netilmicin | | Gram-negative Enterobacteriaceae, including *Pseudomonas* | Broad spectrum, synergy with beta-lactams; enterococci are resistant |
| Amikacin | | Same as above | Less susceptible to aminoglycoside-inactivating enzymes |
| Streptomycin | | Plague, tularemia, brucellosis (plus tetracycline) | |
| **Other Antibiotics** Imipenem with cilastatin | Thienamycin drug: binds to penicillin-binding proteins; very broad spectrum | Most gram-positive and gram-negative bacteria, *Listeria, Bacillus* sp., *Pseudomonas, Acinetobacter* | *Stenotrophomonas maltophilia,* methicillin-resistant *S. aureus,* enterococci are resistant; requires cilastatin to inhibit renal degradation |
| Meropenem | Same as imipenem | Same as imipenem | Does not require cilastatin |
| Aztreonam | Monobactam drug: binds to penicillin-binding proteins of Enterobacteriaceae only; narrow spectrum | Most gram-negative bacteria | No action against anaerobic or gram-positive bacteria; *B. cepacia* is resistant; does not induce beta-lactamase production |
| Tetracyclines | Inhibition of protein synthesis | *Chlamydia, Mycoplasma,* gonococcus, *Actinomyces,* Lyme disease; pelvic inflammatory disease, Rocky Mountain spotted fever, urethritis, *Brucella* sp., tularemia, plague | Stains teeth, contraindicated before 10 yrs of age |
| Chloramphenicol | Inhibition of protein synthesis | *Salmonella, H. influenzae,* meningococcus, pneumococcus, *Shigella, B. fragilis,* Rocky Mountain spotted fever, typhoid fever | Reversible bone marrow suppression, aplastic anemia, gray baby syndrome (rarely used in United States) |
| Rifampin | Inhibition of DNA-dependent RNA polymerase | *S. aureus, Mycobacterium tuberculosis, H. influenzae, Meningococcus* | Red discoloration of secretions; increases metabolism of drugs (e.g., oral contraceptives); resistance develops if used alone |
| Metronidazole | Damage of DNA by free radicals | *Bacteroides* sp., *Clostridium difficile,* anaerobic bacteria, *Gardnerella vaginalis, Capnocytophaga, Giardia, Entamoeba histolytica* | Seizures, encephalopathy, disulfiram reaction, metallic taste |
| Erythromycin | Macrolide: inhibits protein synthesis | *Corynebacterium diphtheriae, Mycoplasma, Chlamydia, Bordetella pertussis, Haemophilus ducreyi, Legionella* sp., *Campylobacter* | Often used as an alternative to penicillin G; nausea, hepatoxicity (estolate ester); increases theophylline and carbamazepine blood levels |
| Azithromycin | Macrolide | Less active than erythromycin against *S. aureus,* pneumococcus, streptococci, more active against *H. influenzae, Mycoplasma, Chlamydia,* gram-negative bacilli; active against *M. catarrhalis, C. pneumoniae, Legionella pneumophila, Borrelia burgdorferi, Neisseria gonorrhoeae* | Possible efficacy for *Mycobacterium avium,* toxoplasma encephalitis, cryptosporidiosis; long half-life: single-dose treatment for uncomplicated *Chlamydia* urethritis or cervicitis Prolonged use may cause hearing loss |

**TABLE 10–12.** Commonly Used Antibiotics for Bacterial Infection *(Continued)*

| Antibiotic | Mechanism of Action/Activity | Sensitive Bacteria/Indications | Comments |
|---|---|---|---|
| Clarithromycin | Macrolide | More active than erythromycin for *S. aureus*, pneumococcus, *Streptococcus* | Similar to azithromycin |
| Clindamycin | Similar to erythromycin | *S. aureus*, *Streptococcus*, most anaerobic bacteria, *Actinomyces* (penicillin-allergic patients) | Pseudomembranous colitis toxicity |
| Vancomycin | Inhibits cell wall synthesis | Methicillin-resistant *S. aureus*, *S. epidermidis*, JK diphtheroids, *C. difficile*, *Enterococcus*, anaerobic bacteria | Red man syndrome if injected too fast, nephrotoxic<br>Resistance in enterococci a major problem |
| Trimethoprim/ sulfamethoxazole | Inhibition of bacterial folate synthesis at two separate sites of the folate pathway | *E. coli*, *Proteus mirabilis*, *Salmonella*, *Shigella*, *H. influenzae*, *Yersinia*, *Pneumococcus*, *S. aureus*, *Pneumocystis carinii*, *M. catarrhalis*, *Nocardia* | Group A streptococci may be resistant; *P. aeruginosa* and enterococci resistant, Stevens-Johnson syndrome—anemia, neutropenia, glucose-6-phosphate dehydrogenase hemolysis |
| Ciprofloxacin | Similar to nalidixic acid; inhibition of bacterial DNA gyrase; broad spectrum | *P. aeruginosa*, *Shigella*, *Salmonella*, *E. coli*, *Klebsiella*, *Proteus* sp., *S. aureus*, *H. influenzae*, gonococcus, *Chlamydia*, *Listeria monocytogenes* | May be given by mouth; arthritis; CNS toxicity; not approved for children <17 yr of age but widely used |

Data from Med Clin North Am 71:1051–1216, 1987; and Med Lett 34:49, 1992.
CNS = central nervous system; CSF = cerebrospinal fluid; DNA = deoxyribonucleic acid; RNA = ribonucleic acid.

1. Presence of a foul-smelling exudate or discharge.
2. Evidence of necrotic tissue, gangrene, or fasciitis.
3. Infection located in proximity to a mucosal surface.
4. Gas in tissue.
5. Gram stain of material that reveals multiple types of organisms.
6. Infection associated with tissue destruction (trauma or malignancy).
7. Failure to respond to antibiotics, especially aminoglycosides.
8. Septic thrombophlebitis.
9. Abscess formation.

Added clues that suggest anaerobes include no growth on routine cultures (sterile pus); failure to grow but presence of bacteria on Gram stain; growth in thioglycollate broth or on media containing kanamycin, neomycin, or paromomycin; production of gas and foul odor in culture; and development of characteristic colonies on agar plates incubated anaerobically.

Rapid diagnosis is possible with indirect immunofluorescence assay and gas-liquid chromatography identification of specific bacterial fermentation profiles from purulent material.

***Treatment.*** The pathogen usually can be predicted from the site of infection (above or below the diaphragm), and most anaerobes have predictable susceptibilities to antibiotic agents. Penicillin G is useful against gram-positive and most gram-negative anaerobes (except *Bacteroides fragilis*) and can be used to treat orofacial and pulmonary infections, unless beta-lactamase–producing anaerobes are present. Cefoxitin, amoxicillin/clavulanate, clindamycin, or metronidazole may be used to treat anaerobic infections at other sites. Anaerobes also usually are susceptible to cefotetan, imipenem, or ticarcillin/clavulanate. Metronidazole is very effective in treating anaerobic brain abscesses, whereas clindamycin is excellent for lung abscesses (see Appendix I).

### References

Behrman RE, Kliegman RM, Arvin AM (eds): Nelson Textbook of Pediatrics, 15th ed. Philadelphia, WB Saunders, 1996, Chapter 194.

Styrt B, Gorbach SL: Recent developments in the understanding of the pathogenesis and treatment of anaerobic infections (first of two parts). N Engl J Med 321:240, 1989.

Styrt B, Gorbach SL: Recent developments in the understanding of the pathogenesis and treatment of anaerobic infections (second of two parts). N Engl J Med 321:298, 1989.

## CLOSTRIDIAL INFECTIONS

Clostridial organisms have been associated with tetanus, gas gangrene (clostridial myonecrosis), food poisoning, necrotizing enteritis, antimicrobial-associated colitis, and botulism. Most of these disorders are the result of toxin elaboration by vegetative organisms.

### Tetanus
(Lockjaw)

*Etiology.* *Clostridium tetani* is an anaerobic, spore-forming, gram-positive bacillus. The spores are resistant to many injurious agents and processes, including boiling. The vegetative forms of *C. tetani* are susceptible to heat and many disinfectants. *C. tetani* survive in soil for years and may be found in house dust, salt and fresh water, the oral cavities of mammals, and feces of many animal species. Spores and vegetative organisms may be found in the intestinal contents of humans.

*C. tetani* causes disease by the production of exotoxins, tetanus toxin or tetanospasmin, and tetanolysin, which is thought to potentiate the effect of tetanus toxin. This is a neurotoxin that migrates transsynaptically and inhibits acetylcholine release, particularly from inhibitory synapses, resulting in muscle contraction, characteristic localized spasms and rigidity. The toxin can also block transmission at neuromuscular junctions and cause paralysis. These toxins are produced by the vegetative forms of the bacteria when they propagate under favorable growth conditions (i.e., low oxygen tension as created by poorly perfused tissue following crush injuries).

*Epidemiology.* Tetanus occurs throughout the world and is a major cause of mortality in developing countries, particularly in unvaccinated individuals. Neonatal tetanus follows contamination of the umbilical cord with these organisms. A few cases are reported in the United States and are associated primarily with contaminated wounds, trauma, and intravenous drug use.

In the United States, tetanus is more common among 1–5 yr old boys and older patients with waning immunity. The incubation period is usually 3–14 days after injury but may be as short as 1 day with serious infection or as long as several months. Tetanus is not transmitted from person to person.

*Clinical Manifestations.* There are several clinical forms of tetanus: (1) localized, (2) generalized, (3) cephalic, and (4) tetanus neonatorum. In each, an examination of the actual wound does not reveal an appearance that is different from that of an uninfected wound.

*LOCALIZED TETANUS.* This pattern is uncommon in children but produces pain and continuous rigidity and spasm of muscles in proximity to the injury; symptoms may persist for weeks and resolve without sequelae. Occasionally, localized tetanus precedes the generalized disorder. The fatality rate is about 1%.

*GENERALIZED TETANUS.* This is the most common form. The onset may be insidious, with gradually increasing muscle stiffness; trismus is the presenting symptom in over 50% of cases. Spasm of the masseter muscles may be associated with stiffness of neck muscles and difficulty in swallowing. Restlessness, irritability, and headache are early manifestations. Spasm of facial muscles immobilizes the jaw, producing a fixed sardonic grin (risus sardonicus). Tonic contractions of the somatic musculature become generalized. Voluntary movement or sensory stimulation (cutaneous, auditory, visual) may initiate spasms or convulsions. The lumbar and abdominal muscles may become rigid; persistent spasm of the back muscles results in opisthotonos. Tetanic seizures are characterized by sudden bursts of tonic contractions of various muscle groups. Spasm of the airway or respiratory muscles causes airway obstruction and respiratory insufficiency. Spasm may cause fractures and local hemorrhages. The patient is completely conscious during the clinical course and experiences intense pain. Signs and symptoms increase over 3–7 days, reach a plateau during the second week, and gradually abate. Recovery is complete in 2–6 weeks.

*CEPHALIC TETANUS.* This type of tetanus is rare and may precede generalized tetanus. The incubation period is 1–2 days after otitis media, trauma to the head and face, and the presence of nasal foreign bodies. Involvement of cranial nerves III, IV, VII (most common), IX, X, and XI is the most prominent feature of the disease.

*TETANUS NEONATORUM.* This pattern begins 3–10 days after birth and is generalized. Difficulty in sucking, excessive crying, difficulty in swallowing, rigidity, tonic contractions, and opisthotonos are common.

*Diagnosis and Differential Diagnosis.* The diagnosis of tetanus is made on clinical grounds. A history of a wound or bite, the characteristic facial appearance, and spasms aid in establishing the diagnosis. Most cases occur in unimmunized individuals or in their infants. Wound cultures are positive for *C. tetani* in one third of instances. Gram stains of the wound may show gram-positive rods with terminal, drumstick-like spores. Trismus may be associated with tooth, peritonsillar, or retropharyngeal abscesses. Spasms also may be seen in rabies, hypocalcemia, and strychnine or phenothiazine intoxication. Rabies and, rarely, tetanus may follow animal bites. Rabies causes pain and numbness at the bite, fever (not noted in tetanus), painful esophageal spasm on drinking, CSF pleocytosis, and, eventually, coma and paralysis.

***Treatment.*** The objectives of therapy are to remove the source of tetanospasmin, to neutralize remaining circulating toxin before it reaches the CNS, and to provide supportive care until tetanospasmin, which is fixed to neural tissue, can be metabolized. Supportive care includes meperidine for pain, benzodiazepines, endotracheal intubation and paralysis, if needed, and ventilatory support. Tracheostomy is often required. Human tetanus immune globulin (antitoxin) (3000–6000 U × 1 dose) should be given, part of which is injected directly into the wound. Wounds should be irrigated and débrided. Penicillin therapy is indicated to eradicate vegetative *C. tetani* organisms. There is no transmission to humans, but body substance isolation should be used until rabies is excluded.

***Prevention.*** Immediate and thorough surgical treatment of wounds is mandatory. The indications for active and passive immunoprophylaxis depend on the prior immunization status and the severity of the wound (Table 10–13). *Tetanus toxoid* should also be given following tetanus because the disease does not induce natural immunity.

**TABLE 10–13.** Tetanus Prevention Following Wounds

| Tetanus Immunization History | Clean | Minor | All Others* | |
|---|---|---|---|---|
| | Td† | TIG‡ | Td | TIG |
| Uncertain or incomplete (<3 doses) | Yes | No | Yes | Yes |
| Complete (>3 doses plus booster) | No§ | No | No‖ | No |

Modified from Report of Committee on Infectious Diseases, 1994 Red Book, 22nd ed. Elk Grove Village, IL, American Academy of Pediatrics, 1994.

*Other wounds include those contaminated with soil, dirt, feces, saliva; and punctures, avulsions, crush injuries, burns, frostbite, and wound resulting from missiles. All wounds require appropriate irrigation and débridement.

†If younger than 7 yr old, DT may be given.
‡Tetanus immune globulin (human).
§Yes, if longer than 10 yr since last immunization.
‖Yes, if longer than 5 yr since last immunization.
DT = diphtheria-tetanus vaccine; Td = tetanus-diphtheria toxoid (adult type); TIG = tetanus immune globulin.

***Prognosis.*** Case fatality rates of tetanus are approximately 20–50% despite modern care; rates for neonatal tetanus are 60% or greater. Patients with an incubation period of 8–10 days, those with progression longer than 60 hr, and those who survive for 10 days recover completely. Tetanus does not produce sequelae other than those due to anoxia.

### References

Behrman RE, Kliegman RM, Arvin AM (eds): Nelson Textbook of Pediatrics, 15th ed. Philadelphia, WB Saunders, 1996, Chapter 193.
Gergen JP, McQuillan GM, Kiely M, et al: A population-based serologic survey of immunity to tetanus in the United States. N Engl J Med 332:761, 1995.

### Botulism

***Etiology.*** *Clostridium botulinum* is an anaerobic, gram-positive bacillus that produces heat-resistant spores. When spores survive food processing, they germinate in the container and elaborate neurotoxins. Seven antigenically distinct toxins have been identified (A–G). All except D have been associated with human disease. *C. botulinum* toxins bind irreversibly to the presynaptic nerve terminals, are internalized by endocytosis, and block achetylcholine release. Neural transmission at ganglionic, postganglionic, and neuromuscular junctions is inhibited.

***Epidemiology.*** There are three forms of botulism:

1. **Infant botulism,** the most common cause of botulism in the United States, caused by germination of spores of *C. botulinum* in the gastrointestinal tract accompanied by toxin produced in vivo rather than by the ingestion of preformed toxin.
2. **Food-borne botulism,** an intoxication from preformed botulinum toxin present in improperly preserved food. Home-preserved foods are the most frequent cause of this type of botulism in the United States.
3. **Wound botulism,** a rare botulism resulting from local wound infection and toxin production by *C. botulinum.*

Infant botulism usually occurs in children younger than 6 mo of age, has a peak onset from 1–3 mo, and is caused by type A and B strains. Adults also have had this type of botulism. Sources for spores include soil, house and vacuum cleaner dust, honey, and possibly corn syrup. The majority of patients have been reported from California, Pennsylvania, Hawaii, and Utah, clusters correlating with areas of high soil spore concentration of C.

*botulinum.* Alterations in the normal host intestinal flora, perhaps pH changes, and altered gut motility may predispose the infant to this disease.

### Clinical Manifestations

INFANT BOTULISM. The course varies from mild constipation and poor feeding to severe neurologic deterioration and sudden, at times unexplained, death. Typically, a previously healthy, afebrile infant has constipation, poor sucking and swallowing; a weak cry and smile develop, and bilateral ptosis, hypotonia, and poor head control are present. Symmetric, descending paralysis progresses over hours to days, involving facial muscles, trunk, and limbs. Ileus, bladder atony, nonreactive dilated pupils, and decreased tearing and salivation may be present. Infants require ventilatory support for apnea or hypoventilation. Because the CNS is not affected, the child is awake and may even appear alert.

FOOD-BORNE BOTULISM. Incubation usually takes 12–36 hr but can range from several hours to a week. Nausea, vomiting, diplopia, dysphagia, dysarthria, and dry mouth are common during the course of disease. Weakness, postural hypotension, absent or diminished deep tendon reflexes, urinary retention, and constipation (not diarrhea) also may develop.

WOUND BOTULISM. The course may be similar to that exhibited after ingestion of *C. botulinum* toxin but is usually milder and more prolonged. The incubation period is 4–14 days.

### Diagnosis and Differential Diagnosis.
The diagnosis of botulism is established by identifying *C. botulinum* organisms and/or toxin in feces, blood, or food products.

*Infant botulism* should be differentiated from septicemia, myasthenia gravis, poliomyelitis, Werdnig-Hoffmann disease, spinal cord injury, near-miss sudden infant death syndrome (SIDS), hypothyroidism, and inborn errors of metabolism.

*Food-borne botulism* must be differentiated from myasthenia gravis, poliomyelitis, Guillain-Barré syndrome, drug intoxication, trichinosis, diphtheria, and various forms of electrolyte or mineral imbalances.

The diagnosis of *wound botulism* is made by demonstrating the organisms in the wound and/or the toxin in blood. An electromyogram with brief, small, abundant potentials suggests botulism.

### Treatment.
Antitoxin is of uncertain value in *infant botulism.* Intensive care alone usually is sufficient. Antibiotics do not shorten the clinical course or decrease intestinal colonization. Aminoglycosides exacerbate or accelerate paralysis and produce respiratory failure as a result of synergistic inhibition of neurotransmission at the neuromuscular junction. A cleansing enema may eliminate the site of toxin production.

All children with *food-borne botulism* must be hospitalized. Vomiting should be induced and gastric lavage initiated. Cathartics may be placed in the stomach at the conclusion of lavage and an enema given to facilitate elimination of unabsorbed toxin. Equine antitoxin has been efficacious in treating food-borne disease. The polyvalent preparation is preferred until the toxin type has been identified. Skin sensitivity testing is mandatory prior to administration. Penicillin G is given to kill *C. botulinum,* which may continue to produce toxin.

*Wound botulism* requires débriding and draining the wound. Performing supportive intensive care measures and administering antitoxin and antibiotics also are indicated.

Supportive care includes monitoring cardiorespiratory functions in anticipation of apnea, hypotension, or aspiration resulting from the absence of the gag reflex; managing constipation; and treating urinary retention, inappropriate antidiuretic hormone secretion, and urinary tract infection. Nutritional support by gavage feeding may be indicated if the gag reflex is absent.

### Prevention.
Boiling food for 10 min destroys the toxin. A pressure cooker is required to kill spores of *C. botulinum*; pressure requirements vary with the food being processed. Because 10% of retail honey in the United States may contain *C. botulinum* spores, it should not be fed to infants younger than 6 mo of age. Breast-feeding may lessen the severity of the illness.

### Prognosis.
Most infants recover without sequelae if adequate intensive care and supportive therapy prevent hypoxia. Severity of illness in food-borne botulism is directly related to the titer of toxin ingested and inversely related to the duration of the incubation period. Complete recovery is delayed for many months and requires regeneration of the previously destroyed presynaptic terminals. Because the toxin does not cross the blood-brain barrier, intelligence is normal in the absence of prior hypoxic episodes.

### References

Behrman RE, Kliegman RM, Arvin AM (eds): Nelson Textbook of Pediatrics, 15th ed. Philadelphia, WB Saunders, 1996, Chapter 192.

Hutchinson DN: Foodborne botulism: New techniques for preserving foods bring the need for greater awareness of the risks. BMJ 305:264, 1992.

Schreiner MS, Field E, Ruddy R: Infant botulism: A review of 12 years' experience at the Children's Hospital of Philadelphia. Pediatrics 87:159, 1991.

## INFECTION DUE TO *CORYNEBACTERIUM DIPHTHERIAE*

*Etiology and Pathophysiology.* C. diphtheriae is a gram-positive, nonsporulating bacillus with three colony types (mitis, gravis, and intermedius). Infection of C. diphtheriae by a lysogenic bacteriophage containing the gene for the toxin is required to produce disease. Toxigenic and nontoxigenic strains of C. diphtheriae cause disease, but only strains that produce toxin are responsible for myocarditis and neuritis.

Diphtheria is characterized by local inflammation and the production of a pseudomembrane composed of necrotic epithelium and coagulated inflammatory cells in the upper respiratory tract (nasal or oral pharynx), which may cause airway obstruction. In addition, toxin production causes injury to distant visceral tissues (nerve, heart, kidney). Diphtheria toxin is an extremely potent inhibitor of protein synthesis which acts by adenosine diphosphate (ADP)–ribosylating elongation factor-2 (EF-2).

*Epidemiology.* Humans are the only known reservoir of C. diphtheriae. Many children under 2 yr of age as well as the older adults lack protective levels of antibody; state laws mandating immunization for school entry have protected most children aged 5–15 yr. Outbreaks in the countries of the former Soviet Union have affected more than 100,000 individuals with variable case fatality rates. These outbreaks have been largely attributed to failure to immunize children and waning immunity in adults but not to lack of efficacy of the available vaccine. Most of the recent cases of respiratory diphtheria in the United States have occurred in adults older than 25 yr.

Diphtheria is acquired by close contact with respiratory droplets from either an asymptomatic carrier or a person with the disease. Fomites and dust occasionally are vehicles of transmission. The incubation period is 2–4 days.

*Clinical Manifestations.* The manifestations of diphtheria depend on the location of infection, the immunization status of the host, and whether toxin enters the systemic circulation. Manifestations are classified by the location of the diphtheritic pseudomembrane: nasal, tonsillar, pharyngeal, laryngeal or laryngotracheal, conjunctival, cutaneous, and genital; more than one anatomic site may be involved.

**Tonsillar or pharyngeal diphtheria** is the most common type, beginning insidiously with malaise, low-grade fever, and a mild sore throat. Within 1–2 days, a membrane forms; its size and extent vary according to the host's immune status. The membrane initially is thin, white, and localized; as the disease progresses, it coalesces and extends from the tonsil to the contiguous soft or hard palate, pharyngeal wall, larynx, and trachea. This pattern distinguishes diphtheria from other diseases producing membranous tonsillitis. The membrane becomes gray and the breath may have a foul, garlic odor. Removal of the exudate is followed by bleeding. Bilateral cervical lymphadenitis is variable. Ten percent of patients present with high fever, toxicity, rapid progression of the pseudomembrane, and edema of the soft tissues of the neck (bull neck). The edema is brawny, pitting, warm, and tender; it occurs in children over 6 yr of age and carries a more severe prognosis. In less severe cases, recovery may be complicated by myocarditis or neuritis caused by systemic absorption of toxin.

**Laryngeal diphtheria** usually results when the membrane extends downward from the pharynx. In 10% of cases, only the larynx is involved. Hoarseness and stridor produce acute and potentially fatal obstruction if the membrane occludes the airway. In severe cases, the membrane may extend downward, forming a cast over the entire tracheobronchial tree.

**Cutaneous diphtheria,** which is common in warmer climates, often is indistinguishable from other skin infections (e.g., impetigo). Skin lesions may be an important source of person-to-person transmission. *Conjunctival lesions* usually are limited to the palpebral conjunctiva, which appears red, edematous, and membranous; corneal erosion may occur. **Aural diphtheria** is characterized by otitis externa accompanied by a persistent, purulent, and frequently foul-smelling discharge.

The more extensive the primary lesion and the lower the antitoxin titer, the more severe the toxicity. Cardiac toxicity occurs in 10% of patients, appears between the 7th and 14th day of illness, and is characterized by heart failure, atrioventricular nodal block and arrhythmias. Isolated peripheral neuropathies involving the palate, pharynx, larynx, extraocular muscles, or diaphragm appear in 2–6 wk. Paralysis of the extremities and elevated CSF protein resembling Guillain-Barré syndrome may occur. Hepatitis, nephritis, and gastritis also may occur.

*Diagnosis and Differential Diagnosis.* Determining the diagnosis requires isolating C. diphtheriae from the membrane or the exudate beneath the membrane. The bacillus is readily recovered on selective media (tellurite) using inhibitors that retard the growth of other microorganisms. Microscopic examination of diphtheritic lesions is unreliable. C. diphtheriae should be tested for toxigenicity.

Tonsillar and/or pharyngeal diphtheria must be

differentiated from streptococcal pharyngitis, EBV infection, viral tonsillitis, primary herpetic tonsillitis, thrush, blood dyscrasias (such as agranulocytosis and leukemia), toxoplasmosis, cytomegalovirus, *Francisella tularensis,* and Vincent angina. Laryngeal diphtheria must be differentiated from viral croup, the presence of foreign bodies, retropharyngeal abscesses, and laryngeal tumors (papillomas, hemangiomas, lymphangiomas).

*Treatment.* Treatment of diphtheria requires neutralizing the circulating toxin and eradicating *C. diphtheriae* with antibiotics. Equine antitoxin must be given as soon as possible because once toxin is bound to tissue, antitoxin has no effect. Antibiotics help stop the production of additional toxin. Penicillin and erythromycin are effective against most strains of *C. diphtheriae* but do not alter the evolution of the disease. The diphtheria carrier state can be treated with penicillin G benzathine, penicillin G, or oral erythromycin. The endpoint of antibiotic therapy and infectivity is indicated by three consecutive negative cultures. Supportive care may include endotracheal intubation for respiratory insufficiency due to airway obstruction or paralysis.

*Prevention.* Prevention requires isolation of the patient and treatment of close contacts who are likely to become ill (if nonimmune) or become carriers. Previously immunized carriers should be given a booster injection of diphtheria toxoid and should be treated with penicillin or erythromycin. Nonimmunized asymptomatic carriers should have samples taken for culture, should receive diphtheria toxoid and penicillin or erythromycin, and should be examined carefully for 7 days. Because diphtheria does not always produce persistent immunity, patients should receive toxoid after the illness.

*Prognosis.* Prior to the use of antitoxin and antibiotics, the mortality rate from diphtheria was 30–50%. Death was most common in younger children (<4 yr old) and often resulted from airway obstruction by the diphtheritic pseudomembrane. Today the mortality rate is less than 5%, and death is due to severe myocarditis. Nasopharyngeal persistence of *C. diphtheriae* may be noted in 5–10% of convalescing patients.

References

Behrman RE, Kliegman RM, Arvin AM (eds): Nelson Textbook of Pediatrics, 15th ed. Philadelphia, WB Saunders, 1996, Chapter 180.

Centers for Disease Control and Prevention: Diphtheria epidemic New Independent states of the Former Soviet Union, 1990–1994. MMWR 44:177, 1995.

Rappuoli R, Perugini M, Falsen E: Molecular epidemiology of the 1984–1986 outbreak of diphtheria in Sweden. N Engl J Med 318:12, 1988.

# INFECTION DUE TO *HAEMOPHILUS INFLUENZAE*

## General Considerations

*Etiology.* *H. influenzae* are nonmotile, small, fastidious, pleomorphic gram-negative coccobacilli. Encapsulated strains are classified according to their soluble capsular polysaccharides (polyribosyl ribitol phosphate [PRP]) and are designated as types a through f. Type b produces serious invasive infections (meningitis, septic arthritis, epiglottitis, pericarditis, facial cellulitis, pneumonia) in children. Infants lacking anti-PRP immunoglobulin G (IgG) have deficient opsonization of these encapsulated organisms. Nontypable unencapsulated strains are associated with sinusitis, conjunctivitis, otitis media, and bronchitis. *H. influenzae* organisms also produce IgA protease and pili or fimbriae. Some strains produce beta-lactamase and thus are resistant to ampicillin.

*Epidemiology.* *H. influenzae* is a part of the normal commensal flora of the upper respiratory tract; most children have unencapsulated strains in their pharynx, and 2–5% carry type b organisms. The mode of transmission is by breathing respiratory droplets or by directly contacting secretions. Children with asplenia (from congenital and surgical causes and sickle cell anemia), those with antibody deficiencies (e.g., IgG2), and patients receiving chemotherapy for malignancies are at an increased risk for infection.

Invasive disease due to *H. influenzae* type b is more common in children younger than 4 yr of age and in specific ethnic groups, including the Inuit in Alaska and Native Americans (Navaho and Apaches). Before effective vaccines were available, *H. influenzae* type b caused approximately 10,000 cases of meningitis per year in the United States. The peak incidence of meningitis caused by this organism was in infants younger than 12 mo of age. Children in day care settings were also at risk for outbreaks of disease due to *H. influenzae* type b.

## Infections Caused by *Haemophilus Influenzae* Type B

### Clinical Manifestations

MENINGITIS. *H. influenzae* type b was a common cause of bacterial meningitis in children between ages 1 mo and 4 yr prior to the widespread use of HIB vaccine. Meningitis caused by *H. influenzae* cannot be distinguished from that due to *N. meningitidis* or *S. pneumoniae* on the basis of clinical presentation. The illness may be complicated at the time of presentation or later by other sites of infection with *H. influenzae,* including pneumonia, arthritis, osteomyelitis, pericarditis, cellulitis, and endophthalmitis.

*ACUTE EPIGLOTTITIS.* This potentially lethal condition, which may result in airway obstruction from an acutely inflamed epiglottis, usually occurs in children between 2 and 7 yr old (see Chapter 12).

*PNEUMONIA.* The incidence of *H. influenzae* pneumonia in children is unknown, but it is most common in children under 6 yr of age. The signs and symptoms of pneumonia caused by *H. influenzae* cannot be distinguished from those caused by other microorganisms. Pleural effusions and lobar and patchy infiltrates may be noted. Associated infections include otitis media, meningitis, and epiglottitis.

*SEPTIC ARTHRITIS. H. influenzae* type b was the most common agent producing septic arthritis in children younger than 3 yr of age. Large joints, such as knees, hips, ankles, and elbows, commonly are affected, often in association with infections such as meningitis. Arthritis that appears late in the course of *H. influenzae* meningitis infection may be an antigen-antibody reaction and not a true joint space infection. Septic arthritis caused by *H. influenzae* type b is indistinguishable from that caused by other bacterial pathogens.

*CELLULITIS.* More than 85% of children with *H. influenzae* type b cellulitis are 2 yr of age or younger. Frequently, an upper respiratory tract infection precedes the acute onset of cellulitis. High fever, marked toxicity, bacteremia, and leukocytosis without a prior history of local trauma are present. The face and neck, particularly the cheek (buccal) and the periorbital area, are the most common sites. The lesion has indistinct margins, is tender and indurated, and may have a violaceous or bluish purple color. Meningitis with facial cellulitis may occur.

*PERICARDITIS. H. influenzae* type b causes up to 15% of bacterial pericarditis cases in children. Children are usually 2–4 yr of age and often have had an antecedent upper respiratory tract infection or adjacent pneumonia.

*BACTEREMIA WITHOUT AN ASSOCIATED FOCUS.* Bacteremia caused by *H. influenzae* type b may occur without any apparent focus of infection other than signs of an upper respiratory tract infection or pharyngitis. Although affected children may appear only mildly ill at the initial visit, they are at substantial risk for development of pneumonia or meningitis, a finding that is in marked contrast to occult pneumococcal bacteremia, which has a much lower risk of metastatic foci or infection following bacteremia without a source.

*NEONATAL DISEASE.* In the neonate, nontypable *H. influenzae* is more common than type b. Septicemia, pneumonia, meningitis, and respiratory distress syndrome produced by nontypable *H. influenzae* are indistinguishable from those due to other neonatal bacterial pathogens. Nontypable *H. influenzae* are acquired by the infant from the mother's genitourinary tract.

**Diagnosis.** Specimens of CSF, blood, synovial fluid, cellulitis aspirate, or other material should be obtained for culture on a selective medium, such as chocolate agar. Latex agglutination tests for detecting capsular antigen in CSF, blood, and urine may aid in rapid diagnosis. Beta-lactamase production and antibiotic susceptibility tests should be performed on all isolates to determine resistance to ampicillin and cephalosporins.

**Treatment (see also Central Nervous System Infections).** Invasive infections presumed to be due to *H. influenzae* initially should be treated with intravenous ceftriaxone or cefotaxime. Regionally, the prevalence of ampicillin-resistant strains varies from 10% to 40%. As much of the pathology associated with *H. influenzae* type b meningitis is due to the host inflammatory response, administration of dexamethasone *prior* to the first dose of antibiotic is recommended and appears to be associated with a decrease in neurologic sequelae, *if* given prior to the antibiotic (see Appendix I).

**Prevention.** Conjugate vaccines with PRP covalently linked to diphtheria toxoid or OMP (outer membrane protein of *N. meningitidis*) should be administered to infants at 2, 4, 6, and 15 mo and to unimmunized children 24–60 mo old (see Fig. 10–1). Because the risk for secondary infection caused by *H. influenzae* type b in close contacts is high, rifampin is recommended for all family contacts (adults, index case, plus young children) of individuals with *H. influenzae* disease when there are other susceptible (not fully immunized) children in the household who are younger than 4 yr of age. Close contacts in day care centers also may be candidates for rifampin therapy.

## References

Behrman RE, Kliegman RM, Arvin AM (eds): Nelson Textbook of Pediatrics 15th ed. Philadelphia, WB Saunders 1996, Chapter 177.

Dagan R and the Israeli Pediatric Bacteremia and Meningitis Group: A two-year prospective, nationwide study to determine the epidemiology and impact of invasive childhood *Haemophilus influenzae* type b infection in Israel. Clin Infect Dis 15:720, 1992.

Korones DN, Marshall GS, Shapiro ED: Outcome of children

with occult bacteremia caused by *Haemophilus influenzae* type b. Pediatr Infect Dis J 11:516, 1992.

Odio CM, Faingezicht I, Paris M, et al: The beneficial effects of early dexamethasone administration in infants and children with bacterial meningitis. N Engl J Med 324:1525, 1991.

Santosham M, Wolff M, Reid R, et al: The efficacy in Navajo infants of a conjugate vaccine consisting of *Haemophilus influenzae* type b polysaccharide and *Neisseria meningitidis* outer-membrane protein complex. N Engl J Med 324:1767, 1991.

## MYCOBACTERIAL INFECTIONS

### Tuberculosis

*Etiology.* Tuberculosis is caused by *Mycobacterium tuberculosis*, an aerobic, slow-growing organism with a complex cell wall structure containing mycolic acid, a 70–80 carbon fatty acid, and arabinogalactan, linked to muramic acid. The high lipid content gives the organism its "acid-fast" staining properties (resistance to decolorization with acid–alcohol), as used in the Ziehl-Neelsen or Kinyoun staining methods used to identify these organisms. The cell wall produces delayed sensitivity reactions to tuberculin. *M. tuberculosis* can be differentiated from other mycobacteria by its lack of pigmentation, slow growth rate, requiring 3–6 wk, and by the use of specific DNA probes.

*Epidemiology.* Tuberculosis is a major cause of mortality throughout the world. Reservoirs of tuberculosis include the elderly, immigrants (Asian, African, Latin American), the homeless, and patients with AIDS. Tuberculosis is more common in crowded semi-industrialized societies and among the poor. Infection in children occurs following inhalation of contaminated respiratory droplets (coughing, sneezing) from heavily infected respiratory tract secretions. Infection in children typically is due to prolonged close contact with an individual having untreated, active, cavitary, sputum-positive disease. The incubation period from infection to development of a positive tuberculin skin test is 2–6 wk.

*Immunity.* Following inhalation into the alveolus, the tuberculosis bacillus is ingested but not killed by the pulmonary macrophage. The bacilli multiply, from pulmonary granulomas, spread to local lymph nodes, and disseminate to extrathoracic organs by lymphatic and hematogenous spread. The alveolar macrophage presents the antigenic material to T lymphocytes, producing delayed-type hypersensitivity, which, together with newly activated macrophages, causes intracellular killing of the bacilli and granuloma formation. Genetic factors, age (<3 yr, puberty), immunosuppression (AIDS, malnutrition, pertussis, measles, lymphoma, corticosteroids), pregnancy, and other factors predispose the patient to serious disease because they alter the immune response.

*Clinical Manifestations.* When a nonimmune host inhales organisms, that host develops a primary complex, which involves the lung parenchyma (usually lower or middle lobes) and its draining lymph node. The organism is then disseminated to other body sites (upper lobes, bone, meninges). Acquired immunity in the healthy host usually contains the infection in dormant foci in lungs, regional lymph nodes, and visceral organs. In the lung, this may be noted 1–2 yr after primary infection as calcified lesions, or the **Ghon complex.** Lesions that apparently have healed may contain dormant but viable bacilli. In addition, disease progression may occur in the lungs or at distal sites of infection. Progression of the primary complex to pulmonary disease or miliary tuberculosis, or progression of CNS granulomas to meningitis, is most common in the 1st yr after primary infection and in children younger than 5 yr. Pulmonary progression also is common during puberty. Skeletal lesions often are delayed 2–3 yr after the primary infection. In hosts with subsequent alteration of immunity, reactivation of the foci also can result in pulmonary or extrathoracic symptoms. Hilar adenopathy may compress the bronchus or trachea, producing airway obstruction and wheezing. Compression of the recurrent laryngeal nerve (hoarseness), phrenic nerve (diaphragm palsy), and vena cava (superior vena cava syndrome) causes additional problems.

**Primary pulmonary tuberculosis** in older infants and children is usually an asymptomatic illness. The diagnosis is confirmed only by a positive skin test, often with minimal abnormalities (infiltrate with hilar adenopathy) on the chest roentgenogram. Malaise, low-grade fever, erythema nodosum, phlyctenular keratoconjunctivitis, or symptoms resulting from lymph node enlargement may occur after the development of delayed hypersensitivity. In older children and adolescents, primary illness presents as an upper lobe infiltrate and cavitation without calcification. In children under 3 yr, primary pulmonary infection may be progressive and merge with miliary tuberculosis or progressive CNS disease to produce tuberculous meningitis.

**Progressive pulmonary tuberculosis** occurs when the primary infection is not contained and produces bronchopneumonia or lobar pneumonia (usually middle or lower) and cavitation with associated fever, weight loss, night sweats, malaise, hemoptysis, and productive cough. The tuberculin skin test is positive.

**Reactivation pulmonary tuberculosis,** uncommon in young children but more common in adolescents, usually is confined to apical segments of upper lobes or superior segments of lower lobes. There is usually little lymphadenopathy and no extrathoracic infection as a result of established hypersensitivity. This is a manifestation of a secondary expansion of infection at a site seeded years previously during primary infection. Cavitation and endobronchial spread of bacilli occur and are associated with fever, night sweats, malaise, and weight loss. A productive cough and hemoptysis often herald cavitation and bronchial erosion.

**Tuberculosis in HIV-infected patients** may have a more variable presentation. In adolescents who would be expected to develop reactivation disease with cavity formation, more diffuse infiltrates may be present. In younger infants, hilar adenopathy and nonspecific pulmonary infiltrates may indicate tuberculosis; upper lobe cavitary disease may also be seen.

**Upper respiratory tract tuberculosis,** which involves the larynx (croupy cough, sore throat, hoarseness) or middle ear (hearing loss, otorrhea, thick perforated eardrum), is a complication of advanced pulmonary disease.

**Pleural effusions** are usually a hypersensitivity response to tuberculous antigens. Less often, effusions may be secondary to discharge of tubercle bacilli into the pleural space from subpleural foci during post-primary tuberculosis. Pleural exudative effusions often are unilateral and may be associated with pericarditis and peritonitis. Biopsy of pleural tissue has a higher diagnostic yield than examination of fluid. The fluid is reabsorbed gradually during therapy.

Hilar **lymphadenopathy** is common in primary pulmonary disease. The most common extrathoracic sites of adenitis are the cervical, supraclavicular, and submandibular areas (scrofula). The illness usually is insidious, unilateral more often than bilateral, and associated with a history of exposure to an infected family member. The nodes are nontender and firm. Chest roentgenograms may reveal pulmonary tuberculosis as well. Suppuration of the nodes may lead to fluctuance and draining sinus tracts. Enlargement may cause compression of adjacent structures. Differential diagnosis includes infections caused by atypical mycobacteria, cat-scratch disease, fungal infection, viral or bacterial disease, toxoplasmosis, sarcoidosis, drug reactions, and malignancy. Diagnosis may be confirmed by fine-needle aspiration but may necessitate excisional biopsy accompanied by appropriate histologic and microbiologic studies.

**Miliary tuberculosis** refers to widespread hematogenous dissemination with infection of multiple organs. The lesions are of roughly the same size as that of a millet seed, from which the name miliary is derived. Miliary tuberculosis is characterized by fever, weakness, malaise, anorexia, weight loss, lymphadenopathy, night sweats, and hepatosplenomegaly. Diffuse bilateral pneumonitis is present and meningitis may be noted. Anemia, monocytosis, thrombocytopenia, hyponatremia, hypokalemia, and abnormal liver function tests are common. The chest roentgenogram reveals bilateral miliary infiltrates demonstrating overwhelming infection. The tuberculin skin test may be nonreactive as a result of anergy. Liver or bone marrow biopsy may be needed for the diagnosis.

**Tuberculous meningitis** occurs in recently infected individuals. In developing countries, it usually occurs before age 5 yr and within 6 mo of the primary infection; in developed countries, it has become an illness of adults. Rupture of CNS tubercles, which were seeded during primary infection, results in a severe inflammatory basilar meningitis (brain stem, basal cisterns, blood vessels). This insidious disease progresses through stages:

- The nonspecific influenza-like *stage 1,* lasting 1–2 wk, which is manifested by low-grade fever and subtle personality changes
- *Stage 2,* in which neurologic signs and symptoms develop that may include headache, stiff neck, positive Kernig or Brudzinski sign, and cranial nerve palsies (III, VI, VII, VIII), including aphasia, disorientation, ataxia, hemiplegia, and seizures
- *Stage 3,* which is demonstrated by increasing intracranial pressure (as a result of obstruction of basal cisterns), stupor, coma, decerebrate or decorticate posturing, and death. Without therapy, death is nearly inevitable within several weeks after the onset of symptoms.

There also may be evidence of concurrent pulmonary disease and hyponatremia caused by the syndrome of inappropriate antidiuretic hormone secretion. A CT scan may show periventricular lucencies, edema, infarctions, and hydrocephalus. Lumbar puncture usually reveals increased spinal fluid pressure. CSF studies reveal a modest increase in cells (50–500 cells/$\mu$L), mostly of lymphocytes, although polymorphonuclear leukocytes may predominate early. Glucose levels are low, and protein levels are elevated. The tubercle bacilli are seen in fewer than 30% of patients; the culture requires weeks to grow organisms. The skin test is positive in about two thirds of cases, but in very ill individuals anergy may be present. In such children, often a history of close contact with a person who has active tuberculosis is revealed. Skin testing and chest roentgenograms of close contacts may facilitate diagnosis and recovery of the organism. An early diagnosis improves the outcome; however, sequelae such as deafness, paralysis, retardation, and hydrocephalus may occur.

In some children, an expanding mass presenting as a CNS infection with focal neurologic signs and low-grade fever may be due to a **tuberculoma of the CNS.** The CT scan may reveal a hypodense area surrounded by edema. As in tuberculous meningitis, children often come from endemic areas or have a history of contact with an infected adult, a positive skin test, and concurrent pulmonary disease.

**Tuberculosis of the heart and pericardium** rarely may result from rupture of mediastinal nodes into the pericardial space or from hematogenous dissemination. The signs and symptoms resemble those seen in pericarditis that is due to other causes, and the exudate resembles that of tuberculous pleuritis. The skin test is usually positive. The diagnosis can be confirmed by examination and culture of the pericardial membranes. Constrictive pericarditis is a late complication.

**Abdominal tuberculosis** occurs secondary to swallowing infected material, including contaminated milk or sputum. This is a relatively uncommon complication in developed nations where dairy herds are inspected for tuberculosis. Manifestations include dysphagia, pain, or signs of obstruction, perforation, hemorrhage, fistula formation, or colitis. Tuberculous peritonitis presents as fever, anorexia, and abdominal pain. The diagnosis depends on skin test results and on histology and culture of involved tissue and peritoneal fluid.

**Urogenital tuberculosis** is a late reactivation complication and is rare in children. Symptomatic illness presents as dysuria, frequency, urgency, hematuria, and "sterile" pyuria.

**Tuberculosis of bone** occurs following dissemination or erosion from adjacent caseating lymph nodes. The spine (**Pott disease**) is the most common site, followed by the hip and the fingers and toes (**dactylitis**). Roentgenograms demonstrate cortical destruction.

*Diagnosis.* The *skin test* response to tuberculin antigen is a manifestation of a T cell–mediated delayed hypersensitivity. It is usually positive 2–6 wk after onset of infection (occasionally 3 mo) and at the time of symptomatic illness. Multiple puncture tests (such as the *tine test*) are no longer recommended for screening high-risk populations. The *Mantoux test,* an intradermal injection, usually on the volar surface of the forearm, of 5 TU (tuberculin units) (intermediate test strength) of Tween-stabi-

lized purified tuberculous antigen (purified protein derivative, standard [PPD-S]) is the standard for screening high-risk populations and for diagnosis in all ill patients or contacts. A 10-mm induration reaction after 48 hr traditionally indicated infection, but erythemia has no significance; 5- to 10-mm induration indicates infection in high-risk populations (strong clinical suspicion of TB, close contacts, HIV) but occasionally may be due to atypical mycobacteria or prior bacille Calmette-Guérin (BCG) vaccine vaccination. In northern states, where atypical bacilli are not endemic, 5–9 mm may be more significant. BCG immunization alone rarely can produce induration to PPD-S greater than 10 mm. A 15 mm induration may be positive for low-risk patients older than 4 yr of age. False-negative responses may occur early in the illness, with use of inactivated antigen (as a result of poor storage practice or inadequate administration), or as a result of immunosuppression (secondary to underlying illness, AIDS, malnutrition, or overwhelming tuberculosis). Tests with questionable results should be repeated after several weeks of therapy and adequate nutrition. An antigen panel should be included with the PPD-S to determine a more global state of anergy.

Although *histologic* demonstration of caseous granulomas is not a diagnostic finding, identifying the bacilli in tissue or secretions by acid-fast staining or nonspecific absorption of fluorescent dyes (fluorochrome stain) suggests the diagnosis.

The ultimate diagnostic confirmation relies on *culture* of the organism, a process that usually is more successful when tissue is utilized (e.g., pleural biopsy, pericardial membrane), rather than only the pleural or pericardial fluid. In young infants, gastric material (often mixed with swallowed sputum) may yield positive results when sputum is unobtainable. Large volumes of fluid (CSF, pericardial fluid) yield a higher rate of recovery of organisms, but slow growth of the mycobacteria (3–6 wk) makes culture less helpful in very ill children. Rapid culture methods ($^{14}$C media) facilitate diagnosis and drug susceptibility testing. Once the organism is grown, the drug susceptibilities should be determined because of the increasing incidence of resistant organisms. Antigen detection and DNA probes have expedited diagnosis, especially in CNS disease.

### Treatment
*HOSPITALIZATION.* Hospitalization is not uniformly mandated but is necessary in several situations when the child needs specialized, continuous, or closely supervised care:

1. Therapy for severe or life-threatening disease.

2. Initial evaluation and therapy of a young child (3 yr of age or younger).
3. For acquisition of culture or biopsy by invasive techniques.
4. Use of corticosteroid therapy or surgical intervention.
5. Treatment of severe drug reaction.
6. Treatment of severe coexisting disease.
7. Initial evaluation and therapy when family or social disorganization would interfere with ambulatory management.

ANTITUBERCULOSIS DRUGS. In general, because of the emergence of drug resistance in vivo, most manifestations of tuberculosis, except those associated with the lowest level of replicating organisms (asymptomatic skin test conversions), are treated with at least two drugs to which the organisms are susceptible (Table 10–14). In life-threatening disease, such as meningitis or miliary tuberculosis, in patients with large numbers of organisms (cavitary lesions), or in regions where the incidence of primary drug resistance is high, four agents are ini-

**TABLE 10–14.** Recommended Treatment Regimens for Drug-Susceptible Tuberculosis in Infants, Children, and Adolescents*

| Infection or Disease Category | Regimen* | Remarks |
|---|---|---|
| *Asymptomatic infection* (positive skin test, no disease): | | If daily therapy is not possible, therapy twice a week may be used for 6–9 mo. HIV-infected children should be treated for 12 mo. |
| Isoniazid-susceptible | 6–9 mo of isoniazid once a day | |
| Isoniazid-resistant | 6–9 mo of rifampin once a day | |
| Isoniazid-rifampin-resistant* | Consult a tuberculosis specialist | |
| *Pulmonary* | *6-mo regimens* | If possible drug resistance is a concern (see text), another drug (ethambutol or streptomycin) is added to the initial 3-drug therapy until drug susceptibilities are determined. |
| | 2 mo of isoniazid, rifampin, and pyrazinamide once a day, followed by 4 mo of isoniazid and rifampin daily | |
| | *or* | |
| | 2 mo of isoniazid, rifampin, and pyrazinamide daily, followed by 4 mo of isoniazid and rifampin twice a week | Drugs can be given 2 or 3 times per wk under direct observation in the initial phase if nonadherence is likely. |
| | *9-mo alternative regimens (for hilar adenopathy only):* | Regimens consisting of 6 mo of isoniazid and rifampin once a day, and 1 mo of isoniazid and rifampin once a day, followed by 5 mo of isoniazid and rifampin twice a week, have been successful in areas where drug resistance is rare. |
| | 9 mo of isoniazid and rifampin once a day | |
| | *or* | |
| | 1 mo of isoniazid and rifampin once a day, followed by 8 mo of isoniazid and rifampin twice a week | |
| *Extrapulmonary meningitis, disseminated (miliary), bone/joint disease* | 2 mo of isoniazid, rifampin, pyrazinamide, and streptomycin once a day, followed by 10 mo of isoniazid and rifampin once a day (12 mo total) | Streptomycin is given with initial therapy until drug susceptibility is known. Steroids are added in meningitis. |
| | *or* | |
| | 2 mo of isoniazid, rifampin, pyrazinamide, and streptomycin once a day, followed by 10 mo of isoniazid and rifampin twice a week (12 mo total) | For patients who may have acquired tuberculosis in geographic areas where resistance to streptomycin is common, capreomycin (15–30 mg/kg/d) or kanamycin (15–30 mg/kg/d) may be used instead of streptomycin. |
| *Other (e.g., cervical lymphadenopathy)* | Same as for pulmonary disease. | See *Pulmonary.* |

From American Academy of Pediatrics: Tuberculosis. *In* Peter G (ed): 1997 Red Book: Report of the Committee on Infectious Diseases, 24th ed. Elk Grove Village, IL: American Academy of Pediatrics, 1997, p 555.
*Duration of therapy is longer in HIV-infected persons and additional drugs may be indicated.
HIV = human immunodeficiency syndrome.

tially utilized. Multiple drug therapy may shorten the duration of treatment and prevent emergence of drug resistance. As a result of problems in compliance with multiple drug therapy, directly observed therapy given three times per week has been found to be effective.

*Isoniazid* (INH) is the drug of choice for tuberculosis and is used in all regimens unless the organism is resistant. It is bactericidal, well absorbed orally, and appears in all body fluids, including CSF. The major side effects are hepatotoxicity (uncommon in children) and neuritis secondary to pyridoxine deficiency, which is rare in children but can be prevented in adolescents and adults by simultaneously administering pyridoxine. Mild elevations of serum glutamic oxaloacetic transaminase are common and are not a contraindication for continuing INH. However, if hyperbilirubinemia, hepatomegaly, systemic "flu-like" illness, or a greater than three-fold elevation of serum glutamic pyruvic transaminase (SGPT) occurs, INH should be discontinued.

*Rifampin* is the other drug of choice for tuberculosis therapy. It is also bactericidal (inhibits bacterial RNA polymerase), well absorbed orally, distributed into all body fluids, and accumulates in infected monocytes. Side effects include orange discoloration of body secretions (with permanent discoloration of soft contact lenses). The major side effect is hepatotoxicity, the risk of which is increased by simultaneously administration of INH. Reducing the dosage decreases the risk. Thrombocytopenia, leukopenia, and an influenza-like syndrome are uncommon side effects. Rifampin interferes with metabolism of several drugs (see Appendix I). It is teratogenic in laboratory animals and contraindicated in the first trimester of pregnancy.

*Ethambutol* is a bacteriostatic oral agent that achieves low concentrations in CSF. It is highly active against tuberculosis. Its main limitation is ocular toxicity (blurred vision, color blindness, visual field constriction due to optic neuritis), which is reversible. Because these toxicities are impossible to monitor in a young (<6 yr) child, the use of ethambutol is precluded below this age unless drug resistance or severe disease is present.

*Streptomycin* is bactericidal, administered intramuscularly, and moderately ototoxic and nephrotoxic. It is utilized only in serious illness for a short period of time (up to 12 wk).

*Pyrazinamide* is a bactericidal oral agent distributed into CSF and an important drug used in multidrug short-course regimens. Side effects include hyperuricemia and polyarthralgias.

*Ethionamide* is a bacteriostatic oral agent used occasionally in therapy of drug-resistant organisms.

*Corticosteroids* are useful in the initial therapy of tuberculous meningitis to lower increased intracranial pressure, and in endobronchial tuberculosis and tuberculous pleuritis or pericarditis to speed the resolution of fluid and obstruction. Steroids should never be used in a patient with tuberculosis without concomitant antituberculosis therapy.

*Prevention.* Tuberculosis is prevented by (1) preventing contact with an actively infected person, (2) providing chemoprophylaxis with INH (see earlier), or (3) possibly by vaccinating using BCG vaccine. The use of BCG, a live attenuated mycobacterial vaccine, remains controversial, although it is used throughout much of the world. Controlled studies on its efficacy are variable. It is generally advocated in endemic regions to prevent neonatal tuberculosis, particularly tuberculous meningitis. There are no data to demonstrate protection in older individuals who might be exposed to multiple drug-resistant tuberculosis, and most experts do not recommend its use in the United States for these purposes. BCG vaccine should not be used in patients with altered immunity.

In a recipient of BCG, a tuberculin skin test of greater than 10 mm induration, 3 or more years after vaccination, is more likely to be due to infection with *M. tuberculosis* than a response to the vaccine, and these patients should be evaluated and treated.

*Tuberculosis During Pregnancy.* Pregnancy does not interfere with a positive skin test, and the test is indicated in all pregnant women. Chest roentgenograms should be deferred in the asymptomatic woman until the end of the first trimester. Asymptomatic women with a positive skin test but normal chest roentgenograms should not receive INH until delivery because of the risk of hepatotoxicity. Women with active disease should receive INH, rifampin, ethambutol, and pyridoxine.

*Infants Born to Mothers with Tuberculosis.* Approximately 50% of the infants born to mothers with active disease will have tuberculosis in the 1st yr of life. If congenital tuberculosis is suspected, the infant should be treated promptly with INH, pyrazinamide, streptomycin, plus rifampin. The skin test may not be positive for 6 mo. If the mother is asymptomatic (PPD-positive) and no active disease is present in the family, the infant is tested (5 TU PPD) at 4–6 wk and 3–4 mo of age. If the family cannot be evaluated, INH (10 mg/kg/24 hr) may be started. If the mother has newly diagnosed but noncontagious disease at delivery, the asymptomatic infant should have a chest roentgenogram and 5 TU PPD (Mantoux) test at 4–6 wk,

3–4 mo, and 6 mo of age. INH is begun at birth and discontinued at 3–4 mo if the PPD is negative and there is no active disease in the family. With poor compliance, maternal positive sputum (culture or stain), and supervision unsure, BCG vaccination is indicated in the asymptomatic, PPD-negative infant. The latter measure may not prevent disease acquisition but may reduce severity and dissemination. If the mother is contagious, the mother and child are separated until she is noncontagious.

### References

Bass JB Jr, Farer LS, Hopewell PC, et al: Diagnostic standards and classification of tuberculosis. Am Rev Respir Dis 142:725, 1990.

Behrman RE, Kliegman RM, Arvin AM (eds): Nelson Textbook of Pediatrics, 15th ed. Philadelphia, WB Saunders, 1996, Chapter 199.

Centers for Disease Control and Prevention: Initial therapy for tuberculosis in the era of multidrug resistance. MMWR 42:(RR1)1, 1993.

Hussey G, Chisholm T, Kibel M: Miliary tuberculosis in children: A review of 94 cases. Pediatr Infect Dis J 10:832, 1991.

Starke JR, Jacobs RF, Jereb J: Resurgence of tuberculosis in children. J Pediatr 120:839, 1992.

Waecker NJ Jr, Connor JD: Central nervous system tuberculosis in children: A review of 30 cases. Pediatr Infect Dis J 9:539, 1990.

### Nontuberculous Mycobacterial Infection

*Etiology.* The staining and morphologic characteristics of nontuberculous *Mycobacterium* species (termed "atypical mycobacteria") are similar to those of *M. tuberculosis*, but they differ in a variety of other characteristics, such as growth patterns and pigment production. The five species commonly associated with human disease include:

- Members of the Runyon Group I, the photochromogens, which form pigment on exposure to light (*M. kansasii, M. marinum*)
- Group II, the scotochromogens, which form pigment in the dark (*M. scrofulaceum*)
- Group III, the nonchromogens, which fail to produce pigment (*M. avium-intracellulare* complex [MAC])
- Group IV, the rapid growers (*M. fortuitum-chelonei*).

There are numerous other mycobacteria, but they rarely are associated with human disease.

*Epidemiology.* Mycobacterial agents are distributed worldwide and exist in soil, vegetation, dust, and water. They are pathogens in various animals. Infection occurs by inoculation of the skin or by inhalation. Atypical mycobacterial infections in immunocompetent patients are more common in warm, humid, rural environments, such as the southern states. No evidence exists for person-to-person spread. Nosocomial infection with *M. chelonei* and *M. fortuitum* have occurred, and opportunistic infection with *M. avium-intracellulare* organisms affects patients with advanced AIDS.

*Clinical Manifestations.* The most frequent manifestation of infection in children is lymphadenitis. This is usually a unilateral cervical, submandibular, or preauricular (less commonly axillary and inguinal) swelling in a 1–5 yr old child with a normal chest roentgenogram and no history of exposure to tuberculosis. The node may suppurate and drain but usually is hard and painless. In the United States, lymphadenitis is often due to *M. avium-intracellulare,* particularly in the Southeast. *M. scrofulaceum* or, rarely, *M. kansasii* are also associated with lymphadenitis; however, *M. tuberculosis* is probably more common, particularly in older children (>12 yr), as the prevalence of this disease has increased. Differential diagnosis should rule out infection due to *M. tuberculosis,* fungi, or bacteria as well as cat-scratch disease, toxoplasmosis, sarcoidosis, lymphoma, and drug reaction. Diagnosis and therapy both are made by excisional biopsy. These organisms are usually highly drug-resistant and therapy must be guided by antimicrobial susceptibility tests.

**Cutaneous disease** is usually the result of inoculation with *M. marinum* (swimming pool granuloma or fish tank granuloma) or with *M. fortuitum-chelonei.* The initial papule or nodule may enlarge and ulcerate. Infection in healthy children often is self-limited. *M. marinum* is treated for 3–4 mo with doxycycline, rifampin, and ethambutol, or trimethoprim/sulfamethoxazole. *M. fortuitum-chelonei* infection usually develops secondary to abrasions, puncture wounds, or foreign body placement during surgery and requires débridement, drainage, and often antibiotic therapy (amikacin, cefoxitin, or clarithromycin for *M. chelonei*).

**Pulmonary infection** with these bacterial agents is uncommon in children and resembles tuberculosis. It may occur rarely with *M. kansasii* in adolescent patients.

**Disseminated disease** with bacteremia, pneumonia, diarrhea, and fever usually occurs in immunocompromised individuals and often is due to the *M. avium-intracellulare* complex, especially in patients with AIDS. Disseminated MAC infection in these patients often presents with unremitting fevers in the absence of specific symptoms along with weight loss, night sweats, and evidence of bone marrow suppression; most commonly, it occurs in patients with long-standing HIV infection and severe depletion of CD4+ T cells. Multiple blood cultures should be examined to isolate the organisms. Therapy usually consists of a multidrug regimen, including ethambutol and clarithromycin, plus a third agent (such as clofazimine, rifabutin, ciprofloxacin or amikacin). Rifabutin alone is recommended for prophylaxis for MAC in AIDS patients with low CD4+ cell counts, after active mycobacterial disease has been excluded. Suppression of infection and symptoms is possible but bacteriologic cure is unusual.

***Diagnosis.*** The diagnosis depends on staining and culture of secretions or tissue. The skin test reaction to PPD often is intermediately positive (5–10 mm of induration in the Mantoux test). MAC is often identified by DNA probes.

### References

Behrman RE, Kliegman RM, Arvin AM (eds): Nelson Textbook of Pediatrics, 15th ed. Philadelphia, WB Saunders, 1996, Chapter 200.
Benson C: Treatment of disseminated disease due to *Mycobacterium avium* complex in patients with AIDS. Clin Infect Dis 18(Suppl 3):S237, 1994.
Wolinsky E: Mycobacterial diseases other than tuberculosis. Clin Infect Dis 15:1, 1992.

## INFECTIONS CAUSED BY NEISSERIAE

Neisseriae are gram-negative, spherical or oval diplococci. The bacteria are observed within polymorphonuclear leukocytes obtained from diseased areas of the body. Neisseriae are aerobic and can be cultured on blood agar, but recovery is enhanced by use of appropriate media. Neisseriae normally are found in the nasal mucosa, pharynx, vagina, and lower intestinal tract. Human disease most commonly is due to infection with *N. meningitidis* and *N. gonorrhoeae* (see Chapter 7).

### Meningococcal Infections

***Etiology.*** *N. meningitidis* is a human pathogen that expresses several virulence factors that enable the organism to cause bacteremia, sepsis, and meningitis. Organisms initially colonize the nasopharynx, then express an IgA protease that allows them to reach the epithelial cell surface, where they are ingested by receptor-mediated endocytosis. These pathogens reach the blood stream where, in the absence of preformed antibody, they cause bacteremia. The pathogenic *Neisseria* express siderophores, which enable them to scavenge iron from transferrin and replicate under these conditions. In addition, their lipopolysaccharide (endotoxin) is highly immunogenic, eliciting macrophage and T-cell activation, cytokine expression, and neutrophil recruitment.

Nine serogroups of *N. meningitidis* have been identified (A, B, C, D, X, Y, Z, 29E, and W135) on the basis of specific capsular polysaccharides. Groups B (45%), C (32%), Y (18%), and W135 are the common serogroups in the United States. Group B is noted in sporadic cases and groups A and C occur in epidemic cases.

***Epidemiology.*** The rates of asymptomatic carriers of *N. meningitidis* vary from 2–5% in healthy children to as high as 90% in military personnel during epidemics. Meningococcal meningitis is a disease of young children who acquire *N. meningitidis* from an adult carrier, usually in the same family. Person-to-person transmission is through infected respiratory droplets. Age-specific attack rates are greatest for infants under 1 yr of age; 80% of cases of meningococcal disease occur in children under 10 yr of age. A second peak appears during adolescence. The estimated likelihood of meningococcal disease in family contacts, usually occurring within 1 wk of the first case (incubation period is 3–4 days), is 1%. This is 1000-fold greater than the risk in the community. Persons with deficiency of terminal complement component (C5-9) and IgG2 subclass are at high risk for recurrent disease. Properdin-deficient males may develop fatal meningococcemia. Meningococcal disease often follows viral upper respiratory tract infections. Epidemic *N. meningitidis* is a common problem in sub-Saharan Africa, the "meningitis belt," as well as in other developing countries. These outbreaks may last several years and are usually due to type A organisms; the annual incidence may be up to 400 cases per 100,000.

***Clinical Manifestations.*** Invasive meningococcal infections usually result in septicemic meningococcemia and/or meningitis. Acute meningococcemia initially occurs as an influenza-like illness but becomes fulminant within hours to days, accompanied by the occurrence of morbilliform, petechial, or purpuric lesions and hypotension; DIC; oliguria; renal failure; and coma. Acute meningococcemia may be associated with varying systemic severity. In meningitis, the signs and symptoms of meningeal irritation are similar to those of acute meningitis produced by *H. influenzae* and *S. pneumoniae*. Meningococcemia may be associated with acute endocarditis, myocarditis, pericarditis, and arthritis. Other less common meningococcal diseases include pneumonia, endophthalmitis, vulvovaginitis, urethritis, pelvic inflammatory disease, adrenal hemorrhage (**Waterhouse-Friderichsen syndrome**), and chronic meningococcemia. The latter is characterized by intermittent fever, malaise, maculopapular rash, arthralgias, and arthritis.

*Diagnosis and Differential Diagnosis.* The diagnosis of meningococcal disease is established by stains and culture of blood, CSF, skin lesions, or other usually sterile sites. When meningitis is present, the laboratory characteristics of CSF reflect an acute bacterial meningitis. A poor prognostic sign is a normal CSF profile with no leukocytes but with sheets of gram-negative diplococci. Alternately, the Gram stain and culture may be negative if the patient was pretreated with antibiotics. Blood, CSF, and urine can be tested by latex agglutination, a technique that can allow the detection of capsular antigen from most *N. meningitidis* types.

The petechial or purpuric rash of meningococcemia is similar to that of diseases characterized by generalized vasculitis, including septicemia caused by gram-negative and gram-positive organisms; bacterial endocarditis; gonococcemia; Henoch-Schönlein purpura; Rocky Mountain spotted fever; endemic typhus; atypical measles; and infection with echoviruses and coxsackieviruses. The morbilliform rash occasionally observed may be confused with any macular or maculopapular viral exanthem (see Table 10–2).

*Treatment.* Intravenous penicillin is the drug of choice for patients with invasive disease. Ceftriaxone, cefotaxime, and chloramphenicol are alternative antibiotics (see Appendix I). Penicillin-resistant strains have been reported from all over the world including Europe, Africa, and the United States (less frequently). These strains have mutations in PBP2 (penicillin-binding protein), a transpeptidase normally inhibited by penicillin. Cefotaxime is active against these organisms. Supportive measures include careful monitoring and treatment of shock, myocarditis, pericarditis, septic arthritis, ARDS, DIC, and necrotic cutaneous or extremity lesions.

*Prevention.* Meningococcal vaccine against serogroups A, C, Y, and W135 is available but is not routinely recommended for children. Vaccine should be administered to children over 2 yr of age who have functional or anatomic asplenia and to those with terminal complement component or properdin deficiencies. Household, day care, nursery school, and closely exposed medical contacts should receive rifampin chemoprophylaxis as soon as possible following diagnosis of the primary case. The patient should be placed in respiratory isolation for 24 hr after admission and should receive rifampin prior to discharge.

*Prognosis.* The mortality rate of acute meningococcemia with septic shock may be as high as 20–50%. The mortality rate for patients with isolated meningococcal meningitis is less than 3%, if treated early. Poor prognostic signs include the development of hypotension, coma, rapidly progressive purpura (within 12 hr), DIC, absence of meningitis, absence of leukocytosis, thrombocytopenia, high antigen concentrations in serum and CSF, and a low sedimentation rate. Survival for 48 hr following initiation of therapy is a good prognostic sign. Sloughing of necrotic skin over purpuric areas usually heals uneventfully.

### References

Behrman RE, Kliegman RM, Arvin AM (eds): Nelson Textbook of Pediatrics, 15th ed. Philadelphia, WB Saunders, 1996, Chapter 178.

Hubert B, Watier L, Garnerin P, et al: Meningococcal disease and influenza-like syndrome: A new approach to an old question. J Infect Dis 166:542, 1992.

Mayon-White R, Heath P: Preventative strategies on meningococcal disease. Arch Dis Child 76:128, 1997.

Zangwill K, Schuchat A, Riedo F, et al: School-based clusters of meningococcal disease in the United States. JAMA 277:389, 1997.

## PERTUSSIS
### (Whooping Cough)

*Etiology.* Pertussis, which means "intense cough," is predominantly caused by *Bordetella pertussis*, but a pertussis-like illness has been associated with infection by *B. parapertussis*, *B. bronchiseptica*, and adenovirus. *B. pertussis* organisms are gram-negative, pleomorphic bacilli with fastidious requirements for growth provided by Bordet-Gengou media.

*Epidemiology.* Pertussis is highly contagious, producing attack rates of more than 90% in susceptible populations. Humans are the only known host of *B. pertussis*; transmission is by droplets released during intense coughing. The incubation period has a mean of 6 days and a range of 6–14 days. Patients are most contagious during the preparoxysmal stage. Risk of disease is highest in children under 5 yr of age; 30% of cases in the United States occur in infants under 6 mo of age. Mortality is greatest in infants under 1 yr of age. There is little seasonal variation. *B. pertussis* rarely is isolated from asymptomatic individuals.

Immunization reduces the incidence and mortality rate of pertussis, but immunity is neither complete nor permanent. Outbreaks of pertussis have been common in urban areas, even in children who were fully immunized. Many adolescents and adults, despite previous vaccination or disease, are susceptible to infection and are the major reservoir for infection of infants. In adults, the syndrome often is atypical, becoming manifest as a severe protracted cough without a whoop. Intrafamily spread is common. The younger the child, the more atypical the signs and symptoms of the disease; infants less than 6 mo of age may have apnea, cyanotic spells, and cough but no whoop. Pertussis is increasing in frequency in areas where immunization has declined.

***Clinical Manifestations.*** Symptomatic illness lasts 6–8 wk and generally is divided into three states: (1) *catarrhal* (prodromal, preparoxysmal), (2) *paroxysmal* (spasmodic cough), and (3) *convalescent.* The clinical manifestations depend on the specific pathogen, the patient's age, and the host's immunization status. Illness caused by *B. parapertussis* or *B. bronchiseptica* is less severe and of shorter duration than that caused by *B. pertussis,* an organism that adheres to and causes necrosis of the respiratory epithelium from the nasopharynx to the terminal bronchioles, resulting in bronchitis, atelectasis, and bronchopneumonia. The perihilar infiltrates produce the "shaggy" heart border on chest roentgenograms characteristic of pertussis.

CATARRHAL STAGE (1–2 WK). Rhinorrhea (clear to mucoid), conjunctival injection, lacrimation, mild cough, wheezing, and low-grade fever are noted. Unfortunately, a diagnosis of pertussis usually is not considered during this stage, even though at this time the organisms are present in the greatest concentration, because the manifestations are similar to those of most nonspecific viral upper respiratory tract infections.

PAROXYSMAL STAGE (2–4 WK OR LONGER). Episodes of coughing increase in severity and frequency. Multiple, repetitive series of five to 10 forceful coughs during an expiration are followed by a sudden massive inspiration, producing the whoop, as air is forcefully inhaled against a narrowed glottis. The whoop may be absent in children younger than 6 mo of age or in adults. Facial petechiae and redness, venous engorgement, and cyanosis may be prominent during the attack. Post-tussive vomiting should raise the suspicion of pertussis. Recurrent episodes are exhausting; patients appear apathetic and lose weight. Attacks may be initiated by yawning, sneezing, eating, drinking, and physical exertion. Paroxysms may produce anoxic brain damage; alternately, pertussis may produce encephalopathy.

CONVALESCENT STAGE (1–2 WK). Paroxysmal coughing and vomiting decrease in frequency and severity. During this phase, chronic cough may persist for several months. Rarely, paroxysmal cough recurs accompanied by subsequent upper respiratory tract infections in the ensuing months.

***Diagnosis and Differential Diagnosis.*** Pertussis is recognized readily during the typical paroxysmal stage. A history of incomplete immunization and of contact with a known case is helpful. Leuko-

cytosis (counts of 20,000–100,000 cells/$\mu$L) with an absolute lymphocytosis is characteristic at the end of the catarrhal stage and during the paroxysmal stage of the disease. Lymphocytosis may not be evident in partially immunized or very young infants. Chest roentgenograms may show perihilar infiltrates, atelectasis, or emphysema.

The diagnosis depends on isolation of *B. pertussis,* usually accomplished during the early phases of illness by culture of nasopharyngeal swabs on glycerin-potato-blood agar medium (Bordet-Gengou) to which penicillin has been added to inhibit growth of other organisms. *B. parapertussis* and *B. bronchiseptica,* both morphologically similar to *B. pertussis,* can be differentiated by specific agglutination reactions. Fluorescent antibody staining of pharyngeal specimens provides a rapid specific diagnosis.

Attacks of coughing may be observed in bronchiolitis, pneumonia (due to *Chlamydia*, bacteria, CMV), cystic fibrosis, tuberculosis, asthma, and intrathoracic lymphadenopathy compressing the trachea and bronchi. A foreign body produces similar coughing and can be distinguished by sudden onset of symptoms and by roentgenography and endoscopy.

***Complications.*** The most frequent complication is pneumonia caused by *B. pertussis* itself or resulting from secondary bacterial infection (pneumococcus, *H. influenzae, S. aureus*). Atelectasis may be secondary to mucus plugs. Otitis media and sinusitis are common and usually are due to *S. pneumoniae.* The force of the paroxysm may rupture alveoli and produce pneumomediastinum, pneumothorax, or interstitial or subcutaneous emphysema. Bronchiectasis may develop. Increased intrathoracic pressure and venous engorgement may cause epistaxis, retinal and subconjunctival hemorrhages, intraventricular and subarachnoid hemorrhage, rupture of the diaphragm, and inguinal hernia. Tetanic seizures may be associated with alkalosis related to persistent vomiting. Convulsions and encephalopathy occur in 2.5% and 0.5% of infants, respectively.

***Treatment.*** Erythromycin aborts or eliminates pertussis when administered in the catarrhal stage of the disease but does not affect the duration of the paroxysmal stage. Erythromycin eliminates organisms from the nasopharynx within 3–4 days, thereby shortening the period of communicability (see Appendix I). Azithromycin or clarithromycin may be equally effective. Corticosteroids and salbutamol aerosols may be helpful in severe cases. Supportive care includes warm mist oxygen, nasopharyngeal suctioning, and parenteral fluids.

***Prevention.*** As a result of limited immunity in

adults and lack of transplacental immunity, infants are highly susceptible to infection. Active immunity can be induced with either the traditional pertussis (whole cell) vaccine or with an "acellular" pertussis vaccine (DTaP). Pertussis vaccine has an efficacy of 70–90%; efficacy declines with fewer vaccinations. The rates of moderate side effects attributed to pertussis vaccine include persistent crying (>3 hr) or high fever (105°F or more) at a rate of 1/100–1000 doses; a seizure or a shock-like collapse at a rate of 1/1750 doses, and "severe" side effects, including coma, prolonged seizures, or both, at a rate of 1/110,000–310,000. The rates of these untoward events are still significantly lower than the morbidity associated with the disease. Side effects secondary to the acellular pertussis vaccine are appreciably less frequent than following the whole cell vaccine. The acellular pertussis vaccine was approved for all pertussis immunizations in 1996.

Prematurity is not believed to increase the risk of seizures following pertussis immunization. Erythromycin is effective in preventing disease in newborn infants and adults exposed to pertussis. Close contacts younger than 7 yr of age who have received four doses of vaccine should receive a booster dose of DTaP unless a booster dose has been given within the preceding 3 yr. They also should be given erythromycin. Close contacts older than 7 yr of age should receive prophylactic erythromycin for 10–14 days but not the vaccine. For the primary immunization schedule and contraindications for DPT or DTaP, see Figure 10–1. If pertussis exposure is probable, because of endemic or epidemic disease, the vaccine may be given at 2 wk of age. Patients who have pertussis do not require further pertussis vaccinations because the disease produces lifelong immunity.

*Prognosis.* The mortality rate is less than 1% but may reach 40% in infants under 5 mo of age. Most deaths are due to pneumonia or other pulmonary complications, asphyxia, or encephalopathy.

### References

Aoyama T, Sunakawa K, Iwata S, et al: Efficacy of short term treatment of pertussis with clarithromycin and azithromycin. J Pediatr 129:761, 1996.

Behrman RE, Kliegman RM, Arvin AM (eds): Nelson Textbook of Pediatrics, 15th ed. Philadelphia, WB Saunders, 1996, Chapter 181.

Blumberg D, Lewis K, Mink C, et al: Severe reactions associated with diphteria-tetanus-pertussis vaccine: Detailed study of children with seizures, hypotonic-hyporesponsive episodes, high fevers, and persistant crying. Pediatrics 91:1158, 1993.

Farizo KM, Cochi SL, Zell ER, et al: Epidemiological features of pertussis in the United States, 1980–1989. Clin Infect Dis 14:708, 1992.

Halsey NA, Peter G: New developments with pertussis vaccine. Pediatrics 96:971, 1995.

Hoppe JE and the Erythromycin Study Group: Comparison of erythromycin estolate and erythromycin ethylsuccinate for treatment of pertussis. Pediatr Infect Dis J 11:189, 1992.

## INFECTIONS CAUSED BY
## *STREPTOCOCCUS PNEUMONIAE*
(Pneumococcal Infections)

*S. pneumoniae* (formerly *Diplococcus pneumoniae*) may colonize the upper respiratory tract but also can become an invasive pathogen.

*Etiology.* *S. pneumoniae* is a gram-positive, encapsulated diplococcus. Eighty-three serotypes are identified by their type-specific capsular polysaccharide. The capsule impedes leukocytic phagocytosis and is an important virulence factor. Serotypes 6, 19, and 23 represent almost 50% of all isolates in children. These, plus types 1, 3, 4, 7, 9, 11, 14, 15, and 18, cause 80% of childhood pneumococcal infections. Carriage of a serotype does not induce local or systemic immunity sufficient to prevent later reacquisition of the same serotype. Colonization is greatest up to 2 yr of age and during the winter months.

*Epidemiology.* Males and blacks are more commonly affected than females and whites. Opsonophagocytosis depends on capsule-specific antibody and the reticuloendothelial system. Pneumococcal disease, therefore, has an increased frequency and severity in patients between 6 mo and 2 yr of age and patients with HIV, sickle cell disease, splenic dysfunction, asplenia, Hodgkin disease, nephrotic syndrome, basal skull fractures through a sinus, deficiencies in humoral (B-cell) immunity, and complement deficiencies. Transmission is through person-to-person contact by respiratory droplet.

*Clinical Manifestations.* *S. pneumoniae* is the most frequent bacterial cause of bacteremia, pneumonia, and otitis media; a common cause of sinusitis; and a common cause of meningitis in infants and children. The peak incidence of meningitis occurs among infants 3–5 mo of age, among children 6–12 mo of age who have otitis media, and among children 13–18 mo of age who are hospitalized for pneumonia. Pneumococcal meningitis is also a common cause of bacterial meningitis in older children and adults, and the pneumococcus is a common cause of bacterial pneumonia in all age groups, with or without the need for hospitalization. Local spread may cause empyema, pericarditis, mastoiditis, and epidural abscess. Bacteremia (occult) rarely is followed by meningitis, septic arthritis, osteomyelitis, and endocarditis. Pneumococcal bacteremia in young children with unexplained fever but no localizing signs or symptoms can occur without sequelae. Spontaneous pneumococcal peritonitis is common in patients with the nephrotic syndrome.

*Diagnosis.* The diagnosis is confirmed in older patients by Gram stain and a culture of sputum and in all patients by recovering pneumococci from blood or CSF culture. Isolation of pneumococci from the nose or throat of patients with otitis media, sinusitis, pneumonia, septicemia, or meningitis is not proof of causation because the frequency of the carrier state is high. Latex agglutination of serum, CSF, and urine is very helpful in establishing the diagnosis of pneumococcal meningitis, pneumonia, and bacteremia. The total white blood cell count is elevated (20,000–30,000/$\mu$L), as is the ESR in serious pneumococcal disease. Paracentesis, Gram stain, and culture are required to differentiate pneumococcal from other pathogens (e.g., *Escherichia coli*) in patients with peritonitis.

*Treatment.* Penicillin is the treatment of choice for pneumococcal disease. The dose and duration of treatment vary with the location of infection. Antimicrobial susceptibility (with an oxacillin disc) should be tested on all pneumococcal isolates.

*S. pneumoniae* organisms that are resistant to penicillin are a common cause of infection in children and in certain areas of the United States account for up to 30% of the pneumococcal isolates. These organisms are noted in children who attend day care and are "relatively" resistant if the penicillin MIC is 0.1–1.0 $\mu$g/mL or high-level resistance if it is greater than 2.0 $\mu$g/mL. Penicillin resistance rates in children attending day care may be as high as 61%, whereas national rates range from 4–48%. Resistant organisms have a series of mutations in the genes for PBP2 (penicillin-binding protein), an important target for the penicillins. The "relatively" resistant strains are effectively inhibited by antibiotics such as cefotaxime or ceftriaxone, whereas the highly resistant isolates, which have an MIC to cefotaxime greater than 0.5 $\mu$g/mL, require a non-$\beta$ lactam agent (vancomycin) for effective killing. This is particularly important in the management of pneumococcal meningitis, in which the amount of antibiotic that diffuses into the CSF may not be adequate to clear a resistant organism.

Current recommendations suggest the empiric use of larger doses of cefotaxime and vanomycin (60 mg/kg/24 hr) for children with meningitis, pending susceptibility data, and another lumbar puncture to ensure sterilization of the CSF 24–36 hr after the start of therapy, primarily in patients with cephalosporin-resistant organisms. Rifampin may be used as adjunctive therapy. Meropenem

may be valuable in the treatment of highly resistant organisms. Therapy for otitis media caused by these organisms may include higher doses of amoxicillin, erythromycin, clarithromycin or azithromycin, clindamycin, or intramuscular ceftriaxone. Tympanocentesis and cultures of middle ear fluid should be considered if the child does not respond to the usual empiric therapy to cover antibiotic susceptible pneumococci as well as the possibility of $\beta$-lactamase producing *H. influenzae* or *M. catarrhalis* species.

*Prevention.* A pneumococcal vaccine composed of purified capsular polysaccharide antigens of 23 pneumococcal serotypes has proved to be highly immunogenic and is associated with a low level of untoward reactions. However, responsiveness to pneumococcal polysaccharide vaccine is unpredictable in young children. This vaccine is recommended for children older than 2 yr of age with (1) asplenia, (2) nephrotic syndrome, (3) sickle cell disease, (4) other hemoglobinopathies, (5) HIV infection, (6) immunosuppression, and (7) about to undergo splenectomy for Hodgkin disease. Immunization does *not* prevent pneumococcal disease related to serotypes not found in the vaccine. Therefore, a history of immunization should not eliminate the need for antibiotics in high-risk situations, such as sickle cell anemia.

Administration of gammaglobulin to children with hypogammaglobulinemia (IgG < 200 mg/dL) reduces the risk of pneumococcal bacteremia and meningitis but not necessarily pneumococcal respiratory infections. Oral penicillin (amoxicillin) should be given continuously to all infants with sickle cell anemia and to other patients who are anatomically or functionally asplenic to prevent sepsis.

Clinical trials are in progress to determine the efficacy of protein-carbohydrate conjugate vaccines that include capsular antigens from the most common pneumococcal types and should be immunogenic in young infants.

### References

Behrman RE, Kliegman RM, Arvin AM (eds): Nelson Textbook of Pediatrics, 15th ed. Philadelphia, WB Saunders, 1996, Chapter 176.

Committee on Infectious Disease: Therapy for children with invasive pneumococcal infections. Pediatrics 99:289, 1997.

Hardie W, Bokulic R, Garcia V, et al: Pneumococcal pleural empyemas in children. Clin Infect Dis 22:1057, 1996.

Lehmann D, Gratten M, Montgomery J: Susceptibility of pneumococcal carriage isolates to penicillin provides a conservative estimate of susceptibility of invasive pneumococci. Pediatr Infect Dis J 16:297, 1997.

Tuomanen EI, Austrian R, Masure HR: Pathogenesis of pneumoccocal infection. N Engl J Med 332:1280, 1995.

## INFECTIONS CAUSED BY SALMONELLAE

Salmonellae are important pathogens of animals and humans. Humans become infected by ingesting contaminated water or food, typically beef, poultry, milk, and eggs. Systemic infection with *Salmonella typhi* (typhoid fever) is uncommon in the United States but is endemic and epidemic in other parts of the world. Infections caused by other types of salmonellae are common throughout the United States.

*Etiology.* Salmonellae are gram-negative, nonencapsulated bacilli. The principal antigens are the flagellum (H) antigens, the cell wall (O) antigens, and the envelope (Vi) heat-labile antigens. A typing scheme utilizing O and H antigens permits the differentiation of more than 2200 salmonella serotypes. Salmonellae are divided into serogroups designated A, B, C1, C2, D, and E on the basis of the O antigen. Although *S. typhi* and *S. paratyphi* are human pathogens, most other serotypes are widely distributed in animals.

Organisms are usually ingested from a contaminated source, and a large inoculum is required since salmonellae are killed by gastric acidity. Salmonellae express a number of specific virulence factors that enable them to elude the normal mucosal defenses. These bacteria attach and invade via specific receptors in the intestinal epithelium found on "M" cells, which are in direct contact with intestinal reticuloendothelial cells of the Peyer patches. The organisms are phagocytosed by macrophages but resist normal phagolysosomal fusion, replicate within the macrophages in the mesenteric lymph nodes, and can be released into the blood stream, causing bacteremia or sepsis. Disseminated infection can occur, particularly with *S. cholerasuis* and in immunocompromised patients, including patients with sickle cell disease and HIV infection, and produces bacteremia and metastatic complications.

### Salmonellosis
(Nontyphoidal)

*Epidemiology.* Salmonella gastroenteritis is most common in children younger than 4 yr of age; infants younger than 1 yr of age have the highest rates of infection, although it can occur at any age. Patients with decreased gastric acidity, especially young infants and older people, are particularly at risk. Infected animals are the major reservoir for the nontyphoid salmonellae. Infected poultry, eggs, and egg products as well as contaminated meats and pet reptiles, such as turtles and iguanas, are frequent sources of infection. There is growing concern that the widespread use of antibiotics in animal feeds has contributed to the increasing incidence of antibiotic-resistant salmonellae.

Humans are important carriers of salmonella species and can cause localized epidemics of food poisoning by fecal-oral contamination of food at large gatherings, such as picnics. Intrafamilial transmission of salmonellosis is frequent.

Seventy to 90% of individuals have a positive stool culture 2 wk after infection, about 50% at 4 wk, and 10–25% at 10 wk. The duration of salmonella excretion is longer in infants. The incubation period for gastroenteritis is from 6 to 72 hr but usually is less than 24 hr.

*Clinical Manifestations.* Salmonella gastroenteritis has a peak incidence in the late summer and early fall, correlating with food-borne outbreaks. Epidemics and disease found in small family clusters occur throughout the year. Onset is abrupt and is characterized by nausea, vomiting, and crampy abdominal pain followed by loose, watery stools that may contain mucus, leukocytes, and blood. Systemic signs of malaise, headache, and chills occasionally are noted. Fever of 38.3–38.9°C (101–102°F) is noted in 70% of patients and lasts for 48 hr. Symptoms subside within 2–5 days in healthy individuals. In patients who are compromised because of extremes of age, sickle cell disease, chronic granulomatous disease, AIDS, malignancy, antibiotic therapy, or corticosteroids, the illness may persist and become manifest as bacteremia with metastatic foci (meningitis, osteomyelitis). Septicemia accompanied by toxic appearance and high fever is much more common in the first 3 mo of life. Bacteremia in young infants and older children may clear spontaneously. Nonetheless, salmonella can localize and cause pneumonia, empyema, abscesses, osteomyelitis, septic arthritis, pyelonephritis, and meningitis. Neonates may become infected at birth, and sepsis and meningitis develop.

*Complications.* Enteritis may produce significant dehydration, electrolyte disturbances, and hypovolemic shock. Other complications of nontyphoidal salmonellosis are unusual and are limited to the extraintestinal lesions noted above. In addition, reactive polyarticular arthritis may develop in children about 2 wk after the diarrheal episode. There is a strong association with the presence of histocompatibility antigen human leukocyte antigen (HLA) B27 and the reactive arthritis syndrome following salmonella infection. Full-blown **Reiter disease** (conjunctivitis, urethritis, and polyarthritis) also may be noted. The joint fluid is sterile.

*Diagnosis.* Culture of stool is indicated when there is fever and the presence of blood, mucus, or leukocytes in the stool. Blood specimens should be obtained for culture in young infants and immuno-compromised patients. Cultures of stool, blood, urine, bone marrow aspirate, CSF, and foci of infection should be obtained in more complicated cases. Although three consecutive negative stool cultures suggest that infection has ceased, excretion may be intermittent. Salmonella gastroenteritis must be distinguished from other viral and bacterial causes of diarrhea (see Chapter 11). Rarely, the clinical course and roentgenographic findings suggest ulcerative colitis.

*Treatment.* Correction of shock, dehydration, and electrolyte imbalances are the most important aspects of the therapy of salmonella gastroenteritis. Uncomplicated enteritis in healthy children usually is improving when stool culture results are known; these children require no antibiotics. Antibiotics are indicated for high-risk individuals because of the possibility of dissemination of disease (infants under 3 mo of age, children with immunologic deficiency, malnutrition, or malignancy).

Children with septicemia, enteric fever, or metastatic sites of infection initially should be treated with ceftriaxone or cefotaxime. Alternative antibiotics are determined on antimicrobial resistance patterns; useful agents for susceptible salmonella include amoxicillin, trimethoprim/sulfamethoxazole, or quinolones. Fluoroquinolones are particularly effective for *Salmonella* infections and are considerably safer than alternatives such as chloramphenicol (see Appendix I).

## Typhoid Fever
### (Enteric Fever)

*Epidemiology.* In the United States, 300–500 cases of typhoid fever occur each year. The majority of reported cases occur in persons under 20 yr of age and are imported from other countries (India, Mexico). The typhoid bacillus infects only humans, and chronic carriers therefore are responsible for new cases.

*Pathogenesis.* The upper small bowel is the predominant site of invasion. Monocytes phagocytize but do not kill the bacilli early in the disease, and they carry the organisms from the blood to the mesenteric lymph nodes and other reticuloendothelial sites in which bacteria proliferate to produce inflammation in lymph nodes, liver, and spleen. Secondary septicemia is disseminated from these sites and usually is prolonged, seeding other organs. The gallbladder is particularly susceptible and is infected from the liver via the biliary system or from the blood. Microorganisms that multiply in the gallbladder eventually are discharged into the intestine.

*Clinical Manifestations.* The pattern of typhoid fever in infants ranges from mild gastroenteritis to severe septicemia without diarrhea. Fever, hepatomegaly, jaundice, anorexia, lethargy, and weight loss can be marked.

In older children, the course is characterized by high fever, malaise, lethargy, myalgia, headache, rash, hepatosplenomegaly, and abdominal pain and tenderness. Diarrhea occurs in fewer than half of older children in the early stage, but constipation is noted in the later stages. The patient may become severely obtunded and exhibit delirium and confusion. At this stage of the disease, the spleen generally is enlarged and abdominal tenderness is present. A macular (rose spots) or maculopapular rash is observable on the skin of as many as 80% of patients. The paradoxic relationship of a high temperature and low pulse rate may be observed. Typically, for each degree rise above 38.3°C (101°F), the pulse should rise 10 beats/minute (bpm). Leukopenia is common.

*Complications.* Intestinal perforation at the site of inoculation, usually in the ileum, occurs in 0.5–3%, and severe gastrointestinal hemorrhage occurs in 1–10% of children with typhoid fever. Most complications occur during the second (dissemination) stage of disease and are preceded by a fall in temperature and blood pressure and a rise in pulse rate. Toxic encephalopathy, cerebral thrombosis, acute cerebellar ataxia, optic neuritis, aphasia, deafness, transverse myelitis, and acute cholecystitis may occur. Pneumonia is common during the second stage of illness but is caused by a superinfection. Pyelonephritis, endocarditis, meningitis, osteomyelitis, and septic arthritis are rare in the normal host. Septic arthritis and osteomyelitis are seen in individuals with hemoglobinopathies.

*Diagnosis and Differential Diagnosis.* Examination of stool reveals mononuclear leukocytes. Blood cultures are positive early in the disease, whereas urine and stool cultures become positive following the secondary septicemia. Bone marrow, lymph nodes, and reticuloendothelial tissues often contain organisms after the blood has been sterilized. In suspected cases with negative cultures, a culture of aspirated bone marrow or duodenal fluid (to evaluate possible biliary infection) may be helpful. A four-fold rise in agglutinin titer in a nonimmunized individual usually is diagnostic.

During the initial stage of typhoid fever, the clinical diagnosis may be bronchitis, bronchopneumonia, gastroenteritis, or influenza. Subsequently, other infectious conditions caused by intracellular microorganisms may need to be considered. Concern about an acute abdomen may lead to unnecessary surgical intervention.

**Treatment.** Antibiotic resistance is common. Based on susceptibility, ceftriaxone, ampicillin, chloramphenicol, trimethoprim/sulfamethoxazole, and ciprofloxacin are useful drugs (see Appendix I).

Corticosteroid therapy has been suggested for severe toxemia or prolonged symptoms. Third-generation cephalosporins may cure carriers, particularly drugs that are metabolized in the liver. Cholecystectomy may be indicated.

**Prognosis.** Antimicrobial therapy has reduced the mortality rate to less than 1% in most areas, but the presence of underlying debilitating disease, perforation of the gastrointestinal tract, severe hemorrhage, or coma increases the mortality rate. Meningitis or endocarditis may be associated with high morbidity and mortality rates. Relapse occurs in up to 10% of those who are not treated with antibiotics.

Individuals who excrete *S. typhi* for 3 or more mo are usually excreters at 1 yr and often for life. The risk of becoming a chronic carrier is low in children; fluroquinolones eradicate the carrier state.

**Prevention.** An oral vaccine against *S. typhi* is available and is indicated for children and adults traveling to endemic areas, particularly where antibiotic resistant strains are common.

## References

Behrman RE, Kliegman RM, Arvin AM (eds): Nelson Textbook of Pediatrics, 15th ed. Philadelphia, WB Saunders, 1996, Chapter 182.

Baird-Parker AC: Foodborne salmonellosis. Lancet 336:1231, 1990.

Gupta A: Multidrug resistant typhoid fever in children: Epidemiology and therapeutic approach. Pediatr Infect Dis J 13:134, 1994.

St. Geme JW, Hodes HL, Marcy SM, et al: Consensus: Management of salmonella infection in the first year of life. Pediatr Infect Dis J 7:615, 1988.

## SHIGELLOSIS
### (Bacillary Dysentery)

See also Chapter 11.

**Etiology.** Shigellae are non–lactose-fermenting gram-negative rods. The genus *Shigella* includes *S. dysenteriae* (group A), important worldwide but rarely isolated in the United States; *S. flexneri* (group B); *S. boydii* (group C); and the most common isolate, *S. sonnei* (group D). Unlike the case with salmonellae, it takes a very small inoculum of ingested shigellae to cause disease. The organisms bind to receptors on M cells, specialized intestinal

epithelial cells overlying the Peyer patches. They are propelled within the epithelial cells by their ability to polymerize host cell actin filaments and can invade and spread laterally from one epithelial cell to the next. This invasion triggers host cell cytokine release as well as apoptosis, resulting in the recruitment of polymorphonuclear leukocytes and other inflammatory cells. In addition, some strains of *Shigella* produce shigatoxin, a potent cytotoxin that acts by inhibiting mammalian protein synthesis.

**Epidemiology.** Shigellosis is a common disease occurring primarily in young children between the ages of 1–10 yr, when fecal-oral transmission may be more likely to occur. Humans are the major reservoir of infection. The organisms survive readily on inanimate objects, facilitating transmission in child care settings, in nursery schools, and within families. In developing countries, water supplies are commonly contaminated. The incubation period varies from 1 to 7 days, and infected adults may shed organisms for a month.

**Clinical Manifestations.** Shigellae are prototypic invasive pathogens that destroy the superficial epithelial cells, producing inflammation, edema, microabscess formation, and ulceration with bleeding.

Mild *Shigella* infections result in watery diarrhea with minimal systemic symptoms. In severe cases, crampy abdominal pain, temperature greater than 40°C (104°F) lasting 1–3 days, and diarrhea containing blood and mucus can occur. The child may have nonlocalized lower abdominal tenderness. Shigellosis may mimic CNS diseases such as meningitis, particularly when high fever is associated with seizures. Seizures occur in 30% of children with *Shigella* gastroenteritis and are more common if the temperature exceeds 40°C (104°F).

*Shigella* infrequently may cause conjunctivitis and vaginitis from autoinoculation. Nonsuppurative arthritis and Reiter syndrome have been associated with *Shigella* infection. Hemolytic-uremic syndrome, possibly associated with toxin production, may coincide or follow enteritis.

**Diagnosis.** Stool should reveal leukocytes and red blood cells. The complete blood count displays leukocytosis composed of immature forms. The diagnosis is established by isolating the organism from stool or rectal cultures. Shigellosis must be differentiated from other causes of dysentery, such as infection with invasive *E. coli*, amebae, *Campylobacter jejuni*, *Yersinia enterocolitica*, and *Salmonella* as well as from intussusception and acute appendicitis.

**Treatment.** Particularly in young infants, fluid and electrolyte replacement, using oral rehydration solutions when possible, is critical. Antimicrobial therapy is complicated by widespread antimicrobial resistance. Appropriate treatment decreases further intestinal shedding of the organisms and further transmission of infection to others. Although oral ampicillin (but not amoxicillin, which does not achieve sufficient lumenal concentrations) was recommended, few isolates remain susceptible. Trimethoprim/sulfamethoxazole can be used if isolates are susceptible. Parenteral ceftriaxone is efficacious, as are the fluoroquinolones, which are often the only therapeutic option and have been safely used for this indication (see Appendix I).

### References

Behrman RE, Kliegman RM, Arvin AM (eds): Nelson Textbook of Pediatrics, 15th ed. Philadelphia, WB Saunders, 1996, Chapter 183.

Bennish ML: Potentially lethal complications of shigellosis. Rev Infect Dis 13:S319, 1991.

Eidlitz-Marcus T, Cohen YH, Nussinovitch M, et al: Comparative efficacy of two and five day courses of ceftriaxone for treatment of severe shigellosis in children. J Pediatr 123:822, 1993.

Goren A, Freier S, Passwell JH: Lethal toxic encephalopathy due to childhood shigellosis in a developed country. Pediatrics 89:1189, 1992.

Schaad UB, Salam MA, Aujard Y, et al: Use of fluoroquinolones in pediatrics: Consensus report of an International Society of Chemotherapy commission. Pediatr Infect Dis J 14:1, 1995.

## STAPHYLOCOCCAL INFECTIONS

Staphylococci are a common cause of pyogenic infections in infants and children. These organisms are gram-positive cocci that grow aerobically or as facultative anaerobes and appear in tetrads or grape-like clusters. Strains are classified as *S. aureus* (coagulase protein A and mannitol positive), *S. epidermidis* species (coagulase protein A and mannitol negative and novobiocin sensitive), and *S. saprophyticus* (coagulase-negative, mannitol-positive, novobiocin-resistant).

### Infections Caused by *Staphylococcus Aureus*

***Etiology.*** Staphylococci cause disease by a number of mechanisms:

1. Local destruction by exoenzymes (catalase, hyaluronidase, coagulase, phospholipases), which also interfere with host defense mechanisms.
2. The secretion of toxins, which can act locally or at a distant site (enterotoxins and TSST-1, the toxic shock toxin).
3. Superantigens, which activate T-cell receptor Vβ chains without requiring processing or α-chain specificity (TSST-1).
4. The organism's ability to elude normal host polymorphonuclear killing by binding the Fc portion of IgG and interfering with efficient opsonophagocytosis.

Strains of *S. aureus* can be classified by bacteriophage group typing. Exfoliative toxin, associated with phage group 2 and some non–group 2 staphylococci, is the cause of "scalded skin syndrome" (**Ritter disease**) and bullous impetigo. Staphylococcal enterotoxin is elaborated by most strains of *S. aureus*. Ingestion of preformed enterotoxin is associated with vomiting and diarrhea and, in some cases, with the development of profound hypotension.

***Epidemiology.*** *S. aureus* is part of normal human flora and is present in the anterior nares and moist areas of the body in about 30% of asymptomatic people. Transmission of *S. aureus* generally occurs via hands, nasal discharge, person-to-person contact, and, rarely, through air. Newborn infants are extremely susceptible to staphylococci; the nasopharynx, skin, and umbilical stump are the most common sites of colonization.

*S. aureus* colonizes skin and mucous membranes through its affinity for host glycoconjugates and intracellular matrix components, such as fibronectin, laminin, and collagen. Any break in the epidermis provides a niche for the organism. Infants with a very thin epidermis and impaired host defenses are particularly at risk, as are hospitalized patients with intravascular access devices or decreased polymorphonuclear leukocyte function due to corticosteroids or cancer chemotherapy. Person-to-person transmission of virulent organisms is common because nasal carriage is frequent in hospital personnel and is a potential source of infection.

***Clinical Manifestations.*** *S. aureus* causes a wide variety of suppurative lesions as well as septicemia and toxin-related diseases, including scalded skin syndrome, toxic shock syndrome, and food poisoning.

*SKIN.* Pyogenic skin infections may be primary or secondary to wounds or to a superinfection of other noninfectious skin disease (e.g., eczema) and include impetigo contagiosa, bullous impetigo, pustules, cellulitis, folliculitis, furuncles, and carbuncles. Toxin produces staphylococcal scalded skin syndrome (Ritter disease) and a rash resembling that in scarlet fever. In these conditions, staphylococci are not present in the lesions.

*RESPIRATORY TRACT.* Infections of the upper respiratory tract caused by *S. aureus* are rare, considering the rate of colonization of this area. Sinusitis caused by *S. aureus* may occur. Suppurative parotitis is a rare infection, but *S. aureus* is a common cause. *S. aureus* is a common cause of suppurative cervical adenitis. Tracheitis resembling viral croup but with high fever and toxicity may be caused by *S. aureus*. Pneumonia caused by *S. aureus* is noted in children under 1 yr of age and is associated with pneumatoceles, empyema, and sepsis.

*SEPSIS.* Staphylococcal bacteremia and sepsis may be primary infections without an initiating focus or localized lesion. Later, organisms may localize in the lungs, heart valves, joints, bones, kidneys, and brain.

*MUSCLE.* Localized staphylococcal abscesses in muscle associated with elevation of muscle enzymes have been called **tropical pyomyositis.** Multiple abscesses occur in 30–40% of cases. Surgical drainage and appropriate antibiotic therapy are essential.

*BONES AND JOINTS.* *S. aureus* is the most common cause of osteomyelitis and septic arthritis in children. These diseases are derived from hematogenous dissemination rather than direct extension of infection from an adjacent skin or soft tissue lesion.

*CENTRAL NERVOUS SYSTEM.* Meningitis caused by *S. aureus* is rare but may follow bacteremia or may originate from direct extension of otitis media or osteomyelitis of the skull or vertebrae. Trauma or infection of meningomyelocele also may predispose the patient to *S. aureus* meningitis. Staphylococcal infection following neurosurgical procedures generally is due to *S. epidermidis*. *S. aureus* can be recovered from brain abscesses following CNS trauma and spinal epidural abscess.

*HEART.* Acute bacterial endocarditis in children may follow staphylococcal bacteremia and occur in the absence of valvular heart disease as well as in patients with minimal valvular abnormalities, such as bicuspid mitral valves. Perforation of heart valves, myocardial abscesses, heart block, acute hemopericardium, purulent pericarditis, and sudden death may ensue.

*KIDNEY.* *S. aureus* is a common cause of renal and perinephric abscess. Uncomplicated urinary tract infection caused by *S. aureus* is unusual. Coagulase-negative staphylococci, particularly *S. saprophyticus*, are an important cause of urinary tract infection in adolescent girls.

*INTESTINAL TRACT.* Food poisoning may be caused by ingestion of preformed staphylococcal enterotoxins that contaminate foods. The short (1–7 hr) incubation period, lack of fever, short illness, and profuse emesis help differentiate it from other causes of food poisoning. Enterotoxins A and D are the most common causes in the United States.

*Diagnosis.* The diagnosis of staphylococcal infection follows the isolation of the organisms from skin lesions, abscess cavities, blood, CSF, or other usually sterile sites. Gram stains reveal gram-positive cocci in clusters. Following isolation, identification is made on the basis of Gram stain and coagulase and mannitol reactivity. Patterns of susceptibility to antibiotics should be assessed to guide therapy. Diagnosis of staphylococcal food poisoning is made on the basis of epidemiologic (e.g., unrefrigerated meats, mayonnaise, or creamed foods) and clinical findings. Food suspected of contamination should be examined by Gram stain culture and tested for enterotoxin.

*Treatment.* Loculated collections of purulent material must be incised and drained. Foreign bodies associated with infection may need to be removed. Virtually all staphylococci are resistant to penicillin; therefore, therapy should include a penicillinase-resistant antibiotic, such as methicillin, oxacillin, and nafcillin, or first-generation cephalosporins (cephalothin and cefazolin), or clindamycin. Vancomycin may be used to treat methicillin-resistant *S. aureus* or *S. epidermidis* (see Appendix I). Strains that hyperproduce beta-lactamase may be treated with amoxicillin/clavulanate, ticarcillin/clavulanate, ampicillin/sulbactam, imipenem, first-generation cephalosporins, fluoroquinolones, or vancomycin.

*Prevention.* Staphylococcal infection is transmitted by hand-to-hand contact. Observance of strict hand-washing techniques is the most effective measure for preventing the spread of staphylococci. Local antibiotic ointment (mupirocin), antiseptic dyes, rifampin, or ciprofloxacin may be useful in reducing the carrier state.

*Prognosis.* Mortality rates have been reduced to 20% by appropriate antibiotic treatment. Staphylococcal pneumonia can be fatal and is more likely to produce morbidity and mortality in young infants. A total WBC count below 5000 cells/$\mu$L or a polymorphonuclear leukocyte response of less than 50% is a grave prognostic sign. Endocarditis may require prolonged treatment and eventual valve replacement.

References

Behrman RE, Kliegman RM, Arvin AM (eds): Nelson Textbook of Pediatrics, 15th ed. Philadelphia, WB Saunders, 1996, Chapter 174.

Espersen F, Frimodt-Moller N, Rosdahl VT, et al: *Staphylococcus aureus* bacteraemia in children below the age of one year. Acta Paediatr Scand 78:56, 1989.

Hodes DS, Barzilai A: Invasive and toxin-mediated *Staphylococcus aureus* diseases in children. Adv Pediatr Infect Dis 5:35, 1990.

Marrack P, Kappler J: The staphylococcal enterotoxins and their relatives. Science 248:705, 1990.

## Toxic Shock Syndrome

Toxic shock syndrome is an acute, multisystem disease characterized by high fever, hypotension, an erythematous rash, and other less specific manifestations.

***Etiology and Epidemiology.*** Toxic shock syndrome is due to staphylococcal toxins, which function as superantigens, activating entire subsets of T cells by binding to specific Vβ chains of the T-cell receptor without Vα specificity. The activation of a large number of immune cells results in an outpouring of cytokines with profound physiologic consequences including fever, vasodilation, hypotension, and multisystem organ involvement. The expression of TSST is upregulated by certain environmental conditions. The initial cases of toxic shock syndrome were tampon-associated, described in women who were using hyperabsorbent tampons that chelated local $Mg^{++}$, providing an environment that triggered TSST-1 expression. Recognition that other staphylococcal (and streptococcal) infections could result in this clinical syndrome has led to increased awareness of this disease and more prompt and effective therapy.

***Clinical Manifestations.*** The onset is abrupt, with high fever, vomiting, diarrhea, and myalgias, with or without sore throat, headache, and malaise. A diffuse erythematous sunburn-like macular rash appears within 24 hr and is associated with hyperemia of pharyngeal, conjunctival, and vaginal mucous membranes. Symptoms often include alterations in the level of consciousness, oliguria, and hypotension, which may progress to shock or may be postural in mild cases. Coagulopathy, hypocalcemia, hypoalbuminemia, leukocytosis, and elevated blood urea nitrogen, creatinine, and serum glutamic oxaloacetic transaminase, or CPK may be present. Recovery occurs within 7–10 days and is accompanied by desquamation of the palms and soles; hair and nail loss may be observed.

***Differential Diagnosis.*** Kawasaki disease resembles toxic shock syndrome, but many features of toxic shock syndrome are absent or rare in Kawasaki disease, including diffuse myalgia, vomiting, abdominal pain, diarrhea, azotemia, hypotension, ARDS, and shock. In addition, Kawasaki disease occurs in children under 5 yr of age who often have aneurysms of the coronary artery or other arteries. Scarlet fever, Rocky Mountain spotted fever, leptospirosis, toxic epidermal necrolysis, drug rash, and measles should be considered.

***Treatment and Prevention.*** Fluid replacement should be aggressive to prevent or treat hypotension. Eradication of the source of toxin producing *S. aureus* (e.g., tampon, nasal packing, abscess) is necessary. Parenteral administration of a beta-lactamase–resistant antistaphylococcal antibiotic, such as nafcillin, oxacillin, or methicillin, is indicated in all cases for treatment and prevention of recurrences.

### References

Behrman RE, Kliegman RM, Arvin AM (eds): Nelson Textbook of Pediatrics, 15th ed. Philadelphia, WB Saunders, 1992, Sec. 12.20.
Resnick SD: Toxic shock syndrome: Recent developments in pathogenesis. J Pediatr 116:321, 1990.
Schafer R, Sheil JM: Superantigens and their role in infectious disease. Adv Pediatr Infect Dis 10:369, 1995.

## Infections Caused by Coagulase-Negative Staphylococci

***Etiology.*** Coagulase-negative staphylococci are common, usually nonpathogenic skin flora that are important causes of nosocomial infection as a result of their ability to colonize intravascular venous access devices.

***Epidemiology.*** Coagulase-negative staphylococci are ubiquitous organisms that have affinity for plastic as a result of surface hydrophobicity as well as the elaboration of an extracellular "slime." Although most, if not all, intravascular catheters become colonized by these organisms, large numbers of coagulase-negative staphylococci and the production of this slime are associated with bacteremia and clinical signs of local or systemic infection. These infections assume major clinical importance if they involve small neonates or CNS shunts.

***Clinical Manifestations.*** In premature neonates, infection caused by coagulase-negative staphylococci presents as noscomial sepsis with or without an indwelling line (see Chapter 6). In older children, bacteremia may be accompanied by intermittent fever; patients generally have few other signs of systemic infection. Persistent bacteremia may represent an infected thrombus or endocarditis in patients with prosthetic valves or Dacron grafts. Such infections often are more indolent than those caused by *S. aureus* and may be difficult to diagnose. Often single positive blood cultures with *S. epidermidis* species are considered contaminants, when they may, in fact, represent a significant infection. Coagulase-negative staphylococci are common causes of infection in CNS ventriculoperitoneal shunts.

*Staphylococcus saprophyticus* is a cause of urinary tract infection, particularly in adolescent girls. Urine cultures that grow gram-positive cocci in symptomatic girls should not be dismissed as contaminants.

*Treatment.* These bacteria synthesize beta-lactamases and have altered penicillin-binding proteins, producing resistance to all of the β-lactam antibiotics. Treatment therefore requires vancomycin. Rifampin also may be added to treat CNS infections. Infected intravenous catheters may be treated without removal in many instances, but CNS shunts must be replaced. *S. saprophyticus* may be treated with amoxicillin or one of the quinolones.

### References

Behrman RE, Kliegman RM, Arvin AM (eds): Nelson Textbook of Pediatrics, 15th ed. Philadelphia, WB Saunders, 1996, Chapter 174.2.

Hall SL: Coagulase-negative staphylococcal infections in neonates. Pediatr Infect Dis J 10:57, 1991.

Lyytikainen O, Saxen H, Ryhanen R, et al: Persistence of a multiresistant clone of *Staphylococcus epidermidis* in a neonatal intensive care unit for a four-year period. Clin Infect Dis 20:24, 1995.

## GROUP A STREPTOCOCCAL INFECTIONS

*Etiology.* Streptococci are gram-positive cocci that grow in chains and that are classified by their ability to produce a zone of hemolysis on blood agar: those producing the enzyme hemolysin that causes partial hemolysis (alpha-hemolytic), those causing complete hemolysis (beta-hemolytic), and those with no hemolysis (gamma-hemolytic). Streptococci are further subdivided on the basis of differences in carbohydrate cell wall components; streptococcal Lancefield groups (A–H and K–V) have been identified.

The Lancefield group A streptococci (*S. pyogenes*) are β-hemolytic and express several important virulence factors. The *M protein* is a surface structure that inhibits complement-mediated opsonophagocytosis. It has homology with certain mammalian proteins (tropomyosin) that may be the basis for some of the nonsuppurative complications of group A streptococcal infection.

More than 80 different types of M protein have been identified and are linked to outbreaks. Immunity to one type does not necessarily protect against infection caused by strains with immunologically distinct M proteins; thus, repeated group A streptococcal infections are possible.

These organisms express numerous exotoxins associated with tissue damage, such as streptolysins, hyaluronidase, DNAse, and a lipoproteinase; they also express an erythrogenic toxin (pyrogenic toxin), the product of the *speA* or *speC* genes, which are phage-encoded superantigens functioning by activating entire classes of T cells by binding to specific Vβ chains without antigen processing. This toxin accounts for the rash of scarlet fever, the streptococcal toxic shock syndrome, and many of the manifestations of severe, invasive group A streptococcal disease. This array of virulence factors enables the organism to produce human disease by three distinct mechanisms:

- Locally invasive disease (skin and soft tissue infection)
- Severe multisystem failure associated with toxin expression (streptococcal toxic shock)
- The nonsuppurative sequelae, including rheumatic fever and glomerulonephritis.

*Epidemiology.* Group A streptococci are normal inhabitants of the nasopharynx; colonization occurs in 15–20% of the population throughout the year. The incidence of pharyngeal disease is highest in school-aged children (5–15 yr of age), in the winter, in northern climates, and in settings of crowding and close contact. Person-to-person spread is by droplets from sneezing and coughing. Occasionally, a pet dog or contaminated food may be the source of infection. Streptococcal infection of the skin is most common in children under 6 yr of age and during summer or in warmer climates in which skin abrasions or insect bites become infected.

*Clinical Manifestations.* The incubation period of streptococcal pharyngitis is 2–5 days.

RESPIRATORY TRACT INFECTION. Streptococcal pharyngitis is associated with an acute sore throat with fever, headache, and tender anterior cervical lymph nodes. Occasionally, vomiting, abdominal pain, and rash may be present. The tonsils are hyperemic, edematous, and covered with exudate. The pharynx is inflamed and covered by a membrane in severe cases. The tongue may be edematous and reddened.

SCARLET FEVER. This disease is due to infection with group A streptococci, which elaborate an erythrogenic toxin that produces a characteristic rash appearing 24–48 hr after the onset of pharyngitis. The epidemiology, symptoms, sequelae, and treatment of scarlet fever are the same as those of streptococcal pharyngitis.

The exanthem is red, punctate, or finely papular. In some patients, it may be palpated more readily than it is seen, having the texture of coarse sandpaper (goose flesh). The rash first appears in the axillae, groin, and neck but within 24 hr becomes generalized. Areas of more intense erythema are noted in the creases of the fingers and groin and the antecubital fossae (Pastia lines). The face appears flushed, and there is circumoral pallor. The rash begins to fade 3–4 days after the onset; desquamation of fine flakes from the face and peeling of the palms and fingers may occur after 1 wk. The tongue has a white coat through which the red and edematous papillae project (white strawberry tongue). After several days, the white coat desquamates; the red tongue with prominent papillae persists (red strawberry tongue).

Scarlet fever rarely may follow infection of wounds (surgical scarlet fever), burns, or streptococcal skin infection. Scarlet fever must be distinguished from measles, rubella, erythema infectiosum, infectious mononucleosis, enteroviral infections, roseola, severe sunburn, toxic shock syndrome, drug reactions, and Kawasaki disease.

SKIN INFECTIONS. The most common skin infection caused by group A beta-hemolytic streptococci is superficial pyoderma (**impetigo**), which begins as a single papulovesicular lesion surrounded by erythema that later becomes one or many golden yellow–crusted, weeping lesions. Fever and systemic signs other than regional lymphadenopathy are uncommon. Streptococcal **cellulitis** is a painful, erythematous, indurated infection of the skin and subcutaneous tissues. Lymphangitis and regional lymphadenitis are common. Streptococcal soft tissue **abscesses** are rare. Acute poststreptococcal glomerulonephritis may follow impetigo despite adequate treatment (see Chapter 16).

ERYSIPELAS. This is an acute cellulitis and lymphangitis of the skin with rapid progression to contiguous skin. The lesion is very erythematous and indurated; the margins have a raised firm border. Erysipelas is associated with fever, vomiting, toxicity, and irritability; progression to bacteremia or abscesses is common. Cellulitis caused by S. aureus is characterized by diffuse brawny edema without discrete margins, whereas that caused by H. influenzae appears purple and is usually located on the face.

BACTEREMIA. Streptococcal bacteremia may follow streptococcal disease of the skin, respiratory tract, rectum, or vagina and has been noted without an obvious focus. DIC, shock, and peripheral gangrene can occur. Hematogenous dissemination may result in meningitis, osteomyelitis, arthritis, soft tissue abscesses, pneumonia, or endocarditis.

**Streptococcal toxic shock syndrome** manifests as hypotension, multisystem organ dysfunction, and musculoskeletal complaints, with or without an erythematous macular rash. It may occur after streptococcal superinfection of varicella lesions. Bacteremia resulting from a virulent pyrogenic exotoxin A–producing group A streptococcus is present in many cases.

VAGINITIS. Group A streptococci are a common cause of vaginitis in prepubertal girls. There usually are a serous discharge, marked erythema, and irritation of the vulvar area, accompanied by discomfort on walking and on urination. Proctitis is rare but may be seen in either sex.

*Diagnosis.* The diagnosis of streptococcal infection is suggested by typical but not pathognomonic findings and should be established by isolating organisms from throat, skin, or blood. Rapid diagnostic tests based on identifying group A antigen from throat swabs are available but vary in their sensitivity and specificity. If such tests are positive, a throat culture is not necessary; if they are negative, a throat culture is warranted. The immunologic response to streptococcal antigen can be assessed by measuring titers to antistreptolysin O (ASO), antideoxyribonuclease B (the best serologic test for pyoderma), and antihyaluronidase (elevated with less regularity than ASO titers). Unfortunately they are of no value in the immediate diagnosis and management of acute streptococcal infection. Throat swabs incubated on blood agar demonstrate a zone of hemolysis, with growth inhibited by bacitracin, which typically inhibits only group A streptococci.

The *differential diagnosis* of acute pharyngitis includes infectious mononucleosis, infection due to cytomegalovirus, HSV, adenovirus, diphtheria, tularemia, toxoplasmosis, and, rarely, aplastic anemia. Pharyngitis and scarlatiniform rash in adolescents may be due to *Arcanobacterium haemolyticum*. Streptococcal pyoderma and cellulitis must be differentiated from staphylococcal skin disease. Bullous impetigo is usually staphylococcal, whereas the golden crusted lesions are caused by streptococci.

*Complications.* These are due to extension of streptococcal infection from the nasopharynx, which results in sinusitis, otitis media, mastoiditis, cervical adenitis, retropharyngeal and peritonsillar abscess, or bronchopneumonia. Hematogenous dissemination of streptococci may cause meningitis, osteomyelitis, or septic arthritis. Nonsuppurative complications include rheumatic fever (see Chapter 13) and acute glomerulonephritis (see Chapter 16).

*Treatment and Prevention.* Penicillin is the treatment of choice for all streptococcal infections; if the patient is allergic to penicillin, erythromycin or clindamycin is used. Bacteremia, erysipelas, and bone or joint infection require intravenous therapy (see Appendix I). Penicillin failures in the treatment of pharyngitis are often attributed to local destruction of the drug by β-lactamase–producing commensal flora. These patients often respond to another course of therapy, including a β-lactamase inhibitor (amoxicillin/clavulanate) or clindamycin. Impetigo is treated with oral erythromycin and locally with mupirocin.

Preventive therapy is indicated to avoid rheumatic fever. Administration of daily oral or monthly intramuscular, long-acting penicillin in patients with an episode of rheumatic fever prevents most cases of streptococcal disease and recurrent illness, if the drug is provided prior to the onset of symptoms. Treatment prevents the later occurrence of rheumatic fever, but not glomerulonephritis. Penicillin prevents rheumatic fever if it is initiated 7–14 days after the onset of the antecedent pharyngitis. Patients treated with penicillin for pharyngitis may be considered noncontagious within 48 hr of therapy.

## References

Ayoub E, Ahmed S: Update on complications of group A streptococcal infections. Curr Probl Pediatr 27:90, 1997.

Behrman RE, Kliegman RM, Arvin AM (eds): Nelson Textbook of Pediatrics, 15th ed. Philadelphia, WB Saunders, 1996, Chapter 175.

Bisno AL, Stevens DL: Streptococcal infections of skin and soft tissue. N Engl J Med 334:240, 1996.

Cockerill F, MacDonald K, Thompson R, et al: An outbreak of invasive group A streptococcal disease associated with high carriage rates of the invasive clone among school age children. JAMA 277:38, 1997.

## YERSINIA ENTEROCOLITICA AND YERSINIA PSEUDOTUBERCULOSIS INFECTIONS

*Etiology.* *Y. enterocolitica* and *Y. pseudotuberculosis* are oxidase-negative, gram-negative bacilli. *Y. enterocolitica* has 35 serotypes and *Y. pseudotuberculosis* has five.

*Epidemiology.* The sources of the organisms include wild and domestic animals, raw milk, chitterlings, oysters, and water supplies. Infection from dogs and human-to-human spread occurs. Infants and children appear most susceptible. The incubation period varies from 1 to 3 wk.

*Clinical Manifestations.* *Y. enterocolitica* commonly is associated with enteritis and enterocolitis, which mimic inflammatory bowel disease and become manifest by fever and bloody diarrhea with mucus and abdominal pain. Young infants may have a nonspecific gastroenteritis or dysentery-like disease. Other manifestations include acute mesenteric adenitis, pharyngitis, hepatosplenic abscesses, arthritis, osteomyelitis, hepatitis, carditis, meningitis, Reiter syndrome, septicemia, and erythema nodosum. Septicemia has been associated with iron intoxication and has occurred after accidental overdose of oral iron in previously healthy children. Treatment with deferoxamine, an iron siderophore that chelates iron in hypertransfused patients with chronic anemia or iron intoxication, may present iron to the dormant organism, which requires iron for growth. Septicemia is associated with a case fatality rate of nearly 50%, despite antibiotic treatment. Mesenteric adenitis typically affects older children and adolescents; the severe abdominal pain may simulate appendicitis. The duration of the illness generally is 2–3 wk without treatment, but occasionally diarrhea may persist for several months and simulate inflammatory bowel disease.

*Y. pseudotuberculosis* has been associated with mesenteric adenitis and terminal ileitis. Abdominal pain may be severe and may suggest acute appendicitis. Septicemia is unusual; other findings include diarrhea and erythema nodosum.

*Diagnosis.* The diagnosis may be established by identifying the organism in stool, mesenteric lymph nodes, bowel mucosa at endoscopy, peritoneal fluid, or blood. Because identification requires special techniques, laboratory personnel should be notified. Passive hemagglutination tests also may confirm the diagnosis. Antibodies are detectable 8–10 days after the onset of illness and may persist for several months.

*Treatment.* Most strains of *Y. enterocolitica* and *Y. pseudotuberculosis* are susceptible to aminoglycosides, tetracycline, chloramphenicol, and trimethoprim/sulfamethoxazole. Patients with septicemia or sites of infection outside the gastrointestinal tract should receive therapy. Parenteral ceftriaxone or cefotaxime plus an aminoglycoside, fluroquinolones or trimethoprim/sulfamathoxazole are the drugs of choice for serious infection. The benefits of treating patients with enterocolitis or mesenteric adenitis are unknown (see Appendix I).

## References

Behrman RE, Kliegman RM, Arvin AM (eds): Nelson Textbook of Pediatrics, 15th ed. Philadelphia, WB Saunders, 1996, Chapter 188.

Butler T: *Yersinia* infections: Centennial of the discovery of the plague bacillus. Clin Infect Dis 19:655, 1994.

Lee LA, Taylor J, Carter GP, et al: *Yersinia enterocolitica* 0: 3: An emerging cause of pediatric gastroenteritis in the United States. J Infect Dis 163:660, 1991.

## SPIROCHETAL INFECTIONS

### Syphilis

*Etiology.* Syphilis is caused by *Treponema pallidum,* a long, slender, coiled spirochete. It cannot routinely be cultivated in vitro but can be seen by darkfield microscopy.

*Epidemiology.* Syphilis is acquired through sexual contact, transplacentally from an infected mother to her fetus and, less commonly, at birth, in the postpartum period, or by infected blood. Infants with congenital syphilis often are born to women who are HIV-positive or use crack cocaine. Infection in males is 3 times more common than in females. Sexual abuse should be considered in young children who have acquired syphilis. The incubation period for primary syphilis is 10–90 days after exposure.

### Clinical Manifestations

CONGENITAL SYPHILIS. Early manifestations occurring between birth and the 1st yr of life include fever, anemia, failure to thrive, irritability, local mucocutaneous lesions (maculopapular rash on trunk, palms, and soles; condylomata lata; bullous eruptions), persistent rhinitis (snuffles), hepatosplenomegaly, lymphadenopathy, dactylitis, and pseudoparalysis resulting from osteochondritis. *Laboratory evaluation* may show direct hyperbilirubinemia, elevated liver function tests, multiple sites of osteochondritis, thrombocytopenia, Coombs-negative hemolytic anemia, and leukocytosis.

The moist secretions of early congenital syphilis are highly contagious. In an untreated pregnant woman, syphilis may be transmitted to the fetus at any time; however, transmission to the fetus is more common during the 1st yr after syphilis has been acquired by the mother. Although some newborns demonstrate symptoms of the disease within the first 4–8 wk after birth, many infants are symptomatic at birth and exhibit nonimmune hydrops with anemia; thrombocytopenia; leukopenia; pneumonia; hepatitis, with or without nephrosis; and osteochondritis.

Late congenital syphilis appears many years after birth and becomes manifest as multiple bone signs (frontal bossing, saber shins), Hutchinson teeth (peg or screw-like), mulberry molars, a saddle-nose deformity, rhagades (perioral linear scars), juvenile paresis, juvenile tabes, interstitial keratitis, eighth nerve deafness, and Clutton joints (painless joint effusions). These manifestations are all rare in the modern era in which penicillin therapy is used to control congenital syphilis.

ACQUIRED PRIMARY SYPHILIS. Three to 6 wk following inoculation, a single painless papule appears, becomes indurated, and progresses to a painless ulcer (chancre). This ulcer usually is found on the genitalia but may appear at any other site of inoculation.

SECONDARY SYPHILIS. An influenza-like illness occurs 6–8 wk after the primary chancre, with generalized adenopathy and a generalized erythematous, maculopapular rash, which is present on the palms and soles. Plaque-like skin lesions (condylo-

mata lata) and mucous membrane lesions also occur and are all infectious. Other manifestations of secondary syphilis may include meningitis, hepatitis, glomerulonephritis, bursitis, and periostitis.

OTHER TYPES OF SYPHILIS. *Latent* syphilis has no clinical manifestations, but a history of untreated syphilis and serologic evidence of infection may be discovered. *Late* syphilis, a slowly progressive disease typically involving the CNS and heart, is not seen in children.

*Diagnosis.* Serologic tests for syphilis include the nontreponemal reagin antibody tests, which are directed against a poorly characterized lipoidal antigen. These tests include (1) the Venereal Disease Research Laboratory (VDRL) test, (2) a rapid plasma reagin (RPR) test, and (3) an automated reagin test (ART). The specific tests include (1) the *T. pallidum* immobilization test, which rarely is used; (2) the fluorescent treponemal antibody–absorption (FTA-ABS) test; and (3) the microhemagglutination test for *T. pallidum*. The specific tests are less likely to be falsely reactive in collagen vascular disease, pregnancy, drug addiction, malaria, infectious mononucleosis, and other infectious diseases ("biologic false-positive tests") than the nontreponemal tests. The serologic tests are uniformly positive in secondary and later stages of syphilis. The VDRL test becomes positive within 4–6 wk after infection. Treatment results in declining titers of the VDRL test, RPR test, and ART, but not the FTA-ABS test.

In the process of identifying congenital syphilis, maternal transplacentally passed antibody often confuses the diagnosis. It is frequently difficult to determine whether the infant has only passive acquisition of antibody. This is particularly true in HIV-infected patients, who may have absent or exaggerated antibody responses. Specific Western blot methods or PCR may improve the diagnosis of asymptomatic but infected patients. Positive CSF VDRL or RPR tests warrant therapy for CNS syphilis in congenital or acquired disease. Darkfield examination of chancres, mucous membranes, or cutaneous lesions may reveal motile organisms.

*Treatment.* *T. pallidum* is extremely sensitive to penicillin, which remains the drug of choice for therapy of all forms of syphilis. Alternate therapy includes tetracycline or erythromycin. Dosage regimens vary according to stage of disease and the presence of neurologic involvement and congenital infection. Neonates must be treated with regimens to provide effective concentrations of penicillin in the CNS. Current regimens for therapy of gonorrhea also effectively treat incubating syphilis. Exposure to a documented case of syphilis warrants "prophylactic" therapy and serologic follow-up. A pregnant woman with documented or possible syphilis should be treated with penicillin to prevent illness in the mother and her offspring. HIV-infected patients with evidence of syphilis should have a lumbar puncture to determine whether CNS infection is present. Erythromycin does not treat the fetus. A systemic, febrile reaction (*the Jarisch-Herxheimer reaction*) occurs in 15–20% of syphilitic patients treated with penicillin. Patients with syphilis who also have AIDS may require prolonged therapy.

## References

Azimi PH, Janner D, Berne P, et al: Concentrations of procaine and aqueous penicillin in the cerebrospinal fluid of infants treated for congenital syphilis. J Pediatr 124:64, 1994.

Behrman RE, Kliegman RM, Arvin AM (eds): Nelson Textbook of Pediatrics, 15th ed. Philadelphia, WB Saunders, 1996, Chapter 201.

Dorfman DH, Glaser JH: Congenital syphilis presenting in infants after the newborn period. N Engl J Med 323:1299, 1990.

Hook EW III, Marra CM: Acquired syphilis in adults. N Engl J Med 326:1060, 1992.

Zenker PN, Berman SM: Congenital syphilis: Trends and recommendations for evaluation and management. Pediatr Infect Dis J 10:516, 1991.

### *Borrelia burgdorferi* Infection
(Lyme Disease)

***Etiology.*** Lyme disease is a tick-borne illness caused by a fastidious spirochete, *B. burgdorferi.* Ticks of the *Ixodes* genus and possibly other blood-sucking insects feed off animal reservoirs, such as the white-footed mouse, the deer, and the dog.

***Epidemiology.*** Lyme disease has been reported in most states but is endemic to the coastal northeastern states, Minnesota, Wisconsin, California, Texas, and Nevada; the predominant vector is *I. dammini* in the East and Midwest and *I. pacificus* in the West. In Europe, Lyme disease may be atypical relative to the clinical presentation in the United States and may be associated with other ticks. Because exposure to ticks is more common in warm months, Lyme disease is noted predominantly in summer.

#### Clinical Manifestations

STAGE 1. Although not all patients recall a tick bite, the typical pattern of disease evolves from this bite. Three to 32 days (mean 7 days) after a tick bite, the site forms an erythematous papule that expands to form a red, raised border and a clear center. Multiple rings may form and new areas of this annular lesion may appear distal to the original site. The lesion, *erythema chronicum migrans,* may be 15 cm wide, may be pruritic or painful, and may contain *B. burgdorferi* organisms.

This skin lesion is not present in all patients. The lesions fade within 1 mo. During this early stage, systemic manifestations include malaise, lethargy, fever, headache, arthralgias, stiff neck, myalgias, and lymphadenopathy. All of these early manifestations resolve without treatment in 1 mo.

STAGE 2. *Cardiac manifestations* occur within 5 wk and include myocarditis, atrioventricular node block (occasionally requiring external pacemakers), ST depression, and T wave inversion. Cardiac disease is serious, present in approximately 10% of patients, and reversible.

*Neurologic manifestations* occur within 4 wk and include lymphocytic "aseptic" meningitis, encephalitis, cranial neuritis (Bell palsy of the nerve VII), polyradiculitis, peripheral neuropathy, mononeuritis multiplex, or transverse myelitis. Neurologic manifestations resolve by 3 mo.

STAGE 3. Arthritis may develop in 50–60% of patients within weeks to years of the tick bite. Intermittent arthritis also is noted in stage 2 and may be monoarticular, pauciarticular, or polyarticular, resembling JRA. The knee, shoulder, elbow, and, rarely, the small joints of the hands are involved. Chronic erosive arthritis may persist in 10% of patients, with involvement of the knee more than other joints. The male-to-female ratio is 7:1. Popliteal cysts may develop, and joint fluid is typically inflammatory, with leukocytic predominance and a total WBC between 500 and 100,000 cells/$\mu$L (Table 10–10). These patients are negative for rheumatoid factor and antinuclear antibody (ANA).

***Diagnosis.*** A history of a tick bite and the classic rash are helpful but not present in all cases. The ESR is elevated and complement may be reduced in patients with arthritis. The VDRL test may be falsely positive. Cryoglobulins and circulating immune complexes may precede or coincide with arthritis. CSF reveals a lymphocytic pleocytosis with normal glucose levels and slightly raised protein levels.

The diagnosis is confirmed by serologic tests specific for *B. burgdorferi.* Because of high false-positive rates, the ELISA must be confirmed by a Western blot. The *differential diagnoses* are many and relate to the organ involved, as discussed under aseptic meningitis, arthritis, and myocarditis. In children, JRA must be considered (see Chapter 9).

***Treatment.*** Stage 1 disease, especially erythema chronicum migrans, may be treated with oral amoxicillin or, in older children, doxycycline for 3 wk. Early treatment may prevent carditis and meningitis. Stages 2 and 3 usually are treated with high-dose parenteral ceftriaxone (50–80 mg/kg/24 hr; max. 2 g) or penicillin G (200–400,000 U/kg/24 hr, max. 20 million U/24 hr) for 2–3 wk, if severe complications are present. Oral doxycycline or amoxicillin are effective for milder disease (see Appendix I).

### References

Behrman RE, Kliegman RM, Arvin AM (eds): Nelson Textbook of Pediatrics, 15th ed. Philadelphia, WB Saunders, 1996, Chapter 198.
Cryan B, Wright DJM: Lyme disease in paediatrics. Arch Dis Child 66:1359, 1991.
Gerber M, Shapiro E, Burke G, et al: Lyme disease in children in southeastern Connecticut. N Engl J Med 335:1290, 1996.
Szer IS, Taylor E, Steere AC: The long term course of Lyme arthritis in children. N Engl J Med 325:159, 1991.

## CHLAMYDIAL INFECTION

*Etiology.* Chlamydiae are obligate intracellular parasites that contain DNA and RNA and do not stain with Gram stain. Infected cells contain cytoplasmic Giemsa stain–positive inclusions. There are two subgroups of the genus *Chlamydia.* Group A contains *C. trachomatis* and the agent of lymphogranuloma venereum (LGV). Group B contains the agent of psittacosis/ornithosis and Reiter syndrome as well as several zoonoses.

### *Chlamydia trachomatis* Infection

*C. trachomatis* contains 15 serotypes that are divided into two groups: oculogenital (subtypes A–K) and LGV (subtypes L-1 and L-3). Trachoma is caused by subtypes A-C.

*Epidemiology.* *C. trachomatis* is a common cause of sexually transmitted disease (STD), causing about 40% of cases of nonspecific urethritis, as well as cervicitis, salpingitis, endometritis, epididymitis, and tubal infertility. Infection rates as high as 30% have been observed in certain adolescent groups (see Chapter 7). About 12% of pregnant women are infected, with rates higher in lower socioeconomic status groups. In infants born vaginally to infected mothers, cultures are positive in about 50%, conjunctivitis develops in 35%, and pneumonitis develops in 20%. Approximately 20–30% of infants with the afebrile pneumonitis syndrome are infected with *Chlamydia.* The incubation period varies, depending on the type of infection.

*Clinical Manifestations.* *Conjunctivitis* caused by *Chlamydia* in the neonate may appear from 3 days to 6 wk after delivery, but it usually occurs in the 2nd wk of life. The eyes are inflamed, with purulent discharge issuing from one or both eyes. Recurrences can occur even with appropriate therapy, but residual eye damage is rare. **Trachoma** is a chronic follicular keratoconjunctivitis resulting from repeated infection and may result in blindness in older children or adults because of extensive local scarring and inflammation.

*Pneumonitis* develops at 3–10 wk of age. The child generally appears well, is afebrile, but has tachypnea and a cough. Apnea also may occur. One half of affected patients have concomitant conjunctivitis. Examination reveals rales and wheezing. Roentgenograms of the chest reveal hyperinflation and diffuse interstitial or patchy infiltrates. Mild eosinophilia (about $400/\mu L$), hypergammaglobulinemia, and mild hypoxemia are common. The illness is self-limiting but may last for weeks.

Beyond infancy, *urethritis* in both sexes and cervicitis in females may occur. These infections may be protracted and recurrent, and in females it may result in chronic PID and infertility.

*Diagnosis.* *Chlamydia* can be grown in treated tissue culture cells, which is the standard method of isolation. Monoclonal antibody detection tests have been useful in the evaluation of genital secretions and in pneumonitis or conjunctivitis of infants. If conjunctivitis is present, scraping the eyelid and staining the exfoliated cells to demonstrate cytoplasmic inclusion bodies may be diagnostic.

Conjunctivitis must be differentiated from inflammation (red eye) caused by silver nitrate (chemical), gonococcal infection, or viral infection (Table 10–15). The pneumonitis must be differentiated from that caused by viruses (especially cytomegalovirus and RSV), *Ureaplasma, Pneumocystis carinii,* and, less commonly, other bacteria and mycobacteria.

The adenopathy of LGV must be differentiated from that caused by cat-scratch disease, pyogenic bacteria, chancroid, granuloma inguinale, syphilis, HSV, and neoplasms. Examination of the node may reveal inclusions using Giemsa stain. Chlamydial cultures may be positive. Serology usually is diagnostic.

*Treatment.* Although topical therapy of conjunctivitis using sulfonamides is effective, oral erythromycin or sulfisoxazole also should be administered to treat either conjunctivitis (to eradicate the nasopharyngeal colonization and risk of subsequent pneumonitis) or pneumonitis. Prophylactic therapy of the infected mother and her sexual partner can decrease the rate of infection in the newborn. For uncomplicated genital tract infection caused by *C. trachomatis* in adolescents and adults, tetracycline, doxycycline, or azithromycin is recommended. LGV is treated with tetracycline or sulfonamides (see Appendix I).

TABLE 10–15. The Red Eye

| Condition | Etiology | Signs and Symptoms | Treatment |
|---|---|---|---|
| Bacterial conjunctivitis | *Haemophilus influenzae, Haemophilus aegyptius, Streptococcus pneumoniae* *Neisseria gonorrhoeae* | Mucopurulent unilateral or bilateral discharge, normal vision, photophobia; Conjunctival injection and edema (chemosis); gritty sensation | Topical antibiotics, parenteral ceftriaxone for gonococcus, *H. influenzae* |
| Viral conjunctivitis | Adenovirus, ECHO virus, coxsackievirus | As above; may be hemorrhagic, unilateral | Self-limited |
| Neonatal conjunctivitis | *Chlamydia trachomatis*, gonococcus, chemical (silver nitrate), *Staphylococcus aureus* | Palpebral conjunctival follicle or papillae; as above | Ceftriaxone for gonococcus and erythromycin for *C. trachomatis* |
| Allergic conjunctivitis | Seasonal pollens or allergen exposure | Itching, incidence of bilateral chemosis (edema) greater than that of erythema, tarsal papillae | Antihistamines, steroids, cromolyn |
| Keratitis | Herpes simplex, adenovirus, *S. pneumoniae, S. aureus, Pseudomonas, Acanthamoeba*, chemicals | Severe pain, corneal swelling, clouding, limbus erythema, hypopyon, cataracts; contact lens history with amebic infection | Specific antibiotics for bacterial/fungal infections; keratoplasty, acyclovir for herpes |
| Endophthalmitis | *S. aureus, S. pneumoniae, Candida albicans*, associated surgery or trauma | Acute onset, pain, loss of vision, swelling, chemosis, redness; hypopyon and vitreous haze | Antibiotics |
| Anterior uveitis (iridocyclitis) | JRA, Reiter syndrome, sarcoidosis, Behçet disease, Kawasaki disease, inflammatory bowel disease | Unilateral/bilateral; erythema, ciliary flush, irregular pupil, iris adhesions; pain, photophobia, small pupil, poor vision | Topical steroids, plus therapy for primary disease |
| Posterior uveitis (choroiditis) | Toxoplasmosis, histoplasmosis, *Toxocara canis* | No signs of erythema, decreased vision | Specific therapy for pathogen |

*Table continued on following page*

**References**

Behrman RE, Kliegman RM, Arvin AM (eds): Nelson Textbook of Pediatrics, 15th ed. Philadelphia, WB Saunders, 1996, Chapter 197.
Bell TA, Stamm WE, Pin Wang S, et al: Chronic *Chlamydia trachomatis* infections in infants. JAMA 267:400, 1992.
Brasfield DM, Stagno S, Whitley RJ, et al: Infant pneumonitis associated with cytomegalovirus, *Chlamydia, Pneumocystis*, and *Ureaplasma*: Follow up. Pediatrics 79:76, 1987.
Martin DH, Mroczkowski TF, Dalu ZA, et al: A controlled trial of a single dose of azithromycin for the treatment of chlamydial urethritis and cervicitis. N Engl J Med 327:921, 1992.
Rettig PJ: Infection due to *Chlamydia trachomatis* from infancy to adolescence. Pediatr Infect Dis 5:449, 1986.

### *Chlamydia pneumoniae* Infection

*C. pneumoniae* is an important cause of respiratory disease in children and adults. Serologic studies demonstrate that primary infection usually occurs in school-aged children; reinfections during adulthood are common. Symptoms are indistinguishable from those of infection due to *Mycoplasma*; pharyngitis, hoarseness, bronchitis, and pneumonia are commonly seen. Symptoms are generally mild but prolonged. *C. pneumoniae* has been associated with 6–10% of cases of pneumonia in adults. Treatment with erythromycins or with tetracyclines in older patients is recommended.

**References**

Grayston JT: *Chlamydia pneumoniae* (TWAR) infections in children. Pediatr Infect Dis J 13:675, 1994.
Kauppinen M, Saikku P: Pneumonia due to *Chlamydia pneumoniae*: Prevalence, clinical features, diagnosis and treatment. Clin Infect Dis 21:S44–52, 1995.

### MYCOPLASMAL INFECTION

**Etiology.** Mycoplasmas are the smallest free-living organisms. They lack a cell wall and are distinct

TABLE 10–15.  The Red Eye *Continued*

| Condition | Etiology | Signs and Symptoms | Treatment |
|---|---|---|---|
| Episcleritis/scleritis | Idiopathic autoimmune disease (e.g., SLE, Henoch-Schönlein purpura) | Localized pain, intense erythema, unilateral; blood vessels bigger than in conjunctivitis; scleritis may cause globe perforation | Episcleritis is self-limiting; topical steroids for fast relief |
| Foreign body | Occupational exposure | Unilateral, red, gritty feeling; visible or microscopic size | Irrigation, removal; check for ulceration |
| Blepharitis | *S. aureus, Staphylococcus epidermidis*, seborrheic, blocked lacrimal duct; rarely molluscum contagiosum, *Phthirus pubis*, *Pediculus capitis* | Bilateral, irritation, itching, hyperemia, crusting, affecting lid margins | Topical antibiotics, warm compresses |
| Dacryocystitis | Obstructed lacrimal sac: *S. aureus, H. influenzae*, pneumococcus | Pain, tenderness, erythema and exudate in area of lacrimal sac (inferomedial to inner canthus); tearing (epiphora); possible orbital cellulitis | Systemic, topical antibiotics; surgical drainage |
| Dacryoadenitis | *S. aureus, Streptococcus*, CMV, measles, EBV, enteroviruses; trauma, sarcoidosis, leukemia | Pain, tenderness, edema, erythema over gland area (upper temporal lid); fever, leukocytosis | Systemic antibiotics; drainage of orbital abscesses |
| Orbital cellulitis (postseptal cellulitis) | Paranasal sinusitis: *H. influenzae, S. aureus, S. pneumoniae,* streptococci; Trauma: *S. aureus*; Fungi: *Aspergillus, Mucor* spp. if immunodeficient | Rhinorrhea, chemosis, vision loss, painful extraocular motion, proptosis, ophthalmoplegia, fever, lid edema, leukocytosis | Systemic antibiotics, drainage of orbital abscesses |
| Periorbital cellulitis (preseptal cellulitis) | Trauma: *S. aureus*, streptococci; Bacteremia: pneumococcus, streptococci, *H. influenzae* | Cutaneous erythema, warmth, normal vision, minimal involvement of orbit; fever, leukocytosis, toxic appearance | Systemic antibiotics |

Data from Am J Med 79:545, 1985; BMJ 296:1720, 1988; Infect Dis Clin North Am 2:99, 1988; Lancet 338:1498, 1991; and Pediatr Ann 22:353, 1993.
CMV = cytomegalovirus; EBV = Epstein-Barr virus; JRA = juvenile rheumatoid arthritis; SLE = systemic lupus erythematosus.

from bacteria but grow on artificial media and are not viruses. Pathogenic species of mycoplasmas include *M. pneumoniae* (pneumonia, systemic infection), *M. hominis* (genitourinary tract infection), and *Ureaplasma urealyticum* (genitourinary tract, neonatal pneumonia).

***Epidemiology.*** *M. pneumoniae* is a major cause of illness in school-aged children and young adults. Clinical illness is unusual before 4 yr of age, and the peak attack rate occurs at 6–15 yr of age. *M. pneumoniae* is estimated to cause one-half million cases of pneumonia and more than 11 million cases of tracheobronchitis in the United States annually. Illness occurs at irregular intervals, tending to begin in the fall with smoldering epidemics. Transmission is presumed to be by droplet spread from symptomatic patients. The incubation period is 2–3 wk.

***Clinical Manifestations.*** Onset of illness (**atypical pneumonia**) is gradual, with headache, malaise, fever, sore throat, and cough. Sputum production, rales, and pleural effusions are frequent. Severe pulmonary disease has been reported in children with sickle cell anemia. Other manifestations include skin eruptions (maculopapular rashes, urticaria, erythema nodosum, Stevens-Johnson syndrome) and, less commonly, meningoencephalitis, Guillain-Barré syndrome, hemolytic anemia, thrombocytopenia, myocarditis, and pericarditis. The nonrespiratory tract illnesses are less firmly established as being due to *M. pneumoniae*.

***Diagnosis.*** Cold agglutinin titers tend to reflect the severity of illness and are likely to be positive in the school-aged child with pulmonary infection due to *Mycoplasma*. Confirmation of the diagnosis is demonstrated by an increase of specific antibodies.

***Treatment.*** Erythromycins or doxycycline (in children over 10 yr of age) is the drug of choice (see Appendix I).

References

Behrman RE, Kliegman RM, Arvin AM (eds): Nelson Textbook of Pediatrics, 15th ed. Philadelphia, WB Saunders, 1996, Chapter 196.
Broughton RA: Infections due to *Mycoplasma pneumoniae* in childhood. Pediatr Infect Dis 5:71, 1986.
Editorial: *Mycoplasma pneumoniae*. Lancet 337:651, 1991.

## CAT-SCRATCH DISEASE

*Etiology.* The cat-scratch disease agent *Bartonella henselae* is a small, pleomorphic, gram-negative bacillus that stains with Warthin-Starry silver impregnation of material from aspirated lymph nodes. It also causes bacillary angiomatosis and peliosis hepatis in immunosuppressed (HIV) and, occasionally, in immunocompetent patients.

*Epidemiology.* Cat-scratch disease has a worldwide distribution, is more common in males, and occurs in temperate climates in the fall and winter months. In more than 90% of cases, the disease follows the scratch (rarely, a lick) of a kitten (less often, of an older cat). The cats are not sick but may be bacteremic. Rare cases have occurred in association with dogs, thorns, or wood splinters.

*Clinical Manifestations.* A primary cutaneous papule or conjunctival granuloma develops 3–10 days after the initial contact. Lymphadenopathy localized to the draining regional nodes develops 2 wk (range, 1–7 wk) later, usually on the head, neck, and axilla. The nodes enlarge to 1–8 cm, may suppurate, and are painful in the early stage of the illness. There is no lymphangitis and usually few systemic signs, although fever and malaise may be noted in 30% of patients. Lymphadenopathy lasts 1–4 mo. Additional but rare features include erythema nodosum, osteolytic lesions, encephalitis, sepsis-like appearance, oculoglandular (Parinaud) syndrome, polyneuritis, transverse myelitis, hepatic or splenic granulomas, endocarditis, thrombocytopenia, and pneumonia.

*Diagnosis.* Usually, cat-scratch disease is suspected by a history of exposure to cats, the primary lesion localized at the site of the scratch or bite, and a single, enlarged node. Aspiration of the node with subsequent microscopic evidence of the bacillus by Warthin-Starry silver stain is diagnostic and may be curative.

*Treatment.* Usually, no treatment is required because the lymphadenopathy resolves in 2–4 mo without sequelae. Aspiration is indicated for large, painful, and uncomfortable lesions. Rifampin, ciprofloxacin, gentamicin, or trimethoprim/sulfamethoxazole may enhance resolution of more severe disease. Bacillary angiomatosis, bacillary peliosis, or relapsing bacteremia may respond to erythromycin (clarithromycin, azithromycin) plus rifampin or doxycycline for 4–6 wk. After an illness, immunity is lifelong. The disease is not contagious; therefore, the patient does not need to be isolated.

References

Bass J, Vincent J, Person D: The expanding spectrum of *Bartonella* infections II: Cat-scratch disease. Pediatr Infect Dis J 16:163, 1997.
Behrman RE, Kliegman RM, Arvin AM (eds): Nelson Textbook of Pediatrics, 15th ed. Philadelphia, WB Saunders, 1996, Chapter 205.
Zangwill K, Hamilton D, Perkins B, et al: Cat scratch disease in Connecticut: Epidemiology, risk factors and evaluation of a new diagnostic test. N Engl J Med 329:8, 1993.

# VIRAL DISEASES

## ANTIVIRAL CHEMOTHERAPY

Therapy against viral disease must take into consideration the intracellular nature of viral replication and, to avoid toxicity to the host's cells, must be directed at viral specific proteins. Viral enzymes (e.g., HIV and reverse transcriptase) or enzymes with different substrate specificity compared with the host's enzyme (thymidine kinase, DNA polymerase of herpes viruses) are targets for antiviral chemotherapy. In addition, recombinant human factors that naturally reduce virus replication and kill viruses, such as interferon and high-dose intravenous immunoglobulin, have been used. To date, the most successful antiviral agents are those nucleoside analogs that interfere with viral DNA or RNA synthesis (Table 10–16).

## ADENOVIRAL INFECTION

*Etiology.* Adenoviruses are double-stranded DNA viruses. More than 40 distinct types have been associated with human illness.

*Epidemiology.* Adenoviruses produce respiratory tract disease year-round, with a higher incidence in the spring, early summer, and mid-winter. Infection occurs early in childhood by respiratory, fecal, oral, and, possibly, conjunctival inoculation. Transmission occurs from person to person, usually by respiratory spread. Asymptomatic infections are common. Enteric strains of adenovirus may be transmitted by the fecal-oral route. The period of communicability is highest during the first several days of illness. The incubation period ranges from 2–14 days.

TABLE 10–16.    Antiviral Chemotherapy

| Drugs | Mechanism of Action | Indication | Comments |
|---|---|---|---|
| Acyclovir (valacyclovir, famciclovir—increases absorption of prodrug) | Requires viral thymidine kinase to produce acyclovir monophosphate, which inhibits DNA polymerase | Herpes simplex 1 and 2, varicella-zoster (systemic, mucocutaneous) | Oral, intravenous, topical; varicella requires higher drug levels; toxic encephalopathy, renal dysfunction |
| Amantadine/rimantadine | Inhibits viral replication | Influenza A | Prophylaxis and therapy; CNS toxicity with poor concentration, confusion |
| Ganciclovir | As acyclovir | CMV, herpes viruses | Neutropenia, recurrence when discontinued |
| Foscarnet | Inhibits viral DNA polymerase | CMV retinitis, ganciclovir-resistant CMV; acyclovir-resistant HSV and varicella-zoster virus | Nonmyelosuppressive; nephrotoxic, $\downarrow \uparrow$ $Ca^{2+}$, $Mg^{2+}$ |
| Ribavirin | Inhibits RNA synthesis and reverse transcriptase | Parenteral for influenza, Lassa virus, use for RSV-controversial | Aerosol has few side effects, avoid exposure in pregnancy |
| Zidovudine (azidothymidine [AZT]) | Inhibits viral reverse transcriptase | HIV–AIDS | Bone marrow depression |
| Didanosine (DDI) and dideoxycytosine (DDC) | Inhibits reverse transcriptase | Advanced AIDS if intolerant of or deteriorating on AZT | Painful peripheral neuropathy, pancreatitis |
| Stavudine (d4T) | Nucleoside analog; inhibits reverse transcriptase | HIV–AIDS | Peripheral neuropathy |
| Lamivudine (3TC) | Nucleoside analog | HIV–AIDS | Increases bone marrow suppression with AZT |
| Viramune | Non-nucleoside inhibitor of reverse transcriptase | HIV–AIDS | Rash; must be used in combination (AZT, DDI) |
| Saquinavir | Viral protease inhibitor | HIV–AIDS | GI distress, diarrhea, drug interaction with rifampin |
| Ritonavir | Protease inhibitor | HIV–AIDS | Bad taste, circumoral paresthesias, diarrhea, drug interactions |
| Indinavir | Protease inhibitor | HIV–AIDS | Nephrolithiasis, drug interactions |

Data from Med Lett 34:31, 1992; and Infect Dis Clinic North Am 1:311, 1987.
AIDS = acquired immunodeficiency virus; CMV = cytomegalovirus; CNS = central nervous system; DNA = deoxyribonucleic acid; GI = gastrointestinal; HIV = human immunodeficiency virus; HSV = herpes simplex virus.

### Clinical Manifestations

*PHARYNGOCONJUNCTIVAL FEVER (TYPES 1, 2, 3, AND 5).* Manifestations of this type of infection are high fever, pharyngitis, conjunctivitis, cervical adenopathy, and rhinitis, all of which last 4–5 days and are accompanied by malaise, lethargy, weakness, and headache of longer duration. Epidemics that may spread from contaminated swimming pools have been reported in summer camps. Pharyngitis, one of the most common manifestations of adenovirus, is a typical symptom in young infants.

*OTHER MANIFESTATIONS.* Adenovirus may cause epidemic keratoconjunctivitis (primary in adults), as well as acute follicular conjunctivitis. Conjunctivitis in children often occurs with pharyngitis (see Table 10–15). Of hospitalized children with pneumonia, 7–10% are infected with adenovirus. This infection may be particularly severe or fatal and is associated with high fever, leukocytosis, elevated ESR, or the development of bronchiolitis obliterans. Noncultivatable "enteric" adenoviruses have been associated with a small proportion of the episodes of diarrhea in infants. Adenovirus also has been recovered from lymph nodes of children who have intussusception, mesenteric adenitis, and lymphadenitis, but in these settings it is not clear whether the virus is the etiologic agent. The sudden onset of hematuria, dysuria, and urinary frequency, accompanied by bacteriologically sterile urine, has been associated with adenovirus types 11 and 21. Hemorrhagic cystitis lasts 1–2 wk.

DISSEMINATED ADENOVIRAL DISEASE. This condition commonly occurs in immunocompromised patients, particularly those with T-cell defects and those who have undergone bone marrow or liver transplantation and in neonates. Clinical manifestations include hepatosplenomegaly, liver failure, DIC, shock, and, ultimately, death. Several other manifestations of severe adenoviral infection, including conjunctivitis, pneumonitis, and pharyngitis, may be variably present.

*Diagnosis.* A striking rise in the polymorphonuclear leukocyte count may occur that is unlike that usually seen in viral infection. Most adenoviruses can be grown in tissue culture, whereas a group of "enteric" adenoviruses thought to be responsible for diarrhea in infants are diagnosed by antigen detection methods or tissue culture techniques available only in research laboratories. PCR techniques are also available. Enteric adenoviruses may be identified by electron microscopy of stool specimens.

*Treatment and Prevention.* There are no currently approved antiviral drugs for therapy or prevention of adenoviral infection. Vaccination is recommended for epidemics such as those occurring in military recruits.

### References

Behrman RE, Kliegman RM, Arvin AM (eds): Nelson Textbook of Pediatrics, 15th ed. Philadelphia, WB Saunders, 1996, Chapter 219.
Michaels MG, Green M, Wald ER, et al: Adenovirus infection in pediatric liver transplant patients. J Infect Dis 165:17, 4, 1992.
Ruuskanen O, Meurman O, Sarkkinen H: Adenoviral diseases in children: A study of 105 hospital cases. Pediatrics 76:79, 1985.

## ENTEROVIRUSES

Enteroviruses, a group of RNA viruses, include 23 group A coxsackieviruses (types A1–A24, except type A23), six group B coxsackieviruses (B1–B6), three polioviruses, and 31 echoviruses (types 1–33, except types 10 and 28). More recent isolates are designated enteroviruses (types 68–71).

*Epidemiology.* These hardy viruses maintain activity for days at room temperature. They are spread from person to person, primarily by the fecal-oral route and, possibly, by the respiratory route, especially among susceptible children in lower socioeconomic status groups and in tropical areas where poor hygiene may exist. There is a peak incidence in summer and fall in temperate climates that is less evident in the tropics. Males and females are equally affected by the disease, although males are more likely to become symptomatically ill. Young children frequently are infected; the disease in neonates may be fulminant, whereas older children have more benign illness unless paralysis or significant myocarditis is present. The incubation period is 3–6 days.

*Pathogenesis.* After initial upper respiratory tract viral implantation, viral replication occurs in regional lymph nodes, followed several days later by a low-grade (minor) viremia. This viremia may involve many secondary sites (heart, skin, pericardium, pleura, lung, liver, brain, spinal cord). Viral replication in these sites coincides with clinical illness and the second (major) viremia. Viral replication is halted by the appearance of antibody on approximately the 7th day of infection. Gastrointestinal tract viral replication and shedding are generally of longer duration but do not necessarily produce gastrointestinal symptoms.

*Pathology and Pathophysiology.* Each of the groups of enteroviruses has a predilection for specific organ systems. The pathognomonic finding in **poliomyelitis** is viral multiplication in motor neurons, a process that occurs predominantly in the spinal cord (especially anterior horn cells), but the medulla, mid-brain, thalamus, hypothalamus, pallidum, and motor cortex also may be involved. Typical organ involvement by *coxsackieviruses* includes pharyngitis (herpangina); skin (**hand-foot-mouth disease**); myocarditis; meningoencephalitis; and involvement of adrenals, pancreas, liver, pleura, pericardium, and, at times, the lung. Hepatic necrosis has been observed in some severe *echovirus* infections. Myositis, pneumonia, and adrenal involvement may also occur.

*Clinical Manifestations*

POLIOVIRUSES. As a result of the success of immunization programs the Western Hemisphere has been free of wild type paralytic poliomyelitis since 1994. The only cases of poliomyelitis are the rare vaccine-associated paralytic polio due to reversion of the vaccine-attenuated strain type 3 poliovirus to neurovirulence. The major forms and clinical manifestations of poliomyelitis are outlined in Table 10–17. The clinician must be vigilant regarding respiratory insufficiency resulting from both respiratory muscle and/or central respiratory center involvement. Such involvement may result in anxiety; jerky, breathless speaking; tachypnea; signs of respiratory distress (nasal flaring, use of accessory muscles of respiration); decreased cough; paradoxic abdominal movement; and immobility of in-

TABLE 10–17. Clinical Manifestations of Poliovirus Infection (Poliomyelitis)

| | |
|---|---|
| Asymptomatic infection | 95% of infected persons are asymptomatic |
| Abortive form (nonspecific febrile illness) | Fever, malaise, anorexia, nausea, vomiting, headache, pharyngitis, abdominal pain |
| Nonparalytic form (aseptic meningitis) | Similar to the abortive form plus stiff neck and signs of meningeal inflammation, soreness of back muscles, tripod sign, positive Kernig and Brudzinski signs, and bulging fontanel; decrease in both superficial (cremasteric, abdominal) and deep tendon reflexes heralds paralysis |
| Paralytic form | Similar to the nonparalytic form, plus weakness of skeletal or cranial muscle groups; with deeper brain involvement the signs and symptoms may be pain, spasticity, hypertonia, respiratory and cardiac arrhythmias, blood pressure and vasomotor changes, and bladder and bowel dysfunction; hallmark is asymmetric, flaccid paralysis in spinal, bulbar, and encephalitic forms |
| Spinal form | Axial and extremity muscle weakness that may involve intercostal muscles and diaphragm |
| Bulbar form | Cranial nerve weakness and respiratory and circulatory disturbances |
| Encephalitic form | Irritability, disorientation, drowsiness, and tremors |

tercostal spaces. Arm and deltoid weakness is a clue to impending respiratory paralysis.

In **bulbar poliomyelitis,** a nasal twang in the voice indicates palatal and pharyngeal weakness, as do pooling of saliva; poor cough; nasal regurgitation of saliva and other fluids; deviation of palate, uvula, or tongue; hoarseness; and aphonia. Changes in respiratory and cardiac function or vasomotor function (blood pressure changes, flushing and mottling of the skin) point toward central involvement of the key regulatory nuclei of the brain stem. The differential diagnosis includes Guillain-Barré syndrome, other types of viral encephalitis, botulism, tetanus, demyelinating encephalomyelitis, tick paralysis, CNS tumor, and

trauma. In the United States, most cases of paralytic poliomyelitis are due to the vaccine virus in normal or immunoincompetent hosts.

NONPOLIO ENTEROVIRAL INFECTION. Unlike the rare or declining occurrence of polio in most developed countries resulting from successful vaccination, the nonpolio enteroviruses remain common. Their manifestations may be biphasic, in which the patient experiences several days of well-being that occur between periods of 1–4 days of illness. Fewer than 50% of patients with enteroviral infection are *asymptomatic.*

The most common manifestation of all types of enteroviral infection is *nonspecific febrile illness.* It generally lasts 3 days and is associated with fever, malaise, headache, pharyngitis, and myalgia. In neonates, gastrointestinal tract symptoms may occur.

The enteroviruses have been associated with a variety of *respiratory tract illnesses,* including conjunctivitis, pharyngitis, herpangina, stomatitis, parotitis, croup, bronchitis, pneumonia, and pleurodynia. Pharyngitis is associated with pharyngeal erythema and, at times, with exudate. **Herpangina** (coxsackievirus A) is associated with fever, oral ulcers, and vesicles surrounded by erythema, usually in the posterior pharynx but also the anterior tonsillar pillars, palate, uvula, and posterior buccal surfaces. The duration is 3–6 days. **Pleurodynia** (Bornholm disease, devil's grip), an acute febrile illness, typically is associated with intense pleuritic chest and upper abdominal muscular pain that occurs in spasms and is intensified by breathing or coughing. The pain may mimic acute pulmonary or abdominal surgical processes and is due to intercostal muscle infection. This illness, often caused by a member of the coxsackie B group, generally occurs in outbreaks and may be associated with the other manifestations of enteroviral infection. Chest roentgenograms usually are normal, and the WBC count may be normal or elevated, with an increased percentage of myeloid cells.

*Gastrointestinal manifestations* commonly are associated with outbreaks of enteroviral infection. They include vomiting (in about 50% of cases), diarrhea (without blood), abdominal pain, mesenteric adenitis, and pseudoappendicitis.

*Acute hemorrhagic conjunctivitis,* particularly that associated with coxsackievirus A24 and enterovirus 70, may become manifest as eye pain, photophobia, blurred vision, lacrimation, erythema, congestion of the eye as a result of edema, chemotic eyelids, and eye discharge. Subconjunctival hemorrhages, conjunctivitis, keratitis, and preauricular adenopathy are present. Outbreaks have occurred in tropical and temperate climates.

*Pericarditis* and *myocarditis* commonly are caused by enteroviruses, especially coxsackieviruses B1–B5, and must be distinguished from acute rheumatic fever and acute bacterial endocarditis. Myocarditis carries a significant mortality rate from acute disease, especially in neonates and young infants. Older patients may experience chronic congestive heart failure and dilated cardiomyopathy after coxsackievirus myocarditis.

*Genitourinary tract manifestations* of the group B coxsackieviruses include orchitis and epididymitis. Rare manifestations include glomerulonephritis, pyuria, hematuria, cystitis, and vaginal ulcerative lesions.

*Myositis, arthritis,* and a dermatomyositis-like syndrome occurring in immunodeficient patients (usually with B-cell defects) have been linked to chronic enteroviral infection.

*Hand-foot-mouth syndrome,* often associated with coxsackievirus A16 or enterovirus 7, is characterized by small intraoral ulcers on the tongue and buccal mucosa associated with vesicular or erythematous macular lesions on the hands, feet, and, occasionally, the buttocks. Nonspecific maculopapular and even petechial rashes also are common during enteroviral infection.

The enteroviruses are the most common cause of seasonal *aseptic meningitis syndrome,* which occurs in summer and fall in temperate climates. This syndrome may be associated with other manifestations of enteroviral infection or may be the sole manifestation of the condition. Rash (erythematous, maculopapular, or petechial), sore throat, muscle pain, and signs of meningeal irritation are common, except in infants under 12 mo of age who commonly are infected. CSF usually reveals an early polymorphonuclear cell predominance, shifting to a lymphocytic predominance in 12–24 hr. The median number of cells is 100–150/μL, but occasionally thousands of cells per microliter are seen. The CSF protein level is mildly elevated, and the glucose level is normal. The duration of illness is generally 4–6 days of fever and 7–14 days of neurologic signs or symptoms. The enteroviruses also are probably the most common cause of seasonal *encephalitis* in locales with low arthropod-mediated arboviral activity.

As with poliovirus, the other enteroviruses uncommonly can cause an acute anterior horn cell infection resulting in *paralysis.* Peripheral neuritis and acute hemiplegia also have been associated with enteroviral infection.

*Neonatal nonspecific febrile illness* may be acquired transplacentally from a mildly ill mother or, more usually, at birth from the sick mother, another sick family member, or a nursery contact. The illness is characterized by fever, irritability, anorexia, mild vomiting, or diarrhea and often is indistinguishable from bacterial sepsis. The duration of the illness is 3–4 days. The peripheral WBC count often is elevated, accompanied by a predominance of polymorphonuclear leukocytes. This illness must be differentiated from neonatal bacterial sepsis, and hospitalization is usually required for diagnostic evaluation and empiric antimicrobial therapy. Echovirus 11 has been associated with fulminating neonatal hepatic necrosis.

*Myocarditis* in the neonate often is due to coxsackieviruses B1–B5. Illness begins abruptly with fever, tachycardia, cardiomegaly, electrocardiographic changes, transient systolic murmurs, shock, and respiratory distress. In the newborn, fulminant *encephalomyocarditis* can occur.

**Diagnosis.** Although the season, location, age of the patient, exposure, and clinical manifestations may suggest enteroviral infection, it often is difficult to differentiate this infection from bacterial infection or other viral infections. The definitive diagnosis may be made by culturing enterovirus from a normally sterile site or from biopsy material. Recovering virus from stool or pharyngeal secretions suggests, but does not prove, that infection exists because a significant number of infants may be asymptomatically shedding enterovirus during an epidemic or continue to shed vaccine strains after polio immunization. Viral growth requires 3–7 days in tissue culture. If polio virus is isolated, it should be sent to the Centers for Disease Control and Prevention (CDC) in Atlanta to distinguish wild polio from vaccine strains. Many of the group A coxsackieviruses require suckling mouse inoculation for recovery. Although a four-fold or greater rise in specific antibody titers in serum is diagnostic, most laboratories will not perform serologic tests in the absence of an isolate because there are a multitude of enteroviruses. However, serum collected at the initial presentation of the patient with the illness and 2–4 wk later may confirm or refute infection, especially in the infant with fecal shedding of virus or in one who has an unusual illness. RNA hybridization with complementary DNA (cDNA) probes may identify the viral genome in infected tissues.

**Treatment.** There are no available specific antiviral therapies for enteroviral infections. In immunocompetent patients, therapy is aimed at anticipating and preventing complications and preparing for the more prolonged phases of rehabilitation, when necessary. Corticosteroid therapy is of no value in any form of enteroviral infection and has worsened experimental murine coxsackievirus myocarditis. Supportive therapy of myocarditis and meningitis is essential and includes providing cardiorespiratory care and controlling increased intracranial pressure, respectively.

*Prevention.* Poliovirus infection can be prevented almost entirely by vaccination (live oral or inactivated injected preparations) (see Fig. 10–1). Because of the concern of vaccine-associated paralytic polio (VAPP), in the absence of wild type disease in the United States, the Advisory Committee on Immunization Practices of the CDC suggests that inactivated polio vaccine (IPV) be used for the first two doses, followed by oral polio vaccine (OPV) to decrease the incidence of VAPP while still providing live virus, which is shed in the gastrointestinal tract and serves to induce herd immunity. For underdeveloped countries, the World Health Organization (WHO) recommends the sole use of OPV. The American Academy of Pediatrics has suggested three options: (1) sequential IPV/OPV, (2) IPV only, or (3) OPV only. For immunocompromised patients in whom the use of live virus vaccine is contraindicated, IPV should be used solely. OPV is recommended for patients who prefer not to have so many injections as well as for those who start their primary immunizations late (after 6 mo of age) in whom the number of injections at each visit would be unacceptable. In addition, OPV is recommended in areas of the world where poliomyelitis has *not* been eradicated, where the ease of administration, lower cost, and advantages to excretion of a live virus aid in the development of herd immunity are obvious advantages.

*Prognosis.* In developed countries, the rate of early mortality from poliovirus infection is 5–7%. Residual disability is influenced by acute management and the extent of appropriate rehabilitation. The major sequelae of nonpolio enteroviral infections are related to myocardial and CNS damage. Young infants, especially those with seizures, may be at higher risk for neurologic sequelae.

## References

Behrman RE, Kliegman RM, Arvin AM (eds): Nelson Textbook of Pediatrics, 15th ed. Philadelphia, WB Saunders, 1996, Chapter 209.

Bergman I, Painter MJ, Wald ER, et al: Outcome in children with enteroviral meningitis during the first year of life. J Pediatr 110:705, 1987.

de Quadros C, Andrus JK, Olive J-M, et al: Eradication of poliomyelitis: Progress in the Americas. Pediatr Infect Dis J 10:222, 1991.

McKinney RE, Katz SL, Wilfert CM: Chronic enteroviral meningoencephalitis in agammaglobulinemic patients. Rev Infect Dis 9:334, 1987.

Strebel PM, Sutter RW, Cochi SL, et al: Epidemiology of poliomyelitis in the United States one decade after the last reported case of indigenous wild virus-associated disease. Clin Infect Dis 14:568, 1992.

## HUMAN PARVOVIRUS INFECTION
### (Erythema Infectiosum, or Fifth Disease)

*Etiology.* Erythema infectiosum is the clinical designation given to infection caused by the human parvovirus B19. Although this is a benign viral exanthem in normal children, the affinity of this virus to red blood cell progenitor cells makes it an important cause of aplastic crisis in patients with hemolytic anemias, including sickle cell disease, spherocytosis, and thalassemia (see Chapter 14). It also causes fetal anemia and hydrops fetalis when primary infection occurs during pregnancy. The erythrocyte P antigen is the cellular receptor for parvovirus B19; the virus replicates in actively dividing erythroid stem cells. The virus is acquired via the respiratory tract and causes transient viremia.

*Epidemiology.* This is a common disease; community epidemics usually occur in the spring. The virus is transmitted by respiratory secretions or by blood product transfusions. Virus can be detected by PCR techniques. Patients may shed the virus prior to the onset of the rash. Seroprevalence studies suggest that 40–60% of adults have antibody to parvovirus B19.

*Clinical Manifestations.* Erythema infectiosum becomes manifest by rash, low-grade or no fever, and, occasionally, by pharyngitis and mild conjunctivitis. The rash appears in three stages. The initial stage typically is demonstrated by erythematous cheeks, which gives a "slapped cheek" appearance to the patient as a result of intense facial erythema. One to 4 days later, an erythematous symmetric, maculopapular, truncal rash appears but later fades as central clearing takes place, giving a distinctive lacy-reticulated rash that lasts 2–40 days (mean, 11 days). This rash often is pruritic; does not desquamate; and may recur with exercise, bath, rubbing, or stress. Adolescents may experience myalgia, significant arthralgia or arthritis, headache, pharyngitis, coryza, and gastrointestinal upset. Parvovirus may produce pancytopenia in immunosuppressed patients.

*Diagnosis and Differential Diagnosis.* Serologic tests demonstrating antibody response to parvovirus and the presence of specific IgM antibody to parvovirus are diagnostic. In serum specimens taken during the acute stage, the virus has been detected by immune electron microscopy and DNA hybridization. A mild leukopenia, thrombocytopenia, and reticulocytopenia may be present. This illness is characteristic, although atypical cases may be confused with other viral exanthems (such as measles, rubella, and enterovirus), as well as with drug rashes or SLE.

*Treatment.* There is no specific therapy. Respiratory isolation is advisable for 7 days after the onset of illness. Patients with sickle cell anemia or fetuses with hydrops may require transfusion. Immunosuppressed patients may develop pancytopenia, which may be treated with IVIG.

## References

Behrman RE, Kliegman RM, Arvin AM (eds): Nelson Textbook of Pediatrics, 15th ed. Philadelphia, WB Saunders, 1996, Chapter 210.

Bell LM, Naides SJ, Stoffman P, et al: Human parvovirus B19 infection among hospital staff members after contact with infected patients. N Engl J Med 321:485, 1989.

Brown KE, Hibbs JR, Gallinella G, et al: Resistance to parvovirus B19 infection due to lack of reception (erythrocyte P antigen). N Engl J Med 330:1192, 1994.

Chorba T, Coccia P, Holman RC, et al: The role of parvovirus B19 in aplastic crisis and erythema infectiosum (fifth disease). J Infect Dis 154:383, 1986.

## HEPATITIS

See Chapter 11.

## HERPES VIRUS INFECTIONS

The human herpes virus family consists of cytomegalovirus, EBV, herpes simplex virus, varicella-zoster virus, human herpesvirus-6 (HHV6), human herpesvirus-7 (HHV7), and human herpesvirus-8 (Kaposi sarcoma–associated virus). The herpes viruses cause acute primary infection, maintain a state of latency in lymphoid and neuronal tissues, and may reactivate and occasionally induce a clinical recurrence, especially in immunocompromised individuals.

### Cytomegalovirus Infection

*Etiology.* CMV is a large, enveloped, double-stranded DNA virus with an icosahedral capsid. After fusion of the viral envelope with host cell membranes, viral replication occurs within the cell nucleus and new viral particles bud through the nuclear membrane and are released through the cell membrane. Infection of host mucosal surfaces occurs via the respiratory or genital tract. Following viremia, the virus disseminates to various tissues and is isolated from many sites.

*Epidemiology.* CMV is a ubiquitous virus. It is the most commonly known human virus that is transmitted *vertically* to the fetus (transplacentally, during birth, and by breast milk), but transmission also occurs *horizontally* from person to person (blood, urine, secretions). In addition, CMV persists in a latent form after a primary infection and reactivation may occur, particularly during immunosuppression. Infection rates are inversely correlated with socioeconomic status. In the United States, 20–50% of childbearing-age women are infected; in developing countries, the infection rate approaches 100%. Four to 10% of pregnant women excrete virus in cervical secretions or in their urine, and 5–25% shed it in milk during lactation. From 1–3% of children are infected prior to birth, and 10–20% acquire infection in the neonatal period. Day care centers are important areas of CMV transmission in infants and young children. These infected infants act as a source of infection for their seronegative parents.

The transmission of CMV infection requires close contact. Epidemic outbreaks have not been reported, although transmission is common in families, in day care centers, and among sexual partners. CMV can be isolated from saliva, urine, nasopharyngeal secretions, milk, semen, blood, and donor organs (kidneys, bone marrow). The incidence of CMV excretion in day care centers may reach 50–70% in 1–2 yr olds. Although infection of the fetus can result from either primary or recurrent disease in the mother, it is the primary form in the mother that results in symptomatic neonatal illness, which is estimated to occur in 5–10% of infants of mothers with primary infection. Horizontal transmission probably occurs most commonly via saliva, but urine also may be an important medium, especially in day care centers. Blood transfusion with CMV-infected blood cells may induce a mononucleosis-like syndrome in susceptible individuals, an effect that often is noted in massively transfused patients after cardiopulmonary bypass. Blood transfusions from CMV-seropositive donors to seronegative recipients are another source of infection in premature infants, in immunosuppressed patients, and following transplantation. Immunocompromised patients often experience severe primary infection and usually, less severe recurrent syndromes. Sexually active individuals have a high rate of CMV infection.

*Clinical Manifestations.* These vary according to age and immune status of the host.

NEONATAL INFECTION. More than 90% of congenitally infected infants are asymptomatic. A significant number (15%) of infants born to women with asymptomatic or symptomatic primary infection occurring early in pregnancy will have a **TORCH syndrome** (*t*oxoplasmosis, *o*ther, *r*ubella, CMV, and *h*erpes simplex) (see Chapter 6). Infants infected during maternal reactivation have less severe disease. Premature neonates who are CMV-seronegative and who receive blood from CMV-positive donors may develop a syndrome characterized by respiratory distress, pallor, sepsis-like signs, hepatosplenomegaly, neutropenia, thrombocytopenia, and lymphocytosis. In a small number of term infants with perinatally acquired disease, CMV pneumonitis, petechial rash, intracranial calcifications, and hepatosplenomegaly occur. Some congenitally infected infants who appear to be asymptomatic at birth will have hearing loss or learning disability in infancy or childhood.

OLDER CHILDREN. Asymptomatic infections are the most common type in older children. A characteristic syndrome caused by CMV in healthy children is a heterophil-negative, mononucleosis-like syndrome and hepatitis. The former often includes fever, malaise, myalgia, headache, anorexia, abdominal pain, and hepatosplenomegaly. Atypical lymphocytosis and reversal of the T-cell helper: suppressor cell ratio is characteristic. The degree of pharyngitis and lymphadenopathy generally is less striking than that seen in the EBV-induced mononucleosis syndrome. As occurs in patients with infectious mononucleosis, an ampicillin-induced rash and abnormal serologic reactions, including the presence of cold agglutinins, ANAs, rheumatoid factor, and cryoglobulins, may occur in this CMV syndrome. A CMV hepatitis syndrome without other manifestations of the mononucleosis syndrome may occur.

IMMUNOCOMPROMISED HOSTS. CMV commonly causes serious infection in immunocompromised hosts: In HIV-infected patients, CMV causes retinitis, pneumonia, gastrointestinal ulcers, and encephalitis. The spectrum of disease is different in organ or bone marrow transplant recipients in whom CMV pneumonitis and neutropenia are major problems. Transplantion of CMV-negative tissue into CMV-negative patients is recommended. CMV-positive patients may reactivate endogenous infection or may acquire new strains from CMV-positive donors. Active CMV infection may be associated with organ rejection.

Diagnosis. The diagnosis may be difficult to establish because of the high rate of asymptomatic excretion, the frequency of reactivation infections, and the presence of IgM antibody in some episodes of reactivation.

NEONATAL INFECTION. The diagnosis of congenital disease (TORCH) relies on demonstrating CMV in urine, pharyngeal secretions, or peripheral blood leukocytes during the 1st wk of life or on demonstrating a positive CMV-IgM serologic test. The serologic diagnosis is complicated by maternal transplacental IgG antibody and the common occurrence of perinatally acquired disease, which makes studies after the first few weeks of life inconclusive in establishing the diagnosis. Negative serologic studies of the infant generally exclude the latter diagnosis, as do negative maternal serologic studies.

The differential diagnosis of congenital CMV includes infection with Toxoplasma, syphilis, rubella, HSV, HIV, Listeria monocytogenes, varicella, and enterovirus.

ACQUIRED INFECTION. Diagnosis of CMV depends on viral isolation and seroconversion. Diagnosis is especially complicated in immunosuppressed patients, who may not mount an immune response and in whom the finding of CMV in the urine is so common as to be nondiagnostic. Thus, diagnosis of CMV hepatitis or pneumonitis may rest on isolation of CMV from the specific site by biopsy, bronchoscopy (bronchoalveolar lavage), or other invasive tests. The isolation of CMV from blood or buffy coat cells has been associated with the presence of invasive CMV disease. Appropriate serologic tests should exclude infection caused by hepatitis A and B viruses and EBV. New antigen detection tests by nucleic acid hybridization or ELISA may simplify the diagnosis of CMV if appropriate tissue specimens are available.

Treatment. Serious CMV infections in immunocompromised patients can be treated with ganciclovir or foscarnet (see Table 10–16). CMV pneumonitis has been treated with ganciclovir and intravenous immunoglobulin. Minimally symptomatic immunocompetent patients require no treatment.

Prevention. In several patient populations, including immunocompromised individuals, seronegative premature neonates, or individuals about to receive a renal transplant, use of blood or kidneys from CMV-seronegative donors or glycerol frozen blood can prevent potentially serious primary infection. Seronegative premature infants should not receive fresh human milk from nonmaternal sources because the rate of CMV excretion in milk is high. Prophylactic ganciclovir may reduce infection in transplant recipients.

Prognosis. Symptomatic congenital infection carries a guarded outlook regarding neurologic sequelae, especially in the child with microcephaly or intracranial calcifications. Hearing loss is a common complication of asymptomatic or symptomatic congenital CMV infection. Acquired infection in the healthy host usually is self-limited, whereas it may be fatal in the immunocompromised host as a result of pneumonitis, encephalitis, or secondary opportunistic infections.

## References

Behrman RE, Kliegman RM, Arvin AM (eds): Nelson Textbook of Pediatrics, 15th ed. Philadelphia, WB Saunders, 1996, Chapter 214.

Boppana S, Fowler K, Vaid Y, et al: Neuroradiologic findings in the newborn period and long term outcome in children with symptomatic congenital cytomegalovirus infection. Pediatrics 99:409, 1997.

Boppana SB, Pass RF, Britt WJ, et al: Symptomatic congenital cytomegalovirus infection: Neonatal morbidity and mortality. Pediatr Infect Dis J 11:93, 1992.

Horwitz CV, Henle W, Henle G, et al: Clinical and laboratory evaluation of cytomegalovirus-induced mononucleosis in previously healthy individuals. Medicine 65:124, 1986.

Ljungman P, Engelhard D, Link H, et al: Treatment of interstitial pneumonitis due to cytomegalovirus with ganciclovir and intravenous immune globulin: Experience of European bone marrow transplant group. Clin Infect Dis 14:831, 1992.

Murph JR, Baron JC, Brown CK, et al: The occupational risk of cytomegalovirus infection among day-care providers. JAMA 265:603, 1991.

## Epstein-Barr Virus Infection
### (Infectious Mononucleosis)

*Etiology.* EBV, a double-stranded DNA virus, contains a capsid, a protein tegument, and a lipid outer envelope. The virus infects permissive cells and is maintained as an episome. Pharyngeal epithelial cells are probably the initial target of viral infection and replication. Viral genes are transcribed in a sequential pattern, first the early antigens, which are viral enzymes necessary for DNA replication, followed by DNA replication and expression of the capsid antigen. These specific gene products provide the basis for the serologic diagnosis of primary or reactivation of EBV infection. EBV infects B cells and immortalizes them, maintaining itself within the nucleus. These B cells are widely disseminated until the immune system, particularly natural killer and T cells, is activated. The atypical lymphocytes present during acute EBV infections are cytotoxic T cells, activated in response to EBV-infected B cells. The ability of this virus to transform B cells is also associated with the X-linked lymphoproliferative syndrome and the post-transplant lymphoproliferative syndromes caused by EBV infection.

*Epidemiology.* EBV infection occurs at an early age in persons in developing countries; most children are seropositive by 3 yr of age. In developed countries, age of infection is inversely related to socioeconomic level; 60–80% of adolescents from lower socioeconomic levels are seropositive. In higher socioeconomic levels, infection typically occurs during high school or college attendance. Susceptible Yale University students demonstrated a 15% seroconversion rate per year. Endemic disease in group settings of adolescents is common.

EBV is transmitted by salivary exchange, contact with contaminated objects, or, less commonly, blood transfusions. It is spread by intimate contact, and EBV is shed in the saliva before and during clinically apparent infection. In addition, 10–20% of healthy seropositive individuals and 60% of seropositive immunosuppressed individuals shed virus intermittently; therefore, the period of communicability is not known. The incubation period is 30–50 days.

*Clinical Manifestations.* The clinical manifestations of EBV are age-related and range from asymptomatic to fatal infections. Infants and young children infected with EBV usually are asymptomatic or experience mild disease that may include tonsillitis, fever, or upper respiratory tract disease. In older children and young adults, a typical infectious mononucleosis syndrome (pharyngitis, fever, lymphadenopathy, hepatosplenomegaly, lymphocytosis) may develop after EBV infection.

The prodromal period of infectious mononucleosis includes malaise, fatigue, headache, nausea, and abdominal pain lasting 1–2 wk. The typical symptoms and signs of mononucleosis include pharyngitis (with enlarged tonsils and exudate), an enanthema (pharyngeal petechiae), fever, lymphadenopathy (posterior cervical; epitrochlear; less commonly, generalized), splenomegaly (up to 50% of patients), and hepatomegaly (10–20%). Eyelid edema and maculopapular or urticarial rash occur in 5–15% of cases. Group A streptococci may be recovered from the pharynx in 30% of children. A diffuse, erythematous rash develops in approximately 80% of patients treated with ampicillin. The symptoms last 2–4 wk, then slowly abate.

ONCOGENICITY OF EBV. EBV is probably the initiator of African Burkitt lymphoma in children and of adult nasopharyngeal carcinoma in Asia. Polyclonal B cell lymphoma in immunocompromised patients and X-linked lymphoproliferative disease (see under Complications) have been shown to be associated with EBV.

COMPLICATIONS. As a result of rapid swelling, splenic rupture may occur. The pharyngeal tonsillar hypertrophy may cause airway obstruction. Neurologic complications may occur in the absence of classic features of mononucleosis and include seizures, ataxia, aseptic meningitis syndrome, Bell palsy, transverse myelitis, encephalitis, combative behavior, headache, and Guillain-Barré syndrome. Other complications include hepatitis (85% of cases); myocarditis; interstitial pneumonia; Coombs-positive hemolytic anemia; antibody-mediated thrombocytopenia; hemophagocytic syndrome; and, rarely, aplastic anemia, pancreatitis, parotitis, orchitis, and Reye syndrome.

In several kindreds, a rare syndrome of *X-linked lymphoproliferative disease* (**Duncan syndrome**) following EBV infection has occurred. The affected males may die of overwhelming infection; they may survive and develop B-cell lymphoproliferative disease; or they may develop hypoplastic syndromes, such as aplastic anemia or hypogammaglobulinemia. Rarely, immunocompromised patients (transplantation, AIDS, ataxia–telangiectasia, severe combined immunodeficiency disorders) and apparently healthy patients may have the same fate.

*Diagnosis.* Nonspecific findings often include a leukocytosis of 10,000–20,000 cells/μL, with at least 20–40% being atypical lymphocytes. These lymphocytes are T cells responding to EBV-infected B cells. Children under 5 yr of age have less striking atypical lymphocytosis. Mild thrombocytopenia occurs in 50% of individuals, and elevated liver enzymes occur in approximately 85%.

Nonspecific tests for the heterophil antibody include the Paul-Bunnell test and the slide agglutination reaction, both of which are based on the appearance of IgM antibody against sheep, horse, or oxen red blood cells not absorbable by guinea pig kidney cells. These are present in the serum for up to 6 mo after EBV infection. This antibody response generally is absent in children under 5 yr of age but identifies about 90% of cases in older children and adults. Specific diagnosis of EBV infection involves analysis for several types of antibodies against specific EBV antigens.

SEROLOGIC RESPONSE TO EBV INFECTION. The most commonly performed test is that for detecting antibodies to viral capsid antigen (VCA). At the time of the onset of symptoms, most patients have high IgG anti-VCA and IgM anti-VCA antibodies as well as antibodies to early antigen (EA). The absence or low level of antibody to Epstein-Barr nuclear antigen (EBNA) and the presence of the anti-VCA antibody indicates acute infection. High levels of IgG anti-VCA and anti-EBNA and absence of IgM anti-VCA and anti-EA indicate previous (not acute) infection. Absence of all anti-EBV antibodies indicates a susceptible, uninfected individual. These serologic tests are particularly useful for evaluating young patients who have heterophil-negative infectious mononucleosis or for those with isolated organ manifestations, such as myocarditis, FUO, and encephalitis.

EBV DNA also can be demonstrated in infected cells by DNA hybridization.

DIFFERENTIAL DIAGNOSIS. The differential diagnosis includes cytomegalovirus infection, toxoplasmosis, hepatitis A, lymphoma, and leukemia. Less commonly confused conditions are rubella, lep-tospirosis, Kawasaki syndrome, HIV infection, human herpesvirus-6, and streptococcal infection.

*Treatment.* The typical patient with mononucleosis requires no antiviral therapy. Bed rest is indicated by the patient's needs and does not improve the course. Acyclovir may have some beneficial effects in life-threatening EBV infection. Corticosteroids have been utilized for respiratory distress resulting from tonsillar hypertrophy, thrombocytopenia, hemolytic anemia, and neurologic complications. Although steroids have been shown to shorten the course of the acute illness, they should not be used in uncomplicated cases. Acyclovir combined with prednisolone does not alter the course of mononucleosis.

*Prevention.* There are no measures to prevent EBV infection. Patients with recent EBV infection should not donate blood. Splenic trauma should be avoided by limiting athletics and repeated examinations.

## References

Alpert G, Fleisher GR: Complications of infection with Epstein-Barr virus during childhood: A study of children admitted to the hospital. Pediatr Infect Dis 3:304, 1984.

Behrman RE, Kliegman RM, Arvin AM (eds): Nelson Textbook of Pediatrics, 15th ed. Philadelphia, WB Saunders, 1996, Chapter 215.

Grierson H, Purtillo DT: Epstein-Barr infections in males with the X-linked lymphoproliferative syndrome. Ann Intern Med 106:538, 1987.

Tynell E, Aurelius E, Brandell A, et al: Acyclovir and prednisolone treatment of acute infectious mononucleosis: A multicenter double blind placebo controlled study. J Infect Dis 174:324, 1996.

## Herpes Simplex Virus (HSV) Infection

*Etiology.* HSV (HSV-1 and HSV-2) are large double-stranded DNA viruses that consist of a linear genome contained within an icosahedral capsid. There is significant DNA homology between types 1 and 2. The virus initially infects mucosal surfaces or injured skin and enters cutaneous neurons, where it migrates along the axons to the sensory ganglia. Viral replication occurs in these ganglia and infectious virus then moves down the axon to infect and destroy the epithelial cells. In immunocompromised patients and in the neonate, viral replication persists and disseminates to other organs.

Latency is established within neurons, where virus is maintained but undergoes active replication only at sporadic intervals triggered by undefined events. Although antibody production in response to infection is associated with recovery from primary HSV infection and maternal transmission of antibody to the neonate appears to be protective in neonatal infections, it does not prevent reactivation disease.

Although either virus can be found in any site, nongenital type 1 (HSV-1) usually occurs above the waist (CNS, eyes, mouth), and genital type 2 (HSV-2) generally involves the genitalia and skin below the waist; HSV type 2 generally occurs in the neonate at any site. *Primary infection* occurs in nonimmune individuals who have never been previously infected. This infection often is asymptomatic but may cause a typical clinical syndrome. In most infected individuals, the virus attains a state of *latency* in neural tissue. *Reactivation* of latent virus may result in a characteristic clinical syndrome of herpetic *recurrence.* In addition, another exposure to a second type or even a second strain of the same type can result in exogenous *reinfection.*

*Epidemiology.* The incubation period is 2–12 days, with a mean of 6–7 days. Approximately 85% of infections are asymptomatic. Institutional and family outbreaks have occurred. Close body contact (saliva, kissing, wrestling, sexual) and inoculation of mucous membranes or disrupted skin are required for infection. After the loss of transplacental antibodies, infants and young children begin to be infected with HSV-1. At the onset of sexual activity, HSV-2 infection becomes more common. HSV infection occurs more frequently in individuals from lower socioeconomic status groups. Approximately 2–5% of healthy individuals shed HSV in oral secretions at any time.

*Pathology.* The classic findings are intranuclear inclusion bodies and multinucleated giant cells. Immunity requires T-cell–mediated activity and anti-HSV antibodies.

### Clinical Manifestations

SKIN AND MUCOUS MEMBRANES. Primary infection of the skin in neonates is common. Autoinoculation from another site may cause a localized vesicular eruption on an erythematous base. Healing is complete in 7–14 days. Recurrences occur at the same site. Infection of a digit causes a viral paronychia, referred to as a **herpetic whitlow,** which is painful, erythematous, and occasionally presents with a vesicular eruption. It is found in children who suck their thumbs and bite their nails. In older children, it may be found concomitantly with genital herpes; in health care professionals, it usually is nosocomially acquired. Abraded or burned skin is quite susceptible to HSV infection. In this setting, the lesions often are atypical, with ulcers predominating. Wrestlers and rugby players acquire cutaneous herpes from close body contact with the cutaneous infections of other players (**herpes gladiatorum** and **herpes rugbiaforum**). Erythema multiforme also is associated with HSV.

ACUTE HERPETIC GINGIVOSTOMATITIS. This is the most common clinical manifestation of primary HSV infection in infants and children beyond the neonatal period. It generally occurs in 1–3 yr olds, although it may occur at any age. The onset is abrupt, with mouth pain, salivation, fetor oris, dysphagia, anorexia, and fever. The vesicles usually rupture, and the typical lesion is ulcerative. The anterior and, less commonly, the posterior oropharynx are involved, with lesions in the gingiva, buccal mucosa, tongue, and lips and, following autoinoculation, on the skin of neck and nose. Regional lymphadenopathy is common. The illness lasts 7–14 days. *Herpangina,* an enteroviral infection, may be differentiated by its vesicles and ulcers, which occur predominantly in the posterior pharynx. In adolescents, a severe exudative pharyngitis may be the manifestation of primary oral HSV infection.

*Recurrent stomatitis* is the typical fever blister that occurs on the mucocutaneous junction. These lesions are a recurrence of oral HSV infection and are not associated with systemic signs or symptoms.

ECZEMA HERPETICUM (KAPOSI VARICELLIFORM ERUPTION). This is a serious, usually primary HSV infection that occurs in individuals with eczema. It may be generalized and involve many areas of skin, producing vesicles, ulcers, and hemorrhagic crusts. Fever (40.0–40.5°C [104–105°F]) for 7–10 days and recurrent attacks are common. In severe cases, the widespread infection acts as a burn, causing fluid loss and hyponatremia. Dissemination to visceral organs or the brain may occur. In previous times, this infection had to be differentiated from vaccinia, variola, and varicella.

OCULAR LESIONS. Conjunctivitis and keratoconjunctivitis may be manifestations of primary or recurrent infection at any age. The conjunctiva is erythematous and swollen, without purulence. Corneal lesions may occur as dendritic or ameboid ulcers or more commonly, in recurrent infection, as a deep keratitis. Vesicular lid lesions, if present, should suggest the diagnosis. HSV, along with bacteria and other viruses, always should be included in the differential diagnosis of conjunctivitis (Table 10–15). Steroids, which worsen HSV ocular infection, should not be used in patients with herpes conjunctivitis. Ocular manifestations of neonates infected with HSV may include cataracts, uveitis, and chorioretinitis, in addition to conjunctivitis and keratoconjunctivitis.

ENCEPHALITIS. HSV is the most common cause of fatal, sporadic viral encephalitis. Beyond the neonatal period, it is predominantly caused by HSV-1. It may be a manifestation of primary or recurrent disease. The mortality rate is over 75% if the infection is not treated. Although HSV resembles other forms of encephalitis with alterations of mentation, fever, and seizures, the characteristic features of neonatal HSV encephalitis are clinical signs of *focal* CNS disease, as evidenced by EEG, CT, or MRI or neuroradiologic signs of focality, especially in the temporal lobe. The spinal fluid usually reveals lymphocytosis, an elevated protein level, a normal glucose level, and red blood cells. The CSF culture is negative for bacteria or HSV (HSV may be recovered in neonatal disease). Detection of HSV antigen or more often DNA, by PCR from the CFS, confirms the diagnosis.

GENITAL HERPES. This condition occurs most commonly in adolescents or young adults. It may be a sign of early sexual activity or child abuse in younger children. About 75% of cases are due to HSV-2. Primary symptomatic infection becomes manifest by vesicular, ulcerative, and crusted lesions in the genital areas of males or females. In females, the cervix is involved as well. Systemic symptoms of fever, adenopathy, paresthesia, and dysuria are common. The course of illness lasts 10–20 days. In patients practicing rectal intercourse, a similar syndrome involving the perirectal area occurs.

Recurrent genital tract disease is characterized by localized vesicles, ulcers, and crusts that last for several days without systemic symptoms. Recurrences occur in 50–80% of patients with primary symptomatic genital tract disease.

Complications of primary genital tract herpes infection include a self-limited aseptic meningitis syndrome. HSV infection of the genital tract of pregnant women can result in the transmission of infection to their offspring.

DISSEMINATED (SYSTEMIC) INFECTION OF THE NEONATE. The majority of cases of neonatal HSV are caused by HSV-2 and are acquired when the infant passes through an infected birth canal. Infants also can be infected by nongenital maternal or nosocomial sources. Most infected mothers are asymptomatic, and usually no history of maternal or paternal genital HSV infection is discovered. The incidence of premature birth is higher than expected. Initial symptoms of disseminated neonatal disease generally occur within 1 wk of birth; diseases localized to the CNS or to the skin, eyes, and mouth more often occur 2–3 wk following birth.

Clinical manifestations in the neonate include (1) a vesicular or pustular eruption; (2) a nonfocal meningoencephalitis syndrome; (3) a respiratory distress pneumonic syndrome; and (4) a generalized, systemic infection involving several internal organs, including the CNS and liver. The systemic infection progresses to acidosis, coagulopathy, shock, and death in the majority of untreated cases. Unfortunately, the telltale vesicular eruption often is late in appearing or does not appear at all (20–30%) prior to the infant's death. Of all infants who present with only local signs, such as vesicles, conjunctivitis, and mouth lesions, 70% have infection that disseminates to other organs. Thus, *any* manifestation of HSV infection in the neonate should be treated with antiviral chemotherapy. If the neonate is left untreated, the mortality of neonatal HSV infection is 50%, with 50% of survivors having significant sequelae. Even localized disease of the skin, eyes, and mouth is associated with sequelae in 10–15% of infants.

IMMUNOCOMPROMISED PATIENTS. Patients with T-cell disorders, severe combined immunodeficiency, AIDS, lymphoma, leukemia, or severe malnutrition and those undergoing chemotherapy or transplantation procedures have a significant increase in susceptibility to serious HSV infection. This becomes manifest rarely as disseminated disease but frequently as severe recurrences, which are typically focal, necrotic, painful lesions that heal slowly. Rarely, these lesions disseminate to other areas of skin or visceral organs. In immunosuppressed patients, HSV commonly causes mucositis and esophagitis as a result of local spread from oral infection. Less commonly, pneumonitis, hepatitis, and, rarely, chronic encephalitis occur.

**Diagnosis.** Cytologic examination (Tzanck stain, Papanicolaou stain) may reveal cells with characteristic intranuclear inclusions or giant cells. These indicate either HSV or varicella-zoster virus infection. Antigen detection tests, such as fluorescent antibody and enzyme-linked immunoassays, are rapid and specific but are only 50–80% sensitive. The test of choice is PCR or (if it is not available) tissue culture for viral cytopathic effects, which is rapid (2–5 days), specific, and sensitive.

Acute and convalescent antibody testing may be diagnostic in primary infection but is not helpful for making clinically useful decisions. Most neonates have transplacental anti-HSV antibody, patients with recurrences have high and stable levels of antibody, and severely immunosuppressed children may fail to produce any antibody.

**Treatment.** Therapy for HSV infection depends on the type of the disease (primary, recurrent), the anatomic sites involved, and, most importantly, the immune status of the host. No treatment is needed for mild, self-limited infection in immunocompetent children (gingivostomatitis, "cold sores"). Acyclovir is used either orally for uncomplicated infections (primary genital lesions) or intravenously for more serious (encephalitis) or disseminated (immunocompromised host, neonate) infections. Topical therapy with trifluridine or iododeoxyuridine is indicated for ocular infection.

*Prevention.* Acquisition of HSV in neonates is greatest when mothers have a primary genital infection at the time of delivery; operative delivery is suggested to prevent neonatal disease. Prepartum HSV cultures do not predict the presence of the virus at the time of delivery. Chronic acyclovir occasionally is used in patients with frequent or severe recurrences of herpes infections (particularly HIV-infected patients); acyclovir resistance has occurred in this setting. The use of condoms provides some protection against sexual transmission of herpes simplex.

## References

Behrman RE, Kliegman RM, Arvin AM (eds): Nelson Textbook of Pediatrics, 15th ed. Philadelphia, WB Saunders, 1996, Chapter 211.

Belongia EA, Goodman JL, Holland EJ: An outbreak of herpes gladiatorum at a high-school wrestling camp. N Engl J Med 325:906, 1991.

Gibbs RS, Mead PB: Preventing neonatal herpes: Current strategies. N Engl J Med 326:946, 1992.

Mertz GJ, Benedetti J, Ashley R, et al: Risk factors for the sexual transmission of genital herpes. Ann Intern Med 116:197, 1992.

Whitley R, Arvin A, Prober C, et al: Predictors of morbidity and mortality in neonates with herpes simplex virus infections. N Engl J Med 324:450, 1991.

Whitley RJ: Acyclovir: A decade later. N Engl J Med 327:782, 1992.

## Varicella-Zoster Virus Infection

*Etiology.* Varicella-zoster virus (VZV) is a member of the Herpesviridae family. It is an enveloped, icosahedral, double-stranded DNA virus that causes varicella as a primary infection or an endogenously reactivated recurrent infection (herpes zoster or shingles). The virus infects susceptible individuals by the conjunctivae or respiratory tract and replicates in the nasopharynx and upper respiratory tract. It then disseminates by a primary viremia and infects regional lymph nodes, the liver, the spleen, and other organs. A secondary viremia follows, resulting in a cutaneous infection with the typical vesicular rash. There is one antigenic type of varicella, and humans are the only host. The organism has been found in dorsal root ganglia cells in individuals with herpes zoster infection.

### Varicella (Chickenpox)

*Epidemiology.* Varicella is a highly contagious infection of childhood. The peak age of occurrence is 5–10 yr; 90% of children in temperate climates are infected by age 10. The secondary household attack rates in susceptible individuals is 90%. The peak seasonal infection rate is late winter and spring. Transmission is by direct contact, droplet, and air. The incubation period is generally 14–16 days, with a range of 11–20 days after contact. The period of communicability ranges from 2 days before to 7 days after the onset of the rash, when all lesions are crusted. Patients with zoster may initiate varicella in seronegative contacts.

### Clinical Manifestations

CHICKENPOX. Primary infection with VZV results in chickenpox. Prodromal symptoms (fever, malaise, anorexia) may precede the rash by 1 day. The characteristic rash appears initially as small red papules that rapidly progress to nonumbilicated, oval, "teardrop" vesicles on an erythematous base. The fluid progresses from clear to cloudy, and the vesicles ulcerate, crust, and heal. New crops appear for 3–4 days, usually beginning on the trunk and then the head, the face, and, less commonly, the extremities. In total, there may be 100–300 lesions, with all forms of lesions being present at the same time. Pruritus is almost universal. Lesions may be present on all mucous membranes. Lymphadenopathy may be generalized. The severity of the rash varies, as do systemic signs and fever, which generally abate after 3–4 days.

CONGENITAL VARICELLA. Varicella in the pregnant woman may result in fetal varicella infection, characterized by low birth weight, cortical atrophy, seizures, mental retardation, chorioretinitis, cataracts, microcephaly, intracranial calcifications, and diagnostic cicatricial scarring of the body or extremities.

In mothers with varicella (not shingles) occurring 5 days before or 2 days after delivery, a severe neonatal varicella syndrome develops that is thought to be due to the lack of transplacental antibody. These infants should be treated as soon as possible with zoster immune globulin (ZIG) to attempt to prevent or ameliorate their infection. Children who were exposed in utero to VZV may develop zoster early in life without ever exhibiting varicella.

*Complications.* Although VZV infection is generally a mild disease, complications are common. Varicella is a more severe disease for neonates, adults, and immunosuppressed individuals. HIV-infected children frequently have a prolonged course and may have recurrent episodes of varicella. Secondary infection of skin lesions by streptococci or staphylococci is the most common complication. Such infections may be mild or life-threatening (toxic shock, necrotizing fasciitis). Thrombocytopenia and hemorrhagic lesions or bleeding also may occur (purpura fulminans, varicella gangrenosa). Pneumonia is uncommon in healthy children but occurs in 15–20% of healthy adults and immunosuppressed patients. Myocarditis, pericarditis, orchitis, hepatitis, ulcerative gastritis, glomerulonephritis, and arthritis complicate VZV. Reye syndrome may be preceded by varicella and, therefore, aspirin should be avoided during varicella infection.

Neurologic complications include postinfectious encephalitis, cerebellar ataxia, nystagmus, and tremor. Guillain-Barré syndrome, transverse myelitis, cranial nerve palsies, optic neuritis, and hypothalamic syndrome have been associated with varicella.

In immunodeficient or immunosuppressed children, primary varicella can be a fatal disease as a result of visceral dissemination, encephalitis, and pneumonitis. In children with leukemia who have not received prophylaxis or therapy for varicella, the mortality rate approaches 10%.

*Diagnosis.* Vesicles contain polymorphonuclear leukocytes. Cytology and electron microscopy of vesicular fluid or scrapings may reveal intranuclear inclusions, giant cells, and virus particles. VZV is fastidious and difficult to culture. If the cytology is consistent with either HSV or VZV but is culture-negative, it may indicate VZV. Infection can be confirmed by detection of varicella specific antigen in vesicular fluid with immunofluorescence of monoclonal antibodies or by testing acute and convalescent antibody for VZV antibody.

*Treatment.* Symptomatic therapy of varicella includes nonaspirin antipyretics, cool baths, and careful hygiene. Intravenous acyclovir is effective in treating varicella in immunocompromised patients. Early therapy prevents severe complications, including pneumonia, encephalitis, and death. Oral acyclovir shortens the duration of illness in normal children; however, it is uncertain whether acyclovir's cost justifies its use in otherwise healthy children. ZIG is not effective therapy once the disease has been contracted.

Oral acyclovir must be given within 24 hr of the appearance of the first cutaneous lesion to have clinical benefit in healthy patients. In adolescents as well as adults, early administration of acyclovir may decrease the incidence of varicella pneumonia. In patients receiving corticosteroids or a chronic regimen of salicylates, its use in uncomplicated varicella is recommended. The dose of acyclovir for varicella-zoster infections is higher than for herpes simplex.

*Prevention.* A live attenuated varicella vaccine was licensed for use in 1995 (see Fig. 10–1). A single dose is recommended for use in healthy children ages 1–12 yr. It is effective but not as protective as the measles vaccine; household exposure to varicella within 5 yr of vaccination results in mild disease (>50 skin lesions) in about 20% of exposed children. The major adverse effects of the vaccine are local tenderness at the injection site and a sparse maculopapular rash occurring within 1 mo of immunization in approximately 5% of vacinees. Transmission of the vaccine virus from a healthy vaccinee is possible.

Passive immunity can be induced by use of ZIG, which is indicated within 96 hr of exposure for susceptible individuals at risk for severe illness. Candidates for ZIG include immunocompromised or immunosuppressed individuals, neonates of infected mothers who had onset of chickenpox within 5 days before delivery or 48 hr after delivery, premature infants younger than 28 wk or those born to mothers lacking a prior history of chickenpox, and possibly children older than 15 yr or adults with a close exposure to varicella. Administration of VZIG does not eliminate the possibility of disease in recipients and prolongs the incubation period to 28 days. Children should not return to school until all vesicles have crusted. The hospitalized child with varicella should be isolated in a room that will prevent the air-circulation system from transmitting the virus.

### Herpes Zoster (Shingles)

*Epidemiology.* Shingles is a recurrence of VZV in individuals previously infected. After the episode of chickenpox, VZV remains latent in nerve ganglion cells, but for unknown reasons (other than immunosuppression) a local recurrence occurs. Herpes zoster is unusual in children under 10 yr of age. Infants and young children with herpes zoster often have a history of early or presumed in utero varicella. Immunocompromised or immunosuppressed children have an increased incidence of herpes zoster.

*Clinical Manifestations.* The pre-eruption phase of shingles includes intense localized pain and tenderness along a dermatome, accompanied by malaise and fever. In several days, the eruption of papules, which quickly vesiculate, occurs in the dermatome or in two adjacent dermatomes. Groups of lesions occur for 1–7 days, then progress to crusts and healing. The typical areas involved are dorsal and lumbar, although cephalic and sacral lesions may develop. Lesions generally are unilateral and are accompanied by regional lymphadenopathy. In one third of patients, a few vesicles occur outside the primary dermatome.

Any branch of cranial nerve V may be involved, which also may cause corneal and intraoral lesions. Involvement of the cranial nerve VII may result in facial paralysis and ear canal vesicles (**Ramsay Hunt syndrome**). Ophthalmic zoster may be associated with ipsilateral cerebral angiitis and stroke. Immunocompromised patients may have unusually severe, painful herpes zoster that involves cutaneous and, rarely, visceral dissemination (to liver, lungs, and CNS). Skin lesions may be chronic and hemorrhagic. Postherpetic neuralgia and ocular complications are rare in normal children. Secondary bacterial infections may occur.

*Diagnosis.* The differentiation between VZV and HSV infections is difficult because HSV may cause infection in a dermatome distribution. The previously healthy patient with more than one recurrence probably has HSV infection, which can be confirmed by culture.

*Treatment.* VZV infection in immunocompromised patients is treated with acyclovir, either orally or parenterally depending on the severity of the infection. Acyclovir therapy decreases pain, shortens the duration of viral shedding, and decreases visceral dissemination.

*Prevention.* There is no clinically useful way to prevent herpes zoster. Patients with herpes zoster are infectious to VZV-susceptible individuals.

### References

American Academy of Pediatrics Committee on Infectious Diseases: Recommendations for the use of live attenuated varicella vaccine. Pediatrics 95:791, 1995.

Behrman RE, Kliegman RM, Arvin AM (eds): Nelson Textbook of Pediatrics, 15th ed. Philadelphia, WB Saunders, 1996, Chapter 213.

Brunell PA: Varicella in pregnancy, the fetus, and the newborn: Problems in management. J Infect Dis 166(Suppl 1):S42, 1992.

Dunkle LM, Arvin AM, Whitley RJ, et al: A controlled trial of acyclovir for chickenpox in normal children. N Engl J Med 32:1539, 1991.

Jackson MA, Burry VF, Olson LC: Complications of varicella requiring hospitalization in previously healthy children. Pediatr Infect Dis J 11:441, 1992.

Kelley R, Mancao M, Lee F, et al: Varicella in children with perinatally acquired human immunodeficiency virus infection. J Pediatr 124:271, 1994.

Peterson C, Mascola L, Chao S, et al: Children hospitalized for varicella: A prevaccine review. J Pediatr 129:529, 1996.

## HUMAN HERPESVIRUS-6
### (Exanthem Subitum, Roseola Infantum)

*Etiology.* HHV-6, a member of the herpesvirus family, is a large, enveloped double-stranded DNA virus. It is the infectious agent of roseola, also called exanthem subitum or sixth disease. This virus is ubiquitous and is likely to be transmitted by respiratory secretions. It infects mature T cells, B cells, astrocytes, and macrophages and causes a relatively prolonged (3–5 days) viremia during primary infection. HHV-6 can be detected in the saliva of healthy adults, which suggests that, as with other herpesviruses, there is latent infection and intermittent shedding of virus.

*Epidemiology.* Most children become seropositive for HHV-6 by 2 yr of age, and most primary infections occur in the first year of life after 6 mo of age. HHV-6 is a major cause of acute febrile illnesses in infants and in one study was responsible for 20% of the visits to the emergency department for infants 6–18 mo of age. There is a notable lack of history of exposure to other children with similar illnesses, which suggests that the virus is acquired from asymptomatic adults. HHV-7 has many similarities to HHV-6.

*Clinical Manifestations.* The most reliable characteristic of HHV-6 infection is high fever, often 40°C or more, with an abrupt onset and lasting 3–7 days. In roseola, a maculopapular rash erupts coincident with defervescence, although it may also be present earlier. Respiratory symptoms, nasal congestion, erythematous tympanic membranes, and cough may occur, and gastrointestinal symptoms are often described: most commonly, patients are irritable and appear toxic. CNS findings are common, with a bulging anterior fontanel often associated with roseola; seizures occur in some patients, suggesting that this virus may be responsible for many febrile seizures.

Laboratory findings include a relatively low white blood cell count, particularly reduced numbers of lymphocytes. Infection in immunocompromised hosts, transplant patients, or children infected with HIV can be disseminated and severe. Reactivation of HHV-6 may be a cause of bone marrow suppression following bone marrow transplantation.

*Differential Diagnosis.* The characteristic timing of the onset of rash immediately following defervescence of fever is not typical of other viral exanthems (rubella, rubeola, enteroviral infection). The differential diagnosis of the infant with high fever must include local infections (otitis media, pneumonia, pyelonephritis, meningitis) and nonlocalized bacteremia (especially pneumococcal). Assays for the diagnosis of primary HHV-6 infection are being developed. Serologic tests, including indirect immunofluorescent and enzyme immunosorbent assays, are available.

*Treatment.* Management of HHV-6 infections is primarily supportive, providing control of fever and symptomatic relief. For immunocompromised patients, ganciclovir and foscarnet, which have in vitro activity against the virus, have been tried, but there are no controlled clinical trials available.

### References

Asano Y, Yoshikawa T, Suga S, et al: Clinical features of infants with primary human herpes virus 6 infection (exanthem subitum, Roseola infantum). Pediatrics 93:104, 1994.

Behrman RE, Kliegman RM, Arvin AM (eds): Nelson Textbook of Pediatrics, 15th ed. Philadelphia, WB Saunders, 1996, Chapter 212.

Hall CB, Long CE, Schnabel KC, et al: Human herpesvirus-6 infection in children: Prospective evaluation for complications and reactivation. N Engl J Med 331:432, 1994.

Levy J: Three new human herpesviruses (HHV 6, 7, 8). Lancet 349:558, 1997.

## HUMAN IMMUNODEFICIENCY VIRUS INFECTION
### (Acquired Immunodeficiency Syndrome)

*Etiology.* The cause of AIDS in infants, children, and adults is HIV. HIV is one of several retroviruses that are RNA viruses possessing the enzyme reverse transcriptase that allows viral RNA to act as a template for DNA transcription and incorporation into the host genome.

*Pathogenesis.* HIV selectively infects human helper T cells via an interaction between the CD4 + and a chemokine surface receptor on the T cell and the viral protein gp120. Because helper T cells are important for delayed hypersensitivity, for T cell–dependent B cell antibody production, and for T cell–mediated lymphokine activation of macrophages, their destruction produces a profound combined (B and T cell) immunodeficiency. Lack of T-cell regulation and unrestrained antigenic stimulation results in a nonspecific and ineffective polyclonal hypergammaglobulinemia. Infection of macrophages disseminates the virus throughout the body. Infection of brain tissue accounts for the encephalopathy and cerebral atrophy associated with the condition.

HIV is a chronic, progressive process with a variable period of clinical latency. Although HIV may not always be culturable from the plasma or circulating mononuclear cells, sensitive assays for HIV nucleic acids demonstrate that virtually all patients have evidence of ongoing viral replication. As long as the host continues to replace the CD4 + cells destroyed by infection, there are no overt manifestations of immunodeficiency. When CD4 + cell numbers become progressively depleted, clinical immunodeficiency results. The ability to quantify the viral load has become important in management. Patients with more virus have a more rapid depletion of the CD4 + cells accompanied by the development of the typical opportunistic infections (*P. carinii* and *M. avium-intracellulare* complex).

*Epidemiology.* HIV is transmitted by contaminated blood and blood products, body secretions (semen, breast milk), infected organs, and, in the pregnant woman, vertically to the fetus. Thus, lifestyles (homosexual or heterosexual promiscuity, intravenous drug use, prostitution), conditions requiring multiple or frequent use of blood products (hemophilia, sick neonates), or birth to an infected mother leads to a high risk of HIV infection.

Perinatal transmission of HIV infection is associated with prematurity, rupture of membranes greater than 4 hr, and perhaps with the levels of circulating viral RNA at the time of delivery. Perinatal transmission can be decreased from approximately 25% to 8% with treatment of the mother with zidovudine during pregnancy and delivery and with treatment of the neonate for 6 wk.

In the pediatric population, the mode of acquisition depends on the age of the individual. The neonate and infant (<15 mo old) acquire HIV from vertical transmission as a result of birth to an infected mother (accounting for 80% of pediatric AIDS) or from receipt of infected blood products. As adolescents become sexually active and experiment with intravenous drugs, their modes of acquisition are similar to those of adults.

Currently, pediatric AIDS is predominantly an illness of blacks (58%) and Hispanics (23%) because of the risk factors of maternal drug addiction and heterosexual activity with high-risk males. In Africa, AIDS is transmitted by heterosexual activity and by transfusion of infected blood.

*Clinical Manifestations.* The incubation period may be as long as 7–10 yr, but it is 1–24 mo with a mean of 5 mo after vertical transmission, a much shorter period than seen in adults. The major clinical manifestations (and classifications) of AIDS are related to immunodeficiency, resulting in frequent and often unusual infections (Tables 10–18 and 10–19). In adults and adolescents, a prodromal period of weight loss, fever, malaise, lymphadenopathy, and diarrhea occurs.

PNEUMONIA. Pulmonary manifestations are common and include *P. carinii* pneumonia (PCP), which may present early in infancy as a severe primary infection with tachypnea, retractions, hypoxemia, elevated serum LDH, and fever. All neonates at risk for vertical transmission of HIV should receive PCP prophylaxis routinely until their HIV status is clarified. In older patients, the development of PCP infection may be related to a decrease in CD4 + cells and prophylaxis is begun when the total CD4 + count falls below 500. More than 50% of the reported cases of PCP occur in infants 3–6 mo of age; PCP accounts for 60% of the AIDS-defining illnesses occurring in the 1st year of life.

PNEUMONITIS. Another common cause of pulmonary disease is **lymphoid interstitial pneumonitis** (LIP), which has a more insidious onset, with cough and tachypnea. These infants have lymphoid hyperplasia, hepatosplenomegaly, and sali-

TABLE 10–18.  CDC Classification for Children (Below 13 Years of Age) with Human Immunodeficiency Virus (HIV) Infection

| Clinical Categories | Diagnostic Criteria |
| --- | --- |
| **N: Not Symptomatic:**<br><br>No signs or symptoms of HIV infection or only one of the conditions listed in Category A | If < 18 months of age has two positive results on separate determinations from one or more of the following:<br>(a) HIV culture,<br>(b) HIV PCR or<br>(c) HIV p24 antigen<br><br>If ≥ 18 months is HIV antibody positive by repeatedly reactive ELISA and confirmatory test (e.g., Western blot or IFA) |
| **A: Mildly Symptomatic:**<br><br>Two or more of the conditions listed, but none of the conditions listed in Categories B or C | Lymphadenopathy (≥0.5 cm at more than two sites; bilateral = one site)<br>Hepatomegaly<br>Splenomegaly<br>Dermatitis<br>Parotitis<br>Recurrent or persistent upper respiratory infection, sinusitis, or OM |
| **B: Moderately Symptomatic:**<br><br>Symptoms of HIV infection other than those listed for Categories A or C. Examples include but are not limited to those listed. | Anemia (<8), neutropenia (<1,000), or thrombocytopenia (<100,000) persisting ≥30 days<br>Bacterial meningitis, pneumonia or sepsis (single episode)<br>Candidiasis, oropharyngeal thrush, persisting >2 mo in children > 6 mo old<br>Cardiomyopathy<br>CMV infection, onset before 1 mo of age<br>Diarrhea, recurrent or chronic<br>Hepatitis<br>HSV stomatitis, recurrent (more than 2 episodes within 1 year)<br>HSV bronchitis, pneumonitis or esophagitis with onset before 1 mo of age<br>Herpes zoster (shingles)—two episodes or more than one dermatome<br>Leiomyosarcoma<br>LIP or pulmonary lymphoid hyperplasia (AIDS defining, report to State)<br>Nephropathy<br>Nocardiosis<br>Persistent fever (lasting > 1 mo)<br>Toxoplasmosis, onset before 1 mo of age<br>Varicella, disseminated (complicated chickenpox) |

*Table continued on following page*

vary gland enlargement. Chest radiographs demonstrate bilateral reticulonodular and interstitial infiltrates. Rales may not be prominent; patients are not as hypoxic as those with PCP infection. A definitive diagnosis requires a lung biopsy that demonstrates CD8+ T cells, immunoblasts, and plasma cells. Some of these patients appear to have evidence of EBV infection as a cofactor. Treatment is primarily supportive, although some patients respond well to corticosteroids.

*ACUTE RETROVIRAL SYNDROME.* Patients acutely infected with HIV may present with an illness characterized by fever, sore throat, fatigue, lymphadenopathy, weight loss, and a macular erythematous rash. The "acute retroviral syndrome" coincides with the appearance of anti-HIV antibodies 2–6 wk following an acute infection.

*Diagnosis.* An infant younger than 18 mo of age is considered to be HIV-infected if born to an HIV-infected mother and has two separate direct HIV tests that are positive. Alternatively, an infant is also considered to be HIV-infected when meeting the CDC case definition for AIDS, based on clinical symptoms and immunologic findings. HIV tests include viral culture, PCR detection of HIV-specific DNA or RNA, tests that can quantify the relative viral RNA load, tests for p24 antigen, the HIV major capsid protein, or identification of antibody to HIV proteins by Western hybridization. Detection of HIV infection in the neonate requires the direct evidence of viral infection, as antibody can be passively acquired from the mother.

AIDS-defining illnesses in children are similar to those in adults but also include lymphoid interstitial pneumonia and lymphoid hyperplasia as well as recurrent bacterial infections. For children older than 13 yr of age, the expanded CDC case definition for adolescents and adults can be applied.

The *differential diagnosis* includes primary immu-

TABLE 10–18.   CDC Classification for Children (Below 13 Years of Age) with Human Immunodeficiency Virus (HIV) Infection *Continued*

| Clinical Categories | Diagnostic Criteria |
|---|---|
| **C. Severely Symptomatic:**<br><br>Any condition listed in the 1987 surveillance case definition for AIDS with the exception of LIP | Serious bacterial infection; 2 in 2 yr: sepsis, pneumonia, meningitis, bone or joint infection, abscess of organ or body cavity (excludes OM, skin or mucosal abscesses and indwelling catheter infections)<br>Candidiasis (esophageal, tracheal, bronchial, pulmonary)<br>Coccidioidomycosis, disseminated or extrapulmonary<br>Cryptococcosis, extrapulmonary<br>Cryptosporidiosis or isosporiasis >1 mo duration<br>CMV disease (onset > 1 mo), other than liver, spleen or lymph nodes<br>Encephalopathy: (>1 finding for >2 mo and no illness that explains:<br>  (a) failure to attain or loss of milestones or intellectual ability shown by neuropsychological tests;<br>  (b) impaired brain growth or acquired microcephaly shown by OFC measurements or brain atrophy on CT scan or MRI (serial imaging needed if <2 years old);<br>  (c) acquired symmetric motor deficit with ≥2 of: paresis, pathologic reflexes, ataxia or gait disturbances<br>Herpes simplex (ulcer > 1 mo duration or pneumonia or esophagitis > 1 mo old)<br>Histoplasmosis, disseminated or extrapulmonary<br>Kaposi sarcoma<br>Lymphoma, primary, in brain<br>Lymphoma, B cell, non-Hodgkin lymphoma<br>*Mycobacterium tuberculosis*, disseminated or extrapulmonary<br>*Mycobacterium* infection, noncutaneous, extrapulmonary or disseminated (except leprosy)<br>*Pneumocystis carinii* pneumonia<br>Progressive multifocal leukoencephalopathy<br>*Salmonella* (nontyphoid) sepsis, recurrent<br>Toxoplasmosis of the brain, onset > 1 mo old<br>Wasting syndrome—in absence of other illness that explains:<br>  (a) weight loss >10% of baseline<br>        *or*<br>  (b) downward crossing of ≥ two percentile lines on the weight chart in a child ≥1 yr<br>        *or*<br>  (c) <5th% on weight for height on 2 consecutive measures ≥ 30 days apart<br>        *plus*<br>    (1) chronic diarrhea (≥2 loose stools/day for ≥ 30 days)<br>        *or*<br>    (2) documented fever for ≥30 days, intermittent or constant |

Modified from Centers for Disease Control and Prevention: MMWR 43(RR-12):1–19, 1994.
AIDS = acquired immunodeficiency virus; CMV = cytomegalovirus; CT = computed tomography; HSV = herpes simplex virus; LIP = lymphoid interstitial pneumonia; MRI = magnetic resonance imaging; OFC = occipitofrontal circumference; OM = otitis media; PCR = polymerase chain reaction.

nodeficiency syndromes (usually found in HIV-negative children whose parents have no risk factors for HIV infection) and intrauterine infection caused by other agents.

**Treatment.** Three classes of drugs are available for the treatment of HIV infection. Zidovudine (AZT) has been shown to be effective in decreasing the transmission of HIV from the infected pregnant woman to the neonate when it is given in the perinatal period. Additional nucleoside analogs used in children include didanosine (dideoxyinosine), zalcitabine (dideoxycytidine), stavudine (D4T), and lamivudine (3TC). Non-nucleoside inhibitors of reverse transcriptase (Viramune [nevirapine]) are undergoing therapeutic trials, as are inhibitors of the HIV protease, an enzyme required to cleave the gag-pol precursor protein of HIV, which contains important structural and enzymatic elements required for viral maturation. Three protease inhibitors are currently in use: saquinavir, ritonavir, and indinivir; all have significant side effects but are important in multidrug therapy (Table 10–16).

The ability of HIV to rapidly become resistant

TABLE 10–19. CDC Classification for Children (Below 13 Years of Age) with Human Immunodeficiency Virus (HIV) Infection

**Immunologic Categories Based on Age-Specific CD4+ T-Lymphocyte Counts and Percent of Total Lymphocytes**

| | Age of Child | | | | | |
| | <12 mo | | 1–5 yr | | 6–12 yr | |
| Immunologic Category | μL | % | μL | % | μL | % |
| --- | --- | --- | --- | --- | --- | --- |
| 1. No suppression | ≥1500 | ≥25 | ≥1000 | ≥25 | ≥500 | ≥25 |
| 2. Moderate suppression | 750–1499 | 15–24 | 500–999 | 15–24 | 200–499 | 15–24 |
| 3. Severe suppression | <750 | <15 | <500 | <15 | <200 | <15 |

**Pediatric HIV Classification Based on Degree of Immune Suppression and Clinical Category***

| | Clinical Categories | | | |
| Immunologic Category | N: No Signs/Symptoms | A: Mild Signs/Symptoms | B: Moderate Signs/Symptoms† | C: Severe Signs/Symptoms† |
| --- | --- | --- | --- | --- |
| 1. No suppression | N1 | A1 | B1 | C1 |
| 2. Moderate suppression | N2 | A2 | B2 | C2 |
| 3. Severe suppression | N3 | A3 | B3 | C3 |

From Centers for Disease Control and Prevention: MMWR 43(RR-12):1–19, 1994.

*Children whose HIV infection status is not confirmed are classified by placing the letter E (for perinatally exposed) before the classification code (e.g., EN1).

†Both Category C and lymphoid interstitial pneumonitis in Category B are reportable to state health departments as acquired immunodeficiency virus (AIDS).

to anti-retroviral agents and the development of cross-resistance to several classes of agents at once are also major problems. Therapeutic regimens involve at least two of the above drugs in combination. Viral loads can be significantly reduced when such combination therapy is used with the amelioration of clinical symptoms and opportunistic infection.

The approach to the numerous opportunistic infections in HIV-infected patients involves both prophylaxis and treatment for infections likely to occur as CD4+ cells are depleted. Infection caused by *P. carinii* can be prevented with trimethoprim/sulfamethoxazole and *M. avium-intracellulare* infection can be prevented with prophylactic rifabutin in patients with CD4+ cell counts less than 200. Pneumococcal sepsis is common, and some patients may benefit from IVIG, as normal B-cell function is often impaired. Oral and gastrointestinal candidiasis is common and often responds to imidazole therapy. Varicella-zoster infection may be severe and should be treated with acyclovir. Recurrent herpes simplex infections may also require acyclovir prophylaxis. Other common infections in HIV-infected patients are toxoplasmosis, CMV, EBV, salmonellosis, and tuberculosis.

Opportunistic infections should be treated aggressively, as with any infection in an immunodeficient host. Treatment of PCP is possible with

high-dose trimethoprim/sulfamethoxazole and steroids. Although routine immunizations may result in suboptimal antibody concentrations, they remain indicated except for the use of most live vaccines in symptomatically infected children. Because of the risk of fatal measles in children with AIDS, live measles vaccine is indicated in presymptomatic, HIV-seropositive patients. Children exposed to varicella or measles should receive ZIG or serum immune globulin, respectively. Household contacts of children with AIDS should receive inactivated, not live, poliovirus vaccine.

**Prevention.** Preventing AIDS or HIV infection in adults will decrease the incidence of infection in children. Adult prevention may result from behavior changes ("safe sex," decrease in intravenous drug use, needle exchange), abortion, or avoidance of pregnancy and breast-feeding (in developed countries) in high-risk women. Screening of blood donors already has markedly reduced the risk of transmission from blood products, including those used to treat hemophilia. HIV infection almost never is transmitted in a casual or nonsexual household setting.

References

Balotta C, Colombo C, Colucci G, et al: Plasma viremia and virus phenotype are correlates of disease progression in vertical human immunodeficiency virus type 1 infected children. Pediatr Infect Dis J 16:205, 1997.

Behrman RE, Kliegman RM, Arvin AM (eds): Nelson Textbook of Pediatrics, 15th ed. Philadelphia, WB Saunders, 1996, Chapter 223.

Carpenter CJ, Fischl MA, Hammer SM, et al: Antiretroviral therapy for HIV infection in 1996: A consensus statement. JAMA 276:146, 1996.

Centers for Disease Control and Prevention: 1995 Revised guidelines for prophylaxis against *Pneumocystis carinii* pneumonia for children infected with or perinatally exposed to human immunodeficiency virus. MMWR 44(RR4):1, 1995.

Centers for Disease Control and Prevention: 1994 Revised classification for human immunodeficiency virus infection in children less than 13 years of age. MMWR 43(RR-12):1, 1994.

Forsyth B, Andiman W, O'Connor T: Development of a prognosis based clinical staging system for infants infected with human immunodeficiency virus. J Pediatr 129:648, 1996.

Sperling R, Shapiro D, Coombs R, et al: Maternal viral load, zidovudine treatment, and the risk of transmission of human immunodeficiency virus type 1 from mother to infant. N Engl J Med 335:1621, 1996.

Wilfert CM, Wilson C, Luzuriaga K, Epstein L: Pathogenesis of pediatric human immunodeficiency virus type 1 infection. J Infect Dis 170:286, 1994.

## INFLUENZA VIRAL INFECTION

**Etiology.** Influenza viruses are RNA orthomyxoviruses with a segmented genome. The viruses infect animals, particularly birds and swine, as well as humans, facilitating genetic reassortments among the viruses infecting different species.

There are three major types: A, B, and C. A and B account for major epidemics and consist of (1) a negatively stranded RNA, which encodes 10 proteins including the hemagglutin (HA), which mediates viral binding to epithelial cells, and (2) neuraminidase (N), an enzyme that allows for viral release from the cell surface. Major changes in HA account for *antigenic drift*, responsible for epidemics of disease occurring in a susceptible population. Minor variations in HA (*antigenic shift*) occur more frequently. These antigenic variants cause cycles of disease and allow for the classification of viruses as A/Hong Kong/68 (H3N2), for example, which is distinct from the H1N1 viruses. Specific antibodies to different viruses are important determinants of immunity.

**Epidemiology.** Influenza occurs seasonally in temperate climates, with annual epidemics of influenza A in the winter months. Influenza B causes outbreaks every 3–4 yr; often both influenza A and B are found concurrently. Antigenic shift is responsible for major pandemics of influenza, which occur every 10–40 yr, with antigenic drifts occurring more frequently every 2–3 yr. The virus is shed in infected respiratory secretions and is transmitted from person to person or by articles contaminated with nasopharyngeal secretions. The period of communicability begins 24 hr before symptoms develop and continues until resolution. The incubation period is from 1–3 days.

**Pathogenesis.** During the incubation period, virus is present in the respiratory tract but rarely in blood and other organs. Virus binds to respiratory epithelial cells, replicates, and causes cell death, desquamation, and decreased mucociliary clearance of bacteria. Immunity correlates better with secretory antibody than with serum antibody, although the latter is associated with protection.

### Clinical Manifestations

OLDER CHILDREN AND ADOLESCENTS. In this group, the manifestations are similar to those seen in adults. There is an abrupt onset of high fever, flushed face, headache, myalgia, cough, and chills. Pharyngitis occurs in 50% of patients, and ocular symptoms (tearing, photophobia, burning, pain on eye motion) and nasal stuffiness are common. These symptoms last 2–5 days. As the systemic signs and symptoms resolve, the cough and nasal congestion become more prominent and last 4–10 days. Leukopenia occurs in 25% of patients, and 10% have clinical and roentgenographic evidence of bronchopneumonia.

YOUNGER CHILDREN. The classic influenza illness is less common in younger children, who manifest laryngotracheitis, bronchiolitis, bronchitis, pneumonia, and/or a mild upper respiratory tract syndrome. Influenza B has been associated with myositis. Parotitis has been reported in influenza A infection. Fever tends to be higher in younger children than in older children. In neonates, the sudden fever and nonspecific signs simulate sepsis, although a nasal discharge may suggest the diagnosis of a viral respiratory tract infection. Influenza C infection has been associated with an upper respiratory tract syndrome.

**Complications.** The most important complication is secondary bacterial infection of the respiratory tract, including otitis media, sinusitis, and pneumonia. These complications should be treated with antibiotics effective against *Haemophilus*, pneumococci, and staphylococci. Virus-related complications include pneumonia, rarely neurologic syndromes, myocarditis, myositis with myoglobinuria, and Reye syndrome. Salicylates should be avoided in children and adolescents with influenza.

**Diagnosis.** In communitywide outbreaks of winter respiratory tract disease involving all age groups, influenza is the most likely agent. Virus may be isolated in 2–6 days from nasopharyngeal secretions in tissue culture. Rapid diagnosis may be made by immunofluorescent techniques or ELISA.

Serologic responses are helpful for retrospective diagnosis.

*Treatment.* Amantadine is useful for prophylaxis and, perhaps, very early in the treatment of influenza A. Ribavirin also has activity against influenza A and B but is rarely used in a clinical setting. Antibiotics should be avoided unless a bacterial superinfection is suspected. Non–aspirin-containing antipyretics increase the patient's comfort and do not carry the risk of the development of Reye syndrome.

*Prevention.* Inactivated vaccine, given on a yearly basis, is indicated for children at risk for complications and, probably, for other children and adults who live in a household with high-risk children. The latter include children with cardiovascular, pulmonary (cystic fibrosis, bronchopulmonary dysplasia), metabolic, renal, or neurologic disorders and those who are immunosuppressed or have a hemoglobinopathy, including sickle cell disease.

*Amantadine* is effective as prophylaxis against influenza A and should be used in unimmunized high-risk children during an outbreak.

### References

Behrman RE, Kliegman RM, Arvin AM (eds): Nelson Textbook of Pediatrics, 15th ed. Philadelphia, WB Saunders, 1996, Chapter 216.

Douglas RG Jr: Prophylaxis and treatment of influenza. N Engl J Med 322:443, 1990.

Groothuis JR, Levin MJ, Rabalais GP, et al: Immunization of high-risk infants younger than 18 months of age with split-product influenza vaccine. Pediatrics 87:823, 1991.

Troendle JF, Demmler GJ, Glezen WP, et al: Fatal influenza B virus pneumonia in pediatric patients. Pediatr Infect Dis J 11:117, 1992.

## MEASLES
### (Rubeola)

*Etiology.* Measles virus is an RNA paramyxovirus with one antigenic type. It is stable at room temperature for 1–2 days and can be cultivated in human or monkey cells, with cytopathic changes visible in 5–10 days.

*Epidemiology.* Measles is highly contagious, particularly by droplets during the prodromal (catarrhal) stage. The infected individual is contagious from 1–2 days prior to the development of the characteristic rash. There are very few subclinical cases. Most neonates and young children are protected from measles by transplacental antibody but become susceptible toward the end of the first year of life. Passive immunity may interfere with effective vaccination until 12–15 mo of age.

The incubation period is 8–12 days from exposure to the onset of symptoms and 14 days from exposure to the onset of rash. In areas where measles vaccination is not available, measles is endemic and responsible for about 1 million deaths per year. Since the widespread use of the measles vaccine, the number of cases has declined dramatically. Recent outbreaks have occurred as a result of decreased rates of immunization in susceptible infants and toddlers in crowded urban areas. Outbreaks of measles in adolescents, particularly on college campuses, have also been reported, and have been found to be due to primary vaccine failure. This leads to the institution of a second dose of measles vaccine for American children at age 12 (middle school).

*Pathogenesis.* Viral particles infect the respiratory tract and spread to regional lymph nodes. A primary viremia disseminates the virus. After viral replication, a secondary viremia occurs 5–7 days after the initial infection as virally infected monocytes and other leukocytes spread the virus to the respiratory tract, skin, and other organs. These infected sites are manifested by rash and the classic symptoms of cough, conjunctivitis, and coryza. Histologic evidence includes the presence of multinucleated giant cells and syncytium formation. The virus is found in the respiratory secretions, blood, and urine of infected individuals.

*Clinical Manifestations.* The manifestations of the 3-day prodromal period include cough, coryza, conjunctivitis, and the pathognomonic Koplik spots (gray-white, sand grain–sized dots on the buccal mucosa opposite the lower molars) that last 12–24 hr. The conjunctiva may reveal a characteristic transverse line of inflammation along the eyelid margin (Stimson line). The rash phase often is accompanied by high fever (40.0–40.5°C [104–105°F]). The macular rash begins on the head (often above the hairline) and spreads over most of the body in 24 hr in a descending fashion. It fades in the same manner. The severity of the illness is related to the extent of the rash. It may be petechial or hemorrhagic (**black measles**). As the rash fades, it undergoes desquamation and brownish discoloration.

Cervical lymphadenitis, splenomegaly, and mesenteric lymphadenopathy (with abdominal pain) may be noted. Otitis media, pneumonia, and gastrointestinal tract symptoms are more common in infants. Liver involvement is more common in adults. Leukopenia is characteristic. In patients with acute encephalitis, the CSF reveals an increased protein, a lymphocytic pleocytosis, and normal glucose levels.

*Complications.* Measles often is complicated by otitis media. Interstitial pneumonia may be caused by measles or, more commonly, may be due to a secondary bacterial infection. The anergy associated with measles may activate latent tuberculosis. Myocarditis and mesenteric adenitis are infrequent complications. Encephalomyelitis occurs in 1–2:1000 cases and usually occurs 2–5 days after the onset of the rash. Early encephalitis probably is due to viral activity in the brain, whereas later onset encephalitis is a demyelinating and probably an immunopathologic phenomenon. **Subacute sclerosing panencephalitis** is a late complication of slow measles infection, occurring years after the acute illness.

*Diagnosis.* The clinical presentation is characteristic. Confirmation includes (1) multinucleated giant cells in nasal mucosal smears, (2) virus isolation in culture, and (3) diagnostic antibody rises in convalescent serum.

The rash must be differentiated from exanthem subitum, rubella, enteroviral or adenoviral infection, infectious mononucleosis, toxoplasmosis, meningococcemia, scarlet fever, rickettsial disease, Kawasaki syndrome, serum sickness, and drug rash. The constellation of fever, rash, cough, and conjunctivitis is fairly diagnostic for measles. Measles modified by transplacental or administered antibody may be less characteristic. Koplik spots usually are pathognomonic but are not always present at the time of the most pronounced rash.

*Treatment.* Therapy is supportive. Photophobia is intensified by strong light, which should be avoided. Immunoglobulin and steroids are of no proven value in established disease. Vitamin A improves outcome in infected malnourished infants (100,000 U, IV, × 1 for children 6 mo–1 yr; 200,000 U, IV, × 1 for children older than 1 yr). Vitamin A supplementation should be considered for populations at risk for severe complications, such as (1) infants aged 6 mo–2 yr requiring hospitalization, (2) HIV-infected infants, or (3) infants from endemic areas. Intravenous ribavirin also may be of benefit in severe infections.

*Prevention*

ACTIVE IMMUNIZATION. Live measles vaccine prevents infection and should be administered to children at 12–15 mo and at 4–5 or 11–12 yr of age (see Fig. 10–1). The effects of vaccination are obstructed by transplacental antibody or passive immunization with immunoglobulin (~12 mo in the former case, 3 mo in the latter). A skin test for tuberculosis prior to or concomitant with vaccination is advised because vaccination may induce a state of anergy for 1 mo. The live vaccine is contraindicated in pregnant women, immunodeficient or immunosuppressed children (see Human Immunodeficiency Virus Infection) during a febrile illness, or if immu-

noglobulin has been administered within 3 mo. If inadvertently vaccinated, immunocompromised patients should receive immunoglobulin. Vaccination shortly after exposure to measles may prevent illness.

PASSIVE IMMUNIZATION. Immune serum globulin may prevent or ameliorate measles if given within 5 days of exposure. Protection is indicated for chronically ill, immunosuppressed, or immunodeficient children. The usual dose is 0.25 mL/kg or 0.5 mL/kg for immunocompromised children (maximum, 15 mL).

## References

Behrman RE, Kliegman RM, Arvin AM (eds): Nelson Textbook of Pediatrics, 15th ed. Philadelphia, WB Saunders, 1996, Chapter 206.

Committee on Infectious Diseases, American Academy of Pediatrics: Vitamin A treatment of measles. Pediatrics 91:1014, 1994.

Gindler JS, Atkinson WL, Markowitz LE, et al: Epidemiology of measles in the United States in 1989 and 1990. Pediatr Infect Dis J 11:841, 1992.

Kaplan LJ, Daum RS, Smaron M, et al: Severe measles in immunocompromised patients. JAMA 267:1237, 1992.

## MUMPS

*Etiology.* Mumps is an enveloped, negative-stranded RNA virus of the paramyxovirus family. Humans are the only known host.

*Epidemiology.* Mumps occurs worldwide and spreads by direct contact, aerosolization of respiratory secretions, and fomites. Epidemics are most frequent in late winter and spring. The incidence of natural infection in developed countries has decreased as a result of immunization.

Although the virus may be isolated from saliva 6 days before and 9 days after the onset of parotid swelling, the illness can be transmitted 1 day before until 3 days after swelling. Transplacental antibody protects infants from infection in the first 6 mo of life. Infection is associated with lifelong immunity. The incubation period is usually 16–18 days but may range from 12–25 days after exposure.

*Pathogenesis.* The virus is acquired through infected respiratory secretions, replicates in the upper respiratory tract and regional lymphatics, and is spread systemically by a primary viremia. It has tropism for the salivary glands, where it causes lymphocytic infiltration and edema. CNS infection also occurs with spread along neuronal pathways.

*Clinical Manifestations.* Thirty percent to 40% of the cases of infection are subclinical, but when symptoms occur, the onset is characterized by fever, muscle pain, headache, malaise, and pain and swelling in the parotid glands lasting 3–7 days. The swelling obscures the angle of the mandible and pushes the earlobe upward and outward. Pain is elicited by palpation of the gland and also by agents, such as citrus juice, that stimulate salivary flow. Swelling and erythema also surround the Stensen duct. Swelling also may be present in the pharynx and larynx and over the manubrium and upper chest (probably as a result of lymphatic obstruction). Swelling of the submandibular glands may accompany parotid swelling, and in 10–15% of cases they may be the only glands involved. The sublingual glands are involved less commonly.

MENINGOENCEPHALOMYELITIS. Sixty-five percent of patients with parotitis have CSF pleocytosis, and more than 10% have clinical manifestations of meningoencephalitis. In the preimmunization era, mumps was one of the most common causes of aseptic meningitis. Early-onset meningitis probably is due to direct viral infection of the brain, whereas meningoencephalitis that occurs 10 days or more after the onset of illness is a postinfectious, demyelinating syndrome.

ORCHITIS, EPIDIDYMITIS. These complications occur in 15–35% of adolescents and adults and rarely occur before puberty. They become manifest at the end of the 1st wk of illness. Bilateral illness occurs in 3% of affected patients. The testes are red, swollen, and tender. Atrophy is common as a sequela but infertility is rare.

PANCREATITIS. Mild pancreatitis is common and may become manifest as epigastric pain, tenderness, and vomiting. An elevated serum amylase value usually is present in mumps, with or without clinical pancreatitis. It may indicate pancreatic or salivary gland involvement.

RARE COMPLICATIONS. Examples of rare complications include nephritis (viruria is common but nephritis is rare), thyroiditis, myocarditis, mastitis, deafness, ocular complications, arthritis, and thrombocytopenia. No firm evidence for a fetal mumps syndrome has been discovered.

**Diagnosis.** The diagnosis is made clinically. Elevated serum amylase is typical and its onset parallels parotid swelling. Specific diagnosis can be confirmed by isolation of the virus from saliva, urine, CSF, or blood by routine viral culture. A rise in serum antibody to mumps also is diagnostic.

**Parotitis** also may be caused by other viruses, such as enterovirus, lymphocytic choriomeningitis virus, and influenza A virus. CMV may cause parotitis in immunocompromised children, and infants with AIDS may present with parotitis. The diagnosis of suppurative parotitis, which usually is due to *S. aureus,* can be confirmed by expression of purulent material containing bacteria through

the Stensen duct. Other causes of swelling in the parotid area include salivary calculus, recurrent parotitis (etiology unknown), salivary gland tumors, lymphomas, and cervical adenitis, which may mimic parotitis.

**Treatment.** No therapy is available except for supportive care.

**Prevention.** Live attenuated mumps vaccine has markedly diminished the incidence of mumps and should be administered to children 15 mo of age as part of their measles, mumps, and rubella (MMR) vaccine (Fig. 10–1). Parotitis and meningoencephalitis are rare complications of the highly protective mumps vaccination.

### References

Behrman RE, Kliegman RM, Arvin AM (eds): Nelson Textbook of Pediatrics, 15th ed. Philadelphia, WB Saunders, 1996, Chapter 208.

Briss PA, Fehrs LJ, Parker RA, et al: Sustained transmission of mumps in a highly vaccinated population: Assessment of primary vaccine failure and waning vaccine-induced immunity. J Infect Dis 169:77, 1994.

McDonald JC, Moore DL, Quennec P: Clinical and epidemiologic features of mumps meningoencephalitis and possible vaccine-related disease. Pediatr Infect Dis J 8:751, 1989.

## PARAINFLUENZA VIRAL INFECTION

**Etiology.** Parainfluenza viruses are RNA viruses of the paramyxovirus family. Four major serotypes (1–4) have been identified, although there is antigenic cross-reactivity among these. Types 1–3 occur in seasonal outbreak settings, whereas type 4 is usually endemic.

**Epidemiology.** By age 3 yr, most children have been symptomatically infected with parainfluenza types 1–3. Type 4 infection also is common but usually asymptomatic. Symptomatic reinfection is common. Infection occurs worldwide, with epidemics occurring in the fall and endemic activity occurring throughout the year. Transmission is from person to person by direct contact, aerosolization of respiratory secretions, and articles contaminated by respiratory tract secretions. The period of contagiousness generally is 4–9 days but may last for up to 2–3 wk. The incubation period is 2–4 days. Infection does not provide complete immunity, but reinfections are usually mild.

**Clinical Manifestations.** The major manifestations include laryngotracheitis (croup), bronchitis, bronchiolitis, and, less commonly, pneumonia, particularly in immunodeficient children. Illness lasts approximately 5 days. Less common manifestations include parotitis, Guillain-Barré syndrome, aseptic meningitis, and Reye syndrome. Secondary bacterial infections, including otitis media, tracheitis, and pneumonia, may occur. In the immunocompromised host, progressive pneumonia may occur.

*Diagnosis.* Tissue culture may be used to provide specific diagnosis within 1 wk. Serologic diagnosis is possible, but results may be confused by cross-reactivity with other paramyxoviruses. Rapid identification of viral RNA by PCR or viral antigen in nasopharyngeal secretions through immunofluorescent techniques or ELISA may be used to establish the diagnosis. Differential diagnosis includes infection caused by other respiratory viruses (influenza virus, RSV, adenovirus, rhinovirus) and mycoplasma. In addition, bacterial infection (acute epiglottitis), aspirated foreign bodies, and angioneurotic edema must be differentiated from viral laryngotracheobronchitis.

*Treatment.* No specific antiviral therapy is available for parainfluenza infection. Secondary bacterial infections must be treated.

*Prevention.* No chemotherapeutic or vaccine modalities are available for prevention.

### References

Behrman RE, Kliegman RM, Arvin AM (eds): Nelson Textbook of Pediatrics, 15th ed. Philadelphia, WB Saunders, 1996, Chapter 217.
Knott AM, Long CE, Hall CB: Parainfluenza viral infections in pediatric outpatients: Seasonal patterns and clinical characteristics. Pedatr Infect Dis J 13:269, 1994.

## RESPIRATORY SYNCYTIAL VIRUS INFECTION

*Etiology.* RSV is a single-stranded RNA virus of the paramyxovirus family. Among its products are surface proteins F and G, the major antigenic determinants. The heavily glycosylated G protein binds to the cellular receptor. Antibody to the F (fusion) protein neutralizes infectivity. RSV can be divided into A and B subgroups that are antigenically distinct, and both can be present concurrently in a population. Humans are the only source of infection.

*Epidemiology.* Worldwide outbreaks of respiratory illness caused by RSV occur among infants each winter or early spring. These outbreaks lead to predictable, yearly increases in infant hospitalization for bronchiolitis and pneumonia. The partially protective effect of transplacental antibody probably accounts for the relative lack of severe infection before 4–6 wk of life. Infection is universal by age 2 yr. Reinfections are common and tend to be mild. RSV is responsible for 55–85% of cases of bronchiolitis, 15–25% of cases of childhood pneumonia, and 6–8% of cases of croup. Illness generally is introduced into families by an older sibling, parents with "colds," and infants exhibiting the more severe syndromes. Nosocomial infection is extremely common among infants during RSV epidemics. The virus is spread by large droplets delivered, either airborne or via the hands, to nose or eyes. The period of viral shedding is 3–8 days but may last for up to 4 wk in young infants and longer in immunocompromised patients. The incubation period is 5–8 days.

*Pathogenesis.* RSV infects the respiratory epithelial cell and causes syncytium formation. The disease is involves the small airways with obstruction from edema, mucus secretion, and inflammatory cells. This leads to distal atelectasis and hyperexpansion of the lung. The pathology can be attributed not only to viral destruction of the epithelium but also to the local immune response.

*Clinical Manifestations.* RSV causes acute respiratory tract disease in all ages, but in infants and young children it is the most important cause of bronchiolitis and pneumonia (see Chapter 12). The initial manifestations of RSV infection include rhinorrhea, pharyngitis, cough, tachypnea, and low-grade fever. If the illness progresses, the cough worsens, wheezing ensues, and signs of respiratory distress appear. Chest roentgenograms usually reveal hyperexpansion and, at times, pneumonitis. In young infants, pneumonia may occur alone or concomitantly with bronchiolitis, a combination that often is associated with a paroxysmal cough resembling that of pertussis. In the very young infant, the premature infant, or the child with underlying respiratory or cardiac illness, only apnea and periodic breathing may occur. Long-term abnormalities in pulmonary function and subsequent wheezing that accompany respiratory infections have been reported in children with RSV bronchiolitis or pneumonia. RSV infection is very severe and life-threatening in patients with pulmonary hypertension (congenital heart disease, bronchopulmonary dysplasia), immunosuppression, or immunodeficiency.

*Diagnosis.* The season of the year, the occurrence of community outbreaks, and the presence of a sibling with an upper respiratory tract infection should alert the physician to the likelihood of RSV infection in an infant with bronchiolitis or pneumonia. Routine laboratory tests are of little use in specific diagnosis. Tests of blood gases often reveal a higher level of hypoxemia than expected, and as the infant's condition worsens, hypercapnia ensues. Specific diagnosis can be made by virus isolation from nasopharyngeal secretions (2–5 days) or tests for rapid detection of RSV antigen or RSV RNA by PCR.

The differential diagnosis of RSV pneumonia in young infants must include infection caused by *Chlamydia*, which often is accompanied by conjunctivitis and eosinophilia; infection caused by pertussis, which usually occurs in an unimmunized child with lymphocytosis; or infection caused by other viral or bacterial agents.

*Treatment.* Symptomatic therapy is usually all that is necessary for most children with RSV infection. Oxygen is indicated for hypoxia. In the severely ill child or in high-risk patients, as noted above, the use of aerosolized ribavirin is controversial, and recent studies fail to discern a beneficial effect. Severely ill hospitalized infants are often treated with beta sympathomimetic aerosols.

*Prevention.* No vaccines are available to prevent RSV infection. Breast-feeding has been linked to less severe illness in infants. The use of RSV immune globulin offers protection in young infants at high risk for complications of RSV infection. It is of no value for therapy. In the hospital setting, meticulous hand washing and the use of gown, gloves, and eye and nose protection has been shown to decrease the occurrence of infection in staff and to decrease the nosocomial spread of RSV.

## References

Behrman RE, Kliegman RM, Arvin AM (eds): Nelson Textbook of Pediatrics, 15th ed. Philadelphia, WB Saunders, 1996, Chapter 218.

Committee on Infectious Diseases, Committee on Fetus and Newborn: Respiratory syncytial virus immune globulin intravenous: Indications for use. Pediatr 99:645, 1997.

Hall CB, Walsh EE, Schnabel KC, et al: Occurrence of groups A and B of respiratory syncytial virus over 15 years: Associated epidemiologic and clinical characteristics in hospitalized and ambulatory children. J Infect Dis 162:1283, 1990.

Smith DW, Frankel LR, Mathers LH, et al: A controlled trial of aerosolized ribavirin in infants receiving mechanical ventilation for severe respiratory syncytial virus infection. N Engl J Med 325:24, 1991.

Wheeler JG, Wofford J, Turner RB: Historical cohort evaluation of ribavirin efficacy in respiratory syncytial virus infection. Pediatr Infect Dis J 12:209, 1993.

## RUBELLA

### (German or Three-Day Measles)

*Etiology.* Rubella, a single-stranded positive-sense RNA virus with a glycolipid envelope, is a member of the togavirus family. Although it is a pathogen of humans only, the virus is readily cultivated in a variety of tissue culture systems.

*Pathogenesis.* The virus is acquired from infected respiratory secretions; it invades the respiratory epithelium and is disseminated by a primary viremia. Following replication in the reticuloendothelial system, a secondary viremia ensues and virus can be isolated from peripheral blood monocytes. Virus is then found throughout the body (secretions, CSF, urine). Infection in utero results in significant morbidity. Maternal infection during the first trimester results in fetal infection in more than 90% of cases and in a generalized vasculitis; chronic infection affects virtually all organ systems (see Chapter 6).

*Epidemiology.* In unvaccinated populations, the illness occurs in 5–14 yr olds. In vaccinated populations, it occurs more commonly in teenagers and young adults (especially in large institutions, such as colleges and hospitals). Health care personnel should be screened for rubella antibody and immunized if their status is seronegative. Maximum communicability of postnatal rubella appears to be 2 days before and 5–7 days after onset of the characteristic rash. The incubation period for postnatal rubella ranges from 14 to 21 days but most commonly is 16–18 days. Infants with congenital rubella may shed virus in nasopharyngeal secretions and urine for more than 1 yr after birth and may transmit the virus to susceptible contacts.

Transplacental antibody is protective during the first 6 mo of life. In closed populations, the infection rate approaches 100%, whereas it is 50–60% among susceptible family members. Subclinical cases outnumber clinically apparent cases by a ratio of 2:1. Rubella generally occurs in the spring, with epidemics occurring in cycles of every 6–9 yr in unvaccinated populations. Infection confers lifelong immunity. Surveys indicate that 10–20% of young adults are susceptible to rubella.

*Clinical Manifestations.* The prodromal phase of rubella (mild catarrhal symptoms) may go unnoticed. The characteristic signs of rubella are retroauricular, posterior cervical, and posterior occipital lymphadenopathy accompanied by an erythematous, maculopapular, discrete rash. The rash begins on the face and spreads to the body; it lasts for 3 days. An enanthem consisting of rose-colored spots on the soft palate may appear before the rash. Other signs include mild pharyngitis, conjunctivitis, anorexia, headache, malaise, and low-grade fever. Polyarthritis (usually of the hands) may occur, especially among older women, but it usually resolves without sequelae. Paresthesia and tendonitis may occur. The WBC count usually is normal or low, and thrombocytopenia rarely occurs.

*Diagnosis.* Rubella has a relatively nonspecific appearance. The clinical diagnosis can be made with confidence only during a rubella epidemic. The *differential diagnosis* includes scarlet fever, mild rubeola, roseola, enteroviral infection, infectious mononucleosis, and drug eruptions. Specific diagnosis can be established by viral isolation from nasopharyngeal secretions or by a 4-fold antibody rise from acute to convalescent serum. Blood, urine, and CSF also may yield the virus, especially in infants with congenital infection.

*Treatment.* No antiviral therapy is available for rubella.

*Prevention.* Immunoglobulin should be used in pregnant, nonimmune women exposed to rubella who refuse to have an abortion even if documented infection has occurred. Serology determines the immune status of a pregnant, exposed woman.

Active immunization with a live attenuated vaccine prevents rubella (see Fig. 10–1). Following vaccination, virus is shed from the nasopharynx for several weeks, but it is not readily communicable. In the United States, vaccination is indicated for all children (given at 12–15 mo of age), for all nonimmune prepubescent children, and for all postpubescent females who are nonimmune and will not become pregnant within 3 mo. This regimen has reduced the incidence of rubella and of the congenital rubella syndrome, primarily by preventing epidemics of rubella. In other countries, only pubescent girls are immunized. This policy does not prevent rubella outbreaks but may decrease the percentage of nonimmune pregnant women.

Although highly attenuated and not associated with fetal damage, the vaccine virus has been recovered from fetuses. Therefore, rubella vaccination is contraindicated in pregnant women. Inadvertent use of the vaccine in this setting is not an indication for abortion. Vaccination is contraindicated in patients with an immunodeficiency state, an immunosuppressed condition, vaccine hypersensitivity, or acute febrile illness in patients who has received immunoglobulin within the last 3 mo. Fever, lymphadenopathy, rash, arthralgia, and arthritis (the latter two especially in older girls and women) may follow vaccination.

### References

Behrman RE, Kliegman RM, Arvin AM (eds): Nelson Textbook of Pediatrics, 15th ed. Philadelphia, WB Saunders, 1996, Chapter 207.
Lee SH, Ewert DP, Frederick PD, et al: Resurgence of congenital rubella syndrome in the 1990s. JAMA 267:2616, 1992.
McIntosh EDG, Menser MA: A fifty-year follow-up of congenital rubella. Lancet 340:414, 1992.

## MYCOTIC INFECTIONS

Diseases caused by fungi frequently cause cutaneous (candidiasis, "ringworm," tinea) or mucocutaneous (candidal thrush, vulvovaginitis) infections in immunocompetent patients or systemic illnesses in immunoincompetent and immunosuppressed patients. Localized pulmonary diseases (histoplasmosis, blastomycosis, cryptococcosis) are common among immunocompetent patients, whereas unusual or disseminated disease is more common among neutropenic, lymphopenic, or immunosuppressed patients. These latter infections include invasive mucormycosis or aspergillosis, disseminated candidiasis, and CNS cryptococcosis.

Treatment depends on the presence of underlying immunologic disease, the site of infection, and the specific fungus involved. Treatment of systemic fungal infections usually requires prolonged antifungal therapy using empiric antifungal agents because most laboratories do not routinely perform antifungal susceptibility testing (Table 10–20).

## COCCIDIOIDOMYCOSIS

*Etiology.* Coccidioidomycosis (San Joaquin fever, desert rheumatism) is caused by *Coccidioides imitis*, a dimorphic fungus.

*Epidemiology.* This fungus is present in soil in the southwestern states, including western Texas, Arizona, New Mexico, and California. It also occurs in Mexico and certain areas of Central and South America. The infection is usually a childhood illness and, once contracted, confers permanent immunity. The spores are spread by inhalation or, less commonly, by implantation. Person-to-person spread does not occur. Hot summers, dry soil, and rodent burrows are an ideal environment for preservation of infectious spores. The incubation period is 10–16 days, with a range of 1 wk to 1 mo.

*Clinical Manifestations*

PRIMARY COCCIDIOIDOMYCOSIS. The primary pulmonary infection is asymptomatic in 60% of patients. Symptomatic disease may resemble an influenza syndrome. Skin manifestations may include a diffuse maculopapular rash; urticaria; and, frequently, erythema nodosum or, less often, erythema multiforme. Skin infection can occur following trauma or with dissemination of the fungus and often occurs with arthralgias. Pleural effusions as well as pneumonitis may be present. The chest roentgenograms often are more impressive than the findings on physical examination.

RESIDUAL PULMONARY COCCIDIOIDOMYCOSIS. Infrequently, a cavity or chronic progressive fibrocavitary syndrome occurs.

DISSEMINATED OR PROGRESSIVE COCCIDIOIDOMYCOSIS. The fungus may occasionally disseminate to the skin, bones, and meninges of normal individu-

TABLE 10–20.  Antifungal Agents

| Drug | Mechanism of Action | Indications | Comments/Toxicity |
|---|---|---|---|
| Amphotericin B | Polyene component of drug combines with fungal membrane sterols | Blastomycosis, candidiasis, histoplasmosis, cryptococcosis, aspergillosis, mucormycosis, coccidioidomycosis, sporotrichosis (extracutaneous) | Fever, chills, azotemia, hypokalemia, toxicity; may be combined with flucytosine |
| Liposomal amphotericin B | Soluble (taken up by reticuloendothelial system) | Same as above | Less nephrotoxicity |
| Nystatin | As above | Candidiasis | Topical/oral use only |
| Flucytosine | Conversion to 5-fluorouracil, which interferes with DNA synthesis | Combined with amphotericin B; candidiasis, cryptococcosis, aspergillosis, mucormycosis | Not used as a single drug; neutropenia, thrombocytopenia, hepatitis |
| Ketoconazole | Interferes with membrane sterol formation | Candidiasis (mucosal), nonmeningeal blastomycosis, or histoplasmosis; ringworm, tinea versicolor | Oral drug; gastrointestinal toxicity; inhibits testosterone synthesis; multiple drug interaction (see Appendix I) |
| Fluconazole | As ketoconazole | Candidiasis (oral, esophagitis), cryptococcosis; some candida species are resistant (C. krusei) | Intravenous or oral drug; gastrointestinal toxicity; drug interactions |
| Itraconazole | As ketoconazole | As ketoconazole; higher tissue levels, Aspergillus | Oral drug; headache hypertension, edema; drug interactions |
| Griseofulvin | Disrupts mitotic spindle formation | Ringworm | Headache, gastrointestinal toxicity |

Data from Med Lett 28:41, 1986; 30:30, 1988; 32:57, 1990.

als or in immunocompromised patients. The mortality rate of meningitis without therapy is 100%. Hydrocephalus is a common complication of CNS disease.

*Diagnosis.* Histologic examination of pulmonary or other involved tissue reveals double-contoured spherules accompanied by endospores without budding. Obtaining specimens for culture on appropriate media should be performed cautiously because the fungus is highly contagious. A positive skin test indicates either recent or previous infection. A negative skin test does not exclude infection and typically may be negative in an individual with disseminated disease. In general, the higher the level of antibody in the serum complement fixation test the more severe the illness. In meningitis, the CSF almost always contains specific antibody. The level and persistence of complement fixation titers in serum and CSF are useful for determining the prognosis and for guiding therapy.

*Treatment.* Primary coccidioidal infection is self-limiting, and no specific therapy is required. Persistent cavitary disease may require surgical excision, usually combined with amphotericin B treatment. Amphotericin B is the agent of choice for treatment of disseminated coccidioidomycosis and may be followed by oral fluconazole or itraconazole therapy (see Appendix I). Fluconazole also has been used with success. For meningitis, intrathecal administration usually is utilized in addition to systemic therapy. Relapse, which is heralded by headache or by abnormal CSF chemistries, may occur years after therapy has ceased. Surgical débridement may be indicated for localized, symptomatic, or progressive lesions.

### References

Behrman RE, Kliegman RM, Arvin AM (eds): Nelson Textbook of Pediatrics, 15th ed. Philadelphia, WB Saunders, 1996, Chapter 233.
Catanzaro A, Galgiani JN, Levine BE, et al: Fluconazole in the treatment of chronic pulmonary and nonmeningeal disseminated coccidioidomycoses. Am J Med 98:249, 1995.
Einstein HE, Johnson RH: Coccidioidomycosis: New aspects of epidemiology and therapy. Clin Infect Dis 16:349, 1993.

### HISTOPLASMOSIS

*Etiology.* Histoplasmosis is caused by a dimorphic fungus, *Histoplasma capsulatum.*

*Epidemiology.* The organism grows particularly well in soil containing bird or bat droppings. In the United States, it is endemic in the Mississippi, Missouri, and Ohio river valleys. Infection is acquired by inhalation of airborne spores. Outbreaks have occurred following exploration and dust-raising activities in heavily contaminated areas. It is not transmitted from person to person. The incubation period is variable but is usually a few weeks from the time of exposure.

*Pathogenesis.* Histoplasmosis infection is much like tuberculosis. Inhalation of spores results in primary infection of the lung, with seeding of multiple organs. An effective immune response results in granulomatous containment of the organism, occasionally associated with calcification.

*Clinical Manifestations.* Asymptomatic infection is most common and may be recognized by serologic and skin test conversion.

*ACUTE PULMONARY HISTOPLASMOSIS.* This condition is an influenza-like illness with hilar adenopathy. Splenomegaly and erythema nodosum or erythema multiforme may be present. Chest roentgenograms reveal patchy infiltrates and hilar adenopathy in about 25% of patients. Involved areas eventually may calcify, resulting in the characteristic "buckshot" areas of healed histoplasmosis. This self-limiting illness persists for 3–4 wk.

*SECONDARY (REINFECTION) PULMONARY HISTOPLASMOSIS.* This condition occurs within 3 days of exposure. Signs and symptoms are the same as those that occur in mild primary disease; chest roentgenograms reveal a miliary pattern.

*DISSEMINATED HISTOPLASMOSIS.* This condition is typically an acute illness of infants, young children, and immunocompromised patients. If the illness is left untreated, it is fatal. Beginning as primary pulmonary histoplasmosis, it progresses to involve the reticuloendothelial system, with diffuse adenopathy, hepatosplenomegaly, pneumonitis, and bone marrow involvement, resulting in anemia, leukopenia, and thrombocytopenia. Death is due to respiratory failure, gastrointestinal tract bleeding, or bacterial sepsis.

*Diagnosis.* Diagnosis of acute histoplasmosis generally is made by demonstration of a serologic response. Sputum cultures usually are negative. In disseminated disease, the organism may be recovered and cultured from bone marrow, lymph nodes, or biopsy material. In patients with disseminated disease, the skin test may be nonreactive. Application of skin test antigen may induce a serologic response, and thus it usually is not utilized for diagnostic purposes or is placed after blood for serologic studies has been drawn.

*Treatment.* Acute histoplasmosis in older children and adults is a self-limited disease and does not require therapy. Other forms of histoplasmosis, including symptomatic pulmonary disease in the infant and young child and disseminated disease, are treated with amphotericin B. In immunocompromised children (particularly AIDS), long-term suppressive therapy is required; itraconazole has been successfully used (see Appendix I).

### References

Behrman RE, Kliegman RM, Arvin AM (eds): Nelson Textbook of Pediatrics, 15th ed. Philadelphia, WB Saunders, 1996, Chapter 231.

Weinberg GA, Kleiman MB, Grosfeld JL, et al: Unusual manifestations of histoplasmosis in children. Pediatrics 72:99, 1983.

Wheat LJ, Connolly-Stringfield PA, Baker RL, et al: Disseminated histoplasmosis in the acquired immunodeficiency syndrome: Clinical findings, diagnosis and review of the literature. Medicine 6:361, 1990.

## SUPERFICIAL FUNGAL INFECTIONS

Cutaneous manifestations of infection by relatively nonvirulent fungi are quite common (Table 10–21).

## RICKETTSIAL DISEASE

*Etiology.* Rickettsiae are gram-negative coccobacillary organisms that resemble bacteria but have incomplete cell walls and have lost enzymes, and thus require an intracellular site for replication.

*Epidemiology.* Rickettsiae infect arthropod vectors and, with the exception of louse-borne epidemic typhus, are transmitted to humans only incidentally. Table 10–22 summarizes the agents, epidemiology, and serologic response to the more common rickettsial infections of humans. Rocky Mountain spotted fever is the most common human rickettsial illness in the United States. Rickettsiae have a limited geographic and seasonal occurrence related to arthropod life cycles, activity, and distribution.

*Pathogenesis.* The fundamental characteristic of the condition is infection of the blood vessels of skin, brain, and subcutaneous tissue resulting in vasculitis, increased vascular permeability, edema, and, eventually, decreased vascular volume, altered tissue perfusion, and widespread organ failure.

*Clinical Manifestations.* Local primary lesions are present in many rickettsial infections. Prominent features include fever, rash, headache, myalgias, and respiratory tract signs and symptoms. Patients with Q fever do not exhibit rash but may have pneumonia and hepatitis as part of their clinical presentation.

TABLE 10–21. Superficial Fungal Infections

| Name | Etiology | Manifestations | Diagnosis | Therapy |
|---|---|---|---|---|
| Tinea capitis (ringworm) | Microsporum audouinii, Trichophyton tonsurans, M. canis | Prepubertal infection of scalp, hairshafts; "black dot" alopecia; T. tonsurans common in blacks | M. audouinii fluorescence: blue-green with Wood lamp*; +KOH, culture | Griseofulvin; selenium sulfide shampoo |
| Kerion | Inflammatory reaction to tinea capitis | Swollen, boggy, crusted, purulent, tender mass with lymphadenopathy; secondary distal "id" reaction common | As above | As above, plus steroids for "id" reactions |
| Tinea corporis (ringworm) | M. canis, T. rubrum, others | Slightly pruritic ring-like, erythematous papules, plaques with scaling and slow outward expansion of the border; check cat or dog for M. canis | +KOH, culture; M. canis fluorescence: blue-green with Wood lamp; differential diagnosis: granuloma annulare, pityriasis, rosea, nummular eczema, psoriasis | Local miconazole or clotrimazole |
| Tinea cruris (jock itch) | Epidermophyton floccosum, T. mentagrophytes, T. rubrum | Symmetric, pruritic, scrotal sparing, scaling plaques | +KOH, culture; differential diagnosis: erythrasma (Corynebacterium minutissimum) | Local miconazole, clotrimazole, undecylenic acid, or tolnaftate; wear loose cotton underwear |
| Tinea pedis (athlete's foot) | T. rubrum, T. mentagrophytes | Moccasin or interdigital distribution, dry scales, interdigital maceration with secondary bacterial infection | +KOH, culture; differential diagnosis: C. minutissimum erythrasma | Medications as above; wear cotton socks |
| Tinea unguium (onychomycosis) | T. mentagrophytes, T. rubrum, Candida albicans | Uncommon before puberty; peeling of distal nail plate; thickening, splitting of nails | +KOH, culture | Oral ketoconazole or griseofulvin |
| Tinea versicolor | Malassezia furfur | Tropical climates, steroids or immunosuppressive drugs; uncommon before puberty; chest, back, arms; oval hypopigmented or hyperpigmented in blacks, red-brown in whites; scaling patches | +KOH; orange-gold fluorescence with Wood lamp; differential diagnosis: pityriasis alba | Selenium sulfide shampoo, topical sodium hyposulfite, oral ketoconazole |
| Candidiasis | C. albicans | Diaper area, intense erythematous plaques or pustules, isolated or confluent | +KOH, culture | Topical nystatin; oral nystatin treats concomitant oral thrush |

*Wood lamp examination uses an ultraviolet source in a completely darkened room. Trichophyton usually has no fluorescence.
KOH = potassium hydroxide.

TABLE 10–22. Rickettsial Diseases of Humans: Summary of Pertinent Features

| Group Disease | Causative Agent | Arthropod Vector | Hosts | Incubation Period | Confirmatory Tests* | Geographic Distribution |
|---|---|---|---|---|---|---|
| **Spotted Fever** | | | | | | |
| Rocky Mountain spotted fever | *R. rickettsii* | Tick | Dogs, rodents | 1–8 days | IFA, DFA | Western hemisphere |
| Boutonneuse fever (Mediterranean spotted fever) | *R. conorii* | Tick | Dogs, rodents | 3–15 days | IFA, DFA | Africa, Mediterranean region, India, Middle East |
| Rickettsialpox | *R. akari* | Mite | Mice | 10–24 days | IFA | North America, Russia, Korea, South Africa |
| **Ehrlichiosis** | *E. canis* | Tick | Dogs | 7–28 days | IFA | Southeast, north and south central United States |
| **Typhus** | | | | | | |
| Epidemic typhus/Brill-Zinsser disease | *R. prowazekii* | Body louse | Humans | — | IFA | Highlands of Africa, Asia, Central and South America |
| Flying squirrel–associated typhus fever | *R. prowazekii* | Lice, fleas | Flying squirrels | 10–14 days | IFA | Eastern United States (including Texas) |
| Murine (endemic) typhus | *R. typhi* | Cat or rat flea, rat louse | Rats | 8 days | IFA | Worldwide |
| **Scrub typhus** | | | | | | |
| Scrub typhus | *R. tsutsugamushi* | Mite | Rodents | 8–10 days | IFA, IP | Pacific Islands, Australia, and central, eastern, and southeast Asia |
| **Others** | | | | | | |
| Q fever | *Coxiella burnetii* | Ticks? | Cattle, sheep, goats, cats | 18–20 days | IFA, CF | Worldwide |

Adapted from Behrman RE, Kliegman RM, Arvin AM (eds): Nelson Textbook of Pediatrics, 15th ed. Philadelphia, WB Saunders, 1996, p 954.
*Although not widely available or highly sensitive, a direct fluorescent antibody (DFA) test can be used to detect rickettsiae in skin biopsies or tissue samples. Preferred confirmatory serologic tests include indirect fluorescent antibody or microimmunofluorescent assay (IFA), complement fixation (CF), and immunoperoxidase (IP) assays. Cross-absorption of the patient's serum with specific rickettsial antigens can be done to distinguish the following infections: *R. rickettsii* versus *R. conorii* or *R. akari*; and *R. prowazekii* versus *R. typhi*.

*Diagnosis.* Organisms can be detected in biopsy specimens (usually of skin) and by staining (usually by immunofluorescence). Serologic diagnosis may be accomplished by detection of specific anti-rickettsial antibodies (IgM and IgG). The use of the Weil-Felix reaction is no longer recommended. Although it is useful for etiologic confirmation, serologic response may not be helpful regarding therapeutic decisions. The Weil-Felix reaction is frequently unreliable because of its false-positive and false-negative results. Culturing of rickettsiae is possible in animals or tissue culture; both are hazardous and generally not available. PCR-based diagnostic tests are under development.

*Treatment.* Therapy with tetracycline or chloramphenicol is curative when begun early (see Appendix I). Quinolones are likely to be useful. The relative risks and benefits of tetracyclines and negligible tooth staining over a short course of therapy must be weighed against the known hematologic side effects of chloramphenicol. Most experts recommend tetracyclines.

*Immunity.* Prolonged immunity and some degree of cross-immunity to other rickettsial infections is conferred by infection. Recurrent or recrudescent activation of rickettsial infection years after the first attack (as in Brill disease or scrub typhus) is common. Humoral antibodies are produced during infections, but cell-mediated immunity is probably of greater importance.

*Prognosis.* Mortality is lower in children than in adults. Early diagnosis and therapy markedly reduce the mortality rate. In the United States, the mortality rate is 5–10% in individuals younger than 30 yr of age with Rocky Mountain spotted fever, the most serious form of rickettsiosis. Mortality rates are consistently higher in nonwhites, presumably because of the difficulty in appreciating the characteristic rash. When death occurs, it is usually in the 2nd wk of illness.

## ROCKY MOUNTAIN SPOTTED FEVER

*Epidemiology.* This is the most common rickettsial illness in the United States, occurring primarily in the Eastern coastal, the Southeast, and the Western states, especially among 5–9 yr old children. Although the illness is transmitted by various ticks, 15–20% of infected individuals are not able to describe tick bites or contacts. Most cases occur from April to September following outdoor activity in wooded areas.

*Clinical Manifestations.* The onset is nonspecific, with headache, malaise, and fever. In a few days, a pale, rose-red macular or maculopapular rash appears in 90% of cases. It begins peripherally and spreads to involve the entire body, including palms and soles. The early rash blanches on pressure and is accentuated by warmth. In several days, it progresses to a petechial and purpuric eruption. Fever, headache, myalgia, malaise, splenomegaly (33%), and facial edema become evident. In severe cases, symptoms of CNS inflammation, myocarditis, renal impairment, pneumonitis, and shock occur.

Thrombocytopenia and hyponatremia are common findings and may be important clues to the etiology of this syndrome. DIC is an ominous finding. The fatality rate in untreated patients is 10–40% compared with 5–7% in appropriately treated patients and nearly zero in those treated early.

*Diagnosis.* The epidemiologic data (locale, time of year, evidence of a tick bite) and clinical manifestations (especially the rash) should facilitate diagnosis. Absence of or failure to obtain appropriate information will greatly hinder diagnosis and increase the risk of a fatal outcome. Fever, headache, and myalgias lasting longer than 1 wk are more indicative of Rocky Mountain spotted fever in endemic areas than of the typical influenza that usually has resolved or begins resolving after 1 wk of duration. The *differential diagnosis* includes a broad spectrum of illnesses, such as measles, collagen vascular diseases, viral infections, Henoch-Schönlein purpura, idiopathic thrombocytopenic purpura, infectious mononucleosis, ehrlichiosis (see Table 10–22), and meningococcemia.

*Treatment.* The relative risks and benefits of tetracyclines and negligible tooth staining over a short course of therapy must be weighed against the known hematologic side effects of chloramphenicol. Most recommend tetracyclines (see Appendix I).

*Prevention.* Protection from tick bites and rapid removal of ticks can prevent Rocky Mountain spotted fever. Ticks are best removed by gentle upward traction with forceps to avoid infecting the patient or oneself with material from the crushed tick.

## References

Abramson JS, Givner LB: Should tetracycline be contraindicated for therapy of presumed Rocky Mountain spotted fever in children less than 9 years of age? Pediatrics 86:123, 1990.
Behrman RE, Kliegman RM, Arvin AM (eds): Nelson Textbook of Pediatrics, 15th ed. Philadelphia, WB Saunders, 1996, Chapters 238–243.
Dumler JS, Taylor JP, Walker DH: Clinical and laboratory features of murine typhus in south Texas, 1980 through 1987. JAMA 266:1365, 1991.
Eng TR, Harkess JR, Fishbein DB, et al: Epidemiologic, clinical, and laboratory findings of human ehrlichiosis in the United States, 1988. JAMA 264:2251, 1990.

Kirk JL, Fine DP, Sexton DJ, et al: Rocky Mount spotted fever: A clinical review based on 48 confirmed cases, 1943–1986. Medicine 69:35, 1990.

Kirkland KB, Marcom PK, Sexton DJ, et al: Rocky Mountain spotted fever complicated by gangrene: Report of six cases and review. Clin Infect Dis 16:629, 1993.

# PARASITIC INFECTIONS

Although much attention is focused on bacterial and viral infections, protozoal and helminthic infections are a more significant health problem in most parts of the world. Malaria is estimated to kill more than 1 million individuals a year, mostly children.

## PROTOZOAL DISEASE

Protozoa are the simplest organisms of the animal kingdom. They are unicellular and most are free living, but some have a commensalistic or parasitic existence. Protozoal disease is considered under the groupings of intestinal and systemic protozoal infections.

### Intestinal Protozoal Infections

#### Amebiasis

*Etiology.* Amebiasis is caused by *Entamoeba histolytica*, a protozoan that exists as a resistant infectious cyst (10–18 μm, with four nuclei) or as a motile, invasive trophozoite.

*Epidemiology.* Humans are the natural host and reservoir of *E. histolytica*. It is transmitted via contaminated food or water and by person-to-person contact.

*Pathogenesis.* Once ingested, a cyst becomes a trophozoite that can cause invasive disease and produce a characteristic flask-shaped ulcer in the intestinal mucosa. The amebas may disseminate to the liver or, less commonly, to other areas, such as the pleura, skin, brain, and lungs. The disease is distributed worldwide, although it is more prevalent in areas of poor sanitation. A patient is intermittently infectious if not treated.

*Clinical Manifestations.* Most infected individuals are asymptomatic, but some present with acute, cramping diarrhea. In 2–8% of infected persons, intestinal amebiasis may be associated with diarrhea that contains blood and mucus and that is associated with fever, abdominal pain, headache, and chills. Symptoms last for days to weeks and recur without therapy. *Ameboma* (a mass due to amebas), extraintestinal lesions, or intestinal perforation and hemorrhage may occur. Twenty-five percent of patients have ulcerative lesions that can be visualized by sigmoidoscopy. These lesions may lead to perforation of the colon and subsequent peritonitis.

Hepatic amebiasis is the most common manifestation of disseminated infection. Amebic liver abscess with fever, abdominal pain, distention, and a tender liver occurs in 1% of infected individuals. These patients often do not have a history of intestinal amebiasis, and their stool is negative for amebas.

*Diagnosis.* The diagnosis of intestinal illness relies on demonstration of the organism in stool or biopsy of ulcers or liver abscess tissue. In invasive intestinal amebiasis and in cases of liver abscess, antibody to ameba is present in over 90% of cases. Ultrasound or CT will delineate the liver abscess, which is usually singular and located in the right lobe.

*Treatment.* Therapy of amebiasis depends on the type of illness. Metronidazole or tinidazole is recommended for forms that invade tissue, followed by iodoquinol for intraluminal organisms.

### References

Ahmed L, El Rooby A, Kassem MI, et al: Ultrasonography in the diagnosis and management of 52 patients with amebic liver abscess in Cairo. Rev Infect Dis 12:330, 1990.

Behrman RE, Kliegman RM, Arvin AM (eds): Nelson Textbook of Pediatrics, 15th ed. Philadelphia, WB Saunders, 1996, Chapter 244.1.

#### Cryptosporidiosis

*Etiology.* *Cryptosporidium* is a coccidian protozoan that can produce an acute illness in immunocompetent and immunocompromised hosts (particularly those with AIDS).

*Epidemiology.* The oocysts of *Cryptosporidium* are hardy, withstand routine disinfectants, and survive in moist areas. Both person-to-person and zoonotic transmission is possible; infection from contaminated water sources cause large-scale outbreaks. *Cryptosporidium* frequently is a cause of diarrhea in young children in developing countries. The prevalence of infection may be as high as 4–7% in sporadic outbreaks of enteritis. The incubation period is 2–14 days.

*Clinical Manifestations.* Cryptosporidiosis can appear as an acute and self-limited enteritis in normal individuals who exhibit watery diarrhea, nausea, and cramps lasting 12–14 days. Although most immunocompetent hosts recover within 10–14 days, occasionally the disease is protracted and oocyst shedding persists for 2 wk. In immunocompromised patients (particularly those with HIV), profuse watery diarrhea with profound weight loss may occur. Biliary tract disease is also found.

*Treatment.* In normal hosts, cryptosporidiosis is usually self-limited and supportive care is sufficient. In patients with more severe disease and in immunocompromised hosts, azithromycin and paromomycin along with appropriate fluid and electrolyte replacement have been efficacious.

### References

Behrman RE, Kliegman RM, Arvin AM (eds): Nelson Textbook of Pediatrics, 15th ed. Philadelphia, WB Saunders, 1996, Chapter 244.4.

MacKenzie WR, Hoxie NJ, Proctor ME, et al: A massive outbreak in Milwaukee of *Cryptosporidium* infection transmitted through the public water supply. N Engl J Med 331:161, 1994.

Vargas SL, Shenep JL, Flynn PM, et al: Azithromycin for treatment of severe *Cryptosporidium* diarrhea in two children with cancer. J Pediatr 123:154, 1993.

### Giardiasis

*Etiology.* Giardiasis is due to *Giardia lamblia,* a flagellated protozoan. The hardy cysts are ingested (often in water) and are the infectious form. The trophozoites are liberated after ingestion and are responsible for symptoms. Giardiae live in the duodenum.

*Epidemiology.* *Giardia* has a worldwide distribution and infects humans, dogs, and wild animals (beavers). Transmission occurs from person to person by fecal-oral spread or by drinking or eating contaminated water or food. Outbreaks occur in day care centers, in institutions for the mentally retarded, and in travelers to the former Soviet Union and the Rocky Mountains.

*Clinical Manifestations.* Individuals vary in their response to infection and have the following clinical manifestations: (1) asymptomatic; (2) an acute illness with a sudden onset of explosive, watery, foul-smelling stools, flatulence, abdominal distention, nausea, and anorexia; and (3) chronic diarrhea and malabsorption (including that of antibiotics and iron), with flatulence, abdominal distention, and abdominal pain, often lasting for months.

*Diagnosis.* Examination of several stool specimens is necessary for visualizing the organism, because intermittent excretion occurs. Examining duodenal contents obtained by direct aspiration or by use of a string test (Enterotest) is more sensitive. Rarely, duodenal intubation with fluid aspiration or biopsy may be required for diagnosis. ELISA can be used to detect *Giardia* antigen in stool specimens; PCR and DNA probes are also available to identify infected patients.

*Treatment.* Several drugs, including metronidazole, tinidazole, and furazolidine are effective in the treatment of giardiasis.

### References

Addiss DG, Juranek DD, Spencer HC: Treatment of children with asymptomatic and nondiarrheal *Giardia* infection. Pediatr Infect Dis J 10:843, 1991.

Behrman RE, Kliegman RM, Arvin AM (eds): Nelson Textbook of Pediatrics, 15th ed. Philadelphia, WB Saunders, 1996, Chapter 244.5.

Gunasekaran TS, Hassall E: Giardiasis mimicking inflammatory bowel disease. J Pediatr 120:424, 1992.

Quick R, Paugh K, Addiss D, et al: Restaurant-associated outbreak of giardiasis. J Infect Dis 166:673, 1992.

## Systemic Protozoal Infections

### American Trypanosomiasis (Chagas Disease)

*Etiology.* American trypanosomiasis is a zoonosis caused by *Trypanosoma cruzi,* a protozoan hemoflagellate.

*Epidemiology.* *T. cruzi* is transmitted to humans by blood-sucking insects called reduviid bugs. The trypomastigotes are released as the insect defecates near its bite. The trypanosome gains entry and amastigotes (intracellular forms) and trypomastigotes (vascular forms) are produced. The infected reduviid bugs have adapted to adobe, mud, and cane housing in most of South and Central America. It is estimated that 24 million South Americans are infected with *T. cruzi.* Several endogenous cases have occurred in Texas. Animal reservoirs, including rats, opossums, and raccoons, may be important. Although it is common to encounter infected reduviid bugs in the southwestern United States, infection in humans appears to be rare, possibly because of better housing, low adaptability of North American reduviids to domestic housing, or difference in *Trypanosoma* virulence. *T. cruzi* also may be transmitted congenitally or by infected blood. The incubation period is 1–2 wk.

### Clinical Manifestations

ACUTE INFECTION. Illness generally is asymptomatic or mild in young children in endemic areas. There may be local inflammation at the site of entry of the parasite. Half of infected children have unilateral eye swelling (Romaña sign), which is the first indication of disease. Some patients have a nodular skin lesion (chagoma) at the site of the original inoculation. Hematogenous dissemination results in malaise, fever, muscle pain, adenopathy, rash, hepatosplenomegaly, and, less often, meningoencephalitis. Myocardial involvement is noted in nearly one half of symptomatic patients, accompanied by tachycardia and arrhythmias. Most cases evolve into an asymptomatic chronic stage. The mortality rate is 10%. Congenital disease is characterized by low birth weight, hepatomegaly, and meningoencephalitis.

*CHRONIC TRYPANOSOMIASIS.* In the symptomatic chronic stage, inflammation and fibrosis result in myocarditis, cardiac failure, or enlargement of a hollow viscus, especially of the esophagus (megaesophagus) or the colon (megacolon). This occurs in 10–15% of cases.

***Diagnosis.*** In acute disease, *T. cruzi* can be demonstrated in blood smears. EIA tests are available, and PCR techniques have been developed.

***Treatment.*** Nifurtimox has been used successfully to treat acute trypanosomiasis.

***Prevention.*** Insect control and adequately protected housing are keys to breaking the bug-human cycle. Blood donors in endemic areas must be screened by serology.

### References

Behrman RE, Kliegman RM, Arvin AM (eds): Nelson Textbook of Pediatrics, 15th ed. Philadelphia, WB Saunders, 1996, Chapters 244.10–244.11.

Grant IH, Gold JWM, Wittner M, et al: Transfusion-associated acute Chagas disease acquired in the United States. Ann Intern Med 111:849, 1989.

Viotti R, Vigliano C, Armenti H, Segura E: Treatment of chronic Chagas' disease with benznidazole: Clinical and serological evolution of patients with long-term follow-up. Am Heart J 127:151, 1994.

### Malaria

***Etiology.*** Malaria is caused by one or more of four *Plasmodium* species: *P. falciparum, P. vivax, P. ovale,* and *P. malariae.*

***Epidemiology.*** Malaria usually is acquired from the bite of an infected female *Anopheles* mosquito. Less commonly, it is acquired transplacentally or via an infected blood transfusion. Infection transmitted through blood transfusion or the transplacental route occurs without the pre-erythrocytic hepatic phase. In children with no pre-existing immunity to malaria, the incubation period varies from 6 to 16 days depending on the *Plasmodium* species involved. Endemic malaria has been reported in the southern United States, but most often it is imported by travelers or immigrants.

***Pathology.*** Infected red blood cells rupture, causing hemolytic anemia and pigment deposition in reticuloendothelial cells. The infected red cells also may sludge and stick in organs, interfering with circulation and inducing pneumonia, encephalitis, or enteritis. *P. falciparum* is associated with the heaviest degree of parasitemia and is the most lethal. Serum antibody production seems to be correlated with clearance of the erythrocyte (but not the hepatic) stage of parasites. Sickle cell anemia and glucose-6-phosphate dehydrogenase (G6PD) deficiency are associated with some protection against lethal malaria.

***Clinical Manifestations.*** Malaria is most severe in children lacking antibody and is milder in children having survived initial attacks. The illness is characterized by a nonspecific prodrome prior to the onset of sudden high fevers with chills. An abrupt return to normal temperature occurs after 2–12 hr. Fever is associated with headache, abdominal and back pain, nausea, and, often, splenomegaly. In established *P. vivax* or *P. malariae* infection, fever may occur every 2 or 3 days, respectively. *P. falciparum* infection also may produce encephalitis, pneumonitis, enteritis, and nephritis. The most serious form of malaria is due to severe and sudden intravascular hemolysis (blackwater fever), associated with heavy *P. falciparum* infection as well as with the use of drugs that induce hemolysis in G6PD-deficient individuals.

***Diagnosis.*** The diagnosis of malaria and the species of *Plasmodium* may be confirmed by examining thick and thin blood smears. These smears should be examined at 12-hr intervals because the level of parasitemia fluctuates. In convalescence, there is an antibody response to the parasite.

***Treatment.*** Specific therapy for malaria depends on the species acquired, the mode of acquisition, and the locale of acquisition. Chloroquine is the therapy for malaria acquired in locales that do not have chloroquine-resistant malaria, such as Mexico, Haiti, the Dominican Republic, most of the Northern Middle East, and west of the Panama Canal Zone. In areas with *P. falciparum* known to be chloroquine-resistant, including much of Africa, Oceania, Southeast Asia, the Indian subcontinent, and South America, therapy consists of quinine plus pyrimethamine/sulfadoxine or quinine plus tetracycline or mefloquin. Severe illness may necessitate the intravenous use of quinine or quinidine. To prevent relapse of mosquito-transmitted *P. ovale* and *P. vivax* infection, primaquine is used to eradicate the hepatic phase of the parasite cycle. Because a hepatic phase does not occur with congenital or transfusion-acquired *P. malariae* or *P. falciparum* infection, primaquine is not indicated in these situations. Primaquine induces hemolysis in patients with G6PD deficiency. In severe disease, multisystem support, transfusion, and possibly exchange transfusion are necessary.

***Prevention.*** Malaria can be prevented by administering chemoprophylaxis, which includes the use of weekly dosages of chloroquine (which must also be taken for 6 wk after leaving the endemic area) and possibly the use of primaquine for terminal prophylaxis in order to eradicate hepatic forms. In areas where *Plasmodium* species are chloroquine-resistant, mefloquine or doxycycline may be used. Control of malaria relies on the prevention of mosquito bites by using special clothing, repellents, night netting, and mosquito eradication programs.

### References

Behrman RE, Kliegman RM, Arvin AM (eds): Nelson Textbook of Pediatrics, 15th ed. Philadelphia, WB Saunders, 1996, Chapter 244.7.

Freedman DO: Imported malaria—here to stay. Am J Med 93:239, 1992.

Subramanian D, Moise KJ Jr, White AC Jr: Imported malaria in pregnancy: Report of four cases and review of management. Clin Infect Dis 15:408, 1992.

Weiss WR, Oloo AJ, Johnson A, et al: Daily primaquine is effective for prophylaxis against falciparum malaria in Kenya: A comparison with mefloquine, doxycycline, and choroquine plus proguanil. J Infect Dis 171:1569, 1995.

### Toxoplasmosis

*Etiology.* *Toxoplasma gondii,* an intracellular protozoan parasite, causes toxoplasmosis.

*Epidemiology.* Newly infected cats excrete the infectious oocysts in their feces. The oocysts and tissue cysts are infectious when ingested. High frequency of human infection occurs in warm, humid climates. Infection also occurs from ingesting undercooked meat containing cysts. Less commonly, transmission occurs by blood transfusion or organ transplant, or transplacentally during acute infection of pregnant women. In the United States the incidence of congenital infection is 1–2:1000 live births. The incubation period for acquired infection is about 7 days.

### Clinical Manifestations

CONGENITAL TOXOPLASMOSIS. Most maternal infection is asymptomatic. Among women infected during pregnancy, 40–60% give birth to an infected infant. The later in pregnancy that infection occurs, the more likely it is that the fetus will be infected but the less severe the illness. Severely affected fetuses will be stillborn. In infants, illness may occur at birth and become manifest by poor feeding, fever, rash, petechiae, lymphadenopathy, hepatomegaly, splenomegaly, jaundice, hydrocephalus or microcephaly, microphthalmia, seizures, cerebral calcifications, and chorioretinitis. This illness must be differentiated from other congenital infections included in the TORCH syndrome (rubella, CMV, HSV, syphilis, hepatitis, and VZV). In 67–75% of infants who are asymptomatic at birth, subsequent defects, such as chorioretinitis, retardation, and neurologic disability, will develop years after birth.

ACQUIRED TOXOPLASMOSIS. This condition is usually an asymptomatic infection. Symptomatic infection is characterized as a heterophil-negative mononucleosis syndrome that includes lymphadenopathy, fever, and hepatosplenomegaly. Disseminated infection, including myocarditis, pneumonia, and encephalitis, is more common in immunosuppressed patients, especially those with AIDS. Localized lymphadenopathy that is difficult to differentiate from Hodgkin disease is one of the more common manifestations of toxoplasmosis.

*Diagnosis.* In toxoplasmosis involving the CNS, the parasites may be visualized in CSF by cytocentrifuge preparations or by growth in inoculated infant mice. Typical histopathology or cysts may be identified in biopsy specimens of involved lung, brain, or lymph node.

Serologic diagnosis can be established by several different antibody tests. A four-fold rise in antibody titer or seroconversion from negative to positive indicates the presence of infection. In congenital infection, the diagnosis is complicated by the presence of maternally derived transplacental antibody. If the maternal antibody status is negative, the diagnosis of congenital toxoplasmosis is excluded; if the maternal and neonate levels are positive, serial studies for several months are necessary to distinguish transplacental antibody (levels will fall) from congenital infection (levels will remain stable or rise). Several research laboratories can perform an IgM/anti-*Toxoplasma* antibody study on the serum from newborns; a positive result indicates infection.

*Treatment.* Treatment includes both pyrimethamine and sulfadiazine, which act synergistically against *Toxoplasma* organisms. Because these compounds are folic acid inhibitors, they are used in conjunction with folinic acid. Spiramycin, which is not licensed in the United States, also is utilized in therapy of pregnant women with toxoplasmosis. Corticosteroids are reserved for patients with acute CNS or ocular infection.

*Prevention.* Ingesting only well-cooked meat and avoiding cats or soil in areas where cats defecate are prudent measures for pregnant or immunocompromised patients. Cat litter should be disposed of daily because oocysts are not infectious during the first 48 hr after passage. Administration of spiramycin to infected pregnant women has been associated with lower risks of congenital infection in their babies.

### References

Behrman RE, Kliegman RM, Arvin AM (eds): Nelson Textbook of Pediatrics. 15th ed. Philadelphia, WB Saunders, 1996, Chapter 244.8.

Cohn JA, McMeeking A, Cohen W, et al: Evaluation of the policy of empiric treatment of suspected toxoplasma encephalitis in patients with the acquired immunodeficiency syndrome. Am J Med 86:521, 1989.

Mitchell CD, Erlich SS, Mastrucci MT, et al: Congenital toxoplasmosis occurring in infants perinatally infected with human immunodeficiency virus 1. Pediatr Infect Dis J 9:512, 1990.

## HELMINTHIASES

The helminths are divided into three groups: one group of round worms, the nematodes, and two groups of flat worms, the trematodes (flukes) and the cestodes (tapeworms).

### Infections Caused by Intestinal Nematodes

Infections are normally acquired by inadvertent ingestion of eggs or by larval forms from soil penetrating the skin.

#### Ascariasis
*Etiology.* Ascariasis is the most prevalent type of helminthiasis, involving 1 billion people. It is caused by *Ascaris lumbricoides,* a large nematode.

*Epidemiology.* After humans ingest the eggs, larvae are released and then penetrate the intestine, migrate to the lungs, ascend the trachea, and are reswallowed. On entering the intestines again, they mature and produce eggs that are excreted in the stool and are deposited in the soil, where they survive for prolonged periods. This is a ubiquitous parasite that generally occurs in warm areas. Human fecal soilage, use of human manure for agriculture, and hand-to-mouth spread are the major sources of ascariasis.

*Clinical Manifestations.* Manifestations may be due to migration of the larvae to other sites of the body or due to the presence of adult worms in the intestine. Pulmonary ascariasis occurs as the larvae migrate through the lung. The manifestations of the condition include cough, blood-stained sputum, eosinophilia, and transient infiltrates on chest roentgenograms. Adult larvae in the small intestine may cause abdominal pain and distention. It is rare that intestinal obstruction from adult worms occurs. Migration of worms into the bile duct may result in the rare occurrence of acute biliary obstruction. Steatorrhea and decreased vitamin A absorption may occur in heavily infected children. Asymptomatic infections are common.

*Diagnosis.* Results from examination of stool for characteristic eggs are diagnostic.

*Treatment.* Mebendazole currently is considered the drug of choice; pyrantel pamoate or albendazole are alternatives.

*Prevention.* Effective control of this worldwide parasite depends on adequate sanitary treatment and disposal of infected human feces, especially before it is used as fertilizer.

#### Enterobiasis (Pinworm)
*Etiology.* Pinworm is caused by *Enterobius vermicularis,* a nematode that is distributed worldwide.

*Epidemiology.* Enterobiasis affects individuals at all socioeconomic levels, especially children. Crowded living conditions predispose individuals to infection. Humans ingest the eggs carried on hands or present in house dust or on bedclothes. They hatch in the stomach, and the larvae migrate to the cecum and mature. At night the females migrate to the perianal area to lay their eggs, which are viable for 2 days.

*Clinical Manifestations.* The most common symptoms are nocturnal anal pruritus and sleeplessness, presumably resulting from the migratory female worms. Vaginitis and salpingitis can occur secondary to aberrant worm migration. *Enterobius* has been recovered from the appendix in several cases, although its role in appendicitis is doubtful.

*Diagnosis.* The eggs are detected by microscopically examining adhesive cellophane tape pressed against the anus in the morning to collect eggs. Less commonly, a worm may be seen in the perianal region.

*Treatment.* The drug of choice is pyrantel pamoate or mebendazole given as a single dose and repeated in 2 wk. Alternatives include albendazole. Repeated therapy may be necessary because of reinfection. Therapy for all family members at once is also often used.

#### Hookworm Infections
*Etiology.* Hookworm infection is caused by several species of hookworms; *Ancylostoma duodenale* and *Necator americanus* are the most important. *A. duodenale* is the predominant species in Europe, the Mediterranean region, northern Asia, and the west coast of South America. *N. americanus* predominates in the Western hemisphere, sub-Saharan Africa, Southeast Asia, and several Pacific islands.

*Epidemiology.* More than 9 million humans are infected with hookworms. Optimal soil conditions and fecal contamination are found in many agrarian tropical countries and in the southeastern United States. Infection typically occurs in young children, especially during the first decade of life. The larvae are found in warm, damp soil and infect humans by penetrating the skin. They migrate to the lungs, ascend the trachea, are swallowed, and reside in the intestine. The worms then mature and attach to the intestinal wall, where they suck blood and shed eggs.

*Clinical Manifestations.* Infections usually are asymptomatic. Intense pruritus ("ground itch"), which may include papules and vesicles, can occur at the site of larval penetration, usually the soles of the feet or between the toes. Migration of larvae through the lungs usually is asymptomatic. Symptoms of abdominal pain, anorexia, indigestion, fullness, and diarrhea occur with hookworm infestation. The major manifestation of infection is subsequent anemia. Chronic infection causes hypoalbuminemia and edema, which may lead to heart failure.

*Diagnosis.* Examination of fresh stool reveals hookworm eggs.

*Treatment.* Pyrantel pamoate or mebendazole eradicates hookworm infection. Therapy for anemia may necessitate iron therapy or, in severe cases, transfusion.

*Prevention.* Eradication depends on sanitation of the patient's environment and chemotherapy. Eradication essentially has been achieved in the southeastern United States.

## Systemic Nematodes

### Visceral Larva Migrans (Toxocariasis)

*Etiology.* Visceral larva migrans (VLM) is caused by ingestion of the eggs of the dog or cat tapeworms *Toxocara canis, Toxocara catii,* and *Toxascaris leonina.*

*Epidemiology.* VLM is most common in young children with pica who have dogs or cats as pets. Ocular toxocariasis occurs in older children. Approximately 2% of dogs in the United States excrete *Toxocara* eggs, and up to 25% of soil samples in public parks contain the eggs. The eggs of these roundworms are produced by adult worms residing in the dog and cat intestine. Ingested eggs hatch into larvae that penetrate the gastrointestinal tract and migrate to the liver, lung, eye, CNS, and heart, where they die and calcify.

*Clinical Manifestations.* Symptoms are due to the number of migrating worms and the immune response they elicit. Most persons who are lightly infected are asymptomatic. Symptoms include fever, cough, wheezing, and seizures. Physical findings may include hepatomegaly, rales, rash, and adenopathy. Visual symptoms may include decreased acuity, strabismus, periorbital edema, or blindness. Eye examination may reveal granulomatous lesions near the macula or disc. These must be differentiated from retinoblastoma and other granulomatous infections.

*Diagnosis.* Eosinophilia and hypergammaglobulinemia associated with elevated isohemagglutinin levels suggest the diagnosis, which may be confirmed by serology (ELISA) or, less commonly, by biopsy.

*Treatment.* This is a self-limiting illness. In severe disease, steroids and diethylcarbamazine may be useful. Albendazole or mebendazole are alternatives.

*Prevention.* Avoiding pica and washing the hands after animal contact may help control the illness. Deworming puppies and kittens, the major excretors of eggs, decreases the risk of infection.

## Infections Caused by Trematodes
### (Flukes)

Trematodes include flukes, which infect the intestine, liver, lung, and blood. Eosinophilia is a prominent clinical sign of trematode infection. These infections are uncommon in the United States.

### Schistosomiasis

*Etiology.* The trematodes (flukes) include *Schistosoma haematobium, S. mansoni, S. japonicum,* and, rarely, *S. intercalatum* and *S. mekongi.*

*Epidemiology.* Schistosomiasis affects more than 2 million people, mainly children and young adults. (The maximum incidence of infection is between ages 10 and 20 yr.) Humans are infected in contaminated water by cercariae that emerge in an infectious form from snails. They penetrate intact skin. Each adult worm migrates to specific sites: *S. haematobium* to the bladder plexus, and *S. intercalatum* and *S. mekongi* to the mesenteric vessels. The eggs are deposited by the adult flukes in urine (*S. haematobium*) or stool (*S. mansoni* and *S. japonicum*). Intermediate hosts for these complex parasites are freshwater snails that are infected by miracidia, which hatch from eggs in freshwater. *S. haematobium* is prevalent in Africa and the Middle East; *S. mansoni* in Africa, the Middle East, the Caribbean, and South America; *S. japonicum* in China, the Phillipines, and Indonesia; *S. mekongi* in the Far East; and *S. intercalatum* in West Africa.

*Clinical Manifestations.* The pathogenesis of schistosomiasis is due to eggs that are trapped at the site of depository or at metastatic locations. Within 3–12 wk of infection, while the worms are maturing, a syndrome of fever, malaise, cough, abdominal pain, and rash can occur. This is followed by a resultant inflammatory response that leads to further symptoms. In infection with *S. haematobium,* bladder granulomas may lead to renal failure and cancer of the bladder. In the other schistosomal infections, intestinal and hepatic egg deposition and inflammation lead to ulceration of the intestine, colic, abdominal pain, and bloody diarrhea. Parasinusoidal liver obstruction causes hepatosplenomegaly, portal hypertension, ascites, and hematemesis. *Katayama fever* is an acute condition, with fever, weight loss, hepatosplenomegaly, and eosinophilia.

*Diagnosis.* Eggs may be found in the stool or urine (*S. haematobium*) of infected individuals. Biopsy of the bladder or rectal mucosa may be helpful but usually is not necessary.

*Treatment.* Priziquantel is the drug of choice for therapy of schistosomiasis in children.

*Prevention.* Sanitary measures, molluscicides, and therapy for infected individuals may help control the illness.

## Tissue Tapeworms

*Etiology.* Canines become infected with tapeworms by eating infected sheep or cattle viscera. The larval stage of the canine tapeworm *Echinococcus granulosus* (hydatid disease) infects humans when *Echinococcus* eggs from dog feces or dog feces–contaminated material are ingested. Humans then become an intermediate host. The embryos pass through the intestine to the liver and other visceral organs, forming cysts up to 2 cm in diameter.

The cysticercus stage of *Taenia solium* (pork tapeworm) is responsible for *neurocysticercosis.* Humans are infected after consuming raw or undercooked larva-containing pork from pigs that were fed raw sewage contaminated with human feces containing *T. solium.* Fecal hand contamination is a potential source of infection.

*Epidemiology.* *E. granulosa* has a worldwide distribution but is endemic in sheep-raising and cattle-raising areas of Australia, South America, South Africa, the Soviet Union, and the Mediterranean region. The prevalence is highest in children. *T. solium* is endemic in Asia, Africa, and Latin and South America.

*Clinical Manifestations.* Symptoms due to *E. granulosa* result from space-occupying cysts and are most typical in adults. Pulmonary cysts may cause hemoptysis, cough, dyspnea, and respiratory distress. Brain cysts appear as tumors; liver cysts cause problems as they compress and obstruct blood flow.

Neurocysticercosis presents with generalized or focal seizures, variable eosinophilia, and calcification of cerebral cysts.

*Diagnosis.* Radiologic diagnosis is possible in endemic areas. Ultrasound confirms the cystic nature of the granulosa mass. Neurocysticercosis demonstrates CT findings of calcified cysts. Serologic tests also are helpful.

*Treatment.* Large or asymptomatic granulosa cysts are removed surgically. Treatment with albendazole has shown some benefit. Neurocysticercosis is treated with albendazole, praziquantel, steroids, and anticonvulsant drugs.

## References

Behrman RE, Kliegman RM, Arvin AM (eds): Nelson Textbook of Pediatrics, 15th ed. Philadelphia, WB Saunders, 1996, Chapters 245.3, 245.13.

Despommier DD: Tapeworm infection: The long and the short of it. N Engl J Med 327:727, 1992.

Hall A, Anwar KS, Tomkins AM: Intensity of reinfection with *Ascaris lumbricoides* and its implications for parasite control. Lancet 140:1253, 1992.

The Medical Letter: Drugs for parasitic infections. Med Lett 37:99, 1995.

Vazquez V, Sotelo J: The course of seizures after treatment for cerebral cysticercosis. N Engl J Med 327:696, 1992.

# Chapter 11

# THE GASTROINTESTINAL TRACT

Barbara S. Kirschner

Dennis D. Black

Gastrointestinal complaints are common pediatric problems. A careful history and physical examination are necessary to determine whether the symptoms are due to a primary gastrointestinal illness or to systemic disease states that may produce abdominal complaints. For example, abdominal pain in patients with sickle cell anemia may represent sickle cell pain crisis, transfusion-associated hepatitis, hemolysis-associated bilirubin stones and cholecystitis, renal papillary necrosis, or the usual causes of abdominal pain not associated with sickle cell anemia, such as gastroenteritis, appendicitis, and lactose malabsorption. Knowledge of the family history and questions that determine the relationship of symptoms to feeding, the color of emesis, the number and character of stools, the nature of defecation and the location of maximum pain can help formulate a differential diagnosis and select laboratory tests or diagnostic (roentgenographic, endoscopic) procedures.

It is important to recognize diseases and their manifestations that are associated with particular age groups. Hence, most patients with intestinal obstruction resulting from congenital anomalies of the esophagus, small intestine, and large bowel have symptoms in the 1st wk of life, whereas the age of onset of inflammatory bowel disease is usually during adolescence. Common manifestations of many gastrointestinal illnesses, both benign and serious, include pain, diarrhea, emesis, constipation, and gastrointestinal hemorrhage.

## CLINICAL MANIFESTATIONS OF GASTROINTESTINAL DISEASE

### ABDOMINAL PAIN

Abdominal pain is the most frequent gastrointestinal complaint that brings children and adolescents to the physician. This pain is classified as (1) visceral, (2) somatic, or (3) referred.

The sensation of pain from the abdominal viscera is produced in response to: (1) stretching or distending of the wall of a hollow organ or the capsule of a solid organ, (2) inflammation, or (3) ischemia. *Visceral pain* usually is dull or crampy and is poorly localized along the dermatomes that innervate the organ. Pain originating from the liver, pancreas, biliary tree, stomach, or proximal small intestine is felt in the epigastrium; pain from the distal small intestine, right colon, and appendix is felt in the periumbilical region; and pain from the left colon, urinary tract, or genital organs usually is felt in the suprapubic area.

Parietal or *somatic pain* represents peritoneal inflammation and is localized to the area of the involved viscera. Peritoneal pain is steady and sharp and associated with voluntary guarding or involuntary rigidity of the overlying abdominal muscles, with or without rebound pain.

*Referred pain* is due to local irritation, with referral along the pathway of innervation of the organ. Pain that begins as dull and poorly localized but that becomes more diffuse and severe suggests that a hollow viscus has ruptured and has progressed to peritonitis.

Critical to the evaluation of abdominal pain is both "how ill" the child appears and whether the onset of the complaint is new or recent (*acute*), or recurrent (*chronic*). As part of the history, it is necessary to determine the following (Table 11–1):

1. The age of onset, the location of the pain, its relation to feeding, its severity, time and frequency of occurrence, and duration and nature.
2. The presence or absence of associated symp-

TABLE 11–1.  Distinguishing Features of Abdominal Pain in Children

| Disease | Onset | Location | Referral | Quality | Comments |
|---|---|---|---|---|---|
| Functional: irritable bowel syndrome | Recurrent | Periumbilical splenic and hepatic flexures | None | Dull, crampy, intermittent, duration 2 hr | Family stress, school phobia, diarrhea/constipation |
| Esophageal reflux | Recurrent, after meals, bedtime | Substernal | Chest | Burning | Sour taste in mouth. Sandifer syndrome |
| Duodenal ulcer | Recurrent, before meals, at night | Epigastric | Back | Severe burning, gnawing | Relieved by food, milk, antacids; family history |
| Pancreatitis | Acute | Epigastric/hypogastric | Back | Constant, sharp, boring | Nausea, emesis, marked tenderness |
| Intestinal obstruction | Acute or gradual | Periumbilical—lower abdomen | Back | Alternating cramping (colic) and painless periods | Distention, obstipation, bilious emesis, increased bowel sounds |
| Appendicitis | Acute | Periumbilical or epigastric, localizes to right lower quadrant | Back or pelvis if retrocecal | Sharp, steady | Nausea, emesis, local tenderness, ± fever |
| Meckel diverticulum | Recurrent | Periumbilical—lower abdomen | None | Sharp | Hematochezia; painless unless intussusception, diverticulitis, or perforation |
| Inflammatory bowel disease | Recurrent | Depends on site of involvement | | Dull cramping, tenesmus | Fever, weight loss, ± hematochezia |
| Intussusception | Acute | Periumbilical—lower abdomen | None | Cramping, with painless periods | Guarded position with knees pulled up, "currant jelly" stools |
| Lactose intolerance | Recurrent with milk products | Lower abdomen | None | Cramping | Distention, gaseousness, diarrhea |
| Urolithiasis | Acute, sudden | Back | Groin | Severe colicky pain | Hematuria |
| Pyelonephritis | Acute, sudden | Back | None | Dull to sharp | Fever, costochondral tenderness, dysuria, urinary frequency |
| Cholecystitis/cholelithiasis | Acute | Right upper quadrant | Right shoulder | Severe colicky pain | Hemolysis ± jaundice, nausea, emesis |

Adapted from Andreoli TE, Carpenter CJ, Plum F, et al: Cecil Essentials of Medicine. Philadelphia, WB Saunders, 1986, p 261.

toms, such as weight loss, fever, vomiting, bloating, diarrhea, hematochezia, or urinary symptoms.

3. Whether any intercurrent illness or recent trauma has occurred.

### Acute Abdominal Pain

In children, acute abdominal pain may be due to extra-abdominal diseases (pneumonia; pharyngitis, especially when caused by group A streptococcus; otitis media; upper respiratory tract infections) although acute gastroenteritis is one of the most common abdominal causes of acute abdominal pain. Pain that persists and brings the patient back to the physician is often due to appendicitis, intussusception, urinary tract infections, pneumonia, and pharyngitis as well as gastroenteritis and viral syndromes. In infants younger than 2 yr of age, trauma, incarcerated hernias, intestinal malrotation, and volvulus also must be considered. Between 2 and 5 yr of age, sickle cell anemia, lower lobe pneumonia, and urinary tract infections may mimic intestinal disorders. In the older child and adolescent, appendicitis is more common and may be difficult to distinguish from gastroenteritis. In the adolescent girl, *mittelschmerz*, ectopic pregnancy, ovarian cysts, and pelvic inflammatory disease are important considerations. Less common causes of acute pain include pancreatitis, Henoch-Schönlein purpura, mesenteric adenitis, lead poisoning, diabetic ketoacidosis, renal stones, and cholecystitis. Sudden acute, excruciating pain suggests obstruction (stones), perforation, or ischemia. Complete blood count (CBC) with differential, urinalysis, pregnancy test, bacterial cultures, serum amylase or lipase, ultrasonography, and abdominal plain films support the findings of a careful history and physical examination. Re-examination several hours later may be necessary to help establish the diagnosis.

## Reference

Scholer S, PiTuch K, Orr D, et al: Clinical outcomes of children with acute abdominal pain. Pediatrics 98:680, 1996.

## Chronic Abdominal Pain

Of all children between the ages of 5 and 15 yr, 10–15% experience chronic abdominal pain. *Chronic recurrent abdominal pain* is defined as three or more episodes of pain, severe enough to affect activities, occurring over a period of 3 mo.

In a large percentage, no specific underlying organic cause is found; the pain may be due to dysfunctional bowel with altered motility. The term *irritable bowel syndrome* frequently is applied to this condition. Associated symptoms include pallor, nausea, headaches, vomiting, lethargy, and diarrhea. Disorders such as nocturnal enuresis, fears, and sleep disturbances are seen in 30% of those with this syndrome. The mother, the father, or other siblings often suffer from abdominal pain. Social factors, such as a new school, new teacher, examinations, peer group conflict, moving, family illness or death, sibling rivalry, or parental pressure for achievement, frequently precipitate or are associated with attacks of pain.

An unknown proportion of patients with chronic pain have lactose intolerance, also manifested by bloating, gaseousness, or diarrhea. In infants, chronic abdominal pain also may be due to colic, gastroesophageal reflux and esophagitis, celiac disease, malrotation, and intra-abdominal tumors. Older children may have pain resulting from acid peptic disease (esophagitis, gastritis, gastric or duodenal ulcer), giardiasis, inflammatory bowel

disease, sickle cell anemia, and, rarely, porphyria, hereditary angioedema, systemic lupus erythematosus (SLE) (vasculitis, serositis), and familial Mediterranean fever. Menstruation-related pain is common in adolescence.

*Diagnostic evaluation* includes a CBC, erythrocyte sedimentation rate (ESR), urinalysis, stools for occult blood and ova and parasites, abdominal ultrasound, and upper gastrointestinal series with small bowel follow-through. Breath hydrogen testing after a lactose challenge identifies lactose intolerance. An upper gastrointestinal series or a barium enema is indicated when malrotation or intussusception are suggested, respectively.

*Treatment* of the irritable bowel syndrome should be directed at: (1) explaining the functional and benign nature of this syndrome, (2) identifying sources of stress and providing guidance on how to relieve them, and (3) offering sympathetic reassurance. In some patients, short-term antispasmodic anticholinergic agents may relieve pain, and a high-fiber diet may be beneficial, especially when constipation is present. Formal psychiatric intervention occasionally may be necessary. Specific therapy for other conditions is discussed later in this chapter.

## DIARRHEA AND MALABSORPTION

The small intestinal mucosa is composed of villous epithelium, crypt epithelium, lamina propria, and muscularis mucosa (Fig. 11–1).

### Pathophysiology of Diarrhea

Five mechanisms explain the pathophysiology of diarrhea (Table 11–2). More than one of these may be present at the same time. A number of disease processes directly affect the secretory and absorptive function of the enterocyte. Some of these processes act by increasing cyclic adenosine monophosphate (cAMP) levels (*Vibrio cholerae, Escherichia coli,* heat-labile toxin, vasoactive intestinal peptide–producing tumors); other processes cause secretory diarrhea by unknown mechanisms (*Shigella* toxin, congenital chloridorrhea). Activation of intestinal production of cAMP produces secretory diarrhea by inhibiting free mucosal sodium chloride absorption and stimulating mucosal chloride secretion. Stimulation of cyclic guanosine monophosphate by *E. coli* heat-stable toxin produces the same effect. Virulence factors for various enteropathogens are noted in Table 11–3. Intestinal resection, inflammation, and infection reduce mucosal surface area, which impairs both digestion and absorption. Ab-

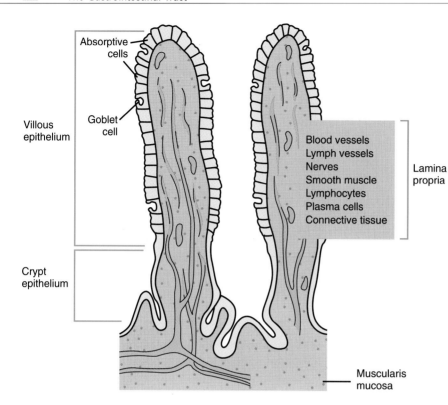

FIGURE 11–1. Anatomy of the mucosa of the small intestine.

TABLE 11–2. Mechanisms of Diarrhea

| Primary Mechanism | Defect | Stool Examination | Examples | Comment |
|---|---|---|---|---|
| Secretory | Decreased absorption, increased secretion | Watery, normal osmolality; osmols = 2 × (Na⁺ + K⁺) | Cholera, toxigenic *E. coli*; carcinoid, VIP, neuroblastoma, congenital chloride diarrhea, *Clostridium difficile, cryptosporidiosis* (AIDS) | Persists during fasting; bile salt malabsorption also may increase intestinal water secretion; no stool leukocytes |
| Osmotic | Maldigestion, transport defects, ingestion of unabsorbable solute | Watery, acidic, + reducing substances; increased osmolality; osmols >2 × (Na⁺ + K⁺) | Lactase deficiency, glucose-galactose malabsorption, lactulose, laxative abuse | Stops with fasting, increased breath hydrogen with carbohydrate malabsorption, no stool leukocytes |
| Increased motility | Decreased transit time or stasis (bacterial overgrowth) | Fecal-like, stimulated by gastrocolic reflex | Irritable bowel syndrome, thyrotoxicosis, postvagotomy dumping syndrome | Infection also may contribute to increased motility |
| Decreased surface area | Decreased functional capacity | Watery | Short bowel syndrome, celiac disease, rotavirus enteritis | May require elemental diet plus parenteral alimentation |
| Mucosal invasion (motile or secretory) | Inflammation, decreased colonic reabsorption, increased motility | Blood and increased WBCs in stool | *Salmonella, Shigella,* amebiasis, *Yersinia, Campylobacter* | Dysentery = blood, mucus, and WBCs |

AIDS = acquired immunodeficiency syndrome; VIP = vasoactive intestinal peptide; WBC = white blood cell.

TABLE 11–3.  Virulence Characteristics of Enteropathogens

| Organisms | Virulence Properties |
|---|---|
| *Campylobacter jejuni* | Invasion; enterotoxin |
| *Clostridium difficile* | Cytotoxin; enterotoxin |
| Cryptosporidium | Adherence |
| Cyclospora | Inflammation |
| *Entamoeba histolytica* | Cyst resistant to physical destruction; invasion; enzyme and cytotoxin production |
| Enteric adenovirus | Mucosal lesion |
| *Escherichia coli* | |
|   Enteropathogenic | Unknown, possibly cytotoxin or adherence |
|   Enterotoxigenic | Enterotoxins (heat stable or labile) |
|   Invasive | Invasion |
|   Enterohemorrhagic (0157:H7) | Cytotoxin |
| *Giardia lamblia* | Cyst resistant to physical destruction; adheres to mucosa |
| Norwalk-like viruses | Mucosal lesion |
| Rotavirus | Damage to microvilli |
| *Shigella* | Invasion; enterotoxin; cytotoxin |
| *Salmonella* | Invasion; enterotoxin |
| *Vibrio cholerae* | Enterotoxin |
| *Vibrio parahaemolyticus* | Invasion; cytotoxin |
| *Yersinia enterocolitica* | Invasion; enterotoxin |

normal intestinal motility reduces mucosal contact time, decreasing both digestion and absorption.

## Acute Diarrhea

A *differential diagnosis* of acute diarrhea in children is presented in Table 11–4. In addition to a complete history, which includes epidemiologic data (day care, travel, single source outbreak, animal and food contact), antibiotic exposure, and a physical examination, the stool should be tested for occult blood and white blood cells (with methylene blue smear). If the stool is negative for both blood and white blood cells, and there is no history to suggest contaminated food ingestion, the cause most likely is viral. Parasitic infestations other than giardiasis, cryptosporidiosis, and, where endemic, amebiasis are not common causes of acute diarrhea. Stool examinations for parasites usually are not helpful unless the diarrhea persists. If the stool is positive for blood and white blood cells, bacterial causes must be excluded first. The absence of bacterial pathogens and toxins suggests the diagnosis of inflammatory bowel disease, particularly in the adolescent patient who demonstrates weight loss, fever, and abdominal pain.

### Specific Causes of Infectious Diarrhea

*Viral Causes.* Viruses associated with gastroenteritis in infants include the rotavirus, calicivirus, enteric adenovirus, astrovirus, and members of the Norwalk agent group. *Rotavirus* is the most frequent cause of diarrhea during the winter months. Primary infection with rotavirus in infancy may cause moderate to severe disease, whereas reinfection in adolescence leads to mild illness. Rotavirus invades the epithelium of upper small intestine; in severe cases, it may extend throughout the small bowel and colon, resulting in villus damage, secondary transient disaccharidase deficiency, and inflammation in the lamina propria. Vomiting may last for 3–4 days, diarrhea for 7–10 days; dehydration is noted in younger patients.

The *diagnosis* may be confirmed on Rotazyme (enzyme-linked immunosorbent assay [ELISA]) testing of the stool. *Treatment* is supportive and consists of supplying fluid and electrolytes to prevent dehydration. Refractory cases featuring protracted diarrhea may benefit from oral immunoglobulins (Ig) or lactobacillus LGG.

### Bacterial Causes

*E. COLI.* Only certain strains of *E. coli* produce diarrhea. *E. coli* is classified by the mechanism of diarrhea: enteropathogenic (EPEC), enterotoxigenic (ETEC), enteroinvasive (EIEC), enteroadherent (EAEC), and enterohemorrhagic (EHEC) (see Table 11–3). EPEC and ETEC adhere to the epithelial cells in the upper small intestine and produce disease by liberating toxins that induce intestinal secretion and limit absorption. EIEC invades the colonic mucosa, producing widespread mucosal damage with acute inflammation. EPEC is responsible for many of the epidemics of diarrhea in nurseries for neonates and day care centers. ETEC plays a major role in **traveler's diarrhea.** EHEC is responsible for a hemorrhagic colitis and most cases of the **hemolytic-uremic syndrome,** especially the *E. coli* 0157:H7 strain. *Treatment* is indicated for infants under 3 mo of age with EPEC and for those patients who remain symptomatic (Table 11–5).

*SALMONELLA.* Salmonellae are transmitted through contact with infected animals (chickens, pet reptiles, turtles) or from contaminated food products, such as milk, eggs, and poultry. The organism produces disease by invading the intestinal mucosa. *Treatment* of mild illness does not shorten the clini-

TABLE 11–4.  Differential Diagnosis of Diarrhea

| | Infant | Child | Adolescent |
|---|---|---|---|
| **Acute** | | | |
| Common | Gastroenteritis<br>Systemic infection<br>Antibiotic associated<br>Overfeeding | Gastroenteritis<br>Food poisoning<br>Systemic infection<br>Antibiotic associated | Gastroenteritis<br>Food poisoning<br>Antibiotic associated |
| Rare | Primary disaccharidase deficiency<br>Hirschsprung toxic colitis<br>Adrenogenital syndrome | Toxic ingestion | Hyperthyroidism |
| **Chronic** | | | |
| Common | Postinfectious secondary lactase<br>  deficiency<br>Cow's milk/soy protein intolerance<br>Chronic nonspecific diarrhea of<br>  infancy<br>Celiac disease<br>Cystic fibrosis<br>AIDS enteropathy | Postinfectious secondary lactase<br>  deficiency<br>Irritable bowel syndrome<br>Celiac disease<br>Lactose intolerance<br>Giardiasis<br>Inflammatory bowel disease<br>AIDS enteropathy | Irritable bowel syndrome<br>Inflammatory bowel<br>  disease<br>Lactose intolerance<br>Giardiasis<br>Laxative abuse (anorexia<br>  nervosa) |
| Rare | Primary immune defects<br>Familial villous atrophy<br>Secretory tumors<br>Congenital chloridorrhea<br>Acrodermatitis enteropathica<br>Lymphangiectasia<br>Abetalipoproteinemia<br>Eosinophilic gastroenteritis<br>Short bowel syndrome<br>Intractable diarrhea syndrome<br>Autoimmune enteropathy | Acquired immune defects<br>Secretory tumors<br>Pseudo-obstruction | Secretory tumor<br>Primary bowel tumor<br>Gay bowel disease |

AIDS = acquired immunodeficiency syndrome.

cal course, but does prolong bacterial excretion. Antibiotic therapy is necessary only for high-risk patients who have symptoms of toxicity, develop metastatic foci, or have *S. typhi* infection (see Table 11–5).

*SHIGELLA.* Shigellae may cause disease by producing toxin either alone or in combination with tissue invasion. Infection is spread by person-to-person contact or by the ingestion of contaminated food. The colon is selectively affected. Antibiotic *treatment* produces a bacteriologic cure in 80% of patients after 48 hr, thus reducing the spread of the disease. Many *S. sonnei*, the predominant strain affecting children, are ampicillin-resistant. Treatment with trimethoprim/sulfamethoxazole generally is effective (see Table 11–5).

*CAMPYLOBACTER JEJUNI.* C. jejuni may account for 15% of episodes of bacterial diarrhea. The infection is spread by person-to-person contact and by contaminated water and food. The organism invades the mucosa of the jejunum, ileum, and colon, producing enterocolitis. Most patients recover spontaneously before the diagnosis is established. *Treatment* speeds recovery and reduces the duration of the carrier state (see Table 11–5).

*YERSINIA ENTEROCOLITICA.* The organism is transmitted by pets and by contaminated food (e.g., chitterlings). Infants and young children characteristically have a diarrheal disease, whereas older children usually have acute lesions of the terminal ileum or acute mesenteric lymphadenitis resembling appendicitis or Crohn disease. Arthritis, rash, and spondylopathy may develop. The course usually is self-limited, lasting 3 days to 3 wk. The efficacy of antibiotic *treatment* is questionable, but children with septicemia or infection in sites other than the gastrointestinal tract should be treated (Table 11–5).

*CLOSTRIDIUM DIFFICILE.* This organism is a common cause of antibiotic-associated diarrhea. *Treatment* includes discontinuation of the prior antibiotic and, if diarrhea is severe, oral vancomycin or metronidazole.

Many bacterial agents may be food contaminants and cause food poisoning. Sudden onset, a common source, epidemic vomiting, and diarrhea should suggest food poisoning (Table 11–6).

**Parasitic Causes.** *Entamoeba histolytica* and *Giardia lamblia* are important parasites found in North America that produce disease. Amebiasis occurs

TABLE 11–5.  Antibiotic Therapy of Diarrhea

| Organism | Treatment* | Comment |
|---|---|---|
| *Salmonella typhi* | Ampicillin§, chloramphenicol§, trimethoprim/sulfamethoxazole, cefotaxime, ciprofloxacin† | Invasive, bacteremic disease |
| Other *Salmonella* | Usually none; amoxicillin, ampicillin, trimethoprim-sulfamethoxazole, cefotaxime, ciprofloxacin† | Treatment indicated if less than 3 mo of age, or if malignancy, sickle cell anemia, AIDS, evidence of nongastrointestinal foci of infection are present |
| *Shigella* | Trimethoprim/sulfamethoxazole, ampicillin | Amoxicillin is not recommended; treatment reduces infectivity and improves outcome |
| *Escherichia coli* Toxigenic | Usually none if endemic; trimethoprim/sulfamethoxazole or ciprofloxacin for traveler's diarrhea | Prevention of traveler's diarrhea with bismuth subsalicylate, doxycycline, or ciprofloxacin† |
| Invasive or pathogenic | Trimethoprim/sulfamethoxazole, neomycin | |
| *Campylobacter* | Mild disease needs no treatment; erythromycin for diarrhea, gentamicin for systemic illness | If started early (days 1–3), treatment reduces symptoms and fecal organisms |
| *Yersinia* | None for diarrhea; gentamicin, chloramphenicol, trimethoprim/sulfamethoxazole for systemic illness | Value of treatment of mesenteric adenitis with antibiotics is not established |
| *Vibrio cholerae* | Tetracycline, trimethoprim/sulfamethoxazole | Fluid maintenance is critical |
| *Clostridium difficile* | Oral vancomycin, metronidazole‡ | *C. difficile* is an agent of antibiotic-associated diarrhea and pseudomembranous colitis |
| *Giardia lamblia* | Quinacrine, furazolidone, metronidazole‡ | Furazolidone only preparation available in liquid form |
| *Cryptosporidium* | None; azithromycin or paromomycin + octreotide in AIDS | A serious infection in immunocompromised patients (AIDS) |
| *Entamoeba histolytica* | Metronidazole‡, tinidazole followed by iodoquinol | |

*All treatment is predicated on knowledge of antimicrobial sensitivities.
†Ciprofloxacin is not indicated for children with growing bones and uncomplicated infections.
‡The safety of metronidazole in children is unknown.
§Often resistant.
AIDS = acquired immunodeficiency syndrome.

in warmer climates, whereas giardiasis is endemic throughout the United States and is common among infants in day care centers.

E. HISTOLYTICA. The site of infection with this organism is the colon, although amebae may pass through the bowel wall and invade the liver, lung, and brain. Diarrhea is of acute onset, is bloody, and contains white blood cells. *Diagnosis* depends on identification of the organism in the stool and may be confirmed serologically. The drug of choice for *treatment* is metronidazole.

G. LAMBLIA. This organism is transmitted through ingestion of cysts either from contact with an infected individual or from food or fresh or well water contaminated with infected feces. It adheres to the microvilli of the duodenal and jejunal epithelium. The onset of the illness usually is insidious but may be acute. *Clinical manifestations* include anorexia, nausea, gaseousness, abdominal distention, watery diarrhea, secondary lactose intolerance, and weight loss. The *diagnosis* may be made by identifying the organism in the stool, in duodenal aspirate, or in the mucosa of a small bowel biopsy. See Table 11–5 for *treatment*.

CRYPTOSPORIDIUM. This causes mild diarrhea in immunocompetent infants attending day care centers. In contrast to the severe diarrhea it produces in patients with acquired immunodeficiency syn-

TABLE 11–6.   Common Causes of Food Poisoning

| Agent | Mechanism | Source | Time of Onset | Signs |
|---|---|---|---|---|
| *Salmonella** | Tissue invasion | Dairy/meat products, eggs | 16–48 hr | Fever, cramps, vomiting, bloody diarrhea |
| *Staphylococcus aureus** | Preformed toxin | Meat, egg salad, pastries | 1–6 hr | Vomiting, diarrhea |
| *Clostridium perfringens** | In vivo toxin production | Meat, gravy | 8–16 hr | Cramps, diarrhea |
| *Clostridium botulinum** | Preformed toxin | Canned food, honey, fish | 18–36 hr | Nausea, vomiting, diarrhea, constipation, paralysis |
| *Escherichia coli* 0157:H7 | Verotoxin | Undercooked meat, cider, water | 24–72 hr | Watery bloody diarrhea: HUS |
| *Bacillus cereus* | | | | |
| Short incubation | Preformed toxin | Fried rice | 1–6 hr | Nausea, vomiting |
| Long incubation | Toxin produced in vivo | Vegetables | 8–16 hr | Vomiting, diarrhea, cramps |
| Cryptosporidiosis | Adherence | Apple cider, water | 24–48 hr | Vomiting, diarrhea, cramps |
| Norwalk agent | Invasion | Waterborne, shellfish | 16–48 hr | Watery diarrhea |
| Heavy metals† | Direct toxicity | Acidic juices in metal containers, lemonade, fruit punch | 1–4 hr | Vomiting, cramps, diarrhea |
| Scombroid | Histamine | Tuna | Minutes | Flushing, dizziness, headache, vomiting, diarrhea |
| Ciguatera | Toxin | Mackerel | 1–6 hr | Paresthesia of lips, tooth pain, cramps, vomiting, diarrhea |
| Paralytic shellfish | Neurotoxin | Dinoflagellates of mollusks | 1–3 hr | Paresthesia of lips and extremities, dysphagia, ataxia |

*Salmonella* (23%), *S. aureus* (18%), *C. perfringens* (8%), and *C. botulinum* (8%) are the most common causes of food poisoning.
†Includes copper, zinc, tin, and cadmium.
HUS = hemolytic uremic syndrome.

drome (AIDS), cryptosporidiosis in normal infants is a self-limited disease (see Table 11–5).

**Management of Diarrhea.** Therapy must be directed to cure the initiating event, to correct dehydration and ongoing fluid and electrolyte deficits, and to manage secondary complications resulting from mucosal injury. Antibiotic treatment is noted in Table 11–5. **Traveler's diarrhea** may be prevented by avoiding uncooked food and untreated drinking water; preventive medication with Pepto-Bismol, tetracycline (8 yr of age or older), or trimethoprim/sulfamethoxazole is controversial. In the near future, **rotavirus diarrhea** may be prevented by vaccination.

*Treatment of fluid deficits* requires an estimation of the degree of dehydration and the determination of any electrolyte imbalance, such as hyperna-

tremia, hyponatremia, or metabolic acidosis (see Chapter 16). Acidosis is due to stool bicarbonate losses, lactic acidosis resulting from fermentation of malabsorbed carbohydrate or shock, and phosphate retention resulting from transient prerenal renal insufficiency. Therapy for severe fluid and electrolyte losses requires intravenous alimentation, whereas less severe degrees of dehydration (<10%) in infants without excessive vomiting may be managed with oral rehydration solutions containing glucose and electrolytes. Jejunal and ileal glucose absorption carry sodium into the enterocyte, thus also drawing in water. Oral rehydration solutions contain 2–2.5% glucose, 75–90 mEq/L $Na^+$, 20–25 mEq/L $K^+$, 45–80 mEq/L $Cl^-$, and 30 mEq/L bicarbonate or citrate.

Severe infections may damage the mucosa, producing a secondary lactase deficiency that causes osmotic diarrhea if a lactose-containing formula is given to an infant. Therefore, a non–lactose-containing formula may be needed during the immediate rehabilitation phase following episodes of *severe* diarrhea. Drugs such as loperamide, paregoric, and diphenoxylate are potentially dangerous and have no place in the management of acute infectious diarrhea in children.

## References

Behrman RE, Kliegman RM, Arvin AM (eds): Nelson Textbook of Pediatrics, 15th ed. Philadelphia, WB Saunders, 1996, Chapters 171, 182–186, 188, 219, 244.

Caprioli A, Pezzella C, Morelli R, et al: Enteropathogens associated with childhood diarrhea in Italy. Pediatr Infect Dis J 15:876, 1996.

Carmeli Y, Samore M, Shoshany O, et al: Utility of clinical versus laboratory tests for the evaluation of acute gastroenteritis. Dig Dis Sci 4:1749, 1996.

Cohen M: Etiology and mechanisms of acute infectious diarrhea in the United States. J Pediatr 118:34, 1994.

Gavin N, Merrick N, Davidson D: Efficacy of glucose based oral rehydration therapy. Pediatrics 98:45, 1996.

Provisional Committee on Quality Improvement, Subcommittee on Acute Gastroenteritis: Practice parameter: The management of acute gastroenteritis in young children. Pediatrics 97:424, 1996.

## Chronic Diarrhea

*Clinical Manifestations.* During infancy, chronic diarrhea may be a manifestation of specific genetic diseases, such as disaccharidase deficiencies, cystic fibrosis, or immunologically mediated diseases (see Table 11–4). *Cow's milk–soy protein intolerance* should be considered in infants younger than 1 yr of age when the stool contains erythrocytes, with or without eosinophils. This can occur even in breast-fed infants if cow's milk proteins enter maternal milk. The mechanism by which milk proteins result in mucosal injury is poorly understood. Immune-mediated disease against gluten (**celiac disease**) begins once the infant is exposed to solid foods containing this protein. Cereals composed of wheat, barley, rye, and, possibly, oats produce the disease, which may necessitate a lifelong withdrawal from these foods.

Chronic diarrhea may also be the only manifestation of **cystic fibrosis**, or this disease may occur in association with meconium ileus, rectal prolapse, hypoalbuminemia, hyponatremic dehydration, and hypoprothrombinemia. The *diagnosis* of cystic fibrosis is confirmed by an elevated sweat chloride content. Primary metabolic disorders of absorption, such as *glucose-galactose malabsorption* and *congenital chloridorrhea*, appear in the neonatal period.

The most common cause of chronic diarrhea during infancy is **chronic nonspecific diarrhea of infancy,** or **toddler's diarrhea**. The onset is between 6 mo and 3 yr of age and is rarely accompanied by pain. Often the first stool in the morning is formed, but stools (four to six per 24 hr) progress during the day to greater liquidity, sometimes containing mucus and food. The infants do not demonstrate fluid and electrolyte abnormalities, dehydration, or failure to thrive. There is often a family history of similar intestinal problems in siblings or in parents. Symptoms may be precipitated by teething or common infectious illnesses. This disorder may be due to ingestion of fruit juices containing large quantities of nonabsorbable sugars that produce diarrhea. In this same age group, a **lactase deficiency** following viral gastroenteritides also is common and may result in secondary lactose malabsorption that may persist for months. Increased breath hydrogen excretion following a standard oral lactose challenge, resulting from colonic bacterial fermentation of malabsorbed lactose, is diagnostic. Bloating, cramping, borborygmus, and flatus also are noted in lactose-intolerant patients during the lactose challenge. A non–lactose-containing formula may be needed until lactase activity regenerates. **Congenital sucrose deficiency** is rare and occurs after sucrose-containing foods (fruits, juices, vegetables) are added to the diet in sufficient quantities to exceed the digestive capacity of the brush border sucrase; treatment consists of avoiding sucrose sugar–containing foods.

Beyond infancy, lactase deficiency and parasitic infection, usually giardiasis, are important common causes of chronic diarrhea (see Table 11–4). Diarrhea as the only manifestation of irritable bowel syndrome is unusual in older children and adolescents. During this older age period, **inflammatory bowel disease** should be considered, especially when diarrhea is associated with fever, hematochezia, abdominal pain, weight loss, rash, arthralgias or arthritis, and uveitis or episcleritis.

When chronic diarrhea persists and is associated with weight loss and global or specific nutritional deficiencies, a **malabsorption syndrome** exists. The usual early manifestations of malabsorption are frequent, bulky-oily, foul-smelling stools (steatorrhea); weight loss; and a ravenous appetite. Late manifestations include failure to thrive, muscle wasting, protuberant abdomen, secondary immune deficiency, and nutritional disorders. Malabsorption of specific nutrients (e.g., vitamin D, which results in rickets; vitamin K, which results in hemorrhage; vitamin $B_{12}$, folate, and iron, which result in anemia; and calcium, which results in hypocalcemic tetany) may develop. Mechanisms of malabsorption include impaired digestion, reduced absorption, decreased surface area, lymphatic obstruction, drugs, infection, collagen vascular disease, and endocrine abnormalities (Table 11–7). Cystic fibrosis, celiac sprue, short bowel syndrome, and giardiasis are common causes of malabsorption. Immune deficiencies usually associated with enteritis include Wiskott-Aldrich syndrome, common variable hypogammaglobulinemia, and AIDS. Certain AIDS-related opportunistic intestinal infections (*Isospora belli, Cryptosporidium, Entamoeba,* and cytomegalovirus) also cause malabsorption and failure to thrive.

**Diagnosis.** The *diagnosis* of a patient with

**TABLE 11–7.** Malabsorption Syndromes

| **Reduced Digestion** | |
|---|---|
| Pancreatic exocrine deficiency | Cystic fibrosis, pancreatitis, Shwachman syndrome |
| Bile salt deficiency | Cholestasis, biliary atresia, hepatitis, cirrhosis, bacterial deconjugation |
| Enzyme defects | Lactase, sucrase, enterokinase, lipase deficiencies |
| **Reduced Absorption** | |
| Primary absorption defects | Glucose-galactose malabsorption, abetalipoproteinemia, cystinuria, Hartnup disease |
| Decreased mucosal surface area | Crohn disease, malnutrition, short bowel syndrome, antimetabolite chemotherapy, familial villous atrophy |
| Small intestinal disease | Celiac disease, tropical sprue, giardiasis, immune/allergic enteritis, Crohn disease, lymphoma, AIDS |
| **Lymphatic Obstruction** | |
| | Lymphangiectasia, Whipple disease, lymphoma, chylous ascites |
| **Others** | |
| Drugs | Antibiotics, antimetabolites, neomycin, laxatives |
| Collagen vascular | Scleroderma |
| **Infestations** | |
| | Hookworms, tapeworm, giardiasis, immune defects |

chronic diarrhea begins with a careful history, including a family and dietary history as it relates to the onset of symptoms. It is important to remember that neither stool odor, which is usually unpleasant, nor stool color, unless blood is seen, has any consistent relationship to the presence of gastrointestinal disease. Physical examination should include a careful assessment of the patient's nutritional status (see Chapter 2) and a check for signs of infection.

Stool should be tested for blood, white blood cells, fat content, and carbohydrate malabsorption. The malabsorption is assessed by identifying an acid stool pH and reducing substances. Fecal fat should not exceed 15% of intake in infants and 10% in older children. To exclude parasitic infection, the clinician must collect three fresh stool specimens for examination. Barium studies should not be done within several days of the stool collection because parasites adhere to the barium. *Roentgenographic findings* may be diagnostic for inflammatory bowel disease; however, for many of the small intestinal mucosal disorders, only a nonspecific "malabsorption pattern," characterized by thickened mucosal folds, edema of the bowel wall, and flocculation of the barium, is present.

A number of studies are available to assess specific types of malabsorption. The D-xylose test provides an index of mucosal carbohydrate absorption. Lactose and sucrose malabsorption can be measured by the breath hydrogen technique. A Sudan stain of the stool may be used as a qualitative assessment of fecal fat, but steatorrhea is best quantitated by a 72-hr fecal fat study. Measurement of the fecal alpha$_1$-antitrypsin level is a screening study for documenting enteric protein loss. Quantitative measurements of protein loss can be made by assessing alpha$_1$-antitrypsin clearance with simultaneous serum and 24-hr stool concentrations. Serum calcium, prothrombin time, and vitamin A and E levels may be determined to assess fat-soluble vitamin deficiencies.

Peroral, *transpyloric biopsy* during gastroduodenoscopy of the small intestinal mucosa may be needed to document diseases such as celiac sprue, lymphangiectasia, giardiasis, abetalipoproteinemia, and tropical sprue.

**Treatment.** Treatment must be directed at the primary disease and at the correction of associated deficiency states, such as rickets and hypoprothrombinemia. Primary therapy for cystic fibrosis requires lifelong pancreatic enzyme replacement, whereas therapy for celiac disease requires strict adherence to a gluten-free diet. Hyperalimentation may be needed for familial enteropathies, short bowel syndrome, or refractory cases of chronic intractable diarrhea.

## References

Behrman RE, Kliegman RM, Arvin AM (eds): Nelson Textbook of Pediatrics, 15th ed. Philadelphia, WB Saunders, 1996, Chapters 252, 284–287.

Goulet O, Kedinger M, Brousse N, et al: Intractable diarrhea of infancy with epithelial and basement membrane abnormalities. J Pediatr 127:212, 1995.

Hyams J, Burke G, Davis P, et al: Abdominal pain and irritable bowel syndrome in adolescents: A community based study. J Pediatr 129:220, 1996.

## CONSTIPATION AND ENCOPRESIS

*Constipation* is defined as infrequent passage of hard, dry stools. *Obstipation* is the absence of bowel movements. The causes of constipation are noted in Table 11–8. Beyond the neonatal period, the most common cause (90–95%) of constipation is voluntary withholding (*functional constipation*), a problem often beginning with the attempt to toilet train the infant (Table 11–9). A family history of similar problems often is obtained. Stool retention may be due to conflicts in toilet training but usually is caused by pain on defecation, which creates a fear of defecation, and further retention. Voluntary withholding of stool increases distention of the rectum, which decreases rectal sensation, necessitating an even greater fecal mass to initiate the urge to defecate. Complications of stool retention include impaction, abdominal pain, overflow diarrhea resulting from leakage around the fecal mass, anal fissure, rectal bleeding, and urinary tract infection caused by extrinsic pressure on the urethra.

*Encopresis*, which is daytime or nighttime soiling by formed stools beyond the age of expected toilet training (4-5 yr), is another complication of constipation (see Chapter 1). In older children, it is important to ask specifically about soiling, because such information may not be expressed because of embarrassment. These children frequently are unable to sense the need to defecate because of stretching of the internal sphincter by the retained fecal mass.

In term infants, meconium should be passed within the first 24 hr of life; failure to pass meconium suggests an underlying disorder. The consistency and frequency of bowel movements vary greatly both in the individual child and among different children. Breast-fed infants usually produce stool with every feeding but may produce stool only one to two times a day. Formula-fed infants usually produce stool daily but may produce stool once every 2 or 3 days. In general, the range of normal for infants is from five stools/day to as few as one every 3rd day.

Stool is produced as the fecal fluid is moved through the colon by three to four mass propulsive movements per day. Water and electrolytes are reabsorbed (95%) in the colon and rectosigmoid, resulting in formed stool. Stool is stored in the rectum until sufficient distention produces the urge to defecate. The internal anal sphincter then relaxes and stool enters the anal canal. The external anal sphincter is a voluntary muscle controlling fecal continence. Failure to defecate may be due to decreased peristalsis (aganglionic segment, spinal cord defect), decreased expulsion (weakened abdominal muscle), and anatomic malformations (anterior dislocation of the anus, neuronal dysgenesis, aganglionic Hirschsprung disease, stenosis). The exclusion of Hirschsprung disease is critical in the *differential diagnosis* of constipation, especially in infants because of the risk of bacterial overgrowth, enterocolitis, and intestinal perforation (see Table 11–9).

*Functional constipation* may be self-perpetuating, often becoming more severe with time; symptomatic treatment is indicated. In infants, increases in

TABLE 11–8.  Causes of Constipation

**Nonorganic (Functional)**

**Organic**

   *Intestinal*

      Hirschsprung disease
      Neuronal dysgenesis
      Anal stenosis
      Anal stricture
      Anterior dislocation of the anus
      Pseudo-obstruction
      Collagen vascular diseases
      Rectal abscess/fissure
      Stricture post-NEC

   *Drugs*

      Lead
      Narcotics
      Antidepressants
      Psychoactive drugs (chlorpromazine [Thorazine])
      Chemotherapeutic agents (vincristine)
      Pancreatic enzymes (fibrosing colonopathy)

   *Metabolic*

      Dehydration
      Cystic fibrosis (meconium ileus equivalent)
      Hypothyroidism
      Hypokalemia
      Hypercalcemia

   *Neuromuscular*

      Infant botulism
      Absent abdominal muscle
      Myotonic dystrophy
      Spinal cord lesions (tumors or spina bifida)
      Chagas disease

NEC = necrotizing enterocolitis.

TABLE 11–9.    Distinguishing Features of Hirschsprung Disease and Functional (Acquired) Constipation

|  | Functional Constipation | Hirschsprung Disease* |
|---|---|---|
| **History** | | |
| Onset of constipation | After 2 yr of age | At birth |
| Encopresis | Common | Very rare |
| Forced bowel training | Usual | None |
| Stool size | Very large | Small, ribbon-like |
| Enterocolitis | None | Possible |
| Abdominal pain | Common | Common |
| Failure to thrive | Uncommon | Common |
| Family history | Variable | Yes but not always |
| **Examination** | | |
| Abdominal distention | Variable | Common |
| Poor growth | Rare | Common |
| Anal tone | Patulous | Tight |
| Rectal examination | Stool in ampulla | Ampulla empty |
| Malnutrition | Absent | Possible |
| **Laboratory** | | |
| Barium enema | Massive amounts of stool, no transition zone | Transition zone, delayed evacuation (greater than 24 hr) |
| Rectal biopsy | Normal | No ganglion cells; ↑ acetylcholinesterase staining |
| Anorectal manometry | Distension of the rectum causes relaxation of the internal sphincter | No sphincter relaxation |

Modified from Behrman RE, Kliegman RM, Arvin AM (eds): Nelson Textbook of Pediatrics, 15th ed. Philadelphia, WB Saunders, 1996, p 1071.
*Note that ultra-short-segment Hirschsprung disease may have clinical features of functional (acquired) megacolon (e.g., constipation).

the intake of juices and fruits, malt extract, or lactulose is effective. For older children, mineral oil, 1–3 oz/24 hr given either in divided doses or as a single dose 2 hr after meals, and increased dietary fiber content usually are successful. If there is marked fecal retention, the rectum must be cleared of impacted stool with enemas and/or cathartics. Once stools are softened, the oil is gradually tapered but the fiber supplements must be continued on a regular basis for several months, during which time the dose gradually is reduced. Psychologic problems leading to or resulting from the constipation may need special attention (see Chapter 1).

## VOMITING

Vomiting occurs in both gastrointestinal and nongastrointestinal diseases in childhood. The forceful ejection of gastric contents is often preceded by nausea and is due to the coordination of gastric atony (except in pyloric stenosis), relaxation of the gastroesophageal junction, and increased intragastric (abdominal) pressure from abdominal wall contractions. Vomiting is mediated by the medullary emesis center in the floor of the 4th ventricle, which is influenced by gastrointestinal (visceral afferent) or nongastrointestinal (chemoreceptive trigger zone) stimuli. The latter elements are affected by various stimuli, including drugs and motion sickness. *Regurgitation* is not vomiting but rather a passive, nonforceful ejection of gastric contents resulting from reflux through a relaxed lower esophageal sphincter. Most infants younger than 3 mo of age regurgitate formula with no apparent ill effects.

The *differential diagnosis* of vomiting should be approached by consideration of age-specific diseases. During the neonatal period, gastrointestinal obstruction often is due to congenital malformations (Table 11–10). In infants, gastroenteritis, overfeeding, and gastroesophageal reflux are the most common causes of emesis and regurgitation. Food allergy and milk protein intolerance also are common. Nongastrointestinal diseases that produce emesis in the infant include systemic infec-

TABLE 11–10.  Causes of Gastrointestinal
              Obstruction

**Esophagus**

| | |
|---|---|
| Congenital | Tracheoesophageal fistula |
| | Isolated esophageal atresia |
| Acquired | Caustic agent esophageal stricture |
| | Peptic stricture |
| | Chagas disease |
| | Collagen vascular disease |

**Stomach**

| | |
|---|---|
| Congenital | Antral webs |
| | Pyloric stenosis |
| Acquired | Bezoars/foreign body |
| | Pyloric stricture (ulcer) |
| | Crohn disease |
| | Eosinophilic gastroenteropathy |
| | Prostaglandin induced |
| | Chronic granulomatous disease |
| | Epidermolysis bullosum |

**Small Intestine**

| | |
|---|---|
| Congenital | Duodenal atresia |
| | Annular pancreas |
| | Malrotation/volvulus |
| | Malrotation/Ladd bands |
| | Ileal atresia |
| | Meconium ileus |
| | Inguinal hernia |
| Acquired | Postsurgical adhesions |
| | Trauma (hematoma) |
| | Crohn disease |
| | Intussusception |
| | Meconium ileus equivalent (cystic fibrosis) |
| | Superior mesenteric artery syndrome |

**Colon**

| | |
|---|---|
| Congenital | Meconium plug |
| | Hirschsprung disease |
| | Colonic atresia, stenosis |
| | Imperforate anus |
| | Rectal stenosis |
| | Malrotation/volvulus |
| Acquired | Ulcerative colitis (toxic megacolon) |
| | Crohn disease |
| | Chagas disease |
| | Stricture post-NEC |
| | Fibrosing colonopathy (cystic fibrosis) |

NEC = necrotizing enterocolitis.

tions, hyperammonemia, associated inborn errors of metabolism, adrenogenital syndrome, rumination, increased intracranial pressure and subdural hemorrhage.

In children and adolescents, vomiting commonly is caused by gastroenteritis, systemic infection, toxic ingestions, and appendicitis. Less common causes are Reye syndrome, hepatitis, ulcers, pancreatitis, malrotation, brain tumor, increased intracranial pressure, cyclic vomiting or abdominal migraine, middle ear infection, and chemotherapy. Children also may have vomiting associated with pertussis syndrome and achalasia. Vomiting also may occur in adolescence as a result of bulimia and inflammatory bowel disease.

A careful history and physical examination are necessary to determine whether the source of vomiting is gastrointestinal or some other systemic disturbance. Neonates with polyhydramnios, drooling, a large amount of gastric aspirate (10–20 mL), persistent emesis, abdominal distention, bile-stained or blood-stained vomitus may be obstructed and should have a contrast study to determine the site of the obstruction. Bile-stained emesis suggests obstruction distal to the ampulla of Vater. Persistent emesis in older children may require endoscopic evaluation, especially in the presence of dysphagia, gastrointestinal hemorrhage, or a foreign body. *Laboratory investigation* should be directed by the information obtained from the history and physical examination in order to determine the presence of infection (culture), reflux (prolonged esophageal pH testing), metabolic disorders (testing for acidosis, hyperammonemia), pancreatitis (testing for amylase and lipase), pyloric stenosis (testing for alkalosis, ultrasound, contrast radiograph) and inflammatory bowel disease (ESR, mucosal biopsy, roentgenographic contrast study).

*Treatment* of emesis is directed toward the underlying disorders and toward correction of dehydration and electrolyte disturbances. Short periods of small frequent feedings of clear fluids may be all that is needed to stop emesis. Rarely, drugs such as promethazine, chlorpromazine, and prochlorperazine by rectal suppository may be useful, but extrapyramidal side effects may ensue. Ondansetron, a serotonin antagonist, is effective treatment for chemotherapy-induced emesis and other causes of refractory vomiting.

## References

Behrman RE, Kliegman RM, Arvin AM (eds): Nelson Textbook of Pediatrics, 15th ed. Philadelphia, WB Saunders, 1996, Chapters 252, 268, 269, 275–281.

Diseth T, Bjørnland K, Nøvik T, et al: Bowel junction, mental health, and psychosocial function in adolescents with Hirschsprung's disease. Arch Dis Child 76:100, 1997.

Fleisher D, Matar M: The cyclic vomiting syndrome: A report of 71 cases and literature review. J Pediatr Gastroenterol Nutr 17:361, 1993.

Madoff RD, Williams JG, Caushaj PF: Fecal incontinence. N Engl J Med 15:1002, 1992.

Partin JC, Hamill SK, Fischel JE, et al: Painful defecation and fecal soiling in children. Pediatrics 89:1007, 1992.

Van der Plas R, Benninga M, Büller H, et al: Biofeedback training in treatment of childhood constipation: a randomized controlled study. Lancet 348:776, 1996.

## GASTROINTESTINAL HEMORRHAGE

Hemorrhage may occur at any location in the gastrointestinal tract, and the differential diagnosis depends to a large extent on the patient's age. **Hematemesis**, blood-stained emesis, results from bleeding proximal to the ligament of Treitz. Less severe upper gastrointestinal bleeding results in a coffee grounds appearance of the emesis. **Melena** refers to soft, usually black or dark-colored stool of a tarry consistency; it usually is suggestive of bleeding from the oropharynx into the proximal small intestine. With stasis of blood in the right colon, bleeding lesions in that area also may appear as melena. **Hematochezia** refers to bright red or maroon-colored stools. Although the lesion is typically colonic, massive upper gastrointestinal bleeding may cause bright red blood per rectum because blood is a cathartic and decreases transit time. *Bright red streaks* of blood coating the surface of a stool suggest a rectal or anal lesion. **Occult gastrointestinal bleeding** is defined as significant, ongoing blood loss in the absence of a discernible change in the color or texture of stools; such loss may produce iron-deficiency anemia if it persists.

Before the evaluation, it is important to be sure that the stool does indeed contain blood and that the blood is from the gastrointestinal tract. A number of commonly ingested substances may simulate hematochezia: noncarbonated drinks (Kool-Aid, Hawaiian Punch), colored gelatins, beets, fruit bars, clingstone peaches, and antibiotics. Similarly, melena is simulated by the ingestion of compounds containing bismuth (Pepto-Bismol), therapeutic iron supplements, charcoal, and spinach. Swallowed blood from a briskly bleeding nasopharyngeal or oral lesion, which is subsequently regurgitated, also may be misinterpreted as upper gastrointestinal bleeding. Rarely, hemoptysis may be confused with hematemesis. Vaginal bleeding and hematuria have been mistakenly interpreted as hematochezia.

The *differential diagnosis* is based primarily on a careful history and a physical examination of the child (Table 11–11) and on the site of bleeding (Table 11–12). Abdominal pain that awakens the patient at night, is relieved by food, and is accompanied by hematemesis is highly suggestive of peptic ulcer disease. Substernal pain suggests esophagitis. Infants and older children with chronic hepatic disease and cirrhosis who exhibit hematemesis probably have bleeding esophageal varices. A history of neonatal omphalitis and subsequent portal vein thrombophlebitis also suggests variceal bleeding secondary to portal vein obstruction; however, for many children who have acute gastrointestinal hemorrhage, no obvious diagnosis is evident at the time of the first episode of bleeding.

If hepatic disease is present, coagulation studies should be performed; if coagulopathy is present, therapy is initiated with parenteral vitamin K and fresh frozen plasma. In newborn infants with bright red bloody emesis or bright red blood passed per rectum, an Apt test should be performed to determine whether the blood is fetal or maternal. Swallowed maternal blood at the time of delivery or from a ruptured lacteal during breast feeding is a common cause of hematemesis or hematochezia in the newborn (see Chapter 6).

TABLE 11–11.  Differential Diagnosis of Gastrointestinal Bleeding in Childhood

|  | Infant | Child | Adolescent |
|---|---|---|---|
| *Common* | Swallowed maternal blood<br>Anal fissure<br>Milk protein allergy<br>Necrotizing enterocolitis<br>Intussusception<br>Bacterial gastroenteritis | Anal fissure<br>Bacterial gastroenteritis<br>Intussusception<br>Ulcer/gastritis (*Helicobacter pylori*)<br>Swallowed epistaxis<br>Juvenile polyp | Bacterial gastroenteritis<br>Inflammatory bowel disease<br>Ulcer/gastritis (*H. pylori*)<br>Polyps<br>Hemorrhoids |
| *Rare* | Volvulus<br>Hemorrhagic disease of newborn<br>Meckel diverticulum | Esophageal varices<br>Esophagitis<br>Coagulopathy<br>Mallory-Weiss syndrome<br>Meckel diverticulum<br>Lymphonodular hyperplasia<br>Foreign body<br>Hemangioma<br>Sexual abuse<br>Hemolytic-uremic syndrome<br>Henoch-Schönlein purpura | Esophageal varices<br>Esophagitis<br>Coagulopathy<br>Mallory-Weiss syndrome<br>Telangiectasia (angiodysplasia)<br>Gay bowel disease |

TABLE 11–12.  Sites and Causes of Gastrointestinal (GI) Bleeding

| Upper GI | Upper and Lower GI | Lower GI |
|---|---|---|
| Epistaxis | Hemorrhagic disease of newborn | Milk/soy protein colitis |
| Esophagitis | Hemangioma | Eosinophilic colitis |
| Gastritis | Osler-Weber-Rendu syndrome | Gastroenteritis |
| Gastric ulcer | Arteriovenous malformation | Intussusception |
| Duodenal ulcer | Tumor | Henoch-Schönlein purpura |
| Esophageal varices | | Polyps |
| Mallory-Weiss syndrome | | Inflammatory bowel disease |
| Foreign body | | Volvulus |
| Caustic ingestion | | Meckel diverticulum |
| | | Lymphonodular hyperplasia |
| | | Pseudomembranous colitis |
| | | Hemolytic-uremic syndrome |

During the initial evaluation, an appropriately sized nasogastric tube should be placed in the stomach to determine whether the bleeding site is above the ligament of Treitz and to monitor the rate of upper gastrointestinal system hemorrhage. If the pylorus is closed, duodenal bleeding may not be detected with a nasogastric tube. If the gastric fluid return is clear, the source of the bleeding probably is below the ligament of Treitz. A small amount of hematemesis or melena may be misleading because a source of major blood loss may be concealed within the intestines. Furthermore, an initial normal hemoglobin and hematocrit value may give a false sense of security, since reequilibration may take 2–4 hr to demonstrate blood losses.

To diagnose the specific cause of upper gastrointestinal bleeding, *endoscopy* should be performed after the hemorrhaging has decreased or stopped. An upper gastrointestinal tract contrast roentgenographic study also may be helpful. Lower intestinal bleeding may be evaluated with proctosigmoidoscopy, colonoscopy, arteriography, or specific scans. The technetium 99m ($^{99m}$Tc) pertechnetate scan, preceded by pentagastrin stimulation, or a histamine $H_2$-receptor antagonist, identifies the ectopic acid–secreting cells creating the hemorrhage in **Meckel diverticulum.**

When the site of bleeding is unclear, arteriography, $^{99m}$Tc sulfur colloid, or $^{99m}$Tc-labeled autologous red blood cells can be infused intravenously. Arteriography and $^{99m}$Tc sulfur colloid detect rapid bleeding, whereas intermittent bleeding is more reliably identified by $^{99m}$Tc-labeled red blood cells.

The goals of *management* of acute gastrointestinal hemorrhage, in order of importance, are

1. To correct hypovolemia.
2. To correct anemia.
3. To stop the bleeding.

4. To prevent recurrence.
5. To diagnose the cause.
6. To apply specific therapy.

The immediate approach to the patient includes:

1. Assessing pulse and blood pressure (both supine and orthostatic changes).
2. Establishing intravenous access for administering fluids.
3. Expanding the intravascular volume in the presence of hypovolemia by providing intravenous crystalloid or colloid fluids.
4. Determining serial blood hemoglobin content.
5. Typing and cross-matching whole blood or packed cells for continued replacement of whole blood or erythrocyte losses.

The *treatment* of gastrointestinal hemorrhage should be specific for the underlying disorder. Anion pump inhibitors (omeprazole), $H_2$-receptor–blocking drugs, and antacids are useful agents for gastritis, esophagitis, and peptic ulcer disease, whereas the Mallory-Weiss syndrome requires the above in addition to close inpatient observation. Acute abdominal crises, such as volvulus and intussusception, require immediate contrast studies, which may be therapeutic for intussusception. Bleeding esophageal varices may be managed with intravenous somatostatin (octreotide), vasopressin, sclerotherapy, or banding. Rarely, emergency transjugular intrahepatic portosystemic shunting or portosystemic shunts are needed to stop variceal hemorrhage in children. Persistent massive hemorrhage that is unresponsive to therapy may require surgical exploration, whether or not a lesion has been identified. New techniques that may avoid emergency surgery include direct intra-arterial infusion of vasopressin, selective embolization of an arteriovenous malformation or isolated bleeding site, and electrocoagulation and laser photocoagulation for a bleeding ulcer or bleeding from angiodysplastic lesions.

## JAUNDICE

Jaundice (icterus) is the yellow discoloration of the skin, mucous membranes, and sclera caused by increased serum bilirubin concentrations that are deposited in tissue. Although indirect hyperbilirubinemia appears on the skin as yellow-brown coloration and direct hyperbilirubinemia gives the skin a yellow-green appearance, laboratory evaluation is needed for diagnosis and classification of the jaundice. Hyperbilirubinemia may be due to overproduction, decreased hepatic uptake or metabolism, and decreased hepatic excretion of bilirubin. Jaundice is the most common physical finding of hepatic dysfunction in children of all ages. Jaundice may be a result of a benign process (as in physiologic jaundice of the newborn), or it may be a sign of serious underlying disease, such as hepatitis. The production and excretion of bilirubin are discussed in Chapter 6.

Jaundice in the neonatal patient is discussed in Chapter 6. In older patients, jaundice always is a sign of significant disease. Icterus in the young infant may not be visible until the bilirubin level is 10 mg/dL; older children and adolescents demonstrate jaundice when the bilirubin is 2.5 mg/dL. Additional signs of underlying hepatic disease include protuberant abdomen, ascites, edema, pruritus with excoriations, dark urine, and acholic white-gray stools.

The *differential diagnosis* and *laboratory evaluation* of a jaundiced infant depend on whether there is indirect or direct hyperbilirubinemia (Fig. 11–2). Patients with indirect hyperbilirubinemia should be evaluated further for evidence of immune-mediated or nonimmune-mediated hemolysis by a CBC, peripheral blood smear, and Coombs test. Nonhemolytic indirect hyperbilirubinemia is common in newborn infants and older children with **Gilbert syndrome.** The remaining patients with indirect hyperbilirubinemia should have an appropriate laboratory assessment based on the history and physical examination (e.g., constipation and a large anterior fontanel should suggest hypothyroidism).

All patients with direct-reacting hyperbilirubinemia (direct bilirubin >1 mg/dL or 20% of total bilirubin), regardless of age, should have a comprehensive diagnostic evaluation to determine potentially serious causes of hepatic dysfunction. The laboratory studies should be based on the following:

- Family history (metabolic or hepatic disease)
- Exposure history (toxins, drugs, infectious agents)
- Age-related diseases (biliary atresia in infancy)
- Physical examination (unusual facies, splenomegaly, psychomotor retardation)
- Screening liver function tests

Screening tests include tests of hepatic synthetic function (i.e., serum albumin, prothrombin time); tests of biliary obstruction (i.e., direct bilirubin, serum alkaline phosphatase, 5'-nucleotidase, gammaglutamyl transpeptidase); and tests of hepatocellular injury (i.e., aspartate aminotransferase, alanine aminotransferase). In many infants, hepatic imaging with ultrasonography, radionucleotide or CT scans, and/or liver biopsy also may be necessary.

### References

Behrman RE Kliegman RM, Arvin AM (eds): Nelson Textbook of Pediatrics, 15th ed. Philadelphia, WB Saunders, 1996, Chapters 252, 282, 302–311.

Caulfield M, Wyllie R, Sivak M, et al: Upper gastrointestinal tract endoscopy in the pediatric patient. J Pediatr 115:339, 1989.

Doig C: Paediatric problems: II. Rectal bleeding. BMJ 305:511, 1992.

Khuroo M, Yattoo G, Javid G, et al: A comparison of omeprazole and placebo for bleeding ulcer. N Engl J Med 336:1054, 1997.

Shields R, Jenkin S, Baxter J, et al: A randomized controlled trial comparing the efficacy of somatostatin with injection sclerotherapy in the control of bleeding esophageal varices. J Hepatol 16:128, 1992.

# GASTROINTESTINAL DISORDERS BY ORGAN

## ORAL CAVITY

Mastication, the primary function of the oral cavity, requires healthy teeth with proper approximation. Two sets of teeth include 20 *primary* or *deciduous* and the 32 *secondary* or *permanent* teeth. The schedule of dental eruption is indicated in Table 11–13. Disorders of tooth development include **enamel hypoplasia,** which appears as enamel fissures, pits, or grooves and which may be due to rickets, serious illness, or the intake of tetracycline. Because enamel formation of permanent teeth is complete between 8 and 10 yr of age, tetracycline given after this age is not incorporated and thus does not stain the teeth. Abnormally shaped teeth are seen in congenital syphilis. Natal, congenital, or prematurely erupted teeth are uncommon and usually not a clinical problem. **Delayed eruption** of all

**Unconjugated Hyperbilirubinemia**

**Hemolysis and Recticuloycytosis**

*Positive Coombs test*
ABO and Rh incompatibility
Autoimmune, systemic lupus erythematosus
Drug induced and idiopathic acquired hemolytic anemia

*Negative Coombs test*
RBC enzyme defect (G6PD deficiency)
Hemoglobinopathy (sickle cell anemia)
RBC membrane defect (hereditary spherocytosis)
Hemolytic-uremic syndrome
Wilson disease

**No Hemolysis**

Gilbert syndrome
Physiologic jaundice of the newborn
Breast milk jaundice
Crigler-Najjar syndrome
Hypothyroidism
Pyloric stenosis
Internal hemorrhage

**Conjugated Hyperbilirubinemia**

**Obstructive**

Biliary atresia
Choledochal cyst
Cholelithiasis
Tumor/neoplasia
Bile duct stenosis
Spontaneous bile duct perforation
Bile-mucus plug

**Infectious**

Hepatitis A, B, C, D, E, G
Cytomegalovirus
Herpes simplex 1,2,6
Epstein-Barr virus
Coxsackievirus
ECHO virus
Measles
Varicella
Syncytial giant cell (paramyxovirus)
Human parvovirus B19
Toxoplasmosis
Syphilis
Leptospirosis
Bacterial sepsis/urinary tract infection (especially gram-negative)
Cholecystitis
Curtis–Fitz-Hugh syndrome

**Metabolic**

Wilson Disease
Alpha-1-antitrypsin deficiency
Galactosemia
Tyrosinemia
Fructosemia
Niemann-Pick disease
Gaucher disease
Zellweger syndrome
Wolman disease
Cystic fibrosis
Neonatal iron storage disease
Indian childhood cirrhosis
Defects in bile acid synthesis

**Toxic**

Total parenteral nutrition
Acetaminophen
Ethanol
Salicylates
Iron
Halothane
Isoniazid
Valproic acid
Veno-occlusive disease (cyclophosphamide)
Herbal teas
Volatile hydrocarbons
*Bacillus cereus* toxin
Phenytoin
Estradiol
Methyldopa

**Idiopathic**

Idiopathic neonatal hepatitis
Alagille syndrome
Nonsyndromic paucity of intrahepatic bile ducts
Progressive familial intrahepatic cholestasis
Familial benign recurrent cholestasis
Cholestasis with lymphedema (Aagenaes syndrome)
Cholestasis with hypopituitarism
Familial erythrophagocytic lymphohistiocytosis

**Autoimmune**

Autoimmune chronic hepatitis
Sclerosing cholangitis
Graft vs. host disease

FIGURE 11-2. Differential diagnosis of jaundice in childhood. G6PD = glucose-6-phosphate dehydrogenase; RBC = red blood cell.

TABLE 11–13. Time of Eruption of the Primary and Permanent Teeth

| Tooth Type | Primary Age (mo) | | Permanent Age (yr) | |
|---|---|---|---|---|
| | Upper | Lower | Upper | Lower |
| Central incisor | 6 ± 2 | 7 ± 2 | 7–8 | 6–7 |
| Lateral incisor | 9 ± 2 | 7 ± 2 | 8–9 | 7–8 |
| Cuspids | 18 ± 2 | 16 ± 2 | 11–12 | 9–10 |
| First bicuspids | — | — | 10–11 | 10–12 |
| Second bicuspids | — | — | 10–12 | 11–12 |
| First molars | 14 ± 4 | 12 ± 4 | 6–7 | 6–7 |
| Second molars | 24 ± 4 | 20 ± 4 | 12–13 | 11–13 |
| Third molars | — | — | 17–21 | 17–21 |

teeth indicates an endocrine or nutritional disturbance, such as hypopituitarism, hypothyroidism, or rickets. Discoloration of the teeth may occur as a consequence of excessive fluoride (>5 ppm), prolonged neonatal hyperbilirubinemia, or the intake of tetracycline.

## Dental Caries

The development of dental caries depends on the interaction of dietary carbohydrate and oral bacteria, specifically *Streptococcus mutans,* on the tooth surface. Organic acids produced by the bacterial fermentation of carbohydrate demineralize the tooth surface, leading to pit formation that progresses to cavity (caries) formation. If unchecked, the process erodes through the tooth, permitting a bacterial invasion of the pulp that becomes painful (toothache). Further spread of the inflammatory process to the alveolar bone results in a dental abscess. Caries in primary teeth may disrupt the development of the permanent teeth.

The best *treatment* for caries is *prevention,* and the most effective preventive measure is fluoridation of the water supply to 1 ppm. In fluoride-deficient areas, supplementation may be necessary. Reducing dietary carbohydrate intake also is important. To prevent the damaging effects of continuous bottle feeding (nursing bottle caries), bedtime bottles, if necessary, should contain only water. Brushing and flossing of teeth should begin by age 3, although most children under 10 yr of age do not have the eye-to-hand coordination to perform either activity properly. The parents must assume this responsibility according to the child's ability. Regular dental visits should begin by age 3.

Early dental *treatment* can salvage most carious

teeth. Dental infection confined to the tooth itself may be managed with filling or extraction. When the infection extends to the adjacent alveolar bone, oral antibiotics (penicillin) should be initiated. More serious spread of infection to the submandibular space (**Ludwig angina**) and to the buccal or orbital spaces, both of which may produce cellulitis, should be managed with intravenous penicillin. The diseased tooth can be identified by localized pain; local treatment (filling or extraction) is needed after the infection is treated.

## Oropharyngeal Candidiasis (Thrush)

Oral candidiasis is common in young infants. The *diagnosis* is made by visual inspection of white plaques covering the oropharyngeal mucosa. Initial *treatment* consists of the topical application of nystatin. All toys and bottle nipples must be boiled daily to prevent reinfection. Refractory cases may require clotrimazole troches or, rarely, intravenous amphotericin. Persistent candidiasis resistant to therapy or the presence of this lesion in older infants who are not receiving broad-spectrum antibiotics suggests an immune disorder, such as AIDS.

### References

Behrman RE, Kliegman RM, Arvin AM (eds): Nelson Textbook of Pediatrics, 15th ed. Philadelphia, WB Saunders, 1996, Chapters 253, 254.
Greene J, Louie R, Wycoff S: Preventive dentistry: I. Dental caries. JAMA 262:3459, 1989.

## CLEFT LIP AND PALATE

### Cleft Lip

Cleft lip, with or without cleft palate, occurs in 1:1000 births and is more common in males. Unilateral cleft lip is due to failure of the ipsilateral maxillary prominence to fuse with the medial nasal prominence, a process that produces a persistent labial groove. Failure of bilateral fusion produces bilateral cleft lip. Multiple genetic as well as environmental factors appear to play a role in the etiology of cleft lip. The recurrence risk in siblings is 3–4%; the risk for a child of a mother with cleft lip is 14%. Associated malformations include hypertelorism and heart, foot, and hand anomalies. Most cleft lips are repaired shortly after birth or once the infant demonstrates steady weight gain. In general, feeding is not a problem with isolated cleft lip deformities.

## Cleft Palate

Development of the palate proper, which includes the hard palate, soft palate, uvula, and maxillary teeth, is completed by the 9th wk of gestation. This region develops from the maxillary bone plates that are initially separated by the tongue. As the tongue descends in the floor of the mouth and moves forward, the two plates fuse. Failure of the tongue to descend produces the midline palatal clefts. The incidence of cleft palate is 1:2500 births.

Genetic factors are important in its *etiology.* The recurrence risks are the same as those for cleft lip. Cleft palates are common in patients with chromosomal syndromes. Surgical repair usually is undertaken between 12 and 24 mo of age. In the immediate newborn period, respiratory and feeding problems may occur. Repositioning the tongue and feeding the baby on his or her side should resolve respiratory difficulties. Most patients do well with a long, soft nipple that has a hole that is larger than usual. Patients with sucking or swallowing difficulty require gavage or gastrostomy feedings. The main problems after cleft palate repair are speech and tooth disturbances and recurrent otitis media. Although two thirds of these patients demonstrate acceptable speech, the voice may have a nasal quality or a muffled tone.

**Pierre Robin syndrome** is an identifiable sporadic or familial condition characterized by high arched or cleft palate, micrognathia, and glossoptosis. Glossoptosis is due to the smallness of the mandible and results in airway obstruction and feeding problems during infancy. As the mandible grows, respiratory and feeding disturbances resolve.

## ESOPHAGUS

### Development

**Tracheoesophageal Fistula.** The esophagus develops as an elongation of the superior portion of the primitive foregut very early in the embryonic process. When the septation between the ventral tube and the dorsal esophagus develops abnormally, **esophageal atresia** results, a condition usually associated with tracheoesophageal fistula (TEF) (see Fig. 11–3).

Forty percent of patients with TEF have associated anomalies; cardiovascular anomalies (patent ductus arteriosus, vascular ring, coarctation of the aorta) are the most frequent. The incidence of imperforate anus, intestinal malrotation, and duodenal anomalies is also increased. **VATER syndrome** describes the association between *v*ertebral defects (hemivertebra), *a*nal atresia, *T*EF, and *r*adial limb dysplasia.

Polyhydramnios and excessive salivation are early *clinical manifestations* of TEF, followed by choking, coughing, and cyanosis after the first feeding. The *diagnosis* may be made by passing a radiopaque catheter and observing coiling in the esophageal pouch on a chest roentgenogram or a

FIGURE 11–3. Various types of tracheoesophageal fistulas (TEF) with relative frequency (%).

pool of contrast dye collected in the atretic esophagus. Infants with TEF without esophageal atresia (H type) may have nonspecific symptoms for several months, but they usually exhibit chronic cough with feeding and recurrent pneumonia.

Primary surgical repair is the *treatment* of choice when the infant's condition is stable. Postoperative anastomotic leak occurs in 5–10% of these infants and requires parenteral or duodenal feedings. Strictures at the anastomotic site require dilating bougienage. In patients with TEF, there is a persistent derangement of esophageal motility. Abnormal lower esophageal sphincter (LES) function results in gastroesophageal reflux, which may lead to esophagitis, stricture formation, wheezing, and recurrent pneumonia. The survival rate for this lesion in term infants without other anomalies or complications is greater than 90%.

**Esophageal Disease.** *Clinical manifestations* of esophageal diseases include a sensation that food is stuck in the esophagus (dysphagia), which may be due to motility disorders or obstruction. Pain on swallowing (odynophagia) may be due to high reflux of acidic stomach contents. *Regurgitation*, rather than forceful emesis, is the most common manifestation of esophageal disease in children.

## Gastroesophageal Reflux
### (Chalasia)

Gastroesophageal reflux (GER) is a common problem during the 1st yr of life. A number of factors alone or in combination may be responsible. These include reduced LES pressure, poor-amplitude esophageal contractions, inappropriate LES relaxation, large hiatal hernia, and delayed gastric emptying. The latter may suggest distal intestinal obstruction.

In older patients, GER is due to neurally mediated episodes of transient relaxation of the lower esophageal sphincter and of the surrounding crural diaphragm. Gastric distention, pharyngeal stimulation, high-fat meals, and upright or right lateral decubitus postures stimulate transient relaxation of the sphincter. In infants, regurgitation, vomiting, and irritability are the most frequent complaints, which, if severe, may result in failure to thrive, aspiration pneumonia, wheezing, or esophagitis with bleeding and anemia. On rare occasions, especially in premature infants, GER may be associated with apnea or bradycardia. **Sandifer syndrome** is GER-associated with the infant manifesting lateral head tilt and back arching resulting from esophagitis. GER in the older child or adolescent may present with regurgitation, retrosternal burning

(esophagitis), dysphagia (stricture), or severe asthma.

The *diagnostic* evaluation of GER often includes a barium swallow with fluoroscopy, but at least 30% of infants have normal esophagrams as a result of the intermittent nature of GER. The study excludes anatomic causes, such as an antral web, duodenal web, pyloric stenosis, or annular pancreas. In patients with recurrent pneumonia, swallowing function should be assessed as part of the upper gastrointestinal series. The definitive test for establishing the presence of GER is the 24-hr esophageal pH probe study. This test documents the percent of time that the esophageal pH is less than 4.0 as well as duration of reflux episodes. Formula or food containing $^{99m}$Tc can be used to assess gastric emptying. Esophageal manometry, which directly measures LES pressure, also may help determine the cause of GER. Finally, when blood loss, anemia, retrosternal burning, or dysphagia is present, endoscopy and esophageal biopsy detects the presence of peptic esophagitis, infection, or stricture formation.

Patients with mild to moderate reflux can be managed with medical *treatment*, which may include feeding cereal-thickened formula and careful burping. Position therapy consisting of a 30-degree prone upright position after feeding has been recommended in the past but is now controversial because prone posturing increases the risk of **sudden infant death syndrome** (SIDS) (see Chapter 12). Most young infants outgrow reflux by 18 mo of age. In cases complicated by esophagitis, $H_2$-blocking agents or omeprazole may be beneficial in reducing acid reflux. Bethanechol, a parasympathomimetic drug, increases esophageal peristalsis and LES tone, whereas metoclopramide, a dopamine antagonist and cholinergic agonist, increases gastric emptying (reducing nausea) and LES tone. The use of both medications is limited by side effects, the most important being a dystonic type of extrapyramidal reaction with metoclopramide. Cisapride, a prokinetic agent, increases lower esophageal sphincter pressure, lower esophageal peristalsis, and gastrointestinal motility by enhancing the release of acetylcholine at the myenteric plexus. It is beneficial in the treatment of GER. However, bradycardia and nodal dysrhythmias have been described when this drug is given concomitantly with macrolide antibiotics or fluconazole-type medications. Infants should receive medications other than theophylline for wheezing because this drug lowers LES pressure. Repeated episodes of pneumonia, failure to thrive, recurrent esophagitis with stricture, severe apnea, and failure to respond to 4–6 wk of medical management are indications for surgery. The most common antire-flux operation is the *Nissen fundoplication*, in which the fundus of the stomach is wrapped 270–360 degrees around the distal esophagus. Gastric distention after a feeding increases pressure around the wrap, thus preventing acid reflux.

## Foreign Bodies

Coins, marbles, disc batteries, and pins are often swallowed and become lodged in the esophagus at one of three sites of narrowing (i.e., the cricopharyngeal muscle, the level of the aortic arch, and the LES at the diaphragm). Symptoms include cough, choking, stridor, odynophagia, retrosternal pain, and excessive salivation. However, many children are asymptomatic. If the foreign body is left in place, ulceration accompanied by bleeding and perforation may occur. Perforation with resultant mediastinitis is heralded by pain, fever, and shock. In experienced hands, smooth objects such as coins, buttons, or marbles may be removed by passing a Foley catheter (8–12 Fr) into the distal esophagus, inflating the balloon, and, by using fluoroscopic guidance, slowly pulling back until the object is obtained. Others favor removing these objects endoscopically or pushing them into the stomach to prevent aspiration. For resistant smooth objects and sharp objects that might penetrate the mucosa, general anesthesia and removal through an eso-phagoscope or bronchoscope are required.

## Corrosive Burns

Corrosive burns are a common cause of esophageal stricture. The most common chemicals producing esophageal damage are the tasteless alkali caustics found in drain cleaners. Household bleaches and ammonia-containing cleaners are much weaker and produce less damage. Alkali agents cause full-thickness penetrating coagulation necrosis, whereas acid burns produce an eschar that coats the mucosa, preventing deeper penetration. Burns in the mouth suggest that the esophagus also is burned. However, the absence of burns on the oral mucosa does not preclude esophageal involvement.

Following a lye ingestion, vomiting should not be induced. Water or milk should be given to dilute the corrosive. Hospitalization, intravenous fluids, and endoscopy are recommended even if there is a doubt about the ingestion. The presence of a burn warrants follow-up with a barium swallow 3–4 wk after the initial injury to check for stricture formation. Strictures need bougienage dilation. Steroids are of no benefit.

## References

Behrman RE, Kliegman RM, Arvin AM (eds): Nelson Textbook of Pediatrics, 15th ed. Philadelphia, WB Saunders, 1996, Chapters 264–273.

Glassman M, George D, Grill B: Gastroesophageal reflux in children: Clinical manifestation, diagnosis, and therapy. Gastroenterol Clin North Am 24:71, 1995.

Lovejoy FJ: Corrosive injury of the esophagus in children: Failure of corticosteroid treatment reemphasizes prevention. N Engl J Med 323:668, 1990.

Schunk J, Harrison M, Corneli H, et al: Fluoroscopic Foley catheter removal of esophageal foreign bodies in children: Experience with 145 episodes. Pediatrics 94:709, 1994.

# STOMACH

## Pyloric Stenosis

After inguinal hernia, hypertrophic pyloric stenosis is the most common condition requiring surgery during the first 2 mo of life. The incidence is 1:150 in males and 1:750 in females. The condition occurs in 5% of siblings and 25% of offspring if the mother was affected. Pylorospasm, secondary to reduced tissue nitric oxide levels (a mediator of relaxation) may lead to hypertrophic pyloric stenosis.

The typical *clinical manifestation* is nonbilious vomiting beginning between the 2nd and 4th wk of life. Emesis increases in frequency and eventually becomes projectile. Clear liquids and/or frequent feedings may lessen the severity of the vomiting temporarily, but weight loss becomes apparent as the obstruction becomes more complete. *Laboratory* abnormalities include hypokalemic metabolic alkalosis with paradoxic aciduria and dehydration. Indirect hyperbilirubinemia also may be present.

The *diagnosis* may be made during or immediately after a feeding by palpating an olive-shaped mass to the right of the umbilicus and witnessing marked peristaltic waves progressing from the left upper quadrant to the epigastrium. The diagnosis is confirmed by ultrasound demonstration of the thick hypoechoic ring in the region of the pylorus. Contrast roentgenographic studies are occasionally necessary.

Pyloromyotomy is the *treatment of choice* once dehydration and electrolyte abnormalities are corrected. Within 1–2 days, most infants can tolerate formula feeding.

## Acid-Peptic Disease

The designation acid-peptic disease refers to a variety of disorders of the proximal gastrointestinal tract resulting from the action of gastric secretions. Local mucosal infection with the urea-splitting bacterium *Helicobacter pylori* also may play an etiologic role. Included under "acid-peptic disease" are gastritis, gastric ulcer, duodenitis, and duodenal ulcer. Strictly speaking, "gastritis" and "duodenitis" refer to inflammatory processes in the mucosa, whereas "ulcer" implies a sharply circumscribed lesion.

**Gastritis.** Acute gastritis may be localized or diffuse. Necrosis of the superficial mucosal cells and damage to the blood vessels of the lamina propria may cause extravasation of blood (acute hemorrhagic gastritis). If erosions form (erosive gastritis) and extend to the submucosa and muscularis, an ulcer may form. Acute gastritis may follow viral infections, the ingestion of aspirin or nonsteroidal anti-inflammatory drugs, cancer chemotherapy, and the ingestion of corrosive agents, such as strong acids. Gastritis also may occur following severe trauma, major surgery, or septic shock.

Hematemesis is the major *clinical manifestation*. Other symptoms include abdominal pain, nausea, and vomiting. Endoscopy is the *diagnostic* method of choice; barium studies usually are not helpful. *Treatment* is similar to that for peptic ulcer disease.

**Gastric Ulcer/Duodenal Ulcer.** Ulcers no longer are considered rare in children because increased rates have been detected by endoscopy. Primary ulcers occur in previously healthy individuals with no history of medication use. They are more duodenal than gastric and tend to have an insidious onset. Gastric ulcers occur in the antrum, whereas primary duodenal ulcers are found in the bulb and usually are solitary. The finding of multiple ulcers either in the 3rd or 4th portion of the duodenum or in the jejunum should raise suspicion of the **Zollinger-Ellison syndrome**. Secondary ulcers are seen in association with underlying systemic disorders (sepsis, burns, raised intracranial pressure) or occur as a consequence of drug therapy. They may hemorrhage or perforate without a prior history of pain, are more common in the stomach and frequently are multiple.

The *etiology* of ulcer disease is closely related to *H. pylori* infection, which is detected in 90% of children with duodenal ulcers and 60–80% of children with gastric ulcers. Drugs such as salicylates and nonsteroidal anti-inflammatory drugs (NSAIDs), genetics, stress, alcohol abuse, and smoking may be contributing factors.

Epigastric burning or gnawing abdominal pain relieved by food or antacids and recurring 1–3 hr after eating is the most common *clinical manifestation*. Nocturnal pain that awakens a child from sleep is typical of peptic ulcer disease and occurs in 30% of children with primary peptic ulcers but is rare in children with psychophysiologic disorders. Vomiting and nausea are other frequent symptoms.

Documentation of an ulcer crater by an upper gastrointestinal roentgenographic series is sufficient to establish the *diagnosis* of peptic ulcer, but the ulcer may be undetected in up to 25% of cases. Endoscopy is often required to identify the lesion.

The goal of *treatment* is to reduce gastric acidity. Antacids are used but have a short duration of action. $H_2$-receptor–blocking agents, such as cimetidine and ranitidine, are effective for 6–12 hr and thus provide sustained relief. Drug interactions are common (see Appendix I). Anions pump inhibitors (omeprazole) effectively reduce acidity by preventing acid release from the parietal cell. Sucralfate has a local coating action and is not absorbed. Therapy should be continued for 6–8 wk. Combination antimicrobial therapy (bismuth salts, amoxicillin or clarithromycin, and metronidazole) for 7–14 days is needed to eradicate *H. pylori*. Indications for surgical vagotomy with pyloroplasty include perforation, obstruction, uncontrolled bleeding, rebleeding in the hospital, and intractable pain.

### Foreign Bodies and Bezoars

Most foreign bodies that reach the stomach pass through to the intestine and should be managed conservatively. Objects without sharp edges should be removed endoscopically if serial roentgenograms show no progress after 3–4 wk. Objects with sharp points, such as safety pins, nails, and needles, should be monitored roentgenographically and should be removed endoscopically if they do not move from the stomach after several days.

Three types of stomach bezoars occur in children: *trichobezoars* (composed primarily of hair), *phytobezoars* (composed of vegetable material), and *lactobezoars* (occurring from milk). Symptoms include abdominal pain, anorexia, vomiting, and weight loss. Children with trichobezoars may be retarded and may have alopecia. Lactobezoars, which may cause gastric outlet obstruction, usually are seen in neonates receiving high-caloric-density formulas by continuous drip.

### References

Behrman RE, Kliegman RM, Arvin AM (eds): Nelson Textbook of Pediatrics, 15th edition. Philadelphia, WB Saunders, 1996, Chapters 274, 275, 282.

Bujanover Y, Reif S, Yahav J: *Helicobacter pylori* and peptic disease in the pediatric patient. Pediatr Clin North Am 43:213, 1996.

Goodwin C, Mendall M, Northfield T: *Helicobacter pylori* infection. Lancet 349:265, 1997.

## DISORDERS OF THE INTESTINE AND COLON

### Congenital Malformations

#### Abdominal Wall Defects

*Omphalocele.* When the abdominal viscera herniate through the umbilical and supraumbilical portions of the abdominal wall into a sac covered by peritoneum and amniotic membrane, the defect is called an omphalocele. It results from a failure of migration of the bowel from the umbilical coelom, and its incidence is 1:6000 births. Large defects may contain the liver and spleen as well as most of the gastrointestinal tract. The sac covering the defect is thin and may rupture in utero or during delivery. Ten percent of infants with omphaloceles are born prematurely; the incidence of associated malformations is high. Thirty-five percent have other gastrointestinal defects; 20%, congenital heart defects; and 10%, the **Beckwith-Wiedemann syndrome** (exophthalmos, macroglossia, gigantism, hyperinsulinemia, hypoglycemia). Primary closure of small defects often is possible. Larger defects require staged repairs that involve covering the sac with a prosthetic material. Survival rates vary and depend on the severity of associated anomalies.

*Umbilical Hernia.* Umbilical hernia results from the incomplete closure of the fascia of the umbilical ring. Herniated omentum or bowel is covered by skin. Umbilical hernia is more common in premature infants and blacks; it is found in up to 40% of black children younger than 1 yr of age. Fascial defects with a diameter of less than 0.5 cm heal spontaneously before age 2 yr. With a ring between 0.5 and 1.5 cm, healing usually is complete by age 4 yr. Surgical closure is advisable if the defect exceeds 1.5 cm at 2 yr of age or if incarceration or symptoms such as abdominal pain have occurred. The practice of manually reducing the hernia and taping some device (such as a coin) over the ring does not accelerate the healing process.

**Gastroschisis.** Gastroschisis is the herniation, without a covering sac, of a variable length of small intestine and, occasionally, of portions of the liver, through an abdominal wall defect located to the right of the umbilical cord. The eviscerated uncovered mass of bowel is adherent, edematous, dark in color, and covered by a gelatinous matrix of greenish material. Sixty percent of these infants are born premature; 14% have associated jejunoileal malformations, usually stenosis or atresias; and 4% have nongastrointestinal malformations. Little evidence supports the notion that genetic factors play a role, and the risk of congenital anomalies in future pregnancies is small. Gastroschisis is a surgical emergency, and a single-stage primary closure is possible in only 10% of patients. Postoperative hypomotility is common.

#### Intestinal Atresia

*Duodenum.* Duodenal obstruction may be complete (atresia), owing to the failure of the lumen to recannalize, or partial (stenosis), owing to a web, band, or annular pancreas. Intrinsic duodenal lesions result from a failure of the lumen to recannalize during the 8th–10th week of gestation. Duodenal atresia is associated with other anomalies (30%), prematurity (25%), and trisomy 21 (20%).

With complete obstruction, bile-stained vomiting begins within a few hours after the first feeding. In utero polyhydramnios may be present. Abdominal roentgenograms usually show gastric and duodenal gaseous distention, which also is called the "double bubble" sign, proximal to the atretic site. The presence of gas in the distal bowel suggests partial obstruction, and a contrast roentgenographic study should be performed.

*Treatment* is surgical. Mortality is related to prematurity and associated congenital anomalies.

*Jejunum and Ileum.* Jejunoileal atresias occur more frequently (2:1) than duodenal atresias and probably are caused by intrauterine infarction. Two thirds of cases involve complete obstruction of either the distal ileum or proximal jejunum, with multiple atresias accounting for only 10–20%. **Meconium ileus** with atresia is due to thick intestinal secretions from cystic fibrosis.

Polyhydramnios is present in 25% of cases. Vomiting of bile-stained material usually begins within 24–48 hr after birth. The abdomen becomes distended, and plain films show dilated loops of small bowel and an absence of colonic gas. Peritoneal calcifications signify **meconium peritonitis**, the result of intrauterine bowel perforation. A barium enema shows a narrowed unused colon (**microcolon**). Surgery is mandatory.

**Malrotation/Volvulus.** Anomalies of intestinal rotation result from failure of the midgut to appropriately re-enter the fetal abdomen. The severity of the malrotation depends on the extent of the rotational arrest. Volvulus occurs when the small intestine is not fixed in the abdomen and becomes suspended by a stalk containing the superior mesenteric artery. Twisting of bowel leads to arterial obstruction, midgut ischemia, and infarction. Further complicating the malrotation is the presence of peritoneal fixation bands (Ladd bands), which may result in partial duodenal obstruction.

Eighty percent of children with this anomaly experience symptoms within the 1st mo of life, although some present during adulthood. Abdominal distention and bilious vomiting suggest obstruction. If volvulus occurs, bloody stools may be followed by perforation and peritonitis. Children who are brought to the physician's attention after the neonatal period may manifest intermittent cramping, abdominal pain, vomiting, and diarrhea (often with hypoalbuminemia and secondary hypogammaglobulinemia) or constipation.

The *diagnosis* of malrotation can be made by demonstrating an abnormal position of the duodenum in an upper gastrointestinal roentgenographic series with small bowel follow-through. Midgut volvulus is a surgical emergency.

**Meckel Diverticulum.** Meckel diverticulum, the vestigial remnant of the omphalomesenteric duct, is the most frequent anomaly of the gastrointestinal tract, is present in 2–3% of the population, is 2–3 cm long, and is located within 100 cm of the ileocecal valve along the antimesenteric border of the small intestine. The peak incidence is 2 yr of age; males predominate (2:1). Heterotopic tissue occurs in 50%; it is usually gastric and is 10 times more common in symptomatic cases because of acid secretion and ulceration.

The *clinical manifestations* include painless rectal bleeding (melena, 84%), intestinal obstruction (intussusception or volvulus, 10%), and painful diverticulitis mimicking appendicitis (6%). *Diagnosis* is discussed in the section on Gastrointestinal Hemorrhage. The definitive *treatment* is surgical resection.

**Congenital Aganglionic Megacolon (Hirschsprung Disease).** The failure of retrograde migration of neural crest–derived ganglion cells in the developing colon results in an aganglionic segment of variable length. This disorder is three times more common among males, may be associated with some syndromes (trisomy 21, Waardenberg), and accounts for 20% of neonatal intestinal obstruction. In 75% of cases, the aganglionic segment is limited to the rectosigmoid colon; 15% extend beyond the splenic flexure. **Neuronal intestinal dysplasia** (hyperganglionosis) demonstrates hyperplasia of the intramural plexus and clinically resembles Hirschsprung disease.

The *diagnosis* should be suspected in any infant who fails to pass meconium within the first 24 hr and who requires repeated rectal stimulation to induce bowel movements. Failure to thrive and abdominal distention may occur. Fever and diarrhea are ominous signs that suggest the presence of coexisting enterocolitis. In some cases, particularly those with short segment (<5 cm) involvement, the diagnosis goes undetected into childhood. These children often are poorly nourished and suffer from massive abdominal distention and anemia. The presence of stool palpable throughout the abdomen and an empty rectum on digital examination are most suggestive of the disease (see Table 11–9).

The *treatment* of Hirschsprung disease is surgical and is performed in two stages. The first stage involves the creation of a colostomy through a section of bowel containing ganglion cells, thus permitting decompression of the dilated colon. In the second stage, the aganglionic segment is removed by pulling the ganglionic segment through the rectum. This procedure is postponed until the infant is 12–14 mo old or delayed for 3–6 mo when the disease has been diagnosed in an older child. The mortality rate is low in the absence of enterocolitis, and the major complications include anal stenosis (5–10%) and incontinence (1–3%).

**Anorectal Malformation/Imperforate Anus.** Anorectal anomalies arise either because of a failure of the urorectal septum to divide the cloaca completely or because of incomplete convergence of the anal tubercles around the termination of the hindgut. The incidence is 1:5000, and 50% of cases demonstrate associated vertebral or genitourinary malformations.

The recognition of anorectal malformations depends on careful inspection of the perianal area at birth. Figure 11–4 illustrates the various types of anomalies. Fistulization between the rectum and surrounding structures may occur. Rectourethral fistulas in males and rectovaginal fistulas in females are associated with "high" lesions, whereas fistulas through to the perineum are associated with "low" lesions. Contrast roentgenograms of a fistula or tube instillation of contrast into the rectum should allow delineation of the anatomy. Anal stenosis may be treated with simple dilation. Other lesions require surgery. Bowel control is achieved in 90% of children with low lesions but in only 50% of those with high lesions.

**Inguinal Hernia.** During fetal development, a peritoneal sac precedes the testicle as it descends from the genital ridge into the scrotum. The lower portion of this sac (processus vaginalis) envelops the testes and forms the tunica vaginalis, whereas the remainder of the sac atrophies. In 50% of patients, the processus vaginalis remains patent. If abdominal contents become trapped in the processus vaginalis, an **indirect hernia** exists. Indirect inguinal hernias are more common in males (4:1), in premature infants, and following increased intra-abdominal pressure (ascites). The hernia becomes manifest as a painless swelling in the inguinal area. Contents of the hernia sac usually can be reduced with gentle pressure. When the contents of the sac cannot be reduced, the hernia is said to be **incarcerated**, necessitating immediate surgery

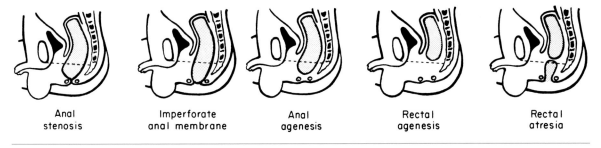

Anal                Imperforate          Anal              Rectal            Rectal
stenosis            anal membrane        agenesis          agenesis          atresia

FIGURE 11–4. Various types of anorectal anomalies. The stippled line is a projection of the puborectalis sling. On a roentgenogram, it is drawn from the lower part of the pubis to the sacrococcygeal junction. (Modified from Silverman A, Roy CE [eds]: Pediatric Clinical Gastroenterology. St. Louis, CV Mosby, 1983.)

to avoid bowel necrosis and testicular infarction. Repair of an asymptomatic reducible hernia should be carried out as soon as possible unless other conditions preclude surgery.

## References

Behrman RE, Kliegman RM, Arvin AM (eds): Nelson Textbook of Pediatrics, 15th ed. Philadelphia, WB Saunders, 1996, Chapters 276–279.
Ford EG, Senac MO, Srikanth MS, et al: Malrotation of the intestine in children. Ann Surg 215:172, 1992.
Martin LW, Torres AM: Hirschsprung's disease. Surg Clin North Am 65:1171, 1985.
St-Vil D, Brandt ML, Panic S, et al: Meckel's diverticulum in children: A 20-year review. J Pediatr Surg 26:1289, 1991.

## Disaccharidase Deficiencies

Primary congenital disaccharidase deficiencies are rare. Sucrase-isomaltase deficiency is the most common form occurring in infancy and is inherited as an autosomal recessive trait. Osmotic diarrhea begins with the introduction of sucrose-containing foods or drinks and may be associated with vomiting, dehydration, abdominal cramping, bloating, and growth failure. The *diagnosis* may be confirmed on breath hydrogen testing and quantitative determination of sucrase-isomaltase activity in jejunal mucosal biopsy. The *treatment* consists of excluding from the diet foods that contain more than 2% sucrose.

Congenital **lactase deficiency** is rare, but late-onset lactase deficiency is common. This inherited form has a striking ethnic variation, being present in 5–10% of whites in contrast to 70% of blacks. The absence of brush border lactase activity causes lactose malabsorption and osmotic diarrhea within hours of lactose ingestion. Symptoms begin between 8 and 15 yr of age and include crampy abdominal pain, bloating, and acidic diarrhea (containing reducing substances). The *diagnosis* may be made on breath hydrogen or lactose tolerance test-

ing. Because the deficiency is relative rather than absolute, some lactose restriction from the diet usually is sufficient to prevent symptoms. Transient secondary lactase deficiency often occurs as a consequence of damage to the small intestinal mucosa following severe viral gastroenteritis. Mucosal recovery occurs in 4–6 wk. *Treatment* consists of a non–lactose-containing formula.

## Protein Intolerance and Sensitivity Syndromes: Cow's Milk and Soy Milk

The proteins in cow's milk and soy milk may cause an immune-mediated inflammatory injury of the small bowel, with villous atrophy, or an injury of the large bowel, producing colitis (inflammation with or without ulceration). The precise immune mechanisms are undetermined. Systemic signs, such as anaphylaxis, wheezing, rhinitis, pulmonary hemosiderosis, and urticaria, may be mediated by IgE antibody. Approximately 4% of all infants are intolerant to cow's milk proteins, and 20–50% of these also are intolerant to soy protein. Milk protein intolerance syndrome usually has an onset within the 1st mo of life. When it causes **enterocolitis**, vomiting, diarrhea, enteric blood loss, and anema are present. Rectal biopsy findings include inflammation, eosinophilic infiltration of the lamina propria and mucosa, ulceration, and crypt abscesses. Another form of this syndrome, **enteropathy**, begins at 2–3 mo of age, and clinical manifestations include prolonged diarrhea, protein-losing enteropathy (edema, hypoproteinemia), malabsorption, and failure to thrive. Small intestinal villous atrophy, at times associated with inflammatory colitis, is present.

The *diagnosis* of cow's or soy milk protein intolerance is usually made by history but may require laboratory tests and mucosal biopsy if the diagnosis is in doubt. Improvement with protein hydrolyzed formula and recurrence of symptoms when milk proteins are reintroduced confirm the diagnosis. Most infants eventually tolerate bovine or soy proteins by 2–3 yr of age. Infants with severe reactions (anaphylaxis) should not undergo challenge. Breast-fed infants may manifest similar symptoms because of the presence of dietary bovine proteins in human breast milk. *Treatment* of the breast-fed infant requires elimination of dairy products by the mother and supplementing her with calcium and vitamin D.

**Eosinophilic gastroenteropathy** is not usually associated with cow's milk sensitivity and is characterized by eosinophilic infiltration of the intestinal mucosa, muscularis, or serosal layers and elevated IgE levels and peripheral eosinophilia. Protein-losing enteropathy, pyloric obstruction (muscular involvement), gastrointestinal bleeding with anemia (mucosal involvement), and ascites (serosal involvement) also may be present. The cause is unknown, but it is a chronic condition that shows a variable response to corticosteroids or oral disodium cromolyn. The *differential diagnosis* includes intestinal parasite infestation.

### Gluten-Sensitive Enteropathy
### (Celiac Disease)

Celiac disease, an immunologically mediated intolerance to gluten-containing grains (wheat, rye, barley, and possibly oats), results in small intestinal villous atrophy with lymphocytic and plasma cell infiltration. The incidence in the United States is 1:3000 births. There is a genetic predisposition: 98% have human leukocyte antigen (HLA)-DQW2 and 80% are HLA-B8 positive. The risk may be increased in patients with IgA deficiency.

*Clinical manifestations* usually begin between 6 and 18 mo and include apathy, irritability, pain, vomiting, chronic diarrhea, steatorrhea, abdominal distention, and failure to thrive; some infants are asymptomatic. A wasted skeletal muscle mass, finger clubbing, and peripheral edema also may occur. Older children may present with unexplained growth failure or may be asymptomatic.

The *diagnosis* is confirmed by an initially abnormal biopsy specimen of the small bowel showing partial or subtotal villous atrophy and improvement in a second specimen with a gluten-free diet. When the diagnosis is in doubt, especially in infants under 1 yr of age, a subsequent biopsy showing reappearance of disease after gluten challenge may be necessary. The presence of serum IgG or IgA against gliadin, reticulin, or endomysial antibodies (the most specific and sensitive) and a low D-xylose absorption are useful screening tests.

A positive IgA endomysial titer is very specific (>95%) but may be negative in affected IgA-deficient children. *Treatment* consists of permanent elimination of gluten-containing foods. Older patients may not have signs when rechallenged with cereals, but they do have mucosal atrophy, which may place them at increased risk for intestinal lymphoma.

### Inflammatory Bowel Disease

**Inflammatory bowel disease** (IBD) includes **ulcerative colitis, Crohn disease**, and **indeterminate colitis.** These conditions result from a genetic predisposition with associated alterations in immunoregulatory action of the gut. They are more common among whites, Jews, and family members; they occur equally in males and females. Most pediatric patients are adolescents, but both diseases have been reported in infancy. Crohn disease may involve any part of the gastrointestinal tract (mouth to anus), whereas ulcerative colitis produces only colonic disease (Table 11–14). Both may have common extraintestinal manifestations, including arthralgias, polyarticular arthritis, primary sclerosing cholangitis (ulcerative colitis primarily), chronic active hepatitis, sacroiliitis, pyoderma gangrenosum, erythema nodosum, nephrolithiasis,

TABLE 11–14.  Comparison of Crohn Disease and Ulcerative Colitis

| Feature | Crohn Disease | Ulcerative Colitis |
|---|---|---|
| Malaise, fever, weight loss | Common | Common |
| Rectal bleeding | Sometimes | Usual |
| Abdominal mass | Common | Rare |
| Abdominal pain | Common | Common |
| Perianal disease | Common | Rare |
| Ileal involvement | Common | None (backwash ileitis) |
| Strictures | Common | Unusual |
| Fistula | Common | Very rare |
| Skip lesions | Common | Not present |
| Transmural involvement | Usual | Not present |
| Crypt abscesses | Variable | Usual |
| Intestinal granulomas | Common | Rarely present |
| Risk of cancer | Increased | Greatly increased |
| Erythema nodosum | Common | Less common |
| Mouth ulceration | Common | Rare |

and uveitis or episcleritis. The pathology of Crohn disease involves transmural inflammation in a discontinuous pattern (skipped lesions): granulomas are present in some specimens. Ulcerative colitis produces superficial diffuse colonic ulceration and crypt abscesses. It involves the rectum in 95% of patients, with or without contiguous extension higher in the colon.

*Clinical Manifestations.* Most children with ulcerative colitis exhibit blood in the stool (100%), abdominal pain (95%), and tenesmus (75%) (see Table 11–14). Ninety percent of patients exhibit mild (<4 stools/day, no fever, anemia, or hypoalbuminemia) to moderate (>6 stools/day, fever, anemia, and hypoalbuminemia) disease. Severe disease may be a fulminant illness accompanied by high fever, abdominal tenderness, distention, tachycardia, leukocytosis, hemorrhage, more than 10 stools/day, and severe anemia. Toxic megacolon and subsequent intestinal perforation are rare complications.

The onset of Crohn disease often is subtle. Cramping abdominal pain, fever of unknown origin, weight loss, and diarrhea are common manifestations. Arthritis may precede gastrointestinal or other extraintestinal manifestations. Perianal disease may produce skin tags, fissures, fistulas, or abscesses. Severe disease is characterized by complications (fever, arthritis, iritis–uveitis, erythema nodosum, anal fissures, abscesses, or fistulas), an abdominal mass, abdominal pain, severe weight loss, and anemia.

*Diagnosis.* The differential diagnosis includes chronic bacterial or parasitic causes of diarrhea, such as *Clostridium difficile, Campylobacter jejuni, Yersinia enterocolitica,* amebiasis, and giardiasis. Because ulcerative colitis involves the rectum in 95% of patients, proctosigmoidoscopy or colonoscopy and biopsy are indicated. Visualization of the mucosa in ulcerative colitis reveals diffuse superficial ulceration and easy bleeding. In Crohn disease, direct visualization and biopsy of the affected area are not always possible.

*Roentgenographic examination* with a double (air)-contrast barium enema demonstrates diffuse colonic lesions and pseudopolyp formation in ulcerative colitis. This examination should not be performed in patients with severely active disease to avoid precipitating toxic megacolon. Crohn disease often reveals focal ileal (upper GI series) and/or colonic involvement with skipped lesions, rectal sparing, segmental narrowing (string sign), and longitudinal ulcers.

*Treatment.* General management includes drug therapy combined with nutritional support (enteral or parenteral); dietary modifications as needed for control of diarrhea, narrowing due to stenotic segments, or lactose intolerance; and transfusion for anemia.

Therapy for ulcerative colitis depends on the severity of the illness. Mild disease may be treated with oral sulfasalazine, which is poorly absorbed and is split by colonic bacteria into sulfapyridine and the active 5-aminosalicylate. Sulfasalazine is active against lipoxygenase and may reduce the elevated mucosal prostaglandin levels. Sulfapyridine may cause headache, hemolytic anemia, and gastrointestinal discomfort. Topical 5-aminosalicylate or hydrocortisone enemas also may be used in mild left-sided disease. They hasten healing but may be refused by children and adolescents. Oral mesalamine (5-aminosalicylate) should be tried in patients who do not tolerate sulfasalazine. Moderate ulcerative colitis is managed with the addition of 1–2 mg/kg/day of prednisone (maximum 60 mg/day) to the above regimen. Sulfasalazine helps to maintain remission. Patients with severe disease require intravenous alimentation, systemic corticosteroids, and close monitoring for hypokalemia, acidosis, anemia, and intestinal perforation. Cyclosporine may be efficacious in severe refractory disease. Emergency colectomy is indicated for refractory toxic megacolon or severe, persistent hemorrhage. Colectomy also is indicated for chronic refractory disease, persistent growth failure, and the presence of moderate or severe dysplasia on biopsy. The risk of colon carcinoma is increased in patients with extensive disease of greater than 10 yr duration. Colonoscopic surveillance is mandatory to determine the presence of dysplasia.

Prednisone is the most effective drug for Crohn disease of the small bowel, although mesalamine is often used concurrently. Colonic involvement also may benefit from the addition of sulfasalazine, whereas perianal disease and fistula formation may respond to metronidazole. Azathioprine and 6-mercaptopurine may permit reduction of corticosteroid dose in children who are dependent on or whose condition is refractory to prednisone. Surgery eventually is needed in approximately 25% of children with ulcerative colitis and 70% of children with Crohn disease because of failure of medical management, intestinal fistula or obstruction, and growth failure.

## Polyps

Most polyps in children are of the juvenile type, although some may occur in association with familial syndromes. These latter include **Peutz-Jeghers syndrome** (mucocutaneous pigmentation;

autosomal dominant), **Gardner syndrome** (soft tissue–bone tumor, rectal cancer; autosomal dominant), and **familial polyposis coli** (carcinoma; autosomal dominant). Juvenile polyps are pedunculated harmartomas, which have a peak incidence between 3 and 5 yr. Seventy percent occur in the rectum or sigmoid colon, and the majority are solitary. The usual presenting symptom is painless rectal bleeding. If the polyp is in the rectum, the *diagnosis* may be made on digital examination; otherwise, the diagnosis depends on a carefully performed air-contrast enema or colonoscopy. The latter procedure affords the opportunity for removal of the polyp at the time of the procedure.

## Appendicitis

Appendicitis is the most common cause of an acute abdomen in older children and adolescents (4:1000 children <16 yr). The cause may be obstruction of the appendiceal lumen by a fecalith or by inflammatory edema produced by lymphatic hyperplasia from a nonspecific infection. Meconium ileus equivalent or ileus-producing drugs (vincristine) are rarer causes of obstruction.

*Clinical manifestations* include a 1–2 day history of periumbilical dull or crampy pain, *followed by* anorexia and nausea, with or without vomiting. The pain remains constant but then localizes in the right lower quadrant (McBurney point) as a result of irritation of the parietal peritoneum. With rupture, the pain initially may subside but then is followed by signs of peritonitis, such as high fever, abdominal wall muscle rigidity resulting from voluntary guarding, and involuntary spasm. Unfortunately, atypical presentations are common among children or patients with retrocecal (less peritoneal irritation: positive psoas sign) or pelvic (less peritoneal irritation: tender rectal examination) appendices. Fever is often 38–38.5°C (100–102°F), and the peripheral white blood cell count usually is normal unless perforation has occurred or peritonitis is present. Urinalysis occasionally may reveal proteinuria and mild pyuria. Abdominal *roentgenograms* may demonstrate a fecalith or acute scoliosis toward the right as a result of psoas muscle spasm. Ultrasonography reveals a noncompressible enlarged appendix surrounded by fluid (donut or target sign) but also excludes ovarian or pelvic disease, mesenteric adenitis, and calculi.

The *differential diagnosis* includes those age-related and sex-related diseases listed in Table 11–1. **Mesenteric adenitis** caused by *Yersinia* species also may mimic appendicitis, whereas **primary peritonitis** may be confused with a ruptured appendix. The latter is noted in patients with ascites, ne-

phrotic syndrome, or, rarely, no underlying illness and is due to *Streptococcus pneumoniae* or *E. coli*

*Treatment* is surgical excision of the acutely inflamed appendix. Peritoneal drainage and broad-spectrum antibiotics effective against anaerobic and gram-negative enteric organisms are added if perforation is present.

## Intussusception

Intussusception occurs when one segment of bowel telescopes into a distal segment. Idiopathic intussusception usually occurs between 6 and 18 mo of life, with only 10% of cases occurring after 3 yr of age. The cause is unknown, but lymphoid hyperplasia (Peyer patches) may form a lead point of the proximal intussusception segment. A lead point is seen in 5% of cases. In older children, Meckel diverticulum, lymphosarcoma, and polyps may form lead points. Intussusception also is seen in cystic fibrosis and in Henoch-Schönlein purpura. The ileocolic form is the most frequent, followed by ilioileal and colocolic. Intussusception causes an acute onset of colicky intermittent abdominal pain. During the episodes of pain the infant will cry, draw up the knees, and perhaps vomit. Lethargy and fever are late findings, as is the passage of currant jelly–colored stools. On physical examination, a sausage-shaped mass may be found in the upper abdomen. Barium enema not only confirms the diagnosis but, with appropriate hydrostatic pressure, may reduce the intussusception in 75% of patients. Surgical reduction should be performed if (1) there are clinical signs of perforation, peritonitis, or shock, (2) medical reduction is unsuccessful, or (3) there is a high likelihood of finding a pathologic lead point.

## References

Behrman RE, Kliegman RM, Arvin AM (eds): Nelson Textbook of Pediatrics, 15th ed. Philadelphia, WB Saunders, 1996, Chapters 283, 286, 289, 290, 292.
Bhisitkul DM, Listernick R, Shkolnik A, et al: Clinical application of ultrasonography in the diagnosis of intussusception. J Pediatr 121:182, 1992.
The European Society for Paediatric Gastroenterology and Nutrition Working Group for the Diagnostic Criteria for Food Allergy: Diagnostic criteria for food allergy with predominantly intestinal symptoms. J Pediatr Gastroenterol Nutr 14:108, 1992.
Hanaver S: Inflammatory bowel disease. N Engl J Med 334:841, 1996.
Hyams JS: Crohn's disease in children. Pediatr Clin North Am 43:255, 1996.
Kerner JA: Formula allergy and intolerance. Gastroenterol Clin North Am 24:1, 1995.
Kirschner BS: Ulcerative colitis in children. Pediatr Clin North Am 235, 1996.
Trier JS: Celiac sprue. N Engl J Med 325:1709, 1991.

Wagnar J, McKinney P, Carpenter J: Does this patient have appendicitis? JAMA 276:1589, 1996.

## LIVER

Manifestations of hepatic disease may include abnormalities of any or all of the specific liver functions. The most common manifestations include jaundice (see Fig. 11–2), hepatomegaly, metabolic disturbances (hypoglycemia, hyperammonemia, encephalopathy, metabolic acidosis, hyperaminoacidemia), portal hypertension (cirrhosis, ascites, varices), and hemorrhage (varices).

*Laboratory tests* of hepatic function (Table 11–15) can be divided into two categories: those that suggest the presence of hepatobiliary disease and those that assess "liver function." Most liver function tests do not quantitatively measure function but instead provide clinical information about the course or severity of disease. In interpreting these tests, one should remember that the liver has a large reserve capacity with the capability for regeneration.

### Acute Viral Hepatitis

A number of agents cause acute hepatic injury (Table 11–16). Characteristics of hepatitis viruses are shown in Table 11–17. The delta agent produces disease only in those patients with hepatitis B infection. Community or parenteral viral hepatitis not due to the agents listed in Tables 11-16 and 11-17 should be considered non-A, non-G hepatitis.

The *clinical course* for HAV, HBV, and HCV is shown in Figure 11–5. A prodromal phase, which lasts approximately 1 wk, is characterized by headaches, anorexia, malaise, nausea, and vomiting and usually precedes the onset of clinically detectable disease. Infants with HBV may have immune complexes accompanied by urticaria and arthritis prior to icterus. Jaundice and a large tender liver are the most common physical findings. However, infants and young children with HAV, HBV, or HCV may not become icteric and mistakenly may be diagnosed as having the "flu." Liver enzymes may increase 15- to 20-fold. Resolution of the hyperbilirubinemia and normalization of the transaminases may take 6–8 wk. While approximately 10% of patients with acute HBV hepatitis develop chronic hepatitis, 60% or more of HCV-infected individuals (from blood transfusions) develop chronic liver disease (see Fig. 11-5). Note the fluctuating transaminase levels characteristic of chronic HCV hepatitis.

A number of *serologic markers* are available to detect the presence of hepatitis A, B, or C. Their appearance and time course also are shown in Figure 11–5. The presence of high-titer IgM-specific antibody to HAV and low or absent IgG antibody titer to the same virus is presumptive evidence for hepatitis A infection. The presence of hepatitis B virus surface antigen (HBsAg) signifies infection with HBV. Antigenemia may appear early in the illness and may be transient. The presence of HBsAg also is diagnostic of the carrier state, and maternal HBsAg status always should be determined when infants less than 1 yr of age are diagnosed with hepatitis B infection. Hepatitis B "e" antigen (HBeAg) appears in the serum with HBsAg. The continued presence of HBsAg and HBeAg in the absence of antibody to e antigen (anti-HBe) is predictive of a high risk of transmission. Clearance of HBsAg from the serum precedes a variable "window" period followed by the emergence of the antibody to surface antigen (anti-HBs), which confers lifelong immunity. Antibody to core antigen (anti-HBc) is a useful marker for recognizing HBV infection during the window phase (i.e., when HBsAg has disappeared but before the appearance of anti-HBs). Anti-HBe is useful in predicting a low degree of infectivity during the carrier state. Seroconversion following HCV infection may occur up to 6 mo after illness. A positive anti-HCV radioimmunoassay (RIA) should be followed with the more specific recombinant immunoblot assay (RIBA), which detects antibodies to multiple HCV antigens. Detection of HCV RNA by polymerase chain reaction (PCR) is a sensitive marker for active infection and may be positive as early as 3 days after inoculation.

Recovery is the rule in most cases of acute viral hepatitis. Less than 1:1000 cases progress to fulminant hepatic necrosis, encephalopathy, and death (see Fulminant Hepatic Failure). The virus-specific risks for chronic hepatitis, carrier state, and hepatocellular carcinoma are noted in Table 11–17.

The *treatment* of acute hepatitis is largely supportive and includes rest, hydration, and adequate dietary intake. Hospitalization is indicated for patients with severe vomiting and dehydration, a prolonged prothrombin time, or evidence of early hepatic encephalopathy. Once the *diagnosis* of viral hepatitis is made, attention should be directed toward preventing its spread. For HAV, careful hygienic measures include hand washing and the careful disposal of excreta, contaminated diapers or clothing, needles, and other blood-contaminated items. As soon as the diagnosis is established, immune serum globulin should be given to all immediate family contacts and, in the case of infants and toddlers, to all close playmates and children at day care centers. Similar hygienic measures are necessary for hepatitis B and C.

TABLE 11–15.  Liver Evaluation Tests

| Test | Mechanism | Significance |
|---|---|---|
| **Hepatic Function** | | |
| Albumin | Decreased synthesis | Decreased hepatic synthesis; increased loss by protein-losing enteropathy or nephrotic syndrome; increased volume of distribution (edema, ascites) |
| Prothrombin time | Decreased synthesis of factors II, VII, IX, and X | Hepatic dysfunction: unresponsive to vitamin K; malabsorption: responsive to vitamin K |
| Ammonia | Decreased ureagenesis; increased portosystemic shunting; increased ammonia load (GI bleeding) | Increased ammonia associated with hepatic encephalopathy; inborn errors of metabolism |
| Indocyanine green clearance | Low dose: indicator of liver blood flow; high dose: indicator of hepatic processing | Particularly sensitive for detecting cirrhosis |
| Galactose elimination test | Hepatic uptake and metabolism | Reflective of functional liver cell mass; useful for following declining hepatic function |
| Aminopyrine breath test | Hepatic uptake; demethylation by cytochrome $P_{450}$; measurement of breath excretion of radiolabel from methyl group | Index of hepatic excretion; useful for detection of cirrhosis; a prognostic indicator in patients with cirrhosis |
| Lidocaine clearance test | Measurement of appearance of MEGX, a major hepatic metabolite | Useful to evaluate liver dysfunction, especially in liver transplantation (before and after) |
| **Cellular Injury** | | |
| Aspartate aminotransferase (AST/SGOT) | Released from damaged hepatocytes | Also in heart, skeletal muscle, kidney, pancreas, RBCs, and brain |
| Alanine aminotransferase (ALT/SGPT) | Released from damaged hepatocytes | More specific for liver injury than AST |
| **Cholestasis** | | |
| Alkaline phosphatase | Greatest elevation usually in extrahepatic obstruction | Also in bone, intestine, placenta, kidney—may need to be fractionated for liver-specific isozyme |
| γ-Glutamyl transpeptidase (GGTP) | Sensitive, but not specific, index of biliary tract disease | Inducible by ethanol, phenobarbital, and other drugs; elevated in diabetes, myocardial infarction, renal failure, and other conditions |
| 5'-Nucleotidase | More specific for liver disease than alkaline phosphatase or GGTP | Biliary disease |
| Direct bilirubin | Decreased hepatic excretion in cholestasis | May also be elevated with hepatocellular injury; may be normal to slightly elevated with cholestasis (primary biliary cirrhosis, chronic cholestatic syndromes) |
| Bile acids | Decreased extraction from portal blood; decreased hepatic excretion in cholestasis | Do not discriminate hepatocellular from obstructive cholestasis |
| **Other** | | |
| α-Fetoprotein | Derepressed fetal gene | Hepatic tumor |
| Anti–smooth muscle, antinuclear, anti–liver-kidney microsomal autoantibodies | Autoimmunity | Autoimmune chronic active hepatitis |

**TABLE 11–15.**  Liver Evaluation Tests *Continued*

| Test | Mechanism | Significance |
|---|---|---|
| ***Imaging*** | | |
| Ultrasonography | Gross anomalies and blood flow using Doppler study | For gallstones, larger masses; can assess hepatic vein or artery, and portal vein thrombosis/obstruction |
| Computed tomography (CT scan) | Greater resolution than with ultrasound | Particularly useful for detecting abscesses and tumors |
| Angiography | Definition of hepatic vessels by contrast injection | Particularly useful for better definition of hepatic vein/portal vein thrombosis/obstruction; defining blood supply to tumors |
| Cholangiography | Definition of biliary tree by contrast injection | Defining biliary tract anatomy for source/site of obstruction |
| $^{99m}$Tc-sulfur colloid scan | Kupffer cell uptake | Large focal lesions |
| $^{99m}$Tc-DISIDA scan | Hepatic uptake and biliary excretion | Discriminating hepatocellular from obstructive cholestasis; confirming presence of choledochal cyst |
| Magnetic resonance imaging (MRI) | Greater resolution than CT | Evaluation of focal lesions (especially hemangiomas) and detecting excess hepatic iron |
| ***Liver Biopsy*** | | |
| Percutaneous, transjugular, laparoscopic, surgical | Obtaining liver tissue for histology, electron microscopy, immunostaining, measurement of copper or iron, and specific enzyme assays | May provide specific diagnosis and prognosis (degree of necrosis/fibrosis) for liver diseases |

The *prevention* of hepatitis may be accomplished by immunization and isolation (Table 11–18). Immune globulin is recommended following exposure to hepatitis. High-risk groups should receive immunization against HBV (e.g., parenteral drug abusers; male homosexuals; prisoners; sexual partners of HBV-infected individuals; infants born to HB$_s$Ag-positive mothers; patients and staff in hemodialysis and oncology units; patients requiring frequent blood or clotting factor concentrates and health care personnel who handle these products; physicians, dentists, and morticians; household contacts of HB$_s$Ag carriers; and patients with Down syndrome). It currently is recommended that all neonates and infants as well as all unvaccinated adolescents be immunized against HBV regardless of risk (see Chapter 10). HAV vaccine may be used in the clinical settings listed in Table 11–18.

### Fulminant Hepatic Failure

Fulminant hepatic failure may occur in patients who have had no pre-existing liver pathology. Massive hepatic necrosis in many cases may be due to viral agents or hepatotoxins. Most cases of fulminant liver failure in childhood are of unknown etiology, although an infectious agent is suspected. Impending acute liver failure should be suspected when transaminase values that initially were elevated 15- to 20-fold fall rapidly as the prothrombin time becomes prolonged (often >100 sec) and unresponsive to parenteral vitamin K. The direct bilirubin level continues to rise (often >15 mg/dL). In severe liver failure, the total bilirubin level continues to rise while the direct fraction decreases as a result of loss of conjugating function. Hepatic encephalopathy is the most dramatic sign of fulminant hepatic failure and progression to cerebral edema with brainstem herniation is often the cause of death. Other complications include hypoglycemia, gastrointestinal hemorrhage, hyponatremia, renal insufficiency (hepatorenal syndrome), and sepsis.

*Treatment* is supportive and includes:

1. Discontinuation of oral feedings and the administration of lactulose by nasogastric tube to trap ammonia in the intestinal lumen as ammonium ion for elimination in the feces.
2. Central venous alimentation with quantities of glucose and fluid sufficient to prevent hypoglycemia and hypovolemia.
3. Central venous pressure monitoring.

TABLE 11–16.    Causes of Acute Liver Disease
in Childhood

### Viral

| | |
|---|---|
| Hepatitis A, B, C, E, G | Herpes simplex 1, 2, 6, 7 |
| Hepatitis D (with B) | Adenovirus |
| Epstein-Barr virus | Lassa fever virus |
| Cytomegalovirus | Dengue |
| Enterovirus | Yellow fever |
| Human parvovirus B19 | Ebola virus |
| | Measles |
| | Varicella-zoster virus |
| | Undefined paramyxovirus (syncytial giant cells) |

### Bacterial

| | |
|---|---|
| Syphilis | Miliary tuberculosis |
| Leptospirosis | Gonococcus (perihepatitis) |
| Bacterial sepsis | *Chlamydia trachomatis* |
| *Coxiella burnetii* | (perihepatitis) |

### Toxic

| | |
|---|---|
| Isoniazid | Iron |
| Oral contraceptives | Erythromycin estolate |
| Androgens | Alcohol |
| Carbon tetrachloride | Mushroom poisoning (*Amanita* |
| Chlorpromazine | *phalloides*) |
| Allopurinol | Valproic acid |
| Acetaminophen | Phenytoin |
| Salicylates | Carbamazepine |
| Hydralazine | Methotrexate |
| Halothane | 6-Mercaptopurine |
| "Ecstasy" drug use | Herbal teas |

### Other

| | |
|---|---|
| Wilson disease | Veno-occlusive disease |
| Inborn errors of metabolism | Tumor |
| (galactosemia, | Infarction |
| tyrosinemia) | Shock |
| Chronic active hepatitis | Heart failure |
| | Anoxia |

From Behrman RE (ed): Nelson Textbook of Pediatrics, 14th ed. Philadelphia, WB Saunders, 1992, p 1018.

4. Intracranial pressure monitoring and, in selected patients with elevated intracranial pressure, administration of mannitol (hyperventilation is not effective in reducing intracranial pressure in these patients).
5. Administration of antacids or $H_2$ receptor antagonists to keep the gastric pH above 4.
6. Administration of intravenous vitamin K or fresh frozen plasma to improve or maintain clotting status. Liver transplantation is an effective therapy. In patients with high serum ammonia levels and worsening encephalopathy, exchange transfusion or plasmapheresis may result in transient improvement while transplantation is awaited.

The short-term *prognosis* is poor, with mortality rates of 80-90%. However, for those who survive, the long-term prognosis is excellent, with full recovery of normal liver function following hepatic regeneration.

## Chronic Liver Disease

Chronic hepatitis is an inflammatory process that lasts more than 6 mo and may become manifest as hepatic failure or chronic liver disease. Viral infections with HBV and HCV are the most frequently identifiable infectious causes. Other causes include drugs (such as alpha-methyldopa, isoniazid, and methotrexate), Wilson disease, alpha$_1$-antitrypsin deficiency, cystic fibrosis, and inflammatory bowel disease.

Chronic hepatitis may be classified as either persistent or active based on the histologic appearance of the liver. In patients with **chronic persistent hepatitis**, the liver architecture is normal and the inflammatory process is confined to the portal area without extension into the periportal region. Patients are usually asymptomatic. Laboratory studies demonstrate fluctuating transaminase levels, minimal or no hyperbilirubinemia, normal prothrombin time, and HBV or HCV seropositivity in most patients. Chronic persistent hepatitis is the most common cause of chronic hepatitis and is a self-limited condition that requires reassurance of the child and family but no specific treatment. Recovery is the rule, but the pathologic lesion and mild biochemical abnormalities may persist for years.

**Chronic active hepatitis** is a more serious form of the disease because the inflammatory process of lymphocytes and plasma cells not only involves the portal area but also extends into the adjacent lobule (periportal hepatitis, piecemeal necrosis). Fibrosis may extend between portal areas (bridging fibrosis). Chronic active hepatitis may progress to cirrhosis and hepatic failure. The *diagnosis* should be considered in any child with persistent or relapsing jaundice 6 mo following an episode of HBV or HCV hepatitis. However, most patients have no evidence of antecedent acute hepatitis. The most common form of chronic active hepatitis in children is the **autoimmune form**, which may have an indolent course. Many patients already have cirrhosis when the diagnosis is made.

*Clinical manifestations* include hepatosplenomegaly, jaundice, malaise, anorexia, and right upper quadrant pain. In addition to the aforementioned features of liver disease, patients with autoimmune chronic active hepatitis also may have extrahepatic manifestations, such as amenorrhea, arthritis, ar-

TABLE 11-17. Characteristics of the Agents Causing Acute Viral Hepatitis

| | Hepatitis A Virus (HAV) (Enterovirus 72) | Hepatitis B* Virus (HBV) | Hepatitis C† Virus (HCV) (Formerly posttransfusion Non-A, Non-B Virus) | Hepatitis D Virus (HDV) | Hepatitis E Virus (HEV) (Formerly Enteral, Non-A, Non-B Virus) | Hepatitis F Virus (HFV) | Hepatitis G Virus (HGV)/(HGBV-C) |
|---|---|---|---|---|---|---|---|
| Agent | 27-nm RNA virus | 42-nm DNA virus | 30-60-nm RNA virus; similar to flaviviruses | 36-nm circular RNA hybrid particle with $HB_sAg$ coat | 27-34-nm RNA virus; similar to Norwalk-type viruses | 27-37-nm DNA virus-like particles | RNA virus; similar to flaviviruses, 25% homology with HCV |
| Transmission | Fecal—oral, Food—water, rare parenteral | Transfusion, sexual, inoculation, vertical | Parenteral, transfusion, vertical (sexual?) | Similar to HBV | Enteral: endemic and epidemic | Enteral | Parenteral, transfusion |
| Incubation period | 15–30 days | 60–180 days | 30–60 days | Similar to HBV | 35–60 days | Unknown | Unknown |
| Serum markers | Anti-HAV | Antigens*, anti-$HB_s$, anti-$HB_c$ | Anti-HCV‖ (IgG, IgM), RIBA, HCV-RNA PCR | Anti-HDV, RNA | Anti-HEV | None | RNA by RT-PCR |
| Fulminant liver failure | Rare | Uncommon unless with δ agent‡ | Uncommon | Yes | Yes in pregnancy | Unknown | Probably no |
| Chronic liver disease | No | Yes | Yes | Yes | Uncommon | Unknown | Persistent infection common; chronic liver disease rare |
| Carrier state | No | Yes§ | Yes | Yes | No | Unknown | Yes |
| Risk of hepatocellular cancer | No | Yes | Yes | No | No | Unknown | Unknown |
| Prophylaxis against | Immune serum globulin vaccine; hygiene | Hepatitis B immune globulin, vaccine Screen blood products for $HB_sAg$ | Screen blood for antibody appearing 4 mo postinfection (6 mo post-transfusion) | Screen blood for HBV markers | Screen blood for IgM, IgG antibody | None | None |

*Hepatitis B whole virus particle is the Dane particle, which consists of a surface antigen $HB_sAg$, a core antigen $HB_cAg$, an e antigen $HB_eAg$, and DNA with a DNA polymerase. Mutant HBV also may produce severe hepatitis.

†An unknown number of posttransfusion hepatitis cases are due to viruses other than HBV, HCV or cytomegalovirus, Epstein-Barr virus, human herpesvirus-6, or known agents and remain designated as caused by a non-A, non-B hepatitis agent.

‡δ Agent or hepatitis D virus requires hepatitis B virus coinfection or superinfection of a chronic HBV carrier for replication.

§Chronic carrier state common in African-Asian, Haitian, Eskimo, and South Pacific immigrants, drug abusers, individuals with Down syndrome, multiply transfused patients, homosexuals, patients on hemodialysis, and dental workers.

‖May be measured by radioimmunoassay (RIA) and confirmed by the more specific recombinant immunoblot assay (RIBA).

PCR = polymerase chain reaction; RT = reverse transcription.

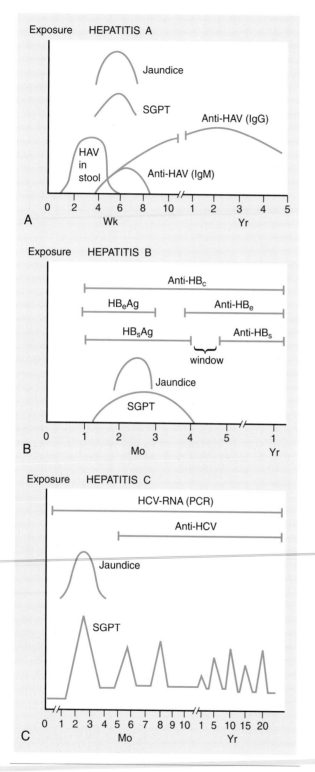

A

B

C

FIGURE 11–5. Clinical course and laboratory findings associated with hepatitis A, B, and C. HAV, hepatitis A virus; HB = hepatitis B; HCV = hepatitis C virus; IgG = immunoglobulin G; PCR = polymerase chain reaction; RNA = ribonucleic acid; SGPT = serum glutamic pyruvic transaminase.

TABLE 11–18.  Prevention of Hepatitis

| Etiology | Clinical Situation | Treatment |
|---|---|---|
| HAV | Before and 1 wk following jaundice | Enteric isolation |
| | Household contacts | IG within 2 wk of exposure |
| | School outbreak | IG only in day care or custodial institutions with high risk of fecal-oral spread |
| | Travel, military, Native Alaskans, Native Americans, homosexuals, IV drug users, epidemics | Vaccination |
| HBV | Perinatal exposure | Vaccination + HBIG |
| | Sexual: acute infection | HBIG ± vaccination |
| | Sexual: chronic carrier | Vaccination |
| | Household contact: chronic carrier | Vaccination |
| | Household contact: acute case | None unless known exposure |
| | Household contact: acute case, known exposure | HBIG + vaccination |
| | Infant (<12 mo): acute case in primary caregiver | HBIG + vaccination |
| | Inadvertent: percutaneous or permucosal exposure | HBIG + vaccination |
| | All neonates and infants | Vaccination |
| HCV | Inadvertent: percutaneous exposure | IG* |

*IG manufactured in the United States contains low antibody titers to HCV and is not likely to be effective.
HAV = hepatitis A virus; HBIG = hepatitis B immune globulin; HBV = hepatitis B virus; IG = immune serum globulin.

thralgia, low-grade fever, and thyroiditis. Patients with autoimmune hepatitis have circulating autoimmune markers. The presence of antinuclear antibodies (ANAs) along with smooth muscle antibodies (SMAs) suggests the diagnosis of autoimmune chronic hepatitis. The isolated presence of liver-kidney microsomal antibodies (LKMs) identifies a second group of patients with autoimmune chronic hepatitis. In chronic active hepatitis, the serum transaminase level is variable, but may not reflect the severity of the liver disease and usually is accompanied by hypergammaglobulinemia. The *diagnosis* is made by liver biopsy, which is a prerequisite for treatment with immunosuppressive agents.

In cases of autoimmune hepatitis, *treatment* with prednisone may lead to a dramatic improvement in the clinical, laboratory, and histologic features as well as a decrease in the mortality rate. Azathioprine is of value because of its steroid-sparing effect. Corticosteroids are contraindicated in patients with viral chronic active hepatitis. In children with autoimmune chronic active hepatitis, 75% respond to therapy but 50% relapse with discontinuation of prednisone. Progression to cirrhosis may occur despite a good response to initial immunosuppression. Patients who are LKM-positive have a poor response to therapy and are unlikely to remain in remission when immunosuppressive drugs are discontinued. Treatment of HBV and HCV chronic active hepatitis with alpha-interferon shows promise, but relapse may occur when therapy is discontinued.

## Cirrhosis

Cirrhosis is the end result of destructive processes producing irreversible fibrosis, scarring, and hepatocellular regeneration, which lead to the formation of regenerative nodules. The nodules cause irreversible distortion of the hepatic vasculature and biliary system. Nodules may be small (<3 mm in micronodular cirrhosis) or large (>3 mm in macronodular cirrhosis). This distortion of the vascular bed leads to portal hypertension and portosystemic shunting. In childhood and adolescence, the *etiology* of cirrhosis includes biliary malformations, alpha$_1$-antitrypsin deficiency, Wilson disease, galactosemia, tyrosinemia, chronic active hepatitis, and prolonged total parenteral nutrition.

*Clinical manifestations* include palmar erythema, spider angiomata, gynecomastia, splenomegaly, ascites, hemorrhoids, cutaneous excoriations from pruritus, and jaundice. The liver may be large and hard (biliary cirrhosis) or small, scarred, and shrunken (postnecrotic cirrhosis). *Laboratory findings* depend on the cause and severity of the process. The major *complications* of cirrhosis in children include portal hypertension with variceal bleeding and hypersplenism, ascites, liver failure with encephalopathy, hepatorenal syndrome, and, rarely, hepatocellular carcinoma.

## Portal Hypertension

Although cirrhosis is an important cause of portal hypertension, any process leading to an increased resistance to portal blood flow into the liver (prehepatic or presinusoidal; e.g., portal vein thrombosis, omphalitis, schistosomiasis), through the liver (intrahepatic or sinusoidal), or from above the liver (suprahepatic or postsinusoidal; e.g., Budd-Chiari syndrome, veno-occlusive disease, pericarditis) re-

sults in portal hypertension. Prehepatic and suprahepatic causes are more likely in children younger than 5 yr of age with no prior history of liver disease. Although rare, lesions such as an arteriovenous malformation, which increases hepatic blood flow, also result in portal hypertension. Portal hypertension leads to the formation of collaterals between the portal and systemic venous circulations. The most important of these connections is that between the portal vein and the azygos vein via submucosal veins (varices) in the stomach and esophagus.

Hemorrhage from *esophageal varices* is associated with hematemesis or melena (see Gastrointestinal Hemorrhage). In children, the bleeding often stops spontaneously but rebleeding may occur. Impaired synthesis of clotting factors, resulting from severe hepatocellular dysfunction or hypersplenism-induced thrombocytopenia, can result in uncontrollable hemorrhage.

*Treatment* consists of replacing blood losses and intravenous infusion of vasopressin or octreotide (somatostatin analog), which causes constriction of the splanchnic arterioles and a reduction of portal pressure and flow. Endoscopic sclerotherapy can be used to arrest acute bleeding and to prevent rebleeding. Repeated sclerosing injections lead to variceal obliteration. Endoscopic banding of varices is another effective technique. Portosystemic shunt surgery may decompress the entire portal system (portocaval anastomosis) or only the varices (distal splenorenal shunt). Transjugular intrahepatic portosystemic shunting (TIPS) is an emergency shunt procedure to avoid surgery but is also used to prevent rebleeding of esophageal varices. Portal hypertension also produces *hypersplenism* that becomes manifest by anemia, neutropenia, and thrombocytopenia.

## Ascites

Ascites is the accumulation of abnormal amounts of fluid in the peritoneal cavity. It results from hypoalbuminemia, portal hypertension, increased hepatic and splanchnic lymph production accompanied by impaired renal sodium and water excretion secondary to hyperaldosteronism and increased levels of antidiuretic hormone. Ascites is clinically detectable as a shifting dullness to percussion when at least 300 mL of fluid is present. Ascites caused by liver disease has the characteristics of a transudate (<3 g protein/dL).

*Treatment* consists of the administration of spironolactone and the restriction of sodium intake. The administration of furosemide may be necessary in refractory cases. Diuresis usually should be accomplished slowly over several days, but aggressive diuresis with abdominal paracentesis or intravenous albumin followed by furosemide is indicated when respiratory function is compromised. The latter approach may lead to plasma volume depletion, hypokalemia, hepatorenal syndrome, and encephalopathy. Spontaneous bacterial peritonitis may be a complication of ascites and should be considered if fever and abdominal pain are present (see Peritoneal Cavity). Abdominal symptoms may be minimal or absent in infants.

## Hepatic Encephalopathy

Progressive deterioration of liver function results in impaired detoxification of metabolic products. This process, along with portosystemic shunting, results in hepatic encephalopathy. Encephalopathy may be acute, as seen in fulminant hepatic failure, or chronic, as seen in slowly progressive liver disease with cirrhosis.

The *etiology* is unknown but may be related to disturbances in neuronal function resulting from the presence of false neurotransmitters in the central nervous system. Ammonia and bacterial products, such as octopamine, mercaptan (fetor hepaticus), or endogenous benzodiazepines and gamma-aminobutyrate, may play important roles. Serum ammonia levels often correlate poorly with the degree of encephalopathy.

The *clinical manifestations* of hepatic encephalopathy are described by four stages: (1) impaired mentation; (2) lethargy, disorientation, and asterixis ("liver flap"); (3) arousable stupor; and (4) coma. *Treatment* of chronic encephalopathy should focus on identification of the precipitating causes, such as intestinal bleeding, infection, central nervous system depressant drugs, and complications of diuretic therapy. Therapy includes maintaining adequate nutrition and reducing ammonia production. Some protein restriction may be needed, but at least 1.0 g/kg/24 hr must be provided to meet metabolic requirements and to prevent endogenous protein breakdown. During acute encephalopathy, no protein should be given; however, glucose infusions are needed to prevent hypoglycemia and proteolysis. Neomycin (oral) reduces the number of bacteria in the intestine available for producing ammonia. Lactulose also should be given to reduce ammonia production; it lowers stool pH, trapping ammonia in the form of the nondiffusible ammonium ion, and is a cathartic, reducing intestinal stasis. Flumazenil, a benzodiazepine antagonist, may reverse hepatic encephalopathy.

## Neonatal Cholestasis

Direct hyperbilirubinemia during the 1st mo of life signifies significant pathology resulting from hepatobiliary structural anomalies, infections, metabolic and genetic disease, drug and nutritional toxicity, and disorders of unknown cause (see Fig. 11–2 and Chapter 6). Except for parenteral alimentation–induced cholestasis in premature infants, the most common disorders in full-term infants that are associated with neonatal cholestasis are extrahepatic biliary atresia and idiopathic neonatal hepatitis. The usual *clinical manifestations* of cholestatic diseases during infancy are jaundice, hepatomegaly, dark urine, and acholic (white) stools.

After specific diagnostic tests are performed, the supportive *treatment* of these patients depends on the extent of the hepatocellular dysfunction and the severity of the cholestasis. Hepatocellular dysfunction predisposes the patient to complications, such as bleeding, encephalopathy, and hepatorenal syndrome, whereas bile salt deficiency may result in fat-soluble vitamin deficiencies, rickets, hypocalcemia (vitamin D deficiency), hemorrhage (vitamin K deficiency), and peripheral neuropathy (vitamin E deficiency). Retention of bile salts may produce pruritus.

*Supportive therapy* includes (1) fat-soluble vitamin supplementation; (2) administration of cholestyramine, to decrease reabsorption of bile salts from the gut; and (3) administration of phenobarbital, to increase the hepatic excretion of bile. The administration of oral ursodeoxycholic acid may improve bile secretion. *Definitive treatment* depends on the underlying process and may involve (1) an exclusion diet (lactose in galactosemia), (2) surgery (in extrahepatic biliary atresia, choledochal cyst), or (3) liver transplantation.

## Biliary Atresia

Biliary atresia is seen in 1:10,000 births and typically involves the extrahepatic bile ducts. In some patients, however, both intrahepatic and extrahepatic biliary structures are affected as a result of an inflammatory process beginning in the perinatal period. The condition is more common in females, and the *etiology* is unknown.

*Clinical manifestations* usually present in a full-term infant in whom jaundice develops during the 2nd or 3rd wk of life. The stools often are acholic, although the shedding of bilirubin-laden intestinal mucosal cells may color the stool. The liver enlarges and becomes quite hard. Splenomegaly usually is detectable by 8 wk. Other than these physical findings, the infants usually appear healthy.

There is an association with the polysplenia syndrome and with trisomy 13 and 18.

*Laboratory tests* demonstrate conjugated hyperbilirubinemia and elevated levels of serum alkaline phosphatase, gamma-glutamyl transferase, and transaminases. Ultrasound examination is helpful in excluding a choledochal cyst. A biliary scan following 5 days of phenobarbital administration (5 mg/kg/day) demonstrates normal hepatocyte uptake but a failure to excrete the isotope into the intestine after 24 hr. This test is less reliable in infants with serum bilirubin levels above 10 mg/dL. Percutaneous liver biopsy shows bile duct proliferation with bile plugging and confirms the diagnosis in 95% of patients.

Ultimately, patients with suspected biliary atresia require exploratory laparotomy. If biliary atresia is found, a *Kasai procedure* (hepatoportoenterostomy) is used to connect the bowel lumen and the porta hepatis containing bile duct remnants. Without surgery, patients usually die from cirrhosis before 2 yr of age. Surgical success is judged by improvement in bile drainage; the earlier the operation (<2 mo of age), the greater the chance of establishing bile flow. Twenty-five percent to 50% of patients survive 5 yr after a successful Kasai procedure, but complications of the procedure include progressive biliary cirrhosis and ascending cholangitis. Another treatment for most infants is liver transplantation, which has an 80–90% survival rate.

## Biliary Hypoplasia

Patients with intrahepatic biliary hypoplasia may be classified as either "syndromic" (**Alagille syndrome**, arteriohepatic dysplasia) or "nonsyndromic." In addition to intrahepatic biliary hypoplasia, infants with Alagille syndrome have facial, cardiac (valvular or peripheral pulmonic stenosis), vertebral (butterfly vertebra), ocular (posterior embryotoxon), and renal (dysplastic kidneys) anomalies. Patients have hypercholesterolemia and associated cutaneous xanthomata. Many of the children have growth failure, and some are mildly mentally impaired.

Alagille syndrome is inherited as an autosomal dominant trait with variable penetrance. The syndrome is associated with microdeletions on the short arm of chromosome 20. Mutations in the Jagged-1 gene on this chromosome have been found in families with the Alagille syndrome. This gene product is involved in intercellular signaling during development and differentiation.

*Treatment* is directed at controlling hypercholesterolemia with diet and cholestyramine and at pre-

venting manifestations of vitamin E deficiency (ataxia, areflexia, loss of vibratory and position sensation, and ophthalmoplegia) with aggressive vitamin E supplementation. Phenobarbital and ursodeoxycholic acid therapy also may help lower serum bilirubin and bile acid levels.

The *prognosis* for hepatic disease of the "syndromic" form is better than that for the nonsyndromic form. Cirrhosis and liver failure usually occur in the nonsyndromic form before adolescence.

## Idiopathic Neonatal Hepatitis

Idiopathic neonatal hepatitis is responsible for most of the cases of intrahepatic cholestasis in infants who are not receiving parenteral nutrition. It usually presents at birth, is more common in males, and may be associated with growth retardation. Idiopathic neonatal hepatitis probably represents more than one disease resulting from infectious or familial causes. It is unusual to have acholic stools and a very high alkaline phosphatase or gamma-glutamyl transferase (GGT) level. Patency of bile ducts may be documented by a biliary scan, although severe cholestasis may cause a false-positive scan. Liver biopsy shows numerous giant cells, lobular disorganization, necrosis, and inflammation without the neoductular proliferation and fibrosis characteristic of extrahepatic atresia.

The *differential diagnosis* includes TORCH (*t*oxoplasmosis, *o*ther, *r*ubella, *c*ytomegalovirus, *h*erpes simplex) infections, biliary atresia (which may be difficult to exclude without biopsy) and other causes of conjugated hyperbilirubinemia (see Fig. 11–2). *Treatment* is as described for Alagille syndrome, and most patients recover within 6–8 mo.

## Progressive Familial Intrahepatic Cholestasis
### (Byler Disease)

Progressive familial intrahepatic cholestasis (PFIC), inherited in an autosomal recessive manner, was first described in an Amish kindred (Byler), and usually presents in the 1st yr of life with progressive cholestasis and pruritus, out of proportion to the level of jaundice. PFIC progresses to cirrhosis, end-stage liver disease, and death by 3 yr without transplantation. PFIC is characterized by low serum GGT and normal cholesterol concentrations, in contrast to other childhood cholestatic disorders. Other than liver transplantation, chronic biliary diversion and ursodeoxycholic acid therapy may reduce pruritus and improve liver function in some patients.

## Reye Syndrome

Reye syndrome is characterized by encephalopathy and the noninflammatory fatty infiltration of the liver and kidney. It has been associated with epidemics of influenza A or B virus and varicella. The administration of aspirin predisposes the patient to this condition. The peak incidence is in children of 6 yr of age, with most cases occurring between 4 and 12 yrs of age.

The *clinical manifestations* begin with intractable vomiting during or immediately following recovery from an upper respiratory tract infection. Over a period of 2–24 hr, the child becomes confused, combative, agitated, stuporous, and, finally, comatose. In addition to the altered level of consciousness, physical findings include dilated pupils, hyperactive deep tendon reflexes, and Kussmaul respirations. Jaundice and fever are absent, and the liver may be normal to moderately enlarged in size. The serum transaminase and ammonia levels are elevated, and the prothrombin time may be prolonged. Hypoglycemia and acidosis also may be present. Cerebrospinal fluid examination is normal, and toxicologic findings of the blood and urine are negative.

The *diagnosis* is made by liver biopsy. Histologic findings include a diffuse microvesicular steatosis, without necrosis or inflammation. The mitochondria are swollen. Infants under 2 yr of age should be evaluated for underlying inborn errors of metabolism, such as medium-chain acyl-coenzyme A dehydrogenase deficiency.

*Treatment* is supportive and similar to that outlined for fulminant hepatic failure. Careful monitoring and treatment of increased intracranial pressure are mandatory.

The *prognosis* correlates best with the depth of coma. Death from Reye syndrome usually is due to increased intracranial pressure because liver regeneration is often present at the time of autopsy.

*Prevention* may be possible by avoidance of salicylates during viral respiratory illnesses.

## Alpha₁-Antitrypsin Deficiency

The glycoprotein alpha$_1$-antitrypsin is produced by hepatocytes under the influence of two autosomally inherited, codominant alleles and makes up 80% of the serum alpha$_1$-globulin fraction. It functions as an inhibitor of trypsin, pancreatic elastase, neutral proteases of leukocytes, and acid proteases of alveolar macrophages. Uninhibited proteolytic activity by these enzymes may cause hepatic or pulmonary injury. There are more than 70 different alleles of this protease-inhibitor (Pi) system. The normal phenotype is MM; Pi ZZ is associated with liver or lung disease. The incidence of the ZZ phenotype is 1:1600–1800, but only 15% of patients with the ZZ phenotype have neonatal cholestasis. The liver disease may be due to the accumulation of an abnormally folded protein within the hepatocyte. Variability in the severity of the liver disease may be related to variations of the endoplasmic reticulum degradative pathway, which removes the abnormal protein.

Cholestatic jaundice that is indistinguishable from neonatal hepatitis during the first 1–3 mo of life may be the initial presenting sign. Hepatosplenomegaly also may be present. Cirrhosis develops in 30–50% of patients, resulting in hepatic failure; progression may be extremely variable (months to years). Older patients may develop pulmonary emphysema, and hepatocellular cancer has developed following cirrhosis. Pancreatitis also may develop.

The *diagnosis* is made by quantifying levels of circulating alpha$_1$-antitrypsin and phenotyping. Liver biopsy reveals the presence of eosinophilic cytoplasmic granules that stain intensely with periodic acid–Schiff (PAS) stain and are resistant to digestion with diastase.

There is no specific *treatment*. Plasma or recombinant alpha$_1$-antitrypsin infusions restore plasma levels but have not yet been demonstrated to cure the hepatic complications. Therapy for cholestasis and the complications of cirrhosis are similar to those previously outlined. In severe cases, transplantation may be necessary.

## Wilson Disease
### (Hepatolenticular Degeneration)

Wilson disease is an autosomal recessive disorder caused by the accumulation of copper in the liver, brain, eyes, kidney, and bone. The defective gene is on chromosome 13 and appears to encode an adenosine triphosphatase (ATPase) involved in copper transport. *Clinical manifestations* are unusual before 5 yr of age and include hepatosplenomegaly and jaundice resembling chronic active hepatitis, hemolytic anemia, deterioration of neurologic function (worsening school performance and handwriting, intention tremor, clumsiness, personality changes), renal tubular acidosis, and the appearance of corneal Kayser-Fleischer rings. Hepatitis is common in younger patients; neuropsychiatric problems are noted in older patients. Wilson disease may present with fulminant liver failure and should be considered, particularly when severe hemolysis is also present.

Low serum copper and low serum ceruloplasmin levels suggest the *diagnosis*, but normal copper values may be found early in the course of the disease. Quantitation of urinary copper output, with or without penicillamine administration or quantitation of hepatic copper levels, confirms the diagnosis.

The goal of *treatment* is to lower tissue copper levels. This has been successfully accomplished with the copper chelating agent D-penicillamine. Foods high in copper, such as chocolate, nuts, and dried fruits, should be avoided. The *prognosis* depends on early diagnosis and successful chelation of the copper.

## References

Balistreri W: Mechanisms and management of pediatric hepatobiliary disease. J Pediatr Gastroenterol Nutr 10:138, 1990.

Behrman RE Kliegman RM, Arvin AM (eds): Nelson Textbook of Pediatrics, 15th ed. Philadelphia, WB Saunders, 1996, Chapters 301–313.

Conjeevaram HS, Di Bisceglie AM: Management of chronic viral hepatitis in children. J Pediatr Gastroenterol Nutr 20:365, 1995.

Czaja A: The variant forms of autoimmune hepatitis. Ann Intern Med 125:588, 1996.

Hardie R, Newton L, Bruce J, et al: The changing clinical pattern of Reye's syndrome, 1982—1990. Arch Dis Child 74:400, 1996.

Hoofnagle J, Di Bisceglie A: The treatment of chronic viral hepatitis. N Engl J Med 336:347, 1997.

Hussein M, Howard E, Mieli-Vergani G, et al: Jaundice at 14 days of life: Exclude biliary atresia. Arch Dis Child 66:1177, 1991.

Jonas MM: Interferon-α for viral hepatitis. J Pediatr Gastroenterol Nutr 23:93, 1996.

Mas A, Rodes J: Fulminant hepatic failure. Lancet 349:1081, 1997.

Miyakawa Y, Mayumi M: Hepatitis G virus: A true hepatitis virus or an accidental tourist? N Engl J Med 336:795, 1997.

Mousseau DD, Butterworth RF: Current theories on the pathogenesis of hepatic encephalopathy. Proc Soc Exp Biol Med 206:329, 1994.

Rössle M, Deibert P, Haag K, et al: Randomized trial of transjugular-intrahepatic-portosystemic shunt versus endoscopy plus propranolol for prevention of variceal rebleeding. Lancet 349:1043, 1997.

Teckman J, Perlmutter DH: Conceptual advances in the pathogenesis and treatment of childhood metabolic liver disease. Gastroenterology 108:1263, 1995.

## PANCREAS

Isolated disease of the exocrine pancreas is uncommon in children. Pancreatic exocrine insufficiency often is part of a genetic or systemic illness. Cystic fibrosis (see Chapter 12) and severe malnutrition are the leading causes of pancreatic disease. **Shwachman syndrome** (neutropenia, dysostosis), an autosomal recessive disorder, accounts for 3–5% of pancreatic insufficiency in childhood.

*Pancreatic function tests* include determination of the levels of serum amylase and lipase (which are increased when pancreatitis is present), and trypsinogen (which is increased in cystic fibrosis); examination of stool for fat droplets or meat fibers (indicating fat and protein maldigestion); and analysis of urine for reduced *para*-aminobenzoic acid (PABA) excretion (which is due to deficient pancreatic chymotrypsin) following ingestion of N-benzoyl-L-tyrosyl-PABA. Cannulation of the pancreatic duct and collection of fluid for enzyme analysis, with and without secretagogue stimulation (endoscopic retrograde cholangiopancreatoduodenoscopy), also may be helpful in evaluating pancreatic insufficiency.

### Annular Pancreas

The annular pancreas is a rare malformation caused by a failure of rotation and fusion of the ventral and dorsal pancreatic buds. A complete pancreatic ring may obstruct the duodenum. **Pancreas divisum** is due to failure of fusion of the dorsal and ventral embryonic pancreas that drains through an accessory papilla. Pancreas divisum is a cause of recurrent pancreatitis.

### Pancreatitis

Pancreatic duct obstruction or nonspecific parenchymal inflammation results in tissue injury from digestive enzymes, which leads to autodigestion and further inflammation and edema. Fat necrosis and hemorrhage are additional complications of acute pancreatitis. The *etiology* is idiopathic in as many as 25% of cases. Other causes include infectious agents (mumps; coxsackievirus, hepatitis virus, influenza virus, *Mycoplasma*), drugs (alcohol, thiazide diuretics, valproic acid, L-asparaginase, acetaminophen, corticosteroids, sulfonamides), cystic fibrosis, alpha$_1$-antitrypsin deficiency, gallstones, biliary "sludge," shock, pancreas divisum, hypertriglyceridemia, hypercalcemia, trauma, renal failure, familial disease, and vasculitis.

The *clinical manifestations* include intense epigastric pain (occasionally radiating to the back), nausea, and vomiting. The abdomen may be tender and rigid, and a mass may be palpable if a pseudocyst has formed. Hemorrhagic pancreatitis may cause shock and produce a blue discoloration around the umbilicus (Cullen sign) or around the flank (Grey Turner sign). Left-sided pleural effusion and ascites are less common manifestations. Poor prognostic features include hyperglycemia (>200 mg/dL), leukocytosis (>16,000), elevated lactic dehydrogenase (>700 IU) and serum glutamic oxaloacetic transaminase (>250 U), and the development of anemia, hypocalcemia, azotemia (blood urea nitrogen >50 mg/dL), metabolic acidosis, hypoxia, and the need for continuous fluid resuscitation.

*Laboratory findings* include elevated serum amylase and lipase levels. Diabetic ketoacidosis, renal failure, parotid gland disease, perforated gastric ulcer, or acidosis may produce false elevations of serum amylase. Pleural or ascitic fluid amylase levels are elevated. Hyperglycemia and hypocalcemia may be present. Abdominal roentgenograms may demonstrate a sentinel loop, pancreatic calcification, or a mass. Ultrasonography demonstrates a swollen pancreas and/or pseudocyst.

*Treatment* includes fluid replacement for hypovolemic shock, bowel rest, nasogastric decompression, and pain medication. Management is also directed toward the relief of complications, such as anemia and hypocalcemia. Pseudocysts that persist beyond 6 wk may require surgery. Endoscopic retrograde cholangiopancreoduodenoscopy may have a role in the management of recurrent pancreatitis to define anatomic abnormalities.

### References

Behrman RE, Kliegman RM, Arvin AM, (eds): Nelson Textbook of Pediatrics, 15th ed. Philadelphia, WB Saunders, 1996, Chapters 293–299.

Dugernier T: Severe acute pancreatitis. The therapeutic dilemma: Medical or surgical intensive care. Intensive Crit Care Digest 10:47, 1991.

Schroder T, Sainio V, Kivisaari L, et al: Pancreatic resection versus peritoneal lavage in acute necrotizing pancreatitis. Ann Surg 214:663, 1991.

Weizman Z, Durie P: Acute pancreatitis in childhood. J Pediatr 113:24, 1988.

## PERITONEAL CAVITY

Primary peritonitis is an acute inflammatory process in the peritoneal cavity attributable to a perforated viscus. It usually occurs in children after splenectomy or in those having chronic ascites, such as that seen in nephrotic syndrome or cirrhosis.

*Clinical manifestations* include the acute onset of fever, severe abdominal pain, and vomiting. The *diagnosis* may be made on abdominal paracentesis. The fluid is an exudate, Gram stain reveals organisms, and many polymorphonucleated leukocytes are present. The responsible bacteria are *Pneumococcus* and gram-negative enteric pathogens. Peritonitis in patients receiving chronic ambulatory peritoneal dialysis includes that caused by *Staphylococcus epidermidis*.

Secondary peritonitis is an inflammatory response to bacteria, bile, or pancreatic enzymes in the abdominal cavity resulting from a ruptured viscus. Necrotizing enterocolitis, appendicitis, and penetrating wounds are common causes. *E. coli, Klebsiella, Proteus, Enterobacter,* and *Bacteroides fragilis* are frequently found pathogens. Combined therapy for anaerobic and gram-negative organisms and appropriate surgery are the treatment of choice.

### Reference

Behrman RE, Kliegman RM, Arvin AM (eds): Nelson Textbook of Pediatrics, 15th ed. Philadelphia, WB Saunders, 1996, Chapters 314–318.

# Chapter 12

# THE RESPIRATORY SYSTEM

Carolyn M. Kercsmar

Disorders of the respiratory system—for example, viral upper respiratory infections, otitis media, pneumonia, asthma, and cystic fibrosis—constitute a substantial part of the pediatrician's clinical practice. Respiratory disease may be insidious because normally a large lung reserve capacity exists and more than half the total lung tissue (or function) may be lost before an individual complains of dyspnea. In addition, the typical symptoms (dyspnea, cough, chest pain) or signs (tachypnea, rales, wheezing) may be overlooked or may be subtle in young children. Fever may be the only symptom of pneumonia, tachypnea the only manifestation of asthma, and cough the only symptom of foreign body aspiration. During a child's development, the pediatrician also must consider genetic (cystic fibrosis), anatomic (congenital anomalies), iatrogenic (oxygen toxicity), immunologic (immunosuppression, immunodeficiency), and extrapulmonary (heart failure) conditions as etiologic variables contributing to pulmonary pathology.

The lung has a tremendous capacity for growth. At birth, the full-term infant has approximately 25 million alveoli; this number increases to nearly 300 million in adulthood. Most of this growth occurs by 8 yr of age; the greatest growth is in the first 3–4 yr.

## ANATOMY OF THE RESPIRATORY SYSTEM

Air enters the nostrils and passes over three turbinates (bony protrusions into the nasal cavity), which are covered by ciliated respiratory epithelium and which increase the total surface area within the nostril. This large surface area and the convoluted patterns the airflow takes as it passes over the turbinates create a high resistance but serve to warm, humidify, and filter the inspired air. Secretions draining from the paranasal sinuses are carried from the nasal cavity to the pharynx by the mucociliary action of the epithelium. The eustachian tubes open from the middle ear into the posterior aspect of the nasopharynx. Lymphoid tissue at this location (the adenoids) may obstruct the orifice of the eustachian tubes.

The epiglottis helps to protect the larynx during swallowing by deflecting swallowed material toward the esophagus. The epiglottis of children has a contour somewhat like the Greek letter *omega* and usually is shaped differently from that of adults. The arytenoid cartilages, which assist in opening and closing the glottis, usually are not very prominent in children. The vocal cords form a V-shaped opening (the glottis), with the apex of the V being anterior, at the base of the epiglottis. Beneath the cords, the walls of the subglottic space converge toward the cricoid ring, a complete ring of cartilage. In children younger than 2 or 3 yr of age, the cricoid ring (in effect, the first tracheal ring) is the narrowest portion of the airway; in older children and adults, the glottis is the smallest part of the airway.

The trachea and main bronchi are supported by rings of cartilage, which extend about 320 degrees around the airway circumference; the posterior wall is membranous. Beyond the lobar bronchi, the cartilaginous support for the airways becomes discontinuous. The more peripheral airways are supported entirely by elastic forces within the lung parenchyma.

The right lung normally has three lobes (upper, middle, and lower) and occupies about 55% of the total lung volume. The left lung normally has two lobes. The left upper lobe has an inferior division (the lingula) that is analogous to the middle lobe on the right.

## PULMONARY PHYSIOLOGY

### PULMONARY MECHANICS

The major function of the lungs is to exchange oxygen ($O_2$) and carbon dioxide ($CO_2$) between the atmosphere and the blood. Factors that influence this function include the anatomy and mechanics of the airways, the mechanics of the respiratory muscles and rib cage, the structure of the blood-gas interface (the alveolar surface), the pulmonary circulation, and the central mechanisms for neuromuscular control of ventilation.

Air enters the lungs via the upper airway whenever the pressure in the thorax is less than that of the surrounding atmosphere. During inspiration at rest, the negative intrathoracic pressure is caused by contraction (and lowering) of the diaphragm. Accessory muscles of respiration may be recruited during labored breathing. The external intercostal, scalene, and sternocleidomastoid muscles lift the rib cage and thus function as muscles of inspiration. During quiet breathing, most exhalation is passive, but during forced exhalation, intrathoracic pressure is increased by the abdominal muscles and by the internal intercostal muscles, which pull the ribs together.

Airway resistance is determined by the diameter of the conducting airway, its length, the viscosity of the gas, and the nature of the airflow. During quiet breathing, airflow (especially in the smaller airways) may be laminar, in which case the resistance is inversely proportional to the 4th power of the radius of the airway. At higher flow rates (as

during exercise), the flow becomes turbulent and the resistance increases even more. Thus, relatively small changes in airway diameter (e.g., increases with normal growth or decreases resulting from mucosal edema or bronchoconstriction) may produce very large changes in airway resistance, a phenomenon more dramatically demonstrated in infants because the same degree of airway narrowing in the smaller airways of an infant produces proportionately greater physiologic effects than it does in the larger airways of an older child or an adult.

When all mechanical forces acting on the lung are at equilibrium (e.g., at the end of a normal relaxed breath), the lung contains a volume of gas known as the *functional residual capacity* (FRC) (Fig. 12–1). This gas volume is important in maintaining exchange of oxygen across the alveolar surface during exhalation. Alterations in pulmonary homeostasis that result in decreased FRC include surfactant deficiency (neonatal respiratory distress syndrome), acute respiratory distress syndrome (ARDS), and restrictive lung diseases. Obstructive lung disease, such as cystic fibrosis, increases FRC.

Normal tidal breathing utilizes the middle range of lung volumes, reaching neither residual volume nor total lung capacity (see Fig. 12–1). Residual volume (RV) is the volume of gas in the lungs at the end of a maximal exhalation, whereas total lung capacity (TLC) is the volume of gas in the lungs at the end of a maximal inhalation. Vital capacity (VC) is the difference between TLC and RV.

With *partial airway obstruction*, airways collapse during exhalation, preventing normal emptying and thus increasing RV while also decreasing VC. Increased degrees of obstruction eventually in-

FIGURE 12–1. Lung volumes and capacities. Although vital capacity and its subdivisions can be measured by spirometry, calculation of residual volume requires measurement of functional residual capacity by body plethysmography, helium dilution technique, or nitrogen washout. (From Andreoli TE, Bennett JC, Carpenter CJ, Plum F [eds]: Cecil Essentials of Medicine, 4th ed. Philadelphia, WB Saunders, 1997, p. 127.)

crease FRC as well. Another manifestation of obstruction is decreased expiratory flow rates. A useful technique to clinically define airway obstruction is measuring the volume of air exhaled during the 1st sec of a forced vital capacity maneuver (forced expiratory volume in 1 sec, $FEV_1$). The forced expiratory flow rate ($FEF_{25-75}$) is the volume of air exhaled per second during the forced expiratory maneuver between 25% and 75% of forced vital capacity. It is more sensitive to obstruction in peripheral airways than is $FEV_1$. VC, $FEV_1$, and $FEF_{25-75}$ are clinically useful measures and can be determined with a simple spirometer. Peak expiratory flow rate (PEFR) measures the most rapid rate of airflow (in liters/second or minute) during a forced expiratory maneuver, is largely a measure of airflow in central airways, and is highly dependent on patient effort. PEFR is best measured with a peak flowmeter, a simple hand-held device readily available in the office or emergency department setting.

Not all the air inspired during each breath reaches the alveoli. Normally, about 30% of each tidal breath fills the anatomic dead space (non–gas-exchanging parts of the respiratory system). The efficiency of ventilation therefore can be enhanced by increasing the tidal volume (because dead space is relatively constant). If tidal volume is decreased (as with central depression of respiratory drive or neuromuscular disease), the ratio of dead space to tidal volume will increase and alveolar ventilation will decrease.

The most common forms of lung disease in children result in airway obstruction. Excess secretions, bronchospasm, mucosal edema, inflammation, stenosis, and airway compression all may produce symptomatic airway obstruction. *Restrictive disease* is less common and is characterized by normal to low FRC and RV, low total lung capacity and VC, decreased lung compliance, and relatively normal flow rates.

## RESPIRATORY GAS EXCHANGE

Gas exchange depends on alveolar ventilation and pulmonary capillary blood flow as well as on the ability of the gases to diffuse across the alveolar-capillary surfaces. Carbon dioxide diffuses 20 times more readily than oxygen. Thus, hypercapnia is a relatively late manifestation of disordered gas exchange, whereas hypoxemia occurs earlier. Under normal circumstances, physiologic matching of ventilation ($\dot{V}_A$) and blood flow ($\dot{Q}$) is maintained by anatomic mechanisms and local constriction of the pulmonary vessels in areas that are hypoventi-

lated. The flow to the pulmonary circulation is capable of increasing at least five-fold. A significant percentage of the capillary bed is not open under normal resting conditions, and blood normally is shunted away from underventilated areas of the lung. However, if hypoxic pulmonary vasoconstriction fails for any reason, the underventilated lung continues to be perfused and the blood returning from that area is unoxygenated, thus producing an intrapulmonary shunt with hypoxemia. Under normal circumstances, the hypoxemia would lead to an increased minute volume and a fall in the arterial carbon dioxide partial pressure ($PaCO_2$) as the shunt increases. Additionally, disorders of unequal ventilation-perfusion matching are much more common causes of hypoxemia than are abnormalities of diffusion, especially in children (Table 12–1).

## CONTROL OF VENTILATION

Ventilation is controlled by central chemoreceptors in the medulla, which respond to the intracellular pH (and, therefore, to the partial pressure of $CO_2$ [$PCO_2$]) (Fig. 12–2). To a lesser extent, ventilation also is controlled by peripheral receptors in the carotid and aortic bodies, which respond predominantly to the partial pressure of oxygen ($PO_2$). The central receptors are very sensitive; small changes in $PaCO_2$ normally result in significant changes in

FIGURE 12–2. Schematic representation of the respiratory control system. The respiratory neurons in the brain stem receive information from the chemoreceptors, peripheral sensory receptors, and cerebral cortex. This information is integrated, and the resulting neural output is transmitted to the chest bellows and lungs. + = Stimulation, − = inhibition. (From Andreoli TE, Carpenter CJ, Plum F, et al [eds]: Cecil Essentials of Medicine, 2nd ed. Philadelphia, WB Saunders, 1986, p 171.)

TABLE 12–1.    Differentiation of Mechanisms of Hypoxia

| Etiology | Example | $Pa_{O_2}$ | $Pa_{CO_2}$ | A-aDO₂ (gradient)* Room Air | A-aDO₂ (gradient)* 100% O₂ | Q̇s/Q̇T (shunt)† Room Air | Q̇s/Q̇T (shunt)† 100% O₂ |
|---|---|---|---|---|---|---|---|
| Hypoventilation | Narcotic overdose, neuromuscular disease | ↓ | ↑ | N | N | N | N |
| Altitude | Mountain climbing | ↓ | ↓ | N | N | N | N |
| Intrapulmonary shunt | Atelectasis | ↓ | N or ↓ | ↑ | ↑ | ↑ | ↑ |
| Cyanotic heart disease | Tetralogy of Fallot | ↓ | N or ↓ | ↑ | ↑ | ↑ | ↑ |
| Pulmonary edema | Cardiomyopathy | ↓ | ↓ N ↑ | ↑ | N or ↑ | ↑ | N or ↑ |
| Adult respiratory distress syndrome | Sepsis, shock | ↓ | N to ↑ | ↑ | N or ↑ | ↑ | ↑ |
| Pneumonia | Lobar pneumococcal pneumonia | N or ↓ | ↓ or N | N or ↑ | N | ↑ | ↑ |
| Pure $\dot{V}_A/\dot{Q}$ mismatch | Bronchopulmonary dysplasia, cystic fibrosis | ↓ | N or ↑ | ↑ | N | ↑ | N |
| Diffusion defect | Scleroderma | ↓ | N | ↑ | N or ↑ | ↑ | N |

*A-aDO₂ = alveolar-arterial O₂ gradient, which is not influenced by changes in minute ventilation and is a measure of gas exchange. The A-aDO₂ can be determined by the *alveolar gas equation:* A-aDO₂ = (P_B − pH₂O) × FiO₂ − Pa_{CO₂}/R, where P_B = atmospheric pressure (usually 760 mm Hg); pH₂O = partial pressure of H₂O (~ 47 mm Hg); R = respiratory exchange ratio (.8); FiO₂ = inspired O₂ (21% for room air). Normal value of A-aDO₂ = 30–50 mm Hg (while breathing 100% O₂). Under normal conditions, alveolar or inspired O₂ should be close to arterial O₂.

†Q̇s/Q̇T = the calculation of venous admixture or shunt. Q̇s = flow through the shunt (area of perfusion but no ventilation). Q̇T = total cardiac output to well-ventilated and poorly ventilated (shunt) areas of the lung. An increased Q̇s/Q̇T is due to shunting or ventilation-perfusion inequality (V̇_A/V̇Q). With 100% O₂, V̇_A/V̇Q is eliminated and the Q̇s/Q̇T represents shunting.

N = normal; Pa_{CO₂} = arterial carbon dioxide partial pressure; Pa_{O₂} = arterial oxygen partial pressure.

minute ventilation. If $Pa_{CO_2}$ is elevated for some time, however, equilibration of the cerebral intracellular space to a higher bicarbonate level may result in relative hypoventilation for the degree of carbon dioxide elevation. The peripheral receptors do not affect ventilation until the arterial oxygen partial pressure ($Pa_{O_2}$) falls to approximately 50 torr. These receptors may become very important when lung disease results in chronic elevation of $Pa_{CO_2}$.

The output of the central respiratory center also is modulated by reflex mechanisms. Full lung inflation inhibits inspiratory effort (the Hering-Breuer reflex) through vagal afferent fibers. Other reflexes from the airways and intercostal muscles may influence the depth and frequency of respiratory efforts (see Fig. 12–2).

## LUNG DEFENSE MECHANISMS

The airways are a direct connection between the lungs and the atmosphere, which is not typically clean or sterile. Large particles are filtered primarily by the nose. The paranasal sinuses and the nasal turbinates are lined with ciliated epithelium, which carries these filtered particles to the pharynx. Particles smaller than 10 μm in diameter may reach the trachea and bronchi, where they are deposited on the mucosa. Particles smaller than 1 μm may reach the alveoli, where they either remain or are exhaled without being deposited. Ciliated cells line the airways from the larynx to the bronchioles; the cilia continuously move a thin layer of mucus toward the mouth, carrying inhaled particulates. Normally, mucociliary transport in the larger airways is fast, with rates averaging 10 mm/min. Alveolar macrophages and polymorphonuclear cells can engulf particles or pathogens opsonized by locally secreted immunoglobulin A (IgA) antibodies or transudated serum antibodies.

Reflex mechanisms also protect the lungs. The most important of these mechanisms is cough, a forceful expiration that removes foreign or infected material from the airways. A cough may be voluntary or may be generated by reflex irritation of the nose, sinus, pharynx, larynx, trachea, bronchi, and bronchioles. During a cough, the person inspires deeply, the glottis closes, the expiratory muscles contract to increase intrathoracic pressure, and the glottis opens suddenly, forcefully releasing air from the system. Loss of the cough reflex leads to aspiration and pneumonia. In young infants, secretions may be swallowed rather than expectorated. Nasal irritation may produce reflex bronchoconstriction to limit the penetration of noxious vapors.

## References

Behrman RE, Kliegman RM, Arvin AM, (eds): Nelson Textbook of Pediatrics, 15th ed. Philadelphia, WB Saunders, 1996, Chapters 320, 321, 323.

Maturation of the respiratory system. *In* Loughlin GM, Eigen H (eds): Respiratory Disease in Children: Diagnosis and Management. Baltimore, Williams & Wilkins, 1994, pp 1–46.

West JB: Respiratory Physiology: The Essentials, 3rd ed. Baltimore, Williams & Wilkins, 1985.

## DIAGNOSTIC MEASURES

### PATIENT EVALUATION, HISTORY TAKING, AND PHYSICAL EXAMINATION

The diagnostic evaluation begins with a careful and complete history and physical examination. Much can be learned by seemingly casual observation of the child during the formal history taking with the parents. The physician should also question the child because children as young as 3–4 yr of age often know things their parents do not ("last week I choked on a peanut"). The signs or symptoms in children with airway disease often appear quite different during sleep, and therefore the physician should inquire specifically about observations of the sleeping child.

To avoid producing anxiety in the child, the physician might recommend that the mother hold the child in her lap during the physical examination. For the observation of the respiratory pattern, rate, depth, and retractions, the child should be quiet and not crying. Clothing should be removed from the upper half of the child's body so that the thorax may be clearly inspected. The observations made during auscultation of the chest may be misleading in young children because they may not take a breath deep enough to produce audible **crackles (rales)** or **rhonchi** (described below) despite the presence of fluid in the alveoli and small airways. With patience, however, most infants can be observed during at least one deep inspiration, whereas the physician may induce older children to take a deep breath by asking them to pretend to blow out a candle.

The *respiratory rate* is an important indicator of respiratory status. Any factor that impairs respiratory mechanics is likely to result in more rapid breathing. Because anxiety or excitement also increases respiratory rates, the sleeping respiratory rate is most reliable. Infants younger than 1 yr of age have sleeping rates ranging from 25 to 35 breaths/min; while awake, the same infants may take from 40 to 80 breaths each min. With increasing maturity, sleeping rates gradually decline toward the adult range of 10–15/min (Table 12–2).

In addition to the rate of respiration, its *pattern* or depth and the degree of effort required for its maintenance are important points to note. *Hyperpnea* (increased depth of respiration) may occur with fever, acidosis, salicylism, pulmonary disease, or extreme anxiety (hyperventilation syndrome, panic attack). Hyperpnea without signs of respiratory distress should suggest a nonpulmonary etiology (acidosis, fever, salicylism). When the degree of effort is increased because of airway obstruction or decreased pulmonary compliance, the intrathoracic pressure may be more negative than usual and intercostal retractions can be observed (see

**TABLE 12–2.** Breathing Patterns

| Pattern | Features | | | | | |
|---|---|---|---|---|---|---|
| Normal rate (breaths/min) | *Preterm:* 40–60 | *Term:* 30–40 | *5 yr:* 25 | *10 yr:* 20 | *15 yr:* 16 | *Adult:* 12 |
| Obstructed | | | | | | |
| Mild | Reduced rate, increased tidal volume | | | | | |
| Severe | Increased rate, increased retraction of accessory muscles, anxiety, cyanosis | | | | | |
| Restrictive | Rapid rate, decreased tidal volume | | | | | |
| Kussmaul respiration | Increased rate, increased tidal volume, regular deep respiration; consider metabolic acidosis or diabetes mellitus | | | | | |
| Cheyne-Stokes respiration | Gradually increasing tidal volume followed sequentially by gradually decreasing tidal volume and apnea; consider central nervous system injury, depressant drugs, heart failure, uremia, or prematurity | | | | | |
| Biot respiration | Ataxic or periodic breathing with a respiratory effort followed by apnea; consider brain stem injury or posterior fossa mass | | | | | |
| Gasping | Slow rate, variable tidal volume; consider hypoxia, shock, sepsis, or asphyxia | | | | | |

Table 12–2). Use of accessory muscles such as the sternocleidomastoids should be apparent on physical examination and should alert the physician to the presence of pulmonary pathology. In children, increased inspiratory effort also results in flaring of the alae nasi, which is a relatively reliable sign of dyspnea. **Grunting** (forced expiration against a partially closed glottis) should suggest hypoxia, atelectasis, pneumonia, or pulmonary edema.

The *sounds of breathing* deserve careful documentation. **Stridor**, usually heard on inspiration, is a harsh sound that emanates from the upper airway and is due to a partially obstructed extrathoracic airway. If stridor is accompanied by signs of respiratory distress or if it is present at rest, immediate investigation and intervention are required. Stridor also may be chronic or congenital in nature, in which case it may be of less importance physiologically unless infection further compromises the airway.

A **wheeze** is produced by partial obstruction of the lower airway and is heard on exhalation. Wheezes may be harsh and low-pitched (usually from large, central airways) or high-pitched and almost musical (from small, peripheral airways). Secretions in the intrathoracic airways may result in wheezing, but more commonly they result in irregular sounds called **rhonchi.** Fluid or secretions in the alveolar spaces or terminal airways may produce a sound that is characteristic of crumpling cellophane (**rales** or **crackles**). This sound may disappear after a few deep inspirations or a cough, but its persistence suggests pneumonitis or pulmonary edema. The quality of breath sounds may be **bronchial**, normally heard over the trachea, with inspiration and expiration clearly auscultated. More peripheral breath sounds are **vesicular,** with a greater proportion of inspiration heard as the expiratory component lessens. Bronchial breath sounds in the lung periphery suggest consolidation or the interface of a pleural effusion.

These physical findings, when combined with inspection for tracheal or cardiac deviation, chest wall motion, percussion, fremitus, voice signs, and the presence or absence of breath sounds, help identify the intrathoracic pathology (Table 12–3). **Digital clubbing** is a sign of chronic pulmonary disease, but it also may be noted in other chronic diseases (cyanotic congenital heart disease, endocarditis, celiac disease, inflammatory bowel disease, chronic active hepatitis, biliary cirrhosis, thalassemia, and Hodgkin disease).

## IMAGING TECHNIQUES

*Chest roentgenograms* are extremely useful in diagnosing respiratory disease in children, but they must be performed in a technically correct manner and be properly interpreted. Failure to obtain satisfactory inspiration, the most common problem, may lead to the erroneous impression of cardiomegaly or the presence of infiltrates. External skinfolds, rotation or other improper position of the chest, or motion also may produce a distorted or unclear image. Whenever possible, chest roentgenograms should be obtained in both the posteroanterior and the lateral projections. Lesions may be apparent on only one of the two views. Expiratory views or fluoroscopy is helpful in detecting the presence of partial bronchial obstruction; a lung or lobe that does not empty on expiration appears hyperinflated.

A *barium esophagram* frequently is of great value in the diagnosis of chest disease in children. Disorders of swallowing or esophageal motility, vascular rings, tracheoesophageal fistulas, or gastroesophageal reflux may lead to aspiration and recurrent or persistent pulmonary disease. When the esophagram reveals that abnormal vascular structures are compressing the esophagus, it may be a major clue that those same vessels are compressing the airways. When searching for an H-type tracheoesophageal fistula, the contrast material should be injected into the esophagus under pressure through a catheter while the injection sites are observed in the lateral projection. Simple barium swallows are much less likely to demonstrate the often small connection between the trachea and esophagus.

*Computed tomography* (CT) is very useful in diagnosing chest disease in children, especially in evaluating lesions in the mediastinum or hilum. Rapid, fine-cut, high-resolution CT provides information about the lumen size or presence of masses within the central intrathoracic airways; bronchiectasis also may be detected.

*Magnetic resonance imaging* (MRI) can identify pathology in the trachea and large central airways. MRI also may visualize the relationships between the great vessels and central airways.

*Ultrasonography* can determine the nature of some intrathoracic masses and the presence of pleural fluid and can identify loculated fluid collections, such as those occurring with empyema or complicated pleural effusion. Diaphragmatic dysfunction (e.g., paralysis or paresis) may also be assessed by ultrasound examination.

## MEASURES OF RESPIRATORY GAS EXCHANGE

A properly performed *arterial blood gas analysis* is one of the most useful measures of lung function, but it is nonspecific in terms of the etiology of

TABLE 12-3. Physical Signs of Pulmonary Disease

| Disease Process | Mediastinal Deviation | Chest Motion | Vocal Fremitus | Percussion | Breath Sounds | Adventitious Sounds | Voice Signs |
|---|---|---|---|---|---|---|---|
| Consolidation | No | Reduced over area | Increased | Dull | Bronchial or reduced | Rales | Egophony,* whispering, pectoriloquy increased† |
| Bronchospasm | No | Hyperexpansion with limited motion | Normal or decreased | Hyperresonant | Normal to decreased | Wheezes, rales | Normal to decreased |
| Atelectasis | Shift toward lesion | Reduced over area | Decreased | Dull | Reduced | None or rales | None |
| Pneumothorax | Tension deviates trachea and PMI to opposite side | Reduced over area | None | Resonant | None | None | None |
| Pleural effusion | Deviation to opposite side | Reduced over area | None or reduced | Dull | None | Friction, rub; splash if hemopneumothorax | None |
| Interstitial process | No | Reduced | Normal to increased | Normal | Normal | Rales | None |

Adapted from Andreoli TE, Bennett JC, Carpenter CJ, Plum F (eds): Cecil Essentials of Medicine, 4th ed. Philadelphia, WB Saunders, 1997, p 115.
* Egophony is present when *e* sounds like *a*.
† Whispering pectoriloquy produces clearer-sounding whispered words.
PMI = point of maximum impulse.

dysfunction. Because of the shape of the oxyhemoglobin dissociation curve, oxygen saturation does not fall appreciably until the $PaO_2$ reaches approximately 60 torr.

The arterial pH and $PCO_2$ also are important measures of respiratory function; $PCO_2$ is regulated almost entirely by ventilation (given a constant carbon dioxide production). Bicarbonate concentration is regulated chiefly by the kidneys. It is important to distinguish between metabolic and respiratory causes of acidosis or alkalosis. At the normal pH of 7.4, the $PaCO_2$ should be about 40 torr, and the bicarbonate about 25 mEq/L. This relationship is governed by the Henderson-Hasselbalch equation:

$$pH = 6.1 + \log\,[(HCO_3)/0.03\ PCO_2]$$

Thus it is the ratio of bicarbonate to $PCO_2$ that governs pH. Metabolic acidosis, which exhibits low bicarbonate, can be compensated by hyperventilation, which lowers the $PCO_2$, whereas respiratory acidosis, which is due to elevated $PCO_2$, can be compensated by renal retention of bicarbonate. Respiratory compensation is a much faster process than renal compensation, which generally requires several days to reach equilibrium.

Noninvasive methods of assessing oxygenation and ventilation are available, although the information provided, while useful, has more limited value than arterial blood gas measurement. *Pulse oximetry* (measurement of oxygen saturation using light absorption) provides a painless, relatively easy, and reliable means of measuring oxygenation. A small probe consisting of a light source and sensor is clipped to a finger or toe, and either continuous or single oxygen saturation measurements are obtained.

*Capnography* (measurement of carbon dioxide by gas analysis) permits a measure of ventilation. Monitoring the content of carbon dioxide in expired air (sampled at end-expiration or averaged over the respiratory cycle) provides an approximate measure of alveolar $PCO_2$. Although most commonly used in intubated and mechanically ventilated patients, capnography units that monitor carbon dioxide content in expired air at the nares are now available. Similarly, transcutaneous electrodes may be used to monitor $PO_2$ and $PCO_2$ at the skin surface, but these techniques are best suited for continuous monitoring in an intensive care unit and for detecting trends rather than for providing absolute numbers.

## PULMONARY FUNCTION TESTING

The simplest clinically useful measures of ventilatory function are *vital capacity* and *expiratory flow rates*, which can be measured with a spirometer. Simple spirometry can be performed in most children 6 yr of age or older. Even an older child cannot be expected to perform reproducibly without training and experience with the technique, and great care must be taken in interpreting the results. Predicted values for lung functions are based on the patient's height. Airway resistance, FRC, and RV (among other measures) require the use of a plethysmograph as well as a spirometer and thus are even more difficult to obtain in young children. An expiratory flow-volume curve can be very informative; flow rates at lower lung volumes are relatively independent of effort and reflect the function of more peripheral airways.

Pulmonary function studies may be useful in evaluating an older child's functional status, although they rarely yield an etiologic diagnosis. Abnormal results may be described in terms of **obstructive disease** (low flow rates, increased RV or FRC) or **restrictive disease** (low VC and TLC, with relative preservation of flow rates and FRC); in addition, the extent of functional impairment often can be estimated.

Pulmonary function testing also can be used to detect reversible airway obstruction characteristic of asthma. In patients with pulmonary function tests consistent with obstructive disease, a significant increase in pulmonary function after the inhalation of a bronchodilator indicates reactive airway disease. These tests are useful not only for determining diagnosis but also for managing therapy. Inhalational *challenge testing* with methacholine or cold, dry air is another useful test for diagnosis of reactive airways disease, but such tests require more sophisticated equipment and special expertise and can be performed only in a formal pulmonary function laboratory.

## ENDOSCOPIC EVALUATION OF THE AIRWAYS

Diagnostic *bronchoscopy* is indicated whenever necessary information about the lungs or airways can be most definitively, safely, or rapidly obtained by this method. Airway structure can be examined, the dynamics of the airways during breathing can be documented, and specimens can be obtained for a variety of diagnostic purposes. For patients of any age, no absolute contraindications to bronchoscopy exist, provided that the proper equipment is available and the physician's skill is adequate. Flexible instruments are advantageous for most diagnostic purposes, whereas rigid instruments must be used for foreign body extraction and for most operative procedures. An airway mucosal biopsy is also possible through pediatric-sized flexible bronchoscopes. Bronchoscopy accompanied by bronchoalveolar lavage assists in the diagnosis of pulmonary infection in the immunocompromised patient.

*Laryngoscopy* often is useful in the diagnosis of stridor and should be performed carefully under appropriate conditions and with the use of sedation, anesthesia, or both. The common technique of *direct* laryngoscopy at the bedside or in the treatment room in an unsedated infant or young child is traumatic to the child, and the results often are misleading. Mirror (*indirect*) laryngoscopy usually can be performed in children 4–5 yr of age or older; in infants and younger children, however, direct laryngoscopy or, preferably, transnasal laryngoscopy using a flexible bronchoscope or nasopharyngoscope yields much better diagnostic information.

## EXAMINATION OF SPUTUM

Sputum specimens, although important in evaluating inflammatory processes in the lower airways, are often difficult to obtain in young children. An expectorated specimen may not provide a representative sample of the lower airway secretions, but microscopic examination helps determine the source of a putative sputum specimen. Sputum should contain macrophages; often ciliated cells also are seen. Material containing large numbers of squamous epithelial cells either is most likely not from the lower airways or is heavily contaminated, so that diagnostic tests performed on such a specimen may yield misleading results. Infected sputum should have many polymorphonucleated leukocytes and one predominant organism in large numbers present on Gram stain. If sputum cannot be obtained, obtaining lung washings by bronchoscopy for microbiologic or cytologic diagnosis may be useful in selected situations (bronchoalveolar lavage).

## LUNG BIOPSY

When less invasive methods have failed in the diagnosis of pulmonary disease, lung biopsy may be required. Although transbronchial lung biopsy through a bronchoscope is useful in adults, a thoracotomy with open biopsy has major advantages in most pediatric patients: thoracotomy allows the surgeon to inspect and palpate the lung and initially to choose the best site for performing the biopsy; and open biopsy provides sufficient mate-

rial for a variety of diagnostic tests. The site of biopsy should be chosen after inspection of the involved lobe on roentgenogram. In most cases, infants and children tolerate open lung biopsy well.

### References

Behrman RE, Kliegman RM, Arvin AM (eds): Nelson Textbook of Pediatrics, 15th ed. Philadelphia, WB Saunders, 1996, Chapters 321, 324.

Effman EL: Basic concepts of lung imaging. *In* Chernik V, Mellins RB (eds): Basic Mechanisms of Pediatric Respiratory Disease. Philadelphia, BC Decker, 1991, pp 383–396.

Fisher MR: Magnetic resonance for evaluation of the thorax. Chest 95:166, 1989.

Naidich DP, Harkin TJ: Airways and lung: Correlation of CT with fiberoptic bronchoscopy. Radiology 197:1, 1995.

Paton J, Bautisa D, Stable W, et al: Digital clubbing and pulmonary function abnormalities in children with lung disease. Pediatr Pulmonol 10:25, 1991.

Schnapp LM, Cohen NH: Pulse oximetry: Uses and abuses. Chest 98:1244, 1990.

Wood RE: Bronchoscopy. *In* Loughlin GM, Eigen H (eds): Respiratory Disease in Children: Diagnosis and Management. Baltimore, Williams & Wilkins, 1994, p 117.

# THERAPEUTIC MEASURES

## OXYGEN ADMINISTRATION

Any child in respiratory distress should be given supplemental oxygen as soon as feasible. Although depressing the respiratory drive is possible if the patient's central chemoreceptors are blunted by chronic hypercapnia, patients in such a state are rare in pediatric practice and should be readily recognized as having chronic, severe respiratory disease (e.g., cystic fibrosis, bronchopulmonary dysplasia). Even in these patients, oxygen therapy may be lifesaving without producing apnea.

In the acute situation, an appropriately sized mask is often the most useful technique for administering oxygen, although some children may become frightened. For a frightened child, a high-flow oxygen source may be held near the child's face until a more satisfactory method can be arranged. For chronic administration of oxygen, a nasal cannula may be helpful because it frees the face and mouth, allowing the patient to eat and speak unhindered by the oxygen delivery system.

The concentration of oxygen administered should be high enough to relieve hypoxemia yet as low as feasible to prevent oxygen toxicity. In general, inspired oxygen concentrations below 40% are safe for long-term use. Determining the concentration of inspired oxygen is more difficult in patients receiving oxygen by nasal cannula; titrating the delivery (in liters/min) according to measurements of $PaO_2$ or by pulse oximetry is best. The safe, acceptable range of oxygen saturation is 92–95%. It is unnecessary to achieve 100% saturation, especially because this may require potentially toxic levels of inspired oxygen. Oxygen, as obtained from tanks or wall sources, is dry and must be humidified to avoid dehydration of the mucosa of the upper respiratory tract.

## AEROSOL THERAPY

Delivering therapeutic agents to the lower respiratory tract often is accomplished by having the patient inhale the agents in aerosol form. Employing aerosol generators that deliver relatively small particles (2–5 μm) is necessary to achieve optimum deposition in the lower airways. The pattern of the patient's breathing greatly influences deposition of the particles. Slow, deep inspirations are needed for maximal effect, but most children, especially infants, cannot perform in this fashion. Therefore, inhaling aerosols from a face mask or mouthpiece for a period of several minutes during quiet tidal breathing is necessary. Metered-dose inhalers produce a high-pressure stream of particles and deposit more of the aerosol on the oral mucosa and posterior pharynx than in the lungs. Infants and children should use spacer devices that trap the respirable aerosol particles issuing from the inhaler into a chamber, from which the patient then breathes more slowly.

The drugs most often given by aerosol are bronchodilators. In certain situations, antibiotics may be given by aerosol.

## PHYSICAL THERAPY

When disease processes impair clearance of pulmonary secretions, physical therapy may help maintain airway patency. Percussion of the thorax over the pulmonary segments while the patient is positioned so that the airways of the percussed segments are directed downward may move secretions toward the central airways, from which they can be expectorated. Chest physiotherapy may also be effectively performed with techniques and devices such as autogenic drainage, the Flutter valve, and percussive vests. A typical therapy session may require 15–30 min; most children with lung disease requiring chest physiotherapy need one to four such sessions daily. In older children, sustained exercise (for 5–15 min) that produces hyperpnea also can be helpful. Chest physiotherapy is most beneficial for children with cystic fibrosis but also may be useful for individuals with neuromus-

cular disease and atelectasis. It generally is not beneficial for pneumonia or asthma.

## INTUBATION

When the natural upper airway is obstructed because of disease, or when assisted ventilation is needed because of disease or anesthesia, it may be necessary to provide an artificial airway for the patient. Intubation alters the physiology of the respiratory tract in a number of ways, not all of which are beneficial: it interferes with humidification, warming, and filtration of inspired air; with phonation; and with transport of secretions by mucocilia and through cough. Intubation also stimulates increased production of secretions. Depending on the reason for the intubation, the airway resistance may be increased or decreased, and the physiologic dead space may be increased.

Endotracheal tubes can easily damage the larynx and the airways if they are of improper size or are not carefully maintained. Because the cricoid ring is the smallest portion of the airway in children and is completely surrounded by cartilage, it is vulnerable to damage, which results in subglottic stenosis. Pressure of the tube that exceeds capillary filling pressure (roughly 35 cm $H_2O$) against the airway mucosa produces mucosal ischemia and, within hours, mucosal necrosis. An endotracheal tube should allow a small air leak at the larynx.

Artificial airways of all types must be kept clear of secretions. Mucus plugs in artificial airways can be fatal. Providing adequate humidification of the inspired air and suctioning the tube will help reduce the probability of occlusion by secretions.

## TRACHEOSTOMY

Tracheostomy is the surgical placement of an artificial airway into the trachea below the larynx. If prolonged intubation is anticipated, elective tracheostomy should be considered to prevent laryngeal trauma and subsequent subglottic stenosis and to increase the patient's comfort and the ease of nursing care. Unfortunately, no clear guidelines are available as to how long a given patient is likely to tolerate an endotracheal tube or when a tracheostomy is necessary. Once laryngeal damage has occurred, the probability of subglottic stenosis is much higher.

Children with **subglottic stenosis** may require a tracheostomy for a prolonged period. Because the tracheostomy tube typically prevents the child from effectively phonating, and thus from communicating distress, special attention must be given to ensure that the child is monitored carefully at all times. As with endotracheal tubes, tracheostomy tubes must be kept clear and clean and vigilant care must be taken to reduce complications. Occlusion of the tube with secretions or accidental dislodgment of the tube can be fatal. Children with tracheostomies may be successfully cared for at home if the caretakers are well trained and adequately equipped.

## MECHANICAL VENTILATION

Patients who are unable to maintain an adequate gas exchange because of airway obstruction, intrapulmonary pathology, neuromuscular disease, or other factors are candidates for mechanical ventilation. Techniques for mechanical ventilation involve inflation of the lungs with compressed gas. Exhalation is always passive. Partial liquid ventilation, an experimental technique using a solution of an oxygen-delivering perfluorocarbon to fill the lungs, followed by application of standard mechanical ventilation has shown promise in improving gas exchange in patients with severe acute respiratory failure. No method accurately mimics the natural breathing mechanisms, and all methods have their drawbacks and complications.

*Positive pressure ventilation* requires intubation or tracheostomy. Positive pressure is transmitted to the entire thorax and may impede venous return to the heart during inspiration (venous return increases during spontaneous inspiration). The airways and lung parenchyma may be damaged by high inflation pressures (as well as by high inspired oxygen concentrations). In general, inflation pressures should be limited to those necessary to provide sufficient lung expansion for adequate ventilation and prevention of atelectasis. Other modes of ventilation include high-frequency jet ventilation and very-high-frequency oscillation; these techniques are used to reduce mean airway pressure and thus the probability of barotrauma (see Chapter 6).

*Pressure-cycled ventilators* frequently are used in infants and deliver an indefinite volume of gas at a fixed inflation pressure. A major disadvantage of this system is that the pressure is sensed in the ventilator circuit rather than in the lung, and increasing degrees of airway resistance (e.g., occlusion of the endotracheal tube) will result in decreasing delivered volumes. *Volume-cycled ventilators* deliver a fixed volume of gas at whatever inflation pressure is necessary (up to a preset maximum). These instruments are more often used in children and adolescents. In either case, the re-

sponse of the patient must be assessed carefully and frequently. Regardless of the method chosen for ventilation, alveolar ventilation (assessed by breath sounds, chest wall excursion, and arterial blood gas measurements) and oxygenation (assessed by arterial blood gas measurements or oximetry) must be adequate.

The normal tidal volume is 5–7 mL/kg body weight; values less than this usually result in hypoventilation and hypercapnia. Patients with lung disease and uneven distribution of ventilation often require larger tidal volumes; most volume-cycled ventilators are operated at tidal volumes of 8–10 mL/kg body weight. Continuous ventilation at smaller volumes results in redistribution of surfactant and atelectasis. An occasional full lung inflation may be provided by a "sigh" on some ventilators or by inflation with an Ambu bag to prevent atelectasis.

### References

Behrman RE, Kliegman RM, Arvin AM (eds): Nelson Textbook of Pediatrics, 15th ed. Philadelphia, WB Saunders, 1996, Chapters 321, 322.

Hirschl RB, Pranikoff T, Wise C, et al: Initial experience with partial liquid ventilation in adult patients with the acute respiratory distress syndrome. JAMA 275:383, 1996.

Lough M: Respiratory treatment and equipment. *In* Blumer JL (ed): A Practical Guide to Pediatric Intensive Care. St. Louis, Mosby-Year Book, 1990, pp 926–996.

# MAJOR PEDIATRIC PULMONARY SYMPTOM COMPLEXES

## UPPER AIRWAY OBSTRUCTION

An upper airway obstruction is defined as blockage of the portion of the airways located above the thoracic inlet; it is manifested during inspiration because the pressure within the upper airway is negative relative to the atmosphere. This negative pressure tends to collapse the upper airway, producing the characteristic sounds associated with upper airway obstruction. Upper airway obstruction ranges from nasal obstruction associated with the common cold to life-threatening obstruction of the larynx or upper trachea. Nasal obstruction is usually more of a nuisance than a danger because the mouth can be used as an airway; however, it may be a serious problem for neonates, who breathe predominantly through the nose. The etiologies of airway obstruction vary with the age of the child (Tables 12–4 and 12–5), and a careful history and physical examination are necessary for the diagnosis.

The *clinical manifestation* most commonly associ-

TABLE 12–4. Age-Related Differential Diagnosis of Airway Obstruction

**Newborn**

Foreign material (meconium, amniotic fluid)
Congenital subglottic stenosis (uncommon)
Choanal atresia
Micrognathia (Pierre Robin syndrome, Treacher Collins syndrome, DiGeorge syndrome)
Macroglossia (Beckwith-Wiedemann syndrome, hypothyroidism, Pompe disease, trisomy 21, hemangioma)
Laryngeal web, clefts, atresia
Laryngospasm (intubation, aspiration, transient)
Vocal cord paralysis (weak cry; unilateral or bilateral, with or without increased intracranial pressure from Arnold-Chiari malformation or other CNS pathology)
Tracheal web, stenosis, malacia, atresia
Pharyngeal collapse (cause of apnea in preterm infant)
Dislocated nasal cartilage
Nasal pyriform aperture stenosis
Nasal encephalocele

**Infancy**

Laryngomalacia (most common etiology)
Subglottic stenosis (congenital, acquired after intubation)
Hemangioma
Tongue tumor (dermoid, teratoma, ectopic thyroid)
Laryngeal dyskinesis
Laryngeal papillomatosis
Vascular rings
Rhinitis

**Toddlers**

Viral croup (most common etiology in children 6 mo–4 yr of age)
Bacterial tracheitis (toxic, high fever)
Foreign body (sudden cough; airway or esophageal)
Spasmodic (recurrent) croup
Laryngeal papillomatosis
Retropharyngeal abscess
Hypertrophied tonsils and adenoids
Diphtheria (uncommon)

**Above 2–3 Yr Old**

Epiglottis (epiglottis, aryepiglottic folds)
Inhalation injury (burns, toxic gas, hydrocarbons)
Foreign bodies
Rhinitis medicamentosa
Angioedema (familial history, cutaneous angioedema)
Anaphylaxis (allergic history, wheezing, hypotension)
Trauma (tracheal or laryngeal fracture)
Peritonsillar abscess (adolescents)
Mononucleosis
Ludwig angina
Diphtheria (uncommon)

CNS = central nervous system.

ated with upper airway obstruction is inspiratory **stridor**, a harsh sound produced usually at or near the larynx by the vibration of upper airway structures. Less commonly, stridor also may be an expiratory noise. Hoarseness suggests involvement of the vocal cords, whereas stridor that changes with position of the child's head or neck suggests a supraglottic etiology. Children with laryngomalacia or pharyngeal hypotonia may exhibit much less stridor while crying because their muscle tone increases. In contrast, an obstructing lesion below the glottis usually produces more stridor during crying because the inspiratory flow rates increase. In many children, stridor decreases during sleep because inspiratory flow rates are lowest at that time. Positional stridor suggests an anatomic problem.

A child with upper airway obstruction usually has some degree of suprasternal retraction as a result of the pressure gradient between the trachea and the atmosphere. Obstruction below the thoracic inlet seldom results in suprasternal retraction because the major pressure drop occurs below the sternal notch.

*Radiographic evaluation* of the child with stridor should include views of the lateral neck and nasopharynx and an anteroposterior (AP) view of the neck taken with the head in extension. The subglottic space on the AP view should be symmetric, and the lateral walls of the airway should fall away steeply. Asymmetry suggests subglottic stenosis or a mass lesion, whereas narrow tapering suggests subglottic edema. An important differential diagnosis is that between supraglottic and subglottic obstruction (Table 12–6).

## LOWER AIRWAY OBSTRUCTION

In contrast to upper airway obstruction, obstruction of the airways below the thoracic inlet produces more expiratory symptoms than inspiratory symptoms. During inspiration, intrathoracic pressure becomes negative relative to the atmosphere. Therefore, the airways tend to increase their diameter during inspiration, and unless substantial, relatively fixed obstruction (or increased airway secretion) is present, few or no abnormal noises may be generated during inspiration. Intrathoracic pressure is increased relative to atmospheric pressure during exhalation, thus tending to collapse the intrathoracic airways and produce wheezing. A **wheeze** is a relatively continuous expiratory sound, generally with a more musical quality than stridor, that is produced by turbulent airflow. Partial airway obstruction may produce wheezing only during the later phase of exhalation.

The *etiology* of wheezing is multiple (Table 12–7), the most common of which is diffuse bronchial obstruction resulting from constriction of bronchial smooth muscle, airway inflammation, or excessive secretions. However, the importance of the aphorism "All that wheezes is not asthma" cannot be

Table 12–5. Differential Diagnosis of Acute Upper Airway Obstruction

| | Laryngotracheobronchitis (Croup) | Laryngitis | Spasmodic Croup | Epiglottitis | Membranous Croup (Bacterial Tracheitis) | Retropharyngeal Abscess | Foreign Body | Angioedema | Peritonsillar Abscess | Laryngeal Papillomatosis |
|---|---|---|---|---|---|---|---|---|---|---|
| Age | 6 mo–3 yr | 5 yr–teens | 3 mo–3 yr | 2–6 yr | Any age (3–10 yr) | <6 yr | 6 mo–5 yr | All ages | >10 yr | 3 mo–3 yr |
| Location | Subglottic | Subglottic | Subglottic | Supraglottic | Trachea | Posterior pharynx | Supraglottic, subglottic, variable | Variable | Oropharynx | Larynx, vocal cords, trachea |
| Etiology | Parainfluenza virus, influenza virus, RSV; rarely *Mycoplasma*, measles, adenovirus | As per croup | Unknown | *Haemophilus influenzae* b | Prior croup or influenza virus with secondary bacterial infection by *Staphylococcus aureus*, *Moraxella catarrhalis*, *H. influenzae* | *S. aureus*, anaerobes | Small objects, vegetables, toys, coins | Congenital C-1 esterase deficiency; acquired anaphylaxis | Group A streptococci, anaerobes | HPV |
| Prodrome onset | Insidious, URI | As per croup | Sudden onset at night; prior episodes | Rapid, short prodrome | Biphasic illness with sudden deterioration | Insidious to sudden | Sudden | Sudden | Biphasic with sudden worsening | Chronic |
| Stridor | Yes | None | Yes | Yes—soft inspiratory | Yes | None | Yes | Yes | No | Possible |
| Retractions | Yes | None | Rare | Yes | Yes | Yes | Yes—variable | Yes | No | No |
| Voice | Hoarse | Hoarse; whispered | Hoarse | Muffled | Normal or hoarse | Muffled | Complete obstruction—aphonic; other variable | Hoarse, may be normal | "Hot potato," muffled | Hoarse |
| Position and appearance | Normal | Normal | Normal | Tripod sitting leaning forward; agitation | Normal | Arching of neck or normal | Normal | Normal; may have facial edema, anxiety | Normal | Normal |
| Swallowing (dysphagia) | Normal | Normal | Normal | Drooling | Normal | Drooling | Variable, usually normal | Normal | Drooling, trismus | Normal |
| Barking cough | Yes | Rare | Yes | No | Yes | No | Variable; brassy if tracheal | Possible | None | Variable |

*Table continued on following page*

471

TABLE 12–5.  Differential Diagnosis of Acute Upper Airway Obstruction *Continued*

| | Laryngotracheo-bronchitis (Croup) | Laryngitis | Spasmodic Croup | Epiglottitis | Membranous Croup (Bacterial Tracheitis) | Retropharyngeal Abscess | Foreign Body | Angioedema | Peritonsillar Abscess | Laryngeal Papillomatosis |
|---|---|---|---|---|---|---|---|---|---|---|
| Toxicity | Rare | No | No | Severe | Severe; may also manifest toxic shock syndrome | Severe | No, but dyspnea | No unless anaphylactic shock or severe anoxia | Dyspnea | None |
| Fever | <101°F | <101°F | None | >102°F | >102°F | >101°F | None | None | >101°F | None |
| X-ray | Subglottic narrowing; steeple sign | Normal | Subglottic narrowing | Thumb sign of thickened epiglottis | Ragged irregular tracheal border; as per croup | Thickened retropharyngeal space | Radiopaque object may be seen | As per croup | None needed | May be normal |
| WBC count | Normal | Normal | Normal | Leukocytosis with left shift | Leukocytosis with left shift | Leukocytosis with left shift | Normal | Normal | Leukocytosis with left shift | Normal |
| Therapy | Racemic epinephrine aerosol, systemic steroids, aerosolized steroids, cool mist | None | Cool mist; occasionally as for croup | Endotracheal intubation, ceftriaxone | Ceftriaxone; intubation if needed | Nafcillin; ampicillin-sulbactam; ceftriaxone; surgical drainage if abscess | Endoscopic removal | Anaphylaxis; epinephrine, IV fluids, steroids; C-1 esterase deficiency; replacement infusion therapy | Penicillin; aspiration | Laser therapy, repeated excision, interferon |
| Prevention | None | None | None | *H. influenzae* b conjugated vaccine | None | None | Avoid small objects; supervision | Avoid allergens; FFP for congenital angioedema | Treat group A streptococci early | Treat maternal genitourinary lesions; possible cesarean section? |

Modified from Arnold IE: Airway obstruction in children. *In* Kliegman RM, Nieder ML, Super DM (eds): Practical Strategies in Pediatric Diagnosis and Therapy. Philadelphia, WB Saunders, 1996, p 126. FFP = fresh frozen plasma; HPV = human papillomavirus; RSV = respiratory syncytial virus; URI = upper respiratory tract infection, coryza, sneezing; WBC = white blood cell.

TABLE 12–6. Differentiating Supraglottic from Subglottic Causes of Airway Obstruction

|  | Supraglottic | Subglottic |
|---|---|---|
| Example | Epiglottitis, peritonsillar and retropharyngeal abscess | Croup, angioedema, foreign body, tracheitis |
| Stridor | Quiet | Loud |
| Voice | Muffled | Hoarse |
| Dysphagia | Yes | No |
| Sitting-up or arching posture | Yes | No |
| Barking cough | No | Yes |
| Fever | High (40°C [104°F]) | Low grade (38–39°C [100.4–102.2°F]) |
| Toxic | Yes | No, unless tracheitis is present |
| Trismus | Yes | No |
| Drooling | Yes | No |
| Facial edema | No | No, unless angioedema is present |

Adapted from Davis H, et al: Acute upper airway obstruction: Croup and epiglottis. Pediatr Clin North Am 28:859, 1981.

overemphasized. Although it often is useful to administer a bronchodilator to determine whether the wheezing is acutely reversible, mere reversibility does not establish a diagnosis of asthma, nor does it eliminate anatomic causes of wheezing. Conversely, the most common cause of wheezing in childhood is reactive airway disease. Wheezing that begins in the first weeks or months of life, or that is persistent despite maximal bronchodilator therapy, is more likely to be due to some other cause, and more extensive diagnostic evaluation may be warranted. Because of their small airways, children under than 2–3 yr of age are more likely to wheeze in response to viral infections. Wheezing that is localized to one area of the chest deserves especially close diagnostic attention (e.g., foreign body, compressing lymph node).

Although a child known to have reactive airway disease certainly does not need *roentgenographic evaluation* with each episode of wheezing, other children with significant respiratory distress, fever, history of aspiration, localizing signs, or persistent wheezing should have chest films included as part of their diagnostic evaluation. Both posterioante-

rior and lateral views should be obtained. Generalized hyperinflation, with flattening of the diaphragm and an increased AP diameter of the chest, suggests diffuse obstruction of small airways. Localized hyperinflation, especially on expiratory films, suggests localized bronchial obstruction, such as with a foreign body or anatomic anomalies.

TABLE 12–7. Causes of Wheezing in Childhood

**Acute**

*Reactive Airway Disease*

Asthma
Exercise-induced asthma
Hypersensitivity reactions

*Bronchial Edema*

Infection
Inhalation of irritant gases or particulates
Increased pulmonary venous pressure

*Bronchial Hypersecretion*

Infection
Inhalation of irritant gases or particulates
Cholinergic drugs

*Aspiration*

Foreign body
Aspiration of gastric contents

**Chronic or Recurrent**

*Reactive Airway Disease* (see above)

*Hypersensitivity Reactions, Allergic Aspergillosis*

*Dynamic Airway Collapse*

Bronchomalacia
Tracheomalacia
Vocal cord adduction

*Airway Compression by Mass or Blood Vessel*

Vascular ring
Anomalous innominate artery
Pulmonary artery dilation (absent pulmonary valve)
Bronchial or pulmonary cysts
Lymph nodes or tumors

*Aspiration*

Foreign body
Gastroesophageal reflux
Tracheoesophageal fistula

*Bronchial Hypersecretion or Failure to Clear Secretions*

Bronchitis, bronchiectasis
Cystic fibrosis
Dysmotile cilia syndrome

*Intrinsic Airway Lesions*

Endobronchial tumors
Endobronchial granulation tissue
Bronchial or tracheal stenosis
Bronchiolitis obliterans
Sequelae of bronchopulmonary dysplasia

*Congestive Heart Failure*

## COUGH

Cough is one of the most common (and sometimes most vexing) respiratory symptoms at all ages. Cough results from stimulation of irritant receptors in the airway mucosa or in other locations, including the ear. It may have many different characteristics, depending on anatomic factors and the cause of the irritation, and significant diagnostic information usually may be derived from the history and physical examination.

Most cases of *acute cough* are associated with respiratory infections (pneumonia, tracheobronchitis, bronchitis, sinusitis, pertussis), and the cough subsides with resolution of the infection. A history of the sudden onset of choking and coughing is often described after aspiration of a foreign body. Other causes include pulmonary edema, thermal or chemical inhalation injury (smoke), and pulmonary embolism or hemorrhage.

*Chronic cough* (daily cough for greater than 6 wk), however, has a more diverse etiology, including allergy (asthma, hypersensitivity pneumonitis, rhinitis), anatomic abnormalities (tracheoesophageal fistula, cysts, gastroesophageal reflux), chronic infection (cystic fibrosis, sinusitis, recurrent aspiration pneumonia, abscess, tuberculosis, fungal pneumonia, histoplasmosis, acquired immunodeficiency syndrome [AIDS]–related infection), environmental exposure to irritants (smoking, drug abuse), foreign body aspiration, psychogenic (habit), and neurologic dysfunction.

Children in the first several years of life often have frequent viral respiratory infections, especially if they are exposed to many other children, as in day care centers. Cough that resolves promptly and clearly is associated with a viral infection does not require further diagnostic evaluation. However, cough that persists beyond 4–6 wk and is not associated with classic viral upper respiratory tract infection symptoms may require investigation.

The circumstances under which chronic cough occurs are important to consider in diagnosis. Nocturnal cough suggests allergy (especially to antigens in the child's bedroom) or drainage from sinuses. Cough associated with exercise suggests reactive airway disease or bronchitis/bronchiectasis. Cough on first arising in the morning frequently is associated with excessive production of tracheobronchial secretions, such as occurs in asthma, bronchitis, bronchiectasis, or cystic fibrosis. Paroxysmal cough should suggest pertussis syndrome, foreign body aspiration, or cystic fibrosis. Chlamydial infections characteristically produce a repetitive, staccato cough. Children with a harsh, brassy cough often have an anatomic problem, such as subglottic edema (croup), tracheomalacia, or tracheal compression, but also may have habit cough. Habit cough disappears with sleep. Cough that arouses a child from sleep is usually the result of a pathologic process. Tumors, mediastinal or parabronchial lymphadenopathy, and pulmonary vasculitis are uncommon causes of chronic cough.

Severe coughing may result in complications such as rib fractures, chest wall pain, pneumothorax, rupture of conjunctival, nasal or anal veins, syncope, hernias, emesis, urinary incontinence, or rectal prolapse. Severe repeated episodes of coughing, as seen in pertussis, may interfere with oral intake and produce malnutrition or may result in cyanosis.

The *diagnostic evaluation* of the child with chronic cough should include a chest roentgenogram and, if possible, an examination of sputum. In children too young to expectorate, a specimen often may be obtained with a throat swab placed deep into the posterior pharynx during coughing. Children with allergies most often produce clear mucoid sputum, although microscopic examination should be performed (see Diagnostic Measures earlier). Some children with allergies may produce apparently purulent sputum that contains numerous eosinophils. Purulent sputum (containing many white blood cells) suggests infection, and a specimen should be obtained for culture. A variety of rapid diagnostic tests (immunofluorescence, enzyme-linked immunosorbent assay [ELISA] utilizing nasal washings or serum) are available to help reach a diagnosis of certain viral pulmonary infections.

### References

Behrman RE, Kliegman RM, Arvin AM (eds): Nelson Textbook of Pediatrics, 15th ed. Philadelphia, WB Saunders, 1996, Chapter 322.1

Munyard P, Bush A: How much coughing is normal? Arch Dis Child 74:531, 1996.

Orenstein DM: Cough. *In* Kliegman RM, Nieder ML, Super DM (eds): Practical Strategies in Pediatric Diagnosis and Therapy. Philadelphia, WB Saunders, 1996, p. 64.

# STRUCTURAL AND DYNAMIC ABNORMALITIES

## THE UPPER AIRWAY

### Adenoidal Tonsillar Hypertrophy

The major abnormalities of the upper airway involve obstructive lesions. The most common is adenoidal tonsillar hypertrophy. The adenoids consist of lymphoid tissue arising from the posterior and superior wall of the nasopharynx in the region of the choanae. Lymphoid hyperplasia may result from recurrent infection, allergy, or nonspecific stimuli and may cause partial or total obstruction of the nasopharynx. The signs of adenoidal hypertrophy include persistent mouth breathing, snoring, and in some patients, obstructive sleep apnea. The eustachian tube enters the nasopharynx at the choanae and may be obstructed by enlarged adenoids, thus promoting recurrent or persistent otitis media.

The *diagnosis* of adenoidal hypertrophy is confirmed by a lateral roentgenogram of the nasopharynx or by nasopharyngoscopy; *treatment* of airway obstruction is by surgical excision. Because the adenoids are not a discrete organ but consist merely of lymphoid tissue, regrowth following adenoidectomy is not uncommon. Tonsils also may enlarge to the point of producing airway obstruction. Obstruction sufficient to produce sleep apnea, retractions, or cor pulmonale may require tonsillectomy.

### Choanal Stenosis
#### (Atresia)

Choanal stenosis or atresia may be bilateral or unilateral and is a relatively rare cause of respiratory distress in the newborn. The neonate is generally an obligate nose breather; thus, nasal obstruction may be fatal. Crying relieves the obstruction, which is worse during quiet activity. Failure to pass a small catheter through the nostrils easily should raise the suspicion of choanal atresia. An oral airway may be lifesaving, but the definitive *treatment* is surgery. The *diagnosis* is confirmed by CT or roentgenographically by instilling a small amount of contrast material or by inspecting the area directly with a nasopharyngoscope or bronchoscope.

### Laryngomalacia

Stridor beginning at birth or shortly thereafter should raise the suspicion of the presence of laryngomalacia (see Table 12–4). This relatively common condition involves the collapse of the epiglottis or arytenoid cartilages during inspiration and usually is benign and self-limiting. In some infants, the epiglottis alone is involved; these patients tend to become asymptomatic during the 1st yr of life. Other infants have very large arytenoid cartilages that prolapse into the glottis during inspiration; in these patients, stridor tends to last longer, sometimes for several years.

Establishing a definitive *diagnosis* in suspected laryngomalacia is important both for its appropriate management and to exclude other, more serious lesions. The *differential diagnosis* should include vocal cord paralysis, laryngeal cysts or other mass lesions (especially when the stridor begins several weeks after birth), congenital subglottic stenosis, tracheomalacia, and compression of the upper trachea by an anomalous innominate artery (see Table 12–4). The child with laryngomalacia will have **inspiratory stridor** but should have no evidence of significant expiratory obstruction. The stridor typically is loudest when the child is feeding or quietly relaxing, or in a supine or neck flexion position, and usually diminishes during sleep or when the child is crying (when increased muscle tone may hold the supraglottic structures out of the air stream). Viral infections may exacerbate laryngomalacia.

No *treatment* is needed unless the infant has hypoxia or growth failure resulting from the airway obstruction; tracheostomy or epiglottoplasty then may be required. Symptoms usually disappear by 18–24 mo of age.

### Subglottic Stenosis

Subglottic stenosis may be congenital or, more commonly, iatrogenic. Aggressive management of premature infants with intubation and mechanical ventilation may produce residual damage to the larynx. Infants with Down syndrome appear to have a smaller larynx than normal and are more susceptible to subglottic stenosis. Subglottic obstruction will produce stridor, and evidence of obstruction will be present on expiration as well as on inspiration. With increasing degrees of respiratory effort, the stridor will worsen (in contrast to laryngomalacia, in which the stridor may lessen with increasing respiratory efforts). Viral infection may exacerbate subglottic stenosis. Definitive *diagnosis* requires endoscopic evaluation.

*Treatment* may necessitate tracheostomy and eventual surgery; however, milder congenital cases improve with age as the larynx grows.

### Mass Lesions

A number of mass lesions affect the larynx, but the most common laryngeal tumor in childhood is the **hemangioma**, which usually is found in the subglottic space. Infants with stridor should be examined head to toe for cutaneous hemangiomas because the presence of such lesions greatly increases the likelihood that the stridor is due to a subglottic hemangioma and mandates endoscopic evaluation. Most patients who have subglottic hemangioma come to the physician's attention prior to 6 mo of age. Subglottic lesions produce asymmetric narrowing of the subglottic space and may be detected on AP roentgenograms of the larynx. The airway obstruction, which usually worsens with crying, may eventually produce pulmonary hypertension and cor pulmonale.

*Treatment* of hemangiomas is controversial, but in many patients tracheostomy is required. Laser therapy, interferon, and steroids have been used with moderate success. As with cutaneous hemangiomas, spontaneous regression is the rule, but this may require many months to several years.

**Juvenile laryngeal papillomatosis,** benign tumors caused by human papillomavirus acquired at birth from maternal genital warts, occurs in infants younger than 2 yr of age. *Treatment* includes laser therapy and interferon, but response to therapy is often poor.

## THE LOWER AIRWAY

### Tracheomalacia

The most common anomaly of tracheal structure and dynamics, although a less common cause of upper airway obstruction, is tracheomalacia. The tracheal cartilage rings normally extend through an arc of approximately 300 degrees, thus maintaining rigidity of the trachea during changes in intrathoracic pressure. In tracheomalacia, the cartilage rings do not extend nearly so far around the circumference, and thus a larger portion of the tracheal wall is membranous. Therefore, the lumen of the intrathoracic portion of the trachea tends to collapse during expiration. This collapse may be apparent in most patients only during forced exhalation or with cough, but coarse, persistent wheezing may be a prominent symptom in other patients. The voice is normal, as is inspiratory effort. Tracheomalacia localized to the cervical trachea may result in inspiratory obstruction. Tracheomalacia almost invariably is present in children who have had esophageal atresia and a tracheoesophageal fistula. Tracheomalacia must be differentiated from extrinsic compressing lesions. In some patients, localized tracheomalacia may result after the trachea has been relieved of compression by a mass lesion or by an abnormal blood vessel. Viral infections may exacerbate the airway obstruction of tracheomalacia. Treatment usually is not necessary, but some patients may require long-term tracheostomy and ventilatory support.

### Tracheosophageal Fistula

Tracheoesophageal fistula is another relatively common anomaly of the trachea, occurring in 1:3000–4500 live births (see Chapter 11).

### Tracheal Compression

**Compression of the trachea by abnormal vessels** may produce persistent wheezing, stridor, or both. The most common of these lesions is anterior compression resulting from an **anomalous innominate artery,** which arises more distally along the arch of the aorta than it normally does. Surgical treatment generally is required only for the most severe cases, especially those complicated by apnea.

A more serious lesion involves complete **encirclement of the trachea** at and just above the carina by a vascular ring. This anomaly may be caused by a double aortic arch or by a right aortic arch with a persisting ligamentum arteriosum. In addition to respiratory symptoms, emesis or dysphagia may be present as a result of esophageal compression.

The *definitive diagnosis* often can be made by barium swallow, although vascular dye contrast study or magnetic resonance angiography (MRA) may be required prior to surgical repair. Less common causes of extrinsic tracheal compression include mediastinal masses and cystic hygromas.

### Endobronchial Mass Lesions

Endobronchial mass lesions are relatively uncommon in children, but when they occur, they most commonly consist of granulation tissue and they result from localized inflammatory lesions. Partial obstruction of an airway by either an intrinsic or an extrinsic mass may result in wheezing or obstructive emphysema if there is more obstruction during exhalation than during inspiration. If the airways become totally obstructed, atelectasis results.

Chest roentgenograms, CT scans, bronchoscopy, or vascular contrast studies may be required for *diagnosis*. Primary tumors of the lungs and airways are rare in children and include nonsecreting carcinoid tumor and congenital bronchial cysts. Metastatic tumors, such as osteogenic sarcoma, may spread to the endobronchial airways from other areas of the body.

### Bronchial Stenosis

Bronchial stenosis may be congenital or acquired and may result in localized wheezing, air trapping, atelectasis, or infection. Acquired stenosis is usually the result of a chronic inflammatory process or localized trauma. *Diagnosis* usually requires bronchoscopy or bronchography on high-resolution CT scan.

## Emphysema

Emphysema, a condition that results when alveolar septa are disrupted or destroyed, is relatively uncommon in children, but generalized or localized overinflation is common and is due to airway obstruction from a variety of causes. Although the term "emphysema" often is used somewhat inaccurately to refer to overinflation or to leakage of air into the interstitial tissues of the lung or into the subcutaneous tissue, this use of the term has become accepted.

**Congenital lobar emphysema** consists of overinflation of one lobe, most often the left upper lobe, which may produce respiratory distress because the surrounding lung tissue has become compressed, shifting the mediastinum. Lobectomy may be required if respiratory distress is severe and progressive. True emphysema develops in the absence of antiproteases (alpha₁-antitrypsin deficiency) but rarely appears before the 3rd decade of life.

## CHEST WALL AND PLEURA

### Scoliosis

Scoliosis, when severe, may result in respiratory dysfunction (see Chapter 19). Marked curvature of the thoracic spine is associated with chest wall deformity and limitation of chest wall movement, which decreases lung volumes (restrictive lung disease). In advanced scoliosis, bronchial obstruction may develop when the bronchi become kinked or compressed by the great vessels that shift to abnormal positions in relation to the airways. Significant loss of inspiratory capacity often leads to pulmonary hypertension, recurrent infection, atelectasis, and respiratory insufficiency.

### Pneumothorax

Pneumothorax is the accumulation of air in the pleural space that may result from external trauma or from leakage of air from the lungs or airways (see Chapter 6, Fig. 6–8). It may occur spontaneously in teenagers and young adults. Predisposing conditions include mechanical ventilation, asthma, cystic fibrosis, disorders of collagen (**Marfan syn-**

**drome**), and exertion with a Valsalva maneuver. The symptoms of pneumothorax include pain, dyspnea, and cyanosis; if the air leak communicates with the mediastinum, subcutaneous emphysema may become apparent. Physical findings may include decreased breath sounds, a tympanitic percussion note, signs of mediastinal shift, and subcutaneous crepitance (see Table 12–3). Few or no physical signs of pneumothorax may be present if the amount of air collection is small, but symptoms may progress rapidly if the air in the pleural space is under pressure ("tension pneumothorax"), with death resulting if the tension is not relieved.

The *diagnosis* is confirmed by chest roentgenogram. In infants, transillumination of the chest wall may help in the rapid diagnosis of pneumothorax.

*Treatment* depends on the amount of intrapleural air and the nature of the underlying disease. Small pneumothoraces often do not need to be treated and may resolve spontaneously. Larger pneumothoraces (and certainly tension pneumothoraces) require immediate drainage of the air. In an emergency situation, a simple needle aspiration may suffice but placement of a chest tube may be required for resolution. Sclerosing the pleural surfaces to obliterate the pleural space may benefit patients with recurrent pneumothoraces.

### Pneumomediastinum

Pneumomediastinum results from the dissection of air from a leak in the pulmonary parenchyma into the mediastinum. The most common cause in children is acute asthma. Symptoms include pain and dyspnea. Physical findings may be absent or may include a crunching noise over the sternum on auscultation. Frequently, subcutaneous emphysema is present in the neck.

The *diagnosis* is confirmed by roentgenogram. *Treatment* is directed toward the underlying lung disease.

### Pleural Effusion

Pleural effusion commonly accompanies inflammatory processes in the lungs and may be heralded by pain, dyspnea, and signs of respiratory insufficiency resulting from compression of the underlying lung. Physical findings include dullness to percussion, decreased breath sounds, mediastinal shift, and decreased tactile fremitus (see Table 12–3).

The *diagnosis* is confirmed roentgenographically; decubitus views or ultrasonography may be helpful to distinguish fluid collections from other densities in the thorax.

Fluid accumulates in the pleural space whenever the local hydrostatic forces pushing fluid out of the vascular space exceed osmotic forces pulling fluid back into the vascular space. The underlying causes of pleural effusion include congestive heart failure, hypoproteinemia, obstruction of lymphatic drainage, malignancy, collagen vascular disease, and inflammation or infection of the pleura. Infection producing a reactive parapneumonic effusion or a more serious purulent **empyema** is the most common cause of pleural effusion in children. The latter often is due to *Streptococcus pneumoniae, Haemophilus influenzae*, streptococci, or *Staphylococcus aureus* (rarely to *Mycobacterium tuberculosis*), whereas anaerobic bacteria produce empyema associated with aspiration pneumonia and dental, lung, or subdiaphragmatic abscesses.

*Diagnostic thoracentesis* may be necessary to establish the cause of the effusion and to exclude infection. Most patients with effusions should undergo diagnostic thoracentesis unless the underlying causes for the effusion are clearly evident (e.g., systemic lupus erythematosus [SLE]), the patient does not have significant respiratory distress, and infection is not suspected. In the absence of inflammation, the fluid should have a low specific gravity (<1.015) and protein content (<2.5 g/dL), low lactic dehydrogenase activity (<200 IU/L), and a low cell count with few polymorphonuclear cells. In contrast, exudative pleural effusions resulting from inflammation have a high specific gravity, high protein (>3.0 g/dL) and lactic dehydrogenase (>250) content, low pH (<7.2) and glucose (<40 mg/dL), and a high cell count with many polymorphonuclear leukocytes.

*Treatment* is directed at the underlying condition that caused the effusion and at relief of the mechanical consequences of the fluid collection. For small effusions, especially if they are transudative, usually no therapy is required. For large effusions, drainage with a chest tube, especially if the fluid is purulent (empyema), is often needed. In this latter case, the fluid is often very thick and may be loculated, which makes simple drainage difficult. All patients with empyema require tube drainage. Drainage of loculated fluid may be facilitated by installation of streptokinase or urokinase into the pleural space via a catheter placed under CT guidance. Surgical removal of organized fibrinous parapneumonic effusions is rarely necessary.

If the underlying condition is treated successfully, the *prognosis* for patients with pleural effusions, including empyema, is excellent.

### References

Behrman RE, Kliegman RM, Arvin AM (eds): Nelson Textbook of Pediatrics, 15th ed. Philadelphia, WB Saunders, 1996, Chapters 331, 332, 365, 370.

Freij BJ, Kusjiesz H, Nelson J, et al: Parapneumonic effusions and emphysema in hospitalized children: A retrospective review of 227 cases. Pediatr Infect Dis 3:578, 1984.

Jay SJ: Diagnostic procedures for pleural disease. Clin Chest Med 6:33, 1985.

Kravitz RM: Congenital malformations of the lung. Pediatr Clin North Am 41:453, 1994.

Prescott C: Nasal obstruction in infancy. Arch Dis Child 72:287, 1995.

Richardson MA, Cotton RT: Anatomic abnormalities of the pediatric airway. Pediatr Clin North Am 31:821, 1984.

Temes RT, Follis F, Kessler RM, et al: Intrapleural fibrinolytics in management of empyema thoracis. Chest; 110:102, 1996.

# GENETIC DISORDERS

## CYSTIC FIBROSIS

Cystic fibrosis (CF), a complex autosomal recessive disorder, is the most common lethal genetic disease affecting Caucasians (1:2500 live births). The gene for cystic fibrosis has been localized to the long arm of chromosome 7 and has been characterized as a large gene (>250 kb of genomic deoxyribonucleic acid (DNA) that encodes a polypeptide of 1480 amino acids, termed *cystic fibrosis transmembrane regulator* (CFTR). The most common mutation, which occurs in approximately 70% of the CF chromosomes, is a specific deletion of three base pairs resulting in a deletion of phenylalanine at position $\Delta$F 508. However, more than 400 other different mutations also have been reported to result in the CF phenotype. Heterozygote detection and prenatal diagnosis of individuals with $\Delta$F 508 deletion is readily accomplished. However, many mutations occur at low frequency; thus present testing identifies only 90% of carriers.

*Etiology.* The major organs involved in CF are epithelial; the secretory and absorptive characteristics of these tissues are affected. The CFTR protein is involved in $Cl^-$ conductance, consistent with the observation that 99% of patients with CF have elevated levels of sweat $Cl^-$. The CFTR is a chloride channel and substantially regulates epithelial $Cl^-$ and possibly $Na^+$ transport. How the abnormal $Cl^-$ conductance accounts for the clinical manifestations of CF is as yet uncertain. It may reduce the function of airway defenses or promote bacterial adhesion to the airway epithelium.

*Clinical Manifestations.* The respiratory epithelium of patients with CF exhibits marked impermeability to chloride and an excessive reabsorption of sodium. These alterations in the bioelectric properties of the epithelium lead to a relative dehydration of the airway secretions, resulting in impaired mucociliary transport and airway obstruction. **Chronic bronchial infection** then develops. Most patients are colonized with *H. influenzae, Staphylo-*

*coccus aureus*, and/or *Pseudomonas aeruginosa* (which predominates in older patients with advanced disease). Chronic bronchial infection leads to cough, which is the most common initial pulmonary manifestation; sputum production; hyperinflation; bronchiectasis; and, eventually, pulmonary insufficiency and death. Digital clubbing is nearly universal in patients with significant lung disease.

Most patients with CF (90%) have exocrine **pancreatic insufficiency** early in life (if not at birth) as a result of inspissation of mucus in the pancreatic ducts and consequent autodigestion of the pancreas. Maldigestion with secondary malabsorption results in steatorrhea (large, fatty, floating, foul-smelling stools), azotorrhea, and a number of secondary deficiency states (vitamins K, D, A, and E) in the untreated patient. Nutrient malabsorption also results in failure to thrive despite a ravenous appetite. Approximately 10% of patients are born with intestinal obstruction resulting from inspissated meconium ("meconium ileus"). In older patients, intestinal obstruction may occur because of maldigestion and thick mucus in the intestinal lumen ("meconium ileus equivalent"). Such events may occur after dietary indiscretions or with inadequate pancreatic enzyme replacement. In adolescent or adult patients, relative insulin deficiency may develop, and **hyperglycemia** may become symptomatic, although ketoacidosis is rare.

As in the respiratory and gastrointestinal tracts, inspissation of mucus in the *reproductive tract* leads to dysfunction. Female fertility is low and the cervical mucus is abnormal, but a number of patients have given birth to children. Secondary amenorrhea often is present as a result of chronic illness and markedly reduced body weight. Males almost universally are azoospermic, with atrophy or absence of the vas deferens.

The failure of the *sweat ducts* to conserve salt may lead to heat exhaustion or to unexplained hypochloremic alkalosis in infants but has relatively little clinical consequence otherwise.

CF is a chronic, insidiously progressive disease exhibiting multiple *complications* related to viscous mucus, malabsorption, and infection (Table 12–8).

*Diagnosis.* The diagnosis of CF should be seriously considered in any patient with chronic or recurring respiratory or gastrointestinal symptoms. Indications for sweat testing are shown in Table 12–9. For the diagnosis to be established, the sweat chloride concentration must exceed 60 mEq/L on two separate sweat tests with adequate sweat volume (at least 75 mg of sweat, and preferably more than 100 mg, must be collected for accurate analysis). In addition to a positive sweat test, the patient must have (1) chronic obstructive lung disease, (2)

**TABLE 12–8.** Complications of Cystic Fibrosis

**Pulmonary**

Bronchiectasis, bronchitis, bronchiolitis, pneumonia
Atelectasis
Hemoptysis
Pneumothorax
Nasal polyps
Sinusitis
Reactive airway disease
Cor pulmonale
Respiratory failure
Mucoid impaction of the bronchi
Allergic bronchopulmonary aspergillosis

**Gastrointestinal**

Meconium ileus
Meconium peritonitis
Meconium ileus equivalent (non-neonatal obstruction)
Rectal prolapse
Intussusception
Volvulus
Fibrosing colonopathy (strictures)
Appendicitis
Intestinal atresia
Pancreatitis
Biliary cirrhosis (portal hypertension: esophageal varices, hypersplenism)
Neonatal obstructive jaundice
Hepatic steatosis
Gastroesophageal reflux
Cholelithiasis
Inguinal hernia
Growth failure (malabsorption)
Vitamin deficiency states (vitamins A, K, E, D)
Insulin deficiency, symptomatic hyperglycemia
Malignancy (rare)

**Other**

Infertility
Delayed puberty
Edema–hypoproteinemia
Dehydration–heat exhaustion
Hypertrophic osteoarthropathy–arthritis
Clubbing
Amyloidosis

exocrine pancreatic insufficiency, or (3) a confirmed family history of classic CF in a sibling or first cousin. Although highly specific for CF, the sweat test is subject to numerous technical problems and is reliable only in laboratories that perform the test frequently and with scrupulous quality control. False-positive and false-negative sweat test results occur in a few well-defined clinical states (Table 12–10). A few patients may have typical but mild symptoms and borderline or even normal sweat $Cl^-$ levels. Other supportive tests, such as measurement of bioelectrical potential differences across respiratory epithelium, low levels of stool trypsin, and detection of the $\Delta F$ 508 genotype (or other known mutation) by DNA analysis may be useful.

## TABLE 12–9.  Indications for Sweat Testing

### Pulmonary

Chronic or recurrent cough
Chronic or recurrent pneumonia
Recurrent bronchiolitis
Atelectasis
Hemoptysis
Staphylococcal pneumonia
*Pseudomonas aeruginosa* in the respiratory tract (in the absence of such circumstances as tracheostomy or prolonged intubation)
Mucoid *P. aeruginosa* in the respiratory tract
Right upper lobe pneumonia

### Gastrointestinal

Meconium ileus
Neonatal intestinal obstruction (meconium plug, atresia)
Steatorrhea, malabsorption
Hepatic cirrhosis in childhood (including any manifestations such as esophageal varices or portal hypertension)
Pancreatitis
Rectal prolapse
Vitamin K deficiency states (hypoprothrombinemia)

### Miscellaneous

Digital clubbing
Failure to thrive
Family history of cystic fibrosis (sibling or cousin)
Salty taste when kissed; salt crystals on skin after evaporation of sweat
Heat prostration, especially under seemingly inappropriate circumstances
Hyponatremic hypochloremic alkalosis in infants
Nasal polyps
Pansinusitis
Aspermia

Prenatal detection of a known CF genotype may be accomplished by amniotic fluid or chorionic villus sampling.

**Treatment.** The complex management of CF is best coordinated by a tertiary referral center. As in the treatment of any chronic disease, the patient-physician relationship is of utmost importance. Physicians, patients, families, and other caretakers must work together to maintain an optimistic, aggressive approach to life and to treatment. Efforts to prevent the occurrence of complications and the progression of lung disease are vital, and immunization to influenza virus and other diseases should be kept up to date. Unfortunately, no universally accepted protocol for treatment exists, and many measures are controversial.

The **electrolyte loss** resulting from the sweat defect is treated by adding more salt to the patient's diet.

**Lung disease** is treated by combining (1) physical measures to help remove mucus from the airways (chest physiotherapy, exercise), (2) pharmaco-

logic measures to clear mucus and improve airway patency (bronchodilators and aerosolized DNAse), and (3) antibiotic therapy to control chronic infection. Monitoring pulmonary bacterial flora and providing aggressive therapy with appropriate antibiotics in full therapeutic doses (oral, aerosolized, and/or parenteral) help to slow the progression of the lung disease. Patients are hospitalized for high-dose intravenous antibiotic therapy whenever necessary, especially when they are infected with organisms resistant to oral agents (e.g., *Pseudomonas*). Under normal circumstances, therapy should last for at least 2 wk; even when using the most aggressive therapy, it is difficult to sterilize the lungs. Infection with *Burkholderia cepacia* is particularly difficult to treat and may be associated with an accelerated clinical deterioration. **Allergic bronchopulmonary aspergillosis** also may complicate CF and require treatment with steroids. Pulmonary complications, such as pneumothorax, hemoptysis (check vitamin K status), and atelectasis, are treated as they are in other patients.

*Pancreatic insufficiency* is treated by replacing pancreatic enzymes, preferably in enteric-coated form, and by encouraging higher caloric intake than normal. Even with the best enzyme replacement, stool losses of fat and protein may be relatively high. Fat is not withheld from the diet, even when significant steatorrhea exists. Instead, enzyme doses are increased to normalize the stools as much as possible; however, lipase concentrations exceeding 2500 U/kg/day have been associated with intestinal obstruction due to fibrosing colonopathy. Fat-soluble vitamins are given in twice-normal doses, preferably in water-miscible form. Meconium ileus often requires surgical intervention but may respond to enemas of hyperosmolar roentgenographic contrast material. Intestinal ob-

## TABLE 12–10.  Causes of False-Positive and False-Negative Sweat Tests

| False Positive | False Negative |
|---|---|
| Adult age | Edema |
| Adrenal insufficiency | Poor technique |
| Ectodermal dysplasia | Atypical cystic fibrosis (uncommon) |
| Nephrogenic diabetes insipidus | |
| Hypothyroidism | |
| Fucosidosis | |
| Mucopolysaccharidosis | |
| Malnutrition | |
| Poor technique | |
| Type I glycogen storage disease | |
| Panhypopituitarism | |

struction in older patients is treated similarly or with oral laxatives.

Therapies under ongoing investigation and showing some benefit are directed toward thinning mucus with inhaled DNAse, anti-inflammatory medications (antiproteases, nonsteroidal anti-inflammatory agents), lung transplantation, and ultimately gene therapy.

*Prognosis.* Pulmonary disease is the major cause of morbidity in CF and is influenced by the inherent severity of disease and by therapy. Patients with meconium ileus have the same prognosis as others with CF if they survive the 1st yr of life. Current data from the Patient Registry of the Cystic Fibrosis Foundation indicate that the median survival age for patients with CF is approximately 27 yr, but patients vary greatly in the severity of their disease.

## IMMOTILE (DYSMOTILE) CILIA SYNDROME

This syndrome is an inherited disorder in which ultrastructural abnormalities in the cilia result in absent or disordered movement. The most classic form of the syndrome, **Kartagener syndrome**, is an autosomal recessive disorder characterized by situs inversus, pansinusitis, and bronchiectasis. Otitis media also is common, and male infertility is universal (as a result of immotile sperm). The cilia lack dynein arms, an ultrastructural feature that represents an ATPase necessary for ciliary motility. Many other variants of the syndrome exist that have a variety of ultrastructural abnormalities of the cilia. In some patients, cilia may move but their beat is abnormal, usually uncoordinated, and ineffective.

Because respiratory tract cilia fail to beat normally, secretions accumulate in the airways and bacterial infection occurs. Chronic infection leads to bronchiectasis by early adulthood. The *diagnosis* should be suspected in individuals with early-onset chronic bronchitis or bronchiectasis; in patients with chronic, recurrent, or persistent pneumonia; and especially in patients with pansinusitis and/or chronic otitis media. Cystic fibrosis should be excluded by sweat testing. The diagnosis is confirmed by electron microscopy of respiratory cilia; the cilia may be obtained from nasal scrapings. Because chronic infection and inflammation may result in ultrastructural abnormalities in nasal cilia, care must be taken in confirming the diagnosis.

*Treatment* is similar to the pulmonary therapy in cystic fibrosis and is directed toward improving clearance of respiratory secretions and controlling infection. Chest physiotherapy, immunoprophylaxis of viral infections (e.g., influenza), and prompt treatment of bacterial infection are helpful, but the course of the disease tends to be slowly progressive, with most patients dying in the 4th to 5th decades.

## ALPHA₁-ANTITRYPSIN DEFICIENCY

Alpha$_1$-antitrypsin deficiency is an inherited absence (relative or absolute) of antiprotease activity. In the respiratory tract, the proteases (especially elastase) released by the normal turnover of phagocytic cells therefore are not inhibited, and, over a period of time (usually two or more decades), emphysema develops. In some forms of the disorder, liver disease appears early in life, but in most children with alpha$_1$-antitrypsin deficiency little evidence for lung disease exists in the 1st decade.

In children or adolescents, dyspnea is the first *clinical manifestation.* Chest roentgenograms may reveal hyperinflation; often the disease may be confused with late-onset asthma. Progressive emphysema or pulmonary cyst formation may be associated with previous pulmonary infection or with exposure to cigarette smoke.

The *diagnosis* is confirmed by demonstrating reduced total alpha$_1$-antitrypsin levels and a ZZ phenotype. Recombinant alpha$_1$-antitrypsin is now available and has some efficacy in *treatment* and *prevention* of the lung disease.

References

Behrman RE, Kliegman RM, Arvin AM (eds): Nelson Textbook of Pediatrics, 15th ed. Philadelphia, WB Saunders, 1996, Chapters 363, 364.
Davis PB, Drumm M, Konstan MW: Cystic fibrosis. Am J Respir Crit Care Med 154:1229, 1996.
Hubbard RC, Brantly ML, Sellers SE, et al: Anti-neutrophilelastase defenses of the lower respiratory tract in α-1-antitrypsin deficiency directly augmented with an aerosol of α-1-antitrypsin. Ann Intern Med 111:206, 1989.

## INFECTIOUS DISORDERS

### THE UPPER AIRWAY

#### Otitis Media

See Chapter 10.

#### Sinusitis

See Chapter 10.

## Croup

The most common syndrome of infectious upper airway obstruction is croup, or acute infectious laryngotracheobronchitis (see Table 12–5 and Chapter 10). Croup is predominantly of viral etiology; parainfluenza types 1 and 2 viruses are the most common agents.

*Clinical Manifestations.* The typical episode begins in a child between 6 mo and 3 yr of age having symptoms of an upper respiratory infection (the common cold) and lasts less than 5 days. A brassy cough (typically characterized as sounding like the barking of a seal), inspiratory stridor, and respiratory distress may develop slowly or acutely. Signs of upper airway obstruction, such as labored breathing and marked suprasternal, intercostal, and subcostal retractions, are evident on examination. Associated lower airway disease accompanied by wheezing and a productive cough may be present. Although the majority of such children are not seriously ill, the airway obstruction may become severe, necessitating placement of an artificial airway. The subglottic space is the major site of obstruction, which is caused by edema resulting from the viral inflammation (see Table 12–6). Roentgenogram reveals the "steeple" sign of a narrowed subglottic space.

*Treatment.* Administration of aerosolized racemic epinephrine may reduce the edema temporarily, producing marked clinical improvement, but the edema and obstruction soon return and the disease runs its course over several days. Epinephrine aerosol treatment may need to be repeated as often as every 20 min in severe cases. During inspiration, the walls of the subglottic space are drawn together, aggravating the obstruction (and probably also the edema), so that children should be kept as calm as possible to reduce their respiratory efforts. The best calming method for a child with croup is to sit in the mother's lap. Sedatives should be used very cautiously and only in the setting of an intensive care unit. Cool mist administered by tent or face mask may help to prevent drying of the secretions around the larynx.

Children with severe croup requiring hospitalization should be monitored carefully. When symptoms subside, it may indicate that the patient either is improving or is becoming fatigued and is in respiratory failure. Because aerosolized epinephrine has a short duration of action, most authorities believe that children requiring such therapy should be hospitalized for observation, even if their obstructive signs clear completely with the first aerosol treatment. Systemically administered corticosteroids are beneficial in treating croup but generally are reserved for seriously ill patients. Topically active inhaled corticosteroids may also be of benefit. If the patient is very young (<4 mo of age) or if symptoms continue for more than 1 wk, the patient should undergo careful laryngoscopy because there is an increased probability that another lesion exists (subglottic stenosis or hemangioma). Sudden worsening (fever, respiratory distress, leukocytosis) suggests a complicating *bacterial tracheitis*. This is a serious and potentially life-threatening condition (see Table 12–5).

Some children have acute episodes of croup-like symptoms without having evidence of a viral infection. These episodes may be severe but usually are of short duration. This acute "spasmodic croup" is not well understood but may involve allergic mechanisms in some patients. It tends to recur and to respond to relatively simple therapies, such as exposure to cool or moist air.

## Epiglottitis

Acute epiglottitis, another syndrome of upper airway obstruction, typically occurs in older children (ages 2–7 yr). The causative agent is predominantly bacterial (*H. influenzae* type b). Immunization of infants and children to *H. influenzae* has made epiglottis extremely rare.

*Clinical Manifestations.* Epiglottitis is characterized by sudden onset, high fever, respiratory distress, fulminant progression, severe dysphagia, and a muffled voice (see Tables 12–5 and 12–6). Patients usually find it easier to breathe sitting erect, and they drool because of the dysphagia. Acute epiglottitis is a true pediatric emergency because the inflamed airway suddenly may become totally obstructed, leading to death. Examination of the pharynx should be discouraged.

*Diagnosis.* In typical cases, epiglottitis should be suspected on observing the patient's clinical presentation. The *differential diagnosis* includes severe croup, bacterial tracheitis, foreign body aspiration, Ludwig angina, and retropharyngeal and peritonsillar abscess (see Table 12–5). Confirmation of the diagnosis is based on direct observation of the inflamed and swollen supraglottic structures and cherry-red enlarged epiglottis, but this procedure should be performed only in the operating room with a competent surgeon and anesthesiologist prepared to place a nasotracheal tube or to perform a tracheostomy. *H. influenzae* may be recovered from the surface of the epiglottis or from blood culture. Epiglottitis may be distinguished from severe croup on the basis of a lateral neck film if there is doubt as to the clinical diagnosis ("thumb sign" of swollen epiglottis). A physician should accompany the patient to the radiology department and be prepared to perform an emergency intubation (which will be much more difficult than under normal circumstances) or tracheostomy.

*Treatment.* Nasotracheal intubation is currently the preferred method of treatment, but the intubated patient requires constant supervision and restraint to decrease the probability of accidental extubation. Tracheostomy is an acceptable alternative. Antibiotics (ceftriaxone) suitable for *H. influenzae* should be given at once. With effective therapy, clinical recovery is rapid, and most patients can be safely extubated within 48–72 hr. The severity of airway obstruction is directly correlated with the rapidity of onset; almost no deaths occur in patients presenting for medical attention more than 24 hr after onset of symptoms.

## THE LOWER AIRWAY

### Bronchiolitis

Bronchiolitis is an acute respiratory illness of young children resulting from inflammation of small airways and characterized by wheezing. Respiratory syncytial virus (RSV) is the principal agent, although other viruses, such as parainfluenza, adenovirus, influenza, rhinovirus, and, infrequently, *M. pneumoniae*, have been associated with the illness.

*Epidemiology.* Bronchiolitis is a common illness of young children; approximately 50% of children experience this illness during the first 2 yr of life, and 95% of children have serologic evidence of previous infection by age 3 yr. Children generally acquire the infection when exposed to family members who typically have symptoms of an upper respiratory tract infection or from infected children in a day care setting. Most cases occur during the winter and early spring, when the associated viral agents are most prevalent in the community.

*Clinical Manifestations.* Affected infants usually have rhinorrhea, sneezing, cough, and low-grade fever, followed in several days by the onset of rapid breathing and wheezing. The child may feed poorly. *Physical examination* is notable for signs of acute respiratory distress, including nasal flaring, tachypnea, intermittent cyanosis, retractions, a prolonged expiratory phase, and wheezes and crackles in the chest. The white blood cell count usually is normal. Chest roentgenograms typically reveal air trapping and may show peribronchial thickening, atelectasis, and infiltrates. The principal physiologic abnormality is hypoxemia secondary to mismatching of ventilation and perfusion. It is unusual for hypercapnia to develop, but it can occur in the severely affected infant with significant airway obstruction or in infants who become fatigued.

*Diagnosis.* The diagnosis of bronchiolitis is based on clinical findings and on knowledge of the epidemiology of viral illnesses prevalent in the community. RSV may be identified on nasopharyngeal secretions by culture or antigen assay. Many other diagnoses should be considered in the young child who presents with an acute **wheezing-associated respiratory illness**. Asthma typically has a recurrent pattern and is responsive to bronchodilators. Pneumonia usually is associated with an infiltrate demonstrated on a chest roentgenogram and, if bacterial infection is present, with a high white blood cell count. In congestive heart failure, an enlarged heart usually is seen on the chest roentgenogram, and either related structural cardiac abnormalities or viral myocarditis may be present. Children with foreign body aspiration often have a history of having aspirated an object and may exhibit localized wheezing or air trapping. Wheezing associated with gastroesophageal reflux is likely to be chronic or recurrent, and the patient may have a history of frequent emesis. Cystic fibrosis may be associated with poor growth, chronic diarrhea, or a family history of the disease.

*Treatment.* The management of the child with bronchiolitis depends on the severity of the illness. Most children have mild symptoms and can be managed with supportive measures at home. Approximately 5% of children with bronchiolitis will require hospitalization. *Indications for hospitalization* include young age (<6 mo), moderate to marked respiratory distress (sleeping respiratory rates of 50–60 or higher), hypoxemia ($Po_2$ <60 mm Hg or oxygen saturation <92% on room air), the occurrence of apnea, inability to tolerate oral feeding, and lack of appropriate care available at home. Children with chronic lung disease, such as bronchopulmonary dysplasia, congenital heart disease (particularly with associated pulmonary hypertension), neuromuscular weakness, and immunodeficiency, are at increased risk of having severe, potentially fatal disease. Consideration should be given to the hospitalization of all of these high-risk children.

*Supportive measures* appropriate to the care of the child with bronchiolitis include administering adequate oral or (in the hospitalized child) parenteral fluids to ensure maintenance of normal hydration in the presence of increased insensible water losses associated with tachypnea. Fever, if high or associated with increased respiratory distress, may be treated with antipyretic agents. Supplemental humidified oxygen should be provided for the hospitalized child in a sufficient concentration to maintain a $PaO_2$ of 70–90 mm Hg (oxygen saturation ≥93%). The use of *bronchodilators*, such as aerosolized beta$_2$-agonists or racemic epinephrine, may be beneficial in selected patients and should be tried in severely affected children. Corticosteroids offer no benefit.

Administering *ribavirin aerosol*, a specific antiviral agent, to children with RSV infection has been demonstrated to be mildly efficacious in clinical trials. This should be considered in severely affected infants and in those at high risk for development of severe, protracted disease (e.g., chronic lung disease, congenital heart disease). Antibacterial therapy is not indicated unless evidence suggests the existence of a concomitant bacterial infection. *Intubation* and *mechanical ventilation* are required to treat respiratory failure or severe apnea. Monthly infusions of RSV hyperimmune gamma globulin confers some protection from severe disease in some high risk groups of infants and toddlers (e.g., those with bronchopulmonary dysplasia, very low birth weight).

*Prognosis.* Complications of bronchiolitis include apnea, respiratory failure, atelectasis, secondary bacterial infection, and pneumothorax or pneumomediastinum (in the child requiring mechanical ventilation). However, the immediate prognosis of most children with bronchiolitis is excellent, with symptoms resolving in 7–10 days. Several studies suggest that some children who experience an episode of bronchiolitis, particularly if they needed to be hospitalized, may be prone to experience further episodes of wheezing, may manifest allergic symptoms, have lower average levels of lung function, and have a modestly higher prevalence of increased airway reactivity later in life. Factors other than the occurrence of bronchiolitis, such as underlying increased bronchial reactivity and exposure to environmental pollutants like cigarette smoke, may contribute to the apparent sequelae of bronchiolitis.

### Bronchiolitis Obliterans

Bronchiolitis obliterans is an uncommon form of chronic bronchiolitis in which there is endobronchiolar granulation tissue and peribronchiolar fibrosis. Most reported cases in young infants have been related to the occurrence of severe viral infection, most commonly adenovirus. Association with influenza, pertussis, measles, and *M. pneumoniae* has been reported. In adults, bronchiolitis obliterans also has been associated with toxic inhalational exposures, connective tissue disorders, and drug administration (such as penicillamine). An interstitial pneumonia may be present. Abnormalities may be diffuse or localized.

*Clinical Manifestations.* The typical illness begins with fever, cough, tachypnea, and wheezing. Notable physical findings include retractions, wheezes, and rales. Chest roentgenograms typically show a nonspecific diffuse infiltrate exhibiting areas of atelectasis, but the roentgenograms may reveal a more miliary pattern. The course of the illness differs from that of acute, uncomplicated bronchiolitis in that the symptoms progress, often after a brief period of improvement, and are accompanied by an increasing shortness of breath, the development of productive cough, hypoxia, and persistent wheezing. Clinically, there is fixed airway obstruction that is poorly responsive to bronchodilators. Increased symptoms can occur as acute exacerbations or more insidiously over a prolonged period. Bronchography reveals obstruction of small airways; arteriography reveals a reduction of the pulmonary bed.

*Complications* include progressive respiratory failure, atelectasis, secondary bacterial infection, and the development of the **unilateral hyperlucent lung syndrome** in those in whom the pathology appears to be confined to one lung. Some patients die early in the course of the disease, whereas others experience a more chronic course.

*Diagnosis.* Bronchiolitis obliterans should be considered in the child who has significant recurrent or persistent respiratory symptoms and evidence of fixed airway obstruction following a severe viral lung infection. Typical bronchographic findings support the diagnosis; confirmation requires lung biopsy. Other diagnoses to consider in a child with recurrent/persistent cough and wheezing with an infiltrate or atelectasis on chest roentgenogram include cystic fibrosis, asthma, gastroesophageal reflux, and foreign body aspiration.

*Treatment.* No specific therapy is available, although corticosteroids often are used in an attempt to mitigate the progressive fibrosis. Appropriate supportive measures include supplemental oxygen, chest physiotherapy, a trial of bronchodilator therapy, and early, aggressive treatment of further lung infections.

### Pneumonia

Pneumonia refers to the inflammation of pulmonary tissue and is associated with consolidation of the alveolar spaces. **Pneumonitis** is a general term for lung inflammation that may or may not be associated with consolidation. **Lobar pneumonia** describes pneumonia localized to one or more lobes of the lung in which the affected lobe or lobes are completely consolidated.

**Bronchopneumonia** refers to inflammation of the lung that is centered in the bronchioles, resulting in the production of a mucopurulent exudate that obstructs some of these small airways and causes patchy consolidation of the adjacent lobules. Bronchopneumonia is usually a generalized process involving multiple lobes of the lung. The distinction between bronchopneumonia and bronchiolitis can be somewhat arbitrary.

**Interstitial pneumonitis** refers to inflammation of the interstitium, which is composed of the walls of the alveoli, the alveolar sacs and ducts, and the bronchioles. Interstitial pneumonitis may be seen acutely with viral infections, but also may be a chronic process.

Anatomic respiratory system malformations, altered systemic or local immunity, and exposure to cigarette smoke predispose the patient to infectious pneumonia. The cause of pneumonia depends on the age, immune status, presence of CF or other chronic lung disease, exposure history, and nosocomial versus community acquisition.

*Etiology.* Pneumonia may be caused by a variety of infectious agents (bacterial, viral, fungal, rickettsial, and parasitic organisms), and inflammatory processes (SLE, sarcoidosis, histiocytosis) as well as by toxic substances (hydrocarbons, smoke, molds, dusts, chemicals, gases, gastric contents) that are inhaled and/or aspirated. The most common cause of pneumonia in children is viral infections; bacterial infections account for only 10–30% of all pediatric pneumonias. Certain infectious

pneumonias are more common at a particular age (Table 12–11).

Microorganisms gain access to the lung by hematogenous dissemination or local spread descending through the respiratory bronchial tree. Although aspiration pneumonia may be seen following seizures or in patients with altered mental status, neuromuscular disease, and gastroesophageal reflux, most cases of pediatric pneumonia are not due to these causes. *H. influenzae* type b pneumonia often is associated with bacteremia, meningitis, and other sites of infection (arthritis, pleural effusion, cellulitis). *S. aureus* is a rare cause of pneumonia in infants; when present, the child is acutely ill with empyema, pneumatoceles, and respiratory failure. Staphylococcal skin infection may precede bacteremia and pneumonia. RSV, influenza viruses, and parainfluenza virus are common causes of viral pneumonia. Viral respiratory infections may precede bacterial pneumonias. Infants between 1 and 3 mo of age often have an **afebrile pneumonia,** which typically is due to congenitally or environmentally acquired agents such as *Ureaplasma urealyticum, Chlamydia trachomatis* (with or without conjunctivitis), cytomegalovirus (CMV), *Pneumocystis carinii,* or RSV. Pneumonia in immunocompromised patients may be due to *P. carinii,* gram-negative enteric bacteria, fungi (aspergillosis, histoplasmosis), mycobacteria (*M. tuberculosis, M. avium*), or CMV, whereas disease in patients with CF usually is due to *S. aureus* (in infancy), *P. aeruginosa,* or *B. cepacia* (in older patients).

Children with immune system dysfunction, malnutrition, or defects in the normal defense mechanisms of the lung are very susceptible to pulmonary infections. The causative agents often are

TABLE 12–11.  Common Causes of Pneumonia at Different Ages*

| Age | Bacterial | Viral | Others |
|---|---|---|---|
| Neonate | Group B streptococci, coliform bacteria | CMV, herpesvirus, enterovirus | *Mycoplasma hominis, Ureaplasma urealyticum* |
| 4–16 wk | *Staphylococcus aureus, Haemophilus influenzae,†  Streptococcus pneumoniae* | CMV, RSV, influenza virus, parainfluenza virus | *Chlamydia trachomatis, U. urealyticum* |
| Up to 5 yr | *S. pneumoniae, S. aureus, H. influenzae,* group A streptococcus | RSV, adenovirus, influenza virus | |
| Over 5 yr | *S. pneumoniae, H. influenzae* | Influenza virus, varicella | *Mycoplasma pneumoniae, Chlamydia pneumoniae, Legionella pneumophila* |

*An increasingly important consideration is *Mycobacterium tuberculosis. Pneumocystis carinii* should always be considered in HIV-infected patients.
†Invasive *H. influenzae,* type b, is now rare in immunized populations.
CMV = cytomegalovirus; HIV = human immunodeficiency virus; RSV = respiratory syncytial virus.

unusual, opportunistic organisms, including gram-negative enteric bacteria, anaerobes, CMV, measles, varicella, *P. carinii*, or fungi.

*Clinical Manifestations.* The typical clinical patterns of viral and bacterial pneumonias usually differ, although the distinction is not always clear for a given patient. Tachypnea, cough, malaise, pleuritic chest pain, and retractions are common to both.

Viral pneumonias more often are associated with cough, wheezing, or stridor; fever is less prominent than in bacterial pneumonia. The chest roentgenogram shows diffuse, streaky infiltrates of bronchopneumonia, and the white blood cell count often is not elevated (lymphocytes are the predominant cell type).

Bacterial pneumonias typically are associated with cough, high fever, chills, dyspnea, and auscultatory findings of lung consolidation (decreased or tubular breath sounds, dullness to percussion, and egophony in a localized region) (see Table 12–3). The chest roentgenogram often shows lobar consolidation and pleural effusion (10–30%), and the peripheral white blood cell count is elevated (>15,000–20,000/mm), with a predominance of neutrophils.

Many cases of pneumonia have characteristics that fall between these two typical patterns of viral and bacterial pneumonia. Lower lobe pneumonia may present with abdominal pain.

*Diagnosis.* The definitive diagnosis of pneumonia requires identification of the causative organism. Sputum for culture is not easily obtained from children. Certain viral agents (RSV, influenza, parainfluenza, adenovirus) may be identified by culture, polymerase chain reaction (PCR), or immunofluorescent staining of infected epithelial cells washed from the nasopharynx. CMV and enterovirus can be cultured from the nasopharynx, urine, or bronchoalveolar lavage fluid. *M. pneumoniae* may be suspected if cold agglutinins are present in peripheral blood samples and confirmed by detecting presence of *Mycoplasma*-specific IgG or IgM in serum. Bacterial agents may be cultured or identified by antigen detection (*Pneumococcus, H. influenzae*) from blood or from an associated pleural effusion. The diagnosis of *M. tuberculosis* may be made by tuberculin skin tests and analysis of sputum or gastric aspirates (culture, antigen detection, or PCR).

Invasive procedures, such as bronchoscopy and bronchoalveolar lavage, lung aspiration, or lung biopsy, may be necessary to obtain culture specimens. These invasive procedures are not used in typical pneumonias, but they may be employed in special instances, such as pneumonia in the immu-nocompromised host or when the clinical picture is unusual.

*Treatment.* The management of pneumonia depends on the age of the patient and the clinical presentation (whether more consistent with viral or with bacterial pneumonia). Neonatal or congenital pneumonia is life-threatening; therefore, infants younger than 2 mo of age with pneumonia should be hospitalized and treated with intravenous antibiotics. If bacterial pneumonia is suspected at birth, antibiotics effective against group B streptococcus and coliform bacteria should be used (see Appendix 1). After the 1st wk of life, antibiotic coverage for *S. aureus* should be included if the roentgenogram demonstrates effusions or pneumatoceles. In older children, drugs effective against *H. influenzae* and *S. pneumoniae* should be used. Appropriate antibiotic choices in older children include amoxicillin, ceftriaxone, erythromycin-sulfamethoxazole, clarithromycin, or trimethoprim-sulfamethoxazole for 10 days. Pneumonia in children 5–10 yr of age frequently is caused by *M. pneumoniae* or *S. pneumoniae* and may be treated with erythromycin or clarithromycin; the latter may be better tolerated. Penicillin-resistant pneumococcus is now common in many communities. These organisms often are resistant to multiple antibiotics and require therapy with ceftriaxone or vancomycin. A small percentage of children with pneumonia require hospitalization. Most children beyond early infancy may be managed as outpatients. Indications for hospitalization include:

1. Moderate to severe respiratory distress.
2. Failure to respond to oral antibiotics.
3. Inability to take oral antibiotics at home because of vomiting or poor compliance.
4. Lobar consolidation in more than one lobe.
5. Immunosuppression.
6. Empyema.
7. Abscess or pneumatocele.
8. Underlying cardiopulmonary disease (e.g., bronchopulmonary dysplasia or pulmonary hypertension).

*Prognosis.* Most children recover from pneumonia rapidly and completely, and the roentgenographic findings should return to normal within 6–8 wk. In a few children, pneumonia may persist longer than 1 mo or may be *recurrent*. In such cases, the possibility of underlying disease must be investigated further (Table 12–12). Evaluation then may include the tuberculin skin test, sweat chloride determination, serum immunoglobulin and IgG subclass determinations, bronchoscopy, and barium swallow.

TABLE 12–12.    Differential Diagnosis of
Recurrent Pneumonia

**Hereditary Disorders**

Cystic fibrosis
Sickle cell disease

**Disorders of Immunity**

AIDS
Bruton agammaglobulinemia
Selective IgG subclass deficiencies
Common variable immunodeficiency syndrome
Severe combined immunodeficiency syndrome

**Disorders of Leukocytes**

Chronic granulomatous disease
Hyperimmunoglobulin E syndrome (Job syndrome)
Leukocyte adhesion defect

**Disorders of Cilia**

Immotile cilia syndrome
Kartagener syndrome

**Anatomic Disorders**

Sequestration
Lobar emphysema
Esophageal reflux
Foreign body
Tracheoesophageal fistula (H type)
Gastroesophageal reflux
Bronchiectasis

AIDS = acquired immunodeficiency syndrome; Ig = immunoglobulin.

## Bronchiectasis

Bronchiectasis, or the dilation of bronchi, may be either *congenital* or *acquired* but most often results from long-standing localized bronchial infection.

*Etiology.* Cystic fibrosis, immotile cilia syndrome, foreign body aspiration, immunodeficiency states, and certain postinfectious conditions (adenovirus, pertussis, measles, tuberculosis) are the most common causes of bronchiectasis. Chronic sinusitis, allergic bronchopulmonary aspergillosis, and, rarely, asthma are other etiologic factors. Chronic infection and inflammation result in destruction of the bronchial wall, with dilation, loss of mucociliary transport, and chronic mucus hypersecretion with obstruction. In its early stages, bronchiectasis may be reversible if the underlying problem can be corrected and the infection controlled.

*Clinical Manifestations.* The presentation of bronchiectasis may be subtle, but often includes productive cough, fever, hemoptysis, digital clubbing, and persistent moist rales over the affected area. Bronchiectasis results in the development of a rich bronchial blood supply to the affected area; thus, **hemoptysis** is a frequent *complication*. Atelec-

tasis is common and is due to obstruction of the affected bronchus. Wheezing is infrequent.

*Diagnosis.* Chest roentgenograms may show dilated airways that usually are manifested as parallel densities ("tram tracks"), and CT scans may show dilated airways appearing as ring shadows. Although bronchography was used to characterize bronchiectasis, it has been replaced by rapid, fine-cut CT. Fusiform dilation ("cylindrical bronchiectasis") may be reversible when the disease is managed aggressively, but saccular dilation usually is irreversible.

*Treatment.* Therapy for bronchiectasis includes antibiotics and chest physiotherapy. Underlying conditions should be treated, if possible. When there is evidence of localized, irreversible bronchiectasis, pulmonary resection should be considered because a focus of infection may spread to other uninvolved areas of the lung. Additional indications for surgery include hemorrhage and resectable disease accompanied by failure to thrive that does not respond to medical therapy.

## Lung Abscess

Lung abscess is an uncommon but serious problem in children and usually is due to aspiration of foreign material into the lung or to infection behind an obstructed bronchus. Occasionally, an abscess develops from hematogenous spread of infection. The most commonly involved sites are the posterior segments of the upper lobes and the superior segments of the lower lobes (into which aspirated material will drain when the child is recumbent). A lung abscess results when there is localized infection that destroys lung tissue, leaving a cavity containing pus and debris. Anaerobic bacteria most often are isolated from abscess cavities, but other organisms also may cause abscesses, including *S. aureus, Klebsiella pneumoniae,* fungi, and mycobacteria.

The *clinical manifestations* initially include fever and other systemic symptoms, but cough usually develops later in the course of the disease. Symptoms may be like those of typical pneumonia (from which abscesses sometimes evolve). Chest roentgenograms reveal a cavitary lesion, often with an air-fluid level, surrounded by parenchymal inflammation. If the cavity communicates with the bronchi, organisms may be isolated from sputum.

Diagnostic bronchoscopy may be indicated to rule out a foreign body and to obtain microbiologic specimens, especially if the patient does not produce sputum. In almost all cases, the lesion will regress when appropriate antimicrobial therapy is administered. Antibiotics should be chosen to cover the most likely organisms (clindamycin or penicillin will cover the majority of anaerobic flora) and should be continued for several weeks until all signs of infection have cleared. In most patients, clinical and roentgenographic resolution is complete within several months. Occasionally, a patient with previously undiagnosed diaphragmatic hernia is suspected of having a lung abscess because air-fluid levels are present on a chest film. If the patient's symptoms do not correspond to the roentgenographic picture, an upper gastrointestinal series may help in the diagnosis.

### Pulmonary Tuberculosis

See Chapter 10.

### Pertussis

See Chapter 10.

### References

American Academy of Pediatrics: Respiratory syncytial virus immune globulin intravenous: indications for use. Pediatrics 99:645, 1997.
Behrman RE, Kliegman RM, Arvin AM (eds): Nelson Textbook of Pediatrics. 15th ed. Philadelphia, WB Saunders, 1996, Chapters 170, 332, 338–340, 357, 358.
Britto J, Habibi P, Walters S, et al: Systemic complications associated with bacterial tracheitis. Arch Dis Child 74:249, 1996.
Epler GR, Colby TV, McLoud TC, et al: Bronchiolitis obliterans organizing pneumonia. N Engl J Med 312:152, 1985.
Everard M: Acute bronchiolitis: A perennial problem. Lancet 348:279, 1996.
Fitzgerald D, Mellis C, Johnson M, et al: Nebulized budesonide is as effective as nebulized adrenaline in moderately severe croup. Pediatr 97:722, 1996.
Lewiston NJ: Bronchiectasis in childhood. Pediatr Clin North Am 31:864, 1984.
Mauro R, Poole S, Lockhart C: Differentiation of epiglottitis from laryngotracheitis in the child with stridor. Am J Dis Child 142:679, 1988.
Nohynek H, Eskola J, Laine E, et al: The causes of hospital-treated acute lower respiratory tract infection in children. Am J Dis Child 145:618, 1991.
Rowe P, Klassen T: Corticosteroids for croup. Arch Pediatr Adol Med 150:344, 1996.
Tan T, Seilheimer D, Kaplan S: Pediatric lung abscess: Clinical management and outcome. Pediatr Infect Dis J 14:51, 1995.

## HYPERSENSITIVITY DISEASES

### ASTHMA

See Chapter 8.

### HYPERSENSITIVITY PNEUMONITIS

Nonasthmatic allergic pulmonary disease, also known as **extrinsic allergic alveolitis**, is due to inhalation of a variety of organic antigens found in dust and may occur as an acute syndrome or as a chronic, progressive disease. The most common antigens are from fungal organisms (such as thermophilic actinomycetes) and avian danders. They often are associated with occupational or agricultural exposure and include thermophilic bacteria found in moldy hay, grain, mushrooms, sugar cane, home or automobile air conditioners, heated humidifiers, *Bacillus subtilis* and amebae found in water, and animal proteins derived from feathers, serum, or excrement.

*Clinical Manifestations.* *Acute symptoms*, which usually begin within 4–8 hr after exposure, include dyspnea, coughing, malaise, fever, and chills. Physical examination reveals tachypnea and diffuse rales without wheezing. There is often marked leukocytosis and elevation of serum immunoglobulins other than IgE. The immune mechanism is similar to a type III or Arthus-like immune response because antigen-antibody complexes are present and the polymorphonuclear leukocytes become activated (see Chapter 8). Chest roentgenograms reveal a diffuse interstitial infiltrate without hyperinflation.

The *chronic form* of hypersensitivity pneumonitis is characterized by persistent and progressive respiratory symptoms (dyspnea, exercise intolerance) without the fever and chills of the acute form. Anorexia and weight loss may be prominent. Fine basilar crackles are heard on physical examination, and the roentgenogram reveals diffuse interstitial fibrosis. Type III and type IV immune responses may be activated in chronic allergic alveolitis.

*Pulmonary function testing* reveals decreased vital capacity, which may be reversible in the acute form but becomes irreversible in the chronic form. $PaO_2$ is decreased as a result of reduced diffusion of oxygen; $PaCO_2$ usually is decreased because of hyperventilation. Precipitating IgG antibodies to the inciting antigen usually are found in the serum but also may be seen in asymptomatic patients.

*Diagnosis.* The diagnosis depends on a high index of suspicion and a careful history and epidemiologic investigation. Often, symptoms subside after hospitalization, only to recur on the patient's return home. Serologic tests for precipitins and cultures of airborne fungi may be helpful; inhalational challenge testing may be necessary for some patients. If a humidifier or air conditioning unit is the source of disease, Legionnaire disease may need to be excluded from the diagnosis.

*Treatment.* Therapy consists of administering steroids and helping the patient avoid exposure to the inciting agent. Proper cleaning of water sources is important. In severe cases, drastic measures to avoid environmental exposure may be necessary. The *prognosis* is usually good if the patient can prevent further exposure.

## ALLERGIC BRONCHOPULMONARY ASPERGILLOSIS

See Chapter 8.

### References

Behrman RE, Kliegman RM, Arvin AM (eds): Nelson Textbook of Pediatrics, 15th ed. Philadelphia, WB Saunders, 1996, Chapters 341–345.
Bierman CW, Pierson WE, Massie FS: Nonasthmatic allergic pulmonary disease. *In* Chernick V, Kendig EL (eds): Disorders of the Respiratory Tract in Children, 5th ed. Philadelphia, WB Saunders, 1990, pp 601–613.

# NEUROLOGIC DISORDERS AFFECTING RESPIRATORY FUNCTION

## APNEA

Apnea is defined as the cessation of breathing resulting from the lack of respiratory effort (**central apnea**) or total airway obstruction (**obstructive apnea**). In many patients, apneic episodes may have both central and obstructive components (**mixed apnea**). Brief respiratory pauses usually lasting up to 10 sec, during which no respiratory effort can be detected, are common in normal infants and children, especially after a sigh. Pauses lasting longer than 15 sec, however, are considered abnormal. Normally, when a child whose airway is occluded tries to breathe, respiratory centers in the brain recruit a progressively greater amount of motor output from the respiratory center until the obstruction is overcome, but if this output fails to overcome the obstruction, an arousal impulse is triggered in the brain that causes the child to involuntarily move his or her head or body in order to relieve the obstruction. If any individual component of this final arousal response system fails, the apneic child will die.

The *etiology* of apnea is diverse and not well understood (Table 12–13). Premature infants commonly exhibit episodes of apnea, which may be associated with cyanosis and bradycardia (see Chapter 6). Apnea occurring in older infants warrants thorough investigation. Surgical therapy (removal of adenoids, tonsils, or other obstructing tissue or bypass of the obstruction by tracheostomy) may be necessary in children who are symptomatic with obstructive apnea.

## SUDDEN INFANT DEATH SYNDROME

Sudden infant death syndrome (SIDS) refers to the unexpected and unexplained death of an infant less than 1 yr of age. In the United States, SIDS occurs in 1.6–2.3/1000 live births and is the most common cause of death between 1 and 12 mo of age. There is a peak incidence between 2 and 3 mo of age. The rates are highest in black and American Indian populations; in children of young, single impoverished mothers; in infants with near-miss SIDS (described below); in premature infants; in infants whose mothers have abused drugs; and during the winter. SIDS is rare prior to 4 wk or after 6 mo of age.

A wide variety of mechanisms have been proposed to explain SIDS. Autonomic dysfunction, aberrations in respiratory control, abnormal upper airway reflexes, cardiac arrhythmias, laryngospasm associated with gastroesophageal reflux, airway obstruction and carbon dioxide rebreathing while prone, and other mechanisms have been considered, but none is widely accepted (see Table 12–13). The pathology of SIDS suggests hypoxia (acute or chronic); intrathoracic petechiae and increased pulmonary artery smooth muscle may be present.

The *risk* of SIDS is increased three to five times in siblings of infants who have died of SIDS. Whether this increased susceptibility is due to genetic or environmental factors is unknown. Monitoring of siblings may be warranted. Because infants who sleep in the prone position are at increased risk for SIDS, current recommendations are that otherwise normal infants sleep supine or on the side. Surveys indicate a decreased incidence of SIDS associated with supine sleeping.

Because SIDS strikes without warning in an infant previously thought to be healthy, the impact on families is especially devastating and psychologic support is needed. Inappropriate investigation for possible child abuse should be avoided. The *differential diagnosis* is noted in Table 12–14.

## ACUTE LIFE-THREATENING EVENTS
("Near-Miss SIDS")

Infants who experience acute life-threatening events, such as prolonged apnea requiring resuscitation, present the physician with challenging problems. Numerous possible *etiologies* (Table 12–14) warrant diagnostic evaluation, which should include an electroencephalogram; chest roentgenogram; electrocardiogram; blood gas analysis; blood chemistries, including glucose, calcium, blood urea nitrogen, and electrolytes; an evaluation for gastroesophageal reflux (barium swallow, pH probe

TABLE 12–13.   Categories of Apnea

| Disease | Example | Mechanism | Signs | Treatment |
|---|---|---|---|---|
| Apnea of prematurity | Premature (<36 wk) | Central control, airway obstruction | Apnea, bradycardia | Theophylline, caffeine, nasal CPAP, intubation |
| Ondine curse | Leigh syndrome | Central control | Apnea | Mechanical ventilation |
| Obesity hypoventilation | Obesity, Prader-Willi syndrome | Airway obstruction, central control | Obesity, somnolence, polycythemia, cor pulmonale | Theophylline, weight loss |
| Obstructive sleep apnea | Chronic tonsil hypertrophy, Pierre Robin syndrome, Down syndrome, cerebral palsy, myotonic dystrophy, myopathy | Airway obstruction by enlarged tonsils/adenoids, choanal stenosis/atresia, large tongue, temporomandibular joint dysfunction, micrognathia, velopharyngeal incompetence; also may be central | Daytime sleepiness, loud snoring, night insomnia and enuresis, hyperactivity, poor school performance, behavior problems, mouth breathing, inspiratory stridor | Tonsillectomy, adenoidectomy, nasal trumpets, CPAP, uvuloveloplasty |
| Cyanotic "breath-holding spells" | Breath-holder younger than 3 yr of age | Prolonged expiratory apnea; hyperventilation; cerebral anoxia | Cyanosis, syncope, brief tonic-clonic movements | Reassurance that the condition is self limiting; must exclude seizure disorder |
| Pallid "breath-holding spells" | Breath holder | Asystole; reflex anoxic seizures | Rapid onset, with or without crying; pallor; bradycardia; opisthotonus; seizures; follows painful stimuli | Atropine (?); must exclude seizure disorder; less benign than cyanotic breath holding |
| SIDS | Previously normal child; increased incidence with prematurity, SIDS in sibling, maternal drug abuse, cigarette smoking, males; may have preceding minor URI | Central respiratory control; cardiac arrhythmia (prolonged QT syndrome) (?); central cardiac control (?); prolonged expiratory apnea (?)<br>Rebreathing (?)<br>*Less common:*<br>(1) Parental-induced airway obstruction–suffocation (accidental or abuse)<br>(2) Chemoreceptor dysfunction<br>(3) Overheating | 2–3 mo old child found cyanotic, apneic, and pulseless in bed | No treatment; prevention with home apnea monitor unproven; supine sleep position reduces risk |

Data from Southall D: Pediatrics 80:73, 1988; Mark J, Brooks J: Pediatr Clin North Am 31:907, 1984; and Gordon N: Dev Med Child Neurol 29:805, 1987.

(?) = unproven contributing factor.

CPAP = continuous positive airway pressure by facial mask or nasal prongs; SIDS = sudden infant death syndrome; URI = upper respiratory infection.

study); and a 12–24 hr recording of heart and respiratory activity (pneumogram).

Parents of infants ascertained to be at high risk for recurrence of such events (or siblings of SIDS victims) may be offered home monitoring with an electronic monitor. No objective guidelines exist for instituting or terminating the monitoring. The ability to predict which infant is at high risk for SIDS on the basis of a pneumogram is not established, but infants with a high percentage of periodic breathing or with apneic spells lasting longer than 15 sec may be at high risk. However, many infants with previously normal pneumograms have subsequently died of SIDS, whereas most infants with abnormal pneumograms have not. The parents of infants who have had acute life-threatening events should be instructed in basic cardiac pulmonary resuscitation.

TABLE 12–14. Differential Diagnosis of Sudden Infant Death Syndrome

Fulminant infection*
Infant botulism†
Seizure disorder
Brain tumor*
Hypoglycemia†
Medium-chain acyl-coenzyme A dehydrogenase deficiency†
Carnitine deficiency*†
Urea cycle defect†
Child abuse*
Hemosiderosis/pulmonary hemorrhage syndrome
Exposure to toxic environmental fungus
Drug intoxication†
Cardiac arrhythmia
Gastroesophageal reflux*
Midgut volvulus/shock*
Laryngospasm

*Obvious or suspected at autopsy.
†Diagnostic test required.

## VOCAL CORD PARALYSIS

Vocal cord paralysis is an important cause of laryngeal dysfunction. Paralysis may be unilateral or bilateral and more often is due to damage of the recurrent laryngeal nerves than to a central lesion. The left recurrent laryngeal nerve passes around the arch of the aorta and thus is more susceptible to damage than the right laryngeal nerve. Trauma such as neck traction during delivery and lesions in the mediastinum are common causes of vocal cord paralysis. Central causes include the Arnold-Chiari malformation, hydrocephalus, intracranial hemorrhage, and dysgenesis of the nucleus ambiguus.

The symptoms of vocal cord paralysis include stridor, a weak cry (in infants), hoarseness, or aphonia. Unilateral paralysis may be relatively asymptomatic. Rarely, the cords are paralyzed in the abducted position, and aspiration results. Patients with such a condition, as well as those with bilateral abductor paralysis resulting in severe airway obstruction, may require tracheostomy. There is no specific treatment. However, patients with traumatic injury to the recurrent laryngeal nerve may have spontaneous improvement over time due, in part, to compensatory movement by the nonparalyzed cord.

The *prognosis* for return of vocal cord function depends on the nature of the injury and whether or not the recurrent laryngeal nerve has been disrupted.

### References

AAP Task Force on Infant Positioning and SIDS: Positioning and SIDS. Pediatrics 89:1120, 1992.

Behrman RE, Kliegman RM, Arvin AM (eds): Nelson Textbook of Pediatrics, 15th ed. Philadelphia, WB Saunders, 1996, Chapters 377, 378, 657.
Holton J, Allen J, Green C, et al: Inherited metabolic diseases in sudden infant death syndrome. Am J Dis Child 66:1315, 1991.
Strollo P, Rogers R: Obstructive sleep apnea. N Engl J Med 334:99, 1996.
Taylor JA, Krieger JW, Reay DT, et al: Prone sleep position and the sudden infant death syndrome in King County, Washington: A case-control study. J Pediatr 128:626, 1996.

# CARDIOVASCULAR DISORDERS

## PULMONARY HYPERTENSION/COR PULMONALE

Diffuse lung disease, upper airway obstruction (such as hypertrophied tonsils or adenoids), pulmonary thromboembolism, or exposure to high altitude may produce pulmonary hypertension. Pulmonary hypertension also may result from excessive pulmonary blood flow when there is a left-to-right cardiac shunt (see Chapter 13). With prolonged hypertension, resulting from either increased flow or hypoxic vasoconstriction, permanent changes occur in the intima and media of the pulmonary artery, making the increased vascular resistance irreversible. Primary pulmonary hypertension is idiopathic, occurs in the absence of parenchymal lung or cardiac disease, may be associated with autoimmune disease (SLE, scleroderma) or anorectic antiobesity drugs, and responds poorly to therapy.

Pulmonary hypertension resulting from *lung disease* leads to hypertrophy and eventually to dilation of the right ventricle, termed cor pulmonale. In advanced states, right heart failure may occur, with limitation of exercise capacity, hepatic congestion, fluid retention, and signs of tricuspid insufficiency. In severe disease, the ventricular septum may be displaced toward the left ventricle, reducing its volume and thus left ventricular function as well.

The most common causes of cor pulmonale in children are diffuse chronic lung diseases, such as CF and bronchopulmonary dysplasia. In these conditions, airway obstruction results in alveolar hypoxia, and parenchymal scarring may increase pulmonary vascular resistance.

The *diagnosis* of pulmonary hypertension should be suspected whenever there is prolonged hypoxemia or severe left-to-right shunting (see Chapter 13). In addition to the physical findings associated with pulmonary or cardiac disease, there may be an accentuated pulmonic component of the second heart sound heard in the left second interspace.

Definitive diagnosis is made by cardiac catheterization, but echocardiography may confirm the presence of significant right ventricular hypertrophy, ventricular dysfunction, and tricuspid insufficiency indicative of increased pulmonary artery pressure.

*Treatment* is directed at the underlying condition. Relief of hypoxemia is essential and usually requires supplemental oxygen therapy. Heart failure may necessitate diuretics and restriction of salt and fluid intake. Vasodilator therapy rarely is successful. Lung or heart-lung transplantation is the treatment for end-stage cor pulmonale.

The *prognosis* is poor once chronic cor pulmonale is present; if left ventricular failure is evident, the prognosis is even worse.

## PULMONARY EDEMA

*Pathophysiology.* At the alveolar-capillary interface, capillary hydrostatic forces and tissue osmotic pressures tend to push fluid into the air spaces, whereas plasma osmotic pressures and tissue mechanical forces tend to force fluid away from the air spaces. Under normal circumstances, the vectorial sum of these forces favors absorption so that the alveolar spaces remain dry. Any fluid entering the alveolus normally is removed by the pulmonary lymphatics. Pulmonary edema forms when transcapillary fluid flux exceeds lymphatic drainage. Reduced left ventricular function accompanied by pulmonary venous hypertension increases capillary hydrostatic pressure, which floods the interstitial spaces and alveoli with fluid, producing pulmonary edema. Fluid initially enters the interstitial space around the terminal bronchioles, alveoli, and arteries (**interstitial edema**), causing increased lung stiffness, premature closure of bronchioles on expiration, and dyspnea and tachypnea as a result of stimulation of lung receptors. If the process continues, fluid enters the alveolar space, reducing compliance and creating a perfused but unventilated area called a *shunt*. Shunting, not the presence of fluid in the alveoli, produces hypoxia.

Pulmonary hypertension as occurs in cor pulmonale rarely produces pulmonary edema, because the site of increased vascular resistance is proximal to the capillary bed. Pulmonary edema may be seen, however, when intrathoracic pressure becomes excessively negative (e.g., upper airway obstruction from hypertrophied tonsils). Pulmonary edema also may occur in patients (1) having decreased serum oncotic pressure, (2) receiving large volumes of intravenous fluid following capillary damage (smoke inhalation, hydrocarbon aspiration), with ascent to high altitude, and (3) having a history of central nervous system injury (neurogenic).

*Clinical Manifestations.* Pulmonary edema typically produces dyspnea, cough (often with frothy, pink-tinged sputum), tachypnea, signs of increased respiratory effort, and diffuse rales. Chest roentgenograms show a diffuse infiltrate that classically is in a perihilar pattern but may be obscured by underlying lung disease. Signs of interstitial edema (Kerley B lines) may be seen, especially at the lung bases.

*Treatment.* Treatment should include positioning the patient in an upright posture and administering oxygen but otherwise is directed toward relieving the underlying problem. Morphine may relieve dyspnea and, by dilating central veins, reduce venous return to the heart. Diuretic therapy (furosemide) and rapid-acting intravenous positive inotropic agents also are helpful. In severe cases, mask continuous positive airway pressure (CPAP) or intubation with positive end-expiratory pressure (PEEP) may be required.

The *prognosis* for patients with pulmonary edema depends on the nature of the underlying cause as well as on the response to therapy.

### Acute (Adult) Respiratory Distress Syndrome (ARDS)

ARDS is a noncardiogenic pulmonary edema that results from increases in the permeability of the alveolar-capillary interface, which allows the alveoli and interstitium to become flooded with transudate. In addition to pulmonary edema produced by classical mechanisms (see above), inflammatory mediators (vasoactive compounds, endotoxin, complement, cytokines, prostaglandins) may increase vascular permeability further and produce chemotactic factors that recruit inflammatory cells to the site of injury. Preformed and newly synthesized mediators (proteases, kinins, prostaglandins) and oxygen-free radicals cause further vascular and parenchymal damage, resulting in hypoxia and hypercapnia, which produce acute pulmonary hypertension. Therefore, ARDS becomes manifested as a composite condition of a pulmonary shunt, decreased pulmonary compliance, and pulmonary hypertension.

The *etiology* of ARDS is varied, but it often results from shock (especially septic shock), aspiration (of hydrocarbons), inhalation of toxic fumes (smoke, nitrogen dioxide, sulfur dioxide, ammonia, phosgene, chlorine gas), pancreatitis, or trauma (burns, near-drowning, head injury, fat emboli from fractures). ARDS also may be associated with pneumonia, pulmonary emboli, disseminated intravascular coagulation, drug overdose, uremia, and multiple transfusions. ARDS is one organ manifestation of **multiple organ dysfunction syndrome** (MODS), which is usually initiated by one of the above etiologic factors during the development of **systemic inflammatory response syndrome** (SIRS) (see Chapter 3).

Patients with ARDS experience severe hypoxemia and respiratory distress. Chest roentgenograms show diffuse alveolar infiltrates, although only interstitial edema may be seen in the early stages. Often, a period of hours to even days may elapse between the original insult and the development of overt respiratory failure.

*Treatment* consists of mechanical ventilation accompanied by the application of PEEP, oxygen, and therapy for the underlying problem. Surfactant and inhaled nitric oxide may also be of some benefit. The mortality rate in patients with ARDS ranges from 50–90%, reflecting the severity of the insult to the lungs and other organ systems that issues both from ARDS itself and from its underlying diseases.

## PULMONARY EMBOLISM

Pulmonary embolism is rare in childhood and may be associated with indwelling vascular catheters, oral contraceptives, lupus anticoagulant or other hypercoagulable states (see Chapter 14), trauma, abortion, or malignancy. Because the pulmonary vascular bed is very distensible, small emboli, even if multiple, usually are not detected unless they are infected, causing pulmonary infection. However, large emboli may result in acute dyspnea, pleuritic chest pain, cough, hemoptysis, and even death. Hypoxia is common, as are right-sided heart strain revealed on the electrocardiogram, an increased $P_2$ heart sound, and occasionally a wedge-shaped pulmonary infiltrate.

Ventilation-perfusion scans are useful in *diagnosis* by showing defects in perfusion without matching ventilation defects. For *definitive diagnosis*, however, a pulmonary angiogram is the procedure of choice.

*Treatment* of proven pulmonary embolism is supportive (oxygen administration) and also should be directed toward the predisposing factors. Heparin may be useful in preventing development of further emboli; thrombolytic therapy or surgery may be helpful in treating massive embolization.

## References

Behrman RE, Kliegman RM, Arvin AM (eds): Nelson Textbook of Pediatrics, 15th ed. Philadelphia, WB Saunders, 1996, Chapters 60.7, 355, 356.

Bernstein D, Coupey S, Schoenberg SK: Pulmonary embolism in adolescents. Am J Dis Child 140:667, 1986.
Macnaughton P, Evans T: Management of adult respiratory distress syndrome. Lancet 339:469, 1992.
Redding GJ: Pulmonary hypertension. *In* Loughlin GM, Eigen H (eds): Respiratory Disease in Children: Diagnosis and Management, Baltimore, Williams & Wilkins, 1994, p 639.
Sarniak AP, Lieh-Lai M: Adult respiratory distress syndrome in children. Pediatr Clin North Am 41:337, 1994.

## ASPIRATION SYNDROMES

Aspiration of material into the lungs is common in children and may be asymptomatic or fatal. When children with depressed levels of consciousness aspirate gastric contents from emesis, it may lead to severe pneumonia or to ARDS. The most common aspiration syndromes include:

1. Foreign body aspiration.
2. Aspiration associated with gastroesophageal reflux.
3. Near-drowning.

### FOREIGN BODY ASPIRATION

Aspiration of foreign bodies into the tracheobronchial tree is more common than usually is recognized. The majority of patients are younger than 4 yr of age, and most of the deaths also occur in this age group. Such children often put virtually anything into their mouths and frequently are out of sight of even the most diligent caretaker. Younger children most commonly aspirate food, balloons and small toys, or other small objects. Older children also may aspirate objects that they have held in their mouths.

*Clinical Manifestations.* A high percentage of children who aspirate foreign bodies present with either a clear-cut history of choking (or witnessed aspiration) or physical or roentgenographic evidence of the foreign body. However, a small percentage of patients with foreign body aspiration will have a negative history because of unobserved or unrecognized events. Physical findings consistent with acute foreign body aspiration include unilateral absence of breath sounds, localized wheezing, stridor, and bloody sputum. Roentgenographic studies may reveal the presence of a radiopaque object or evidence of air trapping on exhalation. When aspiration is suspected, expiratory chest films should be requested, although fluoroscopy may be more helpful.

Because the right main bronchus is a more direct continuation of the trachea than the left main bronchus, foreign bodies tend to enter the right lung preferentially. However, they also may be coughed out more readily from the right side, and, in many large reported series, nearly as many foreign bodies were found on the left as on the right. Some foreign bodies, especially nuts or seeds, may migrate from place to place in the airways and even lodge in the larynx on coughing, totally occluding the airway. Such migratory foreign bodies often are not associated with roentgenographic abnormalities and are difficult to detect.

Foreign bodies also may lodge in the esophagus and compress the trachea, producing respiratory symptoms. An esophageal foreign body should be included in the *differential diagnosis* of infants or young children with persistent stridor or wheezing, particularly if associated with dysphagia.

*Diagnosis.* Most foreign bodies are small and quickly coughed out, but many may remain in the lung for long periods before diagnosis and may come to medical attention because of symptoms of fever, cough, sputum production, or chest pain. Patients with persistent wheezing unresponsive to bronchodilator therapy, persistent atelectasis, recurrent or persistent pneumonia, or persistent cough without other explanation should be suspected of harboring a foreign body. If there is good evidence (in history, physical, or roentgenographic examination) for a bronchial foreign body, the patient should undergo rigid bronchoscopy. Flexible bronchoscopy may be a very useful diagnostic technique when the presentation is not straightforward.

*Prevention and Treatment.* The best approach to foreign body aspiration is to educate parents and caretakers in preventing the event. Before their molar teeth have developed, infants and children should not have nuts, uncooked carrots, and other foods that may be easily broken into small pieces and aspirated. Toys should be free of small parts that also may be aspirated.

## GASTROESOPHAGEAL REFLUX

See Chapter 11.

## NEAR-DROWNING

Near-drowning is a frequent emergency in children that may result in hypoxic organ damage and pulmonary dysfunction. In some cases, laryngospasm prevents the victim from aspirating water into the lungs, and the damage results from hypoxia alone. Usually, however, the victim aspirates water, which disturbs ventilation-perfusion relationships, causes loss of surfactant, and produces pulmonary edema.

The primary goal in *treatment* is to correct acidosis and hypoxia as rapidly as possible. In children, cardiac activity persists long after ventilation ceases, and the most urgent priority is to provide effective ventilation. Under most circumstances, water is absorbed from the lungs quickly, and ventilation should be initiated without delay and without attempting to clear water from the airways. Closed chest cardiac massage is employed, if necessary. Intubation and PEEP often are very helpful in reducing intrapulmonary shunting and improving oxygenation. Once effective ventilation is established, metabolic acidosis often corrects itself but judicious administration of bicarbonate may be necessary in the presence of profound acidosis.

*Cerebral edema* often results from the hypoxic insult and must be managed aggressively. Hyperventilation (to maintain $P_{CO_2}$ in the range of 25–28 torr), fluid restriction, osmotic diuresis, and even drainage of ventricular fluid through a ventriculostomy may be necessary to prevent cerebral ischemia as a result of intracranial hypertension.

The *prognosis* for victims of near-drowning is variable and depends chiefly on the degree of initial hypoxic insult. Children who regain consciousness after they are resuscitated have an excellent prognosis. Submersion for longer than 9 min and cardiopulmonary resuscitation for longer than 25 min in the prehospital setting are associated with a high mortality rate and severe neurologic impairment. Exceptions to this latter observation may occur, however, in persons who have nearly drowned in very cold water, because the cold temperature slows metabolism and limits hypoxic damage.

References

Behrman RE, Kliegman RM, Arvin AM (eds): Nelson Textbook of Pediatrics. 15th ed. Philadelphia, WB Saunders, 1996, Chapters 60.4, 333, 340.

Quan L, Wentz KR, Gore EJ, et al: Outcome and predictors of outcome in pediatric submersion victims receiving prehospital care in King County, Washington. Pediatrics 86:586, 1990.

Rimell F, Thome A, Stool S, et al: Characteristics of objects that cause choking in children. JAMA 274:1763, 1995.

## HEMOSIDEROSIS

Pulmonary hemosiderosis is characterized by the accumulation of hemosiderin in the lungs as a result of bleeding into the lungs. Red blood cells are phagocytosed by alveolar macrophages, and the hemoglobin is converted to hemosiderin; with the use of special iron-staining techniques, the hemosiderin within the alveolar macrophages can be identified microscopically. Hemosiderin-laden macrophages may be found in sputum, gastric aspirate, bronchoalveolar lavage fluid, or a lung biopsy.

*Etiology.* Hemosiderosis may result from bleeding anywhere in the lung, airway, pharynx, nasopharynx, or mouth, but it usually occurs as a result of diffuse alveolar bleeding, which may be of low grade and transient or brisk and massive.

*Clinical Manifestations.* The presentation is variable but often includes iron-deficiency anemia with a history of cough, tachypnea, and wheezing. Occasionally, acute, frank hemoptysis or hematemesis is seen. At the time of acute pulmonary bleeding, fever, leukocytosis, and an elevated erythrocyte sedimentation rate (ESR) may occur. Some cases are associated with eosinophilia. Chest roentgenograms usually show transient infiltrates, but massive infiltrates, atelectasis, and hyperinflation may occur. In the chronic stages, an interstitial pattern suggestive of interstitial fibrosis has been seen.

Many patients are incorrectly diagnosed as having bacterial pneumonia. Iron-deficiency anemia or guaiac-positive stools in a child with pneumonia (particularly if eosinophilia is present) suggests pulmonary hemosiderosis, and sputum, gastric aspirate, and/or bronchoalveolar lavage samples should be obtained to confirm the presence of hemosiderin-laden macrophages.

The *classification* of pulmonary hemosiderosis reflects the associated findings and presumed etiology of the alveolar hemorrhage. In the majority of pediatric cases, no etiology can be identified ("idiopathic pulmonary hemosiderosis"). Cases of pulmonary hemosiderosis associated with glomerular basement membrane disease (glomerulonephritis) may be subdivided into those with circulating antigen-antibody complexes and those with antibody deposited along the basement membrane of the kidney and/or lung (Goodpasture syndrome). These antigen-antibody complexes may be associated with a number of collagen vascular diseases or systemic vasculitis (**Henoch-Schönlein purpura, Wegener granulomatosis**); occasionally, lung involvement with collagen vascular diseases occurs without or prior to renal involvement. Many of these cases are positive for antineutrophil cytoplasm antibodies (ANCAs). Pulmonary hemosiderosis in infants also can be associated with precipitating serum antibodies to cow's milk (**Heiner syndrome**). These infants may exhibit wheezing, eosinophilia, high IgE levels, failure to thrive, and, less often, adenoidal hypertrophy with upper airway obstruction. The role of the milk sensitivity is unclear, but elimination of cow's milk from the diet often decreases the frequency and severity of the alveolar hemorrhage. Certain forms of **heart disease** associated with increased pulmonary venous and capillary pressures also may cause alveolar bleeding and pulmonary hemosiderosis. Acute fulminant pulmonary hemorrhage occurring largely in black male infants has been linked to exposure to the indoor toxin-producing mold, *Stachybotrys atra*, which grows in water-damaged homes.

*Treatment.* Management of the acute episodes of bleeding should include administration of oxygen, blood transfusions, intratracheal epinephrine, and, if necessary, mechanical ventilation accompanied by PEEP to tamponade the bleeding. Attempts should be made to identify the cause of the bleeding; often, an open lung biopsy is necessary (Table 12–15). Idiopathic pulmonary hemosiderosis may respond to corticosteroids. Other immunosuppressant agents, such as azathioprine and cyclophosphamide, have been used when the condition has not responded to the administration of corticosteroids over 2–3 mo. A trial period on a milk-free

TABLE 12–15. Differential Diagnosis of Hemoptysis–Pulmonary Hemorrhage

**Cardiovascular**
  Heart failure
  Eisenmenger syndrome
  Arteriovenous fistula (Osler-Weber-Rendu syndrome)
  Pulmonary embolism

**Pulmonary**
  Respiratory distress syndrome
  Bronchogenic cyst
  Sequestration
  Pneumonia (bacterial, mycobacterial, fungal, parasitic)
  Cystic fibrosis
  Tracheobronchitis
  Bronchiectasis
  Toxic fungus (*Stachybotrys atra*) exposure
  Abscess
  Tumor (adenoma, carcinoid, hemangioma, metastasis)
  Foreign body retention
  Contusion–trauma

**Immune**
  Henoch-Schönlein purpura
  Heiner syndrome
  Goodpasture syndrome
  Wegener granulomatosis
  Systemic lupus erythematosus
  Allergic bronchopulmonary aspergillosis

**Other**
  Hyperammonemia
  Kernicterus
  Intracranial hemorrhage (preterm infant)
  Toxins

diet may be useful, and removal of mold-infested home materials is advised.

*Prognosis.* The outlook depends on the underlying cause of the bleeding. In some children, the course of idiopathic hemosiderosis may be relentless whereas other children bleed only once. Repeated hemorrhage often results in chronic pulmonary fibrosis and respiratory insufficiency.

## RESPIRATORY FAILURE

Respiratory failure occurs when the lungs are unable to deliver sufficient oxygen to the blood to meet metabolic demands. It may develop insidiously or may have an abrupt onset. The *etiology* of respiratory failure is legion. Common causes in children include bronchopulmonary dysplasia, respiratory distress syndrome, ARDS, end-stage cystic fibrosis, neuromuscular disorders, and status asthmaticus. These disorders produce respiratory failure by impairing normal respiratory muscle function due to abnormal metabolic states, nutritional deficiencies, and/or disease of the pulmonary parenchyma, airways, chest wall, or respiratory muscles. The *clinical manifestations* usually include increased respiratory drive, leading to tachypnea, dyspnea, retractions, and the use of accessory muscles. Auscultatory findings vary with the etiology of the problem and may include diminished or absent breath sounds, wheezing or prolonged expiration, crackles and rhonchi, and grunting on exhalation. Because approximately 5 g/dL of circulating deoxygenated hemoglobin is normally required for cyanosis to be evident clinically, patients who are anemic may have seriously impaired oxygen transport without obvious cyanosis. Early in the course of the condition, tachycardia is common. Bradycardia is a late and especially ominous sign and usually is followed rapidly by hypotension and cardiac arrest. Hypoxemia may produce restlessness and irritability, which may progress to confusion, decreased levels of consciousness, seizures, and, eventually, coma. Hypercapnia results in cerebral vasodilation and often severe headache and, in later stages, profound depression of the central nervous system.

*Diagnosis.* The diagnosis of respiratory insufficiency and failure depends on careful observation of the patient, suspicion heightened by knowledge of the history and underlying clinical circumstances, and appropriate laboratory evaluation. The single most useful laboratory study is an arterial blood gas determination. However, when clinical evidence of respiratory insufficiency or failure is present, oxygen therapy should never be withheld while one is awaiting a blood gas study.

*Treatment.* Treatment of respiratory failure should be directed immediately to relieve hypoxemia and hypercapnia. In pediatric patients, it rarely is harmful to administer 100% oxygen for short periods of time, although the patient should be monitored carefully. Rarely, children with chronic respiratory insufficiency have blunted respiratory responses to hypercapnia and function chiefly on their hypoxic drive. In such instances, the administration of high concentrations of oxygen can result in paradoxical respiratory depression.

A careful and systematic search should be made for the underlying (and potentially reversible) causes of the respiratory failure, and appropriate treatment should be instituted. In the presence of refractory hypoxia and/or significant hypercapnia ($Paco_2 > 60$ mm Hg), institution of mechanical ventilation should be considered.

Patients in respiratory failure often are very unstable and must be monitored carefully. Only a few minutes separate apnea from cardiac arrest. In children, most cardiac arrests are the direct result of hypoxemia rather than of a primary cardiac abnormality. If respiratory failure cannot be reversed promptly by specific therapy (e.g., relief of pneumothorax or upper airway obstruction, treatment of bronchospasm), intubation and mechanical ventilation usually will be necessary. In end-stage disease, lung transplantation may be indicated.

*Prognosis.* The outcome for patients with respiratory failure depends almost entirely on the nature of the underlying cause of the failure and the rapidity and efficacy of the therapy initiated. In patients with acute disease, the prognosis should be good. However, in patients with chronic disease such as CF, respiratory failure portends an ominous prognosis, although most patients can survive several episodes if treated vigorously.

## References

Behrman RE, Kliegman RM, Arvin AM (eds): Nelson Textbook of Pediatrics, 15th ed. Philadelphia, WB Saunders, 1996, Chapters 356, 362.

Leatherman JW, Davies SF, Hoidal JR: Alveolar hemorrhage syndromes: Diffuse microvascular lung hemorrhage in immune and idiopathic disorders. Medicine 63:343, 1984.

Montana E, Etzel RA, Allan T, et al: Environmental risk factors associated with pediatric idiopathic pulmonary hemorrhage and hemosiderosis in a Cleveland community. Pediatrics 99(1 Suppl):E51–E58, January 1997.

Panitch H, Schidlow D: Pathogenesis and management of hemoptysis in children. Int Pediatr 4:241, 1989.

# Chapter 13

# THE CARDIOVASCULAR SYSTEM

Michael M. Brook*

Physiologic diagnosis and initial treatment of heart disease in children can usually be determined by careful history and physical examination. Echocardiography is used to determine the exact features of cardiac defects prior to surgery. Cardiac catheterization and angiography are used when specific physiologic or anatomic information is required or when therapeutic catheter interventions are indicated.

The origin of heart disease in children is a combination of genetic and environmental causes. Congenital heart disease may be either genetic (e.g., Down and velocardiofacial syndromes) or acquired (e.g., through maternal rubella) (Table 13–1). Acquired heart disease, such as rheumatic fever or atherosclerosis, may have genetic predispositions or may be due to systemic diseases that directly or indirectly affect the heart or vasculature (Table 13–2). Congenital heart disease is present in about 8 of every 1000 babies. It is slightly more common in premature infants and even more common in fetuses. About half of congenital heart defects are relatively insignificant, but half may result in infant death or disability. Defects such as small ventricular septal defects (VSDs) and bicuspid aortic valves cause little or no disability, but the associated murmurs or clicks may cause substantial parental concern.

Although clinical evaluation is helpful, and usually diagnostic, in *symptomatic infants*, many infants, even those with serious cardiac disease, can initially be asymptomatic in the immediate neonatal period. The same mechanism that results in fetuses with cardiac disease thriving can obscure manifestations in the infant, namely the patent

ductus arteriosus (PDA). For example, coarctation of the aorta often is missed because the pulses and leg blood pressures may be normal for the first day or so until the ductus arteriosus closes and completes the coarctation. Even lethal defects such as hypoplastic left heart syndrome may be inapparent at birth because of the palliative effects of the PDA. Tests performed at the primary level in the newborn nursery, such as electrocardiography and chest roentgenography, may be nonspecific. Results may be normal for the 1st wk or two of life. Many but not all serious congenital cardiac defects are associated with a lower than normal oxygen saturation. However, a normal oxygen saturation ($\geq95\%$), as determined by pulse oximetry, does not guarantee a normal heart. Stenotic valve lesions often have a normal oxygen saturation even if they are severe. Other physical signs, such as tachypnea, hyperpnea, and tachycardia, also are important. Because many nonpathologic heart murmurs are heard at birth, the physician must use good judgment in deciding which require further evaluation by a pediatric cardiologist. The absence of a heart murmur in a neonate is not evidence of the absence of congenital heart disease.

It is vital that the diagnosis of serious congenital cardiac defects be made as early as possible. Virtually every congenital cardiac defect can be treated at least by palliation. If the defect is unrecognized, death, permanent damage, or serious complications (such as stroke) may occur before medical or surgical palliation can be carried out. The physician caring for the infant in the newborn nursery must have a high index of suspicion regarding minor signs and symptoms. It is not the pediatrician's job to make the detailed anatomic or physiologic diagnosis but rather to suspect heart disease, perform initial rapid stabilization, and obtain consul-

---

*Some material in this chapter was originally written by Paul C. Gillette, M.D.

TABLE 13–1.  Congenital Malformation Syndromes Associated with Congenital Heart Disease

| Syndrome | Cardiac Features | Syndrome | Cardiac Features |
|---|---|---|---|
| Trisomy 21 (Down syndrome) | Endocardial cushion defect | Marfan syndrome | Dilated and dissecting aorta, aortic valve regurgitation, mitral valve prolapse |
| Trisomy 18 | VSD, ASD, PDA, PS | Williams syndrome | Supravalvular aortic stenosis, peripheral pulmonary stenosis |
| Trisomy 13 | VSD, ASD, PDA, dextrocardia | | |
| XO (Turner syndrome) | Coarctation of aorta, aortic stenosis | Infant of diabetic mother | Hypertrophic cardiomyopathy, VSD, conotruncal anomalies |
| CHARGE association (*c*oloboma, *h*eart, *a*tresia choanae, *r*etardation, *g*enital and *e*ar anomalies) | TOF, endocardial cushion defect, VSD, ASD | Holt-Oram syndrome | ASD, VSD |
| | | Asplenia syndrome | Complex cyanotic heart lesions, anomalous pulmonary venous return, dextrocardia, single ventricle, single AV valve |
| DiGeorge (velocardiofacial) syndrome | Aortic arch anomalies, conotruncal anomalies* | Polysplenia syndrome | Azygos continuation of inferior vena cava, pulmonary atresia, dextrocardia, single ventricle |
| VACTERL association† (*v*ertebral, *a*nal, *c*ardiac, *t*racheo*e*sophageal, *r*adial and/or renal, *l*imb anomalies) | VSD | | |
| | | Fetal alcohol syndrome | VSD, ASD |
| | | Ellis–van Creveld syndrome | Single atrium |
| Congenital rubella | PDA, peripheral pulmonic stenosis, mitral regurgitation (in infancy) | Zellweger syndrome | PDA, VSD, ASD |

*Conotruncal = TOF, pulmonary atresia, truncus arteriosus, transposition of great arteries.
†VACTERL association is also known as VATER (*v*ertebral, *a*nal, *t*racheoesophageal, *r*adial, *r*enal anomalies) association.
ASD = atrial septal defect; AV = atrioventricular; PDA = patent ductus arteriosus; PS = pulmonic stenosis; TOF = tetralogy of Fallot; VSD = ventricular septal defect.

tation of a pediatric cardiology team. The pediatric cardiologist then determines the physiologic diagnosis and uses echocardiography to make the exact anatomic diagnosis. Magnetic resonance imaging (MRI) and/or cardiac catheterization and angiography may be used to clear up details prior to surgical or catheter palliation or cure.

## DIAGNOSTIC EVALUATION

Congenital heart disease is the major cause of pediatric cardiovascular disease. The diagnostic evaluation of a child suspected of having congenital heart disease should proceed in an organized manner. The diagnosis of congenital heart disease is made accurately by the following:

1. Careful history.
2. Physical examination.
3. Electrocardiography.
4. Chest radiography.
5. Echocardiography and Doppler studies.
6. Cardiac catheterization.
7. Exercise testing.

## HISTORY

In obtaining a history, the examiner must take into account the age of the patient. For example, in the infant, congestive heart failure usually becomes manifest by feeding difficulties, easy fatigability, vomiting, lethargy, increased perspiration, and rapid respirations. Typically, the baby feeds poorly. In the older child, congestive heart failure causes easy fatigability and shortness of breath and dyspnea on exertion, which is usually best described in terms of specific activities such as walking on level ground, walking up steps, and bicycle riding. Orthopnea, paroxysmal nocturnal dyspnea, and edema are uncommon manifestations of heart failure in children. Congenital malformation syndromes (see Table 13–1) and systemic illnesses must be considered (see Table 13–2). The family history of previous congenital cardiac defects also is important.

## PHYSICAL EXAMINATION

A thoughtful, thorough, and careful cardiac examination may provide significant clues to the pres-

TABLE 13–2.   Cardiac Manifestations of
                      Systemic Diseases

| Systemic Disease | Cardiac Complications |
|---|---|
| Hunter-Hurler syndrome | Valvular insufficiency, heart failure, hypertension |
| Fabry disease | Mitral insufficiency, coronary artery disease with myocardial infarction |
| Pompe disease | Short PR interval, cardiomegaly, heart failure, arrhythmias |
| Friedreich ataxia | Myocardiopathy, arrhythmias |
| Duchenne dystrophy | Myocardiopathy, heart failure |
| Juvenile rheumatoid arthritis | Pericarditis |
| Systemic lupus erythematosus | Pericarditis, Libman-Sacks endocarditis; congenital AV block |
| Marfan syndrome | Aortic and mitral insufficiency; dissecting aortic aneurysm |
| Homocystinuria | Coronary thrombosis |
| Kawasaki disease | Coronary artery aneurysm, thrombosis, myocardial infarction, myocarditis |
| Lyme disease | Arrhythmias, myocarditis |
| Graves disease (hyperthyroidism) | Tachycardia, arrhythmias, heart failure |
| Tuberous sclerosis | Cardiac rhabdomyoma |

AV = atrioventricular.

ence of heart disease. The normal *heart rate* varies considerably according to age (Fig. 13–1). Tachycardia may be seen as a manifestation of heart failure or as a dysrhythmia. Bradycardia is seen as a normal finding in patients with high vagal tone, particularly athletes, but may be a manifestation of 2nd-degree or 3rd-degree atrioventricular (AV) block.

The *respiratory rate* in pediatric patients with heart disease may be increased secondary to increased lung stiffness resulting from increased lung water (decreased compliance) from a large left-to-right shunt, associated with pulmonary artery hypertension. Pulmonary venous congestion also may increase the rate. The patient's *height* and *weight* always should be assessed. Failure to thrive is frequently seen in infants with congestive heart failure and may be an important indication for surgery if medical management proves unsuccessful.

The *blood pressure* should be measured in the upper and lower extremities to identify coarctation

of the aorta. If the pressure in only one arm is measured, it should be the right arm because the coarctation may involve the left subclavian artery. The appropriate size cuff for the size of the arm should be used because a cuff that is too small (bladders that encircle less than 90% of the arm and cover less than 75% of the length) will give a blood pressure measurement that is higher than the true intravascular reading. Blood pressure may be measured by the auscultation, oscillometric (Dynamap), or Doppler method. The pulse pressure, determined by subtracting the diastolic pressure from the systolic pressure, normally is less than 50 mm Hg or half the systolic pressure, whichever is less. A wide pulse pressure, as assessed by palpation, usually is seen with aorticopulmonary connections (PDA, aorticopulmonary window, truncus arteriosus) or with aortic insufficiency, fever, anemia, arteriovenous malformations (AVMs), or complete AV block. A narrow pulse pressure is recognized in congestive heart failure, severe aortic stenosis, or pericardial tamponade.

The level of the *jugular vein venous pulsations* in the neck provides a rough assessment of the right atrial pressure. This sign is difficult to ascertain in infants and young children but may be very helpful in the school-aged or older child. The veins are observed with the child sitting or lying in a relaxed manner on an examining table raised to 30 degrees. Greatly increased venous distention then can be recognized because, normally, pulsations are not visible above the clavicle in the sitting position. In complete AV block, the venous pulsations are variable and depend on the position of the tricuspid valve at the time of atrial systole; if the right atrium contracts when the tricuspid valve is closed, a large venous pulsation (cannon wave) will occur.

The presence of *rales (crackles)* in the chest may be a sign of pulmonary edema resulting from increased pulmonary venous pressure; rales also may indicate infection. The absence of rales is a nonspecific sign because the patient in congestive heart failure may breath in a very shallow manner. *Hepatomegaly* is one of the cardinal signs of right-sided heart failure in the infant and child. The liver should be palpated lightly so as not to create a tense abdomen. *Splenomegaly* may be present in some children with long-standing congestive heart failure and may be seen in children with infective endocarditis.

*Cyanosis*, a bluish discoloration of the skin, nails, and mucous membranes, is apparent in infants and children with hypoxemia who have 3–5 g/dL of unsaturated hemoglobin. *Clubbing*, a rounding or convexity of the nails, may begin in infancy; it may become very prominent in hypoxemic adolescents

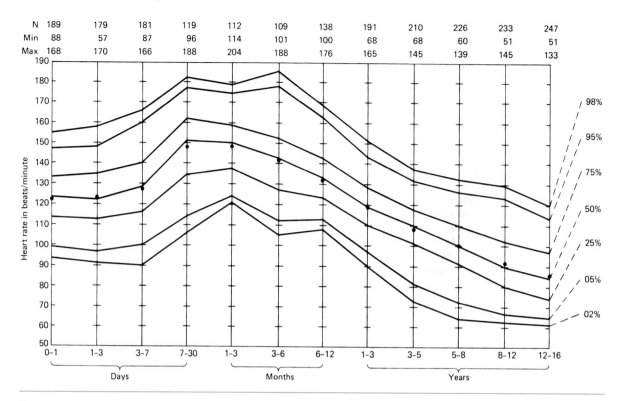

FIGURE 13–1.  Heart rate versus age (● = mean). (From Davignon A, Rautaharju P, Boiselle E: Normal ECG standards for heart rate of infants and children. Pediatr Cardiol 1:123, 1980.)

and young adults. *Edema of the lower extremities* is an uncommon characteristic of heart failure in infants but may be seen in the older child or adolescent.

On inspection, *prominence of the precordial chest wall* frequently is seen in infants and children with cardiomegaly and is especially prominent when the right ventricle is involved. A *hyperdynamic precordium* suggests a volume load, usually caused by a large left-to-right shunt or semilunar or AV valve regurgitation. A *thrill*, the palpable manifestation associated with a loud *murmur*, is felt where the accompanying murmur is loudest.

## AUSCULTATION

The art of auscultation can be improved by a careful, systematic approach, with the examination carried out in a quiet room without distractions. The infant should be examined in whatever position will quiet him or her, and the stethoscope bell should be used first to avoid the startle reaction. The examiner should listen first to the entire cardiac cycle, determining the 1st *heart sound* ($S_1$), systole, the second sound ($S_2$), and diastole. The examiner then should listen carefully for each and

every type of sound and *murmur* possible, concentrating so hard on the sound or murmur in question that nothing else is heard. This technique is called "dissection" and is done at each location over the precordium.

### Heart Sounds

The *1st heart sound*, caused by AV valve closure (Fig. 13–2), is best heard at the lower left sternal border or apex. It may be split, with the second component soft and best recognized at the lower left sternal border.

The *2nd heart sound*, produced by semilunar valve closure, is best heard at the 2nd intercostal space. During inspiration, filling of the right heart is increased and the right ventricular ejection time is increased, resulting in wider splitting of the aortic and pulmonic components of the 2nd heart sound in inspiration than in expiration. Widening of the splitting is seen with right ventricular volume overload, as occurs in an atrial septal defect (ASD) as well as in pulmonic stenosis or right bundle branch block. The pulmonary component of the 2nd heart sound is accentuated when the pulmonary artery pressure is increased, and it is

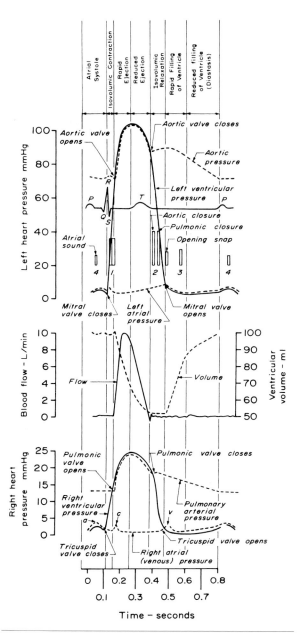

increased when the aortic valve, which is normally the louder component, is closer to the chest than normal. This occurs in transposition of the great arteries. In aortic stenosis, left ventricular systole may be prolonged enough to delay aortic valve closure, causing a narrow split, a single $S_2$, or even a paradoxic split. Advanced left bundle-branch block also may cause a paradoxic split.

The *3rd heart sound* (see Fig. 13–2) is best heard with the stethoscope bell at the apex of the heart one third into diastole, but a right ventricular 3rd heart sound is best heard at the lower left sternal border. A *4th heart sound* (see Fig. 13–2) just before the 1st heart sound, best heard at the 3rd or 4th interspace, may be a sign of poor ventricular compliance.

## Clicks

*Ejection clicks* are heard early in systole and are related to dilation of the ascending aorta or pulmonary artery. *Pulmonary ejection clicks* are heard best at the upper left sternal border and may occur as much as 0.08 sec after the 1st sound; they also may be much closer, even simultaneous with the first sound. They are louder on expiration and may disappear on inspiration. Because $S_1$ normally is soft at the upper left sternal border, an apparent $S_1$ that is loud at the upper left sternal border, especially on expiration, is a clue that the sound is a pulmonary ejection click, not $S_1$. Valvular pulmonic stenosis almost always is associated with a pulmonary ejection click, and pulmonary vascular disease frequently is associated with the condition.

*Aortic ejection clicks*, in contrast, usually are well separated from the 1st sound, do not vary in intensity with respiration, and usually are heard best at the apex (occasionally the lower left sternal border). They usually are associated with a bicuspid aortic valve, valvular aortic stenosis, truncus arteriosus, and tetralogy of Fallot with pulmonary atresia.

FIGURE 13–2. Idealized diagram of temporal events of a cardiac cycle. (From Behrman RE, Kliegman RM, Arvin AM (eds): Nelson Textbook of Pediatrics, 15th ed. Philadelphia, WB Saunders, 1996, p 1268.)

## Murmurs

Murmurs usually are described with regard to their intensity, timing, and pitch. The intensity of the heart sounds can be used as a reference guide for the loudness of a murmur:

A *grade 1* murmur is softer than the heart sounds and is difficult to hear.

A *grade 2* murmur is equal to the heart sounds, and a *grade 3* murmur is louder than the heart sounds. Grade 2 and 3 murmurs are easily heard but are not associated with a thrill.

decreased in intensity when low pulmonary artery diastolic pressure is present, as in pulmonary stenosis. The higher the pulmonary artery diastolic pressure, the earlier the closure of the pulmonic valve. Therefore, when pulmonary hypertension is present, the split is narrow or may be absent. It is obviously single in the presence of pulmonic or aortic valve atresia. The 2nd heart sound is also

A *grade 4* murmur is associated with a precordial thrill.

A *grade 5* murmur is heard with only the edge of the stethoscope on the chest.

A *grade 6* murmur is heard either with the stethoscope off the chest or with the naked ear.

It is important to relate the murmurs to $S_1$ and $S_2$ and to describe their length.

**Systolic ejection murmurs** (Fig. 13–3) typically are associated with obstruction to flow through abnormal semilunar valves or increased flow through normal semilunar valves. They begin after isovolemic contraction, about 0.08 sec after the 1st heart sound. **Holosystolic** or **regurgitant murmurs**, in contrast, typically are seen with a VSD with left-to-right shunt or mitral regurgitation. They begin during isovolumic contraction, obscuring the first heart sound. Ejection murmurs tend to have a crescendo and decrescendo (diamond) shape. Regurgitant murmurs may continue at the same intensity throughout systole, may be decrescendo, may peak late, or may even be of diamond shape. A late systolic murmur, usually crescendo, beginning after a mid-systolic non–ejection click, frequently is heard with mitral valve prolapse, indicating mitral regurgitation.

**Diastolic murmurs** (see Fig. 13–3) are heard when regurgitation occurs across the semilunar valves or when stenosis (real or relative owing to high flow) of the AV valves is present. The murmur of aortic regurgitation usually is very high pitched, decrescendo beginning with the 2nd heart sound, and located along the left sternal border. Pulmonary regurgitation can begin with the 2nd heart sound or may be slightly after it (particularly with right bundle branch block) but is usually of a lower pitch, unless pulmonary hypertension is present, in which case it sounds very much like aortic regurgitation. Stenotic murmurs across the AV valves usually are mid-diastolic and rumbling (very low pitch); the murmur of mitral stenosis occurs at the apex and that of tricuspid stenosis occurs along the lower left sternal border. Murmurs of relative stenosis with anatomically normal AV valves may be associated with an ASD or with high flow across either the tricuspid valve or the mitral valve; these murmurs occur in children with large left-to-right shunts at the level of either the ventricle or the great artery.

**Continuous murmurs** beginning after $S_1$ usually peak in intensity near the end of systole and decrease in intensity a variable time into diastole. This murmur is characteristic of a persistent PDA after the newborn period. The murmur is loudest under the left clavicle and frequently is very harsh and uneven in systole. Other causes of continuous murmurs include cerebral AV fistula, aorticopulmonary collateral vessels, and aorticopulmonary shunts. These latter continuous murmurs tend to be of similar pitch in both systole and diastole, and they have a higher pitch than that of the PDA murmur.

A variety of normal murmurs may be heard throughout childhood. The most common is the **vibratory systolic ejection murmur (Still murmur)**. This left lower sternal border ejection systolic murmur is heard most frequently in preschool-aged children but also can be heard in children near the age of puberty. The murmur rarely is louder than grade 2 or 3, usually lasts about two thirds the length of systole, is heard well in the neck, and rarely is heard in the back. It is believed to originate in the root of the aorta, where everyone of all ages has a normal ejection systolic murmur. Still murmur decreases with the Valsalva maneuver and is often less prominent or less vibratory when one is sitting or standing. Also, a systolic murmur in the root of the pulmonary artery is present, projected onto the chest as the most common normal murmur in adolescents and adults (the normal pulmonary ejection murmur). Another type of common benign murmur is the **venous hum** heard at the right upper or, less commonly, left upper sternal border with particular radiation into the neck. This continuous, medium-pitched murmur disappears when the patient is placed in a supine position, when the jugular vein is compressed, or when the patient looks sharply to the left.

Newborns rarely have any of the aforementioned normal murmurs. For reasons not completely clear, the **patent ductus arteriosus murmur**, present because the baby is premature and/or has a low $P_{O_2}$ from lung disease, often does not sound like that of the congenital patent ductus, which becomes manifest weeks later. The newborn's PDA murmur is usually a nondescript soft systolic murmur.

Another common normal murmur in newborns, often lasting 6 mo or more, is the **peripheral pulmonic stenosis murmur**; it is present because of a normal sharp angle between the main pulmonary artery and each branch. Characteristically, the murmurs are heard at the 1st or 2nd intercostal spaces, both left and right, with transmission to each axilla and to the back. Frequently, the murmurs are louder in the back than in the front. These two murmurs can be very difficult to distinguish from each other.

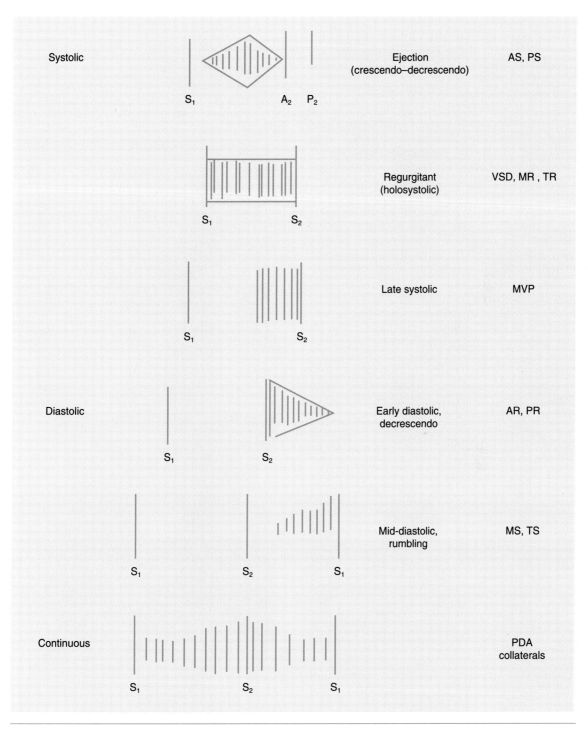

FIGURE 13–3. Types of murmurs. AR = aortic regurgitation; AS = aortic stenosis; MR = mitral regurgitation; MS = mitral stenosis; MVP = mitral valve prolapse; PDA = patent ductus arteriosus; PR = pulmonary regurgitation; PS = pulmonary stenosis; TR = tricuspid regurgitation; TS = tricuspid stenosis; VSD = ventricular septal defect.

## CHEST ROENTGENOGRAMS

The chest roentgenogram can provide a very good estimate of the shape and size of the heart and the size and position of the aorta and pulmonary artery (Fig. 13–4). Frequently, clues to specific cardiac anomalies also are present.

If the roentgenogram has been obtained during maximal inspiration, the cardiothoracic ratio should be less than 55% in infants under 1 yr and less than 50% in older children and adolescents. Interpretation of specific ventricular chamber enlargement is unreliable, but right atrial and left atrial enlargement frequently can be recognized.

Cardiac enlargement can be seen with any lesion that causes increased volume load to the heart or can be secondary to the presence of myocardial dysfunction. The normal large pulmonary arteries are seen in the central one third of the lung fields, with smaller vessels seen in the middle third and no pulmonary vessels seen in the lateral third of the lung fields. In the presence of a large left-to-right shunt (VSD, PDA, truncus arteriosus, or single ventricle without pulmonary stenosis), the increased pulmonary vasculature allows visualiza-tion of medium-sized vessels in the middle third and of small vessels, frequently end on, in the most lateral third of the lung fields. Conversely, congenital cardiac lesions that are associated with a *right-to-left shunt*, where blood destined for the pulmonary circulation is diverted into the systemic circulation, result in diminished pulmonary blood flow, which can be seen as a reduction in size of pulmonary arteries in the middle third of the lung fields.

Elevated pulmonary venous pressure secondary to left-sided congestive heart failure or obstructed pulmonary venous return, as occurs in newborns with total anomalous pulmonary venous connection, results in increased lung water. In the older child, this increase in lung water results in prominence of the pulmonary veins and redistribution of pulmonary flow so that the upper lobe pulmonary arteries are fuller than the lower lobe vessels. In the infant and neonate, however, these signs are absent and the usual pattern is a diffuse haziness or "fluffy" pattern, resulting from increased alveolar water.

Certain other signs on the chest roentgenogram may be helpful in the diagnosis of heart disease.

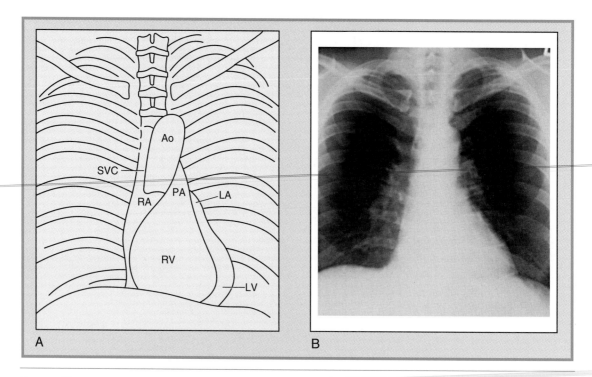

**FIGURE 13–4.** *A,* Schematic illustration of the parts of the heart whose outlines can be identified on a routine chest roentgenogram *(B).* Ao = Aorta; SVC = superior vena cava; RA = right atrium; PA = pulmonary artery; LA = left atrium; RV = right ventricle; LV = left ventricle. *B,* Routine posteroanterior roentgenogram of the normal cardiac silhouette. (From Andreoli TE, Carpenter CCJ, Plum F, et al: Cecil Essentials of Medicine, 2nd ed. Philadelphia, WB Saunders, 1990, p 23.)

For example, **rib notching**, an indentation on the underside of the ribs, may be seen in older children with coarctation of the aorta as a result of large and tortuous intercostal arteries or in children with tetralogy with pulmonary atresia when collateral vessels from the aorta to the intraparenchymal pulmonary arteries provide pulmonary blood flow.

Several "characteristic" roentgenographic patterns are associated with specific cardiac conditions. Severe *tetralogy of Fallot* is associated with the "boot-shaped" heart. The right ventricular hypertrophy causes the apex of the heart to be lifted from the diaphragm, causing the "toe," while the small main pulmonary artery results in a scooped-out left heart border (the "top" of the boot).

*Anomalous drainage of the pulmonary veins* without obstruction results in a "snowman" appearance. The upper circle (the "head") is caused on the left by the vertical vein draining the pulmonary veins and on the right by the enlarged superior vena cava. The lower circle (the "body") is produced by the enlarged heart. When the venous drainage is obstructed a very small heart with severe pulmonary venous congestion is usually present.

*d-Transposition of the great arteries* can be associated with an "egg-on-a-string" pattern. The string is the narrowed upper mediastinum, since the aorta and pulmonary artery are aligned on the posteroanterior projection. The egg is represented by the heart, with a left ventricular apex.

*Ebstein anomaly* of the tricuspid valve often shows a large cardiac shadow that fills the entire chest.

## ELECTROCARDIOGRAPHY

The standard 12-lead electrocardiogram (ECG) is a recording of the electrical activity from cardiac muscle cells onto each lead on the surface of the torso. The ECG is a useful screening test when used along with the chest roentgenogram and a careful physical examination. The ECG also provides insight into the metabolic state of the cardiac cell (e.g., hyperkalemia). Two children with serum potassium levels of 7.0 mEq/L may have different ECGs. One may be normal while the other may have tall peaked T waves, indicating a significant problem. The serum potassium level reflects only what is in the serum. The ECG reflects the state of the cell membrane and may be reflecting both intracellular and extracellular potassium, thus identifying the child in difficulty.

Analysis of the ECG includes the rate, rhythm, P wave, PR interval, QRS complex, QT interval, and ST segment (Fig. 13–5).

### P Wave

The P wave represents atrial depolarization (see Figs. 13–2 and 13–5). The first part of the P wave is due to right atrial depolarization. The best criterion for right atrial enlargement is an increase of the amplitude of the P wave, as is reflected best in lead II. The diagnosis of left atrial enlargement is best made by prolongation of the second portion of the P wave, as usually is exhibited best in the left chest leads.

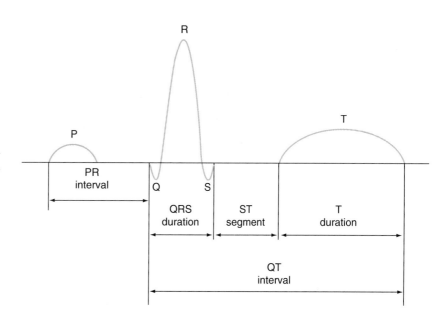

FIGURE 13–5. Nomenclature of electrocardiogram waves and intervals.

### PR Interval

The PR interval is measured from the beginning of the P wave to the beginning of the QRS complex and represents the time it takes for electricity to travel from the high right atrium to the ventricular myocardium (see Figs. 13–2 and 13–5). The greatest time is spent in the AV node. The PR interval increases with age. The conduction time is shortened when conduction velocity is increased, as in glycogen storage disease, or when the AV node is bypassed, as in the Wolff-Parkinson-White syndrome. A prolonged PR interval usually indicates prolonged conduction through the AV node, but disease in the atrial myocardium, bundle of His, or Purkinje system could contribute to this abnormality.

### QRS Complex

The QRS complex represents ventricular depolarization. Unlike the atrium, right and left ventricular activation begins virtually simultaneously in the right and left septa, halfway to two thirds down, as well as in the contiguous left ventricular free wall and right ventricular endocardium. In order to interpret the ventricular ECG properly, it is necessary to understand a number of major concepts:

1. A sequence of activation is present, so that what is being depolarized (and when) must be known.
2. A greater volume of the ventricle causes greater magnitude, as does a greater mass of right or left ventricular muscle.
3. Proximity of the right ventricular wall to the chest surface accentuates that ventricle's contribution.
4. Continued changes occur in the normal ECG with time, beginning with that of the premature or full-term infant and continuing throughout childhood. The spatial magnitudes are very low in the premature infant, become higher in the full-term infant, rise sharply until age 2–3 mo, stabilize until puberty, and then decrease throughout life.
5. Normative data for each age group must be known to make diagnoses.

In the fetus and full-term newborn, the right and left ventricular masses are approximately equal, although the right ventricle may be up to one third thicker. In the premature infant compared with the full-term infant, less right ventricular dominance is exhibited. By the age of 3–6 mo, the left ventricular mass is about twice that of the right ventricle, and when the child reaches school age, the ratio is similar to that of the adult, about 2.5:1 in favor of the left ventricle.

### QT Interval

The QT interval is measured from the beginning of the QRS complex to the end of the T wave (see Fig. 13–5). The corrected QT interval (corrected for rate) should be less than 0.45 sec. It may be prolonged in children with hypocalcemia or hypokalemia (although the latter may be a *QU interval*). It also is prolonged in a group of children at risk for severe ventricular arrhythmias and sudden death (i.e., the prolonged QT syndrome); drugs such as quinidine also may prolong the QT interval.

## ECHOCARDIOGRAPHY AND DOPPLER ULTRASONOGRAPHY

Echocardiography, especially with Doppler and color flow ultrasonography, is the most important noninvasive tool for the evaluation of congenital and acquired heart disease. Many children undergo corrective surgery solely on the basis of echocardiographic assessment of anatomy. The two-dimensional echocardiogram allows visualization of spatial relationships of the cardiac structures in the beating heart. Anatomic details previously requiring angiography are now easily visualized noninvasively, with little or no risk to the patient. Analysis of valve structure and function often is superior to that obtained by angiogram. Ventricular function and cardiac output can also be calculated.

Doppler echocardiography is an adaptation of ultrasound that displays flow in cardiac chambers and vascular structures. The change in frequency imparted to sound waves caused by moving blood can be used to calculate cardiac output, valve and orifice pressure gradients, and directionality of flow within structures. Color flow Doppler encodes the flow direction and velocity in color on the two-dimensional image, allowing easy detection of small septal defects and valve regurgitation. Fetal echocardiography may delineate normal and abnormal function and structure prior to birth.

## CARDIAC CATHETERIZATION AND ANGIOGRAPHY

Catheterization is now reserved for children in whom echocardiography is unclear or unable to provide the specific anatomic information. Children with complicated pulmonary artery anatomy or in whom precise physiologic information (e.g., the magnitude of shunting or the pulmonary artery pressure) is needed, require diagnostic catheterization. Postoperative patients, particularly those doing poorly, may require catheterization for complete determination of the anatomy and physiology. A growing percentage of cardiac catheterizations are performed for therapeutic purposes (thus reducing the need for surgery), such as balloon catheter dilatation of stenotic semilunar valves or pulmonary arteries, and closure of PDAs, ASDs and aorticopulmonary collateral vessels.

Access to the vascular system is usually by percutaneous femoral vein catheterization, with the right-sided chambers entered sequentially. The presence of a patent foramen ovale, especially in infants, frequently allows entrance to the left side of the heart. The left side of heart also can be entered by a transeptal technique or via retrograde arterial catheterization.

Catheterization data include evaluation of the course of the catheter compared with normal, analysis of the oxygen saturation, analysis of the pressures in cardiac structures and blood vessels, various calculations derived from the aforementioned data, and the findings on cineangiography. The normal values are shown in Figure 13–6. The oxygen saturation of the entire right side of the heart reflects the mixed venous saturation and is normally 70–75%; a significant increase in oxygen saturation in a chamber or vessel on the right side indicates a *left-to-right shunt*. The left side of the heart should have a saturation of above 95%; significant decreases below the pulmonary veins suggest the presence of a *right-to-left shunt* resulting from systemic venous blood entering the left side of the heart. A decreased pulmonary venous saturation may be due to hypoventilation, pulmonary disease, or pulmonary venous congestion.

The pressures should be measured in all chambers and vessels entered. Normally, the systolic pressure in the ventricle is equal to the systolic pressure in the great arteries, and the end-diastolic pressure in the atria is equal to the end-diastolic pressure in the ventricle. If a "gradient" in pressure exists, it

FIGURE 13–6. Normal data from cardiac catheterization.

suggests obstruction across the valve. Analysis of the severity of the obstruction requires measurement of both the pressure gradient and the flow across that valve.

Systemic and pulmonary outputs can be measured by the Fick equation, with the cardiac output being equal to the measured oxygen consumption divided by the arteriovenous oxygen content differences between the systemic and pulmonary circulations. The pulmonary-to-systemic flow ratio can be measured by the ratio between the pulmonary and systemic arteriovenous differences, because the same oxygen consumption is in the numerator for both calculations.

Evaluation of the anatomy and physiology of the patient rarely is complete without selective angiocardiograms using a biplane system. Contrast material (~1 mL/kg) is injected rapidly into the cardiac chambers or vessels.

### Exercise Testing

Evaluation of the cardiovascular system normally is done at rest. However, information on cardiac reserve and the adaptation of the normal or abnormal heart to exercise can provide important data on the cardiac status that more closely approximates everyday living.

### References

Behrman RE, Kliegman RM, Arvin AM (eds): Nelson Textbook of Pediatrics, 15th ed. Philadelphia, WB Saunders, 1996, Chapters 380, 381.

Braden DS, Strong WF: Cardiovascular responses to exercise in children. Am J Dis Child 144:1255, 1990.

Brook MM, Silverman NH, Villegas M: Cardiac ultrasound in structural abnormalities and arrhythmias: Recognition and treatment. West J Med 159:286, 1993.

Davignon A, Rautaharju P, Boisselle E, et al: Normal ECG standards for infants and children. Pediatr Cardiol 1:123, 1979/80.

Hansen L, Birkeback N, Oxhøj H: Initial evaluation of children with heart murmurs by the nonspecialist paediatrician. Eur J Pediatr 154:15, 1995.

Higgins CB, et al: Magnetic resonance imaging in patients with congenital heart disease. Circulation 70:851, 1984.

Liebman J: Diagnosis and management of heart murmurs in children. Pediatr Rev 3:321, 1982.

Rosenthal A: How to distinguish between innocent and pathologic murmurs in childhood. Pediatr Clin North Am 31:1229, 1984.

Stümpflen I, Stümpflen A, Wimmer M, et al: Effect of detailed fetal echocardiography as part of routine prenatal ultrasonographic screening on detection of congenital heart disease. Lancet 348:854, 1996.

Wiles HB: Imaging congenital heart disease. Pediatr Clin North Am 37:115, 1990.

## PRENATAL AND NEONATAL CIRCULATION

See Chapter 6.

## MYOCARDIAL FUNCTION AND HEART FAILURE

Myofibril contraction is summated and translated into cardiac work or pump performance. The force generated by the muscle fiber depends on its contractile status and its basal length, which is equivalent to the preload, as noted in the normal Starling curve of Figure 13–7. As the preload (fiber length, left ventricular filling pressure or volume) increases, the myocardial performance (stroke volume, wall tension) increases up to a point. The relationship is the ventricular function curve; alterations in the contractile state of the muscle lower the relative position of the curve but retain the relationship of fiber length to muscle work. Heart rate is another important determinant of cardiac work because the cardiac output equals stroke volume times the heart rate. Additional factors that affect cardiac performance are noted in Table 13–3.

Heart failure results when the cardiac output does not meet the metabolic needs (in terms of oxygen delivery and other factors) of the body. The term "congestive" heart failure refers to increased venous pressure in the pulmonary (left heart failure) or the systemic (right heart failure) veins. Myofibrillar failure is the result of a decline of the myofibril contractility, as noted by a shift of the normal Starling curve (see Fig. 13–7). The compensatory mechanisms used to improve cardiac output include augmented endogenous sympathetic activity (increases inotropy, chronotropy) and the response of the kidney to a perceived reduction of effective plasma volume, leading to salt and water retention. These compensatory mechanisms have beneficial and adverse effects (Table 13–4).

The *etiology* of heart failure is different in various stages of development (Table 13–5). Fetal causes of heart failure include arrhythmias (supraventricular tachycardia, heart block) or severe anemia secondary to hemolysis or blood loss. In the neonate, congenital heart disease, AVMs, cardiomyopathy, and myocarditis are common causes of heart failure; in the older child, myocarditis, acute hypertension (glomerulonephritis, hemolytic-uremic syndrome), and rheumatic fever are important causes of heart failure.

The *treatment* of heart failure is directed toward improving myocardial contractility, preload, and reducing afterload (Table 13–6 and Fig. 13–7).

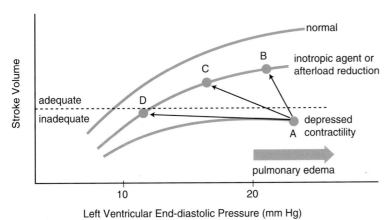

FIGURE 13–7. Ventricular function curve illustrating the effect of inotropic agents or arterial vasodilators. Unlike diuretics, the effect of digitalis or arterial vasodilator therapy in a patient with heart failure is to move onto another ventricular function curve intermediate between the normal and depressed curves. When the patient's ventricular function moves from A to B by the administration of one of these agents, the left ventricular end-diastolic pressure also may decrease because of improved cardiac function; further administration of diuretics or venodilators may shift the function further to the left along the same curve from B to C and eliminate the risk of pulmonary edema. A vasodilating agent that has both arteriolar and venous dilating properties (e.g., nitroprusside) would shift this function directly from A to C. If this agent shifts the function from A to D because of excessive venodilation or administration of diuretics, the cardiac output may fall too low, even though the left ventricular end-diastolic pressure would be normal (10 mm Hg) for a normal heart. Thus, left ventricular end-diastolic pressures of between 15 and 18 mm Hg are usually optimal in the failing heart to maximize cardiac output but to avoid pulmonary edema. (From Andreoli TE, Bennett JC, Carpenter CCJ, Plum F: Cecil Essentials of Medicine, 4th ed. Philadelphia, WB Saunders, 1997, p 34.)

TABLE 13–3. Factors Affecting Cardiac Performance

| **Preload** (left ventricular diastolic volume) | Total blood volume<br>Venous tone (sympathetic tone)<br>Body position<br>Intrathoracic and intrapericardial pressure<br>Atrial contraction<br>Pumping action of skeletal muscle | **Contractility** (cardiac performance independent of preload or afterload) | Sympathetic nerve impulses<br>Circulating catecholamines<br>Digitalis, calcium, other inotropic agents<br>Increased heart rate or postextrasystolic augmentation | } increased contractility |
|---|---|---|---|---|
| | | | Anoxia, acidosis<br>Pharmacologic depression<br>Loss of myocardium<br>Intrinsic depression | } decreased contractility |
| **Afterload** (impedance against which the left ventricle must eject blood) | Peripheral vascular resistance<br>Left ventricular volume (preload, wall tension)<br>Physical characteristics of the arterial tree (for example, elasticity of vessels or presence of outflow obstruction) | **Heart Rate** | Autonomic nervous system<br>Temperature, metabolic rate | |

From Andreoli TE, Bennett JC, Carpenter CCJ, Plum F: Cecil Essentials of Medicine, 4th ed. Philadelphia, WB Saunders, 1997.

TABLE 13–4.    Compensatory Mechanisms in Heart Failure

| Mechanism | Favorable Effects | Unfavorable Effects |
|---|---|---|
| ↑ Sympathetic activity | ↑ Heart rate<br>↑ Contractility<br>↑ Venoconstriction →<br>    ↑ venous return (preload) | ↑ Arteriolar constriction → ↑ afterload<br>↑ $O_2$ requirements |
| Cardiac hypertrophy | ↑ Working muscle mass | ↑ Wall tension<br>↓ Coronary flow<br>↑ $O_2$ requirements<br>Abnormal systolic and diastolic properties of<br>    hypertrophic muscle |
| Frank-Starling mechanism | ↑ Stroke volume for any given amount of<br>venous return | Pulmonary and systemic congestion:<br>    ↑ LV size → ↑ wall tension and $O_2$<br>    requirements |
| Renal salt and water retention | ↑ Venous return | Pulmonary and systemic congestion:<br>    ↑ renin–angiotensin →<br>    ↑ vasoconstriction (afterload) |
| Increased peripheral $O_2$ extraction | ↑ $O_2$ delivery per unit cardiac output | |

From Andreoli TE, Carpenter CCJ, Plum F: Cecil Essentials of Medicine. Philadelphia, WB Saunders, p 34.
LV = left ventricle.

TABLE 13–5.    Etiology of Heart Failure

**Fetus**

Severe anemia (hemolysis, fetal-maternal transfusion, hypoplastic
    anemia)
Supraventricular tachycardia
Ventricular tachycardia
Complete heart block
Congenital cardiac defects
High-output cardiac failure (arteriovenous malformation,
    teratoma)

**Premature Neonate**

Fluid overload
PDA
VSD
Cor pulmonale (BPD)

**Full-Term Neonate**

Asphyxial cardiomyopathy
Arteriovenous malformation (vein of Galen, hepatic)
Left-sided obstructive lesions (coarctation of aorta, hypoplastic left
    heart)
Transposition of great arteries
Large mixing cardiac defects (single ventricle, truncus arteriosus)
Viral myocarditis

**Infant–Toddler**

Left-to-right cardiac shunts (VSD)
Hemangioma (arteriovenous malformation)
Anomalous left coronary artery
Metabolic cardiomyopathy
Acute hypertension (hemolytic–uremic syndrome)
Supraventricular tachycardia
Kawasaki disease
Postoperative repair of congenital heart disease

**Child–Adolescent**

Rheumatic fever
Acute hypertension (glomerulonephritis)
Viral myocarditis
Thyrotoxicosis
Hemochromatosis–hemosiderosis
Cancer therapy (radiation, Adriamycin)
Sickle cell anemia
Endocarditis
Cor pulmonale (cystic fibrosis)
Arrhythmias
Chronic upper airway obstruction (cor pulmonale)
Unrepaired or palliated congenital heart disease
Cardiomyopathy

BPD = bronchopulmonary dysplasia; PDA = patent ductus arteriosus; VSD = ventricular septal defect.

TABLE 13–6.  Treatment of Heart Failure

| Therapy | Mechanism | Therapy | Mechanism |
|---|---|---|---|
| *General Care* | | *Inotropic Agents* Continued | |
| Rest | Reduces cardiac output | Dobutamine | Beta ($\beta_1$)-receptor agent; often combined with dopamine |
| Oxygen | Improves oxygenation in presence of pulmonary edema | Amrinone | Nonsympathomimetic, noncardiac glycosides with inotropic effects; also may produce vasodilation |
| Sodium, fluid restrictions | Decreases vascular congestion; decreases preload | | |
| *Diuretics* | | *Afterload reduction* | |
| Furosemide | Salt excretion by ascending loop of Henle; reduces preload; afterload reduced if hypertension improves; also may cause venodilation | Hydralazine | Arteriolar vasodilator |
| | | Nitroprusside | Arterial and venous relaxation; venodilation reduces preload |
| Combination of distal tubule and loop diuretics | Greater sodium excretion | Prazosin | Oral alpha-adrenergic blocking agent; arterial and venous dilator; venodilation reduces preload |
| | | Captopril/enalapril | Inhibition of angiotensin-coverting enzyme; reduces angiotensin II production |
| *Inotropic Agents* | | *Other* | |
| Digitalis | Inhibits membrane $Na^+$, $K^+$-ATPase and increases intracellular $Ca^{2+}$, improves cardiac contractility, increases myocardial oxygen consumption | Mechanical counterpulsation | Improves coronary flow, afterload |
| | | Transplantation | Remove diseased heart |
| Dopamine | Releases myocardial norepinephrine plus direct effect on beta receptor, may increase systemic blood pressure; at low infusion rates, dilates renal artery, facilitating diuresis | Extracorporeal membrane oxygenation (ECMO) | Bypasses heart |
| | | Partial left ventriculectomy ± mitral valve repair | Improves Laplace relationship by less wall tension |

## References

Behrman RE, Kliegman RM, Arvin AM (eds): Nelson Textbook of Pediatrics, 15th ed. Philadelphia, WB Saunders, 1996, Chapter 399.

Cohn J: The management of chronic heart failure. N Engl J Med 335:490, 1996.

Goldenberg I, Cohn J: New inotropic drugs for heart failure. JAMA 258:493, 1987.

Park M: Use of digoxin in infants and children with specific emphasis on dosage. J Pediatr 108:871, 1986.

Schneeweiss A: Cardiovascular drugs in children: Angiotensin-converting enzyme inhibitors. Pediatr Cardiol 9:109, 1989.

# CONGENITAL HEART DISEASE

## EPIDEMIOLOGY

Congenital heart disease affects 8:1000 births. If congenital dysrhythmias (such as Wolff-Parkinson-White syndrome) are included, the ratio would be 1:100. Most of these lesions occur between 18 and 50 days of gestation. At birth, VSD is the most common lesion, followed in order of decreasing frequency by PDA, tetralogy of Fallot, ASD, coarctation of the aorta, transposition of the great arteries, atrioventricular canal defects (endocardial cushion), and heterotaxias (right and left isomerism). The remaining individual lesions each represent 1–4% of congenital heart defects. Most affected neonates are full-term, appropriate-sized infants of normal pregnancies.

Approximately 30% of infants with heart lesions have extracardiac malformations that also affect their morbidity and mortality (see Table 13–1). Most cases of congenital heart disease (90%) are not associated with identifiable teratogens or single-gene defects. A small number are associated with a teratogen, such as congenital rubella or fetal alcohol syndrome, whereas others may be associated with gross chromosomal disorders (chromosomal deletions, trisomy), congenital anomaly syndromes (VATER, CHARGE), or maternal metabolic disorders (phenylketonuria, diabetes).

The *inheritance* in most patients is multifactorial (polygenetic). The recurrence risk for congenital heart disease in the sibling of an affected infant varies from 2–4%. The risk is greater for the child of a parent with congenital heart disease; in this case, the risk increases to 4–5%.

## HEART DISEASE RESULTING FROM ABNORMAL EMBRYONIC DEVELOPMENT

The heart begins to develop in the very early embryo and circulates blood by the 3rd wk. The initial heart is a straight tube without valves. Because the heart tube grows faster than the organs around it, it loops. Abnormal looping results in abnormal cardiac position, such as dextrocardia, or other anomalies, such as congenitally corrected transposition. When a major abnormality occurs, such as looping in the wrong direction, usually, but not always, one or several smaller abnormalities occur, such as a VSD.

As the heart divides itself into four chambers and as valves develop, many other abnormalities may occur. Sometimes there is a single defect (*d*-transposition of the great arteries) and sometimes there are multiple defects (tetralogy of Fallot). Even a single defect such as transposition can be devastating after birth while having little or no effect antenatally. Conversely, some defects cause fetal death. In addition, one defect can cause another defect by altering blood flow in the fetus. Many fetuses with severe and complex congenital cardiac defects die before birth.

Fetal cardiac diseases also may be iatrogenic. For example, maternal treatment to prevent premature labor may prematurely close the ductus arteriosus, resulting in right ventricular failure. Premature closure of the foramen ovale also can lead to the hypoplastic left heart syndrome.

### Abnormal Development of Venous and Arterial Systems

The development of the venous and arterial systems in the fetus is as complex or perhaps more so than that of the cardiac chambers themselves. The single mature aorta and aortic arch develop from multiple paired aortic arches. Abnormalities in their development, such as a complete interruption of the aorta, may occur at any one of a number of sites. The fact that genetics play a great role in development is underscored by the marked difference in the incidence and site of aortic arch interruption in patients of Chinese or Japanese ancestry versus Caucasians or Filipinos. The influence of fetal hemodynamics on the development of congenital cardiovascular defects is shown by the fact that coarctation of the aorta and interruption of the aortic arch are associated with "upstream lesions" such as aortic or mitral stenosis and certain VSDs that cause less aortic blood flow.

An understanding of *fetal blood flow* is critical to an understanding of fetal and neonatal physiology and the development of congenital cardiovascular defects. The fetus is dependent on placental blood flow. The fetus receives oxygenated, nutrient-loaded blood by way of the umbilical vein. This blood joins with the inferior cava blood and hepatic venous blood to enter the right atrium. It is preferentially but not exclusively shunted across the foramen ovale to the left atrium, the left ventricle, and out the aorta to the upper body and brain. The superior vena cava blood is preferentially but not exclusively directed to the right ventricle, the pulmonary artery, and through the ductus arteriosus to the lower half of the body and the umbilical arteries to the placenta. Only a small amount of blood perfuses the lungs during fetal life. The patent foramen ovale and ductus arteriosus cause the ventricles to work in parallel rather than in series, as they do after birth.

Fetal cardiovascular physiology explains why certain devastating defects, such as transposition of the great arteries, have no effect on the fetus. A similar quantity of blood with a similar oxygen concentration will reach the same organs at the same pressure, no matter which chambers and vessels it passes through. Children with transposition of the great arteries are often large for gestational age. This is partly because the left ventricle, with higher blood glucose, supplies the misplaced pulmonary artery and thus the lower body. The insulin produced in response acts as a growth factor for the infant. Subvalvar or valvar aortic stenosis, particularly in association with a VSD, results in decreased flow through the aortic arch, impairing arch growth and increasing the incidence of coarctation. An anomalous left coronary artery from the pulmonary artery will have the same pressure and a similar oxygen concentration in utero but a markedly lower pressure and lower oxygen saturation shortly after birth. In this situation, the fetal heart does not infarct but the neonatal or infant heart usually does. One congenital heart defect also can protect the neonate from the effects of another. In the infant with a large VSD as well as an anomalous left coronary artery, the increased pressure and oxygen content in the pulmonary artery resulting from the VSD perfuses the myocardium with high-pressure oxygenated blood. If the pulmonary artery resistance drops, or if the VSD spontaneously closes or is closed surgically, the coronary artery perfusion pressure drops and an infarct results.

*At birth and shortly afterward, major changes in the circulation occur.* The manifestation of congenital cardiovascular defects and their timing are dependent on these changes. The umbilical venous and arterial flows are obliterated immediately at birth. The pulmonary blood flow must increase immediately and support the entire organism. It is aided in doing this by the expansion of the lungs, which greatly reduces resistance to pulmonary blood flow. Systemic vascular resistance increases as a result of loss of the low-resistance placental circuit.

Sometimes, because of lung problems such as meconium aspiration, the pulmonary vascular resistance does not decrease. The fetal circulatory pathways may persist in part. Right-to-left shunting may continue to occur at the ductus arteriosus and/or foramen ovale level, resulting in extreme cyanosis. Persistent increase in pulmonary vascular resistance may severely compromise infants with congenital cardiac defects as well. Children with anatomic defects that usually would allow a left-to-right shunt will have a large right-to-left shunt. Children with an anatomically tenuous pulmonary blood flow may have an even further diminished flow. Early aggressive management of this physiology may reverse it or prevent its progression (see Chapter 6).

### Abnormal Positions of the Heart

The location of the heart within the chest may be quite abnormal and the relationships of the chambers may be very confusing. A systematic classification (by Van Praagh) simplifies analysis. In this classification, the heart may be in the right chest (*dextrocardia*) or in the left chest (*levocardia*).

The cardiac chambers are described in terms of their relationship to each other. The atrium may be *solitus*, with the right atrium to the right of the left atrium; *inversus*, with the anatomic right atrium to the left of the anatomic left atrium; or *ambiguous*, when abnormalities of systemic and pulmonary venous return make identification of the two atrial chambers impossible. The ventricles may be in their normal position (*d*) with the right ventricle to the right of the left ventricle, or they may be positioned with the anatomic right ventricle to the left of the anatomic left ventricle (*l*). The great arteries may be normally related, with the pulmonary artery anterior to and to the left of the aorta; *d*-transposed, with the aorta anterior to but still to the right of the pulmonary artery; or *l*-transposed,

if the aorta is anterior to and to the left of the pulmonary artery.

## CLASSIFICATION OF CONGENITAL CARDIAC DEFECTS

Congenital cardiac defects can be classified into four groups based on their physiology (Table 13–7). This classification is an oversimplification and many variations occur. The severity of each lesion is extremely variable. The timing and nature of a patient's clinical presentation are controlled by the physiology of the lesions. In each case, however, there are modifiers. An example is the size of the foramen ovale in complete *d*-transposition of the great arteries. Transposition presents early with cyanosis and tachypnea, but a very small foramen ovale makes it present even earlier.

The simplest lesions are the stenoses, in which usually only one valve or artery is stenotic. In children it is usually the aortic or pulmonic valve, although the mitral and tricuspid valves, rarely, can be stenotic. Valve stenosis usually is isolated, although syndromes (such as **Shone syndrome**) of multiple left heart obstruction occur uncommonly. The right-to-left shunt lesion involves much more complex anatomy and physiology. In most cases, there must also be a left-to-right shunt, which occurs as a simple defect in the septa or arterial walls. Because pulmonary vascular resistance is high at birth, neonates with congenital cardiac defects may have no shunting and thus no physical findings. The "mixing" lesions are those in which there are both right-to-left and left-to-right shunts without significant stenosis, resulting in an arterial saturation in the upper 80th percentile.

TABLE 13–7. Classification of Congenital Cardiac Defects

| | Shunting | | |
| Stenotic | Right→Left | Left→Right | Mixing |
| --- | --- | --- | --- |
| Aortic stenosis | Tetralogy | Patent ductus arteriosus | Truncus |
| Pulmonic stenosis | Transposition | Ventricular septal defect | TAPVR |
| Coarctation of the aorta | Tricuspid atresia | Atrial septal defect | HLH |

HLH = hypoplastic left heart syndrome; TAPVR = total anomalous pulmonary venous return.

## HEMODYNAMIC MEASUREMENTS

Representative oxygen saturations and pressures from catheterization of a child are presented in Figure 13–6. The formulas for calculating pulmonary and systemic *cardiac outputs* are

pulmonary output

$$= \frac{O_2 \text{ consumption in (mL/min)}}{\text{pulmonary arteriovenous difference (mL/L)}}$$

and

systemic output

$$= \frac{O_2 \text{ consumption (mL/L)}}{\text{systemic arteriovenous difference (mL/L)}}$$

where

pulmonary arteriovenous difference
= pulmonary vein
− pulmonary artery oxygen content

and

systemic arteriovenous difference
= systemic artery
− mixed venous oxygen content

Because cardiac output increases with the size of the child, it is related to the patient's surface area in meters. For the resting child, normal cardiac output is about 4 L/min/m². In the absence of cardiac failure, the body's homeostatic mechanisms tend to keep the systemic output near normal, whatever the congenital defect. In the presence of heart failure, the systemic output usually is lowered.

The cardiac outputs and pressures in each side of the heart are critically related to each other. Thus, an elevated systolic pressure of 60 mm Hg in the pulmonary artery in the presence of a VSD is indicative of a greater degree of pulmonary hypertension when the aortic pressure is 90 mm Hg systolic than when the aortic pressure is 120 mm Hg. In the former case, pulmonary hypertension is said to be at two thirds of the systemic level, whereas in the latter, it is one half of the systemic level. When the pressure in the pulmonary artery is equal to that in the aorta, we refer to it as "systemic level" pulmonary hypertension; when it is higher than that of the aorta, it is characterized as "suprasystemic" pulmonary artery pressure.

A calculation of *systemic* (SVR) and *pulmonary* (PVR) *vascular resistance* also can be made. These are the resistances to flow across the resistance vessels, which are mainly small muscular arteries and arterioles. This calculation requires knowledge of the pressures on each side of these resistance vessels. On the systemic side, $\Delta P$ is systemic artery pressure ($P_{sa}$) − right atrial pressure ($P_{ra}$). On the pulmonary side, $\Delta P$ is pulmonary artery pressure ($P_{pa}$) − left atrial pressure ($P_{la}$). The calculation is made from a modification of Poiseuille equation:

$$\text{PVR} = \frac{P_{pa} - P_{la} \text{ [pulmonary } \Delta P]}{\text{pulmonary flow}}$$

and

$$\text{SVR} = \frac{P_{sa} - P_{ra} \text{ [systemic } \Delta P]}{\text{systemic flow}}$$

If the pressure drop is measured in mm Hg and the flow in L/min/m², the calculated resistance is in Wood units. (One Wood unit is equal to 80 dynes·sec/cm⁵/m².) The normal PVR is 2–3 units, whereas the normal SVR is 15–20 units.

An important concept to remember is that *blood flow goes where resistance is least*. Of course, other types of resistance are present besides vascular resistance, such as (1) at valves, where obviously a narrowed valve has a greater resistance to flow than does a wide-open valve; (2) at septal defects, where a small septal defect has a greater resistance to flow than does a large defect; and (3) at ventricles, where a thick-walled, less compliant ventricle has a greater resistance to flow into it than does a thinner-walled, more compliant ventricle.

## ACYANOTIC CONGENITAL HEART LESIONS

### Left-to-Right Shunt Acyanotic Lesions

Acyanotic conditions are those in which the systemic arterial saturation is normal. Left-to-right shunt lesions have communication between the two sides of the heart through which extra blood traverses from the left to the right side. The result is an increase in pulmonary blood flow. A moderate-sized left-to-right shunt has approximately twice as much pulmonary blood flow as systemic blood flow (e.g., a 2:1 pulmonary-to-systemic [P/S] flow ratio). Assuming a normal systemic output of 4 L/min/m², the pulmonary flow is 8 L/min/m².

**Hemodynamics of Common Left-to-Right Shunts**

*Atrial Septal Defect.* Flow from all four pulmonary veins streams through the ASD in both systole and diastole (Fig. 13–8). The result is that very little increase in volume occurs in the left atrium (LA). The right atrium (RA) and the right ventricle (RV) handle twice the normal flow. The roentgenogram shows increased pulmonary artery vascularity and the ECG and echocardiogram show pure right ventricular enlargement (RVE).

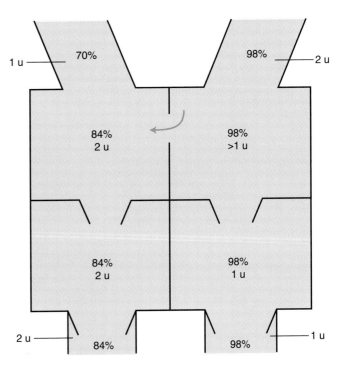

FIGURE 13–8. Atrial septal defect with 2:1 pulmonary-to-systemic (P/S) flow ratio. One unit (u) of cardiac output is 4 L/min/m². % is percent saturation.

No murmur is present from the low-velocity flow across the ASD, but twice the normal flow occurs across the normal tricuspid valve and normal pulmonic valve. The result is that, on the physical examination, in addition to the abnormal right ventricular impulse and widely persistently split $S_2$, a mid-diastolic rumbling murmur is exhibited at the lower left sternal border and a soft systolic ejection murmur is exhibited at the upper left sternal border.

*Patent Ductus Arteriosus.* Figure 13–9 shows normal flow through the right heart until after the blood has reached the pulmonary artery. Twice the normal flow is present in the pulmonary veins, LA, left ventricle (LV), the aorta proximal to the PDA, and pulmonary arteries distal to the PDA. The roentgenogram shows increased pulmonary artery vascularity and may also show increased pulmonary vein size. The ECG and echocardiogram show left atrial enlargement (LAE) and left ventricular hypertrophy (LVH), excluding any effects of increased pulmonary artery pressure.

If the pulmonary artery diastolic pressure is less than the aortic diastolic pressure, a continuous run-off from aorta to pulmonary artery occurs. The result is a continuous murmur. Also, twice the normal flow occurs through the normal mitral and aortic valves. The result is that, in addition to the abnormal left ventricular impulse and hyperdynamic upper left sternal edge and apex, a mid-diastolic rumble is present at that apex and a soft

systolic ejection murmur is present at the upper right sternal border. If the caliber of the PDA is wide, greater transmission of systemic pressure into the pulmonary artery occurs. The wider and shorter the PDA, the higher the right ventricular pressure and the more the right ventricular hypertrophy (RVH) as well as the LVH.

*Ventricular Septal Defect.* Figure 13–10 shows twice as much flow as normal in the pulmonary veins, LA, and LV. The LV sends as much blood through the VSD as into the aorta so that the RV and pulmonary artery also have twice the normal flow. The roentgenogram shows increased pulmonary artery vascularity and may show increased pulmonary vein size. The ECG and echocardiogram show LAE and both LVH and RVH.

A holosystolic murmur is present from left-to-right flow through the VSD. Because LV pressure rises slightly before RV pressure, the left-to-right shunt begins before mitral valve closure, resulting in $S_1$ being obscured by the murmur. Also, twice the flow occurs through the normal mitral and pulmonic valves, so that, in addition to the combined ventricular impulse and the hyperdynamic left sternal edge and apex, a mid-diastolic rumble is exhibited at the apex and a soft systolic ejection murmur is exhibited at the upper left sternal border.

### The Natural History of Acyanotic Lesions with Left-to-Right Shunts

*Atrial Septal Defect.* The most common ASD

FIGURE 13–9. Patent ductus arteriosus with 2:1 pulmonary-to-systemic (P/S) flow ratio (see Fig. 13–8). u = unit.

FIGURE 13–10. Ventricular septal defect with 2:1 pulmonary-to-systemic (P/S) flow ratio (see Fig. 13–8). u = unit.

(6.4:10,000 live births) is of the secundum type and makes up approximately 7% of all cases of congenital heart disease. The ratio of females to males is 2:1. The PVR is lower than normal throughout childhood and heart failure is infrequent. In adulthood, however, a significant number of individuals develop heart failure and/or atrial flutter or pulmonary vascular disease. Therefore, surgery or catheter closure, which is of extremely low risk, should be performed electively at what is deemed the appropriate psychologic age for that child. In most children, this is between 2 and 5 yr of age (Tables 13–8 and 13–9).

*Ventricular Septal Defect.* This is the most common congenital cardiac lesion, making up at least 30% of all cases of congenital heart disease. The incidence in males equals that in females. The most common position of the defect is perimembranous and subaortic, although many muscular defects may be present. VSDs in the endocardial cushion area are not rare, but supracristal defects are quite uncommon except in children of Asian descent, where they are the most common type. VSD is usually a benign disease. The majority of the defects are small, most of which close spontaneously and never need catheterization. VSDs small enough to have normal pulmonary artery pressures and pulmonary-to-systemic flow ratios of less than 2:1 do not need surgery even if closure does not occur. An increase in PVR also does not occur. However, a small percentage of infants with large defects are at risk, and these infants make up a significant percentage of the infants admitted to the hospital with heart failure. Those infants who go into heart failure almost always do so by 2 mo of age.

Patients with large left-to-right shunts can be divided into three groups: (1) those with half-systemic pulmonary hypertension, (2) those with two thirds systemic pulmonary hypertension, and (3) those with systemic-level pulmonary hypertension.

In the first group, medical management is almost invariably without difficulty. The left-to-right shunt also is less, rarely with more than a 2:1 P/S flow ratio, because the defect becomes smaller. Surgery is not necessary. In a few children, a mild amount of pulmonary hypertension (about 40 mm Hg) is still present with a moderate left-to-right shunt. Surgery is recommended for these children.

In the second group, a small number of children are difficult to manage medically, leading to repair of the VSD within a few months after onset of the failure. However, in most, medical management is reasonably successful.

**TABLE 13–8.** Therapy of Congenital Heart Disease: Palliative Procedures

| Procedure | Lesion | Comments |
|---|---|---|
| Blalock-Taussig Teflon tube graft or shunt (subclavian artery to ipsilateral pulmonary artery, usually right-sided) | TOF, pulmonary valve atresia | Improves pulmonary blood flow; most common shunting procedure |
| Balloon atrial septostomy (Rashkind procedure) | TGA, tricuspid atresia | Improves oxygenation with increased atrial mixing |
| Operative atrial septostomy (Blalock-Hanlon operation) | TGA | |
| Catheter balloon dilating valvotomy (balloon valvuloplasty) | Pulmonary valve stenosis; aortic valve stenosis | Increases valve patency |
| Operative valvotomy | As above for balloon plus pulmonary atresia | Increases valve patency; resultant pulmonary valve insufficiency enhances right ventricle growth |
| Prostaglandin $E_1$ infusion | Pulmonary atresia, tricuspid atresia, TOF, coarctation of aorta, interrupted aortic arch, TGA | Maintains pulmonary blood flow via PDA, improves mixing |
| Pulmonary artery banding | Single ventricle | Decreases pulmonary blood flow, prevents heart failure |
| Device occlusion (embolization, umbrella); correction/closure | PDA, VSD, ASD, arteriovenous malformations | Nonsurgical, catheter closure |

ASD = atrial septal defect; PDA = patent ductus arteriosus; TGA = transposition of great arteries; TOF = tetralogy of Fallot; VSD = ventricular septal defect.

TABLE 13–9.    Therapy of Congenital Heart Disease: Corrective Procedures

| Procedure | Lesion | Effect |
| --- | --- | --- |
| Repair of septal defects (patching) | ASD, VSD, endocardial cushion defects | Complete repair |
| Valve replacement, repair | Aortic, mitral, pulmonic stenosis; Ebstein anomaly | Repair but prosthetic valve complications |
| Aortic patch, subclavian flap or end-to-end aortic anastomosis | Interrupted arch, coarctation of aorta | Repair but possible late recoarctation |
| Total correction possible | TOF; anomalous venous return; PDA | Complete repair |
| Mustard or Senning procedure (atrial switch by an intra-atrial baffle) | TGA | Right ventricle remains systemic ventricle |
| Jatene procedure (arterial switch) | TGA | Anatomic correction |
| Fontan procedure (inferior vena cava–to–pulmonary artery anastomosis) | Tricuspid atresia, single ventricle, pulmonary atresia | Alleviates shunting, enhances pulmonary blood flow; atrium functions as right ventricle |
| Norwood procedure | Hypoplastic left heart | Three-staged procedure with variable success |
| Heart transplant | Hypoplastic left heart | Normal heart with risk of immune rejection |
| Heart-lung transplant | Eisenmenger syndrome; cor pulmonale? | Normal organs with risk of rejection |

ASD = atrial septal defect; PDA = patent ductus arteriosus; TGA = transposition of great arteries; TOF = tetralogy of Fallot; VSD = ventricular septal defect.

In the third group, more cases occur in which medical management is unsuccessful, requiring surgery before age 6 mo. As surgery has become progressively safer, the extent of medical management employed has decreased and children are referred for surgical correction earlier, often between 3 and 5 months of age.

**Patent Ductus Arteriosus.** The natural history of the congenital PDA is poorly defined because surgery has been available for a long time. However, three major observations should be noted. First, at the same pulmonary artery pressure, the risk of the development of pulmonary vascular disease is greater in PDA than in VSD. Second, at the same age, the risk of developing infective endocarditis is greater in PDA than in VSD because of jet stream–induced intimal damage. Third, the incidence of spontaneous closure of the congenital PDA is very small. Therefore, because surgery is simple and low risk, all simple congenital PDAs with a left-to-right shunt should be closed. In addition to the standard surgical ligation, occlusion of PDAs using specialized metal coils is an alternative to surgery. There is a slightly higher risk of a tiny residual defect, but the procedure is less invasive and less expensive than surgery. (see Tables 13–8 and 13–9). Those infants who have congestive heart failure and/or large left-to-right shunts with increased pulmonary artery pressure should be operated on at the time of diagnosis.

**Endocardial Cushion Defect (Atrioventricular Canal).** A broad spectrum of endocardial cushion defects have been observed, from varieties of the complete AV canal (including marked deficiency in the ventricular and atrial septa as well as medial portions of tricuspid and mitral valves making a common AV valve) to several varieties of the partial AV canal. The simplest forms are the VSD in the endocardial cushion position and the ostium primum ASD with varying deficiencies of the anteromedial leaflet, causing mitral regurgitation. Equal numbers of males and females are affected. The more complete the defect, the more likely it is that the child has Down syndrome. Approximately one third of children with Down syndrome have some form of AV canal; therefore, all Down syndrome children should receive a cardiac evaluation if symptomatic or before 6 mo of age.

The natural history of the various partial AV canal defects depends on the size of the various atrial and ventricular defects and the amount of mitral regurgitation. The large ostium primum ASD with no mitral regurgitation has the same benign natural history as that of the simple secundum ASD. With a complete AV canal, severe heart failure and/or pulmonary vascular disease is the rule. The clinical and echocardiographic diagnosis depends on the specific anatomy. The characteristic ECG is one showing an abnormally left superior vector (formerly termed "left axis deviation"). A congenital abnormality of the anterior branch of the left bundle results in initial QRS conduction inferiorly, followed by the remainder of the conduction sequence superiorly.

In complete AV canal, left ventricular to right atrial communication is present in addition to the large VSD, leading to an early increase in pulmonary blood flow. If mitral regurgitation is present, early left ventricular failure may occur. The high left ventricular end-diastolic pressure causes the pulmonary venous pressure to be elevated. Therefore, three of the four major factors that slow maturation of the pulmonary resistance vessels are present. In addition, continued high pulmonary blood flow at systemic-level pulmonary artery pressure and high pulmonary venous pressure may be exhibited. Therefore, even when heart failure can be managed, the pulmonary vascular resistance eventually increases and pulmonary vascular disease occurs. Early complete surgical repair, preferably by 3 mo of age, is strongly recommended.

## Obstructive Lesions

**Right-Sided Lesions.** The most common pure right-sided obstructive lesion is **valvular pulmonic stenosis**. Peripheral pulmonic stenosis that is not part of other congenital cardiac lesions (e.g., tetralogy of Fallot) occurs most commonly in association with entities such as congenital rubella, Williams syndrome, Noonan syndrome, Alagille syndrome, cutis laxa, and Ehlers-Danlos syndrome. Isolated pulmonary infundibular stenosis may exist only when a VSD is present or has been present and closed.

The majority of stenotic pulmonic valves have three leaflets with varied leaflet fusion. A less common variety is pulmonary valvular dysplasia, in which the pathology is not of fusion but of a myxomatous tissue that is disorganized, thickened, and immobile. Most patients with dysplastic pulmonary valves have Noonan syndrome.

The *diagnosis* is suggested by a pulmonary ejection click that is maximal on expiration at the upper left sternal border, followed by an ejection systolic murmur and a widely split $S_2$. The more severe the stenosis, the longer the murmur; full-length murmurs are associated with the right ventricular pressures near systemic level. With mild stenosis, the $S_2$ split is not much above normal and pulmonary closure may be of increased intensity. With increasing severity, the split widens and the pulmonary closure softens. In many severe cases, with suprasystemic right ventricular pressure, the murmur may extend across the aortic closure so that no 2nd sound is heard at the upper left sternal border. The ECG shows pure RVH, and the chest roentgenogram shows no significant cardiomegaly and a large dilated (poststenotic) pulmonary artery. In some severe cases, the elevated right atrial pressure may cause the flap of the foramen ovale to open, resulting in a significant right-to-left shunt. Thus, this "acyanotic lesion" would be associated with cyanosis.

Cases have been observed, especially in infancy, in which the pulmonic stenosis is so severe that marked right ventricular failure occurs, associated with venous distention, a large liver, and a large right-to-left shunt at the atrial level. In other infants, the severe stenosis results in cyanosis very shortly after birth from inadequate pulmonary blood flow. These children are dependent on a patent ductus arterious for oxygenation. This condition is termed **critical pulmonic stenosis**.

*Treatment* of valvular pulmonic stenosis is straightforward. Mild pulmonic stenosis with right ventricular pressure of less than 50 mm Hg is very common; it is known not to increase in severity over the years and is associated with normal life expectancy. When the right ventricular pressure is above 60 mm Hg, the treatment is balloon valvuloplasty (see Tables 13–8 and 13–9). The success rate is very high, and the risk is very low. Surgery is performed only in severe cases, such as when the balloon catheter cannot be passed through the stenotic pulmonic valve.

**Left-Sided Lesions**

*Valvular Aortic Stenosis.* Left-sided lesions are very common, particularly if one includes *bicuspid aortic valve without stenosis* in this category. It is not known how common this latter lesion is, although it is known to occur in about half of patients with coarctation of the aorta. The recognition of bicuspid aortic valve (with two sinuses) is important because patients with this abnormality are very susceptible to infective endocarditis. The *diagnosis* is readily made by identifying a sharp sound well separated from $S_1$ and usually maximal at the apex, not varying with respiration, and less well heard at the lower left sternal border and anterior axillary line. This sound is an aortic ejection click.

*Valvular Aortic Stenosis with Systolic Gradient.* This is a major lesion with tremendous variation in severity. In most cases, surgery is not required in childhood. Although it is a potentially progressive lesion, mild cases do not progress until adulthood.

The systolic murmur usually is maximal at the

upper right sternal border or over the sternum and often is associated with suprasternal notch and carotid systolic thrills. When the murmur is significantly less than full length and the split of $S_2$ is normal, indicating no significant prolongation of left ventricular systole, the condition almost certainly is mild. Such patients usually have ECGs that are normal. When the murmur is full length and the split of $S_2$ is narrow, indicating prolongation of left ventricular systole, the condition is significant. Important clues to severity include the initial QRS vector being situated to the left, LVH, and the development of ST-segment and T-wave abnormalities with exercise. Echo-Doppler techniques for predicting severity have become reliable, so that baseline catheterization may no longer be necessary.

If no ST or T abnormalities are present at rest and if the systolic gradient is less than 60 mm Hg, most cardiologists agree that no intervention is indicated (see Tables 13–8 and 13–9). (The presence of ST and T abnormalities at rest, however, provides a clear indication for intervention.) Most advise that children with aortic stenosis should not participate in competitive athletics. When exercise requiring sustained strength is involved (e.g., weightlifting and competitive wrestling), the end-diastolic pressure increases significantly, reducing coronary perfusion. Therefore, this type of exercise especially should be avoided. Sudden unexpected death due to valvular aortic stenosis in childhood or young adulthood is rare. Both surgery and balloon aortic valvuloplasty are palliative and equally successful procedures. For most patients, balloon valvuloplasty is the procedure of choice. Surgery is reserved for those patients unresponsive to balloon dilation or when there is severe valve dysplasia or aortic insufficiency. Even after successful intervention, the stenosis tends to recur over time, with reintervention needed. Repeated interventions often result in the development of aortic insufficiency, which necessitates valve replacement. Prosthetic valve replacement has traditionally been the procedure of choice. The autologous transfer of the pulmonary root (Ross procedure) is another option.

The infants who have *critical aortic stenosis*, sometimes recognized in the 1st wk of life, are very ill. They have very stenotic valves and sometimes abnormal left ventricles. All would die without intervention (see Tables 13–8 and 13–9).

**Coarctation of the Aorta.** Simple coarctation of the aorta is almost always at the level of the ductus arteriosus (or ligamentum arteriosum) and just below the origin of the left subclavian artery. (Occasionally, the origin of the left subclavian is at or below the coarctation.) Because of the position of the ductus, there is no obstruction to flow in the aorta in utero or while the ductus is open in the newborn period. Therefore, simple coarctation often is not recognized in newborns.

The murmur is usually systolic, with a late peak, and can be located anywhere in the anterior chest. It usually is heard well at the apex, left axilla, and left back, but often it is maximal over the left back. The ECG early in infancy may show pure RVH, although later in childhood LVH is expected.

Rarely, coarctation causes heart failure in the 1st mo of life, but often the children are asymptomatic throughout childhood. Eventually, most children have upper extremity systolic pressures in the range of 140–145 mm Hg. Because of the position of the left subclavian artery, the right arm pressure may be higher than that of the left arm. Because the pulse pressure is low below the coarctation, renal endocrine factors work to raise the pressure, both above and below the coarctation.

*Treatment* of *simple* coarctation of the aorta is indicated in Table 13–9. Previously, it had been recommended to wait until 4–5 yr of age for surgery in asymptomatic children because of a higher risk of recoarctation. Advances in surgical techniques have decreased this risk. Therefore, most children should be considered for surgery at the time of diagnosis. Children who are hypertensive should be treated to normalize their blood pressure prior to surgery, which decreases the risk of malignant postoperative hypertension. Special problems arise when the diagnosis is missed or if surgery is not performed until later in life. First, more collateral vessels may be present, leading to increased bleeding during surgery. In addition, by adolescence, the aorta may have stiffened so that end-to-end anastomosis cannot be done. Also, a significantly higher incidence of essential hypertension and death may be present in later life.

*Complicated* coarctation of the aorta, a coarctation in association with another lesion (e.g., PDA arising above the coarctation or, more commonly, a VSD), commonly leads to heart failure by the 2nd wk of life. After treatment of heart failure, surgery must be performed within a few days. For those infants with a PDA, operating on both lesions successfully alleviates the problem. For the more common cases with a VSD, a decision must be made as to whether or not to place a pulmonary artery band as well as to repair the coarctation. Often, only the coarctation is operated on because it is difficult to determine the size of the VSD. If the infant remains very ill, a second operation soon may be necessary to close the VSD.

When a coarctation is corrected, the area of repair may not grow. Consequently, a situation called

TABLE 13–10.  Cyanotic Congenital Heart Disease with Decreased Pulmonary Blood Flow

**Right Ventricular Hypertrophy**

Pulmonary stenosis (severe) with atrial septal defect
Pulmonary atresia (with or without ventricular septal defect)
Tetralogy of Fallot

**Left Ventricular Hypertrophy**

Tricuspid atresia
Pulmonary atresia and hypoplastic right ventricle

**Right, Left, or Combined Ventricular Hypertrophy**

Transposition of great arteries with pulmonary stenosis
Truncus arteriosus with hypoplastic pulmonary arteries

**Neither Ventricle Predominant**

Ebstein anomaly

"restenosis" may develop. Because at the time of the original operation collateral vessels involving spinal cord arterial flow may be lost, a second operation for coarctation may include a risk of spinal cord ischemia. For this reason, balloon arterioplasty is often recommended instead of surgery for restenosis. Balloon arterioplasty is also performed as a treatment for primary coarctation, but the long-term risk of restenosis and aortic aneurysm formation is not yet known.

## CYANOTIC CONGENITAL HEART DISEASE

Cyanotic congenital heart disease can be divided into lesions that have decreased (Table 13–10) or increased (Table 13–11) pulmonary blood flow. Because of persistent cyanosis or right-to-left shunts,

TABLE 13–11.  Cyanotic Congenital Heart Disease with Increased Pulmonary Blood Flow

**Right Ventricular Hypertrophy**

Hypoplastic left heart syndrome
Total anomalous venous return
Transposition of great arteries

**Right, Left, or Combined Ventricular Hypertrophy**

Transposition of great arteries ± ventricular septal defect
Single ventricle
Tricuspid atresia with transposition
Truncus arteriosus

these patients often have characteristic extracardiac complications (Table 13–12).

### Tetralogy of Fallot

The four components of this syndrome are (1) a large nonrestrictive VSD, (2) severe right ventricle outflow tract obstruction, (3) overriding of the aortic root over the ventricular septum, and (4) RVH. The RVH is secondary. Embryologically, there is one defect—hypoplasia of the conus. Because conal tissue provides the major portion of the tissue that closes the membranous ventricular septum and because the conus is hypoplastic, the result is a nonrestrictive VSD and severe infundibular pulmonic stenosis. Flow through the small conus is restricted in utero, resulting in a small annulus and small pulmonary arteries.

Although the location and size of the VSD are relatively constant, the severity of the pulmonary stenosis varies considerably and accounts for the varying age at presentation and the varying clinical course. In a few infants, the pulmonary stenosis may be less severe, associated initially with a left-to-right shunt. A true tetralogy, however, has a right-to-left shunt.

Occasionally, the narrowing is located almost exclusively at the infundibular level, associated with a normal pulmonary valve annulus, normal valve leaflets, and normal distal pulmonary arteries. More commonly, obstruction at the infundibular level is associated with a hypoplastic pulmonary valve annulus and a dysplastic, stenotic pulmonary valve. The main pulmonary artery and distal pulmonary arteries may be hypoplastic, and occasionally discrete stenoses are noted at the takeoff of the right and left pulmonary arteries or even more distally. In the most severe form, there is complete atresia of the infundibulum, the pulmonary valve, and even sometimes the main pulmonary artery. Other intracardiac anomalies are not commonly associated with tetralogy, except that a right aortic arch is present in 25% of the patients.

*Pathophysiology.* Because of the large size of VSD, blood passing through the tricuspid and mitral valves may flow to either the aorta or the pulmonary artery; the degree of intracardiac shunting is a function of the relative outflow resistances (Fig. 13–11). The systemic resistance is composed primarily of the systemic arteriolar resistance, but the pulmonary resistance is due to the anatomic pulmonary stenosis. Because the pulmonary stenosis is severe, there is primarily or exclusively a right-to-left shunt, with blood bypassing the pulmonary artery and going to the aorta. Although the severity of the anatomic abnormal-

TABLE 13–12.  Extracardiac Complications of Cyanotic Congenital Heart Disease

| Problem | Etiology | Therapy |
|---|---|---|
| Polycythemia | Persistent hypoxia | Phlebotomy |
| Relative anemia | Nutritional deficiency | Iron replacement |
| CNS abscess | Right-to-left shunting | Antibiotics, drainage |
| CNS thromboembolic stroke | Right-to-left shunting or polycythemia | Phlebotomy |
| Gum disease | Polycythemia, gingivitis, bleeding | Dental hygiene |
| Gout | Polycythemia, diuretic agents | Allopurinol |
| Arthritis, clubbing | Hypoxic arthropathy | None |
| Pregnancy | Poor placental perfusion, poor ability to increase cardiac output | Bed rest |
| Infectious disease | Associated asplenia, DiGeorge syndrome | Antibiotics |
| | Fatal RSV pneumonia with pulmonary hypertension | Ribavirin, RSV immune globulin |
| Growth | Failure to thrive, increased oxygen consumption, decreased nutrient intake | Treat heart failure; correct defect early |
| Psychosocial adjustment | Limited activity, peer pressure; chronic disease, multiple hospitalizations | Counseling |

CNS = central nervous system; RSV = respiratory syncytial virus.

FIGURE 13–11.  Tetralogy of Fallot.

ity is the primary determinant of the degree of cyanosis, changes in systemic venous oxygen saturation or pulmonary or systemic resistances also influence the degree of right-to-left shunting. For example, exercise or crying, by reducing the systemic arteriolar resistance and increasing systemic venous return, is associated with a large right-to-left shunt, more cyanosis, and a decrease in oxygen saturation. Any agent that increases systemic resistance would have the opposite effect, by decreasing systemic and increasing pulmonary blood flow and, therefore, reducing the right-to-left shunt. The child inherently learns to decrease cyanosis by assuming a squatting position. Squatting increases systemic venous return, resulting in more blood being made available to the pulmonary artery, and increases systemic resistance, driving more venous blood into the lungs.

*Clinical Manifestations.* The clinical findings vary, depending on the degree of right ventricular outflow obstruction. Children with a less severe degree of outflow obstruction may not be cyanotic at birth and initially may have a left-to-right shunt. Usually, the right ventricular outflow tract obstruction is progressive, resulting in increasing hypoxemia and cyanosis over the first few months and years of life. Such children usually do well clinically except for dyspnea and increased cyanosis on exertion. Occasionally, children under 5 yr of age assume a squatting position.

*Hypoxic ("tet") spells* may occur, especially from a few months to 2 yr of life. During such spells, the child typically becomes very restless and agitated and may cry inconsolably. The child is hyperpneic, with gradually increasing cyanosis, which then often leads to a deep sleep. In severe spells, prolonged unconsciousness and even convulsions, hemiparesis, or death may occur. Treatment of these spells consists of administering oxygen, placing the child in the knee-chest position, and giving morphine sulfate. If necessary, the SVR can be acutely increased by intravenous administration of an alpha-adrenergic agonist, such as phenylephrine or methoxamine. Muscular spasm of the infundibulum can be a component of spells and can be decreased by the beta-adrenergic antagonist propranolol. If acidosis is present, intravenous sodium bicarbonate should be given. In severe cases, emergency surgery, either systemic-to-pulmonary artery shunt or total correction, may be necessary.

The volume work of the heart in tetralogy of Fallot is less than normal. Therefore, heart failure does not occur.

On *physical examination*, cyanosis and digital clubbing (in older children) are evident. A quiet heart with a right ventricular impulse is noted.

Because of the very severe pulmonic stenosis, pulmonary closure is not heard. The audible 2nd sound is that of a loud aortic closure at the lower left sternal border resulting from transmission down the descending aorta. Because no murmur occurs from a right-to-left shunt through the VSD, the only murmur heard is that of blood flowing through the pulmonic stenosis. With more severe stenosis, less blood goes through the stenotic right ventricular outflow tract and more goes through the VSD, resulting in a softer, shorter murmur. In maximal tetralogy (pulmonary atresia), there is no systolic murmur, although there may be a loud aortic ejection click (best heard at the apex). Also, a continuous murmur from either a PDA or large collateral artery off the descending aorta (best heard in the back) may be present. In the patient who has a hypoxic spell, the previously heard systolic murmur softens or disappears, returning when the spell is over.

On the *chest roentgenogram*, the heart is not enlarged. Often, a concavity is found in the area usually occupied by the main pulmonary artery ("boot-shaped" heart), and the ascending aorta is large. A right aortic arch may be present.

The *ECG* shows RVH and often right atrial enlargement as well, although in the first weeks of life the ECG may be normal. Echocardiography can define the important features in most patients with tetralogy of Fallot. The extent and anatomy of right ventricular outflow obstruction, the VSD, the proximal branch pulmonary arteries, and the coronary arteries are visualized. Coronary anomalies, specifically a left coronary artery (either left anterior descending or large conal branch) crossing the anterior surface of the right ventricular outflow tract, are present in 5% of patients.

Cardiac catheterization usually is not necessary in the infant, and it is not necessary to take the risk of producing hypoxic spells. On *cardiac catheterization*, equal systolic pressures in the RV and LV and ascending aorta are noted (see Fig. 13–11). The oxygen saturation on the right side of the heart usually is lower than normal because of systemic hypoxemia; however, the pulmonary venous and left atrial saturations are normal.

*Angiography* of the RV, LV, and ascending aorta identifies the anatomy of the VSD(s) and pulmonary arteries. An aortogram can aid in identifying the coronary artery pattern, the presence of a patent ductus arteriosus, or aortopulmonary collateral vessels, which can develop in older children with prolonged cyanosis.

*Complications.* A *cerebrovascular accident* is a devastating complication of cyanotic congenital heart disease (see Table 13–12). In children younger than 2 yr of age, this complication almost invariably is secondary to hypoxemia and anemia rather than to polycythemia, sludging, and in situ thrombosis, and it occurs most commonly in children who are quite hypoxemic, with a relative anemia for the degree of oxygen saturation. Iron deficiency makes the red blood cells somewhat stiffer and results in less oxygen delivery. In older children, in particular, the hematocrit may rise above 65%. Even in this situation, considerable iron deficiency may be present, a diagnosis that cannot be made by examination of the red cells on the blood smear. Serum iron and iron-binding capacity must be measured. When iron therapy is given, the hemoglobin may rise but the hematocrit value usually does not. Conversely, if the iron saturation is normal, the administration of iron can raise the hematocrit to dangerous levels.

Although viscosity of the blood may increase significantly when the hematocrit is above 55%, there is a tradeoff of improved delivery of oxygen to the tissue at the higher hematocrit level. A large number of patients with congenital defects resulting in chronic cyanosis need to maintain their hematocrit level between 60 and 65% for optimal well-being. However, if questions of symptoms of polycythemia at that hematocrit level have arisen or if the hematocrit goes above 65%, partial exchange transfusion is necessary. Withdrawal of blood without continuous exchange is dangerous, the risks being the acute lowering of systemic resistance, more right-to-left shunt, and a cerebrovascular accident.

*Brain abscess* is a less common complication than a cerebrovascular accident. Patients usually are older than 2 yr of age and present with headaches and localizing signs. Any central nervous system event in a cyanotic child over age 2 should be considered a brain abscess until proven otherwise because of the drastic implications. CT scans are diagnostic. Antibiotic therapy occasionally may keep the infection localized, but surgical drainage of the abscess often is required.

*Bacterial endocarditis* is always a risk in children with tetralogy of Fallot prior to complete repair, particularly in patients with systemic-to-pulmonary shunts.

*Treatment.* The treatment of tetralogy of Fallot is surgical (see Tables 13–8 and 13–9). Surgery is indicated if the affected child is significantly symptomatic, hypoxemic with an arterial oxygen saturation of less than 75%, or polycythemic with a hematocrit of more than 60%. *Palliative operations* are performed in patients deemed inappropriate for total correction, because of very young age, severe cyanosis or a protracted spell, or significant coro-

nary abnormality. The *Blalock-Taussig shunt* connecting the subclavian artery to the pulmonary artery is the preferred systemic-to-pulmonary shunt. The Blalock-Taussig shunt is an excellent temporizing procedure, but it does not eliminate right-to-left shunting and has the potential of distorting the pulmonary arteries, making later repair more difficult.

*Total correction* of tetralogy of Fallot is performed under cardiopulmonary bypass. It usually involves closure of the VSD with a Dacron patch and excision of muscle in the right ventricular outflow tract. A right ventriculotomy can be necessary to adequately resect the infundibular muscle, but this procedure can lead to later arrhythmias. Transatrial resection is the preferred method for most patients. If hypoplasia of the pulmonary annulus, main pulmonary artery, or distal pulmonary arteries is present, a patch is placed as a roof over that area. In institutions in which complete repair is frequently done before age 1 yr, the surgical mortality rate is lower than 5%.

Short-term complications include a residual VSD and residual right ventricular outflow tract obstruction because of incomplete relief of the pulmonary stenosis. Pulmonary regurgitation also is expected, even with excellent surgical results. Late complications have included ventricular ectopy and even sudden death resulting from ventricular tachycardia. However, with the ready availability of electrophysiologic studies at catheterization, the identification of those infants at risk of ventricular tachycardia has made pharmacologic preventive therapy very successful. Although long-term data are not available, most children do quite well and remain asymptomatic at least throughout childhood and into young adulthood. Despite pulmonary regurgitation, some patients may do well for much longer periods, the unknown factor being the long-term status of the right ventricle.

### *d*-Transposition of the Great Arteries

Complete transposition of the great arteries (TGA), although less common than tetralogy of Fallot, is the most common lesion seen in the cyanotic infant in the newborn period. In children with this lesion, the great arteries arise off the inappropriate ventricle, the aorta from the right and the pulmonary artery from the left. The systemic venous drainage and pulmonary venous drainage are usually normal, and the right and left atria and the right and left ventricles are in their normal positions. Therefore, desaturated blood from the systemic venous return passes through the RA and RV and out to the aorta, whereas oxygenated pulmonary

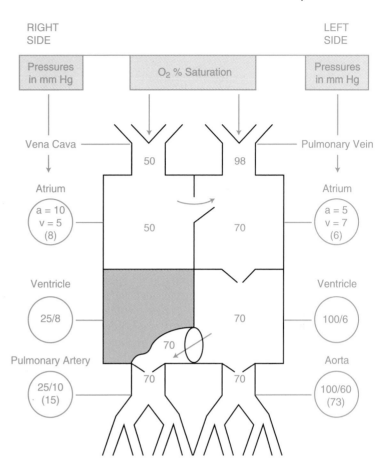

RIGHT SIDE

Pressures in mm Hg

O₂ % Saturation

LEFT SIDE

Pressures in mm Hg

Vena Cava ──── 50

Pulmonary Vein ──── 98

Atrium
a = 10
v = 5
(8)

50          70

Atrium
a = 5
v = 7
(6)

Ventricle
25/8

70

Ventricle
100/6

Pulmonary Artery
25/10
(15)

70

70          70

Aorta
100/60
(73)

FIGURE 13–13. Hypoplastic right ventricle with tricuspid atresia and ventricular septal defect.

Glenn procedure and can result in severe oxygen desaturation or death. The Fontan procedure carries a 5–10% mortality. Over the long term, there is a late mortality rate of 0.5–1% per year from arrhythmias, ventricular failure, or protein-losing enteropathy.

### Truncus Arteriosus

In children with truncus arteriosus, a single arterial trunk from the base of the heart gives rise to the aorta, pulmonary arteries, and coronary arteries. A large VSD invariably is present, and the single semilunar valve has a variable number of leaflets, usually between two and six. The valve may be stenotic, regurgitant or both. The pulmonary arteries may arise as a single trunk before bifurcating (type 1) or may arise separately from the posterior wall of the aorta (type 2).

Because there is a common exit to the aorta and pulmonary artery, the saturation of blood in the systemic arteries is approximately equal to that in the pulmonary arteries. The level of arterial saturation depends on the amount of pulmonary blood flow. If the PVR is high, moderate hypoxemia may result. When the PVR is low, pulmonary blood flow may be torrential, cyanosis minimal, and heart failure severe.

*Clinical Findings.* Initially after birth, the PVR is high and the newborn may do well. As the PVR drops, the pulmonary blood flow increases and the signs and symptoms of heart failure develop. The runoff of blood from truncus into the pulmonary artery in diastole results in a very wide pulse pressure. The heart is hyperdynamic, with loud 1st and 2nd heart sounds, and an aortic ejection click almost always is present. A grade 2 to 3/6 systolic ejection murmur usually is noted at the upper left or right sternal border from increased flow across the semilunar valve; however, if the truncal valve is stenotic, the murmur may be grade 4 and associated with a thrill. An early high-frequency diastolic murmur is present if the truncal valve is regurgitant, and a mid-diastolic rumble at the apex may be present if the pulmonary blood flow (and therefore flow across the mitral valve) is increased. The combination of stenosis and regurgitation results in the characteristic to-and-fro ("washing machine") murmur. In the older child with an increased PVR, progressive cyanosis, polycythemia, and clubbing may occur.

On the chest roentgenogram, the heart usually is large, with increased pulmonary vascularity and pulmonary venous congestion; in 40% of patients, a right aortic arch is found. Because of the association with **DiGeorge syndrome**, the thymus shadow may be absent. When an elevated PVR and diminished pulmonary blood flow are present, the ECG shows RVH, but in the more usual cases, with very increased pulmonary blood flow, biventricular hypertrophy is expected.

On echocardiogram the anatomy usually is seen well, with no demonstrable infundibulum present. At cardiac catheterization and angiography, the catheter usually can pass into the pulmonary arteries from the truncus arteriosus. Right-to-left and left-to-right shunts at the ventricular level are present, with systolic pressures equal in both ventricles.

*Treatment and Prognosis.* Children should be evaluated for hypocalcemia and T-cell deficiencies associated with DiGeorge syndrome. Children with persistent truncus arteriosus usually present early in life, within the first few weeks. The use of vigorous anticongestive measures in an attempt to get the children to grow are usually unsuccessful. A modified *Rastelli procedure* is performed at 2–12 wk of age. The VSD is closed so that the LV passes unimpeded into the truncal valve. The pulmonary artery is removed from the back of the aorta, usually using a button of aortic tissue; the aortic opening is closed, and the RV is connected to the pulmonary arteries with a prosthetic conduit or aortic homograft. At selected centers, the early results have been promising. Successful surgery necessarily requires a later reoperation as the children "outgrow" the conduit.

### Total Anomalous Pulmonary Venous Connection

In children with a total anomalous pulmonary venous connection, there is a failure of incorporation of the common pulmonary vein into the posterior wall of the LA. During embryogenesis, the pulmonary venous return is diverted into one of the early embryonic channels returning to the right side of the heart.

If the left cardinal system persists, pulmonary venous return is to the left superior vena cava, which may drain into the innominate vein or into the coronary sinus and then into the RA. If the right cardinal system persists, the pulmonary veins drain into the right superior vena cava, usually by

way of a persistent ascending LV vein. Drainage directly into the RA is rare.

If the umbilical-vitelline system persists, the common pulmonary veins drain inferiorly through the diaphragm, usually into the portal system of the liver. There is severe obstruction in the liver so that right atrial flow is diminished and pulmonary venous hypertension and congestion are severe. Also, severe pulmonary hypertension is present as a result of a very high PVR. When the drainage is above the diaphragm, pulmonary venous obstruction is not common and PVR usually becomes low. It is uncommon for infants with the latter condition to present before 1 mo of age. Congestive heart failure may be severe. Rarely, these children present late in a manner similar to infants who have an ASD; heart failure and cyanosis are milder than in those infants that present earlier.

*Clinical Manifestations.* Infants who have obstructed pulmonary veins present in the newborn period with severe cyanosis and tachypnea in the first hours of life. Usually, no murmurs are present and the electrocardiogram shows marked RVH. On the chest roentgenogram, the heart is small and interstitial fluid is increased as a result of the marked pulmonary venous congestion, often quite similar in appearance to that of respiratory distress syndrome. For children with only mild or no obstruction who present after the newborn period, cyanosis is subtle but may increase with crying or other exertion. Heart failure may be very severe with a hyperactive right ventricular impulse and a widely split 2nd heart sound that moves little with respiration. The ECG shows severe RVH; cardiac enlargement and increased pulmonary vascularity are apparent on the chest roentgenogram. Rarely, infants in this group are asymptomatic, with the abnormality resembling a simple large ASD.

The echocardiogram is diagnostic and usually sufficient for surgical repair. Cardiac catheterization shows common mixing at the right atrial level, with approximately equal saturations in the RA, RV, and pulmonary artery as well as in the LA, LV, and aorta. Cineangiocardiograms usually can show the sites of drainage by injections either directly into the pulmonary artery or into the common pulmonary vein entered by way of its anomalous connection. Catheterization is contraindicated in infants with obstructed venous return. The angiographic contrast exacerbates the pulmonary edema, increasing the respiratory distress.

*Treatment and Prognosis.* For the newborn with obstructed pulmonary veins, emergency surgery is necessary. For those who present later in infancy or childhood, elective surgery is recommended. The usual operation is to open a wide connection between the common pulmonary vein and the back wall of the LA, after which the previously useful anomalous connection is ligated.

For the infant or older child with low PVR, the prognosis is excellent, with a low surgical risk (under 2%) and a low incidence of postoperative complications. For the newborn with obstructed total veins, surgery is more hazardous (5–15% mortality rate) because of difficult anatomic problems and serious cardiovascular decompensation prior to surgery. Rapid identification and diagnosis result in a lower mortality rate because the surgery is not technically difficult.

### Hypoplastic Left Heart Syndrome

The hypoplastic left heart syndrome (HLHS) includes a number of closely related anomalies that are part of hypoplasia and underdevelopment of the LV. The mitral and aortic valves usually are hypoplastic, and one or both of them may be atretic. The ascending aorta usually is small, although coronary arteries are in the normal position. Discrete coarctation of the aorta is usually present. After birth, the pulmonary venous return from the LA passes across the atrial septum into the RA and then to the RV and the pulmonary artery. The systemic blood flow is via the ductus arteriosus to the ascending and descending aorta. Affected fetuses do well in utero, but after birth the infants become ill very quickly. After birth, the pulmonary venous return comes back to the LA and must go across the atrial septum. If the atrial defect is small, as is usually the case, pulmonary venous pressure increases and the signs and symptoms of left-sided heart failure appear. The entire systemic cardiac output must pass through the ductus arteriosus, so that when this vessel constricts, systemic cardiac output is reduced. Eventually acidosis, hypotension, and death occur.

*Clinical Manifestations.* The usual manifestations are a combination of heart failure resulting from excessive pulmonary blood flow and obstructed pulmonary venous return. Low cardiac output and acidosis occur after constriction of the ductus arteriosus. All peripheral pulses are weak or absent. Cyanosis usually is not prominent, but low cardiac output gives a grayish color to the cool, mottled skin. The cardiac impulse usually is hyperdynamic. Murmurs are not prominent but may be present as a result of increased flow across the tricuspid and pulmonic valves. Because children with HLHS or other left heart obstructive lesions (coarctation, interrupted aortic arch, aortic stenosis) can be asymptomatic before the ductus arteriosus closes, the infant may be discharged

from the nursery without the diagnosis suspected. These children then present in profound cardiovascular collapse within the first weeks of life when the ductus arteriosus closes. $PGE_1$ should be considered in any infant who presents with shock, particularly if there is hepatomegaly or poor response to fluid resuscitation.

The ECG shows severe RVH because of the systemic right ventricular pressure, torrential pulmonary blood flow, and the hypoplastic LV. On the chest roentgenogram, the heart usually is enlarged and there are increased pulmonary vascularity and pulmonary venous congestion. The echocardiogram is diagnostic. The right side of the heart is large. A cardiac catheterization is not necessary because it merely adds undue risk for the infant.

*Treatment and Prognosis.* Without surgery, early death is inevitable. A three-stage palliative approach is most common. The first stage, developed by Norwood, involves creating a large atrial opening by an atrial septectomy, dividing the pulmonary artery, and connecting the proximal segment to the ascending aorta and the distal segment to the descending aorta via a Blalock-Taussig shunt. Thus, the RV serves as the systemic ventricle, pumping blood through the pulmonary valve into the aorta with pulmonary blood flow supplied via a systemic-to-pulmonary artery shunt. The second stage consists of a bidirectional cavopulmonary (Glenn) shunt at 3–12 mo, followed by a Fontan operation at 2–4 yr of age.

After the first stage, most major centers achieve an 80–90% survival. The second and third stages have low (5–10%) mortality, but the longstanding problems of a systemic right ventricle and the underlying difficulties of a Fontan palliation lead to overall survival rates of approximately 50% to late childhood. Cardiac transplantation is an alternative approach. Major transplantation centers report a 30–50% mortality in neonates awaiting transplantation, followed by a 70–80% 5-yr survival. Because of the magnitude of the long-term commitment and relatively poor outcome, some families choose to refuse any surgery.

### THE HIGH-RISK NEWBORN

A myriad of congenital heart diseases are exhibited in the neonatal period, often causing great diagnostic confusion. Despite the large varieties of possible diagnoses, approximately 70% of infants affected by these diseases have one of six lesions:

- Hypoplastic left ventricle syndrome
- Transposition of the great arteries with intact ventricular septum

- Hypoplastic right ventricle with tricuspid atresia
- Hypoplastic right ventricle with pulmonary atresia
- Complicated coarctation of the aorta (with VSD)
- Tetralogy of Fallot.

For completeness, obstructed total anomalous veins also might be added to this list. By systematically assessing the predominant symptoms, one can usually make the physiologic diagnosis from the history, physical examination, chest roentgenogram, and ECG, generating a fairly small differential diagnosis. The important presenting symptoms (Table 13–13) are:

1. *Cyanosis,* with or without respiratory distress.
2. *Hypoperfusion,* with respiratory distress.
3. *Respiratory distress,* without cyanosis or hypoperfusion.

Treatment is summarized in Tables 13–8 and 13–9.

## PRENATAL DETECTION AND TREATMENT OF CONGENITAL CARDIAC DEFECTS

Congenital heart defects can be diagnosed prenatally. Cardiac ultrasound scans usually are performed first by obstetricians. An abnormal four-chamber view of the heart prompts referral to the pediatric cardiac center. Primary pediatric cardiac fetal ultrasound examinations often are performed if the mother or father had congenital heart disease or if the parents had a previous child with a congenital heart defect. Other indications include maternal diabetes (associated with TGA and hypertrophic cardiomyopathy), certain drugs (lithium, phenytoin), major chromosomal anomalies (Down syndrome, other trisomies) and nonimmune hydrops (dysrhythmias, atrioventricular valve regurgitation, cardiomyopathy).

*Fetal echocardiography* is accurate in diagnosis of the most severe types of congenital cardiac defects, such as valve atresia and severe stenosis. It cannot diagnose mild defects, such as PDA or ASD, which are normal in the fetus. It can usually diagnose VSDs or coarctation of the aorta. It has taught us that fetal congenital heart disease is more common than we thought, that fetal wastage is common, and that the defects progress throughout fetal life. Although the usual earliest time at which fetal echocardiography can be performed is now about 16 wk, this time will decrease with improved techniques and technology.

Fetal ultrasonography is useful in the diagnosis of arrhythmias and in following the progression and response to treatment. Both tachyarrhythmias and bradyarrhythmias occur in the fetus and may lead to fetal congestive heart failure and death. Other arrhythmias, such as premature atrial contractions, are common and probably benign. Congenital complete AV block usually is well tolerated in the fetus. The ventricles are able to compensate for the slow rate by increasing their stroke volume. If there is associated congenital heart disease, however, **fetal hydrops** (congestive heart failure) may occur. This diagnosis is made by fetal scalp edema and/or ascites or other fetal edema noted by echocardiography. Congenital complete AV block without associated heart defects often is associated with maternal lupus.

Fetal supraventricular tachycardias cause hydrops more frequently than bradycardias do. Hy-

TABLE 13–13.  Categories of Presenting Symptoms in the Neonate

| Symptom | Physiologic Category | Anatomic Cause | Lesion |
| --- | --- | --- | --- |
| Cyanosis with respiratory distress | Increased pulmonary blood flow | Transposition | *d*-Transposition with or without associated lesions |
| Cyanosis without respiratory distress | Decreased pulmonary blood flow | Right heart obstruction | Tricuspid atresia<br>Ebstein anomaly<br>Pulmonary atresia<br>Pulmonary stenosis<br>Tetralogy of Fallot |
| Hypoperfusion | Poor cardiac output | Left heart obstruction | Total anomalous pulmonary venous return with obstruction<br>Aortic stenosis<br>Hypoplastic left heart syndrome<br>Coarctation of the aorta |
| | Poor cardiac function | Normal anatomy | Cardiomyopathy<br>Myocarditis |

drops can occur within 24 hr or less. Thus, rapid effective treatment is necessary. Initial treatment may be delivery if the fetus is mature. For less mature fetuses, drug treatment through the mother is used. Different antiarrhythmics pass through the placenta to the fetus with different fetal-maternal ratios. Digitalis has the advantages of a virtual 1:1 ratio, increasing contractility, and slowing conduction in the AV node to attempt to stop the tachycardia. It has the disadvantage of a relatively slow onset of action and a small therapeutic-toxic ratio in the fetus and mother. If the mechanism of the tachycardia is atrial re-entry (atrial flutter), digitalis also can result in 2:1 AV block, which tends to prevent hydrops as a result of a slower ventricular rate. If digitalis fails, other drugs may be used by giving them to the mother orally. If the fetus experiences hydrops, the drugs pass the placenta less well. The fetal umbilical vein may be cannulated and drugs given directly to the fetus. Amiodarone is particularly useful in this regard because it has a long half-life even when given intravenously. Very frequent follow-up using fetal ultrasound is used to control therapy.

The diagnosis of a severe congenital cardiac defect presents a bioethical dilemma. Most congenital cardiac defects now can at least be well palliated after birth. The decision between fetal termination and delivery of the infant and treatment of the heart defect is a difficult and individual decision.

## References

Behrman RE, Kliegman RM, Arvin AM (eds): Nelson Textbook of Pediatrics, 15th ed. Philadelphia, WB Saunders, 1992, 1996, Chapters 384–387.

Brook MM, Silverman NH, Villegas M: Cardiac ultrasound in structural abnormalities and arrhythmias: Recognition and treatment. West J Med 159:286, 1993.

Castaneda AR, Jonas RA, Mayer JE, et al: Cardiac Surgery of the Neonate and Infant. Philadelphia, WB Saunders, 1994.

Morban BC: Incidence, etiology, and classification of congenital heart disease. Pediatr Clin North Am 25:721, 1978.

Norwood WI, Pigott JD: Recent advances in congenital cardiac surgery. Clin Perinatol 15:713, 1988.

O'Kelly S, Bove E: Hypoplastic left heart syndrome. BMJ 314:87, 1997.

Perry SB, Keane JF, Locke JE: Pediatric interventions. In Baim DS, Grossman W (eds): Cardiac Catheterization, Angiography and Intervention. Baltimore, Williams & Wilkins, 1996.

Radford DJ, Thong YH: The association between immunodeficiency and congenital heart disease. Pediatr Cardiol 9:103, 1988.

Rao PS: Transcatheter therapy in pediatric cardiology. New York, Wiley-Liss, 1993.

Reddy VM, Liddicoat JR, Brook MM, et al: Results of a protocol of routine primary repair of tetralogy of Fallot in neonates and infants under 3 months of age. Ann Thorac Surg 60:S592, 1995.

Van Hare GF, Soffer LL, Sivakoff MC, et al: 25 year experience with ventricular septal defect. Am Heart J 114:606, 1987.

# CARDIOMYOPATHIES
## (Myocarditis)

The primary cardiomyopathies are conditions involving the myocardium. Invariably the problem for the patient is left ventricular dysfunction; however, biopsy data indicate that the RV also is involved. Most of these cardiomyopathies are of the dilated type, often called *congestive cardiomyopathy*. *Restrictive cardiomyopathies* are rare, as is the slightly more common *hypertrophic cardiomyopathy*.

Although many cases are considered idiopathic, specific etiologic factors are increasingly being discovered. Almost all the dilated cardiomyopathies can be categorized into three types (Table 13–14):

1. Myocarditis.
2. A primary cardiomyopathy, often familial, caused by various abnormalities of mitochondrial energy metabolism.
3. Those induced by drugs, particularly doxorubicin.

*Myocarditis* can occur at any age, including during the newborn period; it frequently is found to be related to a viral infection, such as echovirus or coxsackie B virus. The diagnosis is confirmed during the acute episode by a dilated large heart; severe heart failure, sometimes with shock; and marked ST segment abnormalities on the ECG. Before the era of intensive care units, children often died within 24 hr; if they survived when treated with digitalis and diuretics, they frequently recovered. Today, many patients survive as a result of intensive care with intubation, mechanical ventilation, positive inotropes, and various afterload-reducing drugs (see Table 13–6).

No specific *treatment* is available. Various anti-inflammatory regimens, including steroids, intravenous gamma globulin, and specific autoimmune therapy (such as anti-thymocyte globulin), have met with mixed success. Antiviral therapy is not yet available. Most of these children also appear to recover completely, but some develop severe chronic (dilated) cardiomyopathy. Some patients who gradually develop congestive (dilated) cardiomyopathy may have had asymptomatic viral myocarditis in the past, but others with this disorder have mitochondrial abnormalities and metabolic and familial disorders; fewer cases are being called idiopathic.

Another related concept is **endocardial fibrolastosis** (EFE); it is usually a secondary rather than a primary disorder. Occasionally, it is associated with a small LV and small, very abnormal aortic and mitral valves. However, it is also a nonspecific response to some cardiomyopathies. Primary endo-

TABLE 13–14. Etiology of Myocardial Disease

**Familial–Hereditary**

Duchenne muscular dystrophy
Other muscular dystrophies (Becker, limb girdle)
Myotonic dystrophy
Kearns-Sayre syndrome (progressive external ophthalmoplegia)
Friedreich ataxia
Hemochromatosis
Fabry disease
Pompe disease (glycogen storage)
Carnitine deficiency syndromes
Endocardial fibroelastosis
Mitochondrial myopathy syndromes
Familial restrictive cardiomyopathy
Familial hypertrophic cardiomyopathy
Familial dilated cardiomyopathy (dominant, recessive, X-linked)

**Infections (myocarditis)**

Viral (coxsackievirus, mumps, Epstein-Barr virus, influenza, parainfluenza, measles, varicella, HIV)
Rickettsiae (psittacosis, *Coxiella*, Rocky Mountain spotted fever)
Bacterial (diphtheria, *Mycoplasma*, meningococcus, leptospirosis, Lyme disease)
Parasitic (Chagas disease, toxoplasmosis, *Loa loa*)

**Metabolic, Nutritional, Endocrine**

Beriberi (thiamine deficiency)
Keshan disease (selenium deficiency)
Hypothyroidism
Hyperthyroidism
Carcinoid
Pheochromocytoma
Mitochondrial myopathies and oxidative respiratory chain defects
Type II, X-linked 3-methylglutaconic aciduria

**Connective Tissue—Granulomatous Disease**

SLE
Scleroderma
Churg-Strauss syndrome
Rheumatoid arthritis
Rheumatic fever
Sarcoidosis
Amyloidosis
Dermatomyositis

**Drugs–Toxins**

Doxorubicin (Adriamycin)
Ipecac
Iron overload (hemosiderosis)
Irradiation
Cocaine
Amphetamines

**Coronary Arteries**

Anomalous left coronary artery
Kawasaki disease

**Other**

Sickle cell anemia
Hypereosinophilic syndrome
Endomyocardial fibrosis
Asymmetric septal hypertrophy
Right ventricular dysplasia
Idiopathic

HIV = human immunodeficiency virus; SLE = systemic lupus erythematosus.

cardial fibroelastosis, in rare instances, may be seen in certain families and in infants with an anomalous left coronary artery arising from the pulmonary artery.

Patients with acute myocarditis may die. However, if they survive the difficult early period, they have an excellent chance for complete recovery. In contrast, patients with cardiomyopathy not caused by myocarditis have a poorer prognosis and are not likely to recover. Although some children may stabilize, others rapidly deteriorate. A heart transplant is the only useful therapy after unsuccessful treatment with regimens to manage congestive heart failure.

### References

Behrman RE, Kliegman RM, Arvin AM (eds): Nelson Textbook of Pediatrics, 15th ed. Philadelphia, WB Saunders, 1996, Chapters 392–396.

Burch M, Runciman M: Dilated cardiomyopathy. Arch Dis Child 74:479, 1996.
DeSa DJ: Isolated myocarditis in the first year. Arch Dis Child 60:484, 1985.
Drucker NA, Colan SD, Lewis AB, et al: γ-Globulin treatment of acute myocarditis in the pediatric population. Circulation 89:252, 1994.
Guenthard J, Wyler F, Flowler B, et al: Cardiomyopathy in respiratory chain disorders. Arch Dis Child 74:479, 1996.
Lie J: Myocarditis and endomyocardial biopsy in unexplained heart failure: A diagnosis in search of a disease. Ann Intern Med 109:525, 1988.

## ACUTE RHEUMATIC FEVER

Rheumatic fever was very common in the United States until the late 1960s and early 1970s, when a sharp decline in the incidence was reported; since the mid-1980s, multiple small outbreaks have been reported. Furthermore, acute rheumatic fever (ARF) remains very common in many developing nations. The most commonly affected group is children between 5 and 15 yr of age, but infants and adults also can be affected.

The *pathogenesis* is related to an immune reaction to untreated group A beta-hemolytic streptococcus infection. The serotype of the streptococcus and the genetically determined immune response of the host play a role in the development of acute rheumatic fever.

*Clinical Manifestations.* The wide variety of manifestations of the disease and the similarity to many other diseases may lead to difficulty in diagnosis. The Jones criteria are an attempt to improve diagnosis (Table 13–15). Typically, a child presents 2–6 wk after a pharyngitis with one or more of the major or minor manifestations of ARF as described in these criteria. Arthritis may be difficult to establish. Chorea and erythema marginatum usually are easy to identify, but subcutaneous nodules are not likely to be present unless the disease is obvious and chronic. Evidence of carditis

TABLE 13–15.    Major Criteria in the Jones System for Acute Rheumatic Fever*†

| Sign | Comments |
| --- | --- |
| Polyarthritis | Common: swelling, limited motion, very tender, erythema; migratory: involves large joints but rarely small or unusual joints, such as vertebrae |
| Carditis | Common: pancarditis, valves, pericardium, myocardium; tachycardia greater than explained by fever; new murmur of mitral or aortic insufficiency; Carey Coombs mid-diastolic murmur; heart failure |
| Chorea (Sydenham disease) | Uncommon: presents long after infection has resolved; more common in females; antineuronal antibody positive |
| Erythema marginatum | Uncommon: pink macules on trunk and proximal extremities, evolving to serpiginous border with central clearing; evanescent, elicited by application of local heat; nonpruritic |
| Subcutaneous nodules | Uncommon: associated with repeated episodes and severe carditis; present over extensor surface of elbows, knees, knuckles, and ankles or scalp and spine; firm, nontender |

*Minor criteria include fever (101°–102°F [38.2°–38.9°C]), arthralgias, previous rheumatic fever, leukocytosis, elevated erythrocyte sedimentation rate/C-reactive protein, prolonged PR interval.

†One major plus two minor, or two major criteria with evidence of recent group A streptococcal disease (scarlet fever, positive throat culture, or elevated antistreptolysin O or other antistreptococcal antibodies), strongly suggests the diagnosis of acute rheumatic fever.

is very reliable in the hands of experienced physicians. The PR interval widening is a weak minor criterion because it is nonspecific; if it varies with time (hourly), it is helpful. Varying QRS voltage in the chest leads provides a strong minor criterion if the voltages are measured daily. The presence of a new murmur is very strong evidence for carditis, although overdiagnosis is common because auscultation is not always specific.

For carditis of acute rheumatic fever to be diagnosed on the basis of heart murmur, the murmur must be one of the following:

1. The murmur of mitral regurgitation, a murmur that may be as soft as grade 2, is high frequency, does not necessarily start with $S_1$, usually is almost full length, peaks late, and is best heard at the apex.
2. The murmur of aortic regurgitation, a high-frequency diastolic decrescendo murmur at the 3rd–5th left interspace of any intensity or length, with or without a wide pulse pressure.
3. A mid-diastolic rumbling murmur at the apex, the Carey Coombs murmur, believed to result from edema of the mitral valve.

Finally, the erythrocyte sedimentation rate (ESR) usually is elevated in ARF. Proof of streptococcal infection is critical to the diagnosis. The echocardiographic delineation of mild mitral regurgitation is not diagnostic.

Chronic rheumatic heart disease produces a specific lesion: (1) mitral regurgitation, (2) mitral stenosis, (3) mitral stenosis with mitral regurgitation, (4) aortic regurgitation, or (5) aortic regurgitation with aortic stenosis. Rarely, the tricuspid valve is involved. The pulmonary valve is not known to be involved, and pure or dominant aortic stenosis does not occur.

In pure mitral regurgitation, the mid-diastolic low-frequency murmur does not extend into late diastole. When pure mitral stenosis (and sinus rhythm) is present, the diastolic low-frequency murmur extends into late diastole, often with presystolic accentuation. If mitral regurgitation with stenosis is present, a long diastolic murmur extending into late diastole also is present. Aortic regurgitation may distort the anterior leaflet of the mitral valve as the blood leaks back into the LV, resulting in the low-frequency mid-diastolic murmur called the *Austin Flint murmur.*

*Treatment.* Management consists almost entirely of nonspecific measures: (1) bed rest, (2) penicillin to eradicate the beta-hemolytic streptococcus, and (3) aspirin for the arthritic pain. Steroids have not proved effective in minimizing valve damage, and they should not be used except for patients with severe life-threatening carditis.

Once the diagnosis is made, whether or not valvulitis is present, permanent penicillin prophylaxis is essential. Intramuscular penicillin G benzathine (Bicillin) given every 28 days is more reliable than low-dose oral penicillin given twice a day. Patients following a continuous Bicillin regimen for 10 yr usually improve; only 30% of patients with mitral regurgitation on initial evaluation still have a murmur, although fewer patients with aortic regurgitation lose the murmur. Few treated patients develop mitral stenosis, but poor compliance is associated with the development of mitral stenosis. The development of a stenotic valvular lesion probably is usually due to repeated episodes of acute rheumatic fever. Prevention of such attacks with penicillin should eliminate this late sequela.

Treatment of valve disease includes balloon valvotomy, valve replacement, and vigilant antimicrobial prophylaxis to prevent bacterial endocarditis.

### References

Behrman RE, Kliegman RM, Arvin AM (eds): Nelson Textbook of Pediatrics, 15th ed. Philadelphia, WB Saunders, 1996, Chapter 392.

Guidelines for the diagnosis of rheumatic fever. Jones Criteria, 1992 update. Special Writing Group of the Committee on Rheumatic Fever, Endocarditis, and Kawasaki Disease of the Council on Cardiovascular Disease in the Young of the American Heart Association. JAMA 268:2069, 1992.

Markowitz M: Rheumatic fever in the eighties. Pediatr Clin North Am 33:1141, 1986.

Veasy L, Wiedmeier S, Orsmond G, et al: Resurgence of acute rheumatic fever in the intermountain area of the United States. N Engl J Med 316:421, 1987.

## PERICARDITIS

Pericardial diseases and inflammatory responses of the pericardium may be caused by common and

**TABLE 13–16.**  Etiology of Pericarditis and Pericardial Effusion

| | |
|---|---|
| **Idiopathic (Presumed Viral)** | **Traumatic** |
| **Infectious Agents** | Cardiac contusion (blunt trauma) |
| *Bacteria:* group A streptococcus, *Staphylococcus aureus*, pneumococcus, meningococcus,* *Haemophilus influenzae*,* *Salmonella* species, *Mycoplasma pneumoniae*, *Borrelia burgdorferi*, *Mycobacterium tuberculosis*, rickettsia, tularemia | Penetrating trauma  Postpericardiotomy syndrome  Radiation |
| | **Contiguous Spread** |
| *Viral:*† coxsackievirus (group A, B), echovirus, mumps, influenza, Epstein-Barr, cytomegalovirus, herpes simplex, herpes zoster, hepatitis B | Pleural disease  Pneumonia  Aortic aneurysm (dissecting) |
| *Fungal:* *Histoplasma capsulatum*, *Coccidioides immitis*, *Blastomyces dermatitidis*, *Cryptococcus neoformans*, *Candida* species, *Aspergillus* species | **Metabolic**  Hypothyroidism  Uremia  Gaucher disease  Fabry disease |
| *Parasitic:* *Toxoplasma gondii*, *Entamoeba histolytica*, schistosomes | Chylopericardium |
| **Collagen Vascular–Inflammatory and Granulomatous Diseases** | **Neoplastic** |
| Rheumatic fever | Primary |
| Systemic lupus erythematosus (idiopathic and drug-induced) | Contiguous (lymphoma) |
| Rheumatoid arthritis | Metastatic |
| Kawasaki disease | Infiltrative (leukemia) |
| Scleroderma | |
| Mixed connective tissue disease | **Others** |
| Reiter syndrome | Drug reaction |
| Inflammatory bowel disease | Pancreatitis |
| Wegener granulomatosis | After myocardial infarction |
| Dermatomyositis | Thalassemia |
| Behçet syndrome | Central venous catheter perforation |
| Sarcoidosis | Heart failure |
| Vasculitis | Hemorrhage (coagulopathy) |
| Familial Mediterranean fever | Biliary-pericardial fistula |
| Serum sickness | |
| Stevens-Johnson syndrome | |

From Sigman G: Chest pain. *In* Kliegman RM, Nieder ML, Super DM (eds): Practical Strategies in Pediatric Diagnosis and Therapy. Philadelphia, WB Saunders, 1996, p 192.

*Infectious or immune complex.

†Common (viral pericarditis or myopericarditis is probably the most common cause of acute pericarditis in a previously normal host).

## TABLE 13–17.  Manifestations of Pericarditis

**Symptoms**

Chest pain (worsened if lying down or with inspiration)
Dyspnea
Malaise
Patient assumes sitting position

**Signs**

*Nonconstrictive*

Fever
Tachycardia
Friction rub (accentuated by inspiration, body position)
Enlarged heart by percussion
Distant heart sounds

*Tamponade: as above plus*

Distended neck veins
Hepatomegaly
Pulsus paradoxus (greater than 10 mm Hg with
 inspiration)
Narrow pulse pressure
Weak pulse, poor peripheral perfusion

*Constrictive Pericarditis*

Distended neck veins
Kussmaul sign (inspiratory increase of jugular venous
 pressure)
Distant heart sounds
Pericardial knock
Hepatomegaly
Ascites
Edema
Tachycardia

uncommon disorders. Inflammatory processes, such as viral or bacterial infections and immune-mediated disease (postinfectious immune complexes, connective tissue diseases, the presence of autoantibody), are the most common pathogenic

## TABLE 13–18.  Laboratory Evidence of Pericarditis

| ECG | Elevated ST segments, T wave inversion (late), tachycardia, reduced QRS voltage, electrical alternans (variable QRS amplitudes) |
|---|---|
| Chest roentgenogram | Cardiomegaly ("water bottle heart") |
| Echocardiogram | Pericardial fluid |
| Pericardiocentesis | Gram and acid-fast stains, culture (virus, bacteria, mycobacteria, fungus). Cytology, cell count, glucose, protein, pH |
| Blood tests | ESR, viral titers, ANA, ASO titers, EBV titers |

ANA = antinuclear antibodies; ASO = antistreptolysin O; EBV = Epstein-Barr virus; ECG = electroencephalogram; ESR = erythrocyte sedimentation rate.

mechanisms in pediatric patients. Other causes include uremia, hypothyroidism, trauma, postpericardiotomy, and malignancy (Table 13–16).

The *clinical manifestations* of pericarditis as it progresses from a simple inflammatory response of the pericardium with no cardiovascular compromise to cardiac tamponade and constrictive pericarditis are noted in Table 13–17. *Laboratory diagnosis* is obtained by evaluation of the ECG and chest roentgenogram but is confirmed by echocardiography and eventually by examination of the pericardial fluid obtained by pericardiocentesis (Table 13–18).

*Treatment* is directed at the underlying disease process, alleviation of pericardial fluid accumulation by pericardiocentesis or pericardial drainage, or surgical stripping of the pericardium in patients with constrictive pericarditis.

### References

Behrman RE, Kliegman RM, Arvin AM (eds): Nelson Textbook of Pediatrics, 15th ed. Philadelphia, WB Saunders, 1996, Chapter 397.
Brook I, Frazier E: Microbiology of acute purulent pericarditis. Arch Intern Med 156:1857, 1996.
Sinzobahamvya N, Ikeogu MO: Purulent pericarditis. Arch Dis Child 62:696, 1987.

## INFECTIVE ENDOCARDITIS
(See Chapter 10)

Bacterial endocarditis is infrequent in pediatric patients and occurs on native valves, valves damaged by rheumatic fever, congenitally abnormal valves, acquired valvular lesions (mitral valve prolapse), and prosthetic replacement valves and as a consequence of jet streams of turbulent blood (PDA, VSD, systemic-to-pulmonary shunts). A listing of predisposing factors for the preceding bacteremia, laboratory tests, and *clinical manifestations* of bacterial endocarditis is presented in Table 13–19. Because of the endovascular nature of endocarditis, bacteremia is usually of a continuous nature, may be low grade (few bacteria per milliliter of blood) and is not necessarily altered during episodes of fever or chills. Therefore, the volume of the blood culture probably is more important than the frequency of obtaining specimens for culture. The pathogens responsible for endocarditis depend on the status of the heart valve and the presence or absence of a predisposing procedure. Because some bacterial agents have unusual nutritional requirements and others may need longer than the usual incubation period to demonstrate growth in vitro, the blood samples should be labeled, so that when endocarditis is suspected, the sample can be

**TABLE 13–19.** Manifestations of Infective
Endocarditis

**History**

Prior congenital or rheumatic heart disease
Preceding dental, urinary, or intestinal procedure
Intravenous drug abuse
Central venous catheter
Prosthetic heart valve

**Symptoms**

Fever
Chills
Chest pain
Arthralgia/myalgia
Dyspnea
Malaise

**Signs**

Fever
Tachycardia
Embolic phenomena (Roth spots, petechiae, Osler
nodes, CNS lesion)
Janeway lesions
New or changing murmur
Splenomegaly
Arthritis
Heart failure
Arrhythmias

**Laboratory Tests**

Positive blood culture
Elevated ESR, C-reactive protein
Leukocytosis
Immune complexes
Rheumatoid factor
Hematuria
Echocardiographic evidence of valve vegetations

CNS = central nervous system; ESR = erythrocyte sedimentation
rate.

observed for a longer time. Despite adequate blood culture techniques, 10–15% of cases of endocarditis are culture negative.

*Treatment* of culture-negative patients requires knowledge of the epidemiology and historic risk factors for that patient. Treatment of culture-positive patients is directed against the particular bacteria (e.g., *Staphylococcus aureus, Streptococcus viridans,* enterococcus, HACEK group bacteria) using bactericidal antibiotics. Therapy is continued for 4–8 wk. Surgery is indicated if medical treatment is unsuccessful or for an unusual pathogen, myocardial abscess formation, refractory heart failure, serious embolic complications, or refractory prosthetic valve disease.

*Prevention* of endocarditis is necessary for all patients with (1) structural congenital heart disease, (2) rheumatic valve lesions, (3) prosthetic heart valves, (4) mitral valve prolapse with a regurgitant valve, (5) idiopathic hypertrophic subaortic stenosis, (6) transvenous pacemaker leads, (7) surgical systemic-to-pulmonary shunts or (8) previous endocarditis. Antimicrobial prophylaxis is not indicated for an isolated secundum ASD, a repaired secundum ASD 6 mo after patch placement, or a divided and ligated PDA 6 mo after repair. Antibiotic regimens to prevent endocarditis during dental or respiratory procedures include oral amoxicillin or parenteral ampicillin plus gentamicin. The latter recommendation is for high-risk patients, such as those with prosthetic heart valves, systemic-to-pulmonary shunts, or previous endocarditis. Preventive treatment for gastrointestinal or genitourinary manipulation includes parenteral ampicillin and gentamicin or oral amoxicillin. Vancomycin can be added to gentamicin in patients who are allergic to penicillin (see Appendix I).

## References

Behrman RE, Kliegman RM, Arvin AM (eds): Nelson Textbook of Pediatrics, 15th ed. Philadelphia, WB Saunders, 1996, Chapter 390.
Hogevik H, Olaison L, Andersson R, et al: Epidemiologic aspects of infective endocarditis in an urban population. Medicine 74:324, 1995.
Kavey RE, Frank DM, Byrum CJ, et al: Two-dimensional echocardiographic assessment of infective endocarditis in children. Am J Dis Child 137:851, 1983.
Sanyal SK, Saleh MA, Abu-Melha A: Infective endocarditis during infancy and childhood: Current status. Indian J Pediatr 55:51, 1988.
Van Hare G, Ben-Shachar G, Liebman J, et al: Infective endocarditis in infants and children during the past 10 years: A decade of change. Am Heart J 107:1235, 1984.

# DYSRHYTHMIAS

Cardiac dysrhythmias are a frequent occurrence in children. A dysrhythmia is an abnormal rhythm; the term *arrhythmia* often is used as a synonym. The diverse causes are presented in Table 13–20 and the common types and their treatment in Table 13–21. Many pediatric dysrhythmias do not present a risk to the patient and are normal variants.

Some cardiac abnormalities are subtle, such as the prolonged QT interval, arrhythmogenic right ventricular dysplasia, and mild cardiomyopathy or myocarditis. Ventricular dysrhythmias that require treatment usually are treated with antiarrhythmic drugs (Table 13–22). A specific treatable etiology rarely is found. Infants and young children ($\leq 4$ yr) are the exception, often having small tumors that can be treated with surgery.

## SINUS ARRHYTHMIA AND WANDERING ATRIAL PACEMAKER

These are phasic variations with respiration that are heard in virtually all normal children. They are

## TABLE 13–20.  Etiology of Arrhythmias

**Drugs**

   Intoxication (cocaine, tricyclic antidepressants, others)
   Antiarrhythmic agents (proarrhythmic agents, e.g.,
      quinidine)
   Sympathomimetic agents (caffeine, theophylline,
      ephedrine, others)
   Digoxin

**Infection/Postinfection**

   Endocarditis
   Lyme disease
   Diphtheria
   Myocarditis
   Guillain-Barré syndrome
   Rheumatic fever

**Metabolic–Endocrine**

   Cardiomyopathy
   Electrolyte disturbances ($\downarrow$ $\uparrow K^+$, $\downarrow$ $\uparrow Ca^{2+}$,
      $\downarrow Mg^{2+}$)
   Uremia
   Thyrotoxicosis
   Pheochromocytoma
   Porphyria
   Mitochondrial myopathies

**Structural Lesions**

   Mitral valve prolapse
   Ventricular tumor
   Ventriculotomy
   Pre-excitation/aberrant conduction system (Wolff-
      Parkinson-White syndrome)
   Congenital heart defects
   Arrhythmogenic right ventricle (dysplasia)

**Other Causes**

   Adrenergic-induced
   Prolonged QT interval
   Maternal SLE
   Idiopathic
   Central venous catheter

SLE = systemic lupus erythematosus.

accentuated in athletic children and diminished during most illnesses. Sinus arrhythmia is differentiated from wandering atrial pacemaker by the continuous normal morphology of the P wave preceding each QRS complex in the former compared to the continuously changing P wave morphology in the latter (see Fig. 13–5). These two arrhythmias are thought to be controlled by an interaction of the vagal and sympathetic divisions of the autonomic nervous system.

## PREMATURE BEATS

*Premature atrial contractions* (PACs) are common in fetuses, neonates, and infants and less so in children. They often are of little concern. If they are extremely frequent or early in the cardiac cycle,

they may predispose the neonate to atrial flutter. PACs often decrease in frequency very rapidly after birth; thus a short period of observation plus parental counseling about the presentation and significance of atrial flutter in a neonate may be all that is necessary. If a PAC occurs after each sinus beat and if it fails to conduct to the ventricle (a blocked PAC), a relative bradycardia develops. Thus, the ST segment and T wave should be searched for blocked PACs in bradycardic neonates. If the PACs do not stop or decrease, treatment with digoxin may suppress them. In any case, it does not worsen the bradycardia.

*Premature ventricular contractions* (PVCs) are more common in adolescents and are found infrequently in neonates or infants. Benign PVCs are single (i.e., not two or three consecutively), uniform, disappear with exercise, and occur in patients with normal hearts. Any deviations require extensive evaluation. Bigeminal patterns and frequent PVCs are not considered deviations from benignness, nor is the R-on-T phenomenon. Benign PVCs of childhood do not cause serious dysrhythmias but are present at 5 yr follow-up in 50% of patients. Multiform PVCs, triplets or longer runs, and any type of cardiac abnormality are associated with more sustained dysrhythmias and symptoms, syncope, and death.

## SUPRAVENTRICULAR TACHYCARDIA

Supraventricular tachycardia (SVT) is the most frequent sustained dysrhythmia in pediatrics. Although SVT is not immediately life-threatening, it can lead to serious symptoms if it persists. It most commonly occurs in neonates and infants but also is common in fetuses and older children. The mechanism is usually re-entry, although enhanced automaticity accounts for 5–10% of cases. Re-entry most often involves an accessory connection (bundle of Kent) but may occur in the AV node, sinus node, or atrial muscle (atrial flutter).

Pediatric SVT is characterized by a rate of greater than 210 bpm, a normal narrow QRS complex, and extreme regularity. If the QRS complex is even slightly wide or abnormal in morphology, the diagnosis is likely ventricular tachycardia. There is usually a 1:1 relationship between the atrium and ventricle, but the atrium can be either faster (atrial flutter) or slower (junctional automaticity).

The initial *treatment* of pediatric SVT involves enhancing vagal tone by the diving reflex (see Table 13–21). This involves applying a cold stimulus to the face. If this fails to convert, intravenous adenosine usually is effective at a dose of 100–250

TABLE 13–21.    Arrhythmias in Children

| Type | ECG Characteristics | Treatment |
|---|---|---|
| Complete heart block | Atria and ventricles have independent pacemakers; atrioventricular (AV) dissociation; escape-pacemaker is at atrioventricular junction if congenital | Awake rate <55 beats/min in neonate or <40 beats/min in adolescent or hemodynamic instability requires permanent pacemaker |
| First-degree heart block | Prolonged PR interval for age | Observe, obtain digoxin level if on therapy |
| Mobitz type I (Wenckebach) second-degree heart block | Progressive lengthening of PR interval until P wave is not followed by conducted QRS complex | Observe, correct underlying electrolyte or other abnormalities |
| Mobitz type II second-degree heart block | Sudden nonconduction of P wave with loss of QRS complex without progressive PR interval lengthening | Consider pacemaker |
| Sinus tachycardia | Rate less than 240 beats/min | Treat fever, remove sympathomimetic drugs |
| Supraventricular tachycardia | Rate usually greater than 200 beats/min (180–320); abnormal atrial rate for age; ventricular rate may be slower due to AV block; P waves usually present and are related to QRS complex; normal QRS complexes unless aberrant conduction is present | Increase vagal tone (bag of ice water to face, Valsalva maneuver); adenosine; digoxin; electrical cardioversion if acutely ill; catheter ablation |
| Atrial flutter | Atrial rate usually 300 beats/min, with varying degrees of block; sawtooth flutter waves | Digoxin, cardioversion |
| Premature ventricular contraction (PVC) | Premature, wide, unusually shaped QRS complex, with large inverted T wave | None if normal heart and PVCs disappear on exercise; Lidocaine, procainamide, quinidine |
| Ventricular tachycardia | Three or more premature ventricular beats; AV dissociation; fusion beats, blocked retrograde AV conduction; sustained if longer than 30 sec; rate 120–240 beats/min | Lidocaine, cardioversion, procainamide, propranolol, bretylium, phenytoin |
| Ventricular fibrillation | No distinct QRS complex or T waves; irregular undulations with varied amplitude and contour; no conducted pulse | Nonsynchronized cardioversion |

TABLE 13–22.    Classification of Drugs for Antiarrhythmia

| Class | Action | Examples |
|---|---|---|
| I | Depresses phase O depolarization (velocity of upstroke of action potential); sodium channel blockers | |
| Ia | Prolongs QRS complex and QT interval | Quinidine, procainamide, disopyramide |
| Ib | Significant effect on abnormal conduction | Lidocaine, mexiletine, phenytoin, tocainide |
| Ic | Prolongs QRS complex and PR interval | Flecainide, propafenone, moricizine? |
| II | Beta-blockade, sinus rate slowing, prolonged PR interval | Propranolol, atenolol, acebutolol |
| III | Prolonged action potential; prolonged PR, QT intervals, QRS complex; sodium and calcium channel blocker | Bretylium, amiodarone, sotalol |
| IV | Calcium channel blockade; reduced sinus and AV node pacemaker activity and conduction; prolonged PR interval | Verapamil and other calcium channel blocking agents |

μg/kg. In patients in whom the AV node or sinus node is not part of the re-entry circuit, adenosine may only temporarily (5–10 sec) slow the rate by creating AV block. Atrial overdrive pacing (intra-atrial or transesophageal) often is effective in atrial re-entry tachycardia. Pacing also can be used to create temporary AV block and stabilize the blood pressure. Direct-current synchronized cardioversion at 0.25–1 W·S/kg is the gold standard for converting resistant re-entrant tachycardias.

Once SVT is converted in a child, there is an approximately 90% chance it will recur; therefore, prophylactic pharmacologic therapy is warranted for 6–12 mo. In patients with manifest **Wolff-Parkinson-White syndrome**, digitalis often is not used for fear of precipitating a worse dysrhythmia; otherwise, it is the drug of choice. Propranolol and verapamil also may be used orally in older children.

In cases of SVT that are resistant to medical therapy or that have life-threatening components (Wolff-Parkinson-White syndrome), or when the patient does not want to take medication, the dysrhythmogenic substrate frequently (90%) can be destroyed by catheter ablation.

### BRADYDYSRHYTHMIAS

These dysrhythmias may be congenital, surgically acquired, or, rarely, caused by infection (see Table 13–20). The surgically acquired type is by far the most common. Despite improving knowledge of the location of the heart's electrical system in various heart defects and improving surgical results, both acute and chronic abnormalities of the conduction system and the sinus node occur. Modern pacemakers and leads have greatly improved treatment of these problems.

Congenital complete AV block is often due to maternal systemic lupus erythematosus, with antibodies to the fetal cardiac conduction system crossing the placenta. Association with morphologic cardiac defects is the other common etiologic factor.

#### References

Behrman RE, Kliegman RM, Arvin AM (eds): Nelson Textbook of Pediatrics. 15th ed. Philadelphia, WB Saunders, 1996, Chapters 388–389.

Campbell R, Jammon J, Echt D, Graham T: Surgical treatment of pediatric cardiac arrhythmias. J Pediatr 110:501, 1987.

Committee on Sports Medicine and Fitness: Cardiac dysrhythmias and sports. Pediatrics 95:786, 1995.

Dick M, Scott WA, Serwer GS, et al: Acute termination of supraventricular tachyarrhythmias in children by transesophageal atrial pacing. Am J Cardiol 61:925, 1988.

Kugler J, Danford D: Management of infants, children, and adolescents with paroxysmal supraventricular tachycardia. J Pediatr 129:324, 1996.

Zales VR, Dunnigan A, Benson DW, Jr: Clinical and electrophysiologic features of fetal and neonatal paroxysmal atrial tachycardia resulting in congestive heart failure. Am J Cardiol 62:22, 1988.

### SUDDEN DEATH

Sudden death is a rare but important problem in pediatrics. Most pediatric sudden deaths occur in patients with known heart disease. Unoperated congenital heart disease used to be a prime cause. Because most congenital heart defects now are repaired or palliated early in life, postoperative dysrhythmias are assuming increasing importance. A combination of earlier, more precise repairs with improved myocardial protection and postoperative screening for dysrhythmias, together with pacemaker and medical treatment, has improved the outlook for postoperative patients.

Infrequently, a child without known heart disease dies suddenly from anomalous coronary arteries, aortic stenosis, arrhythmias, myocarditis, or cardiomyopathy (usually hypertrophic). This often occurs in relation to athletics. Many of these deaths probably could be prevented by including a screening ECG with a proper preparticipation history (syncope, dizziness, chest pain, external dyspnea) and physical examination, although this would be expensive. Attention to the symptoms of exercise-related symptoms could prevent many others. Drug use (cocaine, alcohol, tricyclic antidepressants, heroin) must also be considered.

### CHEST PAIN IN CHILDHOOD AND ADOLESCENCE

Chest pain among pediatric patients usually does not represent serious cardiovascular disease as it does in adult patients. Many patients are preadolescents or adolescents who have pain at rest of noncardiac origin (Table 13–23). A careful history (including family history), physical examination, and screening laboratory tests are indicated to reassure the patient and family. These tests should be based on the history and physical findings and should be directed to musculoskeletal, pulmonary, gastrointestinal, or cardiac signs and symptoms. Chest pain suggestive of cardiac pain that is associated with syncope, exertional dyspnea, or an irregular pulse requires more detailed evaluation, such as 24-hr continuous ECG monitoring (Holter monitor).

Chest pain is a very frequent symptom in chil-

TABLE 13–23. Differential Diagnosis of Pediatric Chest Pain

| Musculoskeletal (common) | Gastrointestinal (rare) | Idiopathic (common) |
|---|---|---|
| Trauma (accidental, abuse) | Esophagitis (gastroesophageal reflux) | Anxiety, hyperventilation |
| Exercise, overuse injury (strain, bursitis) | Esophageal foreign body | Panic disorder |
| Tietze syndrome | Esophageal spasm | **Other** (rare) |
| Costochondritis | Esophageal rupture | Spinal cord or nerve root compression |
| Herpes zoster (cutaneous) | Cholecystitis | Breast-related pathology |
| Pleurodynia | Subdiaphragmatic abscess | Castleman disease (lymph node neoplasm) |
| Sickle cell anemia vaso-occlusive crisis | Perihepatitis (Fitz-Hugh–Curtis syndrome) | |
| Osteomyelitis (rare) | Peptic ulcer disease | |
| Primary or metastatic tumor (rare) | Pancreatitis | |
| Fibrositis | **Cardiac** (rare) | |
| Slipping rib | Pericarditis (see Table 13-16) | |
| **Pulmonary** (common) | Postpericardiotomy syndrome | |
| Pneumonia | Endocarditis | |
| Pleurisy | Mitral valve prolapse (uncertain cause) | |
| Asthma | Aortic stenosis (angina) | |
| Chronic cough | Arrhythmias | |
| Pneumothorax, pneumomediastinum | Hypertrophic cardiomyopathy | |
| Infarction (sickle cell anemia) | Marfan syndrome (dissecting aortic aneurysm) | |
| Foreign body | Anomalous coronary artery (angina) | |
| Embolism (rare) | Kawasaki disease (angina) | |
| Pulmonary hypertension (rare) | Cocaine, sympathomimetic ingestion (angina) | |
| Tumor (rare) | Familial hypercholesterolemia (angina) | |

From Sigman G: Chest pain. *In* Kliegman RM, Nieder ML, Super DM (eds): Practical Strategies in Pediatric Diagnosis and Therapy. Philadelphia, WB Saunders, 1996, p 184.

dren as it is in adults. The most frequent cause of cardiac chest pain may be pericarditis. It usually is associated with a febrile illness, and the young age of a patient may result in the chest pain being expressed nonspecifically. Exercise-induced chest pain may indicate exercise-induced asthma, but it rarely may indicate cardiac disease, including coronary artery anomalies. The chest wall is a common cause of chest pain in children. The diagnosis of **costochondritis** may be confirmed by a finding of tenderness of one or more costochondral joints. Esophagogastritis is another frequent cause of chest pain in children. The "pleuritic catch" may be the most frequent benign cause of chest pain in children; it is brief but may recur for years. The popularization of this important symptom in the mass media in an attempt to help recognize coronary artery disease also may confuse children and their parents. Children with chest pain may be mimicking their parents or grandparents.

## CARDIAC PAIN IN INFANCY

Cardiac pain may be due to an **anomalous origin of the left coronary artery** from the pulmonary artery.

The *clinical manifestations* include marked irritability, pallor, diaphoresis, apnea, or shock during or following nursing. These paroxysmal episodes of discomfort are similar to attacks of angina pectoris in adults. Heart failure may develop from poor myocardial performance. There usually is no murmur unless mitral regurgitation is present as a result of papillary muscle ischemia. If there are large collateral vessels (a left-to-right shunt through the coronary artery to the pulmonary arteries), a continuous murmur may be present, but these children usually are not ill. Thus, the *diagnosis* often is made after infancy.

*Laboratory evidence* reveals ECG signs of myocardial ischemia or infarction. Cardiomegaly is present on chest roentgenogram, and the echocardiogram and angiography reveal the anomalous coronary artery. The *differential diagnosis* includes SVT, myocarditis, and cardiomyopathy.

*Treatment* of the acute condition includes oxygen, intravenous inotropic agents, and morphine. Surgical ligation of the artery at its origin from the pulmonary artery may be successful if there are a large left-to-right shunt during systole and diastole, absence of ischemic ECG changes, and large collateral vessels. Other operative procedures in-

TABLE 13–24. Syncope and Dizziness: Etiology

| Diagnosis | History | Symptoms | Description | Heart Rate/Blood Pressure | Duration | Postsyncope | Recurrence |
|---|---|---|---|---|---|---|---|
| **Neurocardiogenic (Vasodepressor)** | At rest | Pallor, nausea, visual changes | Brief ± convulsion | ↓/↓ | <1 min | Residual pallor, sweaty, hot; recurs if child stands | Common |
| **Other Vagal** | | | | | | | |
| Vasovagal | Needlestick | Pallor, nausea | Brief; convulsions rare | ↓/↓ | <1 min | Residual pallor; may recur if child stands | Situational |
| Micturition | Post-voiding | Pallor, nausea | Brief ± convulsion | ↓/↓ | <1 min | Fatigue or baseline | (+) |
| Cough (deglutition) | Paroxysmal cough | Cough | Abrupt onset | May not change | <5 min | Fatigue or baseline | (+) |
| Carotid sinus | Tight collar, turned head | Vague, visual changes | Sudden onset, pallor | Usually ↓/↓ | <5 min | | (+) |
| **Hypoglycemia** | Fasting, insulin use | Gradual hunger, weakness, sweating | Pallor, sweating, loss of consciousness rare | No change or mild tachycardia | Variable | Relieved by eating only | (+) |
| **Neuropsychiatric** | | | | | | | |
| Hyperventilation | Anxiety | SOB, fear, claustrophobia | Agitated, hyperpneic | Mild ↓/→ | <5 min | Fatigue or baseline | (+) |
| Syncopal migraine | Headache | Aura, migraine, nausea | ± Pallor | No change | <10 min | Headache, often occipital | (+) |
| Seizure disorder | Anytime | ± Aura | Convulsion ± incontinence | No change or mild tachycardia | Any duration | Postictal lethargy + confusion | (+) |
| Hysterical | Always an "audience" present | Psychologic distress | Gentle, graceful swoon | No change | Any duration | Normal baseline | (+) |
| Breath-holding (hypoxic) | Agitation or injury | Crying | Cyanosis ± convulsion | ↓/↓ Frequent asystole | <10 min | Fatigue, residual pallor | (+) |
| **Cardiac Syncope** | | | | | | | |
| LVOT obstruction | Exercise | ± Chest pain, SOB | Abrupt during or after exertion, pallor | ↑/→ | Any duration | Fatigue, residual pallor, and sweating | (+) |
| Pulmonary hypertension | Anytime, especially exercise | SOB | Cyanosis and pallor | ↑/→ | Any duration | Fatigue, residual cyanosis | (+) |
| Myocarditis | Post-viral exercise | SOB, chest pain, palpitations | Pallor | ↑/→ | Any duration | Fatigue | (+) |
| Tumor or mass | Recumbent, paroxysmal | SOB ± chest pain | Pallor | ↑/→ | Any duration | Baseline | (+) |
| Coronary artery | Exercise | SOB ± chest pain | Pallor | ↑/→ | Any duration | Fatigue, chest pain | (+) |
| Dysrhythmia | Anytime | Palpitations ± chest pain | Pallor | ↑ or ↓/→ | Usually <10 min | Fatigue or baseline | (+) |

From Lewis DA: Syncope and dizziness. In Kliegman RM, Nieder ML, Super DM (eds): Practical Strategies in Pediatric Diagnosis and Therapy. Philadelphia, WB Saunders, 1996, p 680. LVOT = left ventricular outflow obstruction; SOB = shortness of breath; ± = with or without.

clude transplantation of a cuff of the pulmonary artery with the coronary ostium to the subclavian artery or aorta. The *prognosis* is poor because of myocardial ischemia and severe heart failure.

## SYNCOPE

Syncope is an increasingly important symptom in cardiologic and neurologic evaluation. It has been estimated that two thirds of children will have syncope. Most importantly, it can be a precursor to sudden death. In this instance, there usually is associated diagnosable heart disease. The second type of important syncope is *vasodepressor (neurocardiogenic) syncope*, which, although it does not lead to death, is very frequent. There are many other causes of syncope (dehydration, viral illness), and the presence of heart disease and exercise induction of the syncope are helpful to distinguish the rare patient who needs treatment from the majority with benign transient syncope (Table 13–24).

When the heart ceases effective function, either syncope or seizures may develop. Thus, some pediatric patients with seizures also should be evaluated for syncope. Several cardiological diseases, including the *long QT syndrome* and *hypertrophic cardiomyopathy*, frequently cause syncope. The evaluation of syncope should include a detailed history, including family history. Physical examination may reveal signs of heart disease. ECG and echocardiography are useful in diagnosing electrical and structural heart disease.

In the patient having recurrent syncope with a normal heart, testing of the response of the autonomic nervous system to assuming the upright posture is useful. If a cardiac cause of syncope is found, it should be treated directly. If vasodepressor syncope is diagnosed by autonomic testing, it may be treated by salt and fludrocortisone or beta-blockers. Treatment of vasodepressor syncope usually is temporary. The rare form of autonomic syncope, *cardioinhibitory syncope*, may require a combination of pacemaker and medical treatment.

### References

Brenner JI, Ringel RE, Berman MA: Cardiologic perspectives of chest pain in childhood: A referral problem? To whom? Pediatr Clin North Am 31:1241, 1984.

Liberthson R: Sudden death from cardiac causes in children and young adults. N Engl J Med 334:1039, 1996.

Selbst S: Chest pain in children. Pediatrics 75:1068, 1985.

# HEMATOLOGY

J. Paul Scott

Hematologic disorders are caused by quantitative or qualitative abnormalities of the formed elements of the blood, of the circulating proteins, or of the vascular wall. Diseases of the blood are either congenital or acquired. Hereditary abnormalities in molecular structure may lead to decreased stem cell production (Fanconi anemia), abnormal cell membrane function (hereditary spherocytosis, Glanzmann thrombasthenia), deficiency of an essential enzyme (glucose-6-phosphate dehydrogenase [G6PD] deficiency, chronic granulomatous disease), or dysfunction of a cytosolic (sickle cell anemia) or plasma (hemophilia) protein. Secondary causes of hematologic disease include infiltration of normal structures (leukemia, neuroblastoma), nutritional deficiency (iron, folate, vitamins K, E, and $B_{12}$), autoimmune disease (immune thrombocytopenic purpura), exogenous drugs (antimetabolites, penicillin, anti-inflammatory agents), and altered vascular matrix (thrombosis with vasculitis).

Hematologic disorders have characteristic clinical presentations related to the specific affected blood component or factor (Table 14–1). These manifestations are not diagnostic of the cause of the disorder, but certain characteristic signs and symptoms point to a likely diagnosis, such as spoon-shaped nails or pica with iron deficiency, mental and neurologic manifestations with anemia in vitamin $B_{12}$ deficiency, vaso-occlusive crises in sickle cell anemia, and progressive pancytopenia in association with congenital abnormalities in Fanconi anemia.

## DEVELOPMENTAL HEMATOPOIESIS

Hematopoiesis begins by the 3rd wk of gestation with erythropoiesis in the yolk sac. By 2 mo gesta-

tion, the primary site of hematopoiesis has migrated to the liver. Red blood cells, platelets, and leukocytes are synthesized at that site. By 5–6 mo gestation, the process of hematopoiesis shifts from the liver to the bone marrow. Therefore, an extremely premature infant may have significant **extramedullary hematopoiesis** with limited bone marrow hematopoiesis. During infancy, virtually all marrow cavities are actively hematopoietic, and the proportion of hematopoietic to stromal elements is very high. As the child grows, hematopoiesis moves to the central bones of the body (vertebrae, sternum, ribs, pelvis), and the marrow of the extremities and the skull is replaced with fat. This replacement of marrow with fat is a gradual and partially reversible process. Hemolysis or marrow damage may result in marrow repopulation of cavities where hematopoiesis had previously ceased or cause a delay in the shift of hematopoiesis. Children with thalassemia and other chronic hemolytic diseases may have large head circumferences and prominent skull bones as a result of increased erythropoiesis within the medullary cavities of the skull. Furthermore, hepatosplenomegaly in patients with chronic hemolysis may represent extramedullary hematopoiesis. Because of the extensive utilization of all bone marrow cavities, very young children do not have the marrow reserves of older children and adults. When a patient with cytopenia is being evaluated, a bone marrow examination provides valuable information about processes that result in underproduction of circulating cells. Additionally, bone marrow infiltration by neoplastic elements or storage cells often occurs in concert with similar infiltration in the spleen, liver, and lymph nodes.

The hematopoietic cells consist of (1) a small compartment of pluripotential progenitor stem

TABLE 14–1.  Presentation of Hematologic Disorders

| Condition | Symptoms and Signs | Common Examples |
|---|---|---|
| Anemia | Pallor, fatigue, heart failure, jaundice | Iron deficiency, hemolytic anemia |
| Polycythemia | Irritability, cyanosis, seizures, jaundice, stroke, headache | Cyanotic heart disease, infant of diabetic mother |
| Neutropenia | Fever, pharyngitis, oral ulceration, cellulitis, lymphadenopathy, bacteremia | Congenital or drug-induced agranulocytosis, leukemia |
| Thrombocytopenia | Petechiae, ecchymosis, gastrointestinal hemorrhage, epistaxis | ITP, leukemia |
| Coagulopathy | Bruising, hemarthrosis, mucosal bleeding | Von Willebrand disease, hemophilia, DIC |
| Thrombosis | Pulmonary embolism, deep venous thrombosis | Lupus anticoagulant; protein C, protein S, or antithrombin III deficiency, factor V Leiden |

DIC = disseminated intravascular coagulation; ITP = idiopathic thrombocytopenic purpura.

cells that morphologically resemble small lymphocytes and are capable of forming all myeloid elements; (2) a large compartment of committed, proliferating cells of myeloid, erythroid, and megakaryocytic lineage; and (3) a large compartment of postmitotic maturing cells (Fig. 14–1). The bone marrow is the major storage organ for mature neutrophils and contains about 7 times the intravascular pool of neutrophils; it contains 2.5–5 times as many cells of myeloid lineage as that of erythroid lineage. In addition, smaller numbers of megakaryocytes and plasma cells, histiocytes, lymphocytes, and stromal cells are stored in the marrow.

*Erythropoiesis* (red blood cell production) is controlled by erythropoietin, a hormone made by the juxtaglomerular apparatus of the kidney in response to local tissue hypoxia (see Fig. 14–1). Control of erythropoiesis by erythropoietin begins at the time of hepatic hematopoiesis in early gestation. The normally high hemoglobin level of the fetus is due to fetal erythropoietin production in the liver in response to low $Po_2$ in utero. Erythropoietin is a glycoprotein that stimulates the primitive pluripotent stem cell to differentiate along the erythroid line, leading to production of what is recognized in vitro as the erythroid colony-forming unit (CFU-E). The earliest recognizable erythroid cell in vivo is the erythroblast, which forms eight or more daughter cells. During maturation, the immature red cell nucleus becomes gradually pyknotic as the cell matures and eventually is extruded before the cell is released from the marrow as a reticulocyte. The reticulocyte maintains residual mitochondrial and protein synthetic capacity. These highly specialized red cell precursors are engaged primarily in the production of globin chains, glycolytic enzymes, and heme. Iron is taken up via transferrin receptors and incorporated into the heme ring, which then combines with globin chains synthesized within the immature red blood cell. Once the messenger ribonucleic acid (mRNA) and mitochondria are gone from the red cell, it is no longer capable of heme or protein synthesis but continues to function for its normal life span of about 120 days in older children and adults.

During embryonic and fetal life, the globin genes are sequentially activated and inactivated. The control mechanism of globin chain switching remains incompletely understood. Embryonic hemoglobins are produced during yolk sac erythropoiesis and then are replaced by fetal hemoglobin (hemoglobin F, $\alpha_2\gamma_2$) during the hepatic phase. During the 3rd trimester, ($\gamma$) chain production gradually diminishes and is replaced by ($\beta$) chains, resulting in hemoglobin A ($\alpha_2\beta_2$). Some fetal factors (e.g., being an infant of a diabetic mother) delay onset of beta chain production, but premature birth does not affect its timing. Just after birth, with the expansion of the lungs and establishment of normal neonatal cardiorespiratory function, the oxygen saturation rapidly rises from 65% in utero to nearly 100%. Erythropoietin production ceases and shuts down erythropoiesis. In normal circumstances, there is a gradual decline in hemoglobin levels, with a nadir at 6–8 wk of life. This nadir is accentuated in premature infants; it is reached in a short time because fetal red blood cells have a short survival time compared with that of red cells of older children (60 versus 120 days). Fetal red cells have less deformable membranes and have enzymatic differences from the cells of older children. Senescent red cells are destroyed in the liver and spleen, where they are recognized as abnormal

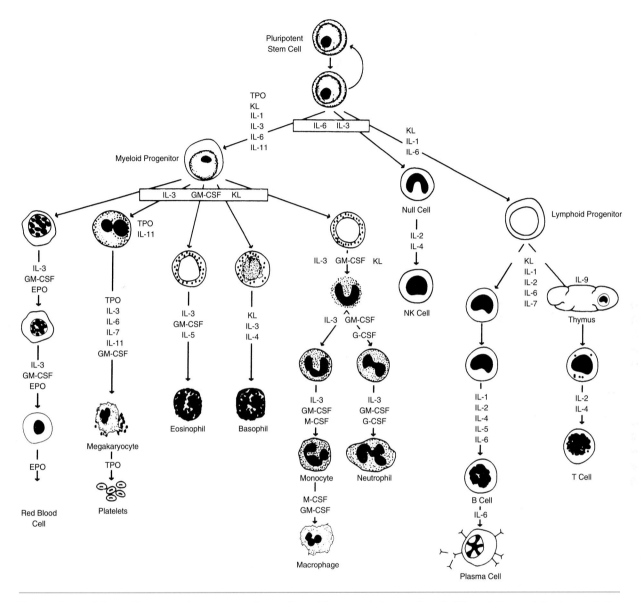

FIGURE 14–1. Schema illustrating the current understanding of hematopoietic growth and differentiation and the hemopoietins that control each step. EPO = erythropoietin; G-CSF = granulocyte colony-stimulating factor; GM-CSF = granulocyte-macrophage colony-stimulating factor; IL = interleukin; KL = kit ligand (also called stem cell growth factor or mast cell growth factor); M-CSF = macrophage colony-stimulating factor; NK = natural killer; TPO = thrombopoietin. (Adapted from Furman WL, Crist WM: Biology and clinical applications of hemopoietins in pediatric practice. Pediatrics 90:716, 1992.)

by changes in their membrane sialic acid content and by the metabolic depletion that occurs as they age. In response to decreased oxygen delivery, erythropoietin is produced and there is a subsequent resumption of erythropoiesis with a rise in the reticulocyte count and a gradual rise in hemoglobin, accompanied by the synthesis of increasing amounts of hemoglobin A. By 6 mo of age in healthy infants, only trace γ chain synthesis occurs.

*Production of neutrophil precursors* is controlled by two different colony-stimulating factors (see Fig. 14–1). The most immature neutrophil precursors are controlled by granulocyte-monocyte colony-stimulating factor (GM-CSF), which is produced by monocytes and lymphocytes. GM-CSF increases the entry of primitive precursor cells into the myeloid line of differentiation. Granulocyte colony-stimulating factor (G-CSF) augments the production of more mature granulocyte precursors. Both, working in concert, can augment production of neutrophils, shorten the usual baseline 10–14 day production time from stem cell to mature neutrophil, and stimulate functional activity. The rapid increase in neutrophil count that occurs with infection is due to release of stored neutrophils from the bone marrow; this is also under the control of GM-CSF. During maturation, a mitotic pool of neutrophil precursors exists: myeloblasts, promyelocytes, and myelocytes possessing primary granules. The postmitotic pool consists of metamyelocytes, bands, and mature polymorphonuclear leukocytes that contain secondary or specific granules that define the cell type. Only bands and mature neutrophils are fully functional with regard to phagocytosis, chemotaxis, and bacterial killing. Eosinophil production is under the control of a related glycoprotein hormone, interleukin-3 (IL-3).

Neutrophils migrate from the bone marrow, circulate for 6–7 hr, and then enter the tissues, where they become end-stage cells that do not recirculate (Fig. 14–2). The ability to adhere to endothelium is controlled by the interaction of adhesive molecules/receptors on the endothelial and leukocyte membrane modulated by cytokines. Neutrophils respond to chemotactic stimuli, especially C5a, and then migrate toward inflammatory stimuli, where they ingest and kill invading microorganisms. Monocytes migrate into tissues, where they become macrophages and may live from months to years. Eosinophils, which play a role in host defense against parasites, also are capable of living in tissues for prolonged periods and, like monocytes, are less streamlined but more durable than neutrophils, which form the first line of defense against infection.

*Megakaryocytes* are giant, multinucleated cells that derive from the primitive stem cell and are polyploid (16–32 times the normal deoxyribonucleic acid [DNA] content) because of nuclear but not cytoplasmic cell division. Platelets form by invagination of the megakaryocytic cell membrane and bud off from the periphery. Thrombopoietin is the primary regulator of platelet production. Platelets function by adhering to damaged endothelium and subendothelial surfaces via specific receptors for the adhesive proteins, von Willebrand factor, and fibrinogen. Platelets also have specific granules that readily release their contents following stimulation and trigger the process of platelet aggregation. Platelets circulate for 7–10 days and, like red cells, have no nucleus.

*Lymphocytes* are particularly abundant in the bone marrow of young children, although they are a significant component of normal bone marrow of all ages. These are primarily B lymphocytes arising in the spleen and lymph nodes, but T lymphocytes also are present (see Chapter 8).

The stroma of the bone marrow is of major importance for the marrow's normal function. Less is known about details of its function than about the function of the other hematopoietic components because of difficulties in growing these cells in culture.

An essential element to the understanding of the hematology of pediatric patients is a detailed knowledge of normal hematologic values during infancy and childhood. These values vary according to age and according to sex after puberty (Table 14–2).

The *coagulation factors* and *anticoagulant proteins* are synthesized primarily in the liver, although factor VIII and von Willebrand factor are synthesized at other sites. Levels of most of these factors increase throughout gestation, although levels of factor VIII, von Willebrand factor, and fibrinogen reach adult normal values by the 2nd trimester.

## ANEMIA

Anemia may be defined either quantitatively or functionally (physiologically). The presence of anemia usually is determined by comparison of the patient's hemoglobin with age-specific and sex-specific normal values. The data presented in Table 14–2 provide the normal ranges, and hemoglobin values below those ranges would represent a perfectly acceptable definition of anemia in most circumstances. However, under certain pathologic states, anemia may be present when the hemoglobin level is within the "normal range," such as in cyanotic cardiac or pulmonary disease or when a hemoglobin with an abnormally high affinity for oxygen is present. In these circumstances, the physiologic definition is more appropriate. It is important to recognize that anemia is not a disease per se, but rather a manifestation of some other primary process. Anemia is a common complication that may accentuate other organ dysfunction. The easiest quantitative definition of anemia is any value for the hemoglobin or hematocrit 2 standard deviations (95% confidence limits) below the mean for age and sex. This value is less easily determined in young children than in adults because the normal range varies considerably with age. The normal hemoglobin concentration is higher at high altitudes (lower inspired oxygen content) than at sea level and in males after puberty because high levels of androgen result in greater red cell synthesis.

*Pathophysiology.* The physiologic consequences of anemia can be determined from the history and physical examination. Acute onset of

FIGURE 14–2. The neutrophil-mediated inflammatory response. *A*, Unstimulated neutrophils expressing L-selectin enter a postcapillary venule. *B*, Gram-negative bacteria invade the subendothelium, release lipopolysaccharide, and stimulate macrophages to secrete inflammatory cytokines IL-1 and TNF, which then activate endothelial cells to express E-selectins and P-selectins. Selectins have a high affinity for sugar molecules (Lewis X) on neutrophils and cause low avidity neutrophil rolling. *C*, Activated endothelial cells express ICAM-1, which serves as a counter receptor for neutrophil β2-integrin receptors, leading to high avidity leukocyte spreading and the start of trans-endothelial migration. Trans-endothelial migration is stimulated by chemotactic factors, which promote neutrophil activation with release of L-selectin and an increase in β2 integrin affinity for ICAM-1 and other counter-receptors. *D*, Neutrophils invade through the vascular basement membranes with release of proteases and reactive oxidative intermediates. (Redrawn from Smolen JE, Boxer LA: Functions of neutrophils. *In* Williams WJ, Beutler E, Erslev AJ, et al [eds.]: Hematology, 5th ed. New York, McGraw-Hill, 1994, p 779. Reprinted in Bennett JC, Plum F (eds): Cecil Textbook of Medicine, 20th ed. Philadelphia, WB Saunders, 1994, p 899.)

anemia is often poorly compensated for and may be manifested by an elevated pulse rate, hemic flow murmur, poor exercise tolerance, headache, excessive sleeping (especially in infants), poor feeding, and syncope. Chronic anemia often is exceptionally well tolerated in children because of their cardiovascular reserve. Anemia that would induce angina in an adult may be asymptomatic in a young child. The extent of cardiovascular or functional impairment, more so than the absolute level of hemoglobin, should dictate the urgency of diagnostic and therapeutic intervention, especially the use of packed red blood cell transfusion to correct a low hemoglobin level.

*Etiology.* Common etiologies and mechanisms leading to anemia and an approach to their organization are presented in Figure 14–3. The causes for anemia can often be suspected from a careful history and physical examination. Often the focus of the history is dictated by the patient's age (Table 14–3). In a newborn, a history of jaundice, pallor, previously affected siblings, drug ingestion by the mother, or excessive blood loss at the time of birth provides important clues to the diagnosis. In a young infant, a careful *dietary history* is crucial. A history of jaundice, blood loss, drug ingestion, or acute or chronic illnesses also will indicate probable causes of anemia. In later childhood and in

TABLE 14–2.   Hematologic Values During Infancy and Childhood

| Age | Hemoglobin (g/dL) | | Hematocrit (%) | | Reticulocytes (%) | Leukocytes (mm³) | | Differential Counts | | | | | | Nucleated Red Cells/100 WBC |
|---|---|---|---|---|---|---|---|---|---|---|---|---|---|---|
| | | | | | | | | Neutrophils (%) | | Lymphocytes (%) | Eosinophils (%) | Monocytes (%) | | |
| | Mean | Range | Mean | Range | Mean | Mean | Range | Mean | Range | Mean | Mean | Mean | | Mean |
| Cord blood | 16.8 | 13.7–20.1 | 55 | 45–65 | 5.0 | 18,000 | (9–30,000) | 61 | (40–80) | 31 | 2 | 6 | | 7.0 |
| 2 wk | 16.5 | 13.0–20.0 | 50 | 42–66 | 1.0 | 12,000 | (5–21,000) | 40 | | 48 | 3 | 9 | | (3–10) |
| 3 mo | 12.0 | 9.5–14.5 | 36 | 31–41 | 1.0 | 12,000 | (6–18,000) | 30 | | 63 | 2 | 5 | | 0 |
| 6 mo–6 yr | 12.0 | 10.5–14.0 | 37 | 33–42 | 1.0 | 10,000 | (6–15,000) | 45 | | 48 | 2 | 5 | | 0 |
| 7–12 yr | 13.0 | 11.0–16.0 | 38 | 34–40 | 1.0 | 8,000 | (4,500–13,500) | 55 | | 38 | 2 | 5 | | 0 |
| Adult | | | | | | | | | | | | | | |
| Female | 14.0 | 12.0–16.0 | 42 | 37–47 | 1.6 | 7,500 | (5–10,000) | 55 | (35–70) | 35 | 3 | 7 | | 0 |
| Male | 16.0 | 14.0–18.0 | 47 | 42–52 | | | | | | | | | | |

From Behrman RE (ed): Nelson Textbook of Pediatrics, 14th ed. Philadelphia, WB Saunders, 1992, p 1232.
*Relatively wide range.
WBC = white blood cells.

**ANEMIA**

↓

**HEMOGLOBIN AND INDICES
RETIC COUNT AND MORPHOLOGY**

**Inadequate Response (RPI < 2)**

**Adequate Response (RPI > 3)
R/O Blood loss**

*Hypochromic, Microcytic*

*Normochromic, Normocytic*

*Macrocytic*

*Hemolytic Disorders*

*Iron deficiency*
- Chronic blood loss
- Poor diet
- Cow's milk protein intolerance
- Menstruation

*Thalassemia*
- β major, minor
- α minor

*Chronic inflammatory disease*

*Copper deficiency*

*Sideroblastic anemia*

*Aluminum, (?) lead intoxication*

*Chronic inflammatory disease*
- Infection
- Collagen-vascular disease
- Inflammatory bowel disease

*Recent blood loss*

*Malignancy/marrow infiltration*

*Chronic renal failure*

*Transient erythroblastopenia of childhood*

*Marrow aplasia/hypoplasia*

*HIV infection*

*Hemophagocytic syndrome*

*Vitamin B$_{12}$ deficiency*
- Pernicious anemia
- Ileal resection
- Strict vegetarian
- Abnormal intestinal transport
- Congenital intrinsic factor or transcobalamin deficiency

*Folate deficiency*
- Malnutrition
- Malabsorption
- Antimetabolite
- Chronic hemolysis
- Phenytoin
- Trimethoprim/sulfa

*Hypothyroidism*
*Oroticaciduria*
*Chronic liver disease*
*Lesch-Nyhan syndrome*
*Down syndrome*

*Marrow failure*
- Myelodysplasia
- Fanconi anemia
- Aplastic anemia

*Drugs*
- Alcohol
- Azidothymidine (zidovudine)

*Hemoglobinopathy*
- Hemoglobin SS, S-C, S-β thalassemia

*Enzymopathy*
- G6PD deficiency
- Pyruvate kinase deficiency

*Membranopathy*
- Hereditary spherocytosis
- Elliptocytosis
- Ovalocytosis

*Extrinsic factors*
- DIC, HUS, TTP
- Abetalipoproteinemia
- Burns
- Wilson disease
- Vitamin E deficiency

*Immune hemolytic anemia*
- Autoimmune
- Isoimmune
- Drug-induced

FIGURE 14–3. Use of the complete blood count, reticulocyte count, and blood smear in the diagnosis of anemia. DIC = disseminated intravascular coagulation; HUS = hemolytic-uremic syndrome; HIV = human immunodeficiency virus; R/O = rule out; RPI = reticulocyte production index; TTP = thrombotic thrombocytopenic purpura.

teenagers, the presence of constitutional symptoms, unusual diets, drug ingestion, or blood loss, especially from menstrual bleeding, often will point to a diagnosis. Congenital red cell disorders (e.g., enzyme deficiencies and membrane problems) often present in the first 6 mo of life and frequently are associated with neonatal jaundice, although they often go undiagnosed. A careful drug history is essential for detecting problems that may be drug-induced (hemolysis in G6PD deficiency, bone marrow suppression, antibody-mediated hemolysis). Pure dietary iron deficiency is rare except in infancy, when cow's milk protein intolerance causes gastrointestinal blood loss, further complicating an inadequate iron intake. A careful history justifies providing replacement therapy without performing an extensive search for blood loss (see Table 14–3).

*Clinical Manifestations.* The *physical examination* also suggests the presence of anemia and may point to the potential causes of the anemia (Table 14–4). Presence of jaundice suggests hemolysis. Pe-

TABLE 14–3.  Historical Clues in Evaluation of Anemia

| Variable | Comments |
|---|---|
| Age | Iron deficiency rare in the absence of blood loss prior to 6 mo in term or prior to doubling birth weight in preterm infants |
| | Neonatal anemia with reticulocytosis suggests hemolysis or blood loss; with reticulocytopenia, it suggests bone marrow failure |
| | Sickle cell anemia and β-thalassemia appear as fetal hemoglobin disappears (4–8 mo of age) |
| Family history and genetic considerations | X-linked: G6PD deficiency |
| | Autosomal dominant: spherocytosis |
| | Autosomal recessive: sickle cell, Fanconi anemia |
| | Family member with early age of cholecystectomy (bilirubin stones) or splenectomy |
| | Ethnicity (thalassemia with Mediterranean origin; G6PD deficiency in blacks, Greeks, and Middle Eastern individuals) |
| | Race (β-thalassemia in individuals of Mediterranean, African, or Asian descent; α-thalassemia in blacks and those of Asian descent; SC and SS in blacks) |
| Nutrition | Cow's milk diet: iron deficiency |
| | Strict vegetarian: vitamin $B_{12}$ deficiency |
| | Goat's milk: folate deficiency |
| | Pica: plumbism, iron deficiency |
| | Cholestasis, malabsorption: vitamin E |
| Drugs | G6PD: oxidants (e.g., nitrofurantoin, antimalarials) |
| | Immune-mediated hemolysis (e.g., penicillin) |
| | Bone marrow suppression (e.g., chemotherapy) |
| | Phenytoin increasing folate requirements |
| Diarrhea | Malabsorption of vitamins $B_{12}$ or E or iron |
| | Inflammatory bowel disease and anemia of chronic disease with or without blood loss |
| | Milk protein intolerance–induced blood loss |
| | Intestinal resection: vitamin $B_{12}$ deficiency |
| Infection | Giardia: iron malabsorption |
| | Intestinal bacterial overgrowth (blind loop): vitamin $B_{12}$ deficiency |
| | Fish tapeworm: vitamin $B_{12}$ deficiency |
| | Epstein-Barr virus, cytomegalovirus: bone marrow suppression, hemophagocytic syndromes |
| | Mycoplasma: hemolysis |
| | Parvovirus: bone marrow suppression |
| | Human immunodeficiency virus |
| | Chronic infection |
| | Endocarditis |
| | Malaria: hemolysis |
| | Hepatitis: aplastic anemia |

G6PD = glucose-6-phosphate dehydrogenase.

techiae and purpura indicate a bleeding tendency. Hepatosplenomegaly and adenopathy suggest infiltrative disorders. Growth failure or poor weight gain suggests an anemia of chronic disease or organ failure. An essential element of the physical examination in a patient with anemia is the investigation of the stool for the presence of occult blood.

The initial *laboratory evaluation* of anemia includes a hemoglobin or hematocrit test to indicate the severity of the anemia. Once the diagnosis of

TABLE 14–4.  Physical Findings in the Evaluation of Anemia

| System | Observation | Significance |
|---|---|---|
| Skin | Hyperpigmentation | Fanconi, dyskeratosis congenita |
| | *Café-au-lait* spots | Fanconi anemia |
| | Vitiligo | Vitamin $B_{12}$ deficiency |
| | Partial oculocutaneous albinism | Chédiak-Higashi syndrome |
| | Jaundice | Hemolysis |
| | Petechiae, purpura | Bone marrow infiltration, autoimmune hemolysis with autoimmune thrombocytopenia, hemolytic uremic syndrome |
| | Erythematous rash | Parvovirus, Epstein-Barr virus |
| | Butterfly rash | SLE autoantibodies |
| Head | Frontal bossing | Thalassemia major, severe iron deficiency, chronic subdural hematoma |
| | Microcephaly | Fanconi anemia |
| Eyes | Microphthalmia | Fanconi anemia |
| | Retinopathy | Hemoglobin SS, SC disease |
| | Optic atrophy | Osteopetrosis |
| | Blocked lacrimal gland | Dyskeratosis congenita |
| | Kayser-Fleischer ring | Wilson disease |
| | Blue sclera | Iron deficiency |
| Ears | Deafness | Osteopetrosis |
| Mouth | Glossitis | $B_{12}$ deficiency, iron deficiency |
| | Angular stomatitis | Iron deficiency |
| | Cleft lip | Diamond-Blackfan syndrome |
| | Pigmentation | Peutz-Jeghers syndrome (intestinal blood loss) |
| | Telangiectasia | Osler-Weber-Rendu syndrome (blood loss) |
| | Leukoplakia | Dyskeratosis congenita |
| Chest | Shield chest or widespread nipples | Diamond-Blackfan syndrome |
| | Murmur | Endocarditis: prosthetic valve hemolysis; severe anemia |
| Abdomen | Hepatomegaly | Hemolysis, infiltrative tumor, chronic disease, hemangioma, cholecystitis, extramedullary hematopoiesis |
| | Splenomegaly | Hemolysis, sickle cell disease, (early) thalassemia, malaria, lymphoma, Epstein-Barr virus, portal hypertension |
| | Nephromegaly | Fanconi anemia |
| | Absent kidney | Fanconi anemia |
| Extremities | Absent thumbs | Fanconi anemia |
| | Triphalangeal thumb | Diamond-Blackfan syndrome |
| | Spoon nails | Iron deficiency |
| | Beau line (nails) | Heavy metal intoxication, severe illness |
| | Mees line (nails) | Heavy metals, severe illness, sickle cell anemia |
| | Dystrophic nails | Dyskeratosis congenita |
| Rectal | Hemorrhoids | Portal hypertension |
| | Heme positive stool | Gastrointestinal bleeding |
| Nerves | Irritable, apathy | Iron deficiency |
| | Peripheral neuropathy | Deficiency of vitamins $B_1$, $B_{12}$, and E, lead poisoning |
| | Dementia | Deficiency of vitamins $B_{12}$ and E |
| | Ataxia, posterior column signs | Vitamin $B_{12}$ deficiency |
| | Stroke | Sickle cell anemia, paroxysmal nocturnal hemoglobinuria |
| General | Small stature | Fanconi anemia, human immunodeficiency virus, malnutrition |

SLE = systemic lupus erythematosus.

anemia has been substantiated, the work-up should include a complete blood count with differential, platelet count, indices, and reticulocyte count. The blood smear should be studied for morphologic abnormalities (Fig. 14–4). Using data obtained from the indices and reticulocyte count, one can organize the work-up for anemia on the basis of whether there is adequate or inadequate red cell production and whether the cells are microcytic, normocytic, or macrocytic (see Fig. 14–3). Examination of the peripheral blood smear is critical in order to assess the number and morphology of red

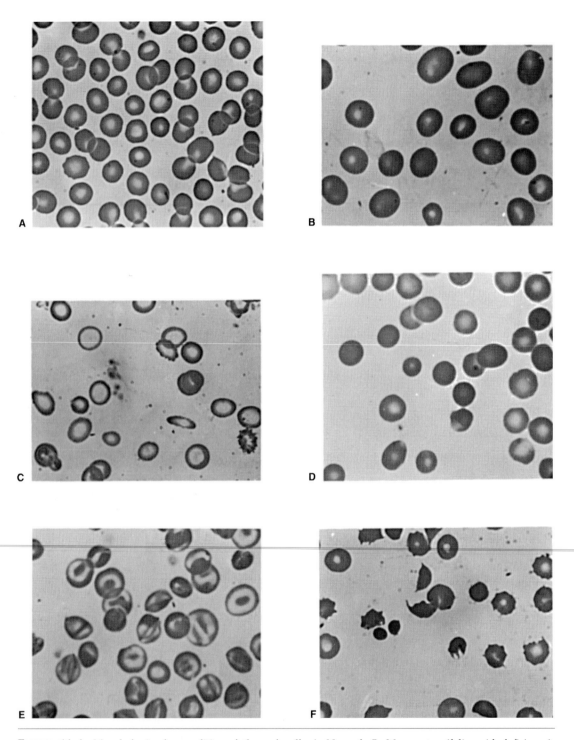

FIGURE 14–4. Morphologic abnormalities of the red cell. *A*, Normal. *B*, Macrocytes (folic acid deficiency). *C*, Hypochromic microcytes (iron deficiency). *D*, Spherocytes (hereditary spherocytosis). *E*, Target cells (Hgb CC disease). *F*, Schistocytes (hemolytic-uremic syndrome). (From Behrman RE [ed]: Nelson Textbook of Pediatrics, 14th ed. Philadelphia, WB Saunders, 1992, p 1237.)

cells, white blood cells (WBCs), and platelets. All cell lines should be scrutinized to determine whether anemia is due to a process limited to the erythroid line or to one that affects other marrow elements.

The reticulocyte production index (RPI), which corrects the reticulocyte count (retic ct) for the degree of anemia, indicates whether the bone marrow is responding appropriately to the anemia. Reticulocytes routinely are counted per 1000 red cells; hence a reduction in the denominator, which occurs in anemia, will falsely increase the reticulocyte count. The formula for calculating the RPI is:

$$\text{RPI} = \text{retic ct} \times \frac{\text{Hgb}_{\text{observed}}}{\text{Hgb}_{\text{normal}}} \times 0.5$$

An RPI greater than 3 suggests increased production and implies either hemolysis or blood loss, whereas an index less than 2 suggests decreased production or ineffective production for the degree of anemia. Reticulocytopenia signifies either that the anemia is so acute in onset that the marrow has not had adequate time to respond, that reticulocytes are being destroyed (antibody mediated), or that intrinsic bone marrow disease is present.

## HYPOCHROMIC, MICROCYTIC ANEMIA WITH INADEQUATE RED CELL PRODUCTION

Hypochromic, microcytic anemia is caused by an inadequate production of hemoglobin (Table 14–5).

## Iron-Deficiency Anemia

Dietary iron-deficiency anemia is most common in bottle-fed infants who are receiving large volumes of cow's milk. They ingest little in the way of dietary substances high in iron, such as meat and green vegetables (see Chapter 2). Iron deficiency is the single most common cause of anemia in the world. Breast-fed infants have iron deficiency less commonly than bottle-fed infants because, although there is less iron in breast milk, this iron is more effectively absorbed. Menstruating adolescents are also at risk for iron deficiency. The sequence of events in the development of iron-deficiency anemia is noted in Table 14–6. In addition to the manifestations of anemia, central nervous system (CNS) abnormalities (apathy, irritability, poor concentration) have been linked to iron deficiency, presumably resulting from alterations of iron-containing enzymes (monoamine oxidase) and cytochromes. Poor muscle endurance, gastrointestinal dysfunction, and impaired white blood cell and T-cell function also have been noted in association with iron deficiency. Increasing evidence has been found that mild iron deficiency in infancy may be associated with later cognitive deficits.

A detailed dietary history usually discloses the child's poor diet. If the dietary history suggests iron deficiency, a therapeutic trial of iron is appropriate with or without laboratory confirmation. In an otherwise healthy child, a therapeutic trial is the best diagnostic study for iron deficiency so long as the child is re-examined and a response is documented. The response to oral iron includes rapid subjective improvement, especially in neuro-

**TABLE 14–5.** Differentiating Features of Microcytic Anemias*

| Tests | Iron-Deficiency Anemia | Thalassemia Minor | Anemia of Chronic Disease† |
|---|---|---|---|
| Serum iron | Low | Normal | Low |
| Serum iron–binding capacity | High | Normal | Low or normal |
| Serum ferritin | Low | Normal or high | Normal or high |
| Marrow iron stores | Low or absent | Normal or high | Normal or high |
| Marrow sideroblasts | Decreased or absent | Normal or increased | Normal or increased |
| Free erythrocyte protoporphyrin | High | Normal or slightly increased | High |
| Hemoglobin A$_2$ or F | Normal | High β-thalassemia; normal α-thalassemia | Normal |
| Red cell distribution width (RDW)‡ | High | Normal | Normal/ ↑ |

*See Table 14–6 for definition of microcytosis.
†Usually normochromic; 25% are microcytic.
‡RDW quantitates the degree of anisocytosis (different sizes) of red blood cells.

TABLE 14–6.   Stages in Development of Iron-Deficiency Anemia

| Hemoglobin (g/dL) | Peripheral Smear | Serum Iron (µg/dL) | Bone Marrow | Serum Ferritin (ng/mL) |
|---|---|---|---|---|
| 13+ (normal) | nc/nc | 50/150 | $Fe^{2+}$ | 40–340 (male) 14–150 (female) |
| 10–12 | nc/nc | ↓ | $Fe^{2+}$ absent, erythroid hyperplasia | <12 |
| 8–10 | hypo/nc | ↓ | $Fe^{2+}$ absent, erythroid hyperplasia | <12 |
| <8 | hypo/micro* | ↓ | $Fe^{2+}$ absent, erythroid hyperplasia | <12 |

From Andreoli TE, Carpenter CCJ, Plum F, et al: Cecil Essentials of Medicine, 3rd ed. Philadelphia, WB Saunders, 1993, p 360.
*Microcytosis, determined by a mean corpuscular volume (in fL) less than 2 standard deviations (SD) below the mean, must be adjusted for age (e.g., −2 SD at 3–6 mo = 74, at 0.5–2 yr = 70, at 2–6 yr = 75, at 6–12 yr = 77, and at 12–18 yr = 78).
nc/nc = normochromic, normocytic; hypo/nc = hypochromic, normocytic; hypo/micro = hypochromic, microcytic.

logic function (24–48 hr), reticulocytosis (48–72 hr), increase in hemoglobin (4–30 days), and repletion of iron stores (1–3 mo). A usual therapeutic dose of 3–6 mg/day of elemental iron will induce an increase in hemoglobin of 0.25–0.4 g/dL/day (1%/day rise in hematocrit). If the hemoglobin fails to rise within 2 wk after the institution of iron treatment, the clinician should carefully re-evaluate the patient for ongoing blood loss, development of infection, poor compliance, or other causes of microcytic anemia (see Fig. 14–3 and Table 14–5).

### Thalassemia Minor

The thalassemia minor syndromes are characterized by a mild hypochromic, microcytic anemia with a low RPI (Table 14–7; see Fig. 14–3). **Alpha-thalassemia** occurs in 1.5% of African-Americans and is a common cause of microcytosis either without anemia or with a mild hypochromic, microcytic anemia. Alpha-thalassemia is common in Southeastern Asians, and an Oriental (Asian) variant is associated with a risk of homozygous alpha-thalassemia, Bart hemoglobin in the newborn (γ4 tetramers), and hemoglobin H (β4 tetramers) in older children. The blood smear is normal in alpha-thalassemia trait except for microcytosis. No basophilic stippling is present. Hemoglobin electrophoresis usually is normal in alpha-thalassemia minor, although Bart hemoglobin may be present in the neonatal period. Homozygous alpha-thalassemia results in hydrops fetalis (Fig. 14–5).

**Beta-thalassemia minor** is prevalent throughout the Mediterranean region, the Middle East, India, and Southeast Asia. The peripheral blood smear shows hypochromic, microcytic red blood cells; target cells and basophilic stippled red cells may also be present. The stippling is caused by precipitation of alpha-chain tetramers. The diagnosis is based on an elevation of hemoglobin $A_2$ and F.

### Lead Poisoning

This may be associated with a hypochromic, microcytic anemia, although most patients have concomitant iron deficiency. The history of a child with pica who lives in an older home with chipped paint or lead dust should raise suspicion of lead poisoning. Basophilic stippling on the blood smear is common. Detection by routine screening, removal from exposure, chelation therapy, and correction of iron deficiency are of utmost importance to the potential development of these children (see Chapter 3). Lead intoxication may rarely also cause hemolytic anemia.

## NORMOCYTIC ANEMIA WITH INADEQUATE RED CELL PRODUCTION

Normocytic anemias include a wide variety of red cell disorders in which the marrow fails to synthe-

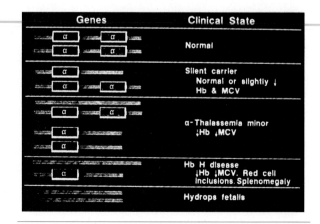

FIGURE 14–5.   Schematic illustration of alpha-globin gene deletions and their clinical consequences. HB = hemoglobin; MCV = mean corpuscular volume. (From Beutler E: The common anemias. JAMA 259:2433, 1988. Copyright 1988, American Medical Association.)

TABLE 14–7.    Comparison of the Thalassemia Syndromes

| Genetic Abnormality | Percent Hemoglobin | | | Other | Clinical Syndrome |
|---|---|---|---|---|---|
| | Hb A | Hb A₂ | Hb F | | |
| Normal αβ | 90–98 | 2–3 | 2–3 | | None |
| **Beta-Thalassemias** | | | | | |
| Thalassemia Major | | | | | |
| β-thalassemia⁰<br>β-thalassemia⁰ | 0 | 2–5 | 95 | — | Severe anemia, abnormal growth, iron overload, needs transfusion, Cooley anemia |
| β-thalassemia⁺<br>β-thalassemia⁺ | Very low | 2–5 | 20–80 | — | Severe hypo/micro anemia with Hb 7–9 g/dL, hepatosplenomegaly, bone changes, iron overload, less need for transfusion |
| Thalassemia Intermedia<br>(varied genetic globin abnormalities) | Overlaps with thalassemia major | | | | |
| Thalassemia Minor<br>β β-thalassemia⁰ or<br>β β-thalassemia⁺ | 90–95 | 5–7 | 2–10 | RBC | Hypo/micro blood smear, mild to no anemia |
| **Alpha-Thalassemias** | | | | | |
| Homozygous α-thalassemia<br>– –/– – | — | — | — | Hb H (β4)<br>Hb Bart (γ4) | Hydrops fetalis, stillborn |
| Hemoglobin H disease<br>– –/– α | 60–70 | 2–5 | 2–5 | Hb H 30–40 | Hypo/micro anemia, Hb 7–10 g/dL, Heinz bodies |
| Alpha-thalassemia trait<br>– α/– α, α α/– – | 90–98 | 2–3 | 2–3 | | Hypo/micro smear, no anemia |
| Silent carrier – α/α α | 90–98 | 2–3 | 2–3 | | Normal |
| **Hemoglobin Lepore**<br>(δβ fusion) | | | | | |
| Heterozygote | 70–80 | 1–2 | 5–20 | Hb Lepore 5–15 | Mild hypo/micro anemia |
| Homozygote | 0 | 0 | 70–90 | Hb Lepore 10–30 | Severe thalassemia major |

From Andreoli TE, Carpenter CCJ, Plum F, et al: Cecil Essentials of Medicine, 3rd ed. Philadelphia, WB Saunders, 1993, p 373.
Hypo/micro = hypochromic, microcytic.

size adequate numbers of red blood cells as a result of a systemic illness. Red cell synthesis fails because of fibrosis, tumor, storage cells, transient or prolonged marrow failure (transient erythroblastopenia of childhood, aplastic anemia), or failure to synthesize erythropoietin (renal failure). Normocytic anemias also occur in the presence of acute blood loss before the marrow has had time to respond. The site of blood loss usually is obvious, commonly in the gastrointestinal tract (see Chapter 11).

Anemia is a common component of **chronic inflammatory disease**, in which cytokines trigger a reticuloendothelial blockade within the marrow. Iron is taken up by the reticuloendothelial cells but is not available for erythroid synthesis. The anemia may be normocytic or, less often, microcytic. At times, this poses a clinical challenge when children with inflammatory disorders that may be associated with blood loss (e.g., inflammatory bowel dis-

ease) present with a microcytic anemia. In these circumstances, the only specific diagnostic test that can clearly differentiate the two entities is a bone marrow aspiration with staining of the sample for iron (see Table 14–5). Serum ferritin levels also may be helpful. A trial of iron therapy is not indicated without a specific diagnosis in children who appear to be systemically ill.

Bone marrow **infiltration by malignant cells** commonly results in a normochromic, normocytic anemia. The mechanism by which neoplastic cells interfere with red cell and other marrow cell synthesis is unclear. The reticulocyte count is low. There may be release of immature myeloid elements into the peripheral blood as a result of the presence of the offending tumor cells. An examination of the peripheral blood may disclose lymphoblasts; when solid tumors metastasize to the marrow, these cells seldom are seen in the peripheral blood. Teardrop cells may be seen in the peripheral blood. Performance of a bone marrow examination frequently is necessary in the face of normochromic, normocytic anemia.

**Congenital pure red cell aplasia** (Diamond-Blackfan syndrome) usually presents in the first few months of life or even at birth (Table 14–8). This is a lifelong disorder. Congenital anomalies are common. Most patients respond to corticosteroid treatment but must receive therapy indefinitely. At the time of presentation, the patient may have mild macrocytosis or may be normocytic. Those who do not respond to steroid treatment are transfusion dependent and are at risk of the multiple complications of chronic transfusion therapy,

TABLE 14–8.  Differentiation of Red Cell Aplasias and Aplastic Anemias

| Disorder | Age of Onset | Characteristics | Treatment |
|---|---|---|---|
| **Congenital** | | | |
| Diamond-Blackfan syndrome (congenital hypoplastic anemia) | Newborn–1 mo; 90% <1 yr age | Pure red cell aplasia, autosomal recessive trait, elevated fetal hemoglobin, fetal i antigen present, macrocytic, thrombosis, short stature, web neck, cleft lip, triphalangeal thumb; late-onset leukemia | Prednisone, transfusion |
| **Acquired** | | | |
| Transient erythroblastopenia | 6 mo–5 yr age; 85% >1 yr age | Pure red cell defect; no anomalies, fetal hemoglobin, or i antigen; spontaneous recovery, normal MCV | Expectant transfusion for symptomatic anemia |
| Idiopathic aplastic anemia (s/p hepatitis, drugs, unknown) | All ages | All cell lines involved; exposure to chloramphenicol, phenylbutazone, radiation | Bone marrow transplant, antithymocyte globulin, cyclosporine, androgens |
| **Familial** | | | |
| Fanconi syndrome | Before 10 yr age; mean is 8 yr | All cell lines; microcephaly, absent thumbs, *café-au-lait* spots, cutaneous hyperpigmentation, short stature; chromosomal breaks, high MCV and hemoglobin F; horseshoe or absent kidney; leukemic transformation; autosomal recessive trait | Androgens, corticosteroids, bone marrow transplant |
| Paroxysmal nocturnal hemoglobinuria | After 5 yr | Initial hemolysis followed by aplastic anemia; increased complement-mediated hemolysis; thrombosis; iron deficiency | Iron, bone marrow transplant, androgens, steroids |
| Dyskeratosis congenita | Mean 10 yr for skin; mean 17 yr for anemia | Pancytopenia; hyperpigmentation, dystrophic nails, leukoplakia; X-linked recessive; lacrimal duct stenosis; high MCV and fetal hemoglobin | Androgens, splenectomy, bone marrow transplant |
| Familial hemophagocytic lymphohistiocytosis | Before 2 yr | Pancytopenia; fever, hepatosplenomegaly, hypertriglyceridemia, CSF pleocytosis | Transfusion; often lethal; VP-16, bone marrow transplantation, IVIg, cyclosporine |
| **Infectious** | | | |
| Parvovirus | Any age | Any chronic hemolytic anemia, typically sickle cell; new-onset reticulocytopenia | Transfusion |
| Epstein-Barr virus (EBV) | Any age; usually <5 yr | X-linked immunodeficiency syndrome, pancytopenia | Transfusion, bone marrow transplantation |
| Viral-associated hemophagocytic syndrome (CMV, HHV-6, EBV) | Any age | Pancytopenia; hemophagocytosis present in marrow, fever, hepatosplenomegaly | Transfusion, antiviral therapy (see Chapter 10), IVIg |

CMV = cytomegalovirus; CSF = cerebrospinal fluid; HHV-6 = human herpesvirus-6; IVIg = intravenous immunoglobulin; MCV = mean corpuscular volume.

including blood-borne virus-associated illnesses and iron overload.

In contrast to the congenital hypoplastic anemias, **transient erythroblastopenia of childhood** (TEC) usually appears after 6 mo of age (see Table 14–8). This is a normocytic anemia caused by bone marrow suppression. Viral infections are thought to be the major cause of TEC, but no specific etiology has been identified. The onset is gradual; however, the anemia may become severe. Recovery usually is spontaneous; transfusion of packed red cells may be necessary pending recovery. Keys to the diagnosis of TEC are a gradual onset of normocytic anemia in a child over 6 mo of age with a normal physical examination. Differentiation from Diamond-Blackfan syndrome, in which erythroid precursors also are absent or diminished in the bone marrow, is noted in Table 14–8.

**Aplastic crises**, which may complicate any chronic hemolytic anemia, are periods of reticulocytopenia during which the usual high rate of red cell destruction leads to an acute exacerbation of the anemia, potentially precipitating cardiovascular decompensation. Human parvovirus B19 (the cause of fifth disease [erythema infectiosum]) infecting erythroid precursors accounts for most of these episodes. Transient erythroid aplasia is without consequence in individuals with normal red cell survival. Recovery from parvovirus infection in hemolytic disease is spontaneous, but patients may need transfusion if the anemia is severe.

## MACROCYTIC ANEMIA

Vitamin $B_{12}$ and folic acid deficiencies lead to macrocytic anemia and are discussed in Chapter 2 (see Figs. 14–3 and 14–4).

## HEMOLYTIC ANEMIAS

Hemolytic diseases are mediated either by intrinsic disorders of the red blood cell or by disorders extrinsic to the red blood cell itself.

### Hemolytic Anemia Caused by Intrinsic Red Cell Disorders

**Membrane Disorders.** The most common red cell membrane disorders are **hereditary spherocytosis** and **hereditary elliptocytosis**. These frequently are associated with neonatal jaundice, although the disorder often goes undiagnosed in the neonate.

*Hereditary Spherocytosis.* This disorder varies greatly in clinical severity, ranging from a severe hemolytic anemia with growth failure, splenomegaly, and chronic transfusion requirements in infancy necessitating early splenectomy to an asymptomatic, well-compensated, mild hemolytic anemia that may be discovered incidentally. The biochemical bases of the defects probably are similar and appear to have in common a defect in the protein lattice (spectrin, ankyrin, protein 4.2) that underlies the red cell lipid bilayer and provides stability of the membrane shape. The amount or the function of the spectrin may be abnormal; the greater the abnormality the more severe the symptoms. When the red cell loses membrane, the shape changes from a biconcave disc to a spherocyte; the spherocyte shape has the lowest ratio of surface area to volume. The red cell, therefore, is less deformable when passing through narrow passages in the spleen. The transmission of this disorder usually is autosomal dominant but occasionally is recessive. There is a high, spontaneous mutation rate. The *diagnosis* should be suspected in patients with even a few spherocytes exhibited on the blood smear because the spherocytes are removed preferentially by the spleen. An incubated osmotic fragility test confirms the presence of spherocytes and increases the likelihood of the diagnosis of hereditary spherocytosis. Nevertheless, the osmotic fragility test result is abnormal in any hemolytic disease in which spherocytes are present, especially antibody-mediated hemolysis.

Splenectomy corrects the anemia and normalizes the red cell survival, but the morphologic abnormalities persist. Splenectomy should be considered for any child with symptoms referable to anemia or growth failure but should be deferred until age 5 yr, if at all possible, to minimize the risk of overwhelming postsplenectomy sepsis and maximize the antibody response to the polyvalent pneumococcal vaccine. Prior to splenectomy, vaccinations against pneumococcus and *Haemophilus influenzae* type B should be given according to current recommendations. Gallstones (bilirubinate), resulting from chronic hemolysis, may be asymptomatic or may be the cause of vague abdominal pain.

*Hereditary Elliptocytosis.* This is a disorder of spectrin dimer interactions that occurs primarily in individuals of African descent. The most common variant is a clinically insignificant, morphologic abnormality without shortened red cell survival. The less common variant is associated with spherocytes, ovalocytes, and elliptocytes and with a moderate, usually compensated, hemolysis. Both variants are transmitted as autosomal dominant traits. Far more significant hemolysis occurs in a very small percentage of patients with elliptocytes, spherocytes, fragmented red cells, and striking microcytosis. This disorder is termed *hereditary pyropoikilocytosis* and is due to a structural abnormality of spectrin. The term "pyropoikilocytosis" refers to the unusual instability of the erythrocytes when exposed to heat (45°C).

**Red Cell Enzyme Deficiencies.** There are numerous red cell enzyme deficiencies, but only a few are clinically important disorders.

*Glucose-6-Phosphate Dehydrogenase Deficiency.* This abnormality in the hexose monophosphate shunt pathway of glycolysis results in the depletion of NADPH and the inability to regenerate reduced glutathione. Reduced glutathione plays a critical role in the reduction of oxidants generated within a red cell; therefore, children with G6PD deficiency develop episodic hemolysis when they are exposed to oxidant stress.

The severity of the hemolysis depends on the enzyme variant. In many G6PD variants, the enzymes become unstable with aging. Young red cells have normal G6PD activity that is lost as the cell ages and cannot be replaced because the cell is anucleated. Older cells are most susceptible to oxidant-induced hemolysis. In other variants, the enzyme is kinetically abnormal. The most common variants of G6PD have been found in areas where malaria is endemic. G6PD deficiency protects against parasitism of the erythrocyte. The most common variant with normal activity is termed type B and is defined by its electrophoretic mobility. The approximate gene frequencies in African-Americans are 70% type B, 20% type A+, and 10% type A−. Only the A− variant is unstable. The A− variant is termed the "African" variant, and 10% of black males are affected. A group of variants found in Sardinians, Sicilians, Greeks, Sephardic and Oriental Jews, and Arabs is termed the "Mediterranean" variant and is associated with chronic hemolysis and potentially life-threatening hemolytic disease. The gene for G6PD is carried on the X chromosome. Clinical hemolysis is most common in males, who will possess a single abnormal X chromosome. Heterozygous females who have randomly inactivated a higher percentage of the normal gene may become symptomatic, as may homozygous females with the A− variant, which occurs in 1% of females of African descent.

When a patient with G6PD is exposed to significant oxidant stress, hemoglobin is oxidized and the sulfhemoglobin is denatured and forms Heinz bodies visible on specially stained preparations. The morphology of acute hemolysis is striking. Red cells appear to have "bites" (cookie cells) taken out of them. These are areas of absent hemoglobin caused by phagocytosis of Heinz bodies by splenic macrophages; as a result, the red cells appear blistered. Jaundice, dark urine resulting from both bilirubin pigments and hemoglobinuria when hemolysis is intravascular, and decreased haptoglobin are common during hemolytic episodes. Because 5% of African-Americans lack haptoglobin, absent haptoglobin is meaningful only in the context of the other abnormalities. Early on, the hemolysis usually exceeds the ability of the bone marrow to compensate, so the reticulocyte count may be low for 3–4 days.

The *diagnosis* of G6PD deficiency is based on decreased NADPH formation. However, G6PD levels may be normal in the setting of acute, severe hemolysis because the most deficient cells have been destroyed. Repeating the test at a later time when the patient is in a steady-state condition, testing the mothers of boys with suspected G6PD deficiency, or performing electrophoresis to identify the precise variant present will facilitate early diagnosis.

The *treatment* of G6PD deficiency is supportive, including transfusion when significant cardiovascular compromise is present and protecting the kidneys against damage from precipitated free hemoglobin by maintaining hydration and urine alkalization. *Prevention* of hemolysis is achieved by avoiding known oxidants, particularly long-acting sulfonamides, nitrofurantoin, primaquine, and dimercaprol; fava beans (favism) have triggered hemolysis, particularly in patients with the Mediterranean variant. Infection also is a major precipitant of hemolysis in G6PD-deficient young children. Patients with the most severe degrees of G6PD deficiency not only have chronic hemolysis, but their neutrophils demonstrate defective oxidative killing because of depletion of NADPH, which serves as an electron donor to the membrane-bound oxidase that produces bactericidal oxygen species (see Chapter 8).

*Pyruvate Kinase Deficiency.* This disorder is much less common than G6PD deficiency and also represents a clinical spectrum of disorders caused by the functional deficiency of pyruvate kinase (Pk). Some individuals have a true deficiency state, and others have abnormal enzyme kinetics. This enzyme in the Embden-Meyerhof pathway of glycolysis is important for the production of two moles adenosine triphosphate (ATP)/mole of glucose metabolized. The metabolic consequence of PK deficiency is ATP depletion, thus impairing red cell survival.

PK deficiency is an autosomal disorder, and most children who are affected (and are not products of inbreeding) are double heterozygotes for two abnormal enzymes. Hemolysis is not aggravated by oxidant stress because these patients tend to have a profound reticulocytosis. Aplastic crises potentially are life-threatening. The spleen is the site for red cell removal in PK deficiency. Most patients experience amelioration of the anemia and a reduction of transfusion requirements after splenectomy.

**Major Hemoglobinopathies.** Because alpha chains are needed for fetal erythropoiesis and production of hemoglobin F ($\alpha_2 \gamma_2$), alpha chain hemoglobinopathies present in utero. There are a total of four alpha genes present on the two number 16 chromosomes (see Fig. 14–5 and Table 14–7). Single-gene deletions produce no disorder (the silent carrier state) but can be detected by measuring the rates of alpha and beta synthesis or by using molecular biologic techniques. Deletion of two genes produces alpha-thalassemia minor with mild or no anemia and microcytosis. In the black population, the gene deletions occur on different chromosomes (*trans*) and the disorder is benign, with virtually no individuals of African descent having more than two genes deleted. In the Oriental (Asian descent) population, deletions may occur on the same chromosome (*cis*) and, therefore, infants may inherit two number 16 chromosomes lacking three or even four genes. Deletion of all four genes results in hydrops fetalis, severe intrauterine anemia, and death unless intrauterine transfusions are administered. Deletion of three genes produces a mild to moderate hemolytic anemia with $\gamma4$ tetramers (Bart hemoglobin) in the fetus and $\beta4$ tetramers (hemoglobin H) in older children and adults (see Table 14–7).

A greater number of disorders occur in beta chain hemoglobinopathies because these abnormalities are not symptomatic in utero. In contrast, severe gamma chain abnormalities would be expected to be lethal. The major group of beta-hemoglobinopathies include those that alter hemoglobin function, including hemoglobins S, C, E, D, and G, and those that alter beta chain production—the beta-thalassemias. Because each red cell has two copies of chromosome 11 and the beta-globin genes are both expressed, most of the disorders of beta chains are not clinically severe unless both beta chains are abnormal. Disorders of the beta chain usually manifest between 6 and 12 mo of age unless they have been detected prenatally or by cord blood screening.

*Beta-Thalassemia Major (Cooley Anemia).* This hemoglobinopathy is caused by mutations that alter beta chain synthesis (see Table 14–7); excess gamma and beta chains do not damage the red cells, whereas excess alpha chains are toxic. Alpha chains precipitate within the cells, resulting in cell destruction either in the bone marrow or in the spleen once the cell is released. The clinical severity of the illness varies to some extent on the basis of the molecular defect; however, most patients are transfusion-dependent from infancy. An uncommon mutation that results in deletion of both beta and delta chains results in **hereditary persistence of fetal hemoglobin** (HPFH), in which gamma chain synthesis represents about 30% of non–alpha chain synthesis in adult life. HPFH usually is asymptomatic.

*Clinical manifestations* of beta-thalassemia major result from the combination of chronic hemolytic disease, decreased production of normal hemoglobin, and ineffective erythropoiesis in the marrow. The anemia is severe and results in growth failure and heart failure. Ineffective erythropoiesis causes increased expenditure of energy and expansion of the bone marrow cavities of all bones, resulting in osteopenia, pathologic fractures, extramedullary erythropoiesis, and an increase in the rate of iron absorption. Patients usually are transfusion-dependent from the end of the 1st yr of life. Adolescents are subject to complications from iron overload (*hemochromatosis*), including non-immune diabetes mellitus, cirrhosis, heart failure, bronzing of the skin, and multiple endocrine abnormalities (thyroid, gonad). The amount of iron the patient acquires from transfusion may be estimated by the formula that each milliliter of packed red blood cells contains approximately 1 mg of iron.

*Treatment* of beta-thalassemia major is based on a hypertransfusion program that corrects the anemia and suppresses the patient's own inadequate erythropoiesis, thus limiting the stimulus for increased iron absorption. This suppression permits the bones to heal, decreases the metabolic expenditures, increases growth, and limits dietary iron absorption. Splenectomy may reduce the transfusion volume but adds to the risk of serious infection. Chelation therapy with desferioxamine, which removes excess iron and prolongs life, should start when laboratory evidence of iron overload is present and prior to clinical manifestations. Bone marrow transplantation in childhood prior to organ dysfunction induced by iron overload has had a high success rate in beta-thalassemia major and is the treatment of choice.

*Sickle Cell Disease.* The common sickle cell syndromes include hemoglobin SS disease, hemoglobin S–hemoglobin C disease, hemoglobin S–beta-thalassemia, and rare variants (Table 14–9). It is important to identify the specific hemoglobin phenotype because the clinical complications differ in frequency, type, and severity.

TABLE 14–9.  Comparison of Sickle Cell Syndromes

| Genotype | Clinical Condition | Percent Hemoglobin | | | | | Other Findings |
|---|---|---|---|---|---|---|---|
| | | Hb A | Hb S | Hb A₂ | Hb F | Hb C | |
| SA | Sickle cell trait | 55–60 | 40–45 | 2–3 | — | — | Usually asymptomatic |
| SS | Sickle cell anemia | 0 | 85–95 | 2–3 | 5–15 | — | Clinically severe anemia; Hb F heterogeneous in distribution |
| S-β⁰ thalassemia | Sickle cell–beta⁰ thalassemia | 0 | 70–80 | 3–5 | 10–20 | — | Moderately severe anemia; splenomegaly in 50%; smear: hypo, micro anemia |
| S-β⁺ thalassemia | Sickle cell–beta⁺ thalassemia | 10–20 | 60–75 | 3–5 | 10–20 | | Hb F distributed heterogeneously; mild microcytic anemia |
| SC | Hb SC disease | 0 | 45–50 | — | — | 45–50 | Moderately severe anemia; splenomegaly; target cells |
| S-HPFH | Sickle—hereditary persistence of Hb F | 0 | 70–80 | 1–2 | 20–30 | — | Asymptomatic; Hb F is uniformly distributed |

From Andreoli TE, Carpenter CCJ, Plum F, et al: Cecil Essentials of Medicine, 3rd ed. Philadelphia, WB Saunders, 1993, p 371.

Sickle cell disease manifests as a chronic hemolytic anemia on which is superimposed sudden, occasionally severe, and life-threatening complications caused by the acute intravascular sickling of the red cells, with resultant pain or organ dysfunction.

PATHOPHYSIOLOGY. As a result of a single amino acid substitution (valine for glutamic acid at the β6 position), hemoglobin S cells change from a normal biconcave disc when oxygenated to a sickled form, with resultant decreased deformability in deoxygenated conditions. Sickle hemoglobin crystallizes and forms a gel in the deoxy state. When reoxygenated, the sickle hemoglobin is normally soluble. The so-called reversible sickle cell is capable of entering the microcirculation. However, as the oxygen saturation falls, sickling may occur with resultant occlusion of the microvasculature. The surrounding tissue undergoes infarction, inducing pain and/or dysfunction. This sickling phenomenon is accentuated by hypoxia, acidosis, increased or decreased temperature, and dehydration (increased concentration of erythrocyte hemoglobin S). The clinical manifestations may be due to infection, anemia, or vaso-occlusion (Table 14–10).

CLINICAL MANIFESTATIONS. The child with sickle cell anemia is vulnerable to life-threatening infection as early as 4 mo of age because of properdin deficiency and splenic dysfunction caused by sickling of the red cells within the spleen, with resultant inability of the spleen to filter microorganisms from the blood stream. Splenic dysfunction is followed eventually by splenic infarction, usually by 2–4 yr of age. In the absence of normal splenic function, the patient is susceptible to overwhelming infection by encapsulated organisms, especially Streptococcus pneumoniae and other pathogens (see Table 14–10). The hallmark of infection is fever. The patient with a sickle cell syndrome who has a temperature greater than 38.5°C (101.5°F) must be evaluated immediately (see Chapter 10). Current precautions to prevent infections include prophylactic daily oral penicillin begun at diagnosis and vaccinations against pneumococcus, H. influenzae type b, hepatitis B virus, and influenza virus.

The anemia of SS disease is usually a chronic, well-compensated, severe anemia that is not routinely transfusion-dependent. The severity depends in part on the patient's phenotype (see Table 14–9). Decisions about transfusion should be made on the basis of the patient's clinical condition, the hemoglobin level, and the reticulocyte count. Manifestations of chronic anemia include jaundice, pallor, variable splenomegaly in infancy, a cardiac flow murmur, and delayed sexual maturation and growth (see Table 14–10).

In three different clinical situations, an acute, potentially life-threatening decline in hemoglobin may be superimposed on the chronic compensated anemia. Splenic sequestration crisis is a life-threatening hyperacute fall in hemoglobin (blood volume) secondary to splenic pooling of the patient's red cells and sickling within the spleen. The spleen is moderately to markedly enlarged, and the reticulo-

TABLE 14–10. Clinical Manifestations of Sickle Cell Anemia*

| Manifestation | Comments |
|---|---|
| Anemia | Chronic, onset 3–4 mo of age; may require folate therapy for chronic hemolysis; hematocrit usually 18–26% |
| Aplastic crisis | Parvovirus infection, reticulocytopenia; acute and reversible; may need transfusion |
| Sequestration crisis | Massive splenomegaly (may involve liver), shock; treat with transfusion |
| Hemolytic crisis | May be associated with G6PD deficiency |
| Dactylitis | Hand-foot swelling in early infancy |
| Painful crisis | Microvascular painful vaso-occlusive infarcts of muscle, bone, bone marrow, lung, intestines |
| Cerebrovascular accidents | Large- and small-vessel occlusion → thrombosis/bleeding (stroke); requires chronic transfusion |
| Acute chest syndrome | Infection, atelectasis, infarction, fat emboli, severe hypoxemia, infiltrate, dyspnea, rales |
| Chronic lung disease | Pulmonary fibrosis, restrictive lung disease, cor pulmonale |
| Priapism | Causes eventual impotence; treat with transfusion, oxygen, or corpora cavernosa–to–spongiosa shunt |
| Ocular | Retinopathy |
| Gallbladder disease | Bilirubin stones; cholecystitis |
| Renal | Hematuria, papillary necrosis, renal-concentrating deficit; nephropathy |
| Cardiomyopathy | Heart failure (fibrosis) |
| Skeletal | Osteonecrosis (avascular) of femoral or humoral head |
| Leg ulceration | Seen in older patients |
| Infections | Functional asplenia, defects in properdin system; pneumococcal bacteremia, meningitis, and arthritis; deafness from meningitis in 35%; *Haemophilus influenzae* sepsis, *Salmonella,* and *Staphylococcus aureus* osteomyelitis; severe *Mycoplasma* pneumonia; risk for transfusion-acquired viral infection† |
| Growth failure, delayed puberty | May respond to nutritional supplements |
| Psychologic problems | Narcotic addiction (rare), dependence unusual; chronic illness, chronic pain |

*Clinical manifestations with sickle cell trait are unusual but include renal papillary necrosis (hematuria), sudden death on exertion, intraocular hyphema extension, and sickling in unpressurized airplanes.
†CMV, EBV, HIV, hepatitis B.
CMV = cytomegalovirus; EBV = Epstein-Barr virus; HIV = human immunodeficiency virus; G6PD = glucose-6-phosphate dehydrogenase.

cyte count is elevated. In an *aplastic crisis,* parvovirus B19 infects red cell precursors in the bone marrow and induces transient red cell aplasia with reticulocytopenia and a rapid worsening of anemia. In the *hyperhemolytic crisis,* there may be an acute fall in hemoglobin associated with medications or infection. There is an increase in bilirubin, reticulocytosis, and accentuated jaundice. These patients usually have G6PD deficiency. For sequestration, aplastic, and hemolytic crises, simple transfusion therapy is indicated when the anemia is symptomatic.

*Vaso-occlusive crises* may occur in any organ of the body, where they are manifested by pain or significant dysfunction (see Table 14–10). The acute chest syndrome is a vaso-occlusive crisis within the lungs, often in association with infection and infarction. The patient may present with pain but within a few hours develops cough, increasing respiratory and heart rates, hypoxia, and progressive respiratory distress. Physical examination of the chest reveals areas of decreased breath sounds, rales, and dullness to percussion. Treatment includes early recognition and prevention of arterial hypoxemia. Oxygen, fluids, judicial use of analgesic medications, antibiotics, and blood transfusion (occasionally exchange transfusion) usually are indicated in therapy of acute chest syndrome. Incentive spirometry reduces the incidence of acute chest crisis in patients having pain in the chest or abdomen.

Patients also may develop vaso-occlusive events within the central nervous system causing clinical or "silent" stroke. They may present with the sudden onset of an altered state of consciousness, seizures, or focal paralysis. Priapism occurs most typically in boys between 6 and 20 yr of age. The child experiences sudden, painful onset of a tumescent penis that will not relax. Therapeutic steps for stroke, priapism, and other potentially life-threatening complications include administration of oxygen, fluids, transfusion to achieve a hemoglobin S less than 30% (often by partial exchange transfusion), and analgesia when appropriate. Fluid management requires recognition that renal medullary infarction results in loss of the ability to concentrate urine. Vaso-occlusive crises may result in avascular necrosis of the femoral head and chronic hip disease.

*Pain crisis* is the most common type of vaso-occlusive event. The pain usually localizes to the long bones of the arms or legs but may occur in smaller bones of the hands or feet in infancy. These painful crises usually last 2–7 days. The treatment of a pain crisis includes fluids, analgesia usually with narcotics or nonsteroidal anti-inflammatory agents, oxygen if the patient is hypoxic, and monitoring of arterial oxygen saturations. The clinician must maintain a sympathetic attitude toward the patient in pain crisis because pain is impossible to quantitate and the risk for drug dependency is highly overrated.

TREATMENT. Direct therapy of sickle cell anemia is evolving. Hydroxyurea has been shown in adults and children to decrease the number and severity of vaso-occlusive events. Bone marrow transplantation has cured a number of children with sickle cell disease.

DIAGNOSIS. The diagnosis is made by the presence of a positive sickle cell solubility test (Sickledex) demonstrating that the patient's red cells sickle (change shape at low oxygen tension) and by a precise characterization of the hemoglobin abnormality using hemoglobin electrophoresis. Every member of an at-risk population should have a precise hemoglobin phenotype (electrophoresis) performed at birth (preferentially) or during early infancy.

*Methemoglobinemia.* Methemoglobinemia, in which ferrous iron has been oxidized to the ferric state, may be either congenital or acquired. Congenital methemoglobinemia may be a result of abnormalities in either the alpha or beta chain. Homozygosity is lethal, whereas heterozygotes usually have a level of 20–30% methemoglobin and are cyanotic in the face of normal $PaO_2$. Homozygous deficiency of NADH reductase (diaphorase) is common in Navajo Indians and results in chronic methemoglobinemia. Infants under the age of 3 mo, whose antioxidant mechanisms are poorly developed, are especially vulnerable.

Acquired methemoglobinemia is seen with ingestion of certain oxidants. Nitrates and nitrites, derived from fertilizer and disinfectants in well water and foods or from enteric bacteria during diarrhea, are major etiologic factors. If sufficiently severe, this condition may be life-threatening. Methemoglobinemia should be suspected in a deeply chocolate-colored cyanotic infant without cardiopulmonary disease in whom metabolic acidosis, a high $PaO_2$, and unsaturated hemoglobin are present. The methemoglobin levels should be measured; treatment with methylene blue or ascorbate usually rapidly reduces $Fe^{3+}$ to $Fe^{2+}$, correcting this condition.

### Hemolytic Anemia Caused by Disorders Extrinsic to the Red Cell

Immune-mediated hemolysis may be extravascular when red cells coated with antibodies or complement are phagocytized by the reticuloendothelial system or may be intravascular when antibody binding leads to complement fixation and lysis of red blood cells.

**Isoimmune hemolysis** is caused by active maternal immunization against fetal antigens that the mother's erythrocytes do not express (see Chapter 6). Examples include antibody to the A, B, and Rh D antigens, other Rh antigens, and the Kell, Duffy, and other blood groups. Anti-A and anti-B hemolysis is caused by the placental transfer of naturally occurring maternal antibodies from mothers who lack A or B antigen (usually blood type O). Positive results of the direct antiglobulin (Coombs) test on the baby's red cells (Fig. 14–6) and the indirect antiglobulin test on the mother's serum and the presence of spherocytes and immature erythroid precursors (erythroblastosis) on the infant's blood smear confirm this diagnosis. Isoimmune hemolytic disease may be highly variable in its clinical severity. No clinical manifestations may be present, or the infant may present with jaundice, severe anemia, and hydrops fetalis.

**Autoimmune hemolytic anemia** (AIHA) is usually an acute, self-limited process that develops after an infection (*Mycoplasma*, Epstein-Barr, or other viral infections). More than 80% of children with AIHA spontaneously recover. AIHA also may be the presenting symptom of a chronic autoimmune disease (e.g., systemic lupus erythematosus [SLE], lymphoproliferative disorders, or immune deficiency). Transfusion is challenging because cross-matching is difficult, since the autoantibodies react with virtually all red cells. The peripheral blood smear usually demonstrates spherocytes and occasionally nucleated red cells. The reticulocyte

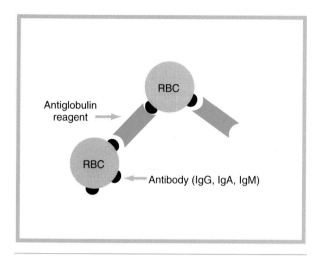

FIGURE 14–6. Coombs or Direct antiglobulin test (DAT). In the Coombs test, an antibody directed against human immunoglobulin (Ig) is used to detect the presence of antibody on the surface of the red blood cells by agglutination. Complement coating on the red blood cells (C3) similarly can be detected by an anticomplement Coombs reagent. Broad-spectrum Coombs reagents can be prepared that detect either immunoglobulin or complement, or both; these are used for screening. (From Andreoli TE, Carpenter CCJ, Plum F, et al: Cecil Essentials of Medicine, 3rd ed. Philadelphia, WB Saunders, 1993, p 367.)

count is variable, because some patients have relatively low reticulocyte counts as a result of autoantibody that cross-reacts with red cell precursors. In addition to transfusion, which may be lifesaving, management of AIHA depends on antibody type and may include administration of corticosteroids and, at times, intravenous immunoglobulin (IVIG). The corticosteroids reduce the clearance of the sensitized red cells in the spleen.

*Drugs* also may induce a Coombs-positive hemolytic anemia. Withdrawal of the drug usually results in resolution of the hemolytic process. Drugs may form a hapten on the red cell membrane (penicillin). Alternatively, drugs may form immune complexes (quinidine) that attach to the red cell membrane. Antibodies then activate complement-induced intravascular hemolysis. The third type of drug-induced immune hemolysis occurs during treatment with alpha-methyldopa and a few other drugs. In this type, prolonged exposure to the drug alters the red blood cell membrane, inducing neoantigen formation. Antibodies are produced that bind to the neoantigen; this produces a positive antiglobulin test far more commonly than it actually induces hemolysis. In each of these conditions the erythrocyte acts as an "innocent bystander."

A second form of acquired hemolytic disease is not immune in nature and is caused by mechanical damage to the membrane of the red cells during circulation. In **microangiopathic hemolytic anemia** (MAHA), the red cells are trapped by fibrin strands in the circulation and physically broken by shear stress as they pass through these strands. Hemolytic-uremic syndrome (HUS), disseminated intravascular coagulation (DIC), thrombotic thrombocytopenic purpura, malignant hypertension, toxemia, and renal graft rejection all produce MAHA. Platelets usually are large, indicating that they are young. These platelets have a decreased survival even if the numbers are normal. Consumption of clotting factors is more prominent in DIC than in the other forms of MAHA. The smear shows red cell fragments (schistocytes), microspherocytes, teardrop forms, and polychromasia. The red cells also may be damaged by exposure to nonendothelialized surfaces (e.g., as in artificial heart valves [the "Waring blender" syndrome]) or as a result of high flow and shear rates in arteriovenous malformations (**Kasabach-Merritt syndrome**).

*Alterations in the plasma lipids*, especially cholesterol, may result in damage to the red cell membrane and shorten red cell survival. Lipids in the plasma are in equilibrium with those in the red cell membrane; high cholesterol levels increase the membrane cholesterol and the total membrane surface without affecting the volume of the cell. This condition produces spur cells. These are seen in abetalipoproteinemia and liver diseases. Hemolysis occurs in the spleen, where poor red cell deformability results in erythrocyte destruction. *Circulating toxins* such as snake venoms and heavy metals that bind sulfhydryl groups (copper, arsenic) may damage the red cell membrane and induce hemolysis. Irregularly spiculated red cells (burr cells) are seen in renal failure. *Vitamin E deficiency* also can cause an acquired hemolytic anemia as a result of abnormal sensitivity of membrane lipids to oxidant stress. Vitamin E deficiency may occur in premature infants who are not being supplemented with vitamin E or who have insufficient nutrition, in severe malabsorption syndromes (including cystic fibrosis), and in transfusional iron overload, which can result in severe oxidant exposure.

## PANCYTOPENIA

Pancytopenia is a decrease in the number of all the formed elements of the blood—erythrocytes, leukocytes, and platelets. Patients present with symptoms of anemia, infection, or bleeding. Individual formed elements, or a combination of elements, may be decreased in numbers because of failure of production (implying intrinsic bone marrow disease), sequestration (as in hypersplenism), or increased peripheral destruction.

*Features that suggest bone marrow failure* and mandate an examination of bone marrow include a low (<2%) RPI, teardrop forms of red cells (implies marrow replacement, not just failure), the presence of abnormal forms of leukocytes or myeloid elements less mature than band forms, small platelets, and an elevated mean corpuscular volume in the face of a low reticulocyte count. Pancytopenia resulting from bone marrow failure is usually a gradual process. Patients may present with one or two involved cell lines but later progress to involvement of all three cell lines.

*Features suggesting increased destruction* include reticulocytosis, jaundice, immature erythroid or myeloid elements on the blood smear, large platelets, and increased serum bilirubin and lactic dehydrogenase.

## APLASTIC ANEMIA

In the child with aplastic anemia, pancytopenia evolves as the hematopoietic elements of the bone marrow disappear and the marrow is replaced by fat. A biopsy is crucial to determine the extent of depletion of the hematopoietic elements. Aplastic anemia may be idiopathic. Alternatively, this disorder may be induced by drugs such as chloramphenicol or by toxins such as benzene. Aplastic anemia also may follow infections, particularly hepatitis and infectious mononucleosis (see Table 14–8).

**Fanconi anemia**, a constitutional aplastic anemia, usually presents in the latter half of the first decade of life and may evolve over a period of years. The repair mechanism for deoxyribonucleic acid (DNA) damage is abnormal in all cells in Fanconi anemia, a finding that facilitates the diagnosis but also may contribute to the development of malignancies (terminal acute leukemia develops in 10% of cases). These patients have a number of characteristic clinical findings (see Table 14–8).

For children with severe aplastic anemia, as defined by an RPI less than 1%, absolute neutrophil count less than 500/mm³, platelet count less than 20,000/mm³, and bone marrow cellularity on biopsy less than 10%, the *treatment* of choice is bone marrow transplantation from a human leukocyte antigen (HLA)–identical, mixed lymphocyte–compatible sibling. With supportive care alone, survival is only about 20% in severe aplastic anemia, although the duration of survival may be years when vigorous blood product and antibiotic

support are provided. When bone marrow transplantation takes place prior to sensitization of the recipient to blood products by repeated transfusion, the survival rate is in excess of 80%. Positive results may be attained by bone marrow transplantation from HLA-compatible, nonrelated donors. Graft-versus-host disease is a complication of bone marrow transplantation (see Chapter 8). The treatment of aplastic anemia without a matched donor for transplantation is evolving with two major options: potent immunosuppressive therapy or unrelated or partially matched bone marrow transplantation. (see Table 14–8). Most patients with Fanconi anemia and about 20% of children with aplastic anemia appear to respond to androgenic therapy, which unfortunately induces masculinization and may cause liver injury and liver tumors. Androgenic therapy increases red cell synthesis and may diminish transfusion requirements. The effect on granulocytes, and especially the platelet count, is less impressive.

Immune suppression of hematopoiesis is postulated to be an important mechanism in patients with postinfectious and idiopathic aplastic anemia. Results of trials using antithymocyte globulin, cyclosporine, and corticosteroids in combination with hematopoietic growth factors have been encouraging. Such therapy is often toxic, and relapses do occur.

## MARROW REPLACEMENT

Marrow replacement may occur as a result of leukemia, solid tumors (especially neuroblastoma), storage diseases, osteopetrosis in infants, and myelofibrosis, which is rare in childhood. The mechanisms by which malignant cells impair marrow synthesis of normal hemopoietic elements are unclear. Bone marrow aspirate and biopsy are needed for precise diagnosis that then determines appropriate therapy.

## PANCYTOPENIA RESULTING FROM DESTRUCTION OF CELLS

This form of pancytopenia may be caused by intramedullary destruction of hemopoietic elements (as occurs in myeloproliferative disorders, folic acid, and vitamin $B_{12}$ deficiency) or as a result of peripheral destruction of mature cells. The usual site of peripheral destruction of blood cells is the spleen, although the liver and other parts of the reticuloendothelial system may participate. *Hypersplenism* may be due to anatomic causes such as portal hypertension or splenic hypertrophy from thalassemia, infections (including malaria), storage diseases such as Gaucher disease, lymphomas, and histiocytosis. Splenectomy is indicated only when the pancytopenia is of clinical significance, causing the patients to have increased susceptibility to bleeding or infection or producing a high transfusion requirement.

## References

Bacigalupo A, Broccia G, Corda G, et al: Antilymphocyte globulin, cyclosporin, and granulocyte colony-stimulating factor in patients with acquired severe aplastic anemia (SAA): A pilot study of the EBMT SAA Working Party. Blood 85:1348, 1995.

Behrman RE, Kliegman RM, Arvin AM (eds): Nelson Textbook of Pediatrics, 15th ed. Philadelphia, WB Saunders, 1996, Chapters 405–425.

Beutler E: Glucose-6-phosphate dehydrogenese deficiency. N Engl J Med; 324:169, 1991.

Boutry M, Needlman R: Use of diet history in the screening of iron deficiency. Pediatrics 98:1138, 1996.

Cherrick I, Karayalcin G, Lanzkowsky P: Transient erythroblastopenia of childhood. Am J Pediatr Hematol Oncol 14:320, 1994.

Eber SW, Armbrust R, Schroter W: Variable clinical severity of hereditary spherocytosis: Relation to erythrocytic spectrin concentration, osmotic fragility, and autohemolysis. J Pediatr 117:409, 1990.

Ehlers KH, Giardina PJ, Lesser ML, et al: Prolonged survival in patients with beta-thalassemia major treated with deferoxamine. J Pediatr 118:540, 1991.

Embury SH, Hebbel RP, Mohandas N, et al (eds): Sickle cell disease: Basic principles and clinical practice, 1st ed. New York, Raven Press, 1994.

Frewin R, Henson A, Provan D: Iron deficiency anemia. BMJ 314:360, 1997.

Goodnough L, Mark T, Andriole G: Erythropoietin therapy. N Engl J Med 336:933, 1997.

Kaushansky K: Thrombopoietin: The primary regulator of platelet production. Blood 86:419, 1995.

Leikin SL, Gallagher D, Kinney TR, et al: Mortality in children and adolescents with sickle cell disease. Pediatrics 84:500, 1989.

Oski FA: Iron deficiency in infancy and childhood. N Engl J Med 329:190, 1993.

Pearson H: Prevention of pneumococcal disease in sickle cell anemia. J Pediatr 129:788, 1996.

Platt OS, Thorington BD, Brambilla DJ, et al: Pain in sickle cell disease: Rates and risk factors. N Engl J Med 325:11, 1991.

Raunikar RA, Sabio H: Anemia in the adolescent athlete. Am J Dis Child 146:1201, 1992.

Scott JP, Hillery CA, Brown ER, et al: Hydroxyurea therapy in children severely affected with sickle cell disease. J Pediatr 128:820, 1996.

Sears DA: Anemia of chronic disease. Med Clin North Am 76:567, 1992.

Steingart R: Management of patients with sickle cell disease. Med Clin North Am 76:669, 1992.

Stewart FM: Hypoplastic, aplastic anemia: Role of bone marrow transplantation. Med Clin North Am 76:683, 1992.

Ware R: Salmonella infection in sickle cell disease: A clear and present danger. J. Pediatr 130:350, 1997.

Walters MC, Patience M, Leisenring W, et al: Bone marrow transplantation for sickle cell disease. N Engl J Med 335:369, 1996.

Weatherall D: The hereditary anemias. BMJ 314:492, 1997.

Webb DKH, Mann JM, Chessells JM: Acquired aplastic anaemia: Still a serious disease. Arch Dis Child 66:858, 1991.

## DISORDERS OF LEUKOCYTES

The major function of phagocytic cells is to ingest and kill pathogens (see Chapters 8 and 10). The major manifestation of neutropenia or neutrophil dysfunction is increased susceptibility to infection with bacteria, fungi, or both.

### NEUTROPENIA

The normal neutrophil count varies with age (see Table 14–2). Neutropenia is defined as an absolute neutrophil count less than $1500/mm^3$ for Caucasion children over 1 yr of age. Black children normally have somewhat lower total and neutrophil counts.

The impact of neutropenia depends on its severity. The susceptibility to infection is unaffected until the absolute neutrophil count (ANC) is less than $1000/mm^3$. Patients do quite well as long as the ANC is greater than $500/mm^3$. At these levels of circulating neutrophils, localized infections are more common than generalized bacteremia. With an ANC less than $200/mm^3$, serious bacterial infections are quite common. Episodes of bacteremia also are associated with the presence of indwelling catheters, mucosal injury secondary to cytotoxic agents, and immunosuppressive agents. The presence of an underlying malignancy, treatment with chemotherapy, or immunodeficiency disorder also increases the risk for serious bacterial or fungal infection. In the absence of an adequate neutrophil count, there is a subsequent delay in migration of neutrophils to areas of damage in the skin and mucous membrane. The major types of infection associated with neutropenia include cellulitis, pharyngitis, gingivitis, lymphadenitis, abscesses (cutaneous or perianal), enteritis (typhlitis), and pneumonia. These sites usually all are colonized heavily with normal bacterial flora that become invasive in the presence of neutropenia. Meticulous attention to oral and skin hygiene and prevention of colonization with fungi are helpful in minimizing such infections.

Neutropenia may be congenital or acquired. Neutropenia may be classified mechanistically (Table 14–11) and commonly may be associated with specific diseases, especially infections (Table 14–12), or drugs (Table 14–13).

*Congenital Neutropenia.* Most congenital neutropenias are caused by an inadequate production

TABLE 14–11.    Mechanisms of Neutropenia

**Abnormal Bone Marrow**

Marrow injury
Drugs: idiosyncratic, cytotoxic (myelosuppressive)
Radiation
Chemicals: DDT, benzene
Hereditary
Immune-mediated: T and B cell and immunoglobulin
Infection: HIV, hepatitis
Infiltrative processes: tumor, storage disease

Maturation defects
Folic acid deficiency
Vitamin $B_{12}$
Glycogen storage disease type Ib
Shwachman syndrome
Organic acidemias
Clonal disorders: congenital
Cyclic neutropenia

**Peripheral Circulation**

Pseudoneutropenia: shift to bone marrow
Hereditary
Severe infection

Intravascular
Destruction: neonatal isoimmune, autoimmune, hypersplenism
Leukoagglutination: lung, after cardiac bypass surgery

**Extravascular Mechanisms**

Increased utilization: severe infection, anaphylaxis
Destruction: antibody-mediated, hypersplenism

Adapted from Bagby G: *In* Andreoli TE, Carpenter, CCJ, Plum F, et al (eds): Cecil Essentials of Medicine, 2nd ed. Philadelphia, WB Saunders, 1990.
DDT = chlorophenothane; HIV = human immunodeficiency virus.

TABLE 14–12.    Infections Associated with Neutropenia

| Bacterial | Rickettsial |
|---|---|
| Typhoid–paratyphoid | Rocky Mountain spotted fever |
| Brucellosis | Typhus |
| Neonatal sepsis | Ehrlichiosis |
| Meningococcemia | Rickettsialpox |
| Overwhelming sepsis | |
| Congenital syphilis | |
| Tuberculosis | |
| **Viral** | |
| Measles | |
| Hepatitis A and B | |
| HIV | |
| Rubella | |
| CMV | |
| Influenza A and B | |
| Epstein-Barr virus | |

CMV = cytomegalovirus; HIV = human immunodeficiency virus.

TABLE 14–13.    Drugs Associated with Neutropenia

**Cytotoxic**
Myelosuppressive, chemotherapeutic agents
Immunosuppressive agents

**Idiosyncratic**
Chloramphenicol
Sulfonamides
Propylthiouracil
Penicillins
Trimethoprim/sulfamethoxazole
Carbamazepine
Phenytoin
Cimetidine
Methyldopa
Indomethacin
Chlorpromazine
Penicillamine
Gold salts

of cells. The most severe clinical disorders are *reticular dysgenesis* (severe combined immunodeficiency with agranulocytosis) and *infantile genetic agranulocytosis* (IGA, or **Kostmann syndrome**). Both are inherited as autosomal recessive disorders and frequently are fatal in infancy. IGA is marked by monocytosis in up to 50% of the circulating leukocytes. Growth of myeloid cultures in vitro is normal, suggesting a defect in control mechanisms; G-CSF levels are undetectable, whereas exogenous G-CSF produces a rise in the neutrophil count. Transfusion of granulocytes and administration of G-CSF during severe infections may be lifesaving. Acute myeloid leukemia has developed in only a few patients who have survived into adolescence. Bone marrow transplantation may be curative.

Other congenital neutropenias caused by deficient production of neutrophils vary in severity and are poorly characterized. *Benign congenital neutropenia* is a functional diagnosis for patients with significant neutropenia in whom major infectious complications do not develop. Many patients whose ANCs range from 100 to 500/mm³ have an increased frequency of infections, particularly respiratory infections, but the major problem is the slow resolution of the infections that develop. These disorders may be sporadic or familial and in some instances are transmitted as an autosomal dominant disorder.

*Cyclic neutropenia* may be transmitted as an autosomal dominant, recessive, or sporadic disorder. This is a stem cell disorder in which all marrow elements cycle. However, the only clinically significant abnormality is neutropenia because of the short half-life of neutrophils (6–7 hr) in comparison with platelets (10 days) and red cells (120 days). The usual neutropenic cycle is 21 days, with agranulocytosis lasting 4–6 days accompanied by monocytosis and often by eosinophilia. Clinical manifestations include stomatitis or oral ulcers, pharyngitis, lymphadenopathy, fever, and cellulitis at the time of neutropenia. Severe debilitating bone pain is common in these patients when the neutrophil count is low. Cyclic neutropenia responds to G-CSF with a reduced number of days of neutropenia and an overall increase of neutrophils.

*Pancreatic insufficiency accompanying bone marrow dysfunction* (**Shwachman-Diamond syndrome**) is also a panmyeloid disorder in which neutropenia is the most prominent manifestation. In this autosomal recessive condition, patients may have all the common complications of neutropenia. A major complication is gingivitis, which may be severe and lead to serious oral infections and alveolar bone destruction. Patients may become edentulous at an early age. Metaphyseal dysostosis and dwarfism also may occur. Patients may respond to G-CSF.

***Acquired Neutropenia.*** Neutropenia may be caused by either marrow hypoplasia or peripheral neutrophil destruction. *Isoimmune neutropenia* occurs in up to 3% of neonates and is due to transplacental transfer of maternal antibodies to fetal neutrophil antigens. In isoimmune neonatal neutropenia, the mother is sensitized to specific neutrophil antigens (NA1, NA2, NB1, and NC1) on fetal leukocytes inherited from the father and not present on maternal cells. Isoimmune neonatal neutropenia, like isoimmune anemia and thrombocytopenia (see Chapter 6), is a transient process. Early treatment of infection (cutaneous is most common; sepsis is rarer) while the infant is neutropenic is the major goal of therapy. Administration of IVIg may decrease the duration of neutropenia.

*Autoimmune neutropenia* usually develops early in childhood (5–24 mo of age) and often persists for prolonged periods. Neutrophil autoantibodies may be immunoglobulin (Ig) M, IgG, IgA, or a combination of these. Usually there is resolution in 6 mo to 4 yr. Clinical symptoms may dictate treatment. Although IVIG or corticosteroids have been used in the past, most patients respond to G-CSF. Most patients do not progress to more generalized autoimmune disorders; however, rarely, autoimmune neutropenia may be an early manifestation of SLE or rheumatoid arthritis. The marrow in autoimmune neutropenia and SLE shows myeloid hyperplasia, except that if antibody is directed against myeloid precursors, it reveals hypoplasia. The *differential diagnosis* of autoimmune neutropenia includes SLE, rheumatoid arthritis (Felty syndrome), bone marrow transplantation, or drug-induced neutropenia.

Neutropenia is common in *stressed neonates.* Virtually any major illness, including asphyxia, may precipitate transient neonatal neutropenia. Significant neutropenia may develop in infected neonates at least in part on the basis of depletion of bone marrow stores. These bone marrow stores, which are 7 times the circulating pool of neutrophils in adults, are far less extensive in neonates. Therefore, their marrow reserve is readily depleted by infectious processes.

***Diagnosis.*** Neutropenia is confirmed by a complete blood count and differential. The evaluation of the neutropenic child depends on associated clinical abnormalities, such as signs of infection, family and medication history, age of the patient, cyclic or persistent nature of the condition, signs of bone marrow infiltration (malignancy, storage disease), and evidence of involvement of other cell lines. An algorithm for the work-up of the child with neutropenia is presented in Figure 14–7.

***Treatment.*** Therapy for neutropenia is dependent on the underlying cause. Patients with severe bacterial infections require broad-spectrum antibiotics; the resolution of neutropenia during an infection is a good prognostic sign. Unfortunately, granulocyte transfusion has been relatively unsuccessful in improving survival in instances of overwhelming infections in neutropenic patients. Chronic mild neutropenia not associated with immunosuppression can be managed expectantly with prompt antimicrobial treatment of soft tissue infections (*Staphylococcus aureus, Streptococcus*). Although past therapy of neutropenia included white blood cell transfusions, corticosteroids, lithium, splenectomy, or IVIg, the current first line of therapy for clinically significant neutropenia is G-CSF.

## LEUKOCYTOSIS
### (Neutrophilia)

Leukocytosis most often is associated with infection (>15,000 WBCs/mm³). When acute infection occurs, particularly bacterial infection, neutrophils are released from bone marrow stores to induce a rapid increase in the circulating WBC count. Chronic infection, such as tuberculosis, osteomyelitis, and abscesses, also may cause neutrophilia. A shift in the distribution of the cells, with a greater number circulating than adhering to blood vessel walls, is a common mechanism for neutrophilia associated with drugs, including corticosteroids and epinephrine. Certain disorders of neutrophil function, especially the lack of the complement receptor CR3 (*Mo-1 deficiency*), are associated with a marked leukocytosis. Leukocytosis also may be a

**NEUTROPENIA**

*WELL CHILD*
**Mucocutaneous Infection**

*Cycles*

Repeat WBC count 2–3 times/wk

*Noncyclic*

1. Antineutrophil antibody (immune, SLE)
2. Nutritional (copper, folate, vitamin B$_{12}$ deficiency)
3. Marrow (arrest, megaloblastic, cellularity)

*SICK CHILD*
**Recurrent Infection**

Neutropenia

1. Bone marrow for congenital disorder
2. Immune globulin levels for Ig deficiency
3. Diepoxybutane test for Fanconi anemia
4. T-cell and B-cell function for reticular dysgenesis
5. Pancreatic function (Shwachman-Diamond syndrome)
6. Colony-stimulating activity
7. Colony-forming unit assay

Pancytopenia

1. Bone marrow for malignancy, aplastic anemia, hemophagocytic disorders
2. Diepoxybutane test for Fanconi anemia
3. Organic acids for methylmalonic acidemia
4. Examine for hypersplenism
5. Bone marrow chromosomes for myelodysplasia

Sepsis, Other infection

1. Bacterial, viral, fungal, TB cultures; rickettsial titers
2. HIV titer

FIGURE 14–7. Algorithm for the evaluation of neutropenia. HIV = human immunodeficiency virus; IgG = immunoglobulin G; SLE = systemic lupus erythematosus; TB = tuberculosis; WBC = white blood cell.

normal variant in some families in which several members have an increase in total neutrophil counts without apparent underlying pathology. Chronic myelogenous leukemia also is characterized by neutrophilia. However, immature forms of granulocytes usually are present.

## DEFECTS IN NEUTROPHIL FUNCTION

These relatively rare inherited disorders tend to be associated with a marked susceptibility to bacterial infection (see Chapter 8). Some acquired functional disorders also occur and may be quite severe. *Leukocyte adhesion deficiency* is due to defective neutrophil chemotaxis, ingestion of particles opsonized with complement, and adherence to surfaces. It is a consequence of lack of CR3, the receptor for C3bi. This disorder presents in early infancy with failure of separation of the umbilical cord, often until as late as 2 mo after birth, with attendant omphalitis and sepsis. The neutrophil count usually is greater than 20,000/mm$^3$ because of failure of the neutrophils to adhere normally to vascular endothelium and to migrate out of blood to the tissues. Cutaneous, respiratory, and mucosal infections occur, and these children usually have severe gingivitis. Sepsis usually leads to death in early childhood. This disorder is transmitted as an autosomal recessive trait that has an unknown frequency. Bone marrow transplantation may be lifesaving.

Defective bacterial killing, because the phagocytes are unable to generate reactive oxygen species such as hydrogen peroxide, hydroxyl radical, and superoxide anion, is the major feature of **chronic granulomatous disease** (see Chapter 8). Nonoxidative killing is abnormal in *secondary granule deficiency*, a rare disorder in which bacterial killing also is delayed. An acquired form of secondary granule deficiency occurs in patients with severe burn injuries; it occurs about 2 wk after the original trauma. This poor killing ability may contribute to the increased susceptibility to bacterial infection of burn patients (see Chapter 3). The acquired defect is reversible.

Another abnormality of secondary granules is **Chédiak-Higashi syndrome,** an autosomal recessive disorder that results in fusion of the primary and secondary granules of the neutrophil. Giant granules are present in many cells, including lymphocytes, platelets, and melanocytes. Patients usually have partial oculocutaneous albinism. Although most patients have frequent fevers in infancy and early childhood, documented bacterial infection is not common. Infection with the Epstein-Barr virus (EBV) produces a loss of natural killer cells and results in a **lymphoproliferative syndrome**, characterized by hepatomegaly, adenopathy, and pancytopenia. This may lead to an "accelerated phase," which usually is rapidly fatal. Children who avoid EBV infection may live into adulthood without major clinical problems, except for gingivitis.

A variety of conditions also are associated with chemotactic defects in neutrophils. **Job syndrome** usually is acquired and may be seen in childhood. The major manifestations are eczema, hyperimmunoglobulinemia E, an extrinsic chemotactic defect, a T-cell defect with reduced interferon production, and recurrent "cold" boils (S. aureus) that do not become markedly red or drain. In some patients, identifying offending allergens or removing them has resulted in resolution of the chemotactic defect as well as the eczema and boils. The "**lazy leukocyte syndrome**" is caused by a chemotactic defect resulting from failure of neutrophil egress from the bone marrow and consequent neutropenia. Several systemic disorders, including uremia, SLE, Hodgkin disease, liver disease, and poorly controlled diabetes mellitus, also have associated chemotactic defects.

### References

Behrman RE, Kliegman RM, Arvin AM (eds): Nelson Textbook of Pediatrics, 15th ed. Philadelphia, WB Saunders, 1996, Chapters 112–131, 428.

Conway L, Clay M, Kline W, et al: Natural history of primary autoimmune neutropenia in infancy. J Pediatr 79:728, 1987.

Dale DC, Bonilla MA, Davis MW et al: A randomized controlled phase III trial of recombinant human G-CSF for treatment of severe chronic neutropenia. Blood 81:2496, 1993.

Jonsson OG, Buchanan GR: Chronic neutropenia during childhood: A 13 year experience in a single institution. Am J Dis Child 145:232, 1991.

Metcalf D: Control of granulocytes and macrophages: Molecular, cellular, and clinical aspects. Science 254:529, 1991.

Smolen JE, Boxer LA: Function of neutrophils and mononuclear phagocytes. In Bennett JC, Plum F (eds): Cecil Textbook of Medicine, 20th ed. Philadelphia, WB Saunders, 1994, p 895–904.

Yang KD, Hill HR: Neutrophil function disorders: Pathophysiology, prevention, and therapy. J Pediatr 119:343, 1991.

## HEMOSTATIC DISORDERS

### NORMAL HEMOSTASIS

Hemostasis is the dynamic process by which coagulation occurs on areas of vascular injury and is limited to areas of injury so that the clot does not extend beyond the initial site of vascular damage. This process involves the carefully modulated interaction of platelets, vascular wall, and procoagulant and anticoagulant proteins. After an injury to the vascular endothelium, subendothelial collagen induces a conformational change in von Willebrand factor, an adhesive protein to which platelets bind via their glycoprotein Ib receptor. Following adhesion, platelets undergo activation and release a number of intracellular contents, including adenosine diphosphate (ADP), that subsequently induce aggregation of additional platelets. Simultaneously, subendothelial collagen and other matrix proteins in the tissue activate the coagulation cascade, leading to the formation of the enzyme thrombin (Fig. 14–8). Thrombin has multiple effects on the coagulation mechanism, including further aggregation of platelets, a positive feedback activation of factors V and VIII, the conversion of fibrinogen to fibrin, and the activation of factor XIII. Thrombin also contributes to the eventual limitation of clot size by binding to the endothelial cell protein thrombomodulin, thereby converting protein C into activated protein C. Thrombin contributes to the eventual lysis of the thrombus by activating plasminogen to plasmin (Fig. 14–9). The platelet plug forms and bleeding ceases usually within 3–7 min. The generation of thrombin results in formation of a permanent clot by the activation of factor XIII, which cross-links fibrin and results in a stable thrombus. These two processes are closely interwoven and occur on the biologic surfaces that mediate coagulation: the platelet, the endothelial cell, and the subendothelium. As a final element to this process, contractile elements within the platelet mediate clot retraction.

Although it is convenient to think of coagulation as having "intrinsic" and "extrinsic" pathways, the reality is that these pathways are closely interactive and do not react independently (see Fig. 14–8). Negatively charged surfaces (glass, collagen, or kaolin) activate factor XII, which then interacts with

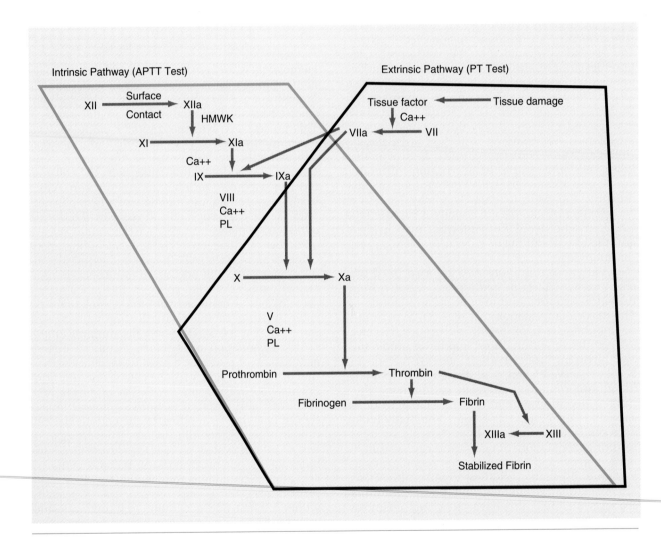

Intrinsic Pathway (APTT Test)

Extrinsic Pathway (PT Test)

FIGURE 14–8.  Simplified pathways of blood coagulation. The area inside the green line is the intrinsic pathway, measured by the activated partial thromboplastin time (APTT). The area inside the black line is the extrinsic pathway, measured by the prothrombin time (PT). The area encompassed by both lines is the common pathway. (From Andreoli, TE, Carpenter CCJ, Plum F, et al: Cecil Essentials of Medicine, 3rd ed. Philadelphia, WB Saunders, 1993, p 409.)

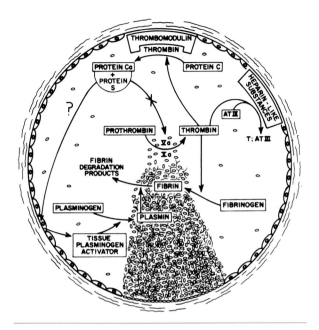

FIGURE 14–9. Formation of the hemostatic plug at the site of vascular injury. Three major physiologic anticoagulant mechanisms—antithrombin III (AT III), protein C, and the fibrinolytic system—are activated to limit clot formation to the site of damage and to prevent generalized thrombosis. T = thrombin. (From Schafer A: The hypercoagulable states. Ann Intern Med 102:814, 1985, p 815.)

prekallikrein and high-molecular-weight kininogen to activate factor XI and initiate the intrinsic system. Tissue factor, in combination with calcium and factor VII, activates the extrinsic pathway. In vivo, factor VIIa, however, most likely activates factor IX, with eventual generation of thrombin, partially explaining why deficiency of factor VIII or IX results in severe bleeding disorders, whereas deficiency of factor XI is usually mild, and deficiency of factor XII is asymptomatic.

As the procoagulant proteins are activated, there are a series of inhibitory factors that serve to tightly regulate the activation of coagulation (see Fig. 14–9). Antithrombin III inactivates thrombin and factors Xa, IXa, and XIa. The protein C and protein S system serves to inactivate activated factors V and VIII, which are cofactors localized in the "tenase" and "prothrombinase" complexes. The tissue factor pathway inhibitor (TFPI), an anticoagulant protein, serves to limit the activation of the coagulation cascade by factors VIIa and Xa. *Fibrinolysis* is initiated by the action of tissue plasminogen activator (urokinase) on plasminogen, producing plasmin, the active enzyme that degrades fibrin into split products (see Fig. 14–9). It is fibrinolysis that eventually dissolves the clot and allows normal flow to resume.

## APPROACH TO THE PATIENT WITH A HEMOSTATIC DISORDER

Patients with hemostatic disorders may present with either complaints of bleeding or clotting. Certain historic variables are paramount in taking the appropriate history. The age at onset of bleeding (acquired, congenital), the sites of bleeding, the amount of trauma required, aspirin (drug) exposure, and the characteristics of symptoms (mucocutaneous or deep bleeding) are critical.

A detailed *family history* is quite important. When one is investigating thrombotic disorders, a personal and family history of early-onset stroke, heart attack, cutaneous thrombosis, and blood clots in the legs or lungs suggests a hereditary predisposition to thromboses. *Physical examination* should characterize the presence of cutaneous, synovial, and mucosal bleeding, in addition to deeper sites of hemorrhage. Evidence of malignancy (lymphadenopathy, hepatosplenomegaly) or chronic hepatic or renal disease also should be sought. The term *petechiae* refers to a nonblanching lesion less than 2 mm in size, *purpura* are groups of adjoining petechiae, *ecchymoses* are isolated lesions larger than petechiae, and *hematomas* are raised ecchymoses.

Screening laboratory studies after the history and physical examination should include those in Table 14–14. No single laboratory test study can confirm all bleeding disorders. Common causes of bleeding are shown in Figure 14–10, and a brief differential diagnosis of hemostatic disorders is outlined in Figure 14–11.

### DISORDERS OF PLATELETS

#### Thrombocytopenia
#### (see Figs. 14–10 and 14–11)

Platelet counts below 150,000/mm$^3$ constitute thrombocytopenia. Mucocutaneous bleeding is the hallmark of platelet disorders, including thrombocytopenia. The risk of bleeding, however, correlates imperfectly with the platelet count. In general, children with platelet counts greater than 80,000/mm$^3$ are able to withstand all but the most extreme hemostatic challenges, such as surgery or major trauma. In contrast, those with platelet counts less than 20,000/mm$^3$ are at risk for spontaneous bleeding. These generalizations are modified by factors such as the age of the platelets (young, large platelets usually function better than old ones) and the presence of inhibitors of platelet function, such as antibodies, drugs (especially aspirin), fibrin degra-

TABLE 14–14.  Screening Tests for Bleeding Disorders

| Test | Mechanism Tested | Normal Values | Disorder |
|---|---|---|---|
| Prothrombin time (PT) | Extrinsic and common pathway | <12 sec beyond neonate; 12–18 sec in term neonate | Defect in vitamin K–dependent factors; hemorrhagic disease of newborn, malabsorption, liver disease, DIC, oral anticoagulants, ingestion of rat poison |
| Activated partial thromboplastin time (APTT; PTT) | Intrinsic and common pathway | 25–40 sec beyond neonate; 70 sec in term neonate | Hemophilia; von Willebrand disease, heparin; DIC; deficient factor XII and XI, lupus anticoagulant |
| Thrombin time (TT) | Fibrinogen to fibrin conversion | 10–15 sec beyond neonate; 12–17 sec in term neonate | Fibrin split products, DIC, hypofibrinogenemia, heparin, uremia |
| Bleeding time (BT) | Hemostasis, capillary and platelet function | 3–7 min beyond neonate | Platelet dysfunction, thrombocytopenia, von Willebrand disease, aspirin |
| Platelet count | Platelet number | 150,000–450,000/mm³ | Thrombocytopenia differential diagnosis (see Fig. 14–10) |
| Blood smear | Platelet number and size; RBC morphology | — | Large platelets suggest peripheral destruction; fragmented, bizarre RBC morphology suggests microangiopathic process (e.g., hemolytic-uremic syndrome, hemangioma, DIC) |

DIC = disseminated intravascular coagulation; RBC = red blood cell.

dation products, and toxins in hepatic or renal disease.

The *etiology* of thrombocytopenia may be organized into disorders of (1) decreased platelet production, (2) increased destruction, and (3) sequestration.

***Thrombocytopenia Resulting from Decreased Platelet Production.*** As a primary disorder, this is rare in childhood, other than as part of an aplastic syndrome. Congenital hypoplastic thrombocytopenia is part of several constitutional disorders. Thrombocytopenia with **absent radii syndrome** is characterized by severe thrombocytopenia in association with orthopedic abnormalities, especially of the upper extremity. The thrombocytopenia usually improves over time. The **Wiskott-Aldrich syndrome** is an X-linked disorder characterized by hypogammaglobinemia, eczema, and thrombocytopenia (see Chapter 8). The platelets on peripheral blood smear are small. Bone marrow transplantation results in a complete cure of the immunodeficiency and thrombocytopenia and resolution of the eczema. X-linked thrombocytopenia is a variant of Wiskott-Aldrich syndrome.

*Acquired thrombocytopenia due to decreased production* is rarely an isolated finding. It is more often seen in the context of *pancytopenia due to bone marrow failure* caused by infiltrative or aplastic processes. Certain chemotherapeutic agents may affect

megakaryocytes selectively more than other marrow elements. *Cyanotic congenital heart disease with polycythemia* often is associated with thrombocytopenia, but this is rarely severe or associated with significant clinical bleeding. Both congenital (TORCH) and acquired *viral infections* (human immunodeficiency virus, [HIV], EBV, measles) and some *drugs* (anticonvulsants, antibiotics, cytotoxic agents heparin, quinidine) may induce thrombocytopenia. Postnatal infections and drug reactions usually cause transient thrombocytopenia, whereas congenital infections may produce prolonged suppression of bone marrow function.

***Thrombocytopenia Resulting from Peripheral Destruction.*** In a well-appearing child, immune-mediated mechanisms are the most common cause of thrombocytopenia. Thrombocytopenia results from increased rates of antibody-dependent platelet destruction. **Neonatal alloimmune thrombocytopenic purpura** (NATP) occurs as a result of sensitization of the mother to antigens present on fetal platelets during gestation. Antibodies cross the placenta and attack the fetal platelet (see Chapter 6). Many platelet alloantigens have been identified and sequenced, permitting prenatal diagnosis of an at-risk fetus. Mothers with **idiopathic thrombocytopenic purpura** (ITP) or with a previous history of ITP may have passive transfer of antiplatelet antibodies that react with fetal platelets, with resul-

**CAUSES OF BLEEDING**

*HEMATOLOGIC*                                    *VASCULAR-NONHEMATOLOGIC*

**Thrombocytopenia**          **Coagulopathy**                    **Child Abuse**

*Primary*                     *Primary*                           Vasculitis
                                                                  Other trauma
   Idiopathic thrombocytopenic    von Willebrand disease          Ulcer
     purpura                      Hemophilia                      Varices
   Neonatal isoimmune             Platelet function defect        Polyps, tumors
   TAR syndrome                                                   Ehlers-Danlos syndrome
   Wiskott-Aldrich syndrome                                       Telangiectasia
                                                                  Angiodysplasia
*Secondary*                   *Secondary*

   Malignancy                     Disseminated intravascular
   Aplastic anemia                  coagulation
   Disseminated intravascular     Anticoagulants
     coagulation                  Vitamin K deficiency, including
   Sepsis                             hemorrhagic disease of the newborn
   Drug-induced                   Hepatic failure
   Hemolytic-uremic syndrome      Renal failure
   Hemangioma                     Maternal anticonvulsants
   Hypersplenism                  Anticoagulant drug ingestion
   Mechanical (artificial heart valve)   (e.g., rat poison)
   Autoimmune (systemic
     lupus erythematosus)
   Human immunodeficiency
     virus

FIGURE 14–10. Common causes of bleeding. TAR = thrombocytopenia with absence of radius.

tant neonatal thrombocytopenia (see Chapter 6). The maternal platelet count is sometimes a useful indicator of the probability the infant will be affected. If the mother had a splenectomy, the maternal platelet count may be normal and is a poor predictor of the likelihood of severe neonatal thrombocytopenia because maternal antibody will trigger destruction of the fetal platelets in the fetal spleen. The infant with NATP is at risk for intracranial hemorrhage both in utero and during the immediate delivery process. In ITP, the greatest risk appears to be during passage through the birth canal, during which molding of the head may induce intracranial hemorrhage. Fetal scalp sampling or percutaneous umbilical blood sampling may be performed to measure the fetal platelet count. Administration of IVIg prior to delivery has been shown to be effective in raising fetal platelet counts and may alleviate thrombocytopenia in the infant in both NATP and ITP. Delivery by cesarean section is recommended to prevent CNS bleeding (see Chapter 6). Those neonates with severe thrombocytopenia (platelet counts <20,000) may be treated with IVIg or corticosteroids until the period of

thrombocytopenia remits. If necessary, infants with NATP may receive washed maternal platelets.

**Autoimmune thrombocytopenic purpura of childhood (childhood ITP)** is a common disorder in children that usually follows an acute viral infection and is caused by an antibody (IgG or IgM) that binds to the platelet membrane and results in splenic destruction of antibody-coated platelets. Rarely, ITP may be the presenting symptom of an autoimmune disease such as SLE. Approximately 80% of children have a spontaneous resolution of ITP within 6 mo following diagnosis. Young children typically present 1–4 wk after viral illness with abrupt onset of petechiae, purpura, and epistaxis. The thrombocytopenia usually is severe. Significant adenopathy or hepatosplenomegaly is unusual, and the red cell and white cell counts are normal. Diagnosis of ITP usually does not require a bone marrow examination. If there are atypical findings, however, marrow examination is indicated to rule out an infiltrative disorder (leukemia) or an aplastic process (aplastic anemia). In ITP, the bone marrow reveals increased megakaryocytes and normal erythroid and myeloid elements.

FIGURE 14–11. Differential diagnosis of childhood thrombocytopenic syndromes. The syndromes are initially separated by their clinical appearance. Clues leading to the diagnosis are presented in italics. The mechanisms and common disorders leading to these findings are shown in the lower part of the figure. Disorders that commonly affect neonates are listed in the shaded boxes. HIV = human immunodeficiency virus; ITP = idiopathic immune thrombocytopenic purpura; NATP = neonatal alloimmune thrombocytopenic purpura; SLE = systemic lupus erythematosus; TTP = thrombotic thrombocytopenic purpura; TAR = thrombocytopenia–absent radius (syndrome); WBC = white blood cell; UAC = umbilical artery catheter; HSM = hepatosplenomegaly. (From Scott JP: Bleeding and thrombosis. *In* Kliegman RM, Nieder ML, Super DM [eds]: Practical Strategies in Pediatric Diagnosis and Therapy. Philadelphia, WB Saunders, 1996, p 849.)

Serious bleeding, especially intracranial bleeding, occurs in fewer than 1% of patients with ITP. Therapy is seldom indicated for platelet counts greater than 30,000/mm³. Therapy does not affect the long-term outcome of ITP but is intended to raise the platelet count acutely. For clinical bleeding or severe thrombocytopenia (platelet count < 20,000/mm³), therapeutic options include prednisone 2–4 mg/kg/24 hr for 2 weeks or IVIG 1 g/kg/24 hr for 1 to 2 days or IV anti-D (RhoGAM) 50 µg/kg/dose for Rh-positive individuals. All of these appear to work by decreasing the rate of clearance of sensitized platelets rather than decreasing production of antibody. IVIG is a preferred therapy. Splenectomy is indicated in acute ITP only for life-threatening bleeding.

The *diagnosis* of *chronic ITP* is confirmed following 6–12 mo of persistent thrombocytopenia. Repeated treatments with IVIG or IV anti-D or high-dose pulse steroids have been effective in delaying splenectomy. Splenectomy is effective in inducing a remission in 70–80% of childhood ITP. The risks of splenectomy (surgery, sepsis from encapsulated bacteria [e.g., pneumococcus]) must be weighed against the risk of severe bleeding.

Microangiopathic hemolytic anemia (MAHA) generally is associated with thrombocytopenia, anemia secondary to intravascular red cell destruction, and depletion of clotting factors. Children with MAHA usually are quite ill (see Anemia). In the child with **DIC**, the deposition of fibrin strands within the vasculature and activation of both thrombin and plasmin result in a wide-ranging hemostatic disorder with activation and clearance of platelets. **Hemolytic-uremic syndrome** occurs as a result of exposure to a toxin that induces endothelial injury, fibrin deposition, and platelet activation and clearance (see Chapter 16). In **thrombotic thrombocytopenic purpura**, platelet consumption precipitated or aggravated by a plasma factor or lack of an inhibitory factor appears to be the primary process, with a modest deposition of fibrin and red cell destruction.

### Disorders of Platelet Function

Disorders of platelet function present with mucocutaneous bleeding and a prolonged bleeding time and may be primary or secondary. Primary disorders of platelet function may involve receptors on the platelet membrane for the adhesive proteins. Glycoprotein (GP) Ib (the von Willebrand factor [vWF] receptor) deficiency causes **Bernard-Soulier syndrome**. GPIIb-IIIa (the fibrinogen receptor) deficiency causes **Glanzmann thrombasthenia**. Mild abnormalities of platelet aggregation and release, detectable by platelet aggregometry, are far more common. Secondary disorders caused by toxins and drugs (uremia, salicylates, nonsteroidal anti-inflammatory agents [NSAIDs], and infections) may cause a broad spectrum of platelet dysfunction.

## DISORDERS OF CLOTTING FACTORS

Hereditary deficiencies of procoagulant proteins result in bleeding. Only deficiencies of prekallikrein and Hageman factor (XII) are not associated with a predisposition toward bleeding. The genes for factors VIII and IX are on the X chromosome, whereas virtually all the other clotting factors are coded on autosomal chromosomes and therefore inherited autosomally. Factor VIII and factor IX deficiencies are the most common severe inherited bleeding disorders. Von Willebrand disease is the most common congenital bleeding disorder.

### Hemophilia

*Hemophilia A* (factor VIII deficiency) occurs in 1 in 5000 males. *Hemophilia B* (factor IX deficiency) occurs approximately one fifth as often. Clinically, the two disorders are indistinguishable other than in their therapy. Because of a lack of factor VIII or IX, there is a delay in generation of thrombin, which is crucial to forming a normal, functional fibrin clot and solidifying the platelet plug that has formed in areas of vascular injury. The severity of the disorder is determined by the degree of clotting factor deficiency. Patients with less than 1% (severe hemophilia) factor VIII or factor IX may have spontaneous bleeding or bleeding with very minor trauma. Patients with 1–5% (moderate hemophilia) factor VIII or factor IX usually require moderate trauma to induce bleeding episodes. In mild hemophilia (>5% factor VIII or IX), significant trauma is necessary to induce bleeding; spontaneous bleeding does not occur. Mild hemophilia may go undiagnosed for many years, whereas severe hemophilia manifests in infancy. In severe hemophilia, spontaneous bleeding occurs, usually in the muscles or joints (hemarthroses).

*Prevention* of long-term crippling orthopedic abnormalities is a major goal of care. Early institution of factor replacement and continuous prophylaxis beginning in early childhood should prevent the chronic joint disease associated with hemophilia.

*Diagnosis.* The diagnosis of hemophilia is based on a prolonged activated partial thromboplastin time (APTT). In the APTT, a surface-active agent activates the intrinsic system of coagulation, of which factors VIII and IX are critical components. With factor VIII or IX deficiency, the APTT is quite prolonged but should correct to normal when the patient's plasma is mixed 1:1 with normal plasma. Once an abnormal APTT is obtained, specific factor assays are needed to make a precise diagnosis, which is critical to decide on the appropriate factor replacement therapy (Table 14–15). Both prenatal diagnosis and carrier diagnosis now are possible using either coagulation-based methods or molecular biologic techniques.

*Treatment.* Early appropriate replacement treatment is the aim of optimal hemophilia care. Acute bleeding episodes are best treated in the home once the patient has attained the appropriate age and the parents have learned home treatment. Bleeding associated with surgery, trauma, or dental extraction often can be anticipated, and excessive bleeding can be prevented with appropriate replacement therapy. For life-threatening bleeding, levels of 80–100% of normal factor VIII or IX are necessary. For mild to moderate bleeding episodes (e.g., hemarthroses), a 40% level for factor VIII or a 30–40% level for factor IX is appropriate. The dose can be calculated by knowing that 1 unit/kg body weight of factor VIII will raise the plasma level 2%, whereas 1 unit/kg of factor IX will raise the plasma level 1%. Therefore, dose = desired level (%) × weight (kg) × 0.5 (for factor VIII) or × 1.0 (for factor IX). Aminocaproic acid and tranexamic acid are inhibitors of fibrinolysis that may be useful for oral bleeding. Desmopressin acetate (DDAVP) is a synthetic vasopressin analog with minimal vasopressor effect. DDAVP triples or quadruples the

TABLE 14–15.   Comparison of Hemophilia A, Hemophilia B, and von Willebrand Disease

|  | Hemophilia A | Hemophilia B | Von Willebrand Disease |
|---|---|---|---|
| Inheritance | X-linked | X-linked | Autosomal dominant |
| Factor deficiency | Factor VIII | Factor IX | Von Willebrand factor and VIIIC |
| Bleeding site(s) | Muscle, joint, surgical | Muscle, joint, surgical | Mucous membranes, skin, surgical, menstrual |
| Prothombin time (PT) | Normal | Normal | Normal |
| Activated partial thromboplastin time (APTT) | Prolonged | Prolonged | Prolonged or normal |
| Bleeding time | Normal | Normal | Prolonged or normal |
| Factor VIII coagulant activity (VIIIC) | Low | Normal | Low or normal |
| Von Willebrand factor antigen (vWF:Ag) | Normal | Normal | Low |
| Von Willebrand factor activity (vWF:Act) | Normal | Normal | Low |
| Factor IX | Normal | Low | Normal or low |
| Ristocetin-induced platelet agglutination | Normal | Normal | Normal, low, or increased at low dose ristocetin |
| Platelet aggregation | Normal | Normal | Normal |
| Treatment | DDAVP* or recombinant VIII | Recombinant IX | DDAVP* or vWF concentrate |

*Desmopressin (DDAVP) for mild to moderate hemophilia A or type 1 von Willebrand disease.

initial factor VIII level of a patient with mild or moderate (not severe) hemophilia A but has no effect on factor IX levels. When adequate hemostatic levels can be attained, DDAVP is the treatment of choice for individuals with mild and moderate hemophilia A.

Patients treated with older factor VIII or IX concentrates were at high risk for hepatitis B, C, and D and HIV. Recombinant factor VIII and factor IX concentrates are safe from virally transmitted illnesses. Older patients who were exposed to factor concentrates or, less often, cryoprecipitate prior to human immunodeficiency virus (HIV) testing have a high prevalence of HIV infection. Acquired immunodeficiency syndrome (AIDS) is the most common cause of death in older patients with hemophilia. Many older patients also have chronic non-A, non-B hepatitis (hepatitis C).

*Inhibitors* are IgG antibodies directed against transfused factor VIII or IX in congenitally deficient patients. Inhibitors arise in 15% of severe factor VIII and much less commonly in factor IX hemophiliacs. They may be high or low titer and demonstrate an anamnestic response to treatment. The *treatment* of bleeding patients with an inhibitor is difficult. For low-titer inhibitors, options include continuous factor VIII infusions or administration of porcine factor VIII. For high-titer inhibitors, it usually is necessary to administer a product that bypasses the inhibitor, such as activated prothrombin complex concentrates or recombinant factor VIIa. The use of frequent high doses of prothrombin complex concentrates, and especially the activated products, paradoxically increases the risks of thrombosis, which has resulted in fatal complications like myocardial infarction. Induction of immune tolerance with continuous antigen exposure plus immunosuppression may be beneficial.

## Von Willebrand Disease

Von Willebrand disease is a common disorder caused by a deficiency of vWF, an adhesive protein that serves two functions: to bridge between subendothelial collagen and platelets and, circulating noncovalently bound to factor VIII, to protect factor VIII from rapid clearance from circulation. Von Willebrand disease usually is inherited as an autosomal dominant trait and rarely as an autosomal recessive trait. vWF is either quantitatively deficient (partial or absolute) or qualitatively (type 2) abnormal (dysproteinemia).

The *clinical manifestations* include mucocutaneous bleeding, epistaxis, gingival bleeding, cutaneous bruising, and menorrhagia. In severe von Willebrand disease, factor VIII deficiency may be profound and the patient also may have manifestations similar to hemophilia A (e.g., hemarthrosis).

Approximately 80% of patients with von Willebrand disease have classic (type 1) disease (i.e., a mild to moderate deficiency of vWF). There are several other clinically important subtypes, each of which requires somewhat different therapy. vWF testing requires measurement of the amount of protein, usually done immunologically as the von Willebrand factor antigen (vWF:ag). Von Willebrand factor activity (vWF:Act) is measured functionally in the ristocetin cofactor assay (vWFR:Co) that utilizes the antibiotic ristocetin to induce vWF to bind to platelets. In Table 14–15, the findings in classic von Willebrand disease are compared with those in hemophilia A and B.

The *treatment* of von Willebrand disease depends on the severity of the bleeding. DDAVP is the treatment of choice for the majority of bleeding episodes in patients with type 1 disease and some patients with type 2 disease. When high levels of vWF are needed and the patient cannot be satisfactorily treated with DDAVP, treatment with a virally attenuated vWF-containing concentrate (e.g., Humate P) may be appropriate, and the dosage can be calculated as for factor VIII in hemophilia. Cryoprecipitate should not be used because it is not virally attenuated. Hepatitis B vaccine should be given prior to exposure to plasma-derived products. As in all bleeding disorders, aspirin should be avoided for patients with von Willebrand disease.

### Vitamin K Deficiency

See Chapters 2 and 6.

### Disseminated Intravascular Coagulation

The term DIC refers to a disorder in which a severely ill patient sustains widespread activation of the coagulation mechanism usually associated with shock. Bleeding and/or clotting manifestations may be present. Normal hemostasis is a balance between hemorrhage and thrombosis. In DIC, this balance is altered by the severe illness so that the patient has activation of both coagulation (thrombin) and fibrinolysis (plasmin). Coagulation factors, especially platelets, fibrinogen, and factors II, V, and VIII, are consumed, as are the anticoagulant proteins, especially antithrombin III, protein C, and plasminogen. Endothelial injury, tissue release of thromboplastic procoagulant factors, or, rarely, exogenous factors (e.g., snake venoms) directly activate the coagulation mechanism (Table 14–16).

The *diagnosis* is a clinical one sustained by laboratory findings (Table 14–17). In some patients, DIC

**TABLE 14–16.** Conditions Associated with Disseminated Intravascular Coagulation

| Acute | Chronic |
|---|---|
| Sepsis | Polycythemia |
| Congenital infection | Hemangioma |
| Asphyxia–hypoxia | Arteriovenous malformation |
| Trauma | Retained dead fetus |
| Shock | Malignancy |
| Burns | Pre-eclampsia |
| Heat stroke | Malignant hypertension |
| Snake bites | Cirrhosis |
| Transfusion reactions | Renal vein thrombosis |
| Promyelocytic leukemia | |
| Respiratory distress syndrome (neonatal) | |
| Acute respiratory distress syndrome | |
| Hepatitis or hepatic failure | |

may evolve more slowly and there may be a degree of compensation. In an acutely ill patient, the sudden occurrence of bleeding from a venipuncture or incision site, gastrointestinal or pulmonary hemorrhage, petechiae, ecchymosis, and/or evidence of peripheral gangrene or thrombosis suggests the diagnosis of DIC.

The *treatment* is problematic. The disorder inducing DIC should be treated effectively, and hypoxia, acidosis, and poor perfusion should be corrected. Depleted blood clotting factors, platelets, and anticoagulant proteins then should be replaced. Heparin may be useful in the presence of significant arterial or venous thrombotic disease unless sites of life-threatening bleeding coexist. In addition, heparin may be useful for the treatment of DIC induced by meningococcemia, purpura fulminans, or acute promyelocytic leukemia. The use of concentrates containing protein C appears promising in treatment of DIC.

**TABLE 14–17.** Laboratory Evidence of Disseminated Intravascular Coagulation

Prolonged prothrombin, partial thromboplastin, and thrombin times
Thrombocytopenia
Low fibrinogen, factors V and VIII
Elevated fibrin degradation (split) products and D-dimers
Microangiopathic RBC morphology

RBC = red blood cell.

## TABLE 14–18.  Hypercoagulable States

**Primary Disorders**

Factor V Leiden (APC resistance)
Antithrombin III deficiency
Protein C deficiency
Protein S deficiency
Dysfibrinogenemia
Plasminogen deficiency

**Secondary Disorders**

*Coagulopathies*

Nephrotic syndrome
Oral contraceptives (estrogen)
Malignancy
Therapy with activated prothrombin complex concentrates
Pregnancy
Lupus anticoagulant (antiphospholipid antibody)
Disseminated intravascular coagulation

*Platelet Disorders*

Diabetes mellitus
Myeloproliferative disorders
Thrombocythemia
Paroxysmal nocturnal hemoglobinuria

*Flow and Vessel Disorders*

Polycythemia-hyperviscosity
Homocystinuria
Marfan syndrome
Vasculitis
Sickle cell anemia
Vessel grafts
Vascular stasis

Adapted from Schafer A: The hypercoagulable states. Ann Intern Med 102:814, 1985.
APC = activated protein C.

## Thrombosis

A hereditary predisposition to thrombosis may be caused either by a deficiency of an anticoagulant protein (protein C or S, antithrombin, or plasminogen) or by an abnormality of a procoagulant protein that makes such protein resistant to proteolysis by its respective inhibitor (factor V Leiden). The functions of the anticoagulant proteins are outlined in Figure 14–9. Deficiency syndromes may present in neonates, especially homozygous protein C deficiency, which presents with purpura fulminans or arterial thrombosis in the major vessels and requires plasma replacement therapy. Patients with heterozygous deficiencies of anticoagulant proteins or factor V Leiden usually present in adolescence or early adulthood. Protein C deficiency that presents in adulthood usually is inherited as an autosomal dominant trait, whereas the homozygous form usually is autosomal recessive. Protein S and AT-III deficiencies are inherited as autosomal dominant traits. Factor V Leiden is the most common hereditary cause of a predisposition to thrombosis appearing in 3–5% of Caucasians. Acquired antiphospholipid antibodies (anticardiolipin, lupus anticoagulant) also produce thrombosis.

*Clinical manifestations* of thromboembolic disease in pediatrics occur most frequently in neonates or in adolescents. Indwelling catheters, vasculitis, sepsis, immobilization, nephrotic syndrome, coagulopathy, trauma, infection, surgery, inflammatory bowel disease, oral contraceptive agents, pregnancy, and abortion all predispose to thrombosis (Table 14–18). The *diagnosis* of venous thrombosis can be made noninvasively by Doppler flow compression studies or plethysmography; however, the gold standard remains the venogram. The manifestations of pulmonary emboli may be highly variable, including sudden chest pain, diminished breath sounds, increased pulmonic 2nd heart sound, cyanosis, tachypnea, and hypoxemia, or minimal, or there may be no findings. Findings on chest roentgenogram vary, but an abnormal ("high

## TABLE 14–19.  Commonly Used Transfusion Products

| Component | Content | Indication | Dose | Expected Outcome |
|---|---|---|---|---|
| Packed RBCs | 250–300 cc RBC/unit | ↓ O₂ carrying capacity* | 10–15 cc/kg | 4 cc/kg → 1 g/dL ↑ in Hg |
| Platelet concentrate | 5.0–7.0 × 10¹⁰ platelets/unit | Severe thrombocytopenia ± bleeding | 1 unit/10 kg | ↑ Platelet count by 50,000/μL |
| Fresh frozen plasma | 1 cc/kg of each clotting factor | Multiple clotting factor deficiency | 10–15 cc/kg | Improvement in prothrombin and partial thromboplastin times |
| Cryoprecipitate | Fibrinogen, factor VIII, vWF, factor XIII | Hypofibrinogenemia, factor XIII deficiency | 1 bag/5 kg | ↑ Fibrinogen by 50–100 mg/dL |

* Should be clinically significant.
RBC = red blood cell, vWF = von Willebrand factor.

TABLE 14–20.  Evaluation of Transfusion Reactions

| Type of Reaction | Clinical Signs | Management of Problems |
|---|---|---|
| Major hemolytic (1:100,000) (incompatibility) | Acute shock, back pain, flushing, early fever, intravascular hemolysis, hemoglobinemia, hemoglobinuria; may be delayed 5–10 days and less severe if anamnestic response is present | 1. Stop transfusion; return blood to bank with fresh sample of patient's blood<br>2. Hydrate IV; support BP, maintain high urine flow, alkalinize urine<br>3. Check for hemoglobinemia, hemoglobinuria, hyperkalemia<br>4. Jaundice, anemia if delayed |
| Febrile (1:100) | Fever at end of transfusion, urticaria (usually due to sensitization to WBC HLA antigens), chills | Pretreat with hydrocortisone, antipyretics, diphenhydramine HCl (Benadryl), or all three; use buffy coat–poor RBC, washed RBC, filtered or frozen RBC |
| Allergic | Fever, urticaria, anaphylactoid reaction (often due to sensitivity to donor plasma proteins) | Benadryl, hydrocortisone; use washed RBC or frozen RBC |

Adapted from Andreoli TE, Carpenter CCJ, Plum F, et al: Cecil Essentials of Medicine, 3rd ed. Philadelphia, WB Saunders, 1993, p 377.
BP = blood pressure; HLA = human leukocyte antigen; RBC = red blood cell; WBC = white blood cell.

probability") ventilation-perfusion scan (V-Q mismatch) is a frequent finding with pulmonary emboli.

*Treatment* of thrombotic disorders depends on the underlying condition and usually includes heparin and then longer term anticoagulation with coumarin. Major vessel thrombosis or life-threatening thrombosis may require treatment with fibrinolytic agents (e.g., streptokinase, urokinase, or tissue plasminogen activator). In the newborn, inherited deficiency syndromes may present as emergencies and require plasma, AT-III concentrates, and protein C concentrates. Symptomatic individuals with protein C, protein S, or AT-III deficiency are usually chronically anticoagulated with coumarin.

## BLOOD COMPONENT THERAPY

Transfusion of red blood cells, granulocytes, platelets, and coagulation factors can be lifesaving or life maintaining (Table 14–19). Whole blood is indicated only when acute hypovolemia and reduced oxygen-carrying capacity are present. Otherwise, packed red blood cells are indicated to treat anemia to increase oxygen-carrying capacity. Blood cell transfusions should not be used to treat asymptomatic nutritional deficiencies that can be corrected by administering the appropriate deficient nutrient (e.g., iron, folic acid). Blood component therapy requires proper anticoagulation of the blood, screening for a variety of infectious agents, and blood group compatibility testing prior to administration. Commonly used blood components are listed in Table 14–19. Typical transfusion reactions are listed in Table 14–20. Long-term complications of transfusions include iron overload, alloimmunization to red and white blood cells or platelets and plasma proteins (1:100), graft-versus-host disease, and infectious diseases (hepatitis [1:250], HIV [<1:250,000] malaria, syphilis, babesiosis, brucellosis, Chagas disease). Transfusional therapy also may result in circulatory overload, especially in the presence of chronic cardiopulmonary deficiency.

## References

Behrman RE, Kliegman RM, Arvin AM (eds): Nelson Textbook of Pediatrics, 15th ed. Philadelphia, WB Saunders, 1996, Chapters 431–440.

Blanchette VS, Imbach P, Andrew M, et al: Randomised trial of intravenous immunoglobulin G, intravenous anti-D, and oral prednisone in childhood acute immune thrombocytopenic purpura. Lancet 344:703, 1994.

Bussel JB: Autoimmune thrombocytopenic purpura. Hematol Oncol Clin North Am 4:179, 1990.

Dahlbäch B: Are we ready for factor V Leiden screening? Lancet 347:1346, 1996.

David M, Manco-Johnson M, Andrew M: Diagnosis and treatment of venous thromboembolism in children and adolescents: On behalf of the Subcommittee on Perinatal Haemostasis of the Scientific and Standardization Committee of the ISTH. Thromb Haemost 74:791, 1995.

Dubansky AS, Boyett JM, Falletta J, et al: Isolated thrombocytopenia in children with acute lymphoblastic leukemia: A rare event in a pediatric oncology group study. Pediatrics 84:1068, 1989.

De Saint Basile G, Lagelouse R, Lambert N, et al: Isolated X-linked thrombocytopenia in two unrelated families is associated with point mutations in the Wiskott-Aldrich syndrome protein gene. J Pediatr 129:56, 1996.

George JN, Woolf SH, Raskob GE, et al: Idiopathic thrombocytopenic purpura: A practice guideline developed by explicit methods for The American Society of Hematology. Blood 88:3, 1996.

Hillarp A, Zoller B, Dahlbäch B: Activated protein C resistance as a basis for venous thrombosis. Am J Med 101:534, 1996.

Katsanis E, Luke K-H, Hsu E, et al: Prevalence and significance of mild bleeding disorders in children with recurrent epistaxis. J Pediatr 113:73, 1988.

Liesner R, Machin S: Platelet disorders. BMJ 314:809, 1997.

Lusher JM, Arkin S, Abildgaard CF, et al: Recombinant factor VIII for the treatment of previously untreated patients with hemophilia A: Safety, efficacy and development of inhibitors. N Engl J Med 328:4532, 1993.

Nichols W, Ginsburg D: Von Willebrand disease. Medicine 76:7, 1997.

Sacher RA, Luban NLC, Strauss RG: Current practice and guidelines for the transfusion of cellular blood components in the newborn. Transfus Med Rev 3:39, 1989.

Schreiber GB, Busch MP, Kleinman SH: The risk of transfusion-transmitted viral infections. N Engl J Med 334:1685, 1996.

Scott JP: Bleeding and thrombosis. *In* Kliegman RM, Nieder ML, Super DM, (eds): Practical Strategies in Pediatric Diagnosis and Therapy. Philadelphia, WB Saunders, 1996, p 839–857.

Van der Born J, Bots M, Haverkate F, et al: Reduced response to activated protein C is associated with increased risk for cerebrovascular disease. Ann Intern Med 125:265, 1996.

# Chapter 15

# ONCOLOGY

Herbert T. Abelson

Childhood cancers represent a group of approximately a dozen common malignancies, each with a distinct epidemiology, pathology, and mortality rate. Malignancy is the most common disease causing death among children between 1 and 16 yr of age; of the approximately 1 million new cases of cancer in the United States each year (exclusive of carcinoma in situ and nonmelanoma skin cancer) about 8000 (<1%) occur in children. It was estimated that 1700 children would die of cancer in 1996, about one third from leukemia. Although the incidence of childhood cancer appears to be increasing, mortality rates have declined (Fig. 15–1). A coordinated multidisciplinary team effort is needed for detecting and managing childhood ma-

lignancies. This should be provided in specialized pediatric cancer centers by staff that include oncologists, surgeons, pathologists, radiotherapists, chemotherapists, psychologists, social workers, epidemiologists, and oncology nurses.

## GENERAL CONSIDERATIONS

*Epidemiology.* The types of childhood cancers tend to differ from those that occur in adults. Adults characteristically develop cancer of solid organs, such as the lung, the colon, the breast, and the genitourinary system. However, leukemia and brain tumors are the predominant malignancies

FIGURE 15–1. Five-year survival rates from childhood cancer in 1960 and 1996. (Adapted from American Cancer Society: Cancer Facts and Figures, 1996. Reprinted with permission of the American Cancer Society, Inc, Atlanta.)

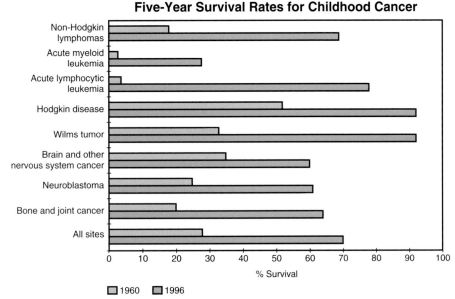

Five-Year Survival Rates for Childhood Cancer

among children (Table 15–1). The annual incidence of all cancers among white children is approximately 12:100,000, whereas the incidence is 9:100,000 among black children. The incidence of cancer is slightly increased among boys compared with girls, with an overall sex ratio of 1.2:1. However, for lymphoma the incidence is higher in boys by 2:1. Leukemia and various embryonal tumors, such as neuroblastoma, Wilms tumor, retinoblastoma, and hepatic tumors, are more common in infancy and early childhood; Hodgkin disease, gonadal malignancy, and bone tumors are seen more commonly during adolescence. It is rare for a newborn infant to have a malignancy; neuroblastoma, congenital leukemia, mesoblastic nephroma, teratoma (sacrococcygeal, mediastinal, gonadal), and the potentially large but nonmalignant lymphangioma or hemangioma (cutaneous, hepatic) are the predominant neonatal neoplasms. Metastasis of malignant disease from the mother to the fetus is very rare and, when present, occurs most often from maternal malignant melanoma.

Most of the common childhood cancers occur sporadically and only rarely are associated with increased host susceptibility resulting from predisposing environmental (Table 15–2) or familial factors (Table 15–3). Nonetheless, environmental risks, single gene or gross chromosomal defects, neurocutaneous or immunodeficiency syndromes, and familial or hereditary conditions associated with malignancy are important disorders to identify among pediatric patients because careful screening, examination, and counseling can detect early signs

**TABLE 15–1.**  Common Childhood Malignancies

| | Percentage of Total Malignancies | |
| --- | --- | --- |
| | *White Children* | *Black Children* |
| Leukemia | 34 | 25 |
| Central nervous system tumors* | 19 | 24 |
| Lymphoma | 11 | 14 |
| Neuroblastoma | 8 | 7 |
| Soft tissue sarcoma† | 7 | 4 |
| Wilms tumor | 6 | 8 |
| Bone tumors‡ | 4 | 5 |
| Retinoblastoma | 3 | 3 |
| Other tumors§ | 8 | 10 |

*Cerebellar astrocytoma, glioblastoma, medulloblastoma, brain stem glioma.

†Rhabdomyosarcoma (embryonal, botryoid, alveolar), fibrosarcoma, primitive neuroectodermal tumors (PNETs).

‡Osteosarcoma, Ewing sarcoma.

§Hepatic, ovarian, testicular, endocrine, melanoma, teratoma.

**TABLE 15–2.**  Environmental Causes of Cancer

| Etiology | Cancer |
| --- | --- |
| *Physical Agents* | |
| Ionizing radiation | Leukemia, thyroid, breast, sarcomas |
| Ultraviolet irradiation | Melanoma, basal and squamous cell in xeroderma pigmentosum |
| *Chemical Agents* | |
| Cigarette, tobacco | Lung, oropharynx, larynx |
| Diethylstilbestrol | Vaginal carcinoma |
| Asbestos | Mesothelioma |
| Androgens | Hepatoma |
| Alkylating agents | Leukemia |
| Topoisomerase II inhibitors | Leukemia |
| Immunosuppressant drugs | Lymphoma |
| Aflatoxin | Hepatic carcinoma |
| Vinyl chloride | Hepatic angiosarcoma |
| Phenytoin | Lymphoma |
| Cyclophosphamide | Bladder cancer |
| Alcohol (fetal alcohol syndrome) | Neuroblastoma |
| Benzene | Leukemia |
| *Microbiologic Agents* | |
| Hepatitis B, C viruses | Hepatic carcinoma |
| HTLV-1 | Lymphoma |
| *Schistosoma haematobium* | Bladder carcinoma |
| Epstein-Barr virus | African Burkitt lymphoma, X-linked immunodeficiency–associated lymphoma, nasopharyngeal carcinoma, post-transplant lymphomas |
| Papillomavirus | Cervical cancer |
| SV40 virus | Possible ependymoma, choroid plexus tumor |
| Human herpes virus 8 | Kaposi sarcoma |
| HIV | Leiomyosarcoma |

HIV = human immunodeficiency virus; HTLV-1 = human T-cell leukemia virus (retrovirus).

of cancer and improve the chance for successful treatment.

*Etiology.* Cancer begins with the onset of unregulated, often rapid growth and proliferation of a single somatic cell. One theory of carcinogenesis,

TABLE 15–3. Familial or Genetic Susceptibility to Malignancy

| Disorder | Tumor/Cancer | Comment |
|---|---|---|
| **Chromosomal Syndromes** | | |
| Chromosome 11p − (deletion) with sporadic aniridia | Wilms tumor | Associated with genitourinary anomalies, mental retardation |
| Chromosome 13q − (deletion) | Retinoblastoma | Associated with mental retardation, skeletal malformations |
| Trisomy 21 | Lymphocytic or nonlymphocytic leukemia | Risk is 15 times normal |
| Klinefelter syndrome (47, XXY) | Breast cancer | |
| Gonadal dysgenesis XO/XY | Gonadoblastoma | Gonads must be removed; 25% chance of gonadal malignancy |
| **DNA Fragility** | | |
| Xeroderma pigmentosum | Basal, squamous cell skin cancers | Autosomal recessive; failure to repair solar-damaged DNA |
| Fanconi anemia | Leukemia | Autosomal recessive; 10% risk for AML; chromosome fragility, positive diepoxybutane test |
| Bloom syndrome | Leukemia, lymphoma | Autosomal recessive; chromosome fragility immunodeficiency; high risk for malignancy |
| Ataxia–telangiectasia | Lymphoma, leukemia | Autosomal recessive; sensitive to x-radiation, radiomimetic drugs; chromosome fragility, immunodeficiency |
| Dysplastic nevus syndrome | Melanoma | Autosomal dominant |
| **Immunodeficiency Syndromes** | | |
| Wiskott-Aldrich syndrome | Lymphoma | Immunodeficiency; X-linked recessive |
| X-linked immunodeficiency (Duncan syndrome) | Lymphoma | Epstein-Barr virus is inciting agent |
| Severe combined immunodeficiency | Leukemia, lymphoma | Immunodeficiency; X-linked recessive |
| **Other Single Gene Defects** | | |
| Neurofibromatosis | Neurofibroma, peripheral nerve sheath, optic glioma, acoustic neuroma, astrocytoma, meningioma, pheochromocytoma | Autosomal dominant |
| Tuberous sclerosis | Fibroangiomatous nevi, myocardial rhabdomyoma | Autosomal dominant |
| Retinoblastoma, genetic form | Sarcoma | Autosomal dominant |
| Wilms tumor, genetic form | Wilms tumor | Autosomal dominant |
| Familial adenomatous polyposis coli | Adenocarcinoma of colon | Autosomal dominant |
| Gardner syndrome | Adenocarcinoma of colon; skull and soft tissue tumors | Autosomal dominant |
| Peutz-Jeghers syndrome | Gastrointestinal carcinoma | Autosomal dominant |
| Tyrosinemia, galactosemia | Hepatic carcinoma | Nodular cirrhosis; autosomal recessive |
| Multiple endocrine neoplasia (MEN) syndrome I (Wermer syndrome) | Parathyroid adenoma, pancreatic islet tumor, pituitary adenoma carcinoid | Autosomal dominant; Zollinger-Ellison syndrome |
| Multiple endocrine neoplasia syndrome II (Sipple syndrome) | Medullary carcinoma of the thyroid, hyperparathyroidism, pheochromocytoma | Autosomal dominant; monitor calcitonin and calcium levels |
| Multiple endocrine neoplasia III (multiple mucosal neuroma syndrome) | Mucosal neuroma, pheochromocytoma, medullary thyroid carcinoma; Marfan habitus; neuropathy | Autosomal dominant |
| von Hippel–Lindau disease | Hemangioblastoma of the cerebellum and retina, pheochromocytoma | Autosomal dominant; mutation of tumor suppressor gene |
| Cancer family syndrome | Colonic, uterine carcinoma | Autosomal dominant |
| Li-Fraumeni syndrome | Bone, soft tissue sarcoma, breast | Autosomal dominant mutation of p53 tumor suppressor gene |
| **Other Congenital Conditions** | | |
| Hemihypertrophy ± Beckwith syndrome | Wilms tumor, hepatoblastoma, adrenal carcinoma | 25% develop tumor, most in first 5 yr of life |

the clonal initiation of malignancy, proposes that the genetic regulation of growth of a single precursor cell becomes abnormal and results in autonomous, uncontrolled proliferation of the transformed cell line. Alternatively, a "two-hit" theory (Knudson hypothesis) has been postulated for initiating the malignant process in many cancers. For example, in familial retinoblastoma, an initial mutation inactivates one copy of the "retinoblastoma" gene in all somatic cells. A subsequent second "hit" in a somatic cell results in the inactivation of the other retinoblastoma gene on the second chromosome. This double-gene mutation produces neoplastic transformation of retinal cells. The second hit may be carcinogen-induced on a spontaneous DNA recombination event in the somatic cell during mitosis. There is probably a sequence of multiple steps needed in the initiation and progression of malignant cell transformation. Unidentified carcinogenic factors, in the presence of unknown genetic susceptibility and a cellular environment favorable to carcinogenesis, may initiate tumor growth in the presence or absence of identifiable extrinsic (see Table 15–2) or familial (see Table 15–3) factors.

Human cellular genes that regulate normal cell growth and that are homologous to the genetic material of transforming ribonucleic acid (RNA) tumor viruses (retroviruses) are called *proto-oncogenes.* Mutagenesis may be initiated by incorporation of the retroviral genome into host DNA (insertional mutagenesis), but more likely tumorigenesis results from unregulated activation of the related endogenous *oncogene* (activated proto-oncogene) present in the host genome. A somatic mutation near a proto-oncogene may cause its uncontrolled expression and amplification as an activated oncogene, which results in neoplastic growth. Alternatively, a mutation involving the expression of anti-oncogenes (tumor suppressor genes) may result in loss of inhibition of an oncogene. Chromosome translocation provides another mechanism for tumorigenesis because it may move one gene from its normal position to an abnormal unregulated site, resulting in uncontrolled cell growth. For example, in Burkitt lymphoma, a break point at the site of the c-myc oncogene occurs, with a translocation between chromosome 8 and the immunoglobulin genes on either chromosome 2, 14, or 22. The c-myc oncogene is now next to the immunoglobulin gene. The end result is B-cell malignant transformation. Familial retinoblastoma is associated with an inherited mutation or deletion of a tumor suppressor gene on one of the pairs of chromosome 13. Subsequently, somatic inactivation of the allele (RB gene) on the other chromosome pair results in carcinogenesis.

During carcinogenesis, the oncogene controls the synthesis of various protein products that contribute to the malignant alteration of the cell. Oncogene products may be proteins that are similar to various growth factors, growth factor receptors, or enzymes that activate these receptors. The end result may be a perpetual signal to the cell to transform and proliferate in the absence of the true growth factor.

Other virus-induced tumors have been associated with deoxyribonucleic acid (DNA) viruses, such as Epstein-Barr virus (EBV), papillomavirus, and hepatitis B virus. The mechanism of action of these viruses may include insertional mutagenesis, point mutation, and oncogene activation. Viral DNA has been recovered in the transformed cells from tumors produced by EBV (Burkitt lymphoma, nasopharyngeal carcinoma), papillomavirus (cancer of the cervix), and hepatitis B virus (HBV) (hepatocellular carcinoma).

*Clinical Manifestations and Diagnosis.* Malignancy may produce nonspecific systemic effects, such as anorexia, weight loss, malnutrition, or fever. Specific manifestations of various malignancies include hematologic, systemic, intracranial, or ocular signs and symptoms (Table 15–4). These manifestations may be a direct effect of local tumor extension (pain, obstruction, pressure) or the results of metastasis. Alternately, tumor products may produce neuroendocrine effects such as hypertension (neuroblastoma, pheochromocytoma), diarrhea (vasoactive intestinal polypeptide, pancreatic tumor), hypoglycemia (islet cell adenoma, sarcoma producing insulin-like growth factor-2 [IGF-2]), or Cushing syndrome (adrenal, lung, pituitary tumors). Signs and symptoms of malignancy may be confused with less severe diseases so that, for example, nasal infections may be confused with nasopharyngeal cancer, lymphadenopathy with lymphoma, anemia or idiopathic thrombocytopenic purpura with leukemia, and diarrhea with neuroblastoma. Leg pain and limp associated with trauma in the athletic adolescent are common manifestations of osteosarcoma and Ewing sarcoma.

Persistent localized pain, unexplained fever, weight loss, persistent painless lymph node swelling, signs of increased intracranial pressure, and soft tissue mass warrant evaluation for suspected malignancy. For most childhood cancers, a tissue biopsy is needed to confirm the diagnosis. This biopsy may include a bone marrow examination for leukemia, malignant histiocytosis, metastatic neuroblastoma, and lymphoma. Tissue obtained at the time of operative resection or during a more limited incisional biopsy of a solid tumor must be classified by histologic type and by the extent to

TABLE 15–4.  Common Manifestations of Childhood Malignancy

| Sign/Symptom | Significance | Example |
|---|---|---|
| *Hematologic* | | |
| Pallor, anemia | Bone marrow infiltration | Leukemia, neuroblastoma |
| Petechiae, thrombocytopenia | Bone marrow infiltration | Leukemia, neuroblastoma |
| Fever, pharyngitis, neutropenia | Bone marrow infiltration | Leukemia, neuroblastoma |
| *Systemic* | | |
| Bone pain, limp, arthralgia | Primary bone tumor, metastasis to bone | Osteosarcoma, Ewing sarcoma, leukemia, neuroblastoma |
| Fever of unknown origin, weight loss, night sweats | Lymphoreticular malignancy | Hodgkin disease, non–Hodgkin lymphoma |
| Painless lymphadenopathy | Lymphoreticular malignancy | Leukemia, Hodgkin disease, non–Hodgkin lymphoma, Burkitt lymphoma |
| Cutaneous lesion | Primary or metastatic disease | Neuroblastoma, leukemia, Langerhans cell histiocytosis, melanoma |
| Abdominal mass | Adrenal-renal tumor | Neuroblastoma, Wilms tumor |
| Hypertension | Sympathetic nervous system tumor | Neuroblastoma, pheochromocytoma, Wilms tumor |
| Diarrhea | Vasoactive intestinal polypeptide (VIP) | Neuroblastoma, ganglioneuroma |
| Soft tissue mass | Local or metastatic tumor | Ewing sarcoma, osteosarcoma, neuroblastoma, thyroid carcinoma, rhabdomyosarcoma, eosinophilic granuloma Askin tumor |
| Diabetes insipidus, galactorrhea, poor growth | Neuroendocrine involvement of hypothalamus or pituitary gland | Adenoma, craniopharyngioma, prolactinoma, Langerhans cell histiocytosis |
| Emesis, visual disturbances, ataxia, headache, papilledema, cranial nerve palsies | Increased intracranial pressure | Primary brain tumor; metastasis |
| *Ophthalmologic Signs* | | |
| Leukokoria | White pupil | Retinoblastoma |
| Periorbital ecchymosis | Metastasis | Neuroblastoma |
| Miosis, ptosis, heterochromia | Horner syndrome: compression of cervical sympathetic nerves | Neuroblastoma |
| Opsoclonus/ataxia | Neurotransmitters? Autoimmunity? | Neuroblastoma |
| Exophthalmos, proptosis | Orbital tumor | Rhabdomyosarcoma |
| *Thoracic Mass* | | |
| Anterior mediastinal | Cough, stridor, pneumonia, tracheal-bronchial compression | Thymoma, teratoma, T cell lymphoma, thyroid |
| Posterior mediastinal | Vertebral or nerve root compression; dysphagia | Neuroblastoma, neuroenteric cyst |

which the tumor mass has invaded adjacent tissue as well as by cytogenetic and molecular biology techniques. After tumor type is identified, staging the tumor and determining metastatic foci are both critical diagnostic principles that will guide the therapeutic approach.

***Principles of Cancer Treatment.*** The choice of cancer therapy is based on the type, stage, and extent of spread of the malignancy. The goal may be curative, palliative, or supportive, but it always involves specific anticancer modalities plus supportive care. Anticancer modalities include surgical excision, radiation therapy, chemotherapy (Table 15–5), or a combination of these three modalities.

TABLE 15–5. Cancer Chemotherapy

| Drug* | Action | Metabolism | Excretion | Indication | Toxicity |
|---|---|---|---|---|---|
| *Antimetabolites* | | | | | |
| Methotrexate | Folic acid antagonist; inhibits dihydrofolate reductase | Hepatic | Renal, 50–90% excreted unchanged; biliary | ALL, lymphoma, medulloblastoma, osteosarcoma | Myelosuppression (nadir 7–10 days), mucositis, stomatitis, dermatitis, hepatitis; renal and CNS with high-dose administration; prevent with leucovorin, monitor levels |
| 6-Mercaptopurine | Purine analog | Hepatic; allopurinol inhibits metabolism | Renal | ALL | Myelosuppression; hepatic necrosis; mucositis; allopurinol increases toxicity |
| Cytosine arabinoside (Ara-C) | Pyrimidine analog; inhibits DNA polymerase | Hepatic | Renal | ALL, lymphoma | Myelosuppression, conjunctivitis, mucositis, CNS dysfunction |
| *Alkylating Agents* | | | | | |
| Cyclophosphamide (Cytoxan) | Alkylates guanine; inhibits DNA synthesis | Hepatic | Renal | ALL, lymphoma, sarcoma | Myelosuppression; hemorrhagic cystitis; pulmonary fibrosis, inappropriate ADH secretion, bladder cancer, anaphylaxis |
| Ifosfamide | Similar to Cytoxan | Hepatic | Renal | Lymphoma, Wilms tumor, sarcoma, germ cell and testicular tumors | Similar to Cytoxan; CNS dysfunction, cardiac toxicity |
| *Antibiotics* | | | | | |
| Doxorubicin (Adriamycin) and daunorubicin (Cerubidine) | Binds to DNA, intercalation | Hepatic | Biliary, renal | ALL, AML, osteosarcoma, Ewing sarcoma, lymphoma, neuroblastoma | Cardiomyopathy, red urine, tissue necrosis on extravasation, myelosuppression, conjunctivitis, radiation dermatitis, arrhythmia |
| Dactinomycin (Actinomycin-D) | Binds to DNA, inhibits transcription | — | Renal, stool, 30% excreted unchanged drug | Wilms tumor, rhabdomyosarcoma, Ewing sarcoma | Tissue necrosis on extravasation, myelosuppression, radiosensitizer, stomatitis |
| Bleomycin | Binds to DNA, cuts DNA | Hepatic | Renal | Hodgkin disease, lymphoma, germ cell tumors | Pneumonitis, stomatitis, Raynaud phenomenon, pulmonary fibrosis, dermatitis |

## Vinca Alkaloids

| Drug | Mechanism | Metabolism/Excretion | Indications | Toxicity |
|---|---|---|---|---|
| Vincristine (Oncovin) | Inhibits microtubule formation | Hepatic | Biliary | ALL, lymphoma, Wilms tumor, Hodgkin disease, Ewing sarcoma, neuroblastoma, rhabdomyosarcoma, brain tumors | Local cellulitis, peripheral neuropathy, constipation, ileus, jaw pain, inappropriate ADH secretion, seizures, ptosis, minimal myelosuppression |
| Vinblastine (Velban) | Inhibits microtubule formation | Hepatic | Biliary | Hodgkin disease; Langerhans cell histiocytosis | Local cellulitis, leukopenia |

## Enzymes

| Drug | Mechanism | Metabolism/Excretion | Indications | Toxicity |
|---|---|---|---|---|
| L-Asparaginase (pegaspargase) | Depletion of L-asparagine | — | Reticuloendothelial system | ALL | Allergic reaction; pancreatitis, hyperglycemia, platelet dysfunction and coagulopathy, encephalopathy |

## Hormones

| Drug | Mechanism | Metabolism/Excretion | Indications | Toxicity |
|---|---|---|---|---|
| Prednisone | Unknown; lymphocyte modification? | Hepatic | Renal | ALL; Hodgkin disease, lymphoma | Cushing syndrome, cataracts, diabetes, hypertension, myopathy, osteoporosis, infection, peptic ulceration, psychosis |

## Miscellaneous

| Drug | Mechanism | Metabolism/Excretion | Indications | Toxicity |
|---|---|---|---|---|
| BCNU (carmustine, nitrosourea) | Carbamylation of DNA; inhibits DNA synthesis | Hepatic; phenobarbital increases metabolism, decreases activity | Renal | CNS tumors, lymphoma, Hodgkin disease | Delayed myelosuppression (4–6 wk); pulmonary fibrosis, carcinogenic, stomatitis |
| Cisplatin | Inhibits DNA synthesis | — | Renal | Gonadal tumors; osteosarcoma, neuroblastoma, CNS tumors, germ cell tumors | Nephrotoxic; myelosuppression, ototoxicity, tetany, neurotoxicity, hemolytic-uremic syndrome; aminoglycosides may increase nephrotoxicity, anaphylaxis |
| Etoposide (VP-16) | Topoisomerase inhibitor | — | Renal | ALL, lymphoma, germ cell tumor | Myelosuppression, secondary leukemia |
| Etretinate (vitamin A analog) and tretinoin | Enhances normal differentiation | Liver | Liver | Some leukemias; neuroblastoma | Dry mouth, hair loss, pseudotumor cerebri, premature epiphyseal closure |

Data from Med Lett 37:25, 1995; and W. Archie Bleyer: Cancer chemotherapy in infants and children. *In* Altman AJ (ed): Pediatric oncology. Pediatr Clin North Am 32:557, 1985.

*Many drugs produce nausea and vomiting during administration, and many cause alopecia with repeated doses.

ADH = antidiuretic hormone; ALL = acute lymphocytic leukemia; AML = acute myelogenous leukemia; CNS = central nervous system; DNA = deoxyribonucleic acid.

Childhood embryonal malignancies and sarcomas are associated with a high rate of micrometastatic disease at diagnosis. Patients with apparently localized osteosarcoma have a greater than 80% risk for development of overt pulmonary metastases if surgical resection of the primary tumor is the only treatment. Similarly, in childhood ALL, if chemotherapy is discontinued when clinical remission is attained, 100% of patients will relapse. Adjuvant chemotherapy or chemotherapy given after surgical removal of the primary tumor is an important part of the treatment of pediatric solid tumors. Likewise, maintenance chemotherapy (chemotherapy given after successful remission induction) plays a critical role in childhood ALL. Other systemic therapies, such as immunotherapy (interleukins, lymphokine-activated killer cells, radiolabeled antibodies) have not yet achieved wide clinical applicability. Bone marrow transplantation (which permits high-dose anticancer therapy) has become the treatment of choice for children with acute myelogenous leukemia in first remission, juvenile chronic myelogenous leukemia, and adult-type chronic myelogenous leukemia in chronic phase. Supportive care includes treatment of malignancy-induced and therapy-induced emergencies (Table 15–6) and infectious complications (Table 15–7) as well as appropriate pain and symptom control.

Tumor growth is governed by the typical cell cycle of normal tissues:

- Phase M: cell division
- Phase G1: normal cell metabolism with protein and RNA synthesis
- Phase G0: a spinoff of the G1 phase and applies to highly differentiated cells or cells that have moved out of the cell cycle for an indeterminate period of time.
- Phase S: DNA synthesis and chromosome replication
- Phase G2: preparative phase for the next cell division in M phase

At any given time, cancer cells in a particular malignancy are usually in different cell phases. Most drugs affect a particular cell phase, usually the S phase. Some drugs affect the cell cycle of tumor cells to a greater extent than the cycle of normal cells. Resistance to the effects of cancer chemotherapy may be due to the fact that the malignant cells are *out of phase* (not synchronized) at the time of exposure to the particular chemotherapeutic agent; resistance to therapy also may be due to the presence of tumor cells in a sanctuary site, such as the brain or testis, which the drugs cannot enter. In addition, tumor cells may develop resistance to drugs by producing enzymes that inactivate the drugs or by creating transport barriers that prevent the penetration of the drug into the cell, or, in the case of P-glycoprotein expression (product of multidrug resistant gene MDR-1), a membrane pump decreases intracellular drug concentration by pumping drug out of the cell.

Resistance to treatment may be overcome by debulking the tumor mass and by bypassing sanctuary barriers (e.g., intrathecal administration of chemotherapeutic agents). Drug resistance also can be reduced by early treatment with multiple agents. The Goldie-Coldman model proposes use of as many drugs as available for the particular cancer at the highest possible doses to prevent cancer cell resistance. Combinations of various drugs acting at different intracellular targets, with treatment lasting for several years, may provide greater success without the emergence of resistant tumor cells.

*Complications.* Most chemotherapeutic agents produce alopecia, nausea and vomiting, and bone marrow suppression because of their effects on rapidly growing cells. In addition, each cancer chemotherapeutic drug may have unique toxicities (e.g., doxorubicin and cardiomyopathy, vincristine and neuropathy) (see Table 15–5). Bone marrow suppression and immunosuppression are responsible for the infectious complications of cancer therapy (see Table 15–7).

Late sequelae also occur in survivors of childhood cancer (Table 15–8). Some complications may be avoided by monitoring the blood level of drugs, by using leucovorin following methotrexate therapy, by using zoster immune globulin (ZIG) as a prophylactic agent when the patient is exposed to varicella (vaccine should be used prior to exposure), or by using trimethoprim/sulfamethoxazole as a prophylactic agent against *Pneumocystis carinii.* More than 60% of childhood malignancies may be cured with a minimum of long-term consequences.

## LEUKEMIA

Each year, 2000–2500 new cases of childhood leukemia develop in the United States; about 40 children per million are affected under age 15 yr. Of these children, 75% will have acute lymphoblastic leukemia (ALL); 15–20%, acute myelogenous leukemia (AML); and the remainder, other forms, including chronic leukemia. (Table 15–9).

*Etiology and Epidemiology.* The acute leukemias are heterogeneous diseases representing the malignant transformation and clonal expansion of hematopoietic cells that are blocked at a particular

TABLE 15–6. Oncologic Emergencies

| Condition | Manifestations | Etiology | Malignancy | Treatment |
|---|---|---|---|---|
| *Metabolic* | | | | |
| Hyperuricemia | Uric acid nephropathy, gout | Tumor lysis syndrome | Lymphoma, leukemia | Allopurinol; alkalinize urine; hydration and diuresis |
| Hyperkalemia | Arrhythmias, cardiac arrest | Tumor lysis syndrome | Lymphoma, leukemia | Kayexalate; sodium bicarbonate, glucose and insulin; check for pseudohyperkalemia from leukemic cell lysis in test tube |
| Hyperphosphatemia | Hypocalcemic tetany; metastatic calcification, photophobia, pruritus | Tumor lysis syndrome | Lymphoma, leukemia | Hydration, forced diuresis; stop alkalinization; oral aluminum hydroxide to bind phosphate |
| Hyponatremia | Seizure, lethargy; asymptomatic | Syndrome of inappropriate ADH (SIADH) secretion; fluid, sodium losses in vomiting, diarrhea, diuresis | Leukemia; CNS tumor | Restrict free water for SIADH; replace sodium if depleted |
| Hypercalcemia | Anorexia, nausea, polyuria, pancreatitis, gastric ulcers; prolonged PR, shortened QT interval | Bone resorption; ectopic parathormone, vitamin D, or prostaglandins | Hodgkin disease; metastasis to bone | Hydration and furosemide diuresis; corticosteroids; mithramycin; calcitonin; diphosphonates |
| *Hematologic* | | | | |
| Anemia | Pallor, weakness, heart failure | Bone marrow suppression or infiltration; blood loss | Any with chemotherapy | Packed red blood cell transfusion |
| Thrombocytopenia | Petechiae, hemorrhage | Bone marrow suppression or infiltration | Any with chemotherapy | Platelet transfusion |
| Disseminated intravascular coagulation | Shock, hemorrhage | Sepsis, hypotension tumor factors | Promyelocytic leukemia; others | Fresh frozen plasma; platelets, correct infection, etc. |
| Neutropenia | Infection | Bone marrow suppression or infiltration | Any with chemotherapy | If febrile, give broad-spectrum antibiotics and G-CSF if appropriate |

*Table continued on following page*

TABLE 15-6. Oncologic Emergencies *Continued*

| Condition | Manifestations | Etiology | Malignancy | Treatment |
|---|---|---|---|---|
| **Hematologic** *Continued* | | | | |
| Hyperleukocytosis ($>50,000/mm^3$) | Hemorrhage, thrombosis; pulmonary infiltrates, hypoxia; tumor lysis syndrome | Leukostasis; vascular occlusion | Leukemia | Leukapheresis; chemotherapy |
| Graft-versus-host disease | Dermatitis, diarrhea, hepatitis | Immunosuppression and nonirradiated blood products; bone marrow transplantation | Any with immunosuppression | Corticosteroids; cyclosporine; antithymocyte globulin |
| **Space-Occupying Lesions** | | | | |
| Spinal cord compression | Back pain ± radicular. *Cord above T10*: Symmetric weakness, increased deep tendon reflex; sensory level present; toes up *Conus medullaris (T10–L2)*: Symmetric weakness, increased knee reflexes, decreased ankle reflexes; saddle sensory loss; toes up or down *Cauda equina (below L2)*: Asymmetric weakness, loss of deep tendon reflex and sensory deficit; toes down | Metastasis to vertebra and extramedullary space | Neuroblastoma; medulloblastoma | Magnetic resonance imaging (MRI) or myelography for diagnosis; corticosteroids; radiotherapy; laminectomy; chemotherapy |
| Increased intracranial pressure | Confusion, coma, emesis, headache, hypertension, bradycardia, seizures, papilledema, hydrocephalus; III and VI nerve palsies | Primary or metastatic brain tumor | Neuroblastoma, astrocytoma; glioma | Computed tomography (CT) or MRI for diagnosis; corticosteroids; phenytoin; ventricular-peritoneal shunt; radiotherapy; chemotherapy |
| Superior vena cava syndrome | Distended neck veins, plethora, edema of head and neck, cyanosis; proptosis; Horner syndrome | Superior mediastinal mass | Lymphoma | Chemotherapy; radiotherapy |

ADH = antidiuretic hormone; G-CSF = granulocyte colony-stimulating factor.

TABLE 15–7.  Infectious Complications of Malignancy

| Predisposing Factor | Etiology | Site of Infection | Infectious Agents |
|---|---|---|---|
| Neutropenia | Chemotherapy, bone marrow infiltration | Sepsis, shock, pneumonia, soft tissue, proctitis, mucositis | *Staphylococcus aureus, Staphylococcus epidermidis, Escherichia coli, Pseudomonas aeruginosa, Candida, Aspergillus,* anaerobic oral and rectal bacteria |
| Immunosuppression, lymphopenia, lymphocyte–monocyte dysfunction | Chemotherapy, prednisone | Pneumonia, meningitis, disseminated viral infection | *Pneumocystis carinii, Cryptococcus neoformans, Mycobacterium, Nocardia, Listeria monocytogenes, Candida, Aspergillus, Strongyloides, Toxoplasma,* varicella-zoster, cytomegalovirus, herpes simplex |
| Splenectomy | Staging of Hodgkin disease | Sepsis, shock, meningitis | Pneumococcus, *Haemophilus influenzae* |
| Indwelling central venous catheter | Nutrition, administration of chemotherapy | Line sepsis, tract or tunnel infection, exit site infection | *S. epidermidis, S. aureus, Candida albicans, P. aeruginosa, Aspergillus, Corynebacterium* JK, *Streptococcus faecalis, Mycobacterium fortuitum, Propionibacterium acnes* |

Data from Englehard D, Marks MI, Good RA: Infections in bone marrow transplant recipients. J Pediatr 108:335, 1986; Bodey GP: Infection in cancer patients: A continuing association. Am J Med 81 (Suppl 1A): 11, 1986; Whimbey E, Kiehn TE, Brannon P, et al: Bacteremia and fungemia in patients with neoplastic disease. Am J Med 82:723, 1987; Pizzo PA: After empiric therapy: What to do until the granulocyte comes back. Rev Infect Dis 9:214, 1987; and Johnson PR, Decker MD, Edwards KM, et al: Frequency of Broviac catheter infections in pediatric oncology patients. J Infect Dis 154:570, 1986.

stage of differentiation and unable to progress to more mature forms. Although much is known about the taxonomy of leukemia, the etiology remains elusive. EBV is associated with African Burkitt lymphoma, whereas a retrovirus, human T-lymphotropic virus I, is associated with some cases of T cell leukemia in adults. Nonetheless, no specific agent has been found for ALL or AML of childhood.

Certain groups of patients, however, are recognized as being at increased risk for leukemia. Those in the increased risk group include the identical twin of a leukemic patient under the age of 4 yr; children with trisomy 21, Fanconi anemia, Bloom syndrome, and ataxia–telangiectasia (see Table 15–3); and children exposed to radiation and some chemotherapeutic agents (see Table 15–2).

*Clinical Manifestations.* Leukemia can be quite varied in its presentation and may mimic other diseases. Most signs and symptoms are due to infiltration of leukemic cells into normal tissues, resulting in either bone marrow failure (anemia, neutropenia, thrombocytopenia) or specific tissue infiltration (lymph nodes, liver, spleen, brain, bone, skin, gingiva, testis) (see Table 15–4). Common presenting symptoms include fever, pallor (anemia), overt signs of bleeding (such as petechiae or ecchymoses), lethargy, malaise, anorexia, and extremity or joint pain. In support of findings suggested by the history, physical examination frequently reveals lymphadenopathy and hepatosplenomegaly. At the time of diagnosis, extramedullary involvement may be present—for example, central nervous system (CNS) involvement, which may result in diffuse or focal neurologic signs and symptoms, including headache, vomiting, papilledema, and nerve VI palsy. In patients with AML, a soft tissue tumor may be found in the spinal cord or in other extramedullary sites. The presence of myeloperoxidase in these tumors may impart a greenish hue; such tumors are known as *chloromas.* The testicle is another common extramedullary site for ALL; a painless enlargement of one or both testes is seen. The CNS and testes are referred to as "sanctuaries" because they are relatively impermeable to treatment with chemotherapeutic agents.

*Diagnosis.* Initial laboratory data provide a broad spectrum of abnormal findings in leukemia. Anemia, abnormal white blood cell and differential counts, and thrombocytopenia are the rule. A reactive eosinophilia may be present. As many as 10% of children with ALL may have normal routine blood counts at diagnosis. Subtle changes may be present in the peripheral smear, however, that identify the underlying abnormality. There may be teardrop-shaped red blood cells, nucleated red

**TABLE 15–8.** Long-Term Sequelae of Cancer Therapy

| Problem | Etiology |
| --- | --- |
| Infertility | Alkylating agents; radiation |
| Second cancers | Genetic predisposition; radiation, alkylating agents, VP16, topoisomerase II inhibitors |
| Sepsis | Splenectomy |
| Hepatotoxicity | Methotrexate, 6-mercaptopurine, radiation |
| Hepatic veno-occlusive disease | High-dose, intensive chemotherapy (busulfan, cyclophosphamide) ± bone marrow transplant |
| Scoliosis | Radiation |
| Pulmonary (pneumonia, fibrosis) | Radiation, bleomycin, busulfan |
| Myocardiopathy pericarditis | Adriamycin (doxorubicin) daunomycin, radiation |
| Leukoencephalopathy | Cranial irradiation ± methotrexate |
| Cognition/intelligence | Cranial irradiation ± methotrexate |
| Pituitary dysfunction (isolated growth hormone deficiency, panhypopituitary) | Cranial irradiation |
| Psychosocial | Stress, anxiety, death of peers; conditioned responses to chemotherapy |

blood cells, and immature myeloid forms, a constellation referred to as "leukoerythroblastic" that strongly suggests leukemia, metastatic disease, myelofibrosis, or infection involving the bone marrow. The differential diagnosis of leukemia includes aplastic anemia, idiopathic thrombocytopenic purpura, other malignancies, collagen-vascular or rheumatologic diseases, virus-induced or familial-hemophagocytic syndromes, and EBV infection.

When the total white blood cell count is less

**TABLE 15–9.** Acute Myeloid Leukemia Subtypes

| | FAB Classification |
| --- | --- |
| Myeloblastic without maturation | M1 |
| Myeloblastic with some maturation | M2 |
| Hypergranular promyelocytic | M3 |
| Myelomonocytic | M4 |
| Monocytic | M5 |
| Erythroleukemia | M6 |
| Megakaryocytic | M7 |

FAB = French-American-British.

than 5000/mm³, blast cells may not be seen in the peripheral blood, a fact that may delay diagnosis. When the white blood cell count is greater than 5000/mm³, some leukemic blasts almost always are seen in the peripheral blood. It is critical to look at the bone marrow in every case because the morphology of blasts in the peripheral blood may not reflect their bone marrow morphology, which is diagnostic. Electrolyte and other biochemical abnormalities, especially hyperuricemia, may be present at diagnosis or after the initiation of therapy (see Table 15–6). It is particularly important to treat existing hyperuricemia with allopurinol and to ensure adequate renal function prior to the onset of antileukemic therapy.

It is possible to recognize stages of human lymphocyte and granulocyte differentiation utilizing specific monoclonal antibodies to define cell surface antigens. When this application is combined with cytochemical histology, with molecular probes, and with morphology (traditional cell surface markers, such as surface membrane immunoglobulin [SmIg], cytoplasmic immunoglobulin [CIg] on B lymphocytes, or sheep erythrocyte receptors on T lymphocytes), the diagnostic classification, treatment, and prognosis become more specific. Precise diagnosis of the type of leukemia is extremely important because it may enable the physician to devise a specific therapy tailored to the particular phenotype (Table 15–10).

Structural chromosomal abnormalities, such as translocations (e.g., t(8;14)(q24;q23) associated with B-cell [SmIg⁺] disease), and increased chromosome number or ploidy (e.g., hyperdiploidy in excess of 50 chromosomes), occur most often in CALLA⁺ early B cells.

*Prognosis.* Factors that have a bearing on the intensity of treatment and on outcome of disease have been identified (Table 15–11). Lower-risk children have the most favorable prognosis and require less intensive therapy. Overall, the initial white blood cell count and age of the child are the most significant variables. French-British-American (FAB) status L2, the presence of massive organomegaly, and CNS disease also may be important factors.

*Treatment.* The principles of treatment for ALL are outlined in Table 15–12. The combination of weekly intravenous vincristine and daily oral prednisone has nonoverlapping toxicities, is not myelosuppressive, and can induce complete remission in more than 90% of patients with ALL within 3–4 wk. All new patients with ALL have a third agent added for induction therapy (e.g., L-asparaginase). Complete remission is defined as disappearance of clinical signs and symptoms of disease, normaliza-

**TABLE 15–10.** Classification of Acute Lymphocytic Leukemia (ALL)

| Cell of Origin | Ia* | CALLA† | CIg‡ | SmIg§ | LEU-9‖ | Incidence (%) | Clinical Characteristics | Prognosis |
|---|---|---|---|---|---|---|---|---|
| T cell | − | − / + | − | − | + | 15 | Mediastinal mass, high WBC count, predominantly males | Good |
| B cell | + | + / − | + / − | + | − | 1 | Burkitt-like | Poor |
| Pre-B cell | + | + | − / + | − | − | 20 | | |
| Early Pre-B cell | + | + | − | − | − | 60–65 | Protean | Good |
| Null cell | + | − | − | − | − | 5–10 | | |

*Immune-associated antigen.
†Common ALL antigen.
‡Cytoplasmic immunoglobulin.
§Surface immunoglobulin.
‖ Monoclonal antibody against T cells.
WBC = white blood cell.

tion of blood counts, and restoration of the bone marrow to normal cellularity, registering 5% or fewer blasts (M1). At this time, about $10^9$–$10^{10}$ leukemic cells remain, which represents a 99–99.9% decrease in tumor cells.

CNS prophylaxis begins at diagnosis and is continued after successful remission induction. This is a crucial part of the treatment because, without routine CNS prophylaxis, approximately 60% of patients with ALL will develop CNS leukemia while they are still in bone marrow remission. CNS leukemia is difficult to treat once it becomes symptomatic because it predisposes the patient to bone marrow relapse. Prophylaxis is accomplished with

**TABLE 15–11.** Prognostic Factors in Acute Lymphoblastic Leukemia of Childhood

| Factor | Favorable (Lower Risk) | Unfavorable (Higher Risk) |
|---|---|---|
| *Demographic* | | |
| Age | 1–9 yr | <1, >10 yr |
| Race | White | Black |
| Sex | Female | Male |
| *Leukemic Burden* | | |
| Initial WBC count | <50 × $10^9$/L | ≥50 × $10^9$/L |
| Adenopathy | Absent | Present |
| Hepatosplenomegaly | Absent to mild (<3 cm) | Marked (>3 cm) |
| CNS disease at diagnosis | Absent | Present |
| LDH | Not high | High |
| *Morphology, Histochemistry, Cytogenetics, and Biochemistry* | | |
| Lymphoblasts* | L1* | L2* or L3* |
| Periodic acid–Schiff stain | Positive | Negative |
| Cytogenetics† | Modal number: 50 | t(1;19), t(8;14), t(9;22) |
| Mitotic and labeling index | Low | High |
| *Immunologic Factors* | | |
| Immunoglobulins | Normal IgG, IgA, IgM | Decreased IgG, IgA, IgM |
| Surface markers | Non-T, non-B cell ALL, CALLA + | B cell ALL *or* Pre-B |
| Glucocorticoid receptors | High number | Lower number |
| *Response to Induction Therapy* | Rapid | Slow |

Modified from Miller DR: Acute lymphoblastic leukemia. Pediatr Clin North Am 27:269, 1980.
*FAB classification: L1 typical (85%) = small cells, little cytoplasm; L2 undifferentiated (15%) = large cells, large cytoplasm; L3 Burkitt type (1%) = cytoplasmic vacuoles.
†Cytogenetics refers to chromosome changes; t is translocation (see Chapter 4).
LDH = lactic dehydrogenase; WBC = white blood cell.

TABLE 15–12.   Treatment of Childhood Acute
              Lymphoblastic Leukemia

**Induction (4 wk)**

1. Hydration
2. Treat hyperuricemia and prevent renal complications by
   using allopurinol
3. Weekly IV vincristine and daily oral prednisone
4. Third agent, such as L-asparaginase or daunorubicin
5. Irradiation for mediastinal mass, spinal tumor, other
   mass-like lesions

**CNS Prophylaxis**

1. Intrathecal methotrexate
   *or*
2. Intrathecal methotrexate, Ara-C, hydrocortisone
   *or*
3. Intrathecal chemotherapy plus cranial irradiation for
   high-risk patients

**Consolidation Treatment for High-Risk Groups (2–4 wk)**

Removes residual or resistant leukemic cells

**Maintenance Therapy (2–5 yr) or Treatment in Remission**

Combinations of drugs with differential modes of activity,
such as vincristine, prednisone, methotrexate, and 6-
mercaptopurine

**Bone Marrow Relapse**

Autologous, purged bone marrow transplant
Allogeneic bone marrow transplant
Multiple drug reinduction, intensive chemotherapy, CNS
irradiation

**Local Tissue Relapse**

CNS: irradiation, intrathecal or intraventricular methotrexate
*plus* reinduction chemotherapy
Testis: irradiation *plus* reinduction chemotherapy

CNS = central nervous system.

intrathecal drugs alone for most patients and with chemotherapy plus cranial radiation for patients at high risk.

Maintenance therapy or treatment during remission is required to completely eliminate the $10^9$–$10^{10}$ leukemic cells remaining after the initial induction of remission. All leukemia cells must be eliminated to prevent relapse. Combinations of active agents are used during maintenance therapy to prevent the development of drug resistance and to exploit the effects of drugs having different mechanisms of action.

Approximately 70% of patients with ALL who are treated with standard therapy achieve long-term disease-free survival. For children between 1 and 9 yr of age who have low white blood cell counts, the rate of survival is 85% with mild to moderately intense therapy; those with a larger tumor burden, evidenced by high white blood cell counts and extramedullary disease, have a 60–80% survival rate with more aggressive therapy. Five-

year survival without relapse is usually considered a cure.

Relapses occur most commonly in bone marrow but also may present in the CNS, testis, or other extramedullary sites. If relapse occurs while the patient is still receiving modern first-line maintenance chemotherapy, the prognosis is worse than for relapse following discontinuation of therapy. Although additional remissions are relatively easy to induce, their duration often is short despite intensive therapy. Bone marrow transplantation has been used in second or subsequent remission for children having matched sibling or unrelated donors with 20–40% long-term disease-free survival.

The treatment of AML entails a very different philosophy from that of ALL. During induction, intensive multiagent chemotherapy (e.g., an anthracycline, 6-mercaptopurine, and cytosine arabinoside) produces transient bone marrow aplasia. Following induction, limited further intensive chemotherapy has been used with allogeneic bone marrow transplantation offered as an alternative if a matched sibling or unrelated donor is available.

*Complications.* Therapy for either ALL or AML may cause (1) bone marrow hypoplasia, resulting in thrombocytopenia and bleeding requiring platelet transfusions; (2) anemia, necessitating blood transfusion; and (3) granulocytopenia, which rarely requires transfusion of white blood cells. Infection also may occur (see Tables 15–5 and 15–7). Metabolic derangements must be anticipated and prevented, if possible, or treated appropriately when present (see Table 15–6). Long-term sequelae are uncommon (see Table 15–8).

# LYMPHOMAS

Malignant lymphomas are the third most common tumor in childhood and are broadly categorized into Hodgkin disease (5.7 cases/million) and non-Hodgkin lymphoma (NHL; 7.4 cases/million).

## NON-HODGKIN LYMPHOMA

*Epidemiology.* NHL occurs at least three times as frequently in boys as in girls. The peak incidence is between ages 7 and 11 yr. Childhood NHL differs from adult NHL in a number of important features. Most cases of NHL in childhood are diffuse, highly malignant, very aggressive, and show little differentiation beyond primitive cells; highly differentiated, nodular lymphomas that occur in adults are rare in children. Distant noncontiguous metastases are common in childhood NHL, making adult staging systems that depend primarily on nodal involvement of little relevance and mandating that systemic therapy be given to all patients. NHL in childhood resembles acute lymphoblastic leukemia more than it resembles adult-onset NHL or Hodgkin disease. Almost half the cases of childhood NHL are of T-cell origin, in contrast to approximately 5% of those in adults.

NHLs have been described in association with congenital or acquired immunodeficiency states following transplantation, chronic immune stimulation, autoimmune disease, and EBV-induced lymphoproliferation (see Tables 15–2 and 15–3). Acquired immunodeficiency syndrome (AIDS) may be associated with B-cell NHL.

*Clinical Manifestations.* The abdomen, head, and neck are the most common sites of the initial manifestation of B-cell NHL, whereas the anterior mediastinum is the primary site for T-cell lymphomas. In the former sites, usually an abdominal mass or evidence of gastrointestinal obstruction or intussusception is present, whereas mediastinal tumors may produce airway or superior vena cava compression and pleural effusion. Painless lymphadenopathy of the cervical, supraclavicular, and axillary nodes often is noted in association with an anterior mediastinal tumor.

The *diagnosis* is established by tissue biopsy. The *differential diagnosis* of lymphadenopathy is extensive and includes infectious, autoimmune, and malignant diseases. Fever and weight loss may be present, and immunosuppressed patients may demonstrate signs and symptoms of primary CNS lymphoma.

No generally agreed on staging classification for childhood NHL is available. It is essential to ascertain whether a patient has local disease (nodal or extranodal) in one site, which has an excellent prognosis, or disseminated disease, which has a less favorable prognosis. Childhood NHL has a high frequency of dissemination to extranodal sites, such as the CNS, bone marrow, or other noncontiguous areas. The progression of disease in childhood NHL does not follow an orderly anatomic sequence of spread as seen with Hodgkin disease. Evaluation prior to therapy should include complete blood count (CBC), bone marrow aspiration and biopsy, chest roentgenograms, lumbar puncture with cerebrospinal fluid cytology, radionuclide bone scan, evaluation of renal and hepatic function, and appropriate computed tomography (CT) and ultrasound studies. Staging laparotomy with splenectomy and liver biopsy is not indicated in childhood NHL. Tumor cells should be obtained for histologic type and for surface and cytoplasmic marker evaluation because this classification may be relevant to therapy and prognosis (Table 15–13).

**TABLE 15–13.** Distribution of Childhood Non-Hodgkin Lymphoma by Histopathologic Type

| Histologic Type | Marker | Incidence (%) |
|---|---|---|
| Lymphoblastic | T cell | 30–50 |
| Histiocytic (large cell) | B cell, non-T, non-B cell | 14–20 |
| Undifferentiated (small cell) | | |
| Burkitt | B cell | 12–20 |
| Pleomorphic | B cell | 15–20 |
| Other | | 1–12 |

*Treatment.* Systemic disease, occult or overt, is present in about 80% of children with NHL. The dramatic improvement in survival for these patients stems in large part from the use of aggressive multidrug combination chemotherapy with agents known to be effective in childhood ALL. Induction produces remission in 90% of affected children, and maintenance chemotherapy reduces the incidence of relapse. CNS prophylaxis is essential. Local radiation therapy and surgery to debulk large tumors may be integrated into the treatment plan. Patients with localized disease have a significantly better survival rate than that of patients with nonlocalized tumors. Patients with a large tumor burden, often identified by hyperuricemia or by a serum lactic dehydrogenase greater than 1000 IU, are at risk for the tumor lysis syndrome (see Table 15–6). When all patients are considered, 50–75% of patients are long-term survivors.

## HODGKIN DISEASE

Hodgkin disease in children is similar to that in adults. It has a bimodal incidence at age 15–30 yr and after the age of 50, and it is rare before 10 yr of age. There is a 3:1 male predominance in early childhood Hodgkin disease; the sex ratio diminishes after puberty to the 1.4:1 ratio seen in adult Hodgkin disease. Hodgkin disease in childhood carries a very good prognosis. The etiology of Hodgkin disease is unknown, but indirect evidence has been uncovered suggesting an infectious agent. Hodgkin disease occurs in clusters and within families.

*Clinical Manifestations.* Painless, firm lymphadenopathy, often confined to one or two lymph node areas, usually the supraclavicular and cervical nodes, is the most common clinical presentation. Mediastinal lymphadenopathy is another frequent initial presentation. Fever, night sweats, occasionally pruritus, and weight loss are noted in 30% of children. Anemia and thrombocytopenia are unusual, but leukocytosis with eosinophilia may occur. Elevation of the erythrocyte sedimentation rate (ESR) and serum copper level are nonspecific but may correlate with disease activity. Cellular immunity, as determined by cutaneous antigen testing, reveals anergy and predisposes the patient to protozoal (*Toxoplasma, P. carinii*), fungal (cryptococcal), or viral (disseminated varicella-zoster) infections. Autoimmune hemolytic anemia or thrombocytopenia and the nephrotic syndrome are rare manifestations.

*Diagnosis and Staging.* The hallmark of diagnosis is the identification of Reed-Sternberg cells in tumor tissue. Histopathologic subtypes in childhood Hodgkin disease are similar to those in adults, with 10–20% lymphocyte predominance, 40–60% nodular sclerosis, 20–40% mixed cellularity, and 1–10% lymphocyte depletion. As in adults, lymphocyte predominance is most favorable and lymphocyte depletion least favorable.

Unlike the case in patients with NHL, it is of critical importance to accurately stage patients with Hodgkin disease because both the type of therapy and the prognosis are directly related to the stage of disease (Table 15–14). Staging is accomplished

**TABLE 15–14.** Ann Arbor Staging Classification for Hodgkin Disease*

**Stage I**
Involvement of a single lymph node region (I), or a single extralymphatic organ or site (I$_E$)

**Stage II**
Involvement of two or more lymph node regions on the same side of the diaphragm (II), or localized involvement of an extralymphatic organ or site and of one or more lymph node regions on the same side of the diaphragm (II$_E$)

**Stage III**
Involvement of lymph node regions on both sides of the diaphragm (III), which may be accompanied by localized involvement of an extralymphatic organ or site (III$_E$), by involvement of the spleen (III$_S$), or both (III$_{SE}$)

**Stage IV**
Diffuse or disseminated involvement of one or more extralymphatic organs or tissues, with or without associated lymph node enlargement

*Each stage is divided into "A" and "B" categories, where A indicates no systemic symptoms and B indicates the presence of one or more of the following: (1) unexplained weight loss greater than 10% of body weight in preceding 6 mo, (2) fever higher than 38°C, and (3) night sweats.
E = extralymphatic; S = splenic involvement.

by clinical (e.g., fever, night sweats) and surgical evaluation. Clinical staging includes the history, physical examination, and initial chest roentgenogram for evaluation of mediastinal, hilar, or pulmonary parenchymal involvement. Evaluation includes determining CBC, ESR, and serum copper level; tests of hepatic and renal function; lymphangiography or CT evaluation of the retroperitoneal nodes; appropriate radionuclide scans; and bone marrow biopsy (rather than an aspiration). The disease may arise in a unifocal node and then spread through contiguous lymph node chains by the lymphatic channels. Right-sided cervical nodal involvement is associated with mediastinal disease, and bilateral or left-sided cervical nodes are associated with splenic disease.

With surgical (exploratory laparotomy) staging in the past, as many as 30% of stage I and II patients are reclassified to higher stages, thus necessitating different therapy (Table 15–15). The most common site of abdominal involvement is the spleen and splenic hilar nodes. At present, surgical staging (including splenectomy) is not indicated for children with Hodgkin disease. It is thought that adequate information is obtained from CT scans of the neck, chest, abdomen, and pelvis; a gallium scan; bone marrow aspirate; and biopsy for those with clinical stage III or IV or B symptoms coupled with the lymph node biopsy for diagnosis.

The major *differential diagnoses* for Hodgkin disease and NHL are lymphadenitis, infectious mononucleosis, tuberculosis, atypical mycobacteria, cat-scratch disease, acquired immunodeficiency syndrome (AIDS), and toxoplasmosis.

*Treatment.* Table 15–15 shows the indicated therapy for various stages of Hodgkin disease. With appropriate therapy, 80–90% of patients survive 5 yr. Irradiation has been the cornerstone of treatment for Hodgkin disease in adults; however, chemotherapy with involved field radiation therapy is utilized to treat prepubertal patients. Radiation fields used in the treatment of the disease are illustrated in Figure 15–2. The majority of children are treated with either ABVD (Adriamycin [doxorubicin], bleomycin, vincristine, and dacarbazine [DTIC]) or a combination of MOPP (nitrogen mustard, vincristine, prednisone, procarbazine) and ABVD (MOPP/ABVD alternating or MOPP/ABV hybrid). Some have replaced nitrogen mustard with Cytoxan. (cyclophosphamide, oncovin, procarbazine, prednisone [COPP]).

*Complications.* Complications include pneumococcal and *Haemophilus influenzae* sepsis in splenectomized patients; growth retardation and restrictive lung disease secondary to irradiation and/or bleomycin; thyroid, testicular, and ovarian dys-

TABLE 15–15.  Recommended Therapy for Children and Young Adults with Hodgkin Disease

| Stage | Patient Features | Therapy |
|---|---|---|
| I, II (favorable) | No bulk disease; no hilar adenopathy | Four cycles of chemotherapy; low-dose radiotherapy to the involved areas |
| Other I, II, and all III | Bulk disease; hilar adenopathy; large mediastinal mass; unfavorable signs | Six cycles of hybrid chemotherapy; low-dose radiotherapy to the involved areas |
| IV | | Six cycles of more aggressive chemotherapy; low-dose radiotherapy to the involved areas |

*Low-dose radiotherapy = 2000–2500 cGy.

function; and development of secondary tumors (see Table 15–3). Although Hodgkin disease is one of the most curable malignant tumors in childhood, concern now must be directed increasingly toward minimizing the serious side effects of successful antitumor treatment.

Splenectomy in young children leaves them susceptible to bacterial sepsis, and for this reason physicians are reluctant to perform staging laparotomies. If splenectomy is anticipated, immunizing all patients with polyvalent pneumococcal vaccine, meningococcal vaccine, and *H. influenzae* vaccine routinely should precede the operation.

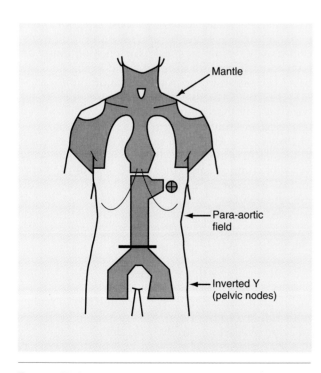

FIGURE 15–2.  Radiation therapy fields used in treatment of Hodgkin disease.

# PRIMARY CENTRAL NERVOUS SYSTEM TUMORS

CNS tumors are the most common solid tumors in children and are second to leukemia in overall incidence of malignant diseases. There are about 1200 new cases per year, or approximately 24 cases per million children under the age of 15 yr. Brain tumors in children differ from those in adults, in that they are predominantly infratentorial tumors (posterior fossae) involving the cerebellum, midbrain, and brain stem (Table 15–16). Childhood brain tumors are differentiated further from those in adults, in that they are usually low-grade astrocytomas or embryonic neoplasms (medulloblastomas, ependymomas, or germ cell tumors), whereas most CNS tumors in adults are malignant astrocytomas and metastatic carcinomas.

*Clinical Manifestations.*  Common presenting signs and symptoms of CNS tumors in childhood often are dismissed initially as signs of intercurrent viral or nonspecific illnesses. Signs of increased intracranial pressure and focal neurologic deficits eventually suggest intracranial pathology (Table 15–17). Headache is not localizing but is suggestive of increased intracranial pressure if it is present at night or on awakening, worsens with cough or straining, and is intermittent but recurs with increasing frequency and intensity. Vomiting without nausea, another nonspecific sign of increased intracranial pressure, usually is intermittent and occurs on arising in the morning. Strabismus with diplopia is the result of nerve VI palsy caused by increased intracranial pressure. Double vision resulting from a nerve VI deficit is not a localizing finding. Papilledema or choked optic discs may be a late but specific sign of increased intracranial pressure. Obstructive hydrocephalus may produce a large cranium if it occurs before the sutures have fused. Focal signs may be present, with or without signs of increased intracranial pressure. Nystagmus usually is due to cerebellovestibular pathway irri-

TABLE 15–16. Location, Incidence, and Prognosis of Central Nervous System Tumors in Children

| Location | Incidence (%) | Five-Year Survival (%) |
|---|---|---|
| *Infratentorial (Posterior Fossa)* | 55–60 | |
| Astrocytoma (cerebellum) | | 90 |
| Medulloblastoma | | 44–55 |
| Glioma (brain stem) | | 0–5 (high grade) 30 (low grade) |
| Ependymoma | | 50–60 |
| *Supratentorial (Cerebral Hemispheres)* | 40–45 25–30 | |
| Astrocytoma | | 10–50 |
| Glioblastoma multiforme | | 0–5 |
| Ependymoma | | 50–60 |
| Choroid plexus papilloma | | 60–80 |
| *Midline* | 15 | |
| Craniopharyngioma | | 70–90 |
| Pineal (germinoma) | | 65–75 |
| Optic nerve glioma | | 50–90 |

tative or destructive lesions, but nystagmus also may be seen with a marked visual deficit (peripheral or cortical blindness). Cranial nerve deficits other than nerve VI deficits localize the lesion to the brain stem. Head tilt, as a compensation for loss of binocular vision, is noted with extraocular muscle weakness.

Personality changes, poor school performance, and change in hand preference should suggest a cortical lesion, whereas ataxia suggests a cerebellar or brain stem lesion. Babinski sign, hyperreflexia, spasticity, and loss of dexterity are suggestive of brain stem or cortical tumors, whereas seizures are noted with cortical lesions. Endocrine abnormalities are noted with pituitary, hypothalamic, or pineal tumors.

*Diagnosis.* History, physical examination, and neurologic examination, including that of visual fields and fundi, are fundamental for evaluation, but CT scan and magnetic resonance imaging (MRI) of the head. They are the procedures of choice for diagnosing and localizing tumors as well as other intracranial masses. MRI may be of additional diagnostic benefit, particularly in posterior fossa and spinal tumors, in which CT scans are

least effective because the surrounding bone often limits resolution. Examination of cerebrospinal fluid (CSF) by cytocentrifuge histology is essential to determine the presence of metastasis in medulloblastoma and pinealoma.

*Differential diagnosis* should include arteriovenous malformation, aneurysm, brain abscess, echinococcal or cysticercosal or other parasite infestation, herpes simplex encephalitis, granulomatous disease (tuberculosis, cryptococcus, sarcoid), intracranial hemorrhage, pseudotumor cerebri, primary cerebral lymphoma, vasculitis, and, rarely, metastatic tumors.

*Treatment.* Once the diagnosis is established, corticosteroids often are administered to reduce tumor edema. With improvements in neurodiagnosis, lessened surgical morbidity, and better chemotherapy programs, an aggressive approach to treatment of pediatric brain tumors has improved outcome (Tables 15–16 and 15–17). Utilizing improved neurosurgical techniques, surgical objectives include biopsy, debulking or complete excision if possible, and treatment of hydrocephalus. Radiation therapy has been the mainstay of treatment of malignant CNS tumors. Medulloblastomas, ependymomas, germ cell tumors, and some low-grade astrocytomas are responsive to radiation in doses of 4500–6500 cGy. About 50% of patients with medulloblastoma are cured by a combination of surgery and radiation therapy to the posterior fossa, whole brain, and spinal axis. Trials of single and multiagent chemotherapy for brain tumors are under way; there is a role for chemotherapy in patients with medulloblastoma and in infants with brain tumors in order to minimize or avoid radiation therapy. Objective tumor responses for a number of chemotherapeutic programs have also been observed in other brain tumors.

*Prognosis.* The 5-yr survival rate associated with all childhood CNS tumors is approximately 50%, resulting in large measure from the high curability of cerebellar astrocytomas and some medulloblastomas (see Table 15–16). The best prognosis is noted following simple surgical total excision of a cystic cerebellar astrocytoma.

## WILMS TUMOR

Wilms tumor is the most common intrarenal malignant tumor of childhood, with a yearly incidence of 7.8 new cases per million children.

*Epidemiology.* The mean age of diagnosis is 3–3 1/2 yr, and no sex predilection is apparent. A hereditary form of Wilms tumor may be associated with a bilateral presentation and with some unilat-

**TABLE 15–17.**  Manifestations and Treatment of Primary Central Nervous System Tumors

| Tumor/Site | Manifestations | Treatment | Comments |
|---|---|---|---|
| Cerebellar astrocytoma | Onset between 5 and 8 yr of age; ↑ ICP, ataxia, nystagmus, head tilt, intention tremor | Surgical excision plus adjuvant radiotherapy if a solid tumor; corticosteroids to ↓ tumor edema | Symptoms present for 2–7 mo; cystic tumors have favorable outcome |
| Medulloblastoma Cerebellar vermis and floor of 4th ventricle | Onset between 3 and 5 yr of age; ↑ ICP, obstructive hydrocephalus, ataxia, cerebrospinal fluid metastasis, and spinal cord compression | Surgical excision and radiotherapy plus adjuvant chemotherapy*; corticosteroids to ↓ tumor edema | Acute onset of symptoms; tumor is radiosensitive; cerebrospinal fluid checked for metastatic cells |
| Ependymoma Floor of 4th ventricle | ↑ ICP, obstructive hydrocephalus; rarely seeds spinal fluid | Surgical excision, radiotherapy, chemotherapy*; corticosteroids to ↓ tumor edema | Onset intermediate between astrocytoma and medulloblastoma |
| Brain stem glioma | Onset between 5 and 7 yr of age; triad of multiple cranial nerve deficit (VII, IX, X, V, VI) pyramidal tract, and cerebellar signs; skip lesions common; ↑ ICP is late | Excision impossible; radiotherapy is palliative; corticosteroids to ↓ tumor edema; experimental chemotherapy* | Small size but critical location makes this tumor highly lethal |
| Pinealoma | Paralysis of upward gaze (Parinaud syndrome); lid retraction (Collier sign); hearing loss; precocious puberty; ↑ ICP; may seed spinal fluid | Radiotherapy, chemotherapy; shunting of CSF | Germ cell line; germinoma, dermoid, teratoma, mixed lesions may calcify or secrete hCG or alpha-fetoprotein |
| Diencephalic glioma Hypothalamus | Onset between 2 and 5 mo of age; alert, euphoric but emaciated appearance; emesis, optic atrophy, nystagmus | Radiotherapy | Patient may become obese after treatment |
| Astrocytoma/glioma Cerebral cortex | Onset between 5 and 10 yr of age; personality changes; headache, motor weakness, seizures, ↑ ICP later | Location determines surgical or radiotherapy; anticonvulsant and corticosteroids; chemotherapy* | *Differential diagnosis:* Abscess, hydatid or porencephalic cyst; herpes simplex encephalitis, granuloma (TB, cryptococcus); arteriovenous malformation; hematoma; lymphoma |
| Optic glioma | Onset before 2 yr of age; poor visual acuity, exophthalmos, nystagmus; ↑ ICP; optic atrophy, strabismus | Surgical resection or radiotherapy; chemotherapy* | Neurofibromatosis in 25% of patients |
| Craniopharyngioma Pituitary fossa | Onset between 7 and 12 yr of age; ↑ ICP, bitemporal hemianopia, sexual and growth retardation; growth hormone and gonadotropic deficiency | Begin cortisol replacement prior to surgery; total excision, adjuvant radiotherapy if extensive | Calcification above sella turcica; diabetes insipidus common postoperatively |

*Chemotherapy may delay need for radiotherapy, thus avoiding treatment-related neurotoxicity. Chemotherapy includes alternating cycles of cyclophosphamide plus vincristine with cisplatin plus etopside.

CSF = cerebral spinal fluid; hCG = human chorionic gonadotropin; ↑ ICP = increased intracranial pressure: headache, vomiting (papilledema, III and VI nerve palsies, wide sutures); TB = tuberculosis.

eral tumors. A number of congenital anomalies frequently are identified in children with Wilms tumor, including sporadic aniridia (1:100 in patients with Wilms tumor versus 1:50,000 in the general population), hemihypertrophy (2:100 in patients with Wilms tumor versus 3:100,000 in the general population), and genitourinary anomalies (5:100 in patients with Wilms tumor), including hypospadias, cryptorchidism, horseshoe or fused kidneys, ureteral duplication, and polycystic kidneys. Wilms tumor with aniridia often is associated with a deletion of part of chromosome 11 [del (11p13)].

*Clinical Manifestations.* More than 80% of children with Wilms tumor present with an abdominal mass, which usually is discovered incidentally by the parents while they are bathing or dressing the child or during a routine well child examination. Associated symptoms and laboratory abnormalities may include abdominal pain, fever, hypertension, and microscopic or gross hematuria. Polycythemia is a rare paraneoplastic complication.

Associated manifestations which suggest an increased risk for Wilms tumor include complete or partial aniridia, hemihypertrophy, and a history of any genitourinary abnormalities. A CBC, urinalysis, liver and renal function studies, and a search for sites of metastases (lung, liver, nodes, kidney, bone, brain) should be performed. Ultrasound studies of the abdomen, plain abdominal roentgenograms, and intravenous pyelograms (IVPs) often reveal a mass that distorts the calyces, displaces the kidney, and does not cross the midline. CT is helpful for identifying metastasis or local spread (to the inferior vena cava and retroperitoneum) and for evaluating the contralateral kidney.

*Diagnosis.* The *differential diagnosis* of Wilms tumor includes benign lesions, such as hydronephrosis, polycystic disease of the kidney, and splenomegaly as well as malignant tumors, such as renal cell carcinoma, neuroblastoma, lymphoma, retroperitoneal rhabdomyosarcoma, and ovarian tumors. Prognostic factors include tumor stage (Table 15–18) and tumor histology (classic nephroblastoma, with a favorable histology and 88% survival, versus anaplastic or sarcomatous variant, with an unfavorable histology and 12% survival). The 4-yr relapse-free survival of patients with tumors of favorable histology is directly related to stage and, with treatment, can be expected to be 97%, 92%, 87%, and 73% for stages I, II, III, and IV, respectively.

*Treatment.* Surgery, either at diagnosis (American Centers) or following preoperative chemotherapy (European Centers), continues to be the cornerstone of therapy. Gentle technique is required to

**TABLE 15–18.** National Wilms Tumor Study Staging System*

**Stage I**

Tumor limited to the kidney and completely excised

The surface of the renal capsule is intact; the tumor is not ruptured before or during removal

No residual tumor is apparent beyond the margins of excision

**Stage II**

Tumor extends beyond the kidney but is completely excised

Regional extension of the tumor is present (i.e., penetration through the outer surface of the renal capsule into the perirenal soft tissues); vessels outside the kidney substance are infiltrated or contain tumor thrombus; the tumor may have been biopsied or local spillage of tumor confined to the flank has occurred; no residual tumor is apparent at or beyond the margins of excision

**Stage III**

Residual nonhematogenous tumor confined to the abdomen
Any of the following may occur:
  a. Lymph nodes on biopsy are found to be involved in the hilus, the periaortic chains, or beyond
  b. Diffuse peritoneal contamination by the tumor has occurred, such as by spillage of tumor beyond the flank before or during surgery, or by tumor growth that has penetrated through the peritoneal surface
  c. Implants are found on the peritoneal surfaces
  d. The tumor extends beyond the surgical margins either microscopically or grossly
  e. The tumor is not completely resectable because of local infiltration into vital structures

**Stage IV**

Hematogenous metastases; deposits beyond stage III (e.g., lung, liver, bone, and brain)

**Stage V**

Bilateral renal involvement at diagnosis

An attempt should be made to stage each side according to the above criteria on the basis of extent of disease prior to biopsy

*The clinical stage is decided by the surgeon in the operating room and is confirmed by the pathologist, who also evaluates the histology. It is done on the basis of gross and microscopic tumor distribution and is the same for tumors with favorable and with unfavorable histologic features. The patient is characterized, however, by a statement of both criteria (e.g., stage II, favorable histology, or stage II, unfavorable histology).

prevent rupture of the tumor during removal. A large transabdominal incision facilitates the search for metastatic disease, examination of the opposite kidney, approach to the inferior vena cava if necessary, and removal of the tumor en bloc when feasible. Radiation, when utilized, is begun postoperatively, with the therapeutic plan dependent on the stage of the disease and age of the patient. In patients with stage III or IV disease, the tumor bed or full abdomen, if necessary, is irradiated with total doses of approximately 1000 cGy. Care must be taken to minimize radiation effects to the liver, because radiation hepatotoxicity is potentiated by subsequent chemotherapy. Chemotherapy utilizing vincristine, dactinomycin, and doxorubicin (Adriamycin) has significantly improved the relapse-free survival rate. The first two drugs are used in all stages, and Adriamycin is used in stages III and IV. If pulmonary metastases are present, lung irradiation is added to the therapy of the primary tumor.

Bilateral Wilms tumor is present in about 5% of children on initial presentation, whereas recurrent disease affects the opposite kidney in 4–5% of patients. Treatment must be individualized but may require excisional biopsy or heminephrectomy on one side and radical nephrectomy on the more involved side, with the objective to preserve as much normal kidney as possible. Preoperative chemotherapy with dactinomycin and vincristine often aids the surgeon in determining the appropriate procedure.

## NEUROBLASTOMA

Neuroblastoma is the most enigmatic of childhood tumors. It arises from the primitive neural crest cells that form the adrenal medulla and the sympathetic nervous system of the cervical sympathetic nervous system of the cervical sympathetic chain, the thoracic chain, and the abdominal organ of Zuckerkandl. Even though, neuroblastoma is responsive to a variety of aggressive chemotherapy treatment protocols, the outlook for children with this tumor has not changed significantly in the last three decades.

*Epidemiology.* Neuroblastoma is the most common malignant tumor in infancy, with a median age of onset at 20 mo of life. In childhood, it ranks fourth in frequency to leukemia, lymphoma, and CNS tumors. Although neuroblastoma represents fewer than 8% of cases of childhood cancer, it is responsible for 15% of cancer deaths in children. The incidence of neuroblastoma is estimated to be 1:100,000 infants, and it may be associated with fetal hydantoin syndrome, von Recklinghausen disease, and Hirschsprung disease.

*Clinical Manifestations.* The most common presentation is an abdominal mass that is hard, smooth, nontender, and most often palpated in the flank. In the abdomen, 45% of tumors arise in the adrenal gland and 25% in the retroperitoneal sympathetic ganglia. Other sites include the pelvis (4%), the posterior mediastinum (20%), and the neck (4%).

Calcification within the tumor often is observed on plain films of the abdomen, and IVP shows displacement of a kidney with minimal distortion of the calyceal system if the tumor arises in the adrenal gland. The presentation must be differentiated from that of Wilms tumor, which also presents as an abdominal flank mass. In contrast to neuroblastoma, Wilms tumors are often lobulated rather than smooth, and they are seen to displace and distort the urinary collecting system on IVP. Neuroblastoma may become manifest at birth as a flank mass or malignant ascites with nonimmune hydrops fetalis.

Neuroblastoma may spread to the liver, producing hepatomegaly, and may metastasize to bone and bone marrow, producing limp and bone pain. Primary involvement of the cervical sympathetic chain produces ipsilateral Horner syndrome with heterochromia of the iris; posterior mediastinal tumors produce pain, spinal cord compression, and airway obstruction. Esthesioneuroblastoma of the olfactory bulb produces epistaxis and nasal obstruction. Metastasis may produce blanching skin nodules, periorbital ecchymosis, and proptosis. Vasoactive intestinal polypeptide secretion may produce watery diarrhea. Rapid multidirectional eye movements (opsoclonus), myoclonus, and cerebellar ataxia also are noted occasionally.

*Diagnosis.* In addition to the history and the physical examination with blood pressure, evaluation should include a CBC, renal and hepatic function tests, chest roentgenogram, abdominal plain film, radionuclide scan of bone and liver, ultrasonogram and CT scan, and a careful search for products of catecholamine metabolism. Most neuroblastomas secrete one or more catecholamines or their metabolic by-products (vanillylmandelic acid [VMA] and homovanillic acid [HVA]). Bone marrow examination may demonstrate neuroblastoma cells forming typical rosettes.

*Prognosis.* Age at presentation, stage of disease, primary site, site of metastases, cytogenetics, DNA ploidy, amplification of the N-myc oncogene (poor prognosis) or TRK (good prognosis), ferritin concentration, degree of cell differentiation, lymphocyte infiltration of the tumor, and the presence of peripheral lymphocytosis all affect survival. In general, children under 1 yr of age have a good prognosis, whereas children over 2 yr of age have a much poorer prognosis (Table 15–19). Older patients generally have more extensive disease. Children with tumors arising in the neck and posterior mediastinum have a better prognosis than those with abdominal primaries. Metastatic lesions in bone or positive ipsilateral lymph nodes carry a poor prognosis.

*Treatment.* Total surgical excision offers the best

TABLE 15–19. International Neuroblastoma Staging System (INSS)

| Stage | Definition | Incidence (%) | Survival at 5 Yr |
|---|---|---|---|
| 1 | Localized tumor with complete gross excision, with or without microscopic residual disease; representative ipsilateral lymph nodes negative for tumor microscopically (nodes attached to and removed with the primary tumor may be positive). | 5 | 90% or greater |
| 2A | Localized tumor with incomplete gross excision; representative ipsilateral nonadherent lymph nodes negative for tumor microscopically. | 10 | 70–80% |
| 2ß | Localized tumor with or without complete gross excision; with ipsilateral nonadherent lymph nodes positive for tumor. Enlarged contralateral lymph nodes must be negative microscopically. | | |
| 3 | Unresectable unilateral tumor infiltrating across the midline,* with or without regional lymph node involvement; or localized unilateral tumor with contralateral regional lymph node involvement; or midline tumor with bilateral extension by infiltration (unresectable) or by lymph node involvement. | 25 | 40–70% (depending on completeness of surgical resection) |
| 4 | Any primary tumor with dissemination to distant lymph nodes, bone, bone marrow, liver, skin and/or other organs (except as defined for stage 4S) | 60 | More than 60% if age at diagnosis is younger than 1 yr; 20% if age at diagnosis is older than 1 yr and under 2 yr; 10% if age at diagnosis is over 2 yr |
| 4S | Localized primary tumor (as defined for stage 1, 2A or 2B), with dissemination limited to skin, liver, and/or bone marrow† (limited to infants < 1 year of age) | 5 | More than 80% |

Modified from Brodeur GM, et al: Revisions of the International Criteria for Neuroblastoma Diagnosis, Staging, and Response to Treatment. J Clin Oncol 11:1466, 1993.

*The midline is defined as the vertebral column. Tumors originating on one side and crossing the midline must infiltrate to or beyond the opposite side of the vertebral column.

†Marrow involvement in stage 4S should be minimal (i.e., <10% of total nucleated cells identified as malignant on bone marrow biopsy or on marrow aspirate). More extensive marrow involvement would be considered to be stage 4. The MIBG scan (if performed) should be negative in the marrow.

hope of cure and may be the only therapy required, but the presence of metastatic disease in a high percentage of patients at diagnosis limits the effectiveness of this modality alone. The role of radiation therapy is not precisely defined, although it clearly plays a role in the palliative treatment of patients with advanced disease. A wide range of chemotherapeutic agents have been used for patients with extensive local or disseminated disease at diagnosis. Although chemotherapy has significantly increased the tumor response rate, the cure rate for children has remained essentially unchanged. The most active agents include vincristine, cyclophosphamide, doxorubicin, cisplatin, and teniposide (VM-26). Experimental protocols with radiolabeled monoclonal antibodies to the neuroblastoma cell line or with total body irradiation and high-dose chemotherapy, followed by purged autologous bone marrow transplantation, are newer approaches to therapy.

A number of curious issues relate to neuroblastoma. Occasionally, one cannot find evidence of a primary tumor but only evidence of metastases to the orbit. Furthermore, a small percentage of neuroblastomas, especially in very young children, appear to regress spontaneously without any treatment; this regression has been documented more frequently in neuroblastoma than in any other malignancy. In addition, as many as 1:200 neonates demonstrate neuroblastoma in situ at autopsy. Also, numerous reports have been made of tumors initially considered to be malignant neuroblastomas that, after treatment, were found to be clearly benign ganglioneuromas. The stage IV-S designation also is unique, in that it refers to a small primary tumor with disseminated disease but without bone involvement. Symptomatic therapy only is needed (usually to control hepatomegaly), and the outcome may be compromised by aggressive chemotherapy. Screening infants at 6 mo of age for urine spot tests of VMA or HVA has been initiated in an attempt to identify patients before widespread dissemination of the tumor has occurred. Evaluation of screening programs suggests that almost all tumors identified have favorable biological features and an excellent outcome with or without treatment. Screening has not identified patients with tumors possessing unfavorable features in whom early identification might improve outcome. Based on these findings, screening infants for neuroblastoma is not performed in the United States.

## SOFT TISSUE SARCOMAS

### RHABDOMYOSARCOMA

Rhabdomyosarcoma is the most common soft tissue sarcoma in children. The incidence is about 4.5 cases/million (1.3/million black children), with a peak occurrence in children 2–6 yr of age and a second peak in adolescence. The tumor arises primarily in skeletal muscle but may occur in any tissue derived from mesenchyme. The early peak is associated with tumors in the prostate, vagina, bladder, and head and neck; the later peak is associated with tumors in the extremities, trunk, and male genitourinary tract. Tumors of the head and neck (35–40%) occur in the orbit, sinuses, nasopharynx, and soft tissues.

*Clinical Manifestations.* The clinical presentation of rhabdomyosarcoma varies, depending on the site of origin and the subsequent mass effect. For example, in the *orbit,* swelling, proptosis, and limitation of extraocular motion may be exhibited; in *other head and neck sites,* nasal mass, chronic otitis media, hemorrhage, ear discharge, obstruction, dysphagia, hearing abnormalities, and cranial nerve involvement may be noted; in the *retroperitoneum,* symptoms associated with a mass are seen; in the *genitourinary tract,* urethral, vaginal (polypoid) masses, peritesticular swelling, hematuria, and urinary frequency or retention may be exhibited; and in the *extremities and trunk,* painful or asymptomatic masses may be the main features. Evaluation must be directed toward the particular site of involvement but, additionally, should include CBC, liver and renal function tests, urinalysis, radionuclide bone scan, bone marrow biopsy, lumbar puncture with spinal fluid cytology for craniospinal sites, and other tests for identifying occult and metastatic disease.

*Diagnosis.* Tissue biopsy is needed for definitive diagnosis. The staging system has prognostic significance. Histopathology also is important because patients with alveolar histology have a consistently higher mortality rate than patients with embryonal histology, irrespective of the primary site of involvement. Embryonal histopathology predominates, especially in younger patients.

*Treatment.* Treatment must be tailored to the site of involvement, but it includes integration of surgery, radiation therapy, and chemotherapy. If it is possible to remove the tumor completely with a wide margin of resection, the chance of local control is good. Radiation therapy combined with chemotherapy can provide local control of gross residual or microscopic disease in 90% of patients.

The combination of cyclophosphamide, vincristine, dactinomycin, and doxorubicin has dramatically improved survival over that achievable by radiation therapy and surgery alone. Although primary site and histology are strong prognostic indicators, the most important determinant of outcome is the extent of disease at diagnosis. Preliminary data suggest that patients with group I (localized tumor, completely resected, and no lymph node involvement) and II (regional disease, completely or grossly resected) tumors can be treated effectively with vincristine and dactinomycin and have a 2–yr relapse-free survival of 83–87% for group I tumors and 70–81% for group II tumors. Chemotherapy for groups III (incomplete resection or biopsy with residual disease) and IV (distant metastatic disease at onset) is not yet satisfactory despite the addition of doxorubicin to vincristine, cyclophosphamide, and dactinomycin. The 2-yr survival rate for patients with group III tumors treated with all four drugs is 71–79%; for patients with group IV tumors, it is 37–40%.

Less common soft tissue sarcomas of infancy and childhood are fibrosarcoma (11% of soft tissue sarcomas), neurofibrosarcoma (3%), synovial sarcoma (5%), liposarcoma (4%), malignant fibrous histiocytoma (4%), hemangiopericytoma (3%), and leiomyosarcoma (<2%).

## MALIGNANT BONE TUMORS

The two most important malignant bone tumors in children are **osteosarcoma** and **Ewing sarcoma.** Less commonly encountered are chondrosarcoma, fibrosarcoma, reticulosarcoma, reticulum cell sarcoma, non-Hodgkin lymphoma of bone, hemangiosarcoma, and malignant giant cell tumor.

### OSTEOSARCOMA

Osteosarcoma is a rare tumor; in children younger than age 15 yr, only about 300 new cases occur each year in the United States. Males are affected 1 1/2 times more often than females.

*Epidemiology and Etiology.* The disease most commonly affects adolescents, with the peak incidence occurring during the period of maximum growth velocity. The primary tumor most often is located at the epiphysis or metaphysis of anatomic sites that are associated with maximum growth velocity (distal femur, proximal tibia, proximal humerus) but any bone may be involved.

The cause is unknown, but the correlation of the location of most tumors with the period of maximum bone growth suggests some relation to increased osteoblastic activity. Genetic factors may have a role in osteosarcoma; 16 sets of siblings with the disease have been identified. Among patients with hereditary retinoblastoma, the incidence of osteosarcoma is increased 500 times, and deletions on the long arm of chromosome 13, which can occur in patients with retinoblastoma, have been found in some osteosarcoma tumors, implicating the RB allele as in retinoblastoma. Osteosarcoma also may occur following radiotherapy.

*Clinical Manifestations.* Osteosarcomas arise in either the medullary cavity or the periosteum. The tumor occurs most frequently in the femur (43% of cases), followed by the tibia (19%) and the humerus (10%). The tumor is usually noticed as a painful swelling or pain near the knee without other symptoms. Often a history of trauma is noted, but this is only an incidental finding. Gait disturbances and pathologic fractures also may be present.

*Diagnosis.* Evaluation should be based on plain films of the affected area, chest roentgenogram, radionuclide bone scan, and MRI scan of the involved bone. These tests may demonstrate sclerosis, periosteal new bone formation, and soft tissue extension of tumor. Because of the frequent presence of pulmonary metastasis (10–15%), CT of the chest is essential to detect small lesions; these lesions often appear as calcified nodules. Micrometastatic disease is present at diagnosis in 80–90% of patients but is undetectable with any of the present tests available. Serum alkaline phosphatase levels may be elevated and may be used as a marker of the response to treatment. The ESR is normal. Arteriography may be useful when limb-sparing procedures are contemplated. Biopsy is essential for accurate diagnosis. Osteosarcoma must be differentiated from Ewing sarcoma, benign and malignant bone tumors, and chronic osteomyelitis.

*Treatment.* Prior to the onset of effective adjuvant chemotherapy, only about 20% of patients with osteosarcoma survived. Until the early 1980s, treatment of pediatric sarcomas involved initial surgery, followed by adjuvant chemotherapy. It is now standard practice to give chemotherapy first, after a biopsy to establish diagnosis. This neoadjuvant chemotherapy has a number of potential advantages. It provides an immediate attack on presumed micrometastatic disease (the major cause of cancer mortality). Tumor shrinkage induced by neoadjuvant chemotherapy may facilitate limb-sparing procedure or minimize surgical morbidity. Finally, evaluation of the amount of necrosis in the resected tumor provides an in vivo measurement of chemotherapeutic efficacy. Currently, 60–70% of patients with localized osteosarcoma of an extremity are cured with this approach.

Chemotherapy includes the use of high-dose methotrexate, doxorubicin, cisplatin, and ifosfamide. The tumor is not radiosensitive at conventional doses. In addition, about one third of patients can be successfully treated if they experience a limited relapse in the lung after a combination of surgery (to remove each pulmonary metastatic lesion) and additional chemotherapy. Poor prognostic findings include age younger than 10 yr, large tumor (>15 cm), osteoblastic cell type, involvement of the axial skeleton or humerus, an elevated serum lactic dehydrogenase level, presence of symptoms for less than 2 mo, and metastasis.

The improvement in a survival for these patients has generated many attempts to lessen the morbidity of surgery by attempting to resect tumors and implant protheses of various sorts rather than simply amputating or disarticulating an extremity. These limb-sparing procedures include the use of bone grafting and an internal prosthesis in selected patients. Postoperative rehabilitation therapy is critical after amputation.

## EWING SARCOMA

Ewing sarcoma is a highly malignant, nonosseous, small round cell tumor (as in neuroblastoma, primitive neuroectodermal tumor [PNET], lymphoma, and rhabdomyosarcoma) that frequently has metastasized at the time of diagnosis. The clonal nature of the malignant cells is revealed by the consistent t(11;22) chromosomal abnormality. The incidence in white children is about 1.9/million, but the disease is almost unknown in blacks. It occurs in younger children as well as in adolescents. The tumor most often involves the diaphyseal portion of long bones. The femur and pelvis are the most common sites, but lesions of the tibia, fibula, ribs, humerus, scapula, and clavicle also are encountered.

The *clinical manifestations* are similar to those of osteosarcoma; however, systemic symptoms, such as weight loss, fatigue, and fever, are found more commonly in Ewing sarcoma. The *diagnostic evaluation* is similar to that for osteosarcoma. The ESR is elevated. Plain roentgenograms of the bone reveal calcified periosteal elevation ("onion-skin"), osteolytic lesions, and sclerosis. Osteomyelitis and eosinophilic granuloma are part of the *differential diagnosis*. Metastasis to the bone by neuroblastoma or rhabdomyosarcoma should be considered in younger children with a solitary bone lesion.

Because the majority of patients with Ewing sarcoma have micrometastatic disease at the time of diagnosis, chemotherapy is a critical component of the *treatment.* Chemotherapy includes vincristine, cyclophosphamide, dactinomycin, and doxorubicin, with agents such as ifosfamide under evaluation. Local control of the tumor initially is obtained with neoadjuvant chemotherapy, followed by surgery with or without the addition of radiation therapy. If tumors affect expendable bones (e.g., fibula, rib, or clavicle), complete surgical excision may be warranted. If the initial combination treatment and the complete surgical excision are unsuccessful, radiation therapy to the involved bone and chemotherapy result in an 80–90% likelihood of local control. The presence or absence of demonstrable metastatic disease at diagnosis is the most important prognostic variable. Other, less favorable features include soft tissue extension, a low lymphocyte count, and elevated serum lactic dehydrogenase levels. Patients with primary tumors of the pelvis do less well than those with tumors at other sites. Without metastatic disease, 40–70% have long-term survival.

## LANGERHANS CELL HISTIOCYTOSIS

Langerhans cell histiocytosis (LCH) includes a group of diseases in which progression is due to proliferation and tissue infiltration of differentiated Langerhans cell histiocytes, which may mimic malignant neoplasms. The disorders probably are not malignancies and are of unknown *etiology.* Abnormalities of immune regulation, such as reduced suppressor and increased helper T lymphocyte counts, have been reported in association with LCH. The pathology reveals granuloma formation composed of histiocytes with characteristic large cell size, grooved nuclei, absence of an obvious malignant cytology, and the presence of characteristic multilaminar Birbeck granules in electron micrographs.

Three classic disease types occur:

1. *Letterer-Siwe disease* often is noted in young children who exhibit multisystemic involvement, including skin (seborrhea, rash), lung (interstitial pneumonia), hepatosplenomegaly, bone marrow infiltration (pancytopenia), and bone (osteolytic, punched-out lesions).
2. *Hand-Schüller-Christian disease* is less serious, noted in older children, and exhibited as granulomatous lesions in bone, tooth loss (mandible), exophthalmos (orbital), diabetes insipidus, and growth hormone deficiency (both factors, hypothalamus).
3. The solitary *eosinophilic granuloma* carries the most favorable prognosis. Patients have dull pain, a mass in the skull, or a localized lytic lesion of the mandible, mastoid, and proximal long bones. Vertebral involvement and collapse may cause spinal cord compression. Involvement of skin and multiple visceral organs with organ system dysfunction (e.g., jaundice, anemia, or hypoxia) has the poorest prognosis.

The *differential diagnosis* includes primary or metastatic bone tumors; leukemia; viral or familial hemophagocytic lymphohistiocytosis; storage diseases, such as Gaucher or Niemann-Pick disease; chronic or recurrent multifocal osteomyelitis; and granulomatous infections of mycobacterial or fungal origin.

*Treatment* of severe systemic disease with multiorgan involvement consists of chemotherapy. Localized granuloma; if of large size, may be treated with excision and bone grafting; rarely, low-dose radiotherapy also is used. Long-term survival is possible, but bone lesions may recur. Long-term sequelae of the disease or its treatment, such as diabetes insipidus, growth failure, pulmonary fibrosis, and cirrhosis, require ongoing management.

## References

Behrman RE, Kleigman RM, Arvin AM, (eds). Nelson Textbook of Pediatrics; 15th ed. Philadelphia, WB Saunders, 1996, Chapters 291, 291.1, 299, 445–461.

Burnett A, Eden O: The treatment of acute leukemia. Lancet 349:270, 1997.

Canellos GP, Anderson JR, Propert KJ, et al: Chemotherapy of advanced Hodgkin's disease with MOPP, ABVD, or MOPP alternating with ABVD. N Engl J Med 327:1478, 1992.

Gurney H: Dose calculation of anticancer drugs: A review of the current practice and introduction of an alternative. J Clin Oncol 14:259, 1996.

Gurney JG, Davis S, Severson RK, et al: Trends in cancer incidence among children in the U.S. Cancer 73:532, 1996.

Kilpatrick S, Wenger D, Gilchrist G, et al: Langerhans cell histiocytosis (histiocytosis X) of bone. Cancer 76:2471, 1995.

Kohn KW: Beyond DNA cross-linking: History and prospects of DNA-targeted cancer treatment. Fifteenth Bruce Cain Memorial Award Lecture. Cancer Res 56:5533, 1996.

Lashford L, Campbell R, Gattamaneni H, et al: An intensive multiagent chemotherapy regimen for brain tumors occurring in very young children. Arch Dis Child 74:219, 1996.

Levy M: Pharmacologic treatment of cancer pain. N Engl J Med 335:1124, 1996.

Link M, Goorin A, Miser A, et al: The effect of adjuvant chemotherapy on relapse-free survival in patients with osteosarcoma of the extremity. N Engl J Med 314:1600, 1986.

Paulino AC: Current issues in the diagnosis and management of Wilms' tumor. Oncology 10:1553, 1996.

Pizzo PA, Poplack DG (eds): Principles and Practice of Pediatric Oncology, 3rd ed. Philadelphia, Lippincott-Raven, 1997.

Pui C: Childhood leukemias. N Engl J Med 332:1618, 1995.

Roberts W, Estrov Z, Ouspenskaia M, et al: Measurement of residual leukemia during remission in childhood acute lymphoblastic leukemia. N Engl J Med 336:317, 1997.

Saha V, Love S, Eden T, et al: Determinants of symptom interval in childhood cancer. Arch Dis Child 68:771, 1993.

Sandlund JT, Downing JR, Crist WM: Non-Hodgkin's lymphoma in childhood. N Engl J Med 334:1238, 1996.

Tannock IF: Treatment of cancer with radiation and drugs. J Clin Oncol 14:3156, 1996.

# Chapter 16

# NEPHROLOGY: FLUIDS AND ELECTROLYTES

Aaron L. Friedman*

Renal dysfunction is common in children. *Primary* dysfunction may be due to diseases originating in the kidney (pyelonephritis, Wilms tumor, dysplasia, minimal change nephrotic syndrome); *secondary* dysfunction may be due to systemic illnesses that alter renal function, such as systemic lupus erythematosus (SLE), dehydration (acute tubular necrosis), heart failure (prerenal azotemia), hemolysis (hemoglobinuria), or nephrolithiasis (hyperparathyroidism). Renal involvement may be one manifestation of a systemic disorder (galactosemia, hemolytic-uremic syndrome), or the kidney may be the target organ for immune-mediated injury (poststreptococcal glomerulonephritis), but a limited number of manifestations of either primary or secondary renal disease exist (Table 16–1). Abnormalities of the many functions of the kidney appear predominantly as alterations in urine appearance or volume, and/or disturbances of fluid and electrolyte or acid-base balance. Renal malformations and tumors (see Chapter 15) may be noted as flank or abdominal masses.

Because fetal urine production contributes to amniotic fluid volume, renal anomalies often are associated with reduced amniotic fluid volume (oligohydramnios) and less often with increased amniotic fluid volume (polyhydramnios). Renal and ureter anomalies are present in 3–4% of infants.

## RENAL PHYSIOLOGY

The major functions of the kidney are to maintain body fluid and electrolyte homeostasis and to re-

---

*Adapted from the chapter of John E. Lewy in the second edition.

**TABLE 16–1.** Common Manifestations of Renal Disease

| Neonate | |
|---|---|
| Flank mass | Dysplasia, polycystic disease, hydronephrosis, tumor |
| Hematuria | Asphyxia, malformation, trauma, renal vein thrombosis |
| Anuria/oliguria | Agenesis, obstruction, asphyxia, vascular thrombosis |

| Child and Adolescent | |
|---|---|
| Cola-red colored urine | Hemoglobinuria (hemolysis); myoglobinuria (rhabdomyolysis); pigmenturia (porphyria, urate, beets, drugs); hematuria (glomerulonephritis, Henoch-Schönlein purpura, hypercalciuria) |
| Gross hematuria | Glomerulonephritis, benign hematuria, trauma, cystitis, tumor, nephrolithiasis |
| Edema | Nephrotic syndrome, nephritis, acute/chronic renal failure, cardiac or liver disease |
| Hypertension | Acute glomerulonephritis, acute/chronic renal failure, dysplasia, coarctation of the aorta, renal artery stenosis |
| Polyuria | Diabetes mellitus, central and nephrogenic diabetes insipidus, hypokalemia, hypercalcemia, psychogenic polydipsia, sickle cell anemia, polyuric renal failure, diuretic abuse |
| Oliguria | Dehydration, acute tubular necrosis, interstitial nephritis, acute glomerulonephritis, hemolytic uremic syndrome |
| Urgency | Urinary tract infection, vaginitis, foreign body, hypercalciuria |

609

move waste products of metabolism. This organ system has metabolic (gluconeogenesis) and endocrine functions (vitamin D activation, erythropoietin production) that also are important.

The major homeostatic functions of the kidney are carried out by the processes of glomerular ultrafiltration, tubular reabsorption, and secretion. *Glomerular ultrafiltration* is the net result of opposing pressures acting within the glomeruli, those pressures moving fluid across the glomerular capillary wall from blood to urinary space and those opposing this filtration.

Glomerular capillary hydrostatic pressure results from the systemic arterial pressure, which is modified by the afferent and efferent arteriolar tone. Because only minimal amounts of protein are filtered by the glomerulus, the oncotic pressure of the urinary space at the beginning of the proximal tubule generally is zero, and thus the pressure favoring filtration is essentially that of the capillary hydrostatic pressure. The hydrostatic pressure within the lumen of the urinary space of the early proximal tubule, plus the mean glomerular capillary oncotic pressure, opposes filtration. The hydrostatic pressure remains constant, but the oncotic pressure of the glomerular capillary progressively rises from the afferent to the efferent end as a result of the removal of fluid during filtration. Thus, the pressures favoring filtration are maximal at the afferent end of the glomerulus and minimal at the efferent end. Alterations in systemic blood flow or in the internal regulation of glomerular pressures also alter the *glomerular filtration rate* (GFR). Obstruction of the renal tubules, ureter, or bladder may raise intratubular pressure and retard filtration. Changes in glomerular capillary protein concentration or in the permeability of the capillary wall also affect the glomerular filtration rate.

Glomerular filtration begins during the 3rd mo of gestation. Glomerulogenesis is completed at about 34 wk of gestation, and subsequently the glomerular filtration rate increases more rapidly than body size.

The GFR is measured most accurately by the infusion of a substance that is freely filtered by the glomerulus but is not metabolized, reabsorbed or secreted, as is inulin. Clinically, creatinine is used to approximate GFR because it is excreted primarily through glomerular filtration and has little tubular reabsorption or secretion except in renal insufficiency. The GFR is calculated as

$$GFR = \frac{UV}{P} \times \frac{1.73}{SA}$$

where U = urine creatinine (mg/dL), V = volume collected over time (mL/min), P = serum creatinine (mg/dL), and SA = body surface area.

This equation must be corrected for body surface area to achieve the standard nomenclature of mL/min/1.73 m². Creatinine clearance is therefore approximately 40 mL/min/1.73 m² in the full-term newborn. GFR increases during the first 2 yr of life more rapidly than body size and achieves adult values/1.73 m² at this time (110–125 mL/min/1.73 m²). Subsequently, GFR and body size increase proportionately, and thus GFR/1.73 m² remains stable throughout the remainder of childhood to adulthood (95–105 mL/min/1.73 m²).

Plasma creatinine concentration alone is not an adequate measure of renal function. The "normal" levels of creatinine in most laboratories vary from 0.3 to 1.5 mg/dL, a range that encompasses individuals of all ages and sizes. The plasma creatinine concentration in a newborn equals the maternal value at delivery because of equilibration across the placenta. The neonate's own plasma creatinine is achieved by 2 wk of age in full-term infants.

Plasma creatinine depends on body mass as well as on renal function; hence, normal creatinine concentration is a gradually increasing absolute value throughout childhood. To determine the relationship between plasma creatinine and GFR in any given child, one classically must measure creatinine clearance or another indicator of GFR. Because urine collections are somewhat difficult to obtain in the young child, another method is used to estimate the GFR; it has been demonstrated that plasma creatinine ($P_{CR}$), length in centimeters (L), and a constant of proportionality (k) reflect the relationship between urinary creatinine excretion and units of body size. The formula is

$$GFR\ (mL/min/1.73\ m^2) = k \times L\ (cm)\ /\ P_{CR}\ (mg/dL)$$

The value for k is 0.33 in preterm infants, 0.45 in full-term infants, 0.55 in children and adolescent girls, and 0.7 in adolescent boys. This formula is useful only in infants and children whose body habitus is reasonably normal and whose renal function is stable.

## FUNCTIONAL MORPHOLOGY

The *proximal tubule* is characterized by iso-osmotic reabsorption of the glomerular ultrafiltrate (Fig. 16–1). Normally, approximately two thirds of the glomerular ultrafiltrate is reabsorbed from the proximal tubule; a number of solutes, such as glucose and amino acids, are reabsorbed completely, and potassium is reabsorbed nearly completely. Most phosphate is reabsorbed from the proximal tubule, and calcium is absorbed in parallel with sodium reabsorption. The straight portion of the proximal tubule is responsible for secreting organic acids, including drugs such as penicillin.

The *loop of Henle* serves a major role, in that 25% of filtered sodium chloride is absorbed in this segment (Fig. 16–1). Differential permeabilities convert the isotonic fluid entering the loop of Henle from the proximal tubule into a hypotonic fluid delivered to the distal tubule. Preferential sodium chloride absorption (associated with active chloride transport) is the principal mechanism by which the countercurrent multiplier is activated and by which the medullary interstitial hypertonicity, required for urinary concentration, is accomplished. This principally occurs in the thick ascending limb. Salt and water movement across the thin limbs is driven primarily by osmotic gradients.

The *distal tubule* is made up of the *distal convoluted tubule*, which is water impermeable and continues to carry out the dilution of luminal fluid by way of active sodium chloride absorption, and the *collecting ducts*, which are the primary sites of *antidiuretic hormone* (ADH) activity. These distal segments are the site of potassium and hydrogen ion secretion, which is responsible for the final acidification of the urine. The processes of sodium reabsorption and potassium and hydrogen ion secretion are all stimulated by aldosterone.

The maximum *urinary concentrating capacity* is less in the newborn (600–800 mOsm/L in the full-term newborn and approximately 400 mOsm/L in the preterm infant) than in children older than 1 yr of age (>1200 mOsm/L). The neonate's ability to dilute the urine is fully developed, but the capacity to excrete a water load is quantitatively less. The newborn exhibits numerous other quantitative limitations, which include the rate of excretion of sodium, potassium, hydrogen ion, and phosphate, but renal functions are qualitatively operative.

### References

Behrman RE, Kliegman RM, Arvin AM (eds): Nelson's Textbook of Pediatrics, 15 ed. Philadelphia, WB Saunders, 1996, Chapter 462.

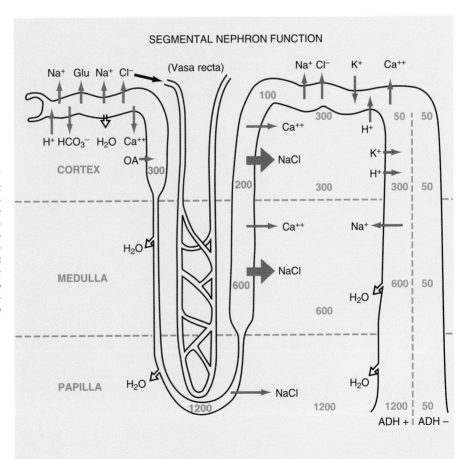

FIGURE 16–1. Major transport functions of each nephron segment, including representative osmolalities in vasa recta, interstitium, and tubule at different levels within the kidney. ADH = antidiuretic hormone. Glu-glucose; OA = organic acid. (From Andreoli TE, Carpenter CCJ, Plum F, et al: Cecil Essentials of Medicine. Philadelphia, WB Saunders, 1986, p 185.)

Jones DP, Chesney RW: Development of tubular function. Clin Perinatol 19:33, 1992.

Robillard JE, Segar JL, Smith FG, et al: Regulation of sodium metabolism and extracellular fluid volume during development. Clin Perinatol 19:15, 1992.

# CONGENITAL AND DEVELOPMENTAL ABNORMALITIES OF THE URINARY TRACT

*Bilateral renal agenesis,* which occurs in 1:4000 births, is due to failure of development of or degeneration of the ureteric bud. Features associated with this condition are **Potter syndrome** (flat facies, clubfoot, pulmonary hypoplasia) resulting from oligohydramnios and fetal compression by the uterus (see Chapter 19). Infants with bilateral renal agenesis usually die of respiratory insufficiency in the 1st wk of life as a result of pulmonary hypoplasia, pneumothoraces, and pulmonary hypertension. *Unilateral renal agenesis* (1:1000 births) is associated with compensatory hypertrophy in the contralateral kidney and normal or minimally reduced renal function. Although this condition is compatible with normal renal function and normal life expectancy, an associated incidence of other abnormalities exists with unilateral renal agenesis, including abnormalities of the genital tract, skeletal system, and cardiovascular system. Unilateral renal agenesis also has been described as a component of the VATER* association, Turner syndrome, and Poland syndrome.

*Renal hypoplasia* refers to kidneys that are present but small in size and that, because of their reduced nephron number, over time predispose a child to progressive renal insufficiency. Hypoplastic kidneys frequently are scarred and difficult to distinguish from those that are chronically infected. Renal hypoplasia also may be associated with poor growth, which is most common in the second decade of life.

*Renal dysplasia* usually is unilateral and may be associated with hypoplasia. It is a developmental abnormality with abnormal organization and ductal differentiation. Most children with this disorder have obstructive anomalies of the urinary tract. It has been suggested that ureteric or urethral obstruction early in gestation is the primary factor that leads to the dysplastic changes. Dysplastic (cystic) kidneys may, with time, resemble renal aplasia and lead to urinary tract infections, hypertension, or, less often, malignancy.

---

*VATER = *Vertebral defects, imperforate *a*nus, *t*racheo-*e*sophageal fistula, *r*adial and *r*enal dysplasia.

## CYSTIC DYSPLASIAS OF THE KIDNEY

*Polycystic kidney disease* is an inherited disease affecting both kidneys. The two major forms include an autosomal recessive type ("infantile" polycystic kidney disease) and an autosomal dominant type ("adult" polycystic disease [ADPKD]). The two conditions differ morphologically and clinically, although both may occur in infancy or in older children.

### Autosomal Recessive Disease

The infantile type is characterized by marked enlargement of both kidneys with innumerable cysts throughout the cortex and medulla, which are dilated collecting ducts. Interstitial fibrosis and tubular atrophy may not be present at birth but progress with time, frequently to renal failure. Hepatic fibrosis is present and may lead to portal hypertension. Bile duct ectasia and biliary dysgenesis also occur. The kidneys of the newborn with the autosomal recessive form are spongy and markedly enlarged and maintain the usual renal configuration; older children demonstrate less severe cyst formation but still show progressive renal fibrosis and tubular atrophy.

Although the *diagnosis* can be made in utero by ultrasonography, many of the live-born infants die in the neonatal period, often from respiratory distress resulting from pulmonary hypoplasia. Eighty percent of infants have clinical manifestations, such as flank mass, hepatomegaly, pneumothorax, proteinuria, or hematuria. Intravenous pyelography (IVP) reveals opacification of dilated collecting ducts, which appear as radial streaks.

*Treatment* is supportive, including the management of hypertension and renal failure. The *prognosis* is poor, in terms of both renal insufficiency and hepatic fibrosis. Renal transplantation and portosystemic shunts (for hepatic fibrosis) may be beneficial.

### Autosomal Dominant

The adult type of polycystic kidney (ADPKD) disease characteristically appears in the fourth or fifth decade of life, but also occurs in infancy or childhood. Infants have a clinical picture similar to that of autosomal recessive polycystic kidney disease, but older children may show a pattern similar to that of adults. Renal pathology shows glomerular and tubular cysts. Family history is positive. Hepatic cysts are present in this disease, but they usually are not of clinical significance, whereas cerebral aneurysms are present; splenic and pancreatic cysts also occur. The gene for ADPKD is on chromosome 6p21-cen. The location or function of the ion pump may contribute to cyst formation.

Renal cysts are also observed in von Hipple-Lindau syndrome and tuberous sclerosis.

## References

Behrman RE, Kliegman RM, Arvin AM (eds): Nelson's Textbook of Pediatrics, 15th ed. Philadelphia, WB Saunders, 1996, Chapters 475.1, 475.2.
Kissane JM: Renal cysts in pediatric patients; A classification and overview. Pediatr Nephrol 4:69, 1990.
Woolf A, Winyard P: Unravelling the pathogenesis of cystic kidney disease. Arch Dis Child 72:103, 1995.

## VESICOURETERAL REFLUX

Vesicoureteral reflux, the abnormal backflow of urine from the bladder to the ureter or kidney, usually results from a congenital incompetence of the vesicoureteral junction or, less often, from incompetence of the junction secondary to obstruction or infection. Reflux may be familial.

*Pathophysiology.* Reflux is potentially harmful because of the exposure of the kidney to *increased hydrodynamic pressure* during voiding. In addition, the incomplete emptying of the ureter and bladder on voiding predisposes the patient to **urinary tract infection** because, in the presence of lower urinary tract infection, reflux allows bacteria to gain access easily to the pelvocalyceal system. **Reflux nephropathy** refers to the development and/or progression of *renal scarring*, often secondary to prolonged reflux, particularly if associated with infection or obstruction (bladder neck obstruction or posterior urethral valves). A significant number of children have end-stage renal disease as a result of reflux nephropathy, which also may be an important precursor to hypertension.

The normal vesicoureteral junction prevents reflux because of the oblique entry of the ureter into the bladder, the length of the ureteral tunnel traversing the bladder wall, and the 4–5:1 ratio of the length of this tunnel to the ureteral diameter. Primary reflux results from a short intramural tunnel ratio, as low as 1.5:1, and is characteristically associated with a lateral position of the ureteral orifice and an underdeveloped trigone. The shortened intramural tunnel decreases the efficiency of the valvular mechanism, allowing reflux to occur. Less often, duplications of the ureters that also exhibit ureteroceles may obstruct the upper collecting system. Reflux may be associated with ureteral diverticulum. Abnormalities of the neurogenic bladder associated with myelomeningocele are complicated by reflux in approximately one third

to one half of affected children. Reflux also may be secondary to increased intravascular pressure when the bladder outlet is obstructed, to inflammation of the bladder (cystitis), or to surgical procedures performed on the bladder.

*Clinical Manifestations.* Reflux is characteristically discovered during radiologic evaluation following a urinary tract infection. Severe reflux may begin in utero and may be associated with neonatal renal insufficiency resulting from renal parenchymal loss. In neonates with urinary tract infection, the incidence of reflux is high. Reflux may resolve with time.

Reflux and infection lead to the serious complication of renal scarring and may eventually result in renal insufficiency or failure. The younger the patient, the more likely reflux will be present and, therefore, a *voiding cystourethrogram* (VCUG) should be performed in all infants and children with a urinary tract infection. The *diagnosis* of previous renal scars can be made by nuclear medicine renal scan with Tc-dimercaptosuccinic acid (DMSA). This scan defines the renal parenchyma and can diagnose acute pyelonephritis, chronic pyelonephritis, and scarring. The VCUG should be performed after the infection has been treated, although the necessity of waiting 4–6 wk before performing a VCUG has been challenged. An international grading system has been used to describe reflux (Fig. 16–2). The incidence of scarring associated with the lowest grades of reflux is quite low (15%) but is very high with the higher grades of reflux (grade 4 or 5), where scarring may occur in two thirds of the patients. Long-term follow-up suggests that reflux is likely to stop without surgical intervention in the low grades, specifically grades 1 and 2, but is far less likely to stop (in fewer than half the patients) in grade 4 or 5.

*Treatment.* The finding of reflux indicates the need for long-term prophylactic antibiotic therapy that includes trimethoprim/sufamethoxazole, sulfisoxazole, or nitrofurantoin. A urine specimen should be obtained for culture at regular (1–3 mo) intervals until three consecutive cultures are negative; after that, the frequency can be further reduced. As noted above in grade 1 to grade 3 reflux, reflux generally disappears with time. More severe reflux, which is associated with significant ureteral dilation or upper tract changes on IVP, *renal ultrasound*, or radioisotope scan, often requires surgical intervention. In general, reflux of any grade found on *voiding cystourethrography* associated with a normal nephrosonogram or scan can be treated medically with long-term prophylactic antibiotics and serial urine cultures. However, if the IVP or renal scan reveals renal scarring and dilation or clubbing

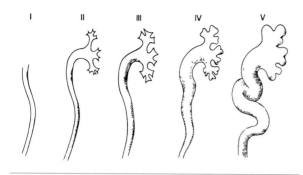

FIGURE 16–2. International Classification of Vesicoureteral Reflux: Grade I, ureter only. Grade II, ureter, pelvis, and calyces. No dilation, normal calyceal fornices. Grade III, mild to moderate dilation and/or tortuosity of the ureter, and mild to moderate dilation of the renal pelvis; slight or no blunting of the fornices. Grade IV, moderate dilation or tortuosity of the ureter and moderate dilation of the renal pelvis and calyces. Complete obliteration of sharp angle of fornices but maintenance of the papillary impressions in the majority of calyces. Grade V, gross dilation and tortuosity of the ureter. Gross dilation of the renal pelvis and calyces. The papillary impressions are no longer visible in most of the calyces. Some authors consider grade IV or V with intrarenal reflux into the collecting ducts a high risk for scarring. (From Duckett JW, Bellinger MF: Cystographic grading of primary reflux as an indicator of treatment. *In* Johnston JH [ed]: Management of Vesicoureteral Reflux. International Perspectives in Urology. Vol 10. Baltimore, Williams & Wilkins, 1984.)

of the pelvocalyceal system, surgical intervention most likely is indicated at the outset. Surgical intervention is employed commonly if reinfection occurs while the patient is receiving antibiotics. Surgical intervention clearly is needed if the reflux is associated with a ureterocele or other urinary tract obstruction. The presence of grade 4 to grade 5 reflux and the failure of time to resolve reflux over several years remain controversial indications for medical or surgical treatment.

*Complications* of reflux nephropathy include hypertension and end-stage renal disease. The latter is predicted by proteinuria (>1 g/day) and is due to the development of focal and segmental *glomerulosclerosis* and interstitial scarring.

## URINARY TRACT OBSTRUCTION

Obstruction of the urinary tract may occur at any anatomic level of the genitourinary system (Table 16–2). Severe obstruction early in gestation is thought to result in **renal dysplasia.** Ureteral obstruction later in fetal life or after birth results in dilation of the ureter and collecting system, often with alterations in renal parenchyma that may range from dilation to scarring and glomerular at-

rophy. The obstructed urinary tract is susceptible to infections, which may further worsen renal injury.

***Clinical Manifestations.*** Obstructions may be silent but usually are discovered as a urinary tract infection or flank masses. In a newborn, bilateral abdominal masses frequently are hydronephrotic obstructed kidneys.

***Diagnosis.*** *Intravenous urography* and *voiding cystourethrography* have been the standard tests for diagnosis of urinary tract obstruction, but a marked reduction in renal function often is associated with poor or nonvisualization of the kidney on the IVP. *Renal ultrasound* studies facilitate the identification of renal agenesis, renal hypoplasia, or cystic changes in the presence of obstruction, scarring, and dilation. The dilated upper urinary

TABLE 16–2.    Site and Etiology of Urinary Tract Obstruction

| Site | Etiology |
|---|---|
| Infundibula | Congenital<br>Calculi<br>Infection<br>Trauma<br>Tumor |
| Pelvis | Congenital stenosis<br>Infection<br>Calculi<br>Tumor |
| Ureteropelvic junction | Congenital stenosis*<br>Calculi<br>Tumor<br>Trauma |
| Ureter | Obstructive megaureter*<br>Ectopic ureter<br>Ureterocele<br>Valves<br>Calculi*<br>Primary renal tumor (Wilms tumor)<br>Retroperitoneal tumor (lymphoma)<br>Inflammatory bowel disease<br>Retroperitoneal fibrosis<br>Chronic granulomatous disease |
| Bladder | Neurogenic dysfunction*<br>Tumor (rhabdomyosarcoma)<br>Diverticula<br>Ectopic ureter |
| Urethra | Posterior valves*<br>Diverticula<br>Strictures<br>Atresia<br>Ectopic ureter<br>Foreign body<br>Phimosis*<br>Priapism |

*Relatively common.

tract may or may not be obstructed. The radioisotope renogram, particularly used in conjunction with a diuretic agent frequently can allow differentiation of patients with a dilated urinary tract, which empties normally, from those with obstruction. Tc-DMSA scans are the most useful test for evaluation of the presence of renal scars.

Obstruction of the urinary tract may be at multiple anatomic levels (see Table 16–2). An obstruction of the ureteropelvic junction is the most common lesion in childhood. Such an obstruction may present as a palpable renal mass, urinary tract infection, hematuria (with or without trauma), or flank pain or may be discovered on routine fetal ultrasonography. Twenty percent of ureteropelvic junction obstructions are bilateral.

*Treatment.* An obstructed ureteropelvic junction requires surgery. The success rate of pyeloplastics in relieving obstruction is high, although dilation may persist.

*Obstructions of the ureter* also may occur at the mid-ureter or at the lower ureter in association with a ureterocele or with an ectopic ureteral orifice, which, in turn, frequently is associated with reflux. Ectopic ureters may drain a single collecting system or may drain the upper portion of a duplicated collecting system. Ectopic ureters frequently are obstructed, and prompt surgical intervention is required.

## PRUNE-BELLY SYNDROME
### (Eagle-Barrett Syndrome)

The absence or severe reduction in abdominal musculature associated with undescended testes and urinary tract abnormalities occurs in approximately 1:40,000 births. The characteristic dilation of the prostatic urethra without posterior urethral valves suggests severe, but possibly transient, urethral obstruction in fetal life. The reduced abdominal musculature may be due to transient tense fetal ascites. Oligohydramnios and pulmonary hypoplasia may be present.

Urinary abnormalities include marked dilation of the ureters and calyceal system, a large bladder, and often a patent urachus. The kidneys may be dysplastic, and the testes usually are undescended in the abdomen. Anomalies of the bowel, heart, and musculoskeletal system may occur. The condition is rare in females. There usually is no demonstrable obstruction of the urinary tract at birth.

Initial *treatment* consists of stabilization of the cardiopulmonary status and prevention of urinary tract infection. Renal ultrasound, measurement of renal function, radioisotope scan, and voiding cystourethrogram facilitate full assessment of the abnormalities. Therapy then is individualized in order to maintain renal function and prevent infection.

## POSTERIOR URETHRAL VALVES

The posterior urethral valve is the most common cause of **bladder outlet obstruction** in males, present in 1:50,000 boys. The valves are sail-shaped membranes that arise from the verumontanum and attach to the contralateral wall of the urethra. In the presence of persistent valves, the prostatic urethra becomes dilated, vesicoureteral reflux may be present, and a small bladder with hypertrophied walls develops. Renal dilation varies in degree from mild hydronephrosis to severe hydronephrosis with dysplasia. Severe obstruction may be associated with oligohydramnios and subsequent lethal pulmonary hypoplasia. The male infant may present in the newborn period with a urinary tract infection, bilateral flank masses (hydronephrosis and hydroureter), a poor voiding stream, or little urinary output. Rupture of the renal pelvis produces **urinary ascites,** the most common cause of ascites in the newborn period. A child may come to medical attention later in infancy with a poor urinary stream, failure to thrive secondary to renal failure, urinary tract infection, or renal tubular acidosis. Infants with pulmonary hypoplasia often die early in infancy.

The *diagnosis* and extent of renal damage are established by ultrasonography and by voiding cystourethrography. In many cases, the diagnosis is made before birth by fetal ultrasonography. Once the infant is stabilized, *treatment* consists of either preliminary decompression and/or valve ablation, depending on the individual circumstances. Valve ablation is successful in most infants, and the serum creatinine level may return to normal by 1 yr of age. Children having persistent elevated creatinine levels also may have associated renal dysplasia. Immediately after relief of the obstruction, a marked diuresis resulting from a defect in urine concentrating ability may be present. Careful follow-up to prevent urinary tract infection is essential.

## References

Behrman RE, Kliegman RM, Arvin AM (eds): Nelson Textbook of Pediatrics, 15th ed. Philadelphia, WB Saunders, 1996, Chapters 492–498.
Jakobsson B, Söderlundhs S, Bert U: Diagnostic significance of $^{99m}$Tc-dimercaptosuccinic acid (DMSA) scintigraphy in urinary tract infections. Arch Dis Child 67:1138, 1992.
Schwartz GW, Brion LT, Spitzer A: The use of plasma creatinine

concentration for estimating glomerular filtration rate in infants, children and adolescents. Pediatr Clin North Am 34:571, 1987.

## DISTURBANCES OF ELECTROLYTES, ACID-BASE BALANCE, AND FLUIDS

Because sodium is the principal extracellular cation, regulation of extracellular fluid parallels regulation of sodium balance. Intrarenal sodium conservation is regulated by the juxtaglomerular apparatus and the macula densa, which sense decreased effective renal blood flow and respond by releasing renin. Renin acts on angiotensinogen to produce angiotensin I. Angiotensin-converting enzyme then converts angiotensin I to angiotensin II, which stimulates the release of aldosterone. Aldosterone increases distal tubule sodium reabsorption. In conditions of severe sodium restriction, decreased intravascular volume (hemorrhage, sepsis), or decreased effective renal blood flow (heart failure), the urinary excretion of sodium approaches zero. In addition, baroreceptors in the atria, aortic arch, carotid bifurcations, and pulmonary vessels also sense volume depletion and signal the brain via cranial nerves IX and X. This signaling results in increased central nervous system (CNS) efferent sympathetic discharge, which regulates renal blood flow, vascular resistance, angiotensin II, and, thus, aldosterone release; the net result is sodium conservation.

The ADH system also senses volume changes. In conditions of hypovolemia, ADH, which increases renal reabsorption of water, is released. In normal day-to-day life this system functions to maintain osmolality within a narrow range because ADH secretion is stimulated during normovolemic states by high serum osmolality.

Atrial natriuretic peptide is synthesized in the cardiac atria and regulates sodium (and intravascular volume) by increasing the glomerular filtration rate and hydrostatic pressure, dilating afferent and constricting efferent arterioles. The hormone also blocks the tubular reabsorption of sodium and chloride.

### PARENTERAL FLUID THERAPY

Illnesses that result in imbalances in fluids and electrolytes pose a greater risk to children than adults. The younger the child, the greater the vulnerability to such disturbances because of the larger daily turnover of water relative to the total body water, the large extracellular fluid space, and in the neonate, the developmental limitations of renal function. The untoward effects of vomiting (reduced intake) and diarrhea (increased losses) appear much more rapidly in the infant than in the adult.

Fluid and electrolyte requirements and their provision are conveniently considered in terms of *maintenance, deficit,* and *supplemental therapy.* Therapeutic plans based on calculations of these needs must be modified constantly based on a continuing clinical reassessment of the child's physical and mental status and the serial monitoring of serum electrolytes, acid-base balance, blood urea nitrogen, and serum creatinine.

### Maintenance Therapy

Ongoing obligatory normal and abnormal losses of fluids and electrolytes from urine, sweat, feces, and lung must be replaced so that deficits do not occur. Disease states may modify the amount and type of such losses. Protein and calories also must be replaced when oral intake is restricted for a protracted time (see Chapter 2). Losses should be replaced orally, when possible, or intravenously.

Maintenance requirements of fluid and electrolytes are directly related to metabolic rate. An increased metabolic rate increases catabolism of metabolic fuels. This leads to increases in the rate of production of water of oxidation from carbohydrate, fat, and protein; in urinary excretion of solute and water; and in heat production, which increases water loss in insensible water loss, sweat, and respiratory gases. The turnover rates of electrolytes also are related closely to water loss and metabolic rate. Thus, maintenance requirements for fluid and electrolytes can be calculated from a child's caloric expenditures.

**Calculation of Normal Maintenance Requirements.** A child's metabolic rate or caloric expenditure depends on age, body weight, degree of activity, temperature, and any pathologic state. Adjustments above basal caloric expenditures for activity are made by observing the patient. The usual hospitalized patient burns calories at a rate 20–30% above basal caloric expenditures. Fever increases caloric expenditures by about 12%/1°C rise in temperature, and salicylism and hyperthyroidism increase caloric expenditures by 25–75%. Conversely, hypothermia results in similar decreases in caloric expenditure per incremental fall in temperature, and hypothyroidism results in a 10–25% decrease in basal metabolism.

Table 16–3 provides a simplified means of calculating expenditure for the average hospitalized child (non-neonate) engaged in the usual bed activity. Additional adjustments should be made for

**TABLE 16–3.** Calculation of Caloric Expenditure from Body Weight

| Body Weight (kg) | Caloric Expenditure* |
|---|---|
| Up to 10 | 100 kcal/kg |
| 11–20 | 1000 kcal + 50 kcal/kg for each kg above 10 kg |
| Above 20 | 1500 kcal + 20 kcal/kg for each kg above 30 kg |

Modified from Behrman RE (ed): Nelson Textbook of Pediatrics, 14th ed. Philadelphia, WB Saunders, 1992, p 196.
*1 kcal (kilocalorie) = 1000 calories.

further activity, temperature, and disease states. The usual fluid and electrolyte losses that occur for each 100 kcal metabolized then also can be estimated. With this approach for replacing losses resulting from ongoing metabolism, 100 mL of fluid should be provided for every 100 kcal expended, and the solution should contain 35 mEq/L of sodium, 20 mEq/L of potassium, and 5% dextrose. This approach to providing maintenance requirements assumes that there is no kidney damage or disease state that would limit renal capacity to adjust urine flow rates and electrolyte excretion over wide ranges.

**Modification of Maintenance Therapy as a Result of Disease.** Maintenance requirements are decreased (30–45 mL/100 kcal of exogenous water to replace insensible water losses, such as sweat and water expired with breathing, is required) in conditions of anuria or extreme oliguria or when excessive or inappropriate release of ADH occurs, such as during meningitis; and for children who are in congestive heart failure. Requirements for fluid and electrolytes are increased as a result of abnormal losses from gastrointestinal drainage, heat stress, adrenal insufficiency, diabetes mellitus, hyperventilation, loss of renal concentrating and diluting ability, diabetes insipidus, and burns. The amount and nature of the losses depend on the underlying disorder and the site of the loss.

## Deficit Therapy

Deficits in body water and electrolytes occur from decreased intake and continuing normal losses, from increased losses with or without the usual intake, or from a combination of these events. Because deficits reflect ongoing physiologic readjustments as well as direct losses, the amount of the deficits often is similar for a variety of precipitating conditions; therefore, they usually can be treated in a similar manner. Fluid and electrolyte

treatment is related to a greater extent to the severity and type of deficit than to the underlying cause. The etiology also must be addressed specifically.

**Severity.** An acute loss of body weight greater than 1%/day reflects a loss of body water. The more rapidly a deficit develops, the less well it will be tolerated. Severe dehydration is frequently associated with shock, but even moderate deficits may cause circulatory instability if they develop over the course of a day (Table 16–4).

**Pathophysiologic Types of Dehydration.** Deficits from dehydration are classified as *isonatremic* (130–150 mEq serum $Na^+/L$), *hyponatremic* (<130 mEq $Na^+/L$), or *hypernatremic* (>150 mEq $Na^+/L$). Because plasma osmolality is reflected in sodium concentration, these forms usually are isotonic, hypotonic, and hypertonic, respectively. This may not be the case when another serum solute (such as glucose) is elevated, as occurs in diabetic ketoacidosis, which may result in hyponatremia and hypertonicity.

*Isonatremic Dehydration.* Approximately proportional fluid and electrolyte losses occur from the extracellular compartment, and because no resulting osmotic gradient across the cell walls takes place, intracellular fluid volume is not significantly changed.

*Hypernatremic Dehydration.* More water than sodium is lost from the extracellular space, or excess sodium is provided, increasing the osmolality of the extracellular fluid and causing water to move out of cells, a movement that adds to the extracellular volume so that extracellular volume depletion is not as clinically severe as expected.

*Hypotonic Dehydration.* Relatively more sodium than water is lost from the extracellular space, or excess water is provided. This leads to movement of water into cells, which further depletes the extracellular fluid, aggravating circulatory insufficiency.

Salt (sodium) poisoning or water intoxication may occur in the absence of dehydration and may produce hypernatremia and hyponatremia, respectively.

**Clinical Assessment of Deficit.** The patient history is the first critical step in this evaluation. Table 16–5 indicates some of the important information that should be sought. For example, a history of fever and high-solute feedings in the presence of watery diarrhea favors hypernatremic dehydration. Physical examination may be complementary to the history and may be particularly helpful in characterizing the severity of dehydration (Table 16–6). Laboratory data may reflect hemoconcentration, although this may be masked by pre-existing anemia or malnutrition. Blood urea nitrogen may

TABLE 16–4.  Assessment of Degree of Dehydration

| | Mild | Moderate | Severe |
|---|---|---|---|
| Infant | 5% | 10% | 15% |
| Adolescent | 3% | 6% | 9% |
| Infants/young children | Thirsty; alert; restless | Thirsty; restless or lethargic but irritable or drowsy | Drowsy; limp, cold, sweaty, cyanotic extremities; may be comatose |
| Older children | Thirsty; alert; restless | Thirsty; alert (usually) | Usually conscious (but at reduced level), apprehensive; cold, sweaty, cyanotic extremities; wrinkled skin on fingers/toes; muscle cramps |

*Signs and Symptoms*
*General Appearance and Condition*

| | | | |
|---|---|---|---|
| Tachycardia | Absent | Present | Present |
| Palpable pulses | Present | Present (weak) | Decreased |
| Blood pressure | Normal | Orthostatic hypotension | Hypotension |
| Cutaneous perfusion | Normal | Normal | Reduced/mottled |
| Skin turgor | Normal | Slight reduction | Reduced |
| Fontanel | Normal | Slightly depressed | Sunken |
| Mucous membrane | Moist | Dry | Very dry |
| Tears | Present | Present/absent | Absent |
| Respirations | Normal | Deep, may be rapid | Deep and rapid |
| Urine output | Normal | Oliguria | Anuria/severe oliguria |

Modified from World Health Organization Guide.

be increased as a result of decreased blood flow and enhanced recycling of urea if the circulation is compromised, and creatinine levels usually are increased as a result of a decrease in glomerular filtration. Urine usually is concentrated and may transiently contain abnormal amounts of protein, casts, and cells. Serum electrolytes and acid-base data reflect specific deficits and their causes.

## Supplemental Therapy

In certain disorders, specific fluids and electrolytes may be needed in addition to those required to replace deficits and maintain homeostasis. For example, in pyloric stenosis, sodium and potassium should be replaced as chloride salts because of gastric losses of hydrochloric acid, and burns may require special replacement of the plasma lost by surface oozing, ultrafiltrate sequestrations around the burn site, and renal nitrogen losses.

TABLE 16–5.  Historic Data for Evaluating Deficits

Weight change (pre-illness versus dehydrated weight)

Intake: quantity and composition of fluids and solids (including drugs) taken during illness

Output: quantity and pattern of output of urine, emesis, diarrhea, sweating, and drainage during illness

General medical status: respiratory function, cardiovascular status, renal function, central nervous system disease, and metabolic state (temperature) are especially relevant

Modified from Behrman RE (ed): Nelson Textbook of Pediatrics, 14th ed. Philadelphia, WB Saunders, 1992, p 199.

## Principles of Therapy

Shock always must be treated as a medical emergency, with intravenous or, rarely, with intraosseous infusions (see Chapter 3). *Oral rehydration* may be appropriate in patients with mild to moderate dehydration (Table 16–7); this decision re-

TABLE 16–6.  Typical Patterns of Physical Signs in Moderate–Severe Dehydration

| Sign | Isonatremic | Hyponatremic | Hypernatremic |
|---|---|---|---|
| Skin | | | |
| Color | Gray | Gray | Gray |
| Temperature | Cold | Cold | Cold |
| Turgor | Poor | Very poor | Fair |
| Feel | Dry | Clammy | Thick, doughy |
| Mucous membrane | Dry | Dry | Parched |
| Eyeball | Sunken and soft | Sunken and soft | Sunken |
| Fontanel | Sunken | Sunken | Sunken |
| State of consciousness | Lethargic | Very lethargic | Hyperirritable |
| Pulse | Rapid | Rapid | Moderately rapid |
| Blood pressure | Low | Very low | Moderately low |

Modified from Behrman RE (ed): Nelson Textbook of Pediatrics, 14th ed. Philadelphia, WB Saunders, 1992, p 200.

quires judgment about the etiology of the illness, the child's condition, and the capacity of the care givers to provide adequate supervision of care.

Intravenous therapy should be provided for children when there is shock, severe dehydration, uncontrollable vomiting, diarrhea exceeding 10 mL/kg/hr, extreme fatigue, stupor, coma, severe gastric distention, or other serious complications. The goal of *initial therapy* is to treat or prevent shock by rapidly expanding the vascular volume by administering 10–30 mL/kg of an electrolyte solution, such as isotonic saline (0.9%; $Na^+$ and $Cl^-$ both 155 mEq/L) or Ringer's lactate. This solution is given immediately, even before electrolyte values are known, because it is equally appropriate for isonatremic, hyponatremic, or hypernatremic dehydration and usually returns the serum sodium level toward normal. It is given as rapidly as possible for shock or over 1–3 hr for less severely ill patients. Ordinarily, 20 mL/kg restores circulatory stability; if signs of shock persist, a second or third infusion of fluid (10–30 mL/kg) may be needed.

When the circulation is stabilized, *subsequent treatment* is directed at correcting the remaining water and sodium deficits and replacing ongoing abnormal and obligatory losses. Treatment usually is based on knowing the serum electrolytes concentrations. Unless hypokalemia is demonstrated or a condition known to be associated with severe potassium losses is present (pyloric stenosis, prolonged diarrhea, diabetic acidosis), potassium losses are not replaced until urinary output is established.

TABLE 16–7.  Oral Rehydration*

| Status† | Mild Dehydration | Moderate Dehydration |
|---|---|---|
| Initial | 50 mL/kg (over 4 hr) | 100 mL/kg (over 6 hr) |
| Subsequent‡ | 100 mL/kg/24 hr | 100 mL/kg/24 hr |

*Amounts and rates should be increased or decreased based on evaluation of patient. Breast-feeding or plain water should be offered as needed.

†World Health Organization oral rehydration solution (ORS) is composed of 2 g glucose (CHO)/100 mL, 90 mEq $Na^+$/100 mL, 20 mEq $K^+$/100 mL, and 30 mEq $HCO_3^-$/100 mL. In the United States, commercially available oral rehydration solutions for the first 12 hr contain 2.0–2.5 g CHO/100 mL, 75 mEq $Na^+$/100 mL, 20 mEq $K^+$/100 mL, and 30 mEq $HCO_3^-$/100 mL. Solutions for subsequent use contain 2.0–2.5 g CHO/100 mL, 45–50 mEq $Na^+$/100 mL, 20 mEq $K^+$/100 mL, and 30 mEq $HCO_3^-$/100 mL.

‡Continue until diarrhea stops. Volume of ORS ingested should equal volume of stool losses. If losses cannot be measured, administer 10–15 mL ORS/kg/hr. Weigh child for best estimate of loss and repair.

## ISONATREMIC DEHYDRATION

In a patient with the isonatremic form of dehydration, sodium is lost from the extracellular space to the external environment and to the intracellular space, where it moves to compensate for intracellular potassium losses. To avoid subsequent overexpansion of the extracellular space after replacement of potassium as a result of sodium shift from the cells, one half of the deficit is replaced in the first 12-hr period, one quarter in the second, and one quarter in the third. In addition, the child should receive replacements for both ongoing normal losses (maintenance water, sodium, and potassium) and continuing abnormal losses during this 24-hr period.

Subsequently, there should be 100% replacement of losses. Careful monitoring of weight is the best guide to successful fluid replacement. Serum electrolytes should be monitored. Potassium losses should be replaced slowly (over 36–48 hr) to avoid hyperkalemia. Potassium concentration in intravenous fluids should usually not exceed 40 mEq/L at a rate not greater than 3 mEq/kg/24 hr.

## DISTURBANCES OF SODIUM BALANCE

### Hyponatremia
### (Na⁺ < 130 mEq/L)

*Etiology and Pathophysiology.* Reduced serum sodium content usually is associated with one of three mechanisms (Fig. 16–3). Because sodium is the main extracellular fluid cation, hyponatremia usually is associated with hypo-osmolality. Occasionally, *pseudohyponatremia* is noted with isotonicity when plasma protein or triglyceride levels are elevated or with hyperosmolality when hypertonic infusions (mannitol, diatrizoate sodium) are given or during hyperglycemia. For every 100 mg/dL increment of glucose, sodium levels decline by 1.6 mEq/L. *Hyperosmolar hyponatremia* is a result of osmotic fluid shifts from the intracellular space to the extracellular space; *isosmolar hyponatremia* is due to an artifact of the laboratory analysis of sodium that measures the sodium content in serum drawn off after centrifugation, which contains both the plasma water and that component represented by excess lipid (hyperlipidemia) or protein (macroglobulinemia). Because sodium is present only in

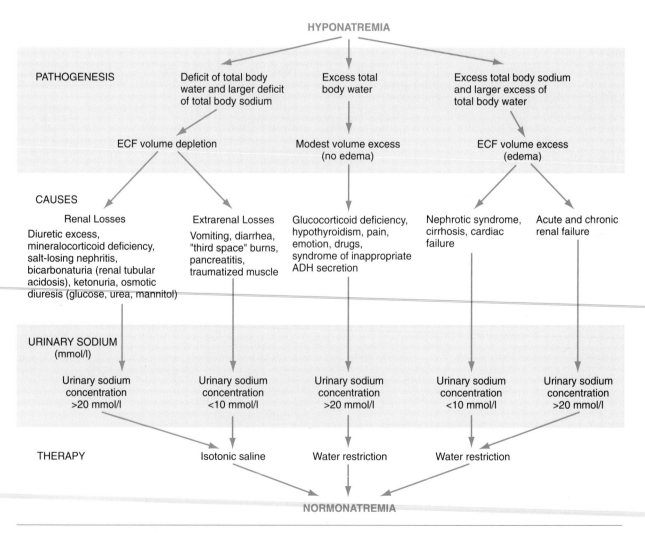

**FIGURE 16–3.** Diagnostic and therapeutic approach to the hyponatremic patient. ADH = antidiuretic hormone; ECF = extracellular fluid. (From Schrier RW, Berl T: Disorders of water metabolism. *In* Schrier RW [ed]: Renal and Electrolyte Disorders, 2nd ed. Boston, Little, Brown & Co, 1980.)

plasma (or serum) water and not in the lipid phase, measurements based on total volume (flame ionization) but not on plasma water yield pseudohyponatremia.

One frequent etiologic factor in true hyponatremia is the **syndrome of inappropriate ADH (SIADH) secretion**, which may be due to a variety of disorders, including unregulated tumor production of ADH-like peptides, pulmonary disorders (pneumonia, positive end-expiratory pressure ventilation, asthma, cystic fibrosis, pneumothorax), drugs (vincristine, opiates, carbamazepine, cyclophosphamide), and direct irritation of the CNS (meningitis, encephalitis, hemorrhage, hypoxia, trauma).

*Hyposmolal hyponatremia* accompanied by increased extracellular volume is also common in various edematous states, such as cardiac failure and cirrhosis. In these states, water retention may be due to a combination of reduced effective plasma volume, which is sensed by the aortic and carotid baroreceptors, and increased activity of the juxtaglomerular apparatus, signaling both ADH and renin secretion. The net result is both water and sodium retention and, thus, the formation of edema. Water retention in excess of sodium produces hyponatremia. This often is intensified when natriuretic (diuretic) agents are prescribed and the fluid intake is hyponatremic.

Hyponatremia without dehydration occurs in infants fed an inappropriately dilute formula due to errors in formula preparation or intentional formula dilution for the treatment of diarrhea or for reasons of financial difficulty. Hyponatremic dehydration may result during diarrhea when fluid replacement is more hypotonic than the diarrheal losses.

*Clinical Manifestations.* The symptoms of hyponatremia may include lethargy, apathy, disorientation, muscle cramps, anorexia, and agitation. The signs may include reduced mental status, decreased deep tendon reflexes, hypothermia, seizures, and pseudobulbar palsies. No clinical manifestations may be apparent. The more severe symptoms rarely occur unless the serum sodium level rapidly falls below 120 mEq/L.

*Treatment.* The treatment depends on the mechanism of hyponatremia and on the presence or absence of serious clinical manifestations (see Fig. 16–3). Acute-onset hyponatremia is more likely to be symptomatic than chronic stable hyponatremia. Initial therapy should be calculated to raise the serum $Na^+$ to 120 mEq/L rapidly, which usually stops seizures. Subsequent correction to 130 mEq $Na^+$/L can be carried out over the next 24–36 hr. Rapid correction to levels greater than 130 mEq/L

may be associated with severe adverse effects, such as central pontine myelinolysis. As a rule, serum sodium should not be raised or lowered more rapidly than 15 mEq/24 hours. Most patients with *acute SIADH* respond to fluid restriction, although sodium chloride (NaCl) infusion may be needed if hyponatremia is symptomatic.

*Hyponatremic dehydration* requires both sodium and fluid replacement in addition to the provision of supplements for ongoing losses and maintenance. Therapy is similar to that for isonatremic dehydration except that, when the sodium value to be infused is calculated, the extra loss of this ion should be taken into account. This replacement usually should be spread over 36 hr. The sodium deficit in hyponatremic dehydration can be estimated by the following equation:

$$(\text{desired } Na^+ - \text{current } Na^+) \times 0.6 \times \text{wt (kg)} = \text{mEq required}$$

Symptomatic hyponatremia may be treated with hypertonic (3%) saline (or normal saline) to raise the serum level to 120 mEq/L.

In situations of symptomatic hyponatremia without edema but with excess total body water, water diuresis may be helpful (diuretics). The volume of diuresis needed to correct hyponatremia may be calculated by the following equation:

$$TBW = 0.6 \times \text{wt (kg)}$$

$$\text{excess water} = TBW - \frac{\text{current } Na^+}{\text{desired } Na^+} \times TBW$$

where TBW = total body water. With this regimen, urine electrolytes also must be replaced with 3% or normal saline and sufficient potassium chloride to avoid additional electrolyte depletion.

### Hypernatremia
### ($Na^+ > 150$ mEq/L)

*Etiology and Pathophysiology.* The serum sodium level is regulated by both ADH secretion and thirst. A high serum sodium level may be due to (1) water loss in excess of sodium loss (increased insensible water losses), (2) insufficient ADH production (central diabetes insipidus) or reduced renal response to ADH (nephrogenic diabetes insipidus), (3) poor response to thirst (hypodipsia), (4) salt poisoning, or less likely, excessive sodium retention (Fig. 16–4).

**Central diabetes insipidus** (absent ADH release) may be acquired (CNS trauma, tumor, auto-

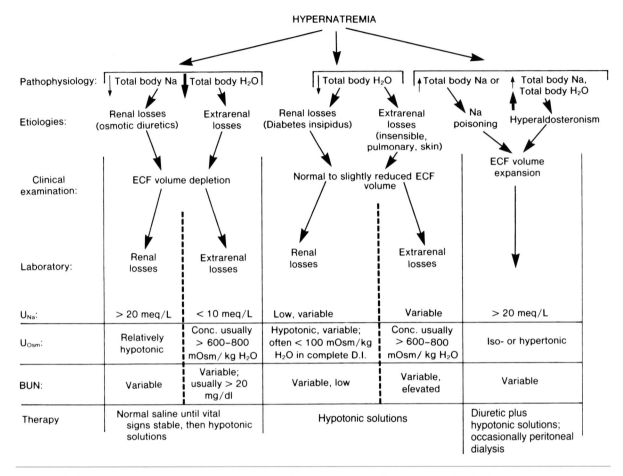

FIGURE 16–4. Approach to hypernatremia. BUN = blood urea nitrogen; ECF = extracellular fluid; $U_{Na}$ = urinary sodium; $U_{Osm}$ = urinary osmolality; ↓ Less reduction; ↓ more severe reduction. (From Norman M: *In* Fleisher G, Ludwig S [eds]: Textbook of Pediatric Emergency Medicine. Baltimore, Williams & Wilkins, 1983, p 423.)

immunity, infection, hypoxia, histiocytosis) or hereditary and associated with craniofacial anomalies. **Nephrogenic diabetes insipidus** (absent or reduced renal response to ADH) may be due to renal pathology (interstitial nephritis, acute tubular necrosis), electrolyte disorders (hypercalcemia, hypokalemia), or drugs (lithium, demeclocycline) or may be hereditary. The hereditary illness appears in infants and is associated with polyuria, polydipsia, dehydration, fever, and growth and developmental retardation; males have a complete deficit, whereas females have a partial disorder. This defect is the result of mutations in the gene that encodes for the aquaporin 2 water channel.

Hypernatremic dehydration may occur in infants with a poor thirst mechanism or in breast-fed neonates of mothers whose milk supply is inadequate if these children have limited supplemental fluid intake. Failure to thrive, dehydration, hyper-

glycemia, hypocalcemia, acidosis, and prerenal azotemia are common associated findings. Infants with diarrhea and fever or those exposed to excessive environmental heat lose water in excess of sodium, placing them at risk for hypernatremia, especially if fluid replacement is hypertonic to losses.

*Clinical Manifestations.* The signs and symptoms relate to the primary disorder, dehydration. In hypernatremic dehydration, intravascular volume is conserved as a result of the hyperosmotic state, which results in a shift of water from the intracellular to the extracellular space. Therefore, the signs of dehydration are not as apparent as they are for an equivalent degree of isotonic dehydration. Based on skin turgor, tachycardia, and blood pressure, the severity of dehydration may be underestimated. Weight change remains the most reliable indicator of the degree of dehydration. Patients with salt poisoning may present in shock with seizures.

*Treatment. Hypernatremic dehydration* requires replacement of water in excess of sodium, which must be done slowly and carefully, because rapidly lowering serum sodium lowers serum osmolality faster than intracellular osmolality is lowered, resulting in fluid crossing the cell membrane into the cell to re-establish osmotic equilibrium. This produces cellular swelling, which in the brain may result in cerebral edema. Hemorrhage and thrombosis also may occur when the correction is too rapid, further contributing to the risk of seizures, coma, and death. Therefore, the serum sodium level should be lowered slowly toward normal at a rate of not more than 15 mEq/L/24 hr. The water deficit in hypernatremic dehydration can be estimated by using the following equation:

$$\text{normal TBW} = 0.6 \times \text{normal weight (kg)}$$

$$\frac{\text{normal Na}^+}{\text{current Na}^+} \times \text{TBW} = \text{current TBW}$$

$$\text{deficit} = \text{normal TBW} - \text{current TBW}$$

The total fluid deficit should be corrected over 36–48 hr unless the serum sodium level is greater than 175 mEq/L. The most important aspects of treating hypernatremic dehydration are the initial management of shock, which re-establishes the circulation and renal blood flow, and then the slow replacement phase, which enables the now well-perfused kidneys to regulate water and sodium homeostasis. If the serum sodium level declines too quickly after treatment of shock, the rate of fluid replacement should be decreased.

Central **diabetes insipidus** requires ADH replacement. Nephrogenic diabetes insipidus will not respond to ADH and is treated with a low-salt and high-water diet. Thiazide diuretics may reduce urine output in children with nephrogenic diabetes insipidus by reducing intravascular volume, which may enhance proximal tubular salt and water reabsorption.

## DISTURBANCES OF POTASSIUM

### Hypokalemia
($K^+ < 3.0$ mEq/L)

*Etiology and Pathophysiology.* Reduced serum potassium concentration may be due to redistribution between the large intracellular potassium compartment and the smaller extracellular potassium space. Shifts of transcellular potassium from serum to cells are noted with acute alkalosis, insulin therapy, sympathomimetic agents, vitamin $B_{12}$ therapy, and familial hypokalemic periodic paralysis.

Net renal loss of potassium is associated with the use of most diuretics, aminoglycosides, amphotericin B, platinum-containing cancer chemotherapy, excessive mineralocorticoid administration, renal disease such as renal tubular acidosis, **Gitelman syndrome,** and **Bartter syndrome.** The latter is characterized by hypokalemic, hypochloremic metabolic alkalosis, hyperaldosteronism, hyperreninemia, increased urine chloride excretion, growth failure, normal blood pressure, hyperplasia of the juxtaglomerular apparatus, and increased urine prostaglandin $E_2$ excretion. It appears to be a defect in the Na–K–Cl co-transporter in the distal nephron.

Bartter syndrome presents in infancy as failure to thrive, salt craving, polyuria, muscle weakness, tetany, and constipation. *Gastrointestinal losses*, such as vomiting (which also results in renal potassium wasting secondary to alkalosis) and diarrhea in previously healthy children, frequently result in hypokalemia.

Gitelman syndrome is often confused with Bartter syndrome but is characterized by familial (autosomal recessive) hypokalemia and hypomagnesemia. Patients may be asymptomatic or may manifest transient weakness or tetany accompanied by emesis, fever, or abdominal pain.

*Clinical Manifestations.* The manifestations of hypokalemia include ileus, muscle weakness, nephrogenic diabetes insipidus, areflexic paralysis, and, especially with the use of digitalis, arrhythmias. The electrocardiogram in hypokalemia reveals ST-segment depression, T-wave reduction, and the presence of a U wave. An approach to the evaluation of patients with hypokalemia is presented in Figure 16–5.

*Treatment.* The type of treatment selected depends on the underlying cause. Renal and gastrointestinal loss usually can be replaced by providing additional potassium chloride administered orally or intravenously. Bartter syndrome is treated with prostaglandin synthetase inhibitors (indomethacin, ibuprofen) together with potassium chloride and a potassium-sparing diuretic. Potassium losses should be replaced carefully to avoid hyperkalemia because potassium must pass through the extracellular space in order to replete the larger intracellular deficits. Gitelman syndrome responds to treatment with magnesium and does not usually require potassium replacement.

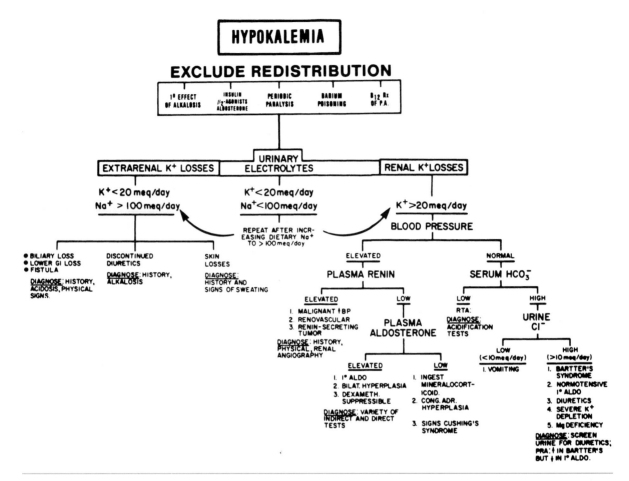

FIGURE 16–5.   Diagnostic approach to hypokalemia. ALDO = aldosteronism; BP = blood pressure; CONG. ADR. = congenital adrenal; GI = gastrointestinal; PA = pernicious anemia; PRA = plasma renin–angiotensin; RTA = renal tubular acidosis; 1° = primary. (From Narins RG, Jones ER, Stom MC, et al: Diagnostic strategies in disorders of fluid, electrolyte, and acid-base homeostasis. Am J Med 72:496, 1982.)

### Hyperkalemia
### ($K^+ > 5.5$ mEq/L)

An increased serum potassium level may be due to transcellular shifts, increased potassium loss from cells, or decreased excretion (Table 16–8). The *clinical manifestations* of hyperkalemia include paresthesias, weakness, flaccid paralysis, and cardiac arrhythmias. The earliest electrocardiographic sign of hyperkalemia is peaked or tented T waves ($K^+$ 5.5–7.0 mEq/L). Higher levels (7.0–8.0 mEq/L) are associated with a prolonged PR interval, ST depression, and the initial widening of the QRS complex. The P wave may flatten as the potassium level increases. When the potassium level exceeds 8.0 mEq/L, the P wave may disappear and the QRS complex widens and merges with the T wave, producing a sine wave pattern. Without treatment, asystole or ventricular fibrillation may occur. Hyponatremia, hypocalcemia, and acidosis intensify hyperkalemic cardiac effects.

The *treatment* of hyperkalemia includes measures to directly antagonize the membrane effects (calcium), redistribute potassium to the intracellular space (sodium bicarbonate, albuterol, glucose, with or without insulin), or remove potassium from the body. The administration of calcium gluconate, sodium bicarbonate, albuterol, and glucose is a temporary measure that must be followed by procedures to remove potassium from the body. This can be accomplished by a forced diuresis or by the oral or rectal administration of a cation exchange resin (Kayexalate) that exchanges sodium for potassium and then binds potassium to be elim-

TABLE 16–8. Etiology of Hyperkalemia

**Transcellular Shift**
Acute acidosis, hyperkalemic familial periodic paralysis

**Increased Endogenous Cell Release**
Hemolysis, rhabdomyolysis, lysis of massive leukocytosis (leukemia)

**Increased Exogenous Administration**
Iatrogenic (intravenous route)

**Decreased Excretion**
Renal failure
Reduced renin-aldosterone production (Addison disease, adrenal genital syndrome, hypoaldosteronism, hyporeninemia)
Reduced tubular excretion (sickle cell anemia, systemic lupus erythematosus, obstructive uropathy, postrenal transplant)
Inhibition of tubular secretion by drugs (digitalis, spironolactone, amiloride, angiotensin-converting enzyme inhibitors)

inated in stool. In situations of renal failure or when there is a need for rapid elimination, hemodialysis or peritoneal dialysis may be necessary.

## DISTURBANCES OF ACID-BASE BALANCE

Maintaining acid-base balance depends acutely on respiratory compensation (Table 16–9) and the tissue-buffering capacity of hemoglobin, albumin, bicarbonate, and bone. More chronic mechanisms involve increased renal excretion or reabsorption of bicarbonate by adding or subtracting bicarbonate molecules to or from the buffering system. Pure acid-base disturbances are due to alterations of only one of these functions, resulting in primary metabolic acidosis or alkalosis or primary respiratory acidosis or alkalosis. Compensating mechanisms rarely completely correct a pure disorder, but they can provide significant improvement of pH. Mixed disturbances involve two or more primary disorders, such as occurs in a patient who has mixed respiratory-metabolic acidosis after a cardiopulmonary arrest.

### Metabolic Alkalosis

A net gain of base or a net loss of acid produces a metabolic alkalosis (Table 16–10). However, unless there is a change in the usual renal mechanisms for reabsorbing bicarbonate or secreting hydrogen ion, the alkalosis will not persist. In situations of persistent extracellular volume depletion (espe-

cially with chloride loss), total body potassium depletion, persistent aldosterone secretion, or a combination of the above, increased proximal tubule reabsorption of bicarbonate develops and metabolic alkalosis becomes sustained. Most patients with metabolic alkalosis have reduced total body potassium stores and hypokalemia, which results in increased hydrogen ion secretion by the distal tubule, maximizing bicarbonate reabsorption along the entire tubule and resulting in a *paradoxical aciduria*.

*Clinical manifestations* include mental confusion, tetany, poor cardiac output, enhanced digitalis toxicity, hypoventilation, and a shift of the hemoglobin oxygen curve to the left. The *treatment* of a metabolic alkalosis depends on the cause. Most cases caused by diuretics, vomiting, bicarbonate therapy, or nasogastric tube losses are "chloride responsive" and can be treated primarily with normal saline, and potassium chloride. Chloride repletion results in enhanced renal bicarbonate excretion. Rarely, ammonium chloride is needed in acutely symptomatic patients. "Chloride-unresponsive" patients may be hypertensive (primary hyperaldosteronism, Cushing syndrome) or normotensive (Bartter syndrome, magnesium deficiency, severe hypokalemia) and require specific therapy for these disease states.

### Metabolic Acidosis

The predominant causes of metabolic aciosis include a loss of bicarbonate (e.g., diarrhea, urinary loss); endogenous production and retention of acids (e.g., inborn errors of metabolism, uremia); and exogenous administration of acid (e.g., salicylate, ethylene glycol). The **anion gap** can be useful to differentiate bicarbonate loss from net acid gain as the *etiology* of acidosis (Table 16–11). In the presence of acidosis, the undetermined anion above the normal range (10–14 mEq/L) is considered to be net acid gained. If the anion gap is normal, bicarbonate loss by the gastrointestinal system or kidney is the probable cause.

**Lactic acidosis** is a frequent cause of a net increase of endogenous acid production and is the result of multiple pathophysiologic mechanisms (Table 16–12).

The *clinical manifestations* of metabolic acidosis may include tachycardia, ventricular arrhythmias, reduced cardiac contractility, Kussmaul respiration, abdominal pain, increased serum uric acid, and hyperkalemia. The *treatment* of increased anion gap acidosis depends on the underlying disease and would include insulin for diabetic ketoacidosis; dialysis for uremia; oxygen for carbon monoxide poi-

**TABLE 16–9.** Characteristics of Primary Acid-Base Disturbances

| Disorder | Etiology | Example | Compensation Mechanisms | Prediction of Pure Compensation |
|---|---|---|---|---|
| **Metabolic** | | | | |
| Acidosis | ↓ $HCO_3^-$ | Hypoxia, drug ingestion, shock | ↓ $P_{CO_2}$ (acute) ↑ renal bicarbonate reabsorption (late) | 1 mEq fall of $HCO_3^-$ = 1–1.3 mm Hg fall of $P_{CO_2}$ |
| Alkalosis | ↑ $HCO_3^-$ ↓ HCl | ↑ Bicarbonate/citrate, pyloric stenosis, gastric tube drainage losses | ↑ $P_{CO_2}$ (acute), renal bicarbonate excretion (late) | $P_{CO_2}$ increases 6 mm Hg for 10-mEq increase of $HCO_3^-$ |
| **Respiratory** | | | | |
| Acidosis Acute (hr) | ↑ $P_{CO_2}$ | Hypoventilation | ↑ $HCO_3^-$ (renal) | $HCO_3^-$ increases 1 mEq/L for each 10 mm Hg $P_{CO_2}$ |
| Chronic (days) | ↑ $P_{CO_2}$ | BPD, cystic fibrosis | ↑ $HCO_3^-$ (renal) | $HCO_3^-$ increases 3–3.5 mEq/L for 10 mm Hg $P_{CO_2}$ |
| Alkalosis Acute (hr) | ↓ $P_{CO_2}$ | Mechanical ventilation for ↑ intracranial pressure, hysteria, hyperammonemia | ↓ $HCO_3^-$ (renal) | $HCO_3^-$ falls 2.5 mEq/L for 10 mmHg of $P_{CO_2}$ |
| Chronic (days) | ↓ $P_{CO_2}$ | Persistent mechanical ventilation | ↓ $HCO_3^-$ (renal) | $HCO_3^-$ falls 5 mEq/L for 10 mmHg of $P_{CO_2}$ |

Data from Narins R: *In* Maxwell M, Kleeman C, Narins R: Clinical Disorders of Fluid and Electrolyte Metabolism, 4th ed. New York, McGraw-Hill, 1987; and DuBose T: Med Clin North Am 67:799, 1983.
BPD = bronchopulmonary dysplasia.

**TABLE 16–10.** Etiology of Metabolic Alkalosis

| Initiation | Maintenance | Maintenance Mechanism | Urine Chloride | Example |
|---|---|---|---|---|
| *Loss of Acid* | | | | |
| GI tract | (1) Volume contraction | (1) ↑ tubular $HCO_3^-$ reabsorption | <10 mEq/L | Pyloric stenosis |
| | (2) Decreased GFR | (2) ↑ fractional $HCO_3^-$ reabsorption | | Congenital chloride diarrhea |
| | (3) Chloride depletion | (3) ↓ GFR, ↓ $Cl^-$ causes ↑ $H^+$ secretion; ↑ renin | | |
| *Renal* sodium delivery to tubule | $K^+$ depletion plus those for GI tract | ↑ Aldosterone, ↑ $H^+$ secretion plus above | >20 mEq/L on diuretics, <10 mEq/L off therapy | Diuretics |
| Hyperreninemic states | As above | As above | >20 mEq/L | Bartter syndrome; primary hyperaldosteronism; licorice ingestion |
| High mineralocorticoid states | | | | Renal artery stenosis |
| *Gain of Base* | | | | |
| Alkalizing salts | Volume contraction Continued base therapy, $K^+$ deficit | As above plus continued source As above | >20 mEq/L | Milk alkali syndrome Citrate in blood products |
| *Posthypercapnic State* | Volume contraction; decreased GFR; $K^+$ and $Cl^-$ depletion | As above | <10 mEq/L | Slow correction of chronic respiratory acidosis |

Data from Cogan M, et al: Med Clin North Am 67:903, 1983; and Sabatin S, Kurtzman N: *In* Maxwell M, Kleeman C, Narins R: Clinical Disorders of Fluid and Electrolyte Metabolism, 4th ed. New York, McGraw-Hill, 1987.
GFR = glomerular filtration rate; GI = gastrointestinal.

TABLE 16–11. Acidosis and the Anion Gap*

**Increased Anion Gap without Acidosis**

Decreased calcium, magnesium, potassium, and other *cations*
Increased albumin, other *anions*; high-dose carbenicillin

**Increased Anion Gap with Acidosis**

Increased endogenous anions: lactate, sulfate, phosphate
(uremia), ketones (diabetes), organic acids (inborn errors
of metabolism)
Increased exogenous acids: salicylate, methanol, ethanol,
paraldehyde

**Normal Anion Gap with Acidosis**

Bicarbonate losses; diarrhea, renal tubular acidosis, carbonic
anhydrase inhibitor, ureterosigmoidostomy, dilutional
acidosis, pancreatic fistula

**Decreased Anion Gap without Acidosis**

Increased calcium, potassium, magnesium, bromide
Decreased albumin

Adapted from Oh W, Carroll H: Current concepts: The anion gap.
N Engl J Med 297:814, 1977.
*Normal anion gap = $Na^+ - (Cl^- + HCO_3^-)$ = 12 mEq/L.

soning; removal of toxins (e.g., salicylate); and provision of sodium bicarbonate when acidosis is
severe or not rapidly corrected by the above measures. The dose of bicarbonate ($HCO_3^-$) may be
calculated by the following equation:

$$\text{dose of bicarbonate} = (\text{normal } HCO_3^- - \text{current } HCO_3^-) \times 0.3 \times \text{wt (kg)}$$

Overalkalinization should be avoided because it
has detrimental effects, such as hypokalemia, reduced oxygen dissociation from hemoglobin, and

TABLE 16–12. Etiology of Lactic Acidosis

| **Type A** | |
|---|---|
| Tissue hypoxia | Shock, asphyxia, carbon monoxide toxicity |
| **Type B** | |
| Systemic disorders | Diabetes mellitus, renal failure, hepatic failure, malignancy, seizures, gut flora that produce D-lactate |
| Drugs | Biguanides, fructose, ethanol, salicylate, methanol, ethylene glycol |
| Inborn errors | Type I glycogen storage disease, pyruvate carboxylase deficiency, pyruvate dehydrogenase deficiency, mitochondrial myopathy, lactic acidemias, and other mitochondrial defects |

further stimulation of lactate production. Partial
correction of the acidosis is preferable while the
underlying cause is being treated. Most children
with diabetic ketoacidosis do not require bicarbonate because ketone body metabolism in the presence of insulin regenerates bicarbonate in the Krebs
cycle. Intravenous bicarbonate in these patients
may produce metabolic alkalosis and complicate
recovery.

### Renal Tubular Acidosis

***Etiology and Classification.*** Renal tubular acidosis (RTA) is a condition characterized by hyperchloremic normal anion gap acidosis, which results
from impaired renal acidification. Three distinctive
types of renal tubular acidosis have been established:

- Type I: distal RTA
- Type II: proximal RTA
- Type IV: RTA associated with a **mineralocorti-coid deficiency**

A type III was proposed but is most likely a variant
of type I.

*PROXIMAL RENAL TUBULAR ACIDOSIS.* The proximal
form results from reduced proximal tubular reabsorption of bicarbonate, either as a result of a failure of hydrogen ion secretion proximally or as
a result of deficient carbonic anhydrase activity.
Normally, 85% of the filtered bicarbonate is reabsorbed in the proximal tubule. In this condition,
reabsorption is reduced. Distal tubular bicarbonate
reabsorption cannot fully compensate for this load,
and, considerable filtered bicarbonate is excreted.
The serum bicarbonate level falls until it reaches
the new bicarbonate threshold, at which time bicarbonate wasting ceases. When the serum bicarbonate reaches this level (~ 15–16 mmol/L), bicarbonate reabsorption now can be considered complete.
The urine may become acidified, because distal
hydrogen ion secretion is normal. Severe hypokalemia is often an associated finding, resulting from
extracellular volume contraction, leading to secondary hyperaldosteronism and distal tubule potassium loss.

Proximal RTA occurs as a primary disease, as a
part of the **Fanconi syndrome,** and in a variety of
other conditions (Table 16–13). Fanconi syndrome
may be idiopathic or secondary to metabolic and/
or toxic conditions, as noted in Table 16–13. In
Fanconi syndrome, a defect exists (sometimes reversible) in proximal tubular reabsorption of glucose, phosphate, and amino acids. This is associated with proximal RTA and a defect in vitamin D

TABLE 16–13.    Etiology of Proximal Renal Tubular Acidosis

**Idiopathic or Primary**
Sporadic
Fanconi syndrome

**Secondary Metabolic Diseases**
Cystinosis
Tyrosinemia
Galactosemia
Hereditary fructose intolerance
Type I glycogen storage disease
Lowe syndrome
Wilson disease
Osteopetrosis (carbonic anhydrase deficiency)

**Drugs and Toxins**
Heavy metals (lead, cadmium, mercury)
Outdated tetracycline
Carbonic anhydrase inhibitors
Vitamin D deficiency or altered metabolism

**Miscellaneous**
Hyperparathyroidism
Dysproteinemic states (monoclonal gammopathy)
Interstitial nephritis (renal transplant rejection, renal vein thrombosis)
Nephrotic syndrome
Prematurity
Pregnancy

metabolism, leading to reduced levels of $1,25\text{-}(OH)_2$ vitamin D.

*DISTAL RENAL TUBULAR ACIDOSIS.* The distal form results from an inability of the distal nephron to secrete hydrogen ion, preventing the reabsorption of the final 15% of bicarbonate (which reaches the distal tubule) and also the final acidification of the urine. In this condition, the urinary pH cannot be reduced below 5.5–6.0, despite severe systemic acidosis. Hyperchloremia and hypokalemia accompany distal RTA. Distal RTA may be an isolated primary defect inherited as either an autosomal dominant or an autosomal recessive trait, or it may occur in association with a variety of disorders (Table 16–14). All forms of distal RTA may be complicated by nephrocalcinosis.

*MINERALOCORTICOID DEFICIENCY.* Type IV RTA results from inadequate production of or reduced responsiveness to aldosterone. It is associated with hyperkalemic and hyperchloremic acidosis. This disorder may be primary or secondary to adrenal disease or parenchymal kidney damage, especially obstructive uropathy. *Hyporeninemic hypoaldosteronism* is another form of type IV RTA that also may result from renal disease associated with interstitial damage.

***Clinical Manifestations.*** Children with RTA

usually present with growth failure and acidosis. If Fanconi syndrome is present, rickets, polyuria, nausea, anorexia, and intermittent vomiting may also occur. Hypokalemia produces muscle weakness and polyuria. Patients with systemic acidosis and alkaline urine whose bicarbonate level is below 15 mEq/L most likely have distal RTA. In children with proximal RTA, the urine becomes acidified when the bicarbonate threshold is attained. Primary RTA must be differentiated from secondary RTA because the latter requires specific therapy of the underlying disorder. For example, removal of galactose (galactosemia) or fructose (hereditary fructose intolerance) from the diet reverses these acquired forms of Fanconi syndrome.

***Diagnosis.*** The diagnosis of RTA consists of determining the ability to secrete hydrogen ion (distal RTA) or the abnormal excretion of bicarbonate (proximal RTA). In a patient with a hyperchloremic metabolic acidosis, a measurement of the urine pH is essential. If the urine pH is less than 5.5 when

TABLE 16–14.    Etiology of Distal Renal Tubular Acidosis

**Primary or Idiopathic**
Sporadic
Familial

**Secondary Inherited Diseases**
Osteopetrosis
Sickle cell anemia
Wilson disease
Hypercalciuria

**Hypercalciuria/Nephrocalcinosis**
Hyperparathyroidism
Hypervitaminosis D
Hyperthyroidism
Medullary sponge kidney

**Drugs and Toxins**
Amphotericin B
Toluene
Amiloride
Lithium

**Interstitial Renal Disease**
Chronic pyelonephritis
Obstructive nephropathy
Renal transplantation rejection
Hyperoxaluria

**Autoimmune and Hypergammaglobulinemic States**
Systemic lupus erythematosus
Chronic active hepatitis
Cryoglobulinemia
Primary biliary cirrhosis
Sjögren syndrome
Thyroiditis
Pulmonary fibrosis

the serum bicarbonate is below normal, and especially if the serum bicarbonate is 16 mEq or less, this is very suggestive of proximal RTA. The provision of bicarbonate, either intravenously or in large doses orally, will increase the serum bicarbonate but will not increase it into the normal range; it will quickly raise the urine pH to >7.5. This means that the threshold for bicarbonate reabsorption has been exceeded despite a filtered load of bicarbonate that is below normal.

To diagnose distal RTA, a measurement of the *urine anion gap* (Na + K −Cl) is helpful. In normal patients under conditions of low serum bicarbonate levels, the gap will be negative because acidification of the urine results in an increase in ammonium chloride excretion. Since the chloride is measured and the ammonium is not measured in the above equation, the anion gap will be negative. Normal individuals will also have a low urine pH (<6). In patients with distal RTA, urinary acidification is not normal and ammonium chloride excretion is low. Therefore, the gap will be zero or positive. Affected patients will not have a urine pH <6.2. This test can be done only when the serum bicarbonate level is low and the patient is not receiving bicarbonate therapy. The gold standard test for urinary acidification is an acid loading test, usually with the use of ammonium chloride. The finding of a further fall in serum bicarbonate without a decline in urine pH below 6.2 and without the development of a negative urine anion gap is proof of distal RTA.

*Treatment.* The goal of therapy is to correct the acidosis and achieve normal childhood growth. A sodium bicarbonate solution (1 mEq/mL) or tablet (8 mEq/tablet) or a sodium citrate–citric acid combination (Shohl solution; Bicitra) containing 1 mEq of Na citrate/mL of solution is administered. Alkali therapy plus potassium supplementation can be given in the form of Polycitra, which contains 1 mEq/mL of sodium citrate and 1 mEq/mL of potassium citrate. Patients with distal RTA require a smaller dose of alkalinizing agents, which is equal to endogenous acid production (1–2 mEq/kg/24 hr). However, because the urine cannot be acidified, nephrocalcinosis is common. Larger doses of alkali are required in proximal RTA to correct the acidosis because of the constant bicarbonate wasting resulting from the inability to reabsorb filtered bicarbonate. Proximal RTA, however, is more likely to resolve than is distal RTA. Type IV RTA most commonly results from obstructive uropathy and may resolve after the the obstruction is corrected. Mineralocorticoid therapy may be needed for type IV RTA associated with aldosterone deficiency.

## References

Arnold WC, Kallen RJ. Fluid and electrolyte therapy. Pediatr Clin North Am 37(2), 1990.

Bartter F, Schwartz W: The syndrome of inappropriate secretion of antidiuretic hormone. Am J Med 42:790, 1967.

Battle D, Hizon M, Cohen E, et al: The use of the urinary anion gap in the diagnosis of hyperchloremic metabolic acidosis. N Engl J Med 318:594, 1988.

Behrman RE, Kliegman RM, Arvin AM (eds): Nelson Textbook of Pediatrics. 15 ed. Philadelphia, WB Saunders, 1996, Chapters 46–50, 482–485.

Carvana R, Buckalew V: The syndrome of distal (type 1) renal tubular acidosis. Medicine 67:84, 1988.

Gill JR Jr, Frolich JC, Bowden RE, et al: Bartter's syndrome: A disorder characterized by high urinary prostaglandins and a dependence of hyperreninemia on prostaglandin synthesis. Am J Med 61:43, 1976.

Narins R (ed): Maxwell and Kleeman Clinical Disorders of Fluid and Electrolyte Metabolism, 5th ed. New York, McGraw-Hill, 1994.

Oh M, Cavrol H: Anion gap. N Engl J Med 297:814, 1977.

Rodriguez-Soriano J, Vallo A: Renal tubular acidosis. Pediatr Nephrol 4:268, 1990.

# RENAL DISEASES

## APPROACH TO THE CHILD WITH HEMATURIA

When hematuria is a chief complaint, it generally is gross hematuria (seen with the naked eye), but microscopic hematuria may be the initial manifestation observed during routine urinalysis. Microscopic hematuria is defined as greater than three to five red blood cells per high-power field in freshly voided and centrifuged urine.

The child who presents with gross hematuria needs prompt evaluation. The child with the combination of microscopic hematuria, no proteinuria, normal blood pressure, and normal renal function should have the urinalysis repeated. If the hematuria persists, further evaluation is appropriate. The first step in evaluating the child with hematuria is taking a careful history, performing a physical examination, and examining the urine. *The presence of red urine but a negative microscopic examination and negative dipstick reaction for blood* suggests that the red urine has been caused by a substance that has colored the urine, as might occur from the child's ingesting a medication such as acetophenetidin, which has a metabolite that produces a dark wine-brown color; from a toxin such as benzene or carbon tetrachloride, both of which produce a red-brown color; from food dyes (beets); or from rifampin (orange-red color). The color also might be due to the side effects of treatment, such as occurs after deferoxamine administration, or due to poisoning with a heavy metal, such as lead, which produces a red-brown coloration of the urine. Urates are a common cause of an orange-red discoloration on the diaper of infants.

If the *urine tests positive for blood but no red blood cells are seen* when the urine is promptly examined, the presence of free hemoglobin or myoglobin should be suspected. **Hemoglobinuria** may be present secondary to hemoglobin excretion from acute intravascular hemolysis (e.g., glucose-6-phosphate dehydrogenase deficiency or paroxysmal nocturnal hemoglobinuria) or from intravascular coagulation (e.g., sepsis, hemolytic-uremic syndrome [HUS]). It may be seen in freshwater drowning, mismatched blood transfusions, and other causes of hemolysis. Rhabdomyolysis and **myoglobinuria** (from a crush injury, burns, myositis, asphyxia) also must be considered.

If *a significant number of red blood cells are present but no casts are observed*, one must consider bleeding beyond the glomerulus and renal tubules. However, it is important to remember that casts as well as red cells will hemolyze on standing, particularly in dilute urine, and they also can be missed if the urine is not examined with reduced light and shortly after voiding.

Another mechanism for localizing hematuria to the glomerulus is by examining the morphology of the red blood cells. Carefully examining the urine by phase contrast microscopy frequently documents altered red cell morphology in glomerular hematuria, whereas morphology characteristically is unaltered when nonglomerular causes are present. However, the absence of casts or the absence of alterations in red blood cell morphology by no means excludes a glomerular etiology.

*The presence of red cells in the absence of casts* is seen in some patients with hematuria associated with sickle cell trait or disease, in some children following marked exercise, or in patients after renal trauma. The presence of a coagulopathy (acute or inherited) may be associated with hematuria, although bleeding from the urinary tract in the absence of bleeding into other organ systems (e.g., skin or joints) is unusual. A family history of hematuria, renal failure, or deafness or the finding of hematuria on a urinalysis performed on siblings or parents suggests the possibility of a familial nephritis. Hypercalciuria is an important cause of isolated hematuria in children; 25–30% of children with isolated hematuria have calcium excretion rates greater than 4 mg/kg/24 hr and/or urinary calcium-to-creatinine ratios greater than 0.2:1.

**Urolithiasis** is one cause of painful hematuria and may be seen in children who have idiopathic hypercalciuria, in children who have been immobilized for long periods of time, and in those with urinary tract malformations and recurrent infections. Idiopathic nephrolithiasis does occur with uric acid, calcium oxalate, and struvite, but it is uncommon. Urolithiasis also occurs in hyperparathyroidism, sarcoidosis, Lesch-Nyhan syndrome, diuretic use, cystic fibrosis, and inflammation bowel disease. Nephrocalcinosis also may be seen in distal RTA, cystinuria, hyperoxaluria, the milk alkali syndrome, and other uncommon conditions.

*Abnormalities of the urinary tract* must be considered in patients with hematuria. *Benign* (hemangioma, hamartoma) or *malignant* (Wilms–kidney, rhabdomyosarcoma–bladder) *tumors must be excluded in patients with hematuria.* Congenital obstruction, cystic disease, severe ureteral reflux, or an infiltrative process may be accompanied by hematuria. Nephrosonogram and/or IVP is an important part of the evaluation to rule out these possibilities. *Urinary tract infection* may present with hematuria, and a urine culture should be part of the initial evaluation of a child with hematuria. *Interstitial nephritis*, which may be drug-induced or idiopathic, may present with hematuria, eosinophilia, and urinary eosinophils with or without casts.

The *differential diagnosis* of hematuria and its association with proteinuria and edema is noted in Table 16–15. The minimal screening evaluation for hematuria is described in Table 16–16.

If the urinalysis reveals the presence of *hematuria and casts*, one of a variety of glomerular diseases should be considered. Glomerular injury may be the result of immunologic injury (e.g., acute poststreptococcal glomerulonephritis), inherited disease (e.g., Alport syndrome), or vascular injury (e.g., acute tubular or cortical necrosis).

### Microscopic Hematuria with Casts or Altered Red Cell Morphology but Little or No Proteinuria

**Immunoglobulin A Nephropathy (Berger Disease).** Microscopic hematuria or recurrent gross hematuria shortly following an upper respiratory infection (1–2 days) and not associated with the signs and symptoms of an acute nephritic syndrome (edema, hypertension, renal insufficiency) suggests the possibility of immunoglobulin A (IgA) nephropathy or idiopathic hematuria (see below). The cause of IgA nephropathy disease is not known, but a consistent finding on renal biopsy is the presence of mesangial proliferation accompanied by mesangial deposits of IgA and variable deposition of IgG and IgM. The course generally is benign in children but may be associated with recurrent bouts of hematuria following or during

TABLE 16–15.  Differential Diagnosis of Proteinuria and Hematuria

| Proteinuria | Hematuria | Edema | Etiology |
|---|---|---|---|
| Yes | No | No | Exercise, orthostatic (intermittent or fixed) fever, dehydration; benign; reflux nephropathy; focal segmental sclerosis; SLE |
| Yes | Yes | No/Mild | Acute glomerulonephritis, IgA nephropathy (Berger disease), Henoch-Schönlein purpura, hemolytic uremic syndrome, endocarditis, hereditary nephritis; interstitial nephritis; SLE, severe exercise |
| Yes | No | Yes | Minimal lesion (change) nephrotic syndrome; focal segmental sclerosis |
| Yes | Yes | Yes | Acute glomerulonephritis, atypical minimal lesion nephrotic syndrome, membranoproliferative (mesangiocapillary) glomerulonephritis, membranous nephropathy |
| No | Yes | No | Benign hematuria, IgA nephropathy, hereditary nephritis, sickle cell anemia, tumor, trauma, interstitial nephritis, nephrolithiasis, idiopathic hypercalciuria |

IgA = immunoglobulin A; SLE = systemic lupus erythematosus.

respiratory infections. IgA nephropathy presents sporadically, with some reports of familial disease, is more common in males than in females, and is characteristically associated with normal renal function and normal serum levels of C3. Although the prognosis is good in children, progressive renal insufficiency and end-stage renal disease have been demonstrated to develop in about 25% of adults. No therapy currently is known that alters the course of the disease. Therapies that have been tried include: glucocorticoids, immunosuppressive agents (cyclophosphamide, cyclosporine, azathioprine), and fish oil.

**Idiopathic Hematuria.** Idiopathic hematuria may be familial or nonfamilial. *Benign familial hematuria* is a common nonprogressive, autosomal dominant disorder, demonstrating thinning of the glomerular basement membrane on electron mi-

croscopy; other family members (parent, sibling) will also have hematuria (usually microscopic). Renal biopsy in patients with the nonfamilial form may be normal or reveal only mild mesangial hypercellularity. Patients who have **Alport syndrome** often present with microscopic hematuria. This familial disorder is associated with progressive bilateral neurosensory deafness (high tones) and progressive renal failure during adolescence and young adulthood, particularly in males. Ocular findings include cataracts, keratoconus, and spherophakia. Electron microscopy of the renal biopsy reveals characteristic splitting and layering of the basement membrane of the glomerulus. The prognosis for patients with nonfamilial or the non-Alport form of idiopathic familial hematuria is excellent, but long-term follow-up is required to exclude the progressive forms of familial hematuria.

### Hematuria with Casts and Mild to Moderate Proteinuria

Children who have hematuria associated with casts and less than 1 g of proteinuria/m$^2$/day usually have nephritis.

**Acute Poststreptococcal Glomerulonephritis.** This disorder is the prototype of the acute nephritic syndrome. Acute glomerulonephritis (AGN) is associated with a sudden onset of gross hematuria in approximately two thirds of children, edema in three fourths, and hypertension in one half and with variable degrees of renal insufficiency.

*Etiology and Pathophysiology.* AGN characteristically follows streptococcal pharyngitis or impe-

TABLE 16–16.  Basic Work-up of the Child with Hematuria

1. *History:* Present, past, family
2. *Physical examination:* Height, weight, blood pressure, optic fundi, presence or absence of abdominal mass, skin appearance, genitalia, edema, complete physical examination
3. *Laboratory:* Urinalysis, urine culture, CBC, smear, platelets, serum BUN, creatinine, calcium, streptozyme, serum complement (C3 as screen), quantitative urinary protein, calcium and creatinine, intravenous pyelogram and/or nephrosonogram

BUN = blood urea nitrogen; CBC = complete blood count.

tigo–pyoderma by 7–21 days. Only certain strains of group A beta-hemolytic streptococci are nephritogenic. Acute poststreptococcal glomerulonephritis is immunologically mediated by activation of the complement system, which initiates a glomerular proliferative and inflammatory response. Antigen-antibody complexes in the glomerular basement membrane induce complement activation. Edema is formed as a result of reduced GFR and hence decreased filtration plus enhanced distal $Na^+$ reabsorption. Plasma volume is elevated and plasma renin is suppressed.

*Clinical Manifestations.* Signs and symptoms may be delayed for 5 days to 3 wk (10-day average) after streptococcal infections. Children may have asymptomatic hematuria. Edema and tea- or cola-colored urine are the most common initial signs. Oliguria, edema, and hypertension may induce complications, such as heart failure and encephalopathy.

*Diagnosis.* The diagnosis is based on the typical findings of edema, hematuria, and hypertension. Oliguria may occur, and pulmonary vascular congestion may be apparent on chest roentgenogram. Encephalopathy or seizures may occur. In addition to hematuria, urinalysis reveals mild to moderate proteinuria, concentrated urine, and the presence of many casts, including coarse and fine granular and red cell casts. Previous streptococcal infection should be documented by the streptozyme test. Confirmation of activation of the complement system is determined by low C3 levels. Renal biopsy usually is not indicated in children with typical AGN; it reveals electron-dense deposits in the subepithelial space. The C3 returns to normal by 6–8 wk. Renal failure, if present, usually resolves in 2–3 wk, as do hypertension and gross hematuria.

*Treatment.* Specific therapy includes diuretics for hypertension, heart failure, pulmonary edema, and oliguria; antihypertensive agents, such as calcium channel blockers (nifedipine) angiotensin-converting enzyme inhibitors, or vasodilators (hydralazine) for hypertension alone; or nifedipine, diazoxide, or nitroprusside for severe hypertension or hypertensive encephalopathy. Proteinuria and edema characteristically decline fairly rapidly (5–10 days), but microscopic hematuria may persist for months or occasionally years, a circumstance that does not alter the generally excellent *prognosis* of this disease, from which greater than 95% of children recover completely.

The absence of evidence for a poststreptococcal glomerulonephritis does not exclude the diagnosis of *acute postinfectious glomerulonephritis,* because multiple etiologic factors (*Pneumococcus, Staphylococcus,* endocarditis related pathogens) have been implicated. Hypocomplementemia persisting beyond 8 wk of the illness, however, suggests the diagnosis of mesangiocapillary glomerulonephritis.

**Mesangiocapillary (Membranoproliferative) Glomerulonephritis.** This disorder may present in a manner similar to that of acute poststreptococcal glomerulonephritis, characteristically, however, persistent hypocomplementemia is present. This membranoproliferative disease frequently appears as a nephrotic syndrome, which is present in fewer than 10% of patients with AGN (see Nephrotic Syndrome).

**Hemolytic-Uremic Syndrome.** HUS is characterized by a microangiopathic hemolytic anemia, renal cortical injury (sometimes progressing to renal cortical necrosis), and thrombocytopenia. HUS is a major cause of acute renal failure in children.

*Etiology and Epidemiology.* HUS may be sporadic, epidemic, and, in some countries (e.g., Argentina), endemic. The disease typically occurs between the ages of 6 mo and 4 yr. Circulating toxins have been implicated as one etiologic mechanism, especially if HUS follows *Escherichia coli* or *Shigella* enteritis. HUS following hemorrhagic colitis has been associated with a verotoxin-producing Escherichia coli 0157:H7. Verotoxin is similar to shigatoxin (*Shigella*) and binds to a specific receptor on endothelial cells, producing endothelial swelling. Familial disease may be due to an alteration in the thromboxane-prostacyclin relationship, which favors endothelial platelet activation.

In most cases, the primary event appears to be endothelial cell injury and subsequent localized clotting and platelet activation. Evidence for disseminated intravascular coagulation (DIC) rarely is present. Microangiopathic hemolytic anemia results from mechanical damage to red cells as they pass through the damaged vascular endothelium. Thrombocytopenia results from platelet adhesion.

*Clinical Manifestations and Diagnosis.* The onset usually appears as a gastroenteritis, most often with blood in the stool, followed in 7–10 days by weakness, lethargy, irritability, and oliguria. Physical examination reveals pallor, edema, petechiae, hepatosplenomegaly, and irritability. The diagnosis is supported by the presence of microangiopathic hemolytic anemia, thrombocytopenia, and acute renal failure. Seizures may indicate CNS involvement. A smear of peripheral red blood cells reveals schistocytes, helmet and burr cells, and fragmented erythrocytes. The reticulocyte count is elevated, and plasma haptoglobin levels are diminished. A Coombs test is negative. Leukocytosis is common. Urinalysis reveals microscopic hematuria, proteinuria, and casts. Other causes of microangiopathic hemolytic anemia should be excluded.

*Treatment.* The patient in acute renal failure requires immediate therapy. Many patients (30–50%) require early intervention with dialysis. Most children (85–90%) survive the acute phase and recover normal renal function. Steroids, plasmapheresis heparinizatiation, and streptokinase are not helpful; platelet inhibitors, hyperimmune globulin, and plasma infusions remain of unproven benefit. Although careful medical management with early-onset dialysis frequently is associated with recovery, children nevertheless should be observed for the late development of hypertension proteinuria, or chronic renal failure. Epidemic disease has the best *prognosis*, whereas familial cases, disease in older patients (>10 yr of age) or in very young patients (<8 mo of age), HUS without diarrhea, and sporadic HUS have a poorer outcome.

**Rapidly Progressive Glomerulonephritis.** Rapidly progressive glomerulonephritis (RPGN) is a clinical syndrome of rapidly progressing nephritis accompanied by renal failure, the pathologic hallmark of which is epithelial cell proliferation and *crescent* formation. One histologic pattern is that of linear immunoglobulin and complement deposition (idiopathic, Goodpasture syndrome). The more common type is the appearance of immune complexes in a "lumpy" pattern in the basement membrane (SLE, poststreptococcal AGN, polyarteritis, Henoch-Schönlein purpura, mesangiocapillary or idiopathic glomerulonephritis). RPGN is more common in late childhood, when patients present with edema, gross hematuria, hypertension, and renal failure. Some children with rapidly progressive lupus nephritis respond to pulse prednisone or cyclophosphamide therapy, whereas other children with poststreptococcal glomerulonephritis recover spontaneously. The prognosis for recovery of renal function is poor for the remaining types of RPGN. Fortunately, transplantation benefits most children having end-stage renal disease associated with the "lumpy" immune complex pattern of RPGN, but not in conditions associated with antiglomerular basement membrane antibodies, such as Goodpasture syndrome.

### References

Andreoli S: Chronic glomerulonephritis in childhood: Membranoproliferative glomerulonephritis, Henoch-Schönlein purpura, and IgA nephropathy. Pediatr Clin North Am 42:1487, 1995.

Behrman RE, Kliegman RM, Arvin AM (eds): Nelson Textbook of Pediatrics, 15th ed. Philadelphia, WB Saunders, 1996, Chapters 462–477.

Grimm PC, Ogborn MR: Hemolytic uremic syndrome: The most common cause of acute renal failure in childhood. Pediatr Ann 23:505, 1994.

Lieu TA, Grasmeder HM, Kaplan BS: An approach to the evaluation and treatment of microscopic hematuria. Pediatr Clin North Am 38:579, 1991.

Lim D, Walker D, Ellsworth P, et al: Treatment of pediatric urolithiasis between 1984 and 1994. J Urol 156:702, 1996.

Remuzzi G, Ruggenenti P: The hemolytic uremic syndrome. Kidney Int 47:2, 1995.

Siegler R, Pavia A, Cook J: Hemolytic uremic syndrome in adolescents. Arch Pediatr Adolesc Med 151:165, 1997.

Simekes A, Spitzer A: Poststreptococcal acute glomerulonephritis. Pediatr Rev 7:278, 1995.

### Hematuria with Casts and Marked Proteinuria

Children who present with hematuria and marked proteinuria (greater than 1 g/m²/day) may have a nephrotic syndrome (see Table 16–15).

### APPROACH TO THE CHILD WITH PROTEINURIA
(Table 16–17)

A small amount of protein is found in the urine of healthy children. The normal amount of urine protein is less than 4 mg/m²/hr or less than 100 mg/m²/24 hr. *Nephrotic proteinuria* is defined as greater than 40 mg/m²/hr or greater than 1 g/m²/24 hr. The intermediary amounts are abnormal but not within the nephrotic range. Qualitative proteinuria of 1+ or greater on at least two to three random urine specimens suggest proteinuria that should be confirmed quantitatively. A semiquantitative evaluation of proteinuria is possible by measuring the urine protein-to-creatinine ratio on a

**TABLE 16–17.**   Evaluation of a Child with Proteinuria*

1. Complete history and physical examination

2. Confirmation of presence of proteinuria by repeat urinalysis

3. Twenty-four-hour urine collection to quantitate proteinuria; if quantitatively increased, proteinuria is present

4. Orthostatic test; if orthostatic test reveals persistent proteinuria, continue with tests listed in steps 5–7

5. Serum BUN, creatinine (calculate creatinine clearance), total protein, albumin, cholesterol, electrolytes

6. Streptozyme, C3', ANA

7. Renal ultrasonography or intravenous pyelogram

*If steps 4–7 are abnormal; or there is a family history of renal disease, hematuria, hypertension, edema; or other manifestations of renal or systemic disease is present, biopsy may be needed.
ANA = antinuclear antibody; BUN = blood urea nitrogen.

single voided urine. The normal ratio generally is less than 0.2:1 when measured in the first morning specimen. The nephrotic urine protein:creatinine ratio is generally greater than 3.5:1.

Initially, one must determine whether the proteinuria is transient or persistent. If persistent, one must assess its severity (see Glomerular Proteinuria, below). *Transient proteinuria* is seen following vigorous exercise and occasionally in children with fevers exceeding 38.5°C (101.3°F). The proteinuria usually is mild, transient, and reproducible.

Another type of transient proteinuria is *postural (orthostatic) proteinuria*. Patients excrete normal amounts of protein while recumbent but have significant, although moderate, proteinuria when in the upright position. Hematuria is absent and renal function, complement levels, and renal ultrasound or IVP are entirely normal. This transient proteinuria is best evaluated by collecting a timed urine specimen while the patient is recumbent (usually overnight), followed by a timed urine collection during a normally active day. The presence of significant, moderate proteinuria during the active period and a decrease in the proteinuria to normal or nearly normal levels during recumbency confirm the diagnosis of orthostatic proteinuria. It is important to remember that "fixed" proteinuria associated with renal disease also will have orthostatic accentuation during activity. Orthostatic proteinuria generally is thought to be benign. If proteinuria is *persistent* ("fixed"), renal disease should be considered (see Table 16–15).

## Tubular Proteinuria

Normal children filter low-molecular-weight proteins, which are reabsorbed in the proximal tubule. Proximal tubular injury results in diminished reabsorptive ability (e.g., Fanconi syndrome) that produces mild to moderate proteinuria characteristically unassociated with edema.

## Glomerular Proteinuria

Glomerular proteinuria is classified by its degree. Intermittent or *mild proteinuria* ($<0.5$ g/m$^2$/day) is seen in pyelonephritis, renal cystic diseases, obstructive uropathies (congenital obstructions and reflux nephropathy), and mild glomerulonephritis. *Moderate proteinuria* (0.5–1 g/m$^2$/day) is seen in acute poststreptococcal glomerulonephritis, mild Henoch-Schönlein nephritis, severe pyelonephritis, chronic glomerulonephritis, and HUS. *Severe proteinuria* ($>1$ g/m$^2$/day) characteristically is associated with the nephrotic syndrome.

## NEPHROTIC SYNDROME

The nephrotic syndrome is an accumulation of symptoms and signs and is characterized by *proteinuria* (mainly albuminuria) greater than 1 g/m$^2$/24 hr, by *hypoproteinemia* (mainly albumin) with a total protein less than 5.5 g/dL and serum albumin less than 2.5 g/dL, by *hypercholesterolemia* ($>250$ mg/dL), and by *edema*. The primary disorder is an increase in glomerular permeability to proteins, most likely caused by a loss of the membrane sialoproteins, which, in turn, results in the loss of the negative charge on the basement membrane. This increase in glomerular permeability causes massive proteinuria accompanied by secondary hypoproteinemia. Plasma oncotic pressure is diminished, resulting in a shift of fluid from the vascular to the interstitial compartment and a contraction in plasma volume. Renal blood flow and GFR are not usually diminished, and in some instances GFR may be above normal. With profound hypoalbuminemia, GFR is diminished. In addition to hypoproteinemic reduction of plasma oncotic pressure, formation of edema is enhanced by a reduction in effective blood volume and by an increase in tubular sodium chloride reabsorption produced by the activation of the renin–angiotensin–aldosterone system. Most serum lipids (including cholesterol and triglycerides) and levels of lipoprotein are elevated because hypoproteinemia stimulates hepatic lipoprotein synthesis; lipid metabolism is diminished.

## Minimal Change Nephrotic Syndrome of Childhood

Minimal change nephrotic syndrome (MCNS) is the most common form of the nephrotic syndrome (80% of cases). There is a male preponderance of 2:1. Typical nephrotic syndrome is defined as absence of persistent hematuria, renal insufficiency, hypertension, and hypocomplementemia. Dependent pitting edema (pretibial, pedal, sacral, scrotal, labial, periorbital) with weight gain or ascites is the most common presentation of nephrotic syndrome. Diarrhea (intestinal edema) or respiratory distress (pulmonary edema, pleural effusion) also may be present. Serum cholesterol usually is elevated and often markedly so ($>400$ mg/dL).

Of all childhood patients having MCNS, children 1–7 yr old are very likely to have steroid-responsive MCNS (87%) and, therefore, corticosteroid therapy may be initiated without performing renal biopsy if the presentation is typical. Children 7–16 yr of age still have a 50% chance of having MCNS on the basis of age alone, and if the children in this age group have a "typical" nephrotic syndrome, a trial of steroid therapy is indicated, because prednisone responsiveness increases the chance of MCNS to 86%.

*Management.* If a child has the typical nephrotic syndrome, *treatment* consists of efforts to reduce edema and specific therapy with prednisone. The child who has a newly developed nephrotic syndrome usually requires hospitalization for diagnostic and therapeutic purposes.

The **edema** of the nephrotic syndrome is treated by restricting salt and water intake; by occasionally optimizing the excretion of these elements with the administration of diuretics; and, if the patient is refractory to diuretics alone, by increasing plasma volume. Sodium chloride intake should be restricted beyond a "no added salt" diet (<2 g Na per 24 hr). This salt restriction may be relaxed when the edema has resolved. At times, moderate fluid restriction is helpful. Diuretics may be required but should be given carefully because their overzealous use may further diminish plasma volume, resulting in hypotension and a fall in GFR.

Potassium supplementation may have to be provided if GFR is normal because considerable urine potassium can be lost as a result of a combination of secondary hyperaldosteronism and diuretic therapy. Hydrochlorothiazide often is effective in treating edema of the nephrotic syndrome unless the serum albumin is quite low or the GFR is impaired. If the GFR is normal, spironolactone may be added to minimize potassium losses. Furosemide generally is effective in inducing diuresis and natriuresis despite moderately decreased GFR and hypoalbuminemia. The administration of furosemide should be started with relatively small doses (1–2 mg/kg), and the patient should be monitored closely for volume depletion and electrolyte disturbances; occasionally even furosemide may be relatively ineffective in alleviating severe hypoalbuminemia in children. In these children, cautious volume expansion with salt-poor albumin (0.5 g/kg IV over 1–2 hr with furosemide 1–2 mg/kg) intravenously, infused during or immediately following albumin, usually results in diuresis. This therapy may be repeated once or twice as needed. The infused albumin will be excreted rapidly (1–2 days) by patients with the nephrotic syndrome. Once adequate volume expansion has been achieved, further therapy with furosemide alone may suffice. Albumin should be given only in the presence of volume contraction, and the patient should be monitored closely for excessive volume expansion, which could lead to congestive cardiac failure.

*Specific therapy* is the administration of predni-

sone in a dosage of 2 mg/kg/day (60 mg/m²/24 hr) divided into two to four doses per day. Approximately 10% of patients respond (urine protein becoming negative or reduced to trace levels) by the end of 1 wk, 70% by the end of 2 wk, 85% by the end of 3 wk, and 92% by the end of 4 wk of therapy. The basics of therapy include continuing the above dose until the urine protein on dipstick is negative or trace for 4 consecutive days or for up to a full 4 wk, whichever occurs first. At that point, the patient is switched to an every-other-day dosage at 60 mg/m². Prednisone should be given once on the dosage day for 2 to 4 wk, then a tapering schedule should be provided to have the patient discontinue receiving prednisone within another 4 wk.

If a child does not respond to daily prednisone therapy, a renal biopsy is indicated because steroid resistance greatly increases the chance that the underlying pathology is other than MCNS. In these circumstances, the diagnosis most likely will be focal segmental glomerulosclerosis, mesangiocapillary (membranoproliferative) glomerulonephritis, or membranous nephropathy.

The treatment of each relapse of the nephrotic syndrome is similar to that given during the initial therapy. A relapse is defined either as persistent proteinuria for greater than 7 days in the absence of a respiratory infection or other intercurrent infection, or as the recurrence of edema. The definition is not simply the recurrence of proteinuria, because during an upper respiratory infection many children with the nephrotic syndrome will have transient proteinuria that resolves spontaneously. Frequent relapses or steroid resistance may require immunosuppressant therapy (cyclophosphamide, chlorambucil, cyclosporine).

*Complications.* Infection is a major complication in children with the nephrotic syndrome (Table 16–18). Bacteremia and peritonitis, particularly with *Streptococcus pneumoniae* or *E. coli*, may occur. A high index of suspicion and prompt evaluation is indicated in a febrile patient. Side effects of

TABLE 16–18.    Complications of Nephrotic Syndrome

Acute renal failure
Hypertension
Hypercoagulable state (renal vein thrombosis, pulmonary embolism)
Spontaneous bacterial peritonitis
Malnutrition
Exacerbation by immunization
Steroid-related toxicity
Antimetabolite-related toxicity

steroids are most common in initial nonresponders and frequently relapsing patients.

### Focal Segmental Glomerulosclerosis

The presentation of focal segmental glomerulosclerosis (FSGS) may be identical to that of MCNS. In some cases, FSGS is thought to progress from MCNS, but in most circumstances it appears to be a separate entity. A circulating factor that increases glomerular permeability to albumin is found in some patients with FSGS. FSGS accounts for approximately 10% of children with the nephrotic syndrome. More than 80% of these patients are *steroid-resistant*, and even those who initially respond frequently become steroid-resistant subsequently. No clearly effective therapy for FSGS exists, although treatment with intravenous pulse methylprednisolone immunosuppressive agents (cyclophosphamide, cyclosporine, and FK506) may produce remission in some patients and alleviate edema in others. Unfortunately, a considerable number of these patients progress to end-stage renal disease within 2–5 yr. Children with FSGS who have progressed to end-stage renal disease and who have received kidney transplants also are more likely to have a recurrence in the transplanted kidney.

### Membranous Nephropathy

Membranous nephropathy is an infrequent cause of the nephrotic syndrome in childhood. Approximately 1% of children with the nephrotic syndrome have this lesion. It is seen most commonly in adolescents and in children who have potentially curable systemic diseases such as hepatitis B, syphilis, malaria, and toxoplasmosis and as a result of drug therapy (gold salts, penicillamine). These patients may present with the nephrotic syndrome or with proteinuria only. Hematuria is common. The presence of proteinuria in a patient with one of the predisposing diseases indicates a renal biopsy.

### Other Types of Nephrotic Syndrome

The nephrotic syndrome has been diagnosed in patients during therapy with penicillamine, gold, mercury compounds, and other drugs. It also has been described in association with several extrarenal neoplasms, such as lymphomas (particularly Hodgkin disease).

The **congenital nephrotic syndrome** appears in two forms during the first 6 mo of life. The Finnish type is an autosomal recessive disorder most common in persons of Scandinavian descent. Prenatal

diagnosis may be possible by detecting elevated amniotic fluid alpha-fetoprotein; the placenta is enlarged. Proteinuria characteristically is present at birth, and the nephrotic syndrome becomes apparent within the first 3 mo. Unfortunately, most of these children have died as a result of infection or renal failure by the age of 5 yr. Renal transplantation may be of value. The other type of congenital nephrotic syndrome is a heterogeneous group of abnormalities mostly associated with drugs or infections, such as syphilis and toxoplasmosis.

### References

Behrman RE, Kliegman RM, Arvin AM (eds): Nelson Textbook of Pediatrics, 15th ed. Philadelphia, WB Saunders, 1996, Chapters 466, 468, 478, 481.
Brodehl J: The treatment of minimal change nephrotic syndrome. Eur J Pediatr 150:380, 1991.
Cameron JS: Membraneous nephropathy in childhood and its treatment. Pediatr Nephrol 4:193, 1990.
Hebib R: Nephrotic syndrome in the first year of life. Pediatr Nephrol 7:347, 1993.
International Study of Kidney Diseases in Children: Minimal change nephrotic syndrome in children: Deaths during the first 5–15 years of observation. Pediatrics 73:497, 1984.
McAdams A, Valentini R, Welch T: The nonspecificity of focal segmental glomerulosclerosis. Medicine 76:42, 1997.
Melvin T, Bennett W: Management of nephrotic syndrome in childhood. Drugs 42:30, 1991.
Mendoza SA, Ture BM: Management of the difficult nephrotic patient. Pediatr Clin North Am 42:1459, 1995.
Southwest Pediatric Nephrology Study Group: Focal segmental glomerulosclerosis in children with idiopathic nephrotic syndrome. Kidney Int 27:442, 1985.

## ACUTE RENAL FAILURE

A significant decrease in GFR or in tubular function is designated as acute renal failure, which generally is associated with a GFR that is reduced sufficiently so that waste products (urea, phosphate) and water cannot be excreted and body fluid homeostasis is altered. Early recognition and management are critical.

***Etiology and Pathophysiology.*** The major causes of acute renal insufficiency are listed in Table 16–19. *Prerenal renal failure* characteristically occurs when the circulating blood volume decreases, hypotension is present, or the effective blood volume decreases. Under these conditions, dehydration produced by vomiting, diarrhea, or a markedly increased insensible water loss can lead to hypovolemia. However, if the underlying cause of inadequate renal perfusion is reversed, renal function usually returns to normal. If the inadequate circulation persists, intrinsic renal damage supervenes.

*Postrenal renal failure* characteristically is obstruc-

TABLE 16–19.   Causes of Acute Renal Failure

| Prerenal/Hypovolemia/Hypotension | Intrinsic |
|---|---|
| Dehydration | Acute tubular necrosis |
|   Vomiting |   Prolonged hypotension secondary to |
|   Diarrhea |     Vomiting |
|   Febrile illness |     Diarrhea |
|   Massive reduction in colloid oncotic pressure |     Shock |
|     (protein-losing enteropathy, nephrotic syndrome) |   Nephrotoxins (drugs) |
| Septic shock | Glomerulonephritis |
| Heart failure |   Primary (poststreptococcal) |
| Hemorrhage |   Secondary (systemic lupus erythematosus, |
| Burns |     endocarditis) |
| Peritonitis, ascites, cirrhosis | Interstitial nephritis |
| |   Primary |
| **Postrenal (Obstruction)** |   Secondary |
| Urethral obstruction |     Drugs (allergic) |
|   Stricture |     Toxins |
|   Posterior urethral valves | Vascular |
|   Diverticulum |   Renal vein thrombosis |
|   Phimosis |   Arterial thromboemboli (umbilical artery catheter) |
| Ureteral obstruction |   Acute tubular necrosis |
|   Calculi |   Acute cortical necrosis |
|   Crystals (drugs, urate) |   Disseminated intravascular coagulation |
|   Papillary necrosis |   Immune-mediated (scleroderma) |
|   Clotted blood | Pigmenturia |
|   Tumor |   Hemoglobinuria |
| Ureterocele |   Myoglobinuria |
| Solitary renal unit with ureterovesical or ureteropelvic | |
|   junction obstruction | |
| Extrinsic tumor compressing bladder outlet | |
| Extrinsic urinary tract tumors | |
| Neurogenic bladder | |
| Tumor lysis syndrome | |

tive in nature. Correcting or temporarily bypassing the obstruction will restore renal function unless renal parenchymal damage also has occurred. *Intrinsic renal failure* may be caused by vascular, immunologic, inflammatory, ischemic, or toxic injury to the kidney.

***Acute Tubular Necrosis.*** Two principal mechanisms have been suggested to explain the renal failure exhibited in acute tubular necrosis. One hypothesis suggests that tubular injury caused by one of the conditions listed in Table 16–19 results in decreased reabsorption of solutes and water. Thus, increased delivery of salt and water to the distal nephron is present, which stimulates the intrinsic renin-angiotensin system and tubuloglomerular feedback. The release of vasoactive substances produces increased cortical vascular resistance, which decreases cortical blood flow and produces further tubular injury. In addition, the release of vasoactive substances results in a diminished GFR, and, when severe, acute renal failure. A second hypothesis suggests that tubular injury results in tubular cell necrosis. Necrotic materials produce intratubular obstruction, raising intratubular resistance and thereby diminishing net glomerular filtration and

tubular flow, which results in acute renal failure. In addition, the cellular necrosis results in loss of integrity of the renal tubule, with backleak of solute and fluid leading to reabsorption of most of the glomerular ultrafiltrate. Evidence exists for each of these theories, and probably both play a role in the pathophysiology of acute renal failure.

Severe vascular compromise may lead to arterial or venous thrombosis or to *acute cortical necrosis.* Whereas acute tubular necrosis commonly is reversible, acute cortical necrosis results in eventual scarring of the damaged glomeruli and permanent loss of renal function.

***Diagnosis.*** History, physical examination, and laboratory data are helpful in evaluating the child with acute renal failure (Table 16–20).

The child with a *prerenal* cause of renal failure frequently has evidence of a precipitating illness associated with vomiting and diarrhea or an inadequate oral intake, or has a history of one of the predisposing factors (see Table 16–19). The physical examination may show signs of dehydration accompanied by decreased weight, decreased skin turgor, and perhaps tachycardia and hypotension. Mucous membranes of the mouth may be dry, and

TABLE 16–20.  Laboratory Differential Diagnosis of Renal Insufficiency

| | Prerenal | | Renal | | |
|---|---|---|---|---|---|
| | *Child* | *Neonate* | *Child* | *Neonate* | *Postrenal* |
| Urine Na$^+$ (mEq/L) | <20 | <20–30 | >40 | >40 | Variable, may be >40 |
| FE$_{Na}$* (%) | <1 | <2–5 | >2 | >2–5 | Variable, may be >2 |
| Urine osmolality (mOsm/L) | >500 | >300–500 | ~300 | ~300 | Variable, may be <300 |
| RFI† (%) | <1 | <2–5 | >2 | >2–5 | Variable |
| Serum BUN/creatinine | >20 | ≥10 | ~10 | ≥10 | Variable, may be >20 |
| Response to volume | Diuresis | | No change | | No change |
| Response to furosemide | Diuresis | | No change | | No change/diuresis |
| Urinalysis | Normal | | RBC, WBC, casts, proteinuria | | Variable/normal, possible crystals |
| Comments | Hx: diarrhea, vomiting, hemorrhage, diuretics Px: volume depletion | | Hx: hypotension, anoxia, exposure to nephrotoxins Px: hypertension, edema | | Hx: poor urine stream/ output Px: Flank mass, distended bladder |

*FE$_{Na}$ = fractional excretion of sodium (%) = (urine sodium/plasma sodium ÷ urine creatinine/plasma creatinine) × 100.
†RFI = renal failure index = (urine sodium ÷ urine creatinine/plasma creatinine) × 100.
BUN = blood urea nitrogen; Hx = history; Px = physical signs; RBC = red blood cells; WBC = white blood cells.

CNS signs of poor perfusion, such as irritability or lethargy, may be present. Urine volume characteristically is decreased.

*Oliguric renal failure* in adults is defined as less than 500 mL/day; oliguria in children is defined as less than 1–2 mL/kg/hr. *Nonoliguric renal failure* may occur and often is complicated by fluid and electrolyte disturbances in addition to azotemia. Urinary osmolality is significantly greater than serum osmolality. Measurement of urinary sodium usually reveals a sodium concentration between 20 mEq/L and 40 mEq/L, and the fractional excretion of sodium (urine to plasma sodium divided by urine to plasma creatinine multiplied by 100) is usually between 1% and 2%. This is expressed as

$$\frac{U/p\ Na}{U/p\ creatinine} \times 100$$

Urinalysis reveals a high specific gravity and, frequently, the absence or rare finding of cellular elements.

*Postrenal renal failure* often is found in early infancy and is associated with an obstructive lesion. Physical findings of dehydration are absent. Urinary output may be decreased, normal, or increased. Urinary osmolality frequently is similar to that of plasma, urinary sodium concentration often is greater than 50 mEq/L, and fractional excretion of sodium is greater than 10%. Urinalysis reveals no sediment abnormalities. Renal ultrasonography, a voiding cystourethrogram, or a radionuclide scan is a useful test in assessing the possibility of postrenal failure.

The child with *intrinsic renal failure* may have a history compatible with one of the predisposing conditions. Physical examination may show signs of adequate, increased, or decreased fluid balance. Papilledema, hypertension, cardiac enlargement, or a gallop rhythm may be present that suggests vascular overload. Signs of systemic involvement resulting from underlying disease may be noted (e.g., in SLE, Henoch-Schönlein purpura, HUS). Urine output characteristically is decreased. Urinary osmolality may be isotonic, hypotonic, or hypertonic. Urinary sodium concentration generally is increased, frequently greater than 40 mEq/L, and the fractional excretion of sodium is greater than 1%. Urinalysis usually contains red cell and granular casts. Usually, hematuria and proteinuria and, sometimes, leukocyturia are exhibited. C3 complement may be depressed in acute poststreptococcal glomerulonephritis, SLE, or membranoproliferative (mesangiocapillary) glomerulonephritis. Evidence of an earlier infection may be present, which can be demonstrated by the presence of a positive streptozyme or hepatitis B surface antigen. Anemia and thrombocytopenia may be present in conditions such as SLE or HUS. A chest roentgenogram may reveal evidence of pulmonary edema and cardiomegaly, suggesting vascular overload.

*Treatment.* Treatment depends on the cause of acute renal insufficiency, although certain modalities commonly are used for many children with acute renal failure. The first step is to develop a plan of comprehensive monitoring. The patient should be weighed at least at 12-hr intervals to determine fluid balance because acute weight changes reflect water loss or gain. Initial fluid and electrolyte therapy and a plan for frequent re-evaluation should be established. Urine output and electrolyte composition should be determined frequently during the acute phase.

Reversible conditions that can be treated should be given prompt attention. Obstructions of the urinary tract should be corrected or bypassed. Infection and/or shock should be treated. Hypovolemia should be corrected promptly. Dopamine may improve renal blood flow in low doses and is effective in various states of poor cardiac output. In addition, dobutamine may improve renal perfusion by enhancing myocardial contractility. Atrial natriuretic peptide administration may benefit some patients having oliguric acute tubular necrosis. If the presence of severe, intrinsic renal failure is in question, a catheter may be placed into the bladder to assess whether urine is present and to remove the urine promptly. If acute renal failure is present, there is no advantage in monitoring small volumes of urinary output, and a urinary catheter may predispose to infection.

*FLUID REQUIREMENTS.* The degree of dehydration should be estimated. If hypovolemia is apparent, intravascular volume should be expanded by intravenous administration of physiologic saline (0.9% sodium chloride); 20 mL/kg is given intravenously over 30–60 min. Once volume depletion has been corrected, an intravenous dose of furosemide, 2 mg/kg, in the presence of anuria is reasonable. If urinary output is not increased, a second dose of furosemide may be given. If no response occurs, further infusion generally is not helpful and increases the risk of ototoxicity.

If the patient shows evidence of excessive weight gain or fluid overload, fluid intake should be reduced to insensible water loss, plus urinary and stool output, plus any fluid drainage (nasogastric tube), minus a planned weight loss. Patients who have acute renal failure are catabolic and lose approximately 1% of body weight/day in the form of tissue losses and not as fluid losses. When the patient maintains weight in the presence of acute renal failure, this generally indicates fluid retention. Diuretics should be used as initial therapy to mobilize retained fluids. Severe fluid overload in the presence of marked oliguria or anuria is one indication for dialysis.

*HYPERKALEMIA.* This condition is often seen in patients with acute renal failure resulting from the absence of potassium excretion and catabolism. High-potassium–containing foods, fluids, and medications should be restricted until renal function is re-established. Lead II of the electrocardiogram is useful for assessing cardiac changes due to hyperkalemia (see Disturbances of Electrolytes, Acid-Base Balance, and Fluids). The presence of hyperkalemia requires immediate attention. Severe hyperkalemia is an indication for dialysis.

*ACIDOSIS.* Acidosis is common in renal failure as a consequence of catabolism and the inability of the failed kidney to secrete hydrogen ion. When severe, intravenous sodium bicarbonate should be administered as noted above, but should be given cautiously in order to avoid fluid overload, hypernatremia, and hypertension. Severe or unrelenting acidosis is an indication for dialysis.

*HYPOCALCEMIA.* Hypocalcemia is seen commonly in acute renal failure in association with hyperphosphatemia. *Treatment* primarily involves efforts to lower the serum phosphorus level. Milk and other high-phosphorus foods are severely limited, and oral calcium carbonate is given to bind phosphorus. Aluminum hydroxide gels previously used to treat hyperphosphatemia have been associated with aluminum intoxication (dementia, rickets). If the patient shows evidence of tetany, an intravenous infusion of 10% calcium gluconate (0.5 mL/kg) may be given slowly.

*CALORIC NEEDS.* It is important to maintain an adequate caloric intake in patients with acute renal failure in order to minimize catabolism. At least 70% of the recommended daily allowance of calories and 0.5–1.0 g of high-quality protein/kg/day should be provided.

*DIALYSIS.* In children with renal insufficiency, dialysis is indicated in order to treat (1) hyperkalemia unresponsive to medical therapy, (2) acidosis unresponsive to medical therapy, (3) hyperkalemia or acidosis in the presence of hypernatremia, (4) fluid overload unresponsive to fluid restriction or to diuretics, or (5) symptoms and signs of "uremia." The method used may be peritoneal dialysis, hemodialysis, or a modification of hemodialysis, such as hemoperfusion or hemofiltration.

*Complications.* The most serious potential complications of acute renal failure are infections, vascular overload, and hyperkalemia. Other potential complications are uremic encephalopathy, seizures, pericardial effusion, hypertension, peptic ulceration, platelet dysfunction, and anemia. In addition, careful monitoring of blood levels of drugs excreted by the kidney and appropriately adjusting either the total dose or the dosing interval are necessary to avoid toxicity (e.g., acyclovir, aminoglycosides, penicillins, cephalosporins, vancomycin, ranitidine, digoxin). The recovery phase of obstructive renal failure and acute tubular necrosis may be complicated by a polyuric phase associated with poor concentrating ability and hypokalemia, or hyperkalemia. The plan of management that minimizes the use of urinary catheters, avoids fluid overload and electrolyte excess, and effectively treats hyperkalemia generally is rewarded by the patient's recovery.

*Prognosis.* Recovery depends on the etiology of acute renal failure. Prerenal failure, postrenal failure, and intrinsic renal failure are reversible in most types of renal disease. In patients with acute tubular necrosis, the period of anuria/oliguria usually lasts 7–10 days and is followed by 2–7 days of polyuria. With good supportive care and steady monitoring, all patients should recover from acute tubular necrosis. Lack of improvement suggests acute cortical necrosis or some other cause. Renal failure associated with RPGN, renal vascular thrombosis, and cortical necrosis may not be reversible and may require chronic dialysis and eventual renal transplantation.

### References

Allgren R, Marbury T, Rahman S, et al: Anaritide in acute tubular necrosis. NEVM 336:828, 1997.

Behrman RE, Kliegman RM, Arvin AM (eds): Nelson Textbook of Pediatrics, 15th ed. Philadelphia, WB Saunders, 1996, Chapters 487–489.

Gaudio KM, Siegal NJ: Pathogenesis and treatment of acute renal failure. Pediatr Clin North Am 34:771, 1987.

Thadhani R, Pascual M, Bonventre J: Acute renal failure. N Engl J Med 334:1448, 1996.

## CHRONIC RENAL FAILURE

*Etiology.* The cause of chronic renal failure in childhood is closely related to the age of the child at the time that renal failure occurs. Between birth and 10 yr of age, congenital and obstructive abnormalities are the most common causes. After age 10, acquired diseases, such as focal segmental glomerulosclerosis, chronic glomerulonephritis, reflux nephropathy, HUS, and progressive hereditary disorders (Alport syndrome, cystic disease), are likely causes of chronic renal failure. In each category, renal function progressively deteriorates and is accompanied by the contraction of the renal parenchyma with subsequent end-stage renal failure. The progression to end-stage renal failure is vari-

able and depends on features such as hyperfiltration, ongoing immunologic injury, proteinuria, hypertension, secondary hyperparathyroidism, and infection.

*Clinical Manifestations.* *Growth failure* in children with chronic renal failure is prominent. The factors associated with growth retardation include undernutrition, osteodystrophy, hormonal abnormalities, medications (e.g., steroids), and acidosis. Increased calorie intake leads to a slight increase in growth, but considerably more calories are needed than are necessary to achieve comparable growth in children with normal renal function. Children with chronic renal failure also have progressive anemia, frequently are hypertensive, are at increased risk for infection or CNS disturbances, and demonstrate severe osteodystrophy.

*Treatment.* The management of children with chronic renal failure and their complex problems requires a team of pediatric nephrologists, clinical nursing specialists, nutritionists, social workers, psychiatrists, psychologists, recreational and occupational therapists, and various other professionals.

DIET. Children with chronic renal insufficiency have diminished growth velocity and progressive retardation of bone age prior to puberty. They should be provided with more than 80% of the recommended dietary allowance of calories. Infants often require greater than 125% of the recommended daily allowance in order to achieve moderate growth. Protein should be provided at a level of 1.5 g/kg/24 hr and should consist of high-biologic-value proteins. Milk and milk products must be restricted because of its high phosphate content. In infants, a high-quality protein formula, such as PM60/40 (Ross Laboratories), used in conjunction with calcium carbonate as a phosphate binder, may be indicated. Supplemental calcium usually is necessary because the child must avoid milk products. Children with renal insufficiency also need vitamin supplementation because they become deficient in water-soluble vitamins.

To keep the serum bicarbonate in the 19–20 mEq/L range, acidosis should be treated with appropriate doses of sodium bicarbonate or sodium citrate (Bicitra). Water balance usually is maintained reasonably well until dialysis is required, and, therefore, water restriction rarely is necessary. A "no added salt" diet will provide adequate but not excessive sodium intake, although, as a consequence of obstructive uropathies, some children with renal insufficiency may be salt wasters, thus requiring increased salt intake. Patients with intrinsic renal disease usually have hypertension, for which salt restriction is needed. High-potassium foods should be avoided once renal failure is established.

*RENAL OSTEODYSTROPHY.* Renal osteodystrophy (most commonly, osteitis fibrosa) is a nearly constant accompaniment of chronic renal failure and is associated with hyperphosphatemia, high serum alkaline phosphatase activity, and secondary hyperparathyroidism. The initial therapy is to restrict phosphate in the diet, most commonly by restricting milk and milk products. In addition, calcium carbonate may be used to bind phosphate in the gastrointestinal tract. The phosphate level should be kept in the 5–6 mg/dL range to minimize secondary hyperparathyroidism while providing enough phosphate for new bone formation. Because milk restriction leads to inadequate calcium intake, a child should receive approximately 1 g of elemental calcium from all sources per day. Because that is not provided in the diet, calcium gluconate supplements should be given.

Chronic renal failure is associated with an inability of the kidney to convert 25-hydroxycholecalciferol to 1,25-dihydroxycholecalciferol. Therapy with either synthetic vitamin D (dihydrotachysterol) or 1,25-dihydroxycholecalciferol usually is necessary.

*ANEMIA.* Anemia is a common finding in chronic renal failure in children. There is an ongoing debate as to whether the anemia results primarily from toxic depression of erythropoiesis by abnormal or retained metabolites or from a failure of the kidney to produce erythropoietin in response to anemia. Reduced serum iron and elevated iron-binding capacity are common but do not indicate iron deficiency because the anemia is normochromic and normocytic and the ferritin levels are normal or elevated. Tranfusions are rarely needed if recombinant-produced erythropoietin is administered.

*GROWTH.* Therapy with recombinant-produced growth hormone is useful in children having chronic renal failure or receiving dialysis. Accelerated growth occurs with pharmacologic doses of human growth hormone.

***Treatment of End-Stage Renal Failure.*** The principal treatment of end-stage renal failure is *renal transplantation.* Cadaver donors and living related donors have been used extensively for renal transplantation. Children with progressive renal failure should be referred to a center specializing in renal transplantation for children for evaluation. Thoroughly evaluating the cause of chronic renal failure, listing potential donors, and beginning to prepare the family and child for dialysis and transplantation should be begun before the threat of end-stage renal failure becomes immediate.

*Dialysis* is effective for sustaining the patient who is awaiting renal transplantation or in whom renal transplantation is not possible. Few children are given hemodialysis as the preferential mode of dialysis. The development of continuous ambulatory peritoneal dialysis (CAPD) and continuous cycling peritoneal dialysis (CCPD) has made chronic dialysis an effective and well-tolerated technique during the necessary time prior to transplantation. The principal complication of peritoneal dialysis is peritoneal infection, especially with staphylococcus *(S. epidermidis* or *S. aureus).* Because of improved techniques used in dialysis and immunosuppressive drugs used for transplantation (e.g., cyclosporine), the outlook for children with end-stage renal disease is encouraging. Patient and graft survival are highest in pediatric patients beyond infancy.

## References

Behrman RE, Kliegman RM, Arvin AM (eds): Nelson Textbook of Pediatrics. 15th ed. Philadelphia, WB Saunders, 1996, Chapters 489–498.

Bereket G, Fine RN: Pediatric renal transplantation. Pediatr Clin North Am 42:1603, 1995.

Evans ED, Greenough LA, Etterger RB: Principles of renal replacement therapy in children. Pediatr Clin North Am 42:1579, 1995.

Fine R, Salusky I, Ettenger R: The therapeutic approach to the infant, children and adolescent with end-stage renal disease. Pediatr Clin North Am 34:789, 1987.

Warady BA, Johns K: New hormones in the therapeutic arsenal of chronic renal failure: Growth hormone and erythropoietin. Pediatr Clin North Am 42:1551, 1995.

## HYPERTENSION

Systolic and diastolic blood pressure values increase gradually between birth and 18 yr of age. During this period and adulthood, most patients "track" in a constant percentile around the mean. The younger the hypertensive patient, the greater the chance the hypertension will be secondary to another disease rather than being essential.

***Etiology.*** Hypertension in children may be due to renal (Table 16–21), endocrine (Table 16–22), vascular (Table 16–23), and neurologic (Table 16–24) disorders and to miscellaneous disorders, such as essential hypertension, drugs or foods (steroids, licorice), or prolonged immobilization.

***Clinical Manifestations.*** The signs and symptoms of hypertension include heart failure, stroke, seizures, headache, coma, polyuria, oliguria, and blurred vision. However, many patients are asymptomatic, which emphasizes the importance of frequently obtaining a blood pressure reading from every infant and child. In young infants, blood pressure may be measured with the Dynamap ma-

TABLE 16–21.    Renal Causes of Hypertension

**Congenital Anomalies**

Dysplastic kidney
Polycystic disease
Obstructive uropathy

**Acquired Lesions**

Wilms tumor
Acute glomerulonephritis
Hemolytic-uremic syndrome
Henoch-Schönlein purpura
Systemic lupus erythematosus
Familial nephritis (Alport syndrome)
Reflux nephropathy
Segmental hypoplasia (Ask-Upmark kidney)
Drugs, toxins (cyclosporine, steroids, lead)

TABLE 16–23.    Vascular Causes of Hypertension

Coarctation of aorta
Postcoarctation repair
Renal artery embolism (neonate with umbilical artery catheter)
Renal vein thrombosis
Endocarditis
Renal artery stenosis
Fibromuscular dysplasia
Neurofibromatosis
Arteritis (Takayasu, periarteritis nodosa, aortoarteritis)
Sarcoidosis
Essential hypertension (etiology uncertain)

chine; in older patients, standard sphygmomanometry and auscultation are sufficient. Additional physical findings include papilledema, abdominal bruits (renovascular), arm blood pressure greater than leg pressure (aortic coarctation), *café-au-lait* spots (neurofibromatosis), flank masses (hydronephrosis, renal dysplasia, neuroblastoma, Wilms tumor), ataxia, opsoclonus (neuroblastoma), tachycardia, flushing, diaphoresis (pheochromocytoma), and truncal obesity, acne, striae, and buffalo hump (Cushing syndrome).

*Diagnosis.* The diagnostic evaluation of patients with hypertension includes urinalysis, blood urea nitrogen, creatinine, electrolytes, acid-base balance, chest roentgenogram, and renal ultrasound. Clues from the history, physical examination, mode of presentation, initial laboratory data, and age should determine the next sequence of tests. A renal radionuclide scan and the determination of plasma hormone levels (catecholamines, thyroxine, cortisol, renin) and urine hormone levels (vanillylmandelic acid, homovanillic acid, dopamine, steroid hormones) are more specific and noninvasive methods. These should be undertaken if the history or physical examination suggests the possibility. Finally, renal arteriography and renal biopsy are

invasive tests that may provide definitive diagnosis.

*Treatment.* Before treatment is initiated, it is important to determine whether the hypertension is persistent or intermittent; whether the measurements are accurate (appropriate-size blood pressure cuff); and that the hypertension is not compensatory, as occurs with increased intracranial pressure or as a result of a coarctation of the aorta.

For mild hypertension, dietary manipulation (decreased salt intake), weight loss (for obese patients), and exercise should be considered. If drug therapy is desired, starting with a low dose of a diuretic, such as thiazide, might be considered. All diuretic therapy has the drawback of causing potassium loss in the urine, which may necessitate potassium supplementation. Other medications used as first-line therapy for mild to moderate hypertension include calcium channel blockers (nifedipine), angiotensin-enzyme (ACE) inhibitors (captopril or enalapril), and beta blockers (propranolol, atenolol) or combined alpha and beta blockers (labetalol). The beta blockers are associated with the undesired side effects of lethargy and depression.

For severe hypertension, combined therapy (such as a diuretic and a calcium channel blocker), a diuretic and an ACE inhibitor, or perhaps all three options might be appropriate. Renovascular

TABLE 16–22.    Endocrine Causes of Hypertension

Neuroblastoma
Pheochromocytoma
Adrenal genital syndrome (11-hydroxylase deficiency)
Cushing syndrome
Hyperparathyroidism–hypercalcemia
Hyperaldosteronism
Hyperthyroidism
Diabetic nephropathy
Liddle syndrome

TABLE 16–24.    Neurologic Causes of Hypertension

Neurofibromatosis
Guillain-Barré syndrome
Subdural hemorrhage
Dysautonomia (Riley-Day syndrome)
Increased intracranial pressure (with bradycardia)
Poliomyelitis
Quadriplegia
Encephalitis
Stress, anxiety

hypertension, when amenable to treatment, can be managed with angioplasty or surgery on the involved vessel. Primary endocrine abnormalities or other primary diseases (coarctation of the aorta) require specific therapy. Hypertensive emergencies warrant intensive care and therapy with nifedipine, sodium nitroprusside, or labetolol.

*Prognosis.* The prognosis depends on the primary disorder. Essential hypertension, when present in adolescents and not associated with morbidity at presentation, contributes to the cardiovascular, CNS, and renal morbidity associated with hypertension in older patients.

## References

Behrman RE, Kliegman RM, Arvin AM (eds): Nelson Textbook of Pediatrics. 15th ed. Philadelphia, WB Saunders, 1996, Chapter 404.
Harshfield GA, Alpert BS, Pullman DA, et al: Ambulatory blood pressure readings in children and adults. Pediatrics 94:180, 1994.
Sinaiko A: Hypertension in children. N Engl J Med 335:1968, 1996.
Tyagi S, Kaul U, Satsangi D, et al: Percutaneous transluminal angioplasty for renovascular hypertension in children: Initial and long term results. Pediatrics 99:44, 1997.

# GENITAL DISORDERS

## ANOMALIES OF THE PENIS

### Hypospadias

Hypospadias occurs in approximately 1:500 newborn infants. The urethral meatus is located below and proximal to its normal position, an abnormality resulting from a failure of the urethral folds to fuse completely over the urethral groove. The ventral foreskin also is lacking, while the dorsal portion gives the appearance of a hood.

*Chordee* is a term for a ventral curvature of the penile shaft. The meatus may be on the glans or at any point along the penis to the penile-scrotal junction. Rarely, the urethra opens onto the perineum. In this circumstance, the chordee is extreme, and the scrotum is biphid and sometimes extends to the dorsal base of the penis. Testes are undescended in 10% of boys with hypospadias, and inguinal hernias are common.

The *differential diagnosis* of severe hypospadias with undescended testes must include the various causes of ambiguous genitalia (e.g., congenital adrenal hyperplasia, masculinization of females). The frequency of other anomalies of the urinary tract in males with hypospadias is relatively low, except

in those whose urethral opening is very close to the penile-scrotal junction.

Males with hypospadias should not be circumcised because the foreskin often is necessary for later repair. The ideal age of repair remains controversial, although most pediatric urologists tend to operate before the patient is 18 mo of age.

### Phimosis

In 90% of uncircumcised male infants, the prepuce becomes retractable by the age of 3 yr, but after this age, the inability to retract the prepuce is termed phimosis. The condition may be congenital or a sequela to inflammation. Severe phimosis usually requires surgical enlargement of the opening or circumcision. Accumulation of smegma is not pathologic and does not require surgical treatment. *Paraphimosis* occurs when the prepuce is retracted behind the coronal sulcus and cannot be returned to its normal position, which usually is due to venous stasis and edema and leads to severe pain. Occasionally, when the condition is discovered early, reduction of the foreskin is possible with lubrication. In some cases, circumcision is needed.

## DISORDERS AND ABNORMALITIES OF THE SCROTUM AND ITS CONTENTS

### Undescended Testes (Cryptorchidism)

Undescended testes are found in 0.7% of children after 1 yr of age. The frequency is higher in full-term newborn infants (3.4%) than in older children. In cases discovered at birth, the percentage increases with prematurity (17% in infants with birth weights between 2000 and 2500 g and 100% in infants weighing less than 900 g). Although spontaneous testicular descent does not occur beyond the age of 1 yr, failure to find one or both testes in the scrotum does not necessarily indicate undescended testicles.

*Retractile testes,* absent testes, and ectopic testes also may be the cause of cryptorchidism. The true undescended testis is found along the path of normal descent, usually with a patent processus vaginalis. The undescended testis commonly is associated with an *inguinal hernia*; it also is subject to *torsion.* A higher incidence of infertility in adulthood, a risk of development of tumor in the undescended testis, and untoward psychologic effects in adolescence and adulthood are associated with the condition. Cryptorchidism is bilateral in up to 30% of reported cases. Infertility is uniform in adults with untreated bilateral cryptorchidism. Because infertility also is common in adults with a history of unilateral undescended testicle, the contralateral descended testis may also be abnormal.

The undescended testis usually is histologically normal at birth, but atrophy and poor development are found by the end of 1 yr. Although cryptorchidism is still a subject of controversy, reports indicate that surgical correction at an early age results in a greater probability of fertility in adulthood. Stimulation with human chorionic gonadotropin (hCG) results in testosterone release from functioning testes. This helps in consideration of exploration for abdominal testes and often results in descent of retractile testes. The development of a malignant tumor in the cryptorchid testis has been reported to occur 20–44% of the time, usually in the third or four decade of life. The greatest risk seems to be in those who are untreated or who underwent surgical correction during or after puberty.

**Indirect inguinal hernias** accompany undescended testes and also are seen frequently with ectopic testes. Torsion, with or without infarction, may occur and probably is related to excessive mobility of these testes. *Orchidopexy* usually is undertaken in the 2nd yr of life. Most testes that are extra-abdominal can be brought into the scrotum when the associated hernia is corrected. If the testis is not palpable, ultrasonography may determine its location. The closer the testis is to the internal inguinal ring, the better the chance of successful orchidopexy.

### Retractile Testes

Retractile testes are normal testes that have retracted into the inguinal canal as a result of an exaggeration of the cremasteric reflex. The *diagnosis* of retractile testes is likely if testes are palpable in the newborn examination but not at a later examination. Retractile testes frequently can be identified and brought into the scrotum by palpation when the child is warm and relaxed, and they characteristically remain in the scrotum permanently with puberty. The retractile testis does not cause the complications commonly associated with a true undescended testis.

### Torsion of the Testis

Torsion is an emergency that requires prompt diagnosis and treatment. It accounts for approximately 40% of cases of acute scrotal pain and swelling at all ages and is the major etiologic factor in patients under the age of 6 yr. It usually is caused by an abnormal fixation of the testis to the scrotum. If the tunica vaginalis covers both the testis and the epididymis as well as the distal spermatic cord, the testis can rotate freely and torsion is facilitated. On examination, the swelling is apparent, tenderness is severe, and the cremasteric reflex is absent.

The *differential diagnosis* of torsion of the testes includes an incarcerated hernia and torsion of the testicular epididymal appendices. Torsion of the appendices is associated with point tenderness over the lesion and minimal swelling. In adolescence, the differential diagnosis of testicular torsion must also include **epididymitis.** Epididymitis is the most common cause of acute scrotal pain and swelling in older adolescents. The differential diagnosis frequently is helped by an antecedent history of sexual activity (infection with *Chlamydia, gonococcus*) or urinary tract infection (infection with *E. coli*). Testicular torsion must be considered as the principal diagnosis when severe acute testicular pain is present.

If radiologic studies are in doubt, prompt surgical exploration should be performed. If the testis is explored within 6 hr of torsion, the gonads will survive (in up to 90% of cases). The procedure is detorsion and fixation of the testis to the scrotum. The contralateral testis usually is fixed to the scrotum to prevent future torsion. If torsion of the appendices is found at the time of exploration, removal of the necrotic tissue is indicated.

### References

Behrman RE, Kliegman RM, Arvin AM (eds): Nelson Textbook of Pediatrics, 15th ed. Philadelphia, WB Saunders, 1996, Chapters 498–499.

Berkowitz GS, Lapinski RH, Dolgun SE, et al: Prevalence and natural history of cryptorchidism. Pediatrics 92:44, 1993.

Davenport M: Problems with the penis and prepuce. BMJ 312:299, 1996.

Fallon B, Welton M, Hawtrey C: Congenital anomalies associated with cryptorchidism. J Urol 127:91, 1987.

Study Group John Radcliffe Hospital. Cryptorchidism: A prospective study of 7500 consecutive male births 1984–1988. Arch Dis Child 67:892, 1992.

# URINARY TRACT INFECTION

Urinary tract infection (UTI) is the most common genitourinary disease of childhood.

*Clinical Manifestations.* The symptoms and signs of UTI vary markedly with age. *Neonates* commonly present with failure to thrive, feeding problems, diarrhea, vomiting, fever, and hyperbilirubinemia. The *1 mo–2 yr old infant* with a UTI usually has nonurinary tract manifestations, such as feeding problems, failure to thrive, diarrhea, and unexplained fever. This age group also presents with a UTI masquerading as gastrointestinal illness, such as "colic," irritability, and screaming periods. In the 1st mo of life, a male preponderance is seen in patients with UTI. The sex ratio of UTI has a female preponderance from the 2nd mo of life to adulthood. The *2–6 yr old child* may have gastrointestinal symptoms, but in this age group the classic signs of urinary tract infection, such as urgency, dysuria, frequency, and abdominal pain, begin to appear. The *6–18 yr old child* most commonly will have urgency, frequency, dysuria, and abdominal or flank pain. Urinary tract infections occur in 1–2% of school-aged girls. In all children, *unexplained fevers* and sustained abdominal symptoms without explanation are indicators to examine the urine and obtain a urine specimen for culture.

Congenital genitourinary tract abnormalities predispose patients to UTI, and UTI should be suspected when unexplained fevers or other symptoms are found in a child with these problems.

*Diagnosis.* The diagnosis of UTI is made by a *positive culture of bacteria* in the urine. The finding of any bacteria in urine obtained by bladder catheterization or by suprapubic bladder puncture indicates infection. A properly collected voided urine, promptly plated, that grows more than 100,000 colonies/mL of a single organism on quantitative bacterial culture has a 95% positive correlation with suprapubic aspiration. A count of less than $10^5$ bacterial colonies on a voided specimen has diminished value. The presence of *leukocytes* in the urine suggests that infection may be present in the symptomatic child, but an inflammatory disease, such as acute poststreptococcal glomerulonephritis, is associated with leukocyturia. *Blood* in the urine may be present in UTI, particularly in adolescent females, but the presence of blood or leukocytes in the urine is not diagnostic. The presence of numerous motile bacteria in a freshly voided and examined urine (uncentrifuged urine) specimen from symptomatic infants and children has a 94% correlation with a positive culture of a suprapubic aspiration. The presence of even scant bacteria has an 82% correlation with a positive suprapubic aspiration. A delay of 1–2 hr in the examination of a voided specimen frequently will lead to bacterial multiplication and, hence, to a false impression of infection.

The most common cause of bacteriuria in the absence of a UTI is contamination of the urine by periurethral and anterior urethral flora. Colony counts will be low, however, if the urine is plated for culture promptly. In a few cases, bacterial colony counts of less than 100,000 on a voided specimen occur when a UTI is present. This may happen in the very well-hydrated child who is voiding frequently and has a dilute urine. It also may occur if the child has received recent antimicrobial therapy or if bacterial inhibitors are present. Fewer than $10^5$ bacterial colonies also may be seen when UTI is caused by fastidious organisms (e.g., tuberculosis).

*Localization* of a UTI is important because infection of the upper urinary tract is associated more frequently with anatomic abnormalities than is infection of the lower urinary tract. Unfortunately, the clinical presentation is of limited help in determining the site of infection in neonates, infants, and toddlers. Fever and abdominal pain can occur with either lower or upper UTI, although high fevers favor upper tract involvement. Direct methods of investigation, such as bladder washout specimens, usually are contraindicated because of their invasiveness. Indirect methods, including examining the urine for glitter cell and white cell casts (which, if present, indicate upper tract infection), finding evidence of an inability to maximally concentrate the urine, finding antibody-coated bacteria measured by immunofluorescence, beta$_2$-microglobulin excretion in 24-hr urine collections, and performing lactic dehydrogenase differential excretion all have been suggested, but these are of limited practical value in differentiating upper from lower UTIs. A high erythrocyte sedimentation rate (ESR), leukocytosis, and bacteremia are noted in pyelonephritis. Nephromegaly as seen with ultrasonography or renal scan suggests pyelonephritis more than other tests.

*Predisposing Factors.* The short urethra in girls predisposes them to UTI. Uncircumcised male infants are also at risk for UTI. The *E. coli* serotypes from bowel flora frequently are found in UTI. Furthermore, certain strains of bacteria have increased adherence to uroepithelial cells, which correlates with the presence of bacterial pili. A hydronephrotic kidney, vesicoureteral reflux, a poorly emptying bladder, congenital malformations, nephrolithiasis, and other factors leading to *urinary stasis* predispose the patient to UTI. The specific role of vesicoureteral reflux in the pathogenesis of UTI is unclear. A high incidence of vesicoureteral reflux is reported in association with UTI, but its pathogenic significance remains unclear. However, the presence of vesicoureteral reflux and infection is a predisposing factor for chronic infection and renal scarring. Nonetheless, scarring may occur without reflux.

The most common bacteria isolated from symptomatic or asymptomatic children experiencing their first UTI, occurring at any age and in both boys and girls, is *E. coli*. Other organisms, such as

*Klebsiella, Proteus,* enterococci, and *Staphylococcus saprophyticus,* appear more frequently in the presence of obstruction or abnormalities of the urinary tract.

**Treatment.** UTI should be treated promptly. Neonates require 10–14 days of parenteral antibiotic therapy because UTI is often associated with bacteremia. Older children with acute cystitis should receive at least a 5–7 day course of oral antibiotic therapy. The most common therapy is with amoxicillin or trimethoprim/sulfamethoxazole. In children with high fevers, white cell casts, or other symptoms or signs of *acute pyelonephritis,* the initial use of broad-spectrum parenteral antibiotics is indicated. In children with pyelonephritis who do not have toxic symptoms, treatment includes a parenteral antibiotic, such as ampicillin or a cephalosporin. Patients who show evidence of toxicity (chills, high fever) often are treated with ampicillin and gentamicin (or another aminoglycoside) or a third-generation cephalosporin alone. Once systemic toxicity has resolved and the patient is afebrile, oral therapy with an agent to which the cultured organism is sensitive should be administered to complete at least 14 days of therapy. It is important to repeat the urine culture 4–7 days after the therapy is discontinued because many relapses are asymptomatic. UTI has a tendency to recur, even without predisposing factors. Follow-up urine specimens should also be obtained for culture after recurrent cystitis or pyelonephritis, first at 1-mo intervals and subsequently at 3-mo intervals for at least 1 yr.

**Follow-up Evaluation of the Urinary Tract.** The decision as to whether to perform a work-up following UTI depends on the likelihood that complicating abnormalities are present. A history of treatment failure, the presence of unusual organisms, growth disturbances, suspicion of an anomaly or abscess, and frequent recurrences suggest a more complex problem. The indications for radiologic evaluation include

1. All children under 10 yr of age.
2. UTI in any male.
3. UTI in a female over 10 yr of age who has signs of symptoms of pyelonephritis or who responds slowly to treatment.
4. Recurrent UTI in a prepubertal, nonsexually active female.

The timing of evaluation is important. If the patient has toxic symptoms, responds slowly or poorly to therapy, or has a mass or bladder distention, prompt nephrosonography and ultrasound of the bladder are indicated. If the symptoms are those of lower UTI and response is rapid, it is best to wait until the end of the acute therapy to perform a voiding cystourethrogram (VCUG). It is often useful to continue prophylactic therapy until the VCUG is completed (1–3 wk after the onset of the UTI). An experienced nephrosonographer can provide most of the important anatomic information by using renal ultrasound. However, small scars and slight calyceal dilations may be missed. Therefore, some suggest, in addition, a radionuclide study or IVP (see Vesicoureteral Reflux). A voiding cystourethrogram is essential to assess reflux, bladder wall thickness, and bladder emptying.

## References

Behrman RE, Kliegman RM, Arvin AM (eds): Nelson Textbook of Pediatrics, 15th ed. Philadelphia, WB Saunders, 1996, Chapter 492.

Benador D, Benador N, Slosman D, et al: Are young children at highest risk of renal sequelae after pyelonephritis? Lancet 349:17, 1997.

Hellerstein S: Urinary tract infection: Old and new concepts. Pediatr Clin North Am 42:1433, 1995.

Strife C, Gelfand M: Renal cortical scintigraphy: Effect on medical decision making in childhood urinary tract infection. J Pediatr 129:785, 1996.

# ENDOCRINE DISORDERS

Dennis M. Styne

Nicole S. Glaser

Endocrine systems usually operate with feedback loop control, thus allowing the level of endocrine defect to be identified by deduction. Endocrine disorders generally manifest in one of four ways:

1. By excess hormone in thyrotoxicosis, of thyroid hormone; if the excess is secondary to autonomous hormone secretion ($T_4$) by an end organ, the trophic hormone thyroid-stimulating hormone (TSH) will be suppressed.
2. By deficient hormone in hypothyroidism, of thyroid hormone; if the deficiency is at the target organ ($T_4$), the trophic hormone will be elevated (TSH).
3. By an abnormal response of target tissues to hormone (in testicular feminization syndrome, by resistance to male sex hormones).
4. By gland enlargement, which may cause effects as a result of size (in nonfunctioning pituitary adenoma, by neurologic signs and symptoms).

Because hormones are circulating biochemical messengers, the location of action classically is distant from the specialized organ (gland) of origin. Consequently, signs and symptoms of an endocrine disorder usually are related to the peripheral tissue's response to the hormone excess or deficiency. Indeed, functioning endocrine tumors frequently produce profound physiologic changes that reveal the pathologic process long before the appearance of signs and symptoms related to tumor mass. Hormone action also may be *paracrine* (acting on adjacent neighboring cells) or *autocrine* (acting on cell of origin) (Fig. 17–1).

*Peptide hormones* act through specific cell membrane receptors (Fig. 17–2). *Steroid hormones* work by attachment to intracellular receptors, which then translocate the hormone to the nucleus where

they interact with deoxyribonucleic acid (DNA) (hormone response elements upstream to the specific gene), causing appropriate effects (Fig. 17–3). Hormones generally are involved in a feedback loop so that the production of a substance is regulated by its effect; for example, corticotropin-releasing factor (CRF) stimulates adrenocorticotropic hormone (ACTH) to produce cortisol, which in turn feeds back to suppress CRF and ACTH production so that an equilibrium is reached. The equilibrium's set point may change with development; in prepuberty small amounts of sex steroids completely suppress gonadotropin secretion, but during pubertal development the sensitivity of this feedback decreases and increased sex steroid pro-

FIGURE 17–1. Schematic representation of mechanisms of action of hormones and growth factors. Whereas traditional hormones are formed in glands and transported to distant sites of action through the blood stream (endocrine change), peptide growth factors may be produced locally by the target cells themselves (autocrine modality to action) or by neighboring cells (paracrine). (From Wilson JD, Foster DW [eds]: Williams Textbook of Endocrinology, 8th ed. Philadelphia, WB Saunders, 1992, p 1087.)

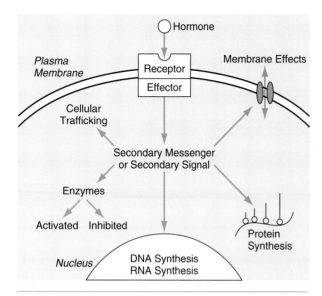

**FIGURE 17–2.** A general model for the action of peptide hormones, catecholamines, and other membrane-active hormones. The hormone in the extracellular fluid interacts with the receptor at the cell membrane and activates an associated effector system, which results in generation of an intracellular signal or second messenger that produces the final effects of the hormone. Abnormalities in the transmembrane domains of the receptors may cause disease (e.g., testotoxicosis). Abnormalities in the secondary messenger region may also cause disease (e.g., McCune-Albright syndrome). (From Wilson JD, Foster DW [eds]: Williams Textbook of Endocrinology, 8th ed. Philadelphia, WB Saunders, 1992, p 92.)

duction is allowed before gonadotropin secretion is inhibited.

Receptor number and avidity may be regulated by hormones as well; excessive continuous exposure to gonadotropin-releasing hormone (GnRH) downregulates GnRH receptor number as well as receptor activity on pituitary gonadotropes.

The interpretation of serum hormone levels must be related to their controlling factors; a given value of parathyroid hormone may be normal in a eucalcemic patient but the same value may be inadequate in a hypocalcemic patient with partial hypoparathyroidism and excessive in a hypercalcemic patient.

The *hypothalamus* controls many endocrine systems. Hypothalamic releasing factors travel down capillaries of the pituitary portal system to stimulate the anterior pituitary gland to release the hormones specific for the releasing factor (Fig. 17–4). These pituitary hormones then circulate and reach their target glands to exert their effect and create other hormones that then feed back to suppress hypothalamic and pituitary secretion (insulin-like growth factor-1 [IGF-1]), cortisol, sex steroids, thy-

roxine). Prolactin is the only pituitary hormone that is suppressed by a hypothalamic factor, prolactin inhibitory factor (dopamine). Hypothalamic deficiency leads to a decrease in most pituitary hormone secretions but may lead to an increase in prolactin secretion.

In childhood, increased *pituitary* secretion of various hormones as a result of an adenoma is rare, although cases of pituitary gigantism (growth hormone excess) are described. Destructive lesions of the pituitary gland or hypothalamus are more common in childhood. A *craniopharyngioma*, a tumor of Rathke pouch, may descend into the sella turcica, causing erosion and calcification and destroying pituitary and hypothalamic tissue as it enlarges. Hypopituitarism in this case will be due to lack of functioning pituitary and or hypothalamic cells. Acquired hypopituitarism also may result from pituitary infections, from infiltration such as with Langerhans cell histocytosis (histiocytosis X), lymphoma, and sarcoidosis, or following radiation therapy and trauma. Congenital hypopituitarism usually is due to absence of hypothalamic releasing factors, even though the pituitary gland can be stimulated by exogenous hypothalamic releasing factors. Congenital hypopituitarism does not indicate a tumor. Congenital defects of pituitary secretion may result from anatomic malformations of the hypothalamus, from pituitary hypoplasia or aplasia, or from more subtle defects of hormone secretion. Congenital defects associated with hypopituitarism include **holoprosencephaly** (cyclopia, cebocephaly, orbital hypotelorism), **septo-optic dysplasia** (optic nerve hypoplasia, absent septum pellucidum), and cleft palate.

Pituitary function testing can be performed directly by measuring the specific pituitary hormone in the basal state or after stimulation. Indirect assessment of pituitary function can be obtained by measuring serum concentrations of the target gland hormones. The most appropriate test depends on the specific hormone in question and the type of information sought (Table 17–1). Several tests of pituitary function are listed in Table 17–2.

## GROWTH

Normal growth is the final common pathway of many factors, including endocrine, environmental, nutritional, and genetic influences (see Chapter 1). Maintenance of a normal linear growth pattern is good evidence of overall health and is considered a bioassay for the whole child. The effects of certain hormones on growth and ultimate height are listed in Table 17–3. Stature influences psychologic, social, and, potentially, economic well-being. Parental

FIGURE 17–3. Proposed mechanism of action of steroid hormones (e.g., glucocorticoids, estrogens, progesterone) in activation of specific gene transcription. The steroid (S) diffuses across the plasma membrane and binds to a cytoplasmic receptor (SR). In the absence of steroid, the receptor resides in the cytoplasm as an inactive complex with heat shock protein (HSP). When the steroid binds to the receptor, the HSP dissociates from it. The steroid-receptor complex is translocated to the nucleus, where it binds to a chromatin receptor consisting of the steroid receptor response DNA element (SRE), thereby activating the transcription of specific genes involved in steroid hormone action. RNA transcripts are translated into proteins that mediate changes in cell function. Some models also suggest the presence of a membrane-associated glucocorticoid receptor. (Adapted from Chan L, O'Malley BW: Mechanism of action of the sex steroid hormones. N Engl J Med 294:1322, 1976; reprinted by permission.)

FIGURE 17–4. Hormonal influences of the hypothalamus and pituitary gland. *Solid line* represents stimulatory influence; *dotted line* represents inhibitory influence. SRIF = somatotropin release inhibiting factor; GHRH = growth hormone–releasing hormone; CRH = corticotropin-releasing hormone; PIF = prolactin inhibitory factor; GnRH = gonadotropin-releasing hormone; TRH = thyrotropin-releasing hormone; GH = growth hormone; ACTH = adrenocorticotropin; FSH = follicle-stimulating hormone; LH = luteinizing hormone; TSH = thyroid-stimulating hormone; $T_4$ = thyroxine; $T_3$ = triiodothyronine.

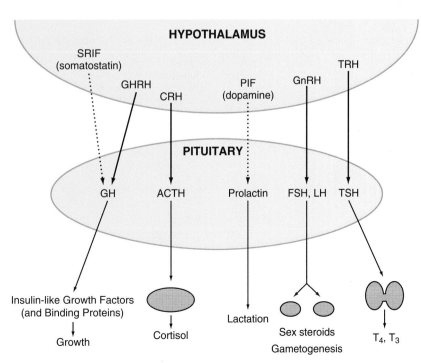

TABLE 17–1. Diagnostic Evaluation of Hypopituitarism

| Manifestation | Cause | Tests* |
|---|---|---|
| Growth failure and/or hypothyroidism | GH deficiency and/or TRH/TSH deficiency | Provocative GH tests, free T$_4$, bone age, IGF-1, IGF BP3 |
| Hypoglycemia | GH deficiency and/or ACTH insufficiency | Provocative GH tests, test of ACTH, IGF-1, IGF BP3 secretion |
| Micropenis, pubertal delay/arrest | Hypogonadotrophic hypogonadism or GH deficiency (penis) | Sex steroids (E$_2$, testosterone), LH, FSH after GnRH administration, provocative GH tests |
| Polyuria, polydipsia | ADH deficiency | Urine analysis (sp. gr.), serum electrolytes, water deprivation test |

* Each patient with hypopituitarism should have a CNS MRI scan as part of evaluation to determine the etiology of the condition.
ADH = antidiuretic hormone; E$_2$ = estradiol; FSH = follicle-stimulating hormone; GH = growth hormone; LH = luteinizing hormone; sp. gr. = specific gravity; T$_4$ = thyroxine; TRH = thyrotropin-releasing hormone; TSH = thyroid-stimulating hormone; IGF-1 = insulin-like growth factor; IGF BP3 = insulin-like growth factor binding protein 3.

concern about the psychosocial consequences of abnormal stature is a common factor that causes a family to seek medical attention.

## MEASUREMENT OF GROWTH

Accurate measurements of height and weight should be plotted on growth charts for the timely diagnosis of growth disorders (see Chapter 1). The correct measurement of an infant requires one adult to hold the baby's head still and one other to extend the feet with the soles perpendicular to the lower leg. A calipers-like device, such as an infantometer, or the movable plates on a baby scale are slid until one rests at the top of the baby's head and the other at the bottom of the baby's feet perpendicular to a ruler so that the exact distance between the two plates can be determined.

After 2 yr of age, a child should be measured in the standing position. A decrease of roughly 1.25 cm in height measurement may occur when the

TABLE 17–2. Anterior Pituitary Hormone Function Testing

| Random Hormone Measurements | Provocative Stimulation Test | Target Hormone Measurement |
|---|---|---|
| GH (useless as a random determination) | Arginine (a weak stimulus)<br>L-dopa (useful clinically)<br>Insulin-induced hypoglycemia (a dangerous test)<br>Clonidine (useful clinically)<br>GRH<br>12–24 hr integrated GH levels (of questionable utility) | IGF-1, IGF BP3 (affected by malnutrition as well as GH deficiency) |
| ACTH (useful only if in high normal range) | Cortisol after insulin-induced hypoglycemia (a dangerous test)<br>11-desoxycortisol after metyrapone<br>CRH<br>ACTH stimulation test may differentiate ACTH deficiency from primary adrenal insufficiency | A.M. cortisol<br><br>24-hr urinary free cortisol |
| TSH* | TRH | FT$_4$ |
| LH, FSH* | GnRH (difficult to interpret in prepubertal subjects) | Testosterone<br>Estradiol |
| Prolactin elevated in hypothalamic disease and decreased in pituitary disease | TRH | None |

*New supersensitive assays allow determination of abnormally low values found in hypopituitarism.
CRH = corticotropin-releasing hormone; FSH = follicle-stimulating hormone; GH = growth hormone; GRH = growth hormone–releasing hormone; L-dopa = L-dihydroxyphenylalanine; LH = luteinizing hormone; FT$_4$ = free thyroxine; TRH = thyrotropin-releasing hormone; TSH = thyroid-stimulating hormone; IGF-1 = insulin-like growth factor; IGF BP3 = insulin-like growth factor binding protein 3.

TABLE 17–3.    Hormonal Effects on Growth

| Hormone | Bone Age | Growth Rate | Adult Height* |
|---|---|---|---|
| Androgen excess | Advanced | Increased | Diminished |
| Androgen deficiency | Normal or delayed | Normal or decreased | Increased slightly or normal |
| Thyroxine excess | Advanced | Increased | Normal or diminished |
| Thyroxine deficiency | Retarded | Decreased | Diminished |
| Growth hormone excess | Normal or advanced | Increased | Excessive |
| Growth hormone deficiency | Retarded | Decreased | Diminished |
| Cortisol excess | Retarded | Decreased | Diminished |
| Cortisol deficiency | Normal | Normal | Normal |

Adapted from Underwood LE, Van Wyk JJ: Normal and aberrant growth. *In* Wilson JD, Foster DW (eds): Textbook of Endocrinology, 8th ed. Philadelphia, WB Saunders, 1992, p 1083.
*Effect in most patients with treatment.

child is standing rather than in the lying position, and many referrals are made incorrectly for a child who appears "not to be growing" when in fact the position and the device of measurement are all that have changed. Children measured in the standing position should be barefoot against a hard surface where they can place their backs with legs straight, bare feet together, and all aspects of the body pressed as far back as possible against the upright surface. Barrettes or hair buns must be removed. A Harpenden stadiometer or eqivalent is optimal for the measurement of stature.

Arm span is a useful measurement of the distance between the tips of the fingers when the patient holds an outstretched arm horizontally while standing against a solid surface. Measurement of arm span is essential when the diagnosis of Klinefelter syndrome, short-limbed dwarfism, or other dysmorphic conditions is considered. The upper-to-lower segment ratio is the result of the division of the measurement from the symphysis pubis to the floor (lower segment) subtracted from the total height by the lower segment; this ratio changes with age. A normal term baby has an upper-to-lower ratio of 1.7:1, a 1-yr-old has a ratio of 1.4:1, and a 10-yr-old has a ratio of 1:1. Conditions of hypogonadism lead to much-decreased upper-to-lower ratio in the adult, whereas hypothyroidism leads to a very high upper-to-lower ratio in the child.

## ENDOCRINE FACTORS AFFECTING GROWTH

*Growth hormone* (GH), or somatotropin, is a 191-amino acid peptide secreted by the pituitary gland under the stimulatory control of hypothalamic growth hormone–releasing factor (GRF) and the inhibitory control of growth hormone–releasing in-

hibitory factor (somatostatin or SRIF) (see Fig. 17–4). GH secretion is enhanced by alpha-adrenergic stimulation, hypoglycemia, starvation, exercise, and stress. GH secretion is inhibited by beta-adrenergic stimulation, hyperglycemia, and GH treatment. GH has direct effects (diabetogenic activity) and indirect effects mediated by the IGFs. Serum concentrations of GH are low throughout the day except for occasional peaks within the 24-hr period. Thus, the determination of a random GH concentration is of little value unless the sample is obtained during an episode of secretion, which is unlikely. The inability to release GH can be determined only by a stimulation test to measure peak GH secretion (see Table 17–2).

Most of the growth effects of GH are due to GH-stimulated production of IGFs. Serum IGF-I is related to GH secretion, rising in GH excess and decreasing in GH deficiency. Malnutrition lowers IGF-I levels. IGF-I is considered to function as a paracrine, autocrine, or endocrine agent (see Fig. 17–1). IGF-I is the agent most closely associated with linear growth. IGF-II levels decrease in GH deficiency but do not rise in GH excess.

*Thyroid hormone* is essential for normal postnatal growth, although a thyroid hormone–deficient fetus will achieve a normal birth length; similarly, a GH-deficient fetus will have a normal birth length. Thyroid hormone is necessary to allow the secretion of GH; thus, hypothyroid patients may falsely appear to be GH-deficient. The effects of other hormones on growth are noted in Table 17–3.

## ABNORMALITIES OF GROWTH

### Short Stature of Nonendocrine Causes
(Tables 17–4 and 17–5)

*Short stature* is defined as subnormal height relative to other children of the same sex, age, ethnic back-

TABLE 17–4.  Causes of Short Stature

**Variations of Normal**

Constitutional (delayed bone age)
Genetic (short familial heights)

**Endocrine Disorders**

GH deficiency
  Congenital
    Isolated GH deficiency
    With other pituitary hormone deficiencies
    With midline defects
    Pituitary agenesis
    With gene deficiency
  Acquired
    Hypothalamic/pituitary tumors
    Histiocytosis X (Langerhans cell histiocytosis)
    CNS infections and granulomas
    Head trauma (birth and later)
    Hypothalamic/pituitary radiation
    CNS vascular accidents
    Hydrocephalus
    Autoimmune
    Psychosocial dwarfism (functional GH deficiency)
    Amphetamine treatment for hyperactivity*
Laron dwarfism (increased GH and decreased IGF-I)
Pygmies (normal GH and IGF-II but decreased IGF-I)
Hypothyroidism
Glucocorticoid excess
  Endogenous
  Exogenous
Diabetes mellitus under poor control
Diabetes insipidus (untreated)
Hypophosphatemic vitamin D–resistant rickets
Virilizing congenital adrenal hyperplasia (tall child, short adult)
  P-450$_{c21}$, P-450$_{c11}$ deficiencies

**Skeletal Dysplasias**

Osteogenesis imperfecta
Osteochondroplasias

**Lysosomal Storage Diseases**

Mucopolysaccharidoses
Mucolipidoses

**Syndromes of Short Stature**

Turner syndrome (syndrome of gonadal dysgenesis)
Noonan syndrome (pseudo–Turner syndrome)
Autosomal trisomy 13, 18, 21
Prader-Willi syndrome
Laurence-Moon or Bardet-Biedl syndromes
Autosomal abnormalities
Dysmorphic syndromes (Russell-Silver, Cornelia de Lange)
Pseudohypoparathyroidism

**Chronic Disease**

Cardiac disorders
  Left-to-right shunt
  Congestive heart failure
Pulmonary disorders
  Cystic fibrosis
  Asthma
GI disorders
  Malabsorption (e.g., celiac disease)
  Disorders of swallowing
  Inflammatory bowel disease
Hepatic disorders
Hematologic disorders
  Sickle cell anemia
  Thalassemia
Renal disorders
  Renal tubular acidosis
  Chronic uremia
Immunologic disorders
  Connective tissue disease
  Juvenile rheumatoid arthritis
  Chronic infection
  AIDS
Hereditary fructose intolerance

**Malnutrition**

Kwashiorkor, marasmus
Iron deficiency
Zinc deficiency
Anorexia due to chemotherapy of neoplasms

Modified from Styne DM: Growth disorder. *In* Fitzgerald PA (ed): Handbook of Clinical Endocrinology. Norwalk, CT, Appleton & Lange, 1986, pp 73–99.
\* = only if caloric intake severely diminished.
AIDS = acquired immunodeficiency syndrome; CNS = central nervous system; GI = gastrointestinal; IGF = insulin-like growth factor.

ground, and for family heights. The 3rd or 5th percentile of the growth curve is selected for demarcation, but pathologic short stature is usually 3.5 standard deviations below the mean. *Growth failure*, however, is a slow growth rate irrespective of stature. Plotted on a growth chart, growth failure appears as a curve that crosses percentiles and is below the 5th percentile of height velocity for age (Fig. 17–5). The corrected midparental height is the average height of the parents; 6.5 cm (2.5 inches) is added for a male patient, and 6.5 cm is subtracted for a female. The resulting number ±8 cm represents a range of expected adult height. The presence of a height 3.5 standard deviations below the mean, a height velocity below the 5th percentile, or a height below the 5th percentile when corrected for midparental height requires a diagnostic evaluation (Table 17–6).

Nutrition is the most important factor affecting growth on a worldwide basis (see Chapter 2). **Failure to thrive** may develop in the infant as a result of **maternal deprivation** (nutritional deficiency or aberrant psychosocial interaction) or as a result of organic illness (anorexia, nutrient losses, hypermetabolism). Psychologic difficulties can affect growth, as in **psychosocial dwarfism.** In this situa-

TABLE 17–5. Differential Diagnosis and Therapy of Short Stature

| | Hypopituitarism Including Gonadotropin Deficiency (Possibly with ACTH or TRF Deficiency) | Constitutional Delay | Familial Short Stature | Deprivational Dwarfism | Turner Syndrome | Hypothyroidism | Chronic Disease |
|---|---|---|---|---|---|---|---|
| Family history | Rare | Frequent | Always | No | No | Variable | Variable |
| Gender | Both | Males > females | Both | Both | Female | Both | Both |
| Facies | Immature or with midline defect (e.g., cleft palate or optic hypoplasia) | Normal | Normal | Normal | Turner facies or normal | Coarse, cretin (if congenital) | Normal |
| Sexual development | Delayed | Delayed | Normal | May be delayed | Female prepubertal | Usually delayed, may be precocious if hypothyroidism is severe | Delayed |
| Bone age | Delayed | Delayed | Normal | Usually delayed; growth arrest lines present | Delayed | Delayed | Delayed |
| Dentition | Delayed | Delay possible | Normal | Variable | Normal | Delayed | Normal or delayed |
| Hypoglycemia | Variable | No | No | No | No | No | No |
| Karyotype | Normal | Normal | Normal | Normal | 45,X or partial deletion of X chromosome or mosaic | Normal | Normal |
| Free $T_4$ | Low (if TRF-deficient) or normal | Normal | Normal | Normal or low | Normal: hypothyroidism may be acquired | Low | Normal |
| Stimulated GH | Low | May be transiently low or normal | Normal | Possibly high | Usually normal | Low | Variable |
| Insulin-like growth factor I | Low | Normal for bone age but low for chronologic age | Normal | Low | Normal | Low | Low or normal (depending on nutritional status) |
| Therapy | Replace deficiencies | Reassurance; sex steroids to initiate secondary sexual development in selected patients | None | Change or improve environment | Sex hormone replacement, GH; oxandrolone appears useful | $T_4$ | Treat malnutrition, organ failure (e.g., dialysis, transplant, cardiotonic drugs, insulin) |

ACTH = adrenocorticotropic hormone; GH = growth hormone; $T_4$ = thyroxine; TRF = thyrotropin-releasing factor.

FIGURE 17–5. Patterns of linear growth. Normal growth percentiles (5th, 50th, 95th) are shown along with typical growth curves for constitutional delay of growth and adolescence (short stature with normal growth rate for bone age and delayed pubertal growth spurt and eventual achievement of normal adult stature) (A), familial short stature (short stature in childhood and as an adult with a normal growth rate) (B), and acquired pathologic growth failure (C) (e.g., acquired untreated primary hypothyroidism).

tion, the child is psychologically abused and develops functional GH deficiency and poor growth.

The common condition known as **constitutional delay in growth** is a variation of normal growth and not a disease (see Fig. 17–5 and Table 17–5). There usually is a family member who has delayed growth and/or puberty during childhood but achieves a normal final height. The bone age is delayed, but the growth is appropriate for bone age. Constitutional delay in growth usually leads to constitutional delay in puberty, so that secondary sexual development is delayed. **Genetic or familial short stature** (see Fig. 17–5 and Table 17–5) refers to a child born to a family with short parents who is expected to reach a lower than average height. The combination of constitutional growth delay and genetic short stature leads to exceptional short stature and brings the child to medical attention sooner.

Recognizable physical syndromes of short stature often combine obesity and decreased height; normal nonsyndromatic obese children are usually taller than average (see Table 17–4). The **Prader-Willi syndrome** includes fetal and infantile hypotonia, small hands and feet (acromicria), postnatal acquired obesity and insatiable appetite, developmental delay, hypogonadism, almond-shaped eyes, and abnormalities of the 15th chromosome. **Laurence-Moon** or **Bardet-Biedl syndromes** include combinations of short stature, obesity, retinitis pigmentosum, polydactyly, and hypogonadism in an autosomally inherited pattern.

### Short Stature Caused by Growth Hormone Deficiency
#### (Tables 17–4 and 17–5)

Classic congenital or idiopathic severe GH deficiency occurs in 1:4000 children. Idiopathic GH deficiency is a hypothalamic disease of inadequate GRF; the pituitary gland manufactures GH but does not secrete it. Less often, GH deficiency is due to anatomic defects of the pituitary gland or, in genetic forms, a portion of the GH gene is missing. Classic GH deficiency indicates virtually no secretion of GH, but intermediate forms of decreased GH secretion (partial GH deficiency or neurosecretory disorder) are described. **Acquired GH deficiency** causing **late onset growth failure** suggests a serious etiology (e.g., tumor).

*Clinical Manifestations.* Infants with congenital GH deficiency achieve a normal birth length at term and weight, but soon the growth rate slows and they become chubby and short. Careful measurements in the 1st yr of life may suggest the diagnosis, but most patients are not diagnosed until several years of age. A patient with classic GH deficiency has the appearance of a cherub (a chubby, immature appearance), with a high-pitched voice resulting from an immature larynx but with intellectually age-appropriate speech unless severe hypoglycemia occurred or facial dysmorphology includes a CNS defect that affects mentation. Male neonates with isolated GH deficiency with or without gonadotropin deficiency may have a **microphallus**, (a stretched penile length of less than 2.0 cm). Severe fasting hypoglycemia leading to seizures in the newborn occurs because of decreased gluconeogenesis. Patients who lack adrenocorticotropic hormone (ACTH) in addition to GH may have more profound hypoglycemia, because cortisol is another factor in gluconeogenesis.

Dysraphism (midline defects) of the head may be associated with hypothalamic deficiency leading to hypopituitarism; 6% of patients with cleft palate

TABLE 17–6.   Growth Failure: Screening Test

| Test | Rationale |
|------|-----------|
| CBC | *Anemia:* nutritional, chronic disease, malignancy<br>*Leukocytosis:* inflammation, infection<br>*Leukopenia:* bone marrow failure syndromes<br>*Thrombocytopenia:* malignancy, infection |
| ESR, CRP | Inflammation of infection, inflammatory diseases, malignancy |
| SMA 20 (electrolytes, liver enzymes, BUN) | Signs of acute or chronic hepatic, renal, adrenal dysfunction; hydration and acid-base status |
| Carotene, folate, and prothrombin time; antiendomesial antibody | Assess malabsorption; detect celiac disease |
| Urinalysis | Signs of renal dysfunction, hydration, water and salt homeostasis; renal tubular acidosis |
| Karyotype | Determines Turner (XO) or other syndromes |
| Cranial imaging (MRI) | Assesses hypothalamic-pituitary tumors (craniopharyngioma, glioma, germinoma) or congenital midline defects |
| Bone age | Compare with height age, and evaluate height potential |
| IGF-I, IGF BP3 | Reflects growth hormone status or nutrition |
| Free thyroxine | Detects panhypopituitarism or isolated hypothyroidism |
| Prolactin | Elevated in hypothalamic dysfunction or destruction, suppressed in pituitary disease |

BUN = blood urea nitrogen; CBC = complete blood count; CRP = C-reactive protein; ESR = erythrocyte sedimentation rate; IGF BP3 = insulin-like growth factor binding protein 3; MRI = magnetic resonance imaging.

are GH deficient. Patients with pendular nystagmus (sign of poor vision) due to optic hypoplasia with or without absence of the septum pellucidum (septo-optic dysplasia) frequently have anterior and, possibly, posterior pituitary hormone deficiencies.

*Diagnosis.* GH testing should be offered to a patient who is short (well below the 5th percentile), usually more than 3.5 standard deviations below the mean, who is growing poorly (< the 5th percentile growth rate for age), and/or who is below the 5th percentile for height when corrected for family heights. After chronic disease is ruled out and routine laboratory testing is completed, (see Table 17–6), two GH stimulatory tests are performed (see Table 17–2).

Classic GH-deficient patients do not show an increase in serum GH levels after stimulation by various secretagogues. Some patients release GH in response to secretagogues but cannot spontaneously release GH during the day. Measuring IGF-1 and its growth hormone–dependent binding protein (IGF-BP3) is helpful but not infallible. In difficult cases, an operational definition of GH deficiency might be that patients who require GH will grow significantly faster when administered a normal dose of GH.

*Treatment.* GH deficiency is treated with biosynthetic recombinant DNA-derived GH, given subcutaneously 6 times/wk or daily. Administration of GH to patients with normal GH responsiveness to secretagogues is controversial. Treatment with GH carries the risk of an increased incidence of slipped capital femoral epiphysis and pseudotumor cerebri. Human cadaver pituitary GH is no longer used because of the risk of contamination with the neurodegenerative infectious **Jakob-Creutzfeldt** agent.

GH is effective in increasing growth rate and final height in Turner syndrome and in chronic renal failure.

Psychologic support of children with severe short stature is important, as they may become the object of ridicule by classmates. Marital status, satisfaction with life, and vocational achievement may possibly be decreased in children of short stature who are not given supportive measures.

### Tall Stature
(Table 17–7)

*Constitutional tall stature* indicates an advancement of bone age and physical development leading to tall stature during childhood but an ultimate normal adult height. Moderate obesity may lead to this situation by advancing the bone age and leading to taller than average stature. *Genetic tall stature* occurs when parents are tall.

TABLE 17–7.    Causes of Tall Stature

| Variations of Normal | Nonendocrine Disorders |
|---|---|
| Constitutional | Marfan's syndrome |
| Genetic | Klinefelter's syndrome |
| Exogenous obesity | XYY syndrome |
| **Endocrine Disorders** | Cerebral gigantism (Sotos syndrome) |
| Pituitary gigantism | Homocystinuria |
| Sexual precocity | Weaver Smith syndrome |
| Thyrotoxicosis | |
| Beckwith-Wiedemann syndrome | |

Modified from Styne DM: Growth disorder. *In* Fitzgerald PA (ed): Handbook of Clinical Endocrinology. Norwalk, CT, Appleton & Lange, 1986, pp 73–99.

**Cerebral gigantism** or **Soto syndrome** manifests in infancy by increased growth rate, prominent forehead, sharp chin, high arched palate, hypertelorism, and, frequently, developmental delay. By mid-childhood, the growth rate normalizes.

**Marfan syndrome** combines tall stature with arm span exceeding height, a very low upper-to-lower segment ratio, long thin fingers (arachnodactyly) and toes, hyperextensibility of the joints, aortic dilation, and superior subluxations of the lens. **Homocystinuria** may present with a phenotype similar to that of Marfan syndrome. Mental retardation is characteristic and there is increased urinary secretion of the homocysteine. The lens subluxation in this condition may be inferior.

**Endocrine Etiology of Tall Stature. Pituitary gigantism** caused by excess GH secretion is quite rare.

*Clinical Manifestations.* If a GH-secreting adenoma occurs after puberty, a patient will have acromegaly, but in infancy the child will grow remarkably because the epiphyses are not closed. Height velocity is increased; leonine faces and acromegalic facial features may occur. Organomegaly may be noted, and glucose intolerance or diabetes mellitus may result. Elevated fasting serum GH or IGF-1 concentrations confirm the diagnosis.

*Diagnosis.* The initial evaluation should include an estimation of the patient's genetic height potential as discussed above. If familial or constitutional tall stature or the noted syndromes are not possibilities or if other signs suggesting pituitary gigantism are present, laboratory tests specific for diagnosis of pituitary gigantism (GH, IGF-I levels, MR imaging) should be performed.

*Treatment.* Treatment of pituitary gigantism is indicated. Usually, therapy is not indicated for a normal child who is predicted to become "too" tall. However, estrogen administration, if the bone age has not reached 10 yr, may reduce the final height in girls who are predicted to be more than 5 ft 10 inches by causing rapid pubertal progression, leading to earlier epiphyseal fusion. Boys may be similarly treated with testosterone. These hormone therapies are rarely indicated.

## References

Behrman RE, Kliegman RM, Arvin AM (eds): Nelson Textbook of Pediatrics, 15th ed. Philadelphia, WB Saunders, 1996, Chapter 512.

Guidelines for the use of growth hormone in children with short stature: A report by the Drug Therapeutics Committee of the Lawson Wilkins Pediatric Endocrine Society. J Pediatr 127:857, 1995.

Neely EK, Rosenfeld RG: Use and abuse of human growth hormone. Ann Rev Med 45:407, 1994.

Rosenbloom AL, Rosenfeld R, Guevano-Aguirre J: Growth hormone insensitivity. Pediatr Clin North Am 44:423, 1997.

Rosenfeld RG, Albertsson-Wikland K, Cassoria F, et al: Diagnostic controversy: The diagnosis of childhood growth hormone deficiency revisited. J Clin Endocrinol Metab 80:1532, 1995.

Schwartz I, Grunt J: Growth, short stature, and the use of growth hormone: Considerations for the practicing pediatrician—an update. Curr Probl Pediatr 27:14, 1997.

Sklar CA: Growth and neuroendocrine dysfunction following therapy for childhood cancer. Pediatr Clin North Am 44:489, 1997.

# PUBERTY AND ITS DISORDERS
(see Chapters 1 and 7)

The staging of pubertal changes and the sequence of events are discussed in Chapter 7 (see Figs. 7–1 to 7–4; Tables 7–1 to 7–3). Control of the onset of puberty involves adrenal maturation (*adrenarche,* the development of pubic and axillary hair), and hypothalamic-pituitary-gonadal maturation (genital development in boys and breast development in girls).

## DELAYED PUBERTY
(Table 17–8)

Puberty is delayed when there is no sign of pubertal development by age 13 yr in girls and 14 yr in boys living in the United States.

### Constitutional Delay in Growth and Adolescence
(see Table 17–5 and Abnormalities of Growth)

Patients who have a significantly delayed bone age (a 1.5- to 2-yr delay as a teenager) but who always have grown at the normal rate for their bone age will have delayed onset of their pubertal develop-

TABLE 17–8.  Classification of Delayed Puberty and Sexual Infantilism

**Constitutional Delay in Growth and Puberty (Delayed Activation of Hypothalamic GnRH Pulse Generator)**

**Hypogonadotropic Hypogonadism**

Central nervous system disorders
    Tumors (craniopharyngioma, germinoma, glioma)
    Congenital malformations
    Radiation therapy
    Other causes
Isolated gonadotropin deficiency
    Kallmann syndrome (anosmia–hyosmia)
    Other disorders
Idiopathic and genetic forms of multiple pituitary hormone deficiencies
Miscellaneous disorders
    Prader-Willi syndrome
    Laurence-Moon-Bardet-Biedl syndromes
    Functional gonadotropin deficiency
        Chronic systemic disease and malnutrition
        Hypothyroidism
        Cushing disease
        Diabetes mellitus
        Hyperprolactinemia
        Anorexia nervosa
        Psychogenic amenorrhea
        Impaired puberty and delayed menarche in female athletes and ballet dancers (exercise amenorrhea)

**Hypergonadotropic Hypogonadism**

Klinefelter syndrome (syndrome of seminiferous tubular dysgenesis) and its variants
Other forms of primary testicular failure
Anorchia and cryptorchidism
Syndrome of gonadal dysgenesis and its variants (Turner syndrome)
Other forms of primary ovarian failure
XX and XY gonadal dysgenesis
    Familial and sporadic XX gonadal dysgenesis and its variants
    Familial and sporadic XY gonadal dysgenesis and its variants
Pseudo-Turner syndrome
Galactosemia

Modified from Grumbach MM, Styne DM: Puberty. *In* Wilson JD, Foster DW (eds): Williams Textbook of Endocrinology, 9th ed. Philadelphia, WB Saunders, 1998.

ment as a variation of normal; this is often familial. Puberty usually begins by the time the bone age reaches 12 yr of age in boys and 11 yr in girls. Patients who have constitutional delay in puberty usually begin pubertal development by 18 yr of age.

## Hypogonadotropic Hypogonadism
### (Table 17–9; see Table 17–8)

Patients with hypogonadotropic hypogonadism have eunuchoid proportions because their long bones grow for a longer than normal period of time, producing an upper-to-lower ratio below 0.9 and an arm span wider than their height. If the patient has concurrent GH deficiency, stature will be exceptionally short.

**Isolated Gonadotropin Deficiency.** If there is an inability to release gonadotropins but no other pituitary abnormality, the patient has isolated gonadotropin deficiency (almost universally a result of absent GnRH). Patients grow normally until the time of the pubertal growth spurt, when they fail to experience accelerated growth.

**Kallmann syndrome** combines isolated gonadotropin deficiency with abnormal olfaction. There is genetic heterogeneity; some patients have a decreased sense of smell, others have abnormal reproduction, and some have both. This disorder is due to mutations in the KAL gene at Xp 22.3 (X-chromosome) and causes the GnRH neurons to remain ineffectually located in the primitive nasal area. Olfactory bulbs are often absent on magnetic resonance imaging (MRI).

**Abnormalities of the Central Nervous System.** Central nervous system (CNS) tumors are a serious cause of gonadotropin deficiency. Craniopharyngiomas have a peak incidence in the teenaged years and may lead to any type of anterior or posterior hormone deficiency. Craniopharyngiomas calcify, erode the sella turcica, and may impinge on the optic chiasm, leading to bitemporal hemianopsia as well as optic atrophy. Germinomas are noncalcifying hypothalamic tumors that frequently produce human chorionic gonadotropin (hCG), causing sexual precocity in boys; they may also be located in the pineal area. Both tumor types may produce headaches.

**Idiopathic Hypopituitarism.** Congenital absence of various combinations of pituitary hormones may produce idiopathic hypopituitarism. Inheritance may be X-linked or autosomal recessive but sporadic types of congenital idiopathic hypopituitarism are more common.

Congenital hypopituitarism may manifest in a male with GH deficiency and/or associated gonadotropin deficiency with a microphallus (stretched neonatal penile length less than 2.5 cm). The concurrent absence of GH and ACTH may lead to hypoglycemia from decreased gluconeogenesis. Patients may have associated midline facial defects, such as cleft palate and optic hypoplasia.

**Syndromes of Hypogonadism.** Weight loss resulting from voluntary dieting, malnutrition, or chronic disease will lead to decreased gonadotropin function when weight falls below 80% of ideal weight. **Anorexia nervosa** is characterized by striking weight loss (see Chapters 2 and 3). Primary or secondary amenorrhea frequently is found in

TABLE 17–9. Differential Diagnostic Features of Delayed Puberty and Sexual Infantilism

| | Stature | Plasma Gonadotropins | GnRH Test: LH Response | Plasma Gonadal Steroids | Plasma DHAS | Karyotype | Olfaction |
|---|---|---|---|---|---|---|---|
| *Constitutional Delay in Growth and Adolescence* | Short for chronologic age, usually appropriate for bone age | Prepubertal, later pubertal | Prepubertal, later pubertal | Low, later normal | Low for chronologic age, appropriate for bone age | Normal | Normal |
| *Hypogonadotropic Hypogonadism* | | | | | | | |
| Isolated gonadotropin deficiency | Normal, absent pubertal growth spurt | Low | Prepubertal or no response | Low | Appropriate for chronologic age | Normal | Normal |
| Kallmann syndrome | Normal, absent pubertal growth spurt | Low | Prepubertal or no response | Low | Appropriate for chronologic age | Normal | Anosmia or hyposmia |
| Idiopathic multiple pituitary hormone deficiencies | Short stature and poor growth since early childhood | Low | Prepubertal or no response | Low | Usually low | Normal | Normal |
| Hypothalamo-pituitary tumors | Decrease in growth velocity of late onset | Low | Prepubertal or no response | Low | Normal or low for chronologic age | Normal | Normal |
| *Primary Gonadal Failure* | | | | | | | |
| Syndrome of gonadal dysgenesis and variants | Short stature since early childhood | High | Hyper-response for age | Low | Normal for chronologic age | XO or variant | Normal |
| Klinefelter syndrome and variants | Normal to tall | High | Hyper-response at puberty | Low or normal | Normal for chronologic age | XXY or variant | Normal |
| Familial XX or XY gonadal dysgenesis | Normal | High | Hyper-response for age | Low | Normal for chronologic age | XX or XY | Normal |

From Grumbach MM, Styne DM: Puberty. *In* Wilson JD, Foster DW (eds): Williams Textbook of Endocrinology, 9th ed. Philadelphia, WB Saunders, 1998. DHAS = dehydroepiandrosterone sulfate; GnRH = gonadotropin-releasing hormone; LH = luteinizing hormone.

affected girls, and pubertal development is absent or minimal, depending on the level of weight loss. Regaining weight may not immediately reverse the condition. Increased physical activity, even without weight loss, can lead to decreased menstrual frequency and gonadotropin deficiency. When physical activity is interrupted, menstrual function may return. **Hypothyroidism** inhibits the onset of puberty and delays menstrual periods. Conversely, severe primary hypothyroidism may lead to precocious puberty.

### Hypergonadotropic Hypogonadism

Hypergonadotropic hypogonadism is characterized by elevated gonadotropin level resulting from primary gonadal failure.

**Ovarian Failure.** The Turner syndrome of gonadal dysgenesis is a common cause of ovarian failure and short stature. The incidence of Turner syndrome is 1:2000–5000 births (see Chapter 4). Patients with variants of Turner syndrome, other types of gonadal dysgenesis, galactosemia, or following radiation therapy or chemotherapy also may have ovarian failure (see Table 17–8).

**Testicular Failure.** Klinefelter syndrome (seminiferous tubular dysgenesis) is the most common cause of testicular failure. The incidence is approximately 1:1000 in males. Testosterone levels may be close to normal because Leydig cell function may be spared; however, seminiferous tubular function characteristically is lost, causing infertility. The age of onset of puberty usually is normal, but secondary sexual changes may not progress because of inadequate Leydig cell function (see Chapter 4).

### Differential Diagnosis

Once it is determined that no secondary sexual development is present after the upper age limits of normal pubertal development, gonadotropin determinations should be obtained to determine whether the patient has hypogonadotropic or hypergonadotropic hypogonadism (see Table 17–9). Differentiation between constitutional delay in growth and hypogonadotropic hypogonadism is difficult if no family history for the former or no CNS or olfactory abnormalities for the latter are identified. Sometimes a period of observation for months or years is necessary before the diagnosis is confirmed by spontaneous pubertal development or lack of it.

### Treatment

If a permanent condition is apparent, replacement with sex steroids is indicated. Girls are given ethinyl estradiol in daily doses until breakthrough bleeding occurs, at which time cycling is started with a dose on the first 21 days of the month; on days 12–21, a progestational agent, such as medroxyprogesterone acetate, is added to mimic a normal menstrual period. In boys, testosterone enanthate once every 4 wk may be started. This regimen is appropriate for patients with either hypo- or hypergonadotropic hypogonadism. Both groups, as well as those with constitutional delay, are at risk for decreased bone density. Patients with hypogonadotropic hypogonadism may be able to achieve fertility by the administration of gonadotropin therapy or hypothalamic-releasing hormone therapy on an appropriate schedule.

Estrogen replacement for patients with Turner syndrome may be offered at the normal age of puberty in low doses to ensure feminization and to improve psychologic function as well as to attempt to decrease the likelihood of osteoporosis. Growth hormone will increase the growth rate and final height of these patients. Patients with Turner syndrome have had successful pregnancies after in vitro fertilization with a donor ovum.

## SEXUAL PRECOCITY
(Tables 17–10 and 17–11)

### Classification

Sexual precocity (precocious puberty) is secondary sexual development occurring before the age of 9 yr in boys or 8 yr in girls. The condition is **true precocious puberty** or central precocious puberty if it emanates from premature reactivation of the hypothalamic-pituitary-gonadal axis (GnRH-dependent), or **incomplete precocious puberty** if the hypothalamic-pituitary-gonadal axis is not involved in the process (GnRH-independent). A boy may have incomplete precocious puberty as a result of autonomous production of testosterone or other androgens from the testes or adrenals or as a result of a tumor that produces hCG, stimulating the testes. A girl might have precocious puberty as a result of autonomous production of estrogens from the ovaries or adrenal glands. Members of some families enter puberty prior to the lower limits of normal (**constitutional** or **familial precocious puberty**). In these cases, every aspect of pubertal development is normal but early.

**Idiopathic Precocious Puberty.** Although the endocrine changes of puberty, such as increased pulsatile gonadotropin secretion and increased response of luteinizing hormone (LH) to GnRH, are the same as in normal puberty, the clinical course

TABLE 17–10.    Classification of Sexual Precocity

| | |
|---|---|
| **True Precocious Puberty or Complete Isosexual Precocity (Premature Reactivation of the Hypothalamic GnRH Pulse Generator)** | Females<br>    Estrogen-secreting ovarian or adrenal neoplasms<br>    Ovarian cysts<br>Males and females<br>    McCune-Albright syndrome<br>    Primary hypothyroidism<br>    Peutz-Jeghers syndrome |
| Idiopathic true precocious puberty<br>CNS tumors<br>    Hamartomas (ectopic GnRH pulse generator)<br>    Other tumors<br>Other CNS disorders<br>True precocious puberty after late treatment of congenital virilizing adrenal hyperplasia | **Iatrogenic Sexual Precocity** |
| | **Variations of Pubertal Development** |
| |     Premature thelarche<br>    Premature menarche<br>    Premature adrenarche<br>    Adolescent gynecomastia |
| **Incomplete Isosexual Precocity (GnRH-Independent Sexual Precocity)** | **Contrasexual Precocity** |
| Males<br>    Chorionic gonadotropin-secreting tumors (hCG-dependent sexual precocity)<br>        CNS tumors (e.g., germinoma, chorionepithelioma, and teratoma)<br>        Tumors in locations outside the CNS (hepatoblastoma)<br>        LH-secreting pituitary adenoma<br>    Increased androgen secretion by adrenal or testis<br>        Congenital adrenal hyperplasia (21-OH deficiency, 11-OH deficiency)<br>        Virilizing adrenal neoplasm<br>        Leydig cell adenoma<br>        Familial testotoxicosis (familial premature gonadotropin–independent Leydig cell and germ cell maturation) | Feminization in males<br>    Adrenal neoplasm<br>    Increased extraglandular conversion of circulating steroids to estrogen<br>Virilization in females<br>    Congenital adrenal hyperplasia<br>        21-OH deficiency<br>        11-OH deficiency<br>        $3\beta$-ol deficiency<br>    Virilizing adrenal neoplasms<br>    Virilizing ovarian neoplasms (e.g., arrhenoblastomas) |

From Grumbach MM, Styne DM: Puberty. *In* Wilson JD, Foster DW (eds): Williams Textbook of Endocrinology, 9th ed. Philadelphia, WB Saunders, 1998.
    CNS = central nervous system; GnRH = gonadotropin-releasing hormone; hCG = human chorionic gonadotropin; LH = luteinizing hormone; OH = hydroxylase.

may be waxing and waning. Idiopathic precocious puberty occurs approximately 9 times more often in girls than boys. Boys have a higher incidence of CNS disorders, such as tumors and hamartomas, precipitating the precocious puberty. Hamartomas of the cinerea have characteristic appearance on computed tomography (CT) or MRI and do not need biopsy for diagnosis. The mass of GnRH neurons acts like an unrestrained ectopic hypothalamus but is not a true neoplasm and does not grow. The resulting precocious puberty is very amenable to medical therapy. Optic or hypothalamic gliomas (with or without neurofibromatosis), astrocytomas, and ependymomas also can cause precocious puberty by exerting mass effects on those areas of the CNS that normally inhibit pubertal development. Almost any condition that affects the CNS, including hydrocephalus, meningitis, encephalitis, suprasellar cysts, head trauma, and irradiation, has been reported to precipitate central precocious puberty. Children with epilepsy and mental retardation have an increased incidence of precocious puberty.

**Incomplete GnRH-Independent or Pseudoprecocious Puberty** (see Tables 17–10 and 17–11). Because of an abnormality in the G-protein system, which causes unregulated constitutive activation of adenyl cyclase, several endocrine organs may autonomously function, creating the **McCune-Albright syndrome.** Characteristically these patients have irregular *café au lait* spots, polyostotic fibrous dysplasia of the long bones, and precocious puberty. They also may have hyperthyroidism, hyperadrenalism, or acromegaly in addition. Boys may have familial premature Leydig and germ cell activation caused by a different genetic defect causing constitutive activation of the LH receptor.

**Evaluation of Sexual Precocity** (see Table 17–11). On physical examination, it should be noted whether changes characteristic of normal puberty are apparent (see Chapter 7) or whether only isolated estrogen or androgen effects are present in girls. In boys it is important to note whether the testes are enlarged over 2.5 cm, which suggests ectopic production of hCG or central (GnRH-dependent) precocious puberty; if the testes are not enlarged but virilization is progressing, the source of the androgens may be the adrenal glands.

Laboratory examinations include sex steroid and

TABLE 17–11.  Differential Diagnosis of Sexual Precocity

| | Serum Gonadotropin Concentration | LH Response to GnRH | Serum Sex Steroid Concentrations | Gonadal Size | Miscellaneous |
|---|---|---|---|---|---|
| **True Precocious Puberty (Premature Reactivation of Hypothalamic GnRH Pulse Generator)** | Prominent LH pulses, initially during sleep | Pubertal | Pubertal values of testosterone or estradiol | Normal pubertal testicular enlargement or ovarian and uterine enlargement (by sonography) | MRI scan of brain to rule out CNS tumor or other abnormality; skeletal survey for McCune-Albright syndrome |
| **Incomplete Sexual Precocity (Pituitary Gonadotropin-Independent)** | | | | | |
| *Males* | | | | | |
| Chorionic gonadotropin–secreting tumor in males | High hCG | Prepubertal | Pubertal values of testosterone | Slight to moderate uniform enlargement of testes | Hepatomegaly suggests hepatoblastoma; MRI scan of brain if chorionic gonadotropin-secreting CNS tumor suspected |
| Leydig cell tumor in males | Prepubertal | Prepubertal | Very high testosterone | Irregular asymmetric enlargement of testes | |
| Familial testotoxicosis | Prepubertal | Prepubertal | Pubertal values of testosterone | Testes symmetric and larger than 2.5 cm but smaller than expected for pubertal development; spermatogenesis occurs | Familial; probably sex-limited, autosomal dominant trait |
| Premature adrenarche | Prepubertal | Prepubertal | Prepubertal testosterone; DHAS or urinary 17-ketosteroid values appropriate for pubic hair stage 2 | Testes prepubertal | Onset usually after 6 yr of age; more frequent in brain-injured children |
| *Females* | | | | | |
| Granulosa cell tumor (follicular cysts may present similarly) | Low | Prepubertal | Very high estradiol | Ovarian enlargement on physical examination, MRI, CT, or sonography | Tumor often palpable on abdominal examination |
| Follicular cyst | Low | Prepubertal | Prepubertal to very high estradiol values | Ovarian enlargement on physical examination, MRI, CT, or sonography | Single or repetitive episodes; exclude McCune-Albright syndrome (skeletal survey) |
| Feminizing adrenal tumor | Low | Prepubertal | High estradiol and DHAS values | Ovaries prepubertal | Unilateral adrenal mass |
| Premature thelarche | Prepubertal | Prepubertal | Prepubertal or early pubertal estradiol | Ovaries prepubertal | Onset usually before 3 yr of age |
| Premature adrenarche | Prepubertal | Prepubertal | Prepubertal estradiol; DHAS or urinary 17-ketosteroid values appropriate for pubic hair stage 2 | Ovaries prepubertal | Onset usually after 6 yr of age; more frequent in brain-injured children |

Modified from Grumbach MM, Styne DM: Puberty. *In* Wilson JD, Foster DW (eds): Williams Textbook of Endocrinology, 9th ed. Philadelphia, WB Saunders, 1998.
CNS = central nervous system; CT = computed tomography; DHAS = dehydroepiandrosterone sulfate; GnRH = gonadotropin-releasing factor; hCG = human chorionic gonadotropin; LH = luteinizing hormone; MRI = magnetic resonance imaging.

gonadotropin levels, usually in the GnRH-stimulated state (see Table 17–11). Thyroid hormone determination is useful. If there is a suggestion of a CNS anomaly or a tumor (CNS, hepatic, adrenal, ovarian, testicular), a CT or MRI scan of the appropriate location is indicated.

### Treatment
#### (Table 17–12)

Long-acting, superactive analogs of GnRH are the treatment of choice for central precocious puberty because they suppress gonadotropin secretion by downregulating GnRH receptors in the pituitary gonadotropes. The early sexual development and increased height of the patient with precocious puberty mandate psychologic counseling for children and families. In patients with incomplete precocious puberty, removal of the hormone-secreting tumor, if possible, is curative. McCune-Albright syndrome is treated with testolactone. Boys with GnRH-independent premature Leydig cell and germ cell maturation do not respond to GnRH analogs but require treatment with ketoconazole (an inhibitor of testosterone synthesis), spironolactone (an antiandrogen), or testolactone (an aromatase inhibitor). After successful therapy of the latter conditions, central precocious puberty may secondarily develop; GnRH agonist administration is effective therapy.

## VARIATIONS IN PUBERTAL DEVELOPMENT

### Inappropriate Breast Development

*Benign premature thelarche* is the isolated appearance of unilateral or bilateral breast tissue in girls, usually at ages 6 mo to 3 yr. There are no other signs of puberty and no evidence of excessive estrogen effect (e.g., thickening of the vaginal secretions, increased height velocity, or bone age acceleration). Ingestion or application of estrogen-containing compounds must be excluded as a cause. Vaginal bleeding is absent, and no acceleration in growth velocity is noted. Laboratory investigations are not usually necessary, but a pelvic ultrasound study may rarely be indicated to exclude ovarian pathology. Girls with this condition should be re-evaluated at intervals of 6–12 mo to ensure that premature thelarche is not the beginning of isosexual precocious puberty. The prognosis is excellent, if no progression occurs, and no treatment other than reassurance is necessary.

In boys, the appearance of breast tissue is referred to as *gynecomastia* (see Chapter 7).

### Isolated Premature Adrenarche (Pubarche)

The appearance of pubic hair before the age of 8 yr in girls or before the age of 9 yr in boys is

TABLE 17–12.    Pharmacologic Therapy of Sexual Precocity

| Disorder | Treatment | Action and Rationale |
|---|---|---|
| GnRH-dependent true or central precocious puberty | GnRH agonists | Desensitization of gonadotropes; blocks action of endogenous GnRH |
| GnRH-independent incomplete sexual precocity | | |
| Girls | | |
|     Autonomous ovarian cysts | Medroxyprogesterone acetate | Inhibition of ovarian steroidogenesis; regression of cyst (inhibition of FSH release) |
|     McCune-Albright syndrome | Medroxyprogesterone acetate* | Inhibition of ovarian steroidogenesis; regression of cyst (inhibition of FSH release) |
| | Testolactone* or fadrozole | Inhibition of P-450 aromatase; blocks estrogen synthesis |
| Boys | | |
|     Familial testotoxicosis | Ketoconazole* | Inhibition of P-450$_{c17}$ (mainly 17,20-lyase activity) |
| | Spironolactone* or flutamide *and* testolactone or fadrozole | Antiandrogen Inhibition of aromatase; blocks estrogen synthesis |
| | Medroxyprogesterone acetate* | Inhibition of testicular steroidogenesis |

Modified from Grumbach MM, Kaplan SL: Recent advances in the diagnosis and management of sexual precocity. Acta Paediatr Jpn 30(Suppl):155, 1988.
* If true precocious puberty develops, a GnRH agonist can be added.
FSH = follicle-stimulating hormone; GnRH = gonadotropin-releasing hormone.

premature adrenarche and is relatively common. If the pubic hair is associated with any other feature of virilization (clitoral enlargement, advanced bone age) or other signs (acne, rapid growth, voice change), a detailed investigation for a pathologic virilizing cause is performed. Measurements of testosterone, 17-hydroxyprogesterone (17-OHP), and dehydroepiandrosterone (DHEA) in basal and ACTH-stimulated states are indicated in heavily virilized patients. Ultrasound studies may reveal a virilizing adrenal or ovarian tumor. Excessive 17-OHP or DHEA levels indicate an enzyme defect of congenital adrenal hyperplasia. Most patients with isolated pubic hair, however, do not have these abnormal signs of progressive virilization and reflect *premature pubarche*. Premature activation of DHEA secretion from the adrenal gland (adrenarche) is postulated to be the etiologic factor. Bone age may be slightly advanced and height slightly increased, but testosterone concentrations are normal, whereas DHEA-S levels usually are high for prepuberty but are consistent with Tanner (Sexuality Maturity Rating) stages II and III (see Figs. 7–1 and 7–4).

### References

Behrman RE, Kliegman RM, Arvin AM (eds): Nelson Textbook of Pediatrics, 15th ed. Philadelphia, WB Saunders, 1996, Chapters 516, 517, 535–539.

Grumbach MM, Styne DM: Puberty. *In* Wilson JD, Foster DW (eds): Williams Textbook of Endocrinology, 9th ed. Philadelphia, WB Saunders, 1997.

Ringel M, Schwindinger W, Levine M: Clinical implications of genetic defects in G proteins. Medicine 75:171, 1996.

Rosenfield RL: The ovary and female sexual maturation. *In* Sperling MA (ed): Pediatric Endocrinology. Philadelphia, WB Saunders, 1996, pp 329–386.

Styne DM. The testes: Disorders of sexual differentiation and puberty. *In* Sperling MA (ed): Pediatric Endocrinology. Philadelphia, WB Saunders, 1996, pp 423–476.

Styne DM: Recent developments in disorders of puberty. Pediatr Clin North Am 44:505, 1997.

## THYROID

Disorders of thyroid function are common endocrine problems in pediatrics. Diagnosis of thyroid disorders is based on an understanding of the hypothalamic-pituitary-thyroid axis (Fig. 17–6).

### THYROID PHYSIOLOGY AND DEVELOPMENT

Thyrotropin-releasing hormone (TRH), a tripeptide synthesized in the hypothalamus, stimulates the release of pituitary thyroid-stimulating hormone (TSH). Pituitary TSH is a glycoprotein that stimulates the synthesis and release of thyroid hormones

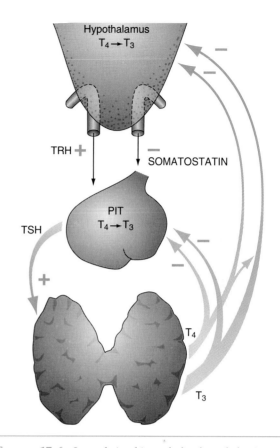

**FIGURE 17–6.** Interrelationships of the hypothalamic-pituitary-thyroid axis. Thyroid-stimulating hormone (TSH) from the pituitary gland (PIT) stimulates the secretion of both thyroxine ($T_4$) and triiodothyronine ($T_3$) from the thyroid gland. These act at the pituitary gland level to control secretion of TSH by a negative feedback mechanism. In addition, $T_4$ is metabolized to the potent $T_3$ within the pituitary gland by a monoiodinase. Secretion of TSH is stimulated by thyrotropin-releasing hormone (TRH) from the hypothalamus and inhibited by somatostatin. Thyroid hormone acts at the hypothalamus to stimulate secretion of somatostatin (somatostatin acts as a negative signal to the pituitary secretion of TSH). (From Wilson JD, Foster DW [eds]: Williams Textbook of Endocrinology, 8th ed. Philadelphia, WB Saunders, 1992, p 169.)

by the thyroid gland. Normal plasma concentrations of TSH are less than 5 $\mu$U/mL. Thyroid function develops in three stages:

1. Embryogenesis occurs from the floor of the primitive oral cavity, and the gland descends to its definitive position in the anterior lower neck by the end of the 1st trimester. This site remains functional (rarely, a lingual or sublingual site may be the only functioning thyroid gland).

2. The hypothalamic-pituitary-thyroid axis becomes functional in the 2nd trimester.

3. Peripheral metabolism of thyroid hormones matures in the 3rd trimester.

Thyroxine ($T_4$), triiodothyronine ($T_3$), and TSH do not appreciably cross the placenta, so their concentration in fetal serum reflects fetal secretion and metabolism. However, antithyroid antibodies, thyroid-stimulating immunoglobulins (TSIs), iodides (including radioactive iodides), propylthiouracil, and methimazole, do cross the placenta and affect fetal thyroid function.

The thyroid gland efficiently concentrates and organifies iodine into tyrosine; with subsequent coupling of two tyrosines, $T_4$ or $T_3$ is synthesized, representing the major thyroid hormones. The major fraction of circulating $T_3$ ($\sim$ two thirds) is derived from peripheral monodeiodination of $T_4$ to $T_3$. Free $T_3$ is the metabolically active form. $T_4$ and $T_3$ are covalently bound to a specific serum carrier protein, thyroxine-binding globulin (TBG), and, to a lesser extent, to albumin. Only the small (<2%) fractions of $T_4$ and $T_3$ not bound to this or to other serum carriers, free $T_4$ and free $T_3$, are biologically active and exert negative feedback on TSH release. The conversion of $T_4$ to $T_3$ requires the removal of one iodine from the outer ring; removing an iodine from the inner ring results in reverse $T_3$ ($rT_3$), which has little biologic effect. Preferential conversion to $rT_3$ occurs in utero and in all forms of severe illness, including respiratory distress syndrome, fevers, anorexia, cachexia, and starvation. In contrast, conversion from $T_4$ to $T_3$ increases immediately after birth and throughout life.

At birth, there are several dramatic changes in thyroid function. Interpretation of thyroid function tests must take into account the influence of TBG as assessed directly or indirectly via the $T_3$ resin uptake test and the age-related changes in circulating thyroid hormone concentrations. Free $T_4$ is the test of choice; however, because screening programs measure total $T_4$, TBG must be considered in the newborn. When TBG concentrations are normal, the $T_3$ resin uptake is increased in hyperthyroidism and decreased in hypothyroidism, reflecting the change in number of unoccupied binding sites. Thus, the thyroid hormone level and $T_3$ resin uptake test results vary in the same direction in disease states. In contrast, with altered TBG capacity (a benign condition), the $T_4$ level and $T_3$ resin uptake move in opposite directions; there is an elevated $T_4$ level with reduced $T_3$ resin uptake when there is TBG excess and a low $T_4$ level with high $T_3$ resin uptake when there is TBG deficiency. Factors increasing TBG capacity (and total but not free $T_4$) are estrogens, oral contraceptives, pregnancy, genetic increased TBG, acute hepatitis, maturity (neonates), narcotic abuse, and acute intermittent porphyria; factors decreasing TBG capacity (and total but not free $T_4$) are competing drugs (phenytoin, salicylates), congenital TBG deficiency, nephrotic syndrome, glucocorticoids, severe nonthyroid illness, androgens, and severe liver failure with cirrhosis.

A summary of laboratory test results in various types of thyroid abnormalities is illustrated in Table 17–13. Thyroid scans rarely are indicated in pediatric thyroid disease. A thyroid scan performed with short-lived $^{123}I$ will indicate the size, shape, and location of the thyroid gland. Agenesis or ectopic glands and hyperfunctioning "hot" nodules or nonfunctioning "cold" nodules may be detected. A solitary nodule is ominous, especially if it is solid and nonfunctional. An ultrasound study may determine whether it is cystic or solid. If solid, an $^{123}I$ scan will indicate its functional status. Solitary nodules are usually subject to excisional biopsy. Scans are not needed in the diagnosis of Hashimoto thyroiditis or thyrotoxicosis.

## THYROID DISORDERS

### Hypothyroidism

Hypothyroidism is considered to be congenital or acquired and, in each instance, as goitrous or nongoitrous.

TABLE 17–13.  Laboratory Test Results in Various Types of Thyroid Function Abnormalities in Children*

|  | Serum Total $T_4$ | Free $T_4$ | Serum TSH | Serum $T_3$ Resin Uptake | Serum TBG |
|---|---|---|---|---|---|
| Primary hypothyroidism | ↓ | ↓ | ↑ | ↓ | N |
| Hypothalamic (TRH) hypothyroidism | ↓ | ↓ | N | ↓ | N |
| Pituitary (TSH) hypothyroidism | ↓ | ↓ | N | ↓ | N |
| TBG deficiency | ↓ | N | N | ↑ | ↓ |
| TBG excess | ↑ | N | N | ↓ | ↑ |

*N = normal; ↓ = decreased; ↑ = increased; $T_3$ = triiodothyronine; $T_4$ = thyroxine; TBG = thyroid-binding globulin; TRH = thyroid-releasing hormone; TSH = thyroid-stimulating hormone.

**Congenital Hypothyroidism.** Congenital hypothyroidism occurs in approximately 1:4000 live births and is usually caused by a dysgenetic (agenesis, aplasia, ectopia) malformation of the thyroid gland. Thyroid tissue usually is not palpable, as these are nongoitrous conditions. The free $T_4$ concentration is low and TSH levels are elevated, documenting primary hypothyroidism. Routine neonatal screening programs are presently available in every state in the United States and in most countries. Typically, $T_4$ is measured in neonates and a subsequent TSH measurement is made if the original $T_4$ value is low. An immediate confirmatory serum sample should be obtained from any infant having a positive screening test (low $T_4$, high TSH); therapy is started in strongly positive cases while the results of the serum test are awaited. Primary TSH screening is gaining favor.

Congenital TBG deficiency occurs in about 1:10,000 live births and is associated with a low total $T_4$ concentration and a normal TSH value. Isolated secondary or tertiary hypothyroidism is rare, occurring in 1:100,000 live births. Secondary (pituitary) or tertiary (hypothalamic) hypothyroidism can be distinguished from TBG deficiency by determining the free $T_4$. When tertiary or secondary hypothyroidism is detected, assessment of other pituitary hormones and investigation of pituitary-hypothalamic anatomy via MRI is indicated.

**Goitrous congenital hypothyroidism** is unusual, occurring in about 1 in 30,000 live births. The goiter reflects an inborn error of metabolism in the pathway of iodide incorporation or thyroid hormone biosynthesis or reflects the transplacental passage of antithyroid drugs.

*Clinical manifestations* of congenital hypothyroidism include gestation greater than 42 wk (50%), birth weight greater than 4 kg (25%), hypothermia (33%), acrocyanosis (33%), respiratory distress (22%), large posterior fontanel (33%), abdominal distention (50%), lethargy and poor feeding (40%), jaundice more than 3 days after birth (75%), edema (70%), umbilical hernia (60%), mottled skin (50%), constipation (45%), large tongue (45%), dry skin (45%), hoarse cry (40%), and congenital anomalies (2–4%). In the immediate newborn period, the symptoms and signs usually are subtle but become more evident weeks or months after birth. Thyroid hormones are crucially important for maturation and differentiation of tissues, such as bone (bone age is often delayed) and brain. Hence, the importance of newborn screening is to make an early diagnosis and initiate thyroid replacement therapy.

When *treatment* is initiated within 1–2 mo of birth, the overall *prognosis* for normal intellectual development is excellent; screening programs usually offer therapy within 1 wk of birth. If therapy is instituted after 6 mo or later, when the signs of hypothyroid cretinism are present, the likelihood of normal intellectual function is markedly decreased; however, growth improves after thyroid replacement.

**Acquired Hypothyroidism.** The *etiology* of acquired hypothyroidism is presented in Table 17–14 and the *clinical manifestations* are summarized in Table 17–15. The signs and symptoms may be subtle, and hypothyroidism should be suspected in any child who has a decline in growth velocity, especially if not associated with weight loss. The most common cause in older children is autoimmune thyroiditis (Hashimoto thyroiditis). The failure of the thyroid gland may be heralded by a rise of TSH before $T_4$ levels fall. Acquired hypothyroidism is not a cause of permanent developmental delay.

**Hashimoto Thyroiditis.** Also known as autoimmune or *lymphocytic thyroiditis*, Hashimoto thyroid-

TABLE 17–14.    Causes of Hypothyroidism in Infancy and Childhood

| Age | Manifestation | Cause |
|---|---|---|
| Newborn | No goiter | Thyroid gland dysgenesis or ectopic location<br>Exposure to iodides<br>TSH deficiency<br>TRH deficiency |
| | Goiter | Inborn defect in hormone synthesis* or effect<br>Maternal goitrogen ingestion, including propylthiouracil, methimazole, iodides<br>Severe iodide deficiency (endemic) |
| 1–10 yr | No goiter | Thyroid gland dysgenesis<br>Cystinosis<br>Hypothalamic-pituitary insufficiency |
| | Goiter | Hashimoto thyroiditis: chronic lymphocytic thyroiditis<br>Inborn defect in hormone synthesis or effect<br>Goitrogenic drugs |
| 10–18 yr | No goiter | Surgical after thyrotoxicosis or other thyroid surgery |
| | Goiter | Hashimoto thyroiditis<br>Inborn defect in hormone synthesis or effect<br>Goitrogenic drugs<br>Infiltrative (sarcoid, lymphoma) |

*Impaired iodide transport, defective thyroglobulin iodination, defective iodotyrosine dehalogenase, defective thyroglobulin, or its coupling to idiotyrosines.

TABLE 17–15.  Symptoms and Signs of Hypothyroidism

| | |
|---|---|
| Ectodermal | Poor growth |
| | Dull facies: thick lips, large tongue,* depressed nasal bridge,* periorbital edema |
| | Dry scaly skin |
| | Sparse brittle hair |
| | Diminished sweating |
| | Carotenemia |
| | Vitiligo |
| Circulatory | Sinus bradycardia/heart block |
| | Cold extremities |
| | Cold intolerance |
| | Pallor |
| | ECG changes: low-voltage QRS complex |
| Neuromuscular | Muscle weakness |
| | Hypotonia: constipation, potbelly |
| | Umbilical hernia* |
| | Myxedema coma ($CO_2$ narcosis, hypothermia) |
| | Pseudohypertrophy of muscles |
| | Myalgia |
| | Physical and mental lethargy |
| | Developmental delay* |
| | Delayed relaxation of reflexes |
| | Paresthesias (nerve entrapment: carpal tunnel syndrome) |
| | Cerebellar ataxia* |
| Skeletal | Delayed bone age* |
| | Epiphyseal dysgenesis,* increased upper to lower segment ratio |
| Metabolic | Myxedema |
| | Serous effusions (pleural, pericardial, ascites)* |
| | Hoarse voice (cry)* |
| | Weight gain |
| | Menstrual irregularity |
| | Arthralgia |
| | Elevated CPK |
| | Macrocytosis (anemia) |
| | Hypercholesterolemia |
| | Hyperprolactinemia |
| | Precocious puberty in severe cases |

*Signs classic for congenital hypothyroidism appearing during infancy.
CPK = creatine phosphokinase; ECG = electrocardiogram.

itis is a common cause of goiter and acquired thyroid disease in older children and adolescents. A genetic predisposition may be present because a family history of thyroid disease is present in 25–35% of patients. The *etiology* is an autoimmune process targeted against the thyroid gland with lymphocytic infiltration, antimicrosomal or antithyroglobulin antibodies, and lymphoid follicle and germinal center formation preceding fibrosis and atrophy.

*Clinical manifestations* include firm, nontender euthyroid, hypothyroid or, rarely, hyperthyroid (Hashitoxicosis) diffuse goiter with a pebble-like feeling, and an insidious onset after 6 yr of age (the incidence peaks in adolescence, with a female predominance); and a pea-sized Delphian lymph node above the thyroid isthmus may be found. Associated autoimmune diseases include diabetes mellitus, adrenal insufficiency (Schmidt syndrome), and hypoparathyroidism; trisomy 21 and Turner syndrome predispose to autoimmune thyroiditis.

The *diagnosis* may be confirmed by serum antimicrosomal, antithyroglobulin antibodies; biopsy is hardly ever indicated. Antimicrosomal or antithyroglobulin antibodies may be present in Hashimoto thyroiditis.

*Treatment* with thyroid hormone sufficient to suppress TSH to a normal level is indicated for hypothyroidism. Patients without manifestation of hypothyroidism require periodic thyroid function testing (TSH, $T_4$). Goiter with a normal TSH is not usually an indication for treatment.

### Hyperthyroidism

**Graves Disease.** Most children with hyperthyroidism have Graves disease, which is produced by autoantibodies (thyroid-stimulating antibodies [TSIs]), which stimulate thyroid gland activity, simulating the effects of TSH. The resulting excessive synthesis, release, and peripheral metabolism of thyroid hormones produce the clinical features. Hashimoto thyroiditis and thyrotoxicosis are on a continuum of autoimmune disease. Antimicrosomal and antithyroglobulin antibodies may be present in thyrotoxicosis; exceptionally high titers may indicate coexistent Hashimoto thyroiditis (Hashitoxicosis), with the eventual risk of delayed hypothyroidism. In Graves disease, $T_4$ and/or $T_3$ levels are elevated while TSH is suppressed. Rare causes of hyperthyroidism include McCune-Albright syndrome, thyroid neoplasm, TSH hypersecretion, subacute thyroiditis, and iodine or thyroid hormone ingestion.

*Clinical Manifestations.* The signs of fully expressed Graves disease consist of hyperthyroidism (Table 17–16), stare (a result of adrenergic activity), exophthalmos, ophthalmopathy, dermopathy, myopathy, and acropachy (clubbing). In children, Graves disease is about five times more common in females than in males, with a peak incidence in adolescence; however, most children rarely exhibit all of these clinical features. Personality changes, mood instability, and poor school performance are common presenting problems. The tremor, anxiety, inability to concentrate, and weight loss may be

TABLE 17–16. Clinical Manifestations
of Hyperthyroidism

| | |
|---|---|
| Increased catecholamine effects | Nervousness<br>Palpitations<br>Tachycardia<br>Atrial arrhythmias<br>Systolic hypertension<br>Tremor<br>Brisk reflexes |
| Hypermetabolism | Increased sweating<br>Shiny, smooth skin<br>Heat intolerance<br>Fatigue<br>Weight loss—increased appetite<br>Increased bowel movement (hyperdefecation)<br>Hyperkinesis |
| Myopathy | Weakness<br>Periodic paralysis<br>Cardiac failure—dyspnea |
| Miscellaneous | Proptosis, stare, exophthalmos, lid lag, opthalmopathy<br>Hair loss<br>Inability to concentrate<br>Personality change (emotional lability)<br>Goiter<br>Thyroid bruit<br>Onycholysis<br>Painful gland*<br><br>*Acute thyroid storm* (hyperpyrexia, tachycardia, coma, high-output heart failure, shock) |

* Unusual except in subacute thyroiditis with hyperthyroid phase.

insidious and confused with a psychologic disorder until thyroid function tests reveal the elevated serum $T_4$ level. $T_4$ may remain near normal while serum $T_3$ is selectively elevated ($T_3$ toxicosis). A firm, homogeneous goiter usually is present. Many patients complain of neck fullness and, in older subjects, a change in the size of their shirt collars. Thyroid gland enlargement is best visualized with the neck extended and with the examiner lateral to the patient; palpation of the thyroid gland is best performed with the examiner's hands around the neck. The patient swallows so the examiner can feel the size, consistency, nodularity, and motion of the gland. A bruit may be auscultated over the gland.

***Treatment.*** Three treatment choices are available: (1) medical, (2) surgical, and (3) radioactive iodine.

*DRUGS.* Medical therapy consists of propylthiouracil (PTU) to block thyroid hormone synthesis (150–450 mg/24 hr PO in divided doses every 8 hr). Propranolol is started if symptoms are severe (2–3 mg/kg/24 hr orally) to control cardiac manifestations and is tapered after 1–2 mo when the pulse rate is reduced to less than 100 beats/min. PTU usually is continued for 1–2 yr, as there is a remission rate of approximately 25% per year. In patients complying with the treatment regimen, the 2-yr course of treatment can be repeated. PTU should suppress thyroid function to the point that thyroid hormone replacement is needed. Complications of PTU include lupus-like syndrome, rash, granulocytopenia, and jaundice. Complications are usually reversible; failure to monitor and then discontinue PTU may be fatal. Methimazole is an alternate agent, and is given in approximately 10% of the dose of PTU. Iodine may also be used for a few weeks to suppress thyroid function but then becomes ineffective and is not recommended.

*SURGERY.* Surgical treatment consists of partial thyroidectomy. Risks associated with thyroidectomy include the use of anesthesia and the possibility that the thyroid removal will be excessive, causing hypothyroidism, or that it will be inadequate, resulting in persistent hyperthyroidism, keloid formation, recurrent laryngeal nerve palsy, and hypoparathyroidism (transient postoperative or permanent). Even with optimal immediate postoperative results, most patients become hypothyroid within 10 yr.

*RADIOIODINE.* Radioiodine ($^{131}I$) is slower in its therapeutic effects, may require repeated dosing, and may cause hypothyroidism. Although studies reveal no long-term consequences, concern remains about possible long-term sequelae in children. Radioiodine is reserved for older (nonpregnant) teenagers. Continued monitoring for the development of hypothyroidism is essential.

**Thyroid Storm.** Thyroid storm (see Table 17–16) is a rare medical emergency consisting of tachycardia and hyperthermia; *treatment* includes reducing the hyperthermia with a cooling blanket and administering propranolol to control tachycardia. Iodine may be given to block thyroid hormone release. Cortisol may be indicated for relative adrenal insufficiency, and therapy for heart failure may include diuretics and digoxin.

**Congenital Hyperthyroidism.** This disorder results from transplacental passage of material TSIs. The *clinical* manifestations in the neonate may be masked for several days until the short-lived effects of transplacental maternal antithyroid medication wear off, at which time the effects of TSIs are observed. Irritability, tachycardia (often with signs of cardiac failure simulating "cardiomyopathy"), polycythemia, craniosynostosis, bone age advancement, poor feeding, and later failure to thrive are the clinical hallmarks. This condition may be anticipated if the mother is known to be thyrotoxic in pregnancy so that timely therapy can be offered. If the mother was cured of her hyperthyroidism before pregnancy by surgery or radioiodine treatment, which limits or curtails $T_4$ production but not the underlying immune disturbance producing TSIs, the infant may still be affected.

*Treatment* for the neonate includes oral propranolol at 2–3 mg/kg/24 hr in divided doses and propylthiouracil approximately 5 mg/kg/24 hr orally in three divided doses. Because the half-life of immunoglobulin is several weeks, spontaneous resolution of neonatal thyrotoxicosis resulting from transplacental passage of TSIs usually occurs by 2–3 mo of life.

## TUMORS OF THE THYROID

Carcinoma of the thyroid is rare in children, but papillary and follicular carcinoma represent 90% of children's thyroid cancers. A history of therapeutic head or neck irradiation or exposure to nuclear accidents predisposes a child to thyroid cancer. Carcinoma usually presents as a firm to hard, painless, nonfunctional solitary nodule and may spread to adjacent lymph nodes. Rapid growth, hoarseness (recurrent laryngeal nerve involvement), and lung metastasis may be present. If the nodule is solid on ultrasound, "cold" on radioiodine scanning, and feels hard, the likelihood of a carcinoid is high. Fine-needle aspiration biopsy may not accurately reveal the cell type, and excisional biopsy is usually performed.

*Treatment* includes total thyroidectomy, selective regional node dissection, and radioablation with $^{131}$I for residual or recurrent disease. The *prognosis* is usually good if the disease is diagnosed early.

**Medullary carcinoma of the thyroid** (MCT) may be asymptomatic except for a mass. *Diagnosis* is based on the presence of elevated calcitonin levels, either in the basal state or following pentagastrin stimulation, or histology. This tumor most often occurs with multiple endocrine neoplasia II (MEN), with pheochromocytoma, or alone in a familial pattern. The presence of the RET oncogene is predictive of the development of MCT, and using DNA probes directed at the affected gene in family members is indicated.

### References

Behrman RE, Kliegman RM, Arvin AM (eds): Nelson Textbook of Pediatrics, 15th ed. Philadelphia, WB Saunders, 1966, Chapters 518–524.

Dayan C, Daniel G: Chronic autoimmune thyroiditis. N Engl J Med 335:99, 1996.

Fisher DA: Clinical review 19: Management of congenital hypothyroidism. J Clin Endocrinol Metab 72:523, 1991.

Foley TP: Disorders of the thyroid in children. *In* Sperling MA (ed): Pediatric Endocrinology. Philadelphia, WB Saunders, 1996, pp 171–194.

Lazarus J: Hyperthyroidism. Lancet 349:339, 1997.

Lindsay R, Toft A: Hypothyroidism. Lancet 349:413, 1997.

Millman B, Pellitteri P: Thyroid cancer in children and adolescents. Arch Otolaryngol Head Neck Surg 121:126, 1995.

Zimmerman D, Gan-Gaisano M: Hyperthyroidism in children and adolescents. Pediatr Clin North Am 37:1273, 1990.

# DISORDERS OF SEXUAL DIFFERENTIATION

## NORMAL SEXUAL DEVELOPMENT

Gender is determined by a combination of karyotype (genotypic or chromosomal sex), which usually determines the morphology of internal organs and gonads (gonadal sex), by the appearance of the external genitalia and the form of secondary sex characteristics (phenotypic sex), by the self-perception of the individual (gender identity), and by the perception of others (gender role). In most children these features blend and conform, but in some patients one or more features may be aberrant, leading to intersex problems.

Ambiguous genitalia in a newborn must be considered an endocrine emergency. Insensitive handling of the situation may lead to a lifelong pattern of gender uncertainty in a patient and confusion in the parents. Complicating matters, the laboratory evaluations required may take days or weeks to be completed before a sex is assigned or a name is given.

*Diagnosis* and *treatment* of disorders of sex differentiation are best understood easily when the embryology and hormonal control of normal sex differentiation is known. The internal and external genitalia are formed between the 9th and 13th wk of gestation. Regardless of karyotype, a fetus is bipotential and has the capacity to develop a normal male or female phenotype. A female phenotype develops unless a specific "male" influence alters development. The male or female phenotype develops internally from bipotential gonads and internal ducts, and externally from bipotential anlage (Fig. 17–7). In the presence of a testes-determining gene for the testes-determining factor (TDF) on the Y chromosome, the primitive fetal gonad differentiates into a testis (Fig. 17–8). The testis secretes testosterone, which has direct effects (stimulation of development of the wolffian ducts) but must be metabolized for other effects. Testosterone is locally converted into dihydrotestosterone (DHT) by 5α-reduction. DHT causes enlargement,

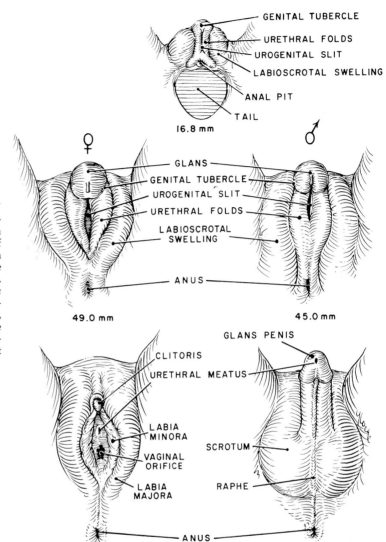

GENITAL TUBERCLE
URETHRAL FOLDS
UROGENITAL SLIT
LABIOSCROTAL SWELLING
ANAL PIT
TAIL
16.8 mm

GLANS
GENITAL TUBERCLE
UROGENITAL SLIT
URETHRAL FOLDS
LABIOSCROTAL SWELLING
ANUS
49.0 mm

45.0 mm

CLITORIS
URETHRAL MEATUS
LABIA MINORA
VAGINAL ORIFICE
LABIA MAJORA
GLANS PENIS
SCROTUM
RAPHE
ANUS

FIGURE 17–7. Differentiation of male and female external genitalia as proceeding from a common anlage. Testosterone acts at 9–13 wk of gestation to virilize the bipotential anlage. In the absence of testosterone action, the female phenotype develops. (From Grumbach MM, Conte FA: Disorders of sexual differentiation. *In* Wilson JD, Foster DW [eds]: Textbook of Endocrinology, 8th ed. Philadelphia, WB Saunders, 1990, p 873. Adapted from Spaulding MH: The development of the external genitalia in the human embryo. Contrib Embryol Carnegie Instit 1921;13:69–88.)

rugation, and fusion of the labia majora into a scrotum; fusion of the ventral surface of the penis to enclose a penile urethra; and enlargement of the phallus with ultimate development of male external genitalia (see Figs. 17–7 and 17–8). Testicular production and secretion of müllerian duct-inhibitory substance causes the regression and disappearance of the müllerian ducts. In the presence of testosterone, the wolffian ducts develop into the vas deferens, seminiferous tubules, and prostate.

In the absence of TDF, an ovary spontaneously develops from the bipotential, primitive gonad. In the absence of fetal testicular secretion of müllerian-inhibitory substance, a normal uterus, fallopian tubes, and posterior third of the vagina develop out of the müllerian ducts as the wolffian ducts degenerate. In the total absence of andro-

gens, the external genitalia appear female. In the absence of adequate virilization because of abnormal development of the testes, biosynthetic defects of testosterone or DHT, or androgen receptor defects, any phenotype between female and male may develop; the patient has ambiguous genitalia or an intersex condition. Every child, regardless of intersexuality, should be raised definitively either as a male or female.

## ABNORMAL SEXUAL DEVELOPMENT

### Virilization of the 46,XX Female (Female Pseudohermaphroditism)

Masculinization of the external genitalia of genotypic females always is due to the presence of

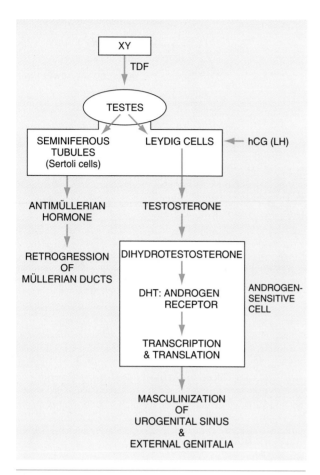

A diagrammatic scheme of male sex determination and differentiation. DHT = dihydrotestosterone; TDF = testis-determining factor. (From Wilson JD, Foster DW [eds]: Williams Textbook of Endocrinology, 8th ed. Philadelphia, WB Saunders, 1992, p 918.)

TABLE 17–17.    Causes of Virilization in the Female

| Condition | Additional Features |
| --- | --- |
| P-450$_{c21}$ deficiency | Salt loss in some |
| 3β-Hydroxysteroid dehydrogenase deficiency | Salt loss |
| P-450 C$_{11}$ deficiency | Salt retention/hypertension |
| Androgenic drug exposure (e.g., progestins) | Exposure between 9th and 12th wk gestation |
| Mixed gonadal dysgenesis or mosaic Turner syndrome | Karyotype = 46,XY/45,X |
| True hermaphrodite | Testicular and ovarian tissue present |
| Maternal virilizing adrenal or ovarian tumor | Rare, positive history |

one production or action (Table 17–18). The penis is small, with various degrees of hypospadias (penile or perineal) and associated chordee or ventral binding of the phallus; unilateral, but more often bilateral, cryptorchidism may be present. The testis (gonad) should be carefully sought in the inguinal canal or labioscrotal folds. Very rarely, a palpable gonad in the inguinal canal or labioscrotal fold

TABLE 17–18.    Causes of Inadequate Masculinization in the Male

| Condition | Additional Features |
| --- | --- |
| P-450$_{scc}$ (STAR) deficiency | Salt loss |
| 3β-Hydroxysteroid dehydrogenase deficiency | Salt loss |
| P-450$_{c17}$ deficiency | Salt retention/hypokalemia/hypertension |
| 17,20-Desmolase deficiency | Adrenal function normal |
| 17β-Hydroxysteroid oxidoreductase deficiency | Adrenal function normal |
| Dysgenetic testes | Possible abnormal karyotype |
| Leydig cell hypoplasia | Rare |
| Testicular feminization or androgen insensitivity (complete) | Female external genitalia, absence of müllerian structures |
| Testicular feminization or androgen insensitivity (partial) | As above with ambiguous external genitalia |
| 5α-Reductase deficiency | Autosomal recessive, virilization at puberty |

excessive androgens during the critical period of development (8–13 wk gestation) (Table 17–17). The magnitude of the changes will reflect the quantity and duration of exposure to androgens. The degree of virilization can range from mild clitoral enlargement to that of a "male" phallus with a penile urethra and fused scrotum with raphe. Ambiguous genitalia in females is most commonly the result of an enzyme deficiency that impairs adrenal cortisol synthesis but does not affect testosterone production (see Adrenal Gland). Under these conditions, ACTH stimulates hyperplasia of the adrenal cortex and excessive adrenal production of androgens.

### Inadequate Masculinization of the 46,XY Male (Male Pseudohermaphroditism)

Underdevelopment of the male external genitalia occurs because of a relative deficiency of testosterrepresents a herniated ovary or an ovotestis in a hermaphrodite. The latter patients have both ovarian and testicular tissue, usually an XX genotype (80%), and ambiguous external genitalia. Production of testosterone by a gonad in utero implies that testicular tissue is present and that some cells carry Y chromosomal DNA.

Testosterone production can be reduced by specific deficiencies of the enzymes needed for androgen biosynthesis or by dysplasia of the gonads. In the latter, if müllerian-inhibiting substance production also is reduced, a rudimentary uterus and fallopian tubes will be present. Enzyme defects in testosterone biosynthesis, which also block cortisol production, produce adrenal hyperplasia. Hypopituitarism with LH deficiency does not result in ambiguous genitalia because placental hCG present in the fetal circulation stimulates fetal gonadal testosterone synthesis during the critical 9 to 13 weeks of gestation to allow a normal male phallus. Later in gestation, fetal LH is needed to normally stimulate the testes to produce androgen to enlarge the fetal penis. Thus, congenital gonadotropin deficiency may produce a microphallus; this condition is often combined with deficiencies of GH and ACTH, causing neonatal hypoglycemia.

The complete form of **testicular feminization syndrome** is the most dramatic example of androgen insensitivity. Absolute resistance of target tissues to the actions of the androgens in some patients occurs because the androgen receptor cannot bind DHT. In others, a postreceptor defect is presumed. Affected patients have a 46,XY karyotype, normally formed testes usually located in the inguinal canal or labia majora, and feminine-appearing external genitalia with a short vagina and no internal müllerian structures. At the time of puberty, testosterone concentrations rise to the normal male range. Because some of the testosterone is converted to estradiol in peripheral tissues, breast development ensues at the normal age of puberty without growth of pubic, facial, or axillary hair or the occurrence of menstruation.

## APPROACH TO THE INFANT WITH GENITAL AMBIGUITY

The major goals of infant care are a rapid determination of the correct sex of rearing and identification of any life-threatening disorders (e.g., salt loss and shock). Sex assignment is based on the feasibility of genital reconstruction and potential fertility rather than on karyotype or gonadal histology. For example, it is usually inappropriate to raise a female infant who is severely virilized from congeni-

tal adrenal hyperplasia as a male. If surgically corrected as a female, she will likely retain fertility because the internal organs are female. Similarly, a 46,XY male with an extremely small phallus that will not increase in size with androgen therapy should probably be raised as a female because surgical construction of a fully functional phallus is very difficult. Although sex assignment should be accomplished as rapidly as possible, the naming of the infant should be delayed until the correct choice is clear.

*Diagnosis.* The first step toward diagnosis is to determine if the disorder represents virilization of a female (androgen excess) or underdevelopment of a male (androgen deficiency) (see Fig. 17–8). Inguinal gonads that are evident on palpation nearly always are testes and indicate that incomplete development of a male has occurred. Similarly, absence of female internal genitalia (detected by ultrasound) implies that müllerian-inhibiting substance was secreted by fetal testes. Karyotype determination, although helpful in diagnosis, is only one of many factors in deciding the sexual identity for rearing purposes.

Most virilized females have adrenal hyperplasia, and 90% have 21-hydroxylase deficiency. The diagnosis is established by measuring the plasma concentration of 17-OHP (see Adrenal Gland), which typically is hundreds of times above the normal range. Other enzymatic defects also can be diagnosed by quantifying the circulating levels of the steroid that serves as the defective enzyme's substrate.

Accurate diagnoses are more difficult to obtain in underdeveloped males. When adrenal hyperplasia coexists, excessive ACTH secretion will elevate levels of specific adrenal steroid precursors substantially. If the defect is restricted to testosterone biosynthesis, the measurement of testosterone and its precursors after stimulation by hCG may be required. Patients with normal levels of testosterone either have persistent androgen resistance or had an interruption of normal morphogenesis at a critical time. Abnormalities of the sex chromosomes may be associated with dysgenetic gonads, as is persistence of müllerian structures.

*Treatment.* Treatment consists of (1) replacing deficient hormones (e.g., cortisol in adrenal hyperplasia and testosterone at the time of puberty in androgen biosynthetic defects); (2) surgical restoration; and (3) psychologic support of the whole family. Gonads and internal organs discordant for the sex of rearing are removed. Dysgenetic gonads should be removed because gonadoblastomas or dysgerminomas may develop in the future. Reconstructive surgery should be started by 2 yr of age so that genital structure will reflect sex of rearing during the time when gender identity is acquired.

### References

Behrman RE, Kliegman RM, Arvin AM (eds): Nelson Textbook of Pediatrics, 15th ed. Philadelphia, WB Saunders, 1996, Chapter 540.

Griffin JE: Androgen resistance: The clinical and molecular spectrum. N Engl J Med 326:611, 1992.

Grumbach M, Conte F: Disorders of sexual differentiation. *In* Wilson J, Forest D (eds): Williams Textbook of Endocrinology, 8th ed. Philadelphia, WB Saunders, 1992, p 853.

McCauley E: Disorders of sexual differentiation and development: Psychological aspects. Pediatr Clin North Am 37:1405, 1990.

Witchel SS, Lee PA: Ambiguous genitalia. *In* Sperling MA (ed): Pediatric Endocrinology. Philadelphia, WB Saunders, 1996, pp 31–50.

## ADRENAL GLAND

The adrenal gland consists of an outer cortex, responsible for the synthesis of steroids, and an inner medulla derived from neuroectodermal tissue, which synthesizes catecholamines. The *adrenal cortex* consists of three zones: an outer glomerulosa whose end product is the mineralocorticoid aldosterone, which regulates sodium balance; a middle zone, the fasciculata, whose end product is cortisol; and an inner reticularis that synthesizes sex steroids. The general scheme of these synthetic steps is shown in Figure 17–9.

The hypothalamic-pituitary-adrenal axis comprises a classic negative feedback system. A hypothalamic corticotropin-releasing hormone (CRH)

FIGURE 17–9. Steroid hormone biosynthetic pathways. (From Styne DM: Sexual differentiation. *In* Fitzgerald PA [ed]: Handbook of Clinical Endocrinology. Norwalk, CT, Appleton & Lange, 1986, pp 73–99.)

stimulates the release of pituitary ACTH, derived by selective processing from pro-opiomelanocortin, which contains the sequences of endorphins. The sequence of melanocyte-stimulating hormone (MSH) is contained within the ACTH molecule. ACTH governs the synthesis and release of cortisol and adrenal androgens. Primary adrenal insufficiency or cortisol deficiency from any defect in the adrenal results in an oversecretion of ACTH; cortisol deficiency (secondary or tertiary) also may occur from CRH or ACTH deficiency, causing low serum ACTH concentrations. Endogenous (or exogenous) glucocorticoids feed back to inhibit ACTH and CRH secretion. The renin-angiotensin system, as well as potassium, regulates aldosterone secretion; except in excess, ACTH has little effect on aldosterone production.

Steroids that are free (i.e., not bound to cortisol-binding protein [transcortin]) may cross the placenta from mother to fetus. Because the fetal CRF–ACTH–adrenal axis is operational in utero, deficiencies in cortisol synthesis lead to excessive ACTH secretion and if a virilizing adrenal enzyme defect is present, the fetal adrenal gland will secrete androgens, thus virilizing the fetus. The normal variation of serum cortisol and ACTH levels (high in early morning, lower at night) may not be established until the end of the 1st to 4th yr of life.

## ADRENAL INSUFFICIENCY

The *clinical manifestations* of inadequate adrenal function result from the inadequate secretion or action of glucocorticoids, mineralocorticoids, or both (Table 17–19). In addition, in the case of enzyme defects that commonly affect the gonad as well as the adrenal gland, overproduction or underproduction of potent androgens can occur, depending on the site of blockade (see Fig. 17–9). Thus, there may be progressive virilization of the external genitalia in females and males or incomplete virilization in males. Ambiguity of the external genitalia is therefore a common manifestation of disordered fetal adrenal enzyme function. Precise *diagnosis* is essential for the prescription of appropriate therapy, long-term outlook, and genetic counseling. Table 17–20 presents a diagnostic classification of adrenal insufficiency in infancy and childhood.

The dominant clinical features of adrenal insufficiency in infancy are related to mineralocorticoid deficiency. Serum electrolyte measurement reveals hyponatremia and hyperkalemia usually developing 5–7 days after birth. Vomiting, dehydration, and acidosis soon follow, as do shock and, if un-

**TABLE 17–19.** Clinical Manifestations of Adrenal Insufficiency

**Cortisol Deficiency**
Hypoglycemia
Inability to withstand stress
Vasomotor collapse
Hyperpigmentation (in primary adrenal insufficiency with excess of adrenocorticotropic hormone)
Apneic spells
Hypoglycemic seizure
Muscle weakness, fatigue

**Aldosterone Deficiency**
Vomiting
Hyponatremia
Urinary sodium wasting
Salt craving
Hyperkalemia
Acidosis
Failure to thrive
Volume depletion
Hypotension
Dehydration
Shock
Diarrhea
Muscle weakness

**Androgen Excess or Deficiency (Caused by Adrenal Enzyme Defect)**
Ambiguous genitalia in certain conditions

treated, death. In females, ambiguous genitalia resulting from excessive androgen secretion is often a major clue. In males, the diagnosis of adrenal insufficiency may be overlooked or confused with pyloric stenosis. However, in pyloric stenosis, the vomiting of hydrochloric acid results in hypochloremia; serum potassium is normal or low and alkalosis is present. This distinction may be lifesaving in preventing unnecessary investigations, inappropriate therapy, or surgery. Scrotal or virilized labial pigmentation suggests the excess ACTH (MSH) secretion of congenital adrenal hyperplasia (**adrenogenital syndrome**).

In patients with congenital adrenal hypoplasia or adrenal hemorrhage, the secretion of all adrenal steroids will be low. In contrast, congenital adrenal hyperplasia, as a result of one of the enzyme defects listed in Figure 17–9, leads to a diagnostic steroid pattern in blood and urine. Deficiency of 21-hydroxylase is the most common (95%) and serves as a paradigm for these disorders.

### 21-Hydroxylase Deficiency

Deficient 21-hydroxylase activity (P-450$_{c21}$ deficiency) results in the decreased conversion of 17-OHP to 11-desoxycortisol and of progesterone to

TABLE 17–20.   Causes of Adrenal Insufficiency in Infancy and Childhood

**Congenital Adrenal Hypoplasia**

Secondary to ACTH deficiency
Autosomal recessive
X-linked

**Adrenal Hemorrhage, Necrosis, Thrombosis**

**Congenital Adrenal Hyperplasia**

$P-450_{scc}$ (Cholesterol side chain cleavage) deficiency
$3\beta$-Hydroxysteroid dehydrogenase deficiency
$P-450_{c21}$ (21-Hydroxylase) deficiency
$P-450_{c11}$ ($11\beta$-Hydroxylase) deficiency
$P-450_{c17}$ (17-Hydroxylase) deficiency

**Isolated Deficiency of Aldosterone Synthesis**

$P-450_{c11}$ (18-Hydroxylase) deficiency
$P-450_{c11}$ (18-Hydroxysteroid dehydrogenase) deficiency

**Pseudohypoaldosteronism—End-Organ Unresponsiveness to Aldosterone**

**Congenital Adrenal Unresponsiveness to ACTH**

**Addison Disease**

Autoimmune adrenal insufficiency*
Infections of the adrenal gland
    Tuberculosis
    Histoplasmosis
    Meningococcosis
Infiltration of the adrenal gland
    Sarcoidosis
    Hemochromatosis
    Amyloidosis
    Metastatic cancer, lymphoma
Adrenoleukodystrophy

**Secondary**

Craniopharyngioma
Histiocytosis
Empty sella syndrome
Pituitary irradiation
Sarcoidosis
Hypothalamic lesions
Postpartum pituitary necrosis
Head trauma

**Drugs (Suppress Adrenal Steroidogenesis)**

Acute withdrawal of steroid therapy given for more than
    7–10 days
Metyrapone
Ketoconazole

---

*Isolated or as part of polyglandular syndrome type I (adrenal, hypoparathyroidism, mucocutaneous candidiasis) or type II (adrenal, thyroid, insulin-dependent diabetes).
ACTH = adrenocorticotropic hormone.

desoxycorticosterone (see Fig. 17–9). The obligatory decreased production of cortisol allows hypersecretion of ACTH, which, in turn, stimulates the synthesis of steroids immediately proximal to the block and causes shunting of precursors to the androgen pathway, leading to the overproduction of testosterone. The latter results in many of the *clinical manifestations*. Virilization of the external genitalia of the female occurs in utero; the development of the ovaries, fallopian tubes, and uterus is unaffected. The degree of virilization in the external genitalia of the female is variable, ranging from mild clitoromegaly to complete fusion of labioscrotal folds, simulating a phallus (see Disorders of Sexual Differentiation). A male infant with this defect appears normal at birth, although penile enlargement may be apparent thereafter. The deficiency in aldosterone found in about 75% of patients causes salt wasting with shock and dehydration unless appropriate treatment is given.

Inadequately treated, $P-450_{c21}$ deficiency (assuming salt loss does not lead to serious complications) demonstrates postnatal virilization, causing excessive growth, early appearance of pubic hair, progressive penile or clitoral enlargement, excessive linear growth, and tall stature due to progressive advancement in the bone age that is accompanied by early epiphyseal fusion, ultimately yielding short adult stature. Nonclassical $P-450_{c21}$ deficiency is noted well after birth and demonstrates similar but milder manifestations.

*Biochemical diagnostic studies* demonstrate elevated levels of serum 17-OHP, the substrate for the defective $P-450_{c21}$ enzyme activity. Serum cortisol and aldosterone levels (in salt losers) are low, whereas the level of testosterone is elevated, as it is derived from 17-OHP.

The incidence of classical 21-hydroxylase deficiency is about 1:12,000 among various Caucasian populations. An incidence of 1:500 occurs in one isolated ethnic population. Nonclassical congenital adrenal hyperplasia may occur with an incidence of 1:50 in certain populations. Two genes on chromosome 6 code for 21-hydroxylase; if there is an affected sibling, the genotype may be determined permitting prenatal diagnosis in a subsequent pregnancy.

The goals of *treatment* are to achieve normal linear growth and bone age advancement. Chronic therapy consists of providing glucocorticoid at a dose of approximately 18 mg/m²/24 hr of hydrocortisone or its equivalent. Other glucocorticoid regimens and dose schedules have been recommended, but we recommend cortisol or hydrocortisone. Mineralocorticoid therapy for salt losers consists of $9\alpha$-fludrocortisone (Florinef) at a dose of 0.1–0.2 mg/24 hr along with sodium chloride supplementation, especially for infants in the 1st yr of life. Surgical correction of ambiguous external genitalia begins by 1 yr of life to permit normal development of gender identity. The adequacy of glucocorticoid replacement therapy is often monitored by determining serum concentrations of adrenal metabolites, but the assessment of linear growth and skeletal age is the best reflection of appropriate therapy. Threefold higher doses of glucocorticoids are given during stressful states, such as febrile illnesses and surgery, to avoid adrenal insufficiency. Mineralocorticoid therapy is monitored with serum sodium and potassium and plasma renin levels. Prenatal treatment with dexamethasone to suppress fetal ACTH-induced androgen production has been reported as successful in eliminating ambiguous genitalia in affected female fetuses, if begun at approximately the 7th wk of gestation.

### Other Enzyme Defects

In patients with some enzyme defects, an elevation in the precursor steroid is present immediately proximal to the enzyme block, a deficiency of steroids is present subsequent to the block, and an excess of precursor is metabolized through remaining normal alternate enzyme pathways (see Fig. 17–9). The excessive secretion of precursor steroids is suppressed by glucocorticoid treatment. The other enzyme defects are rare in contrast to that of 21-OH deficiency.

In **11-OH deficiency**, the next most common condition, virilization occurs but salt retention and hypokalemia, rather than salt wasting, occur as a result of the buildup of desoxycorticosterone (see Fig. 17–9), a potent mineralocorticoid. Hypertension develops as a result of excessive mineralocorticoid production.

A summary of the clinical and biochemical features of adrenal insufficiency in infancy is listed in Table 17–21.

### Addison Disease

Addison disease is a rare acquired disorder of childhood, usually associated with autoimmune destruction of the adrenal cortex. *Clinical manifestations* are hyperpigmentation, salt craving, postural hypotension, fasting hypoglycemia, and episodes of shock during severe illness. Baseline and ACTH-stimulated cortisol values are subnormal, thereby confirming the diagnosis; hyponatremia, hyperkalemia, and elevated plasma renin activity indicate mineralocorticoid deficiency.

Replacement *treatment* with 18 mg/m$^2$/24 hr of hydrocortisone is indicated, with supplementation during stress at three times the normal maintenance dosage. Mineralocorticoid replacement with fludrocortisone is usually required. Associated autoimmune disorders that must be considered include diabetes mellitus, thyroiditis, oophoritis, pernicious anemia and malabsorption, chronic hep-

atitis, vitiligo, alopecia, and mucocutaneous candidiasis (see Table 17–20).

### Cushing Syndrome

Classic *clinical manifestations* of Cushing syndrome in children include progressive central obesity, marked failure of longitudinal growth, hirsutism, weakness, a nuchal fat pat (buffalo hump), acne, striae, hypertension, and often hyperpigmentation (only if ACTH is elevated). Affected children have adrenal adenoma, carcinoma, nodular adrenal hyperplasia, an ACTH-secreting pituitary microadenoma, causing bilateral adrenal hyperplasia (Cushing disease), or a very rare ACTH-secreting tumor. The high-dose dexamethasone suppression test (20 mcg/kg orally every 6 hr for 48 hr) suppresses glucocorticoid secretion in Cushing disease but not in autonomous adrenal production of cortisol or in an ectopic ACTH-secreting tumor. Parenteral glucocorticoid therapy is necessary during and immediately after surgical removal of the cause of the syndrome to avoid acute adrenal insufficiency.

Spontaneous Cushing syndrome is rare in childhood, but iatrogenic Cushing syndrome is far more common and produces similar features; the latter may be induced by the use of potent glucocorticoids for chronic inflammatory, neoplastic, and collagen vascular disorders and for suppression of the immune response. Depending on the potency of glucocorticoid used and its duration of use, both adrenal gland size and secretory ability and pituitary ACTH are suppressed. Recovery of pituitary ACTH secretion precedes that of adrenal gland function. Hence, glucocorticoids should be withdrawn gradually over a number of weeks. During this tapering process, any emergency requires glucocorticoid therapy at triple the physiologic dose. The ability of the adrenal to respond to ACTH with a doubling of plasma cortisol to levels of at least 15–20 μg/dL indicates recovery of pituitary-adrenal function.

*Treatment* of Cushing syndrome includes excision of autonomous adrenal, pituitary, or ectopic ACTH-secreting tumors. Rarely, adrenalectomy or adrenal ablative agents (mitotane-*o,p'*-DDD) are needed to control the symptoms.

### References

Azziz R, Dewailly D, Owerbach D: Clinical review 56—nonclassic adrenal hyperplasia: Current concepts. J Clin Endocrinol Metab 78:810, 1994.

Behrman RE, Kliegman RM, Arvin AM (eds): Nelson Textbook of Pediatrics, 15th ed. Philadelphia, WB Saunders, 1996, Chapters 528–538.

Miller WL: Pathophysiology, genetics and treatment of hyperandrogenism. Pediatr Clin North Am 44:375, 1997.

Table 17-21. Clinical and Biochemical Features in Newborn Adrenal Insufficiency

| | | Ambiguous Genitalia | | Serum | | | | | Urine | | |
|---|---|---|---|---|---|---|---|---|---|---|---|
| | Electrolyte Disturbance* | Virilized Female | Undervirilized Male | Cortisol | 11-Deoxycortisol | 17-OHP | DHEA | Aldosterone | 17-OHCS | 17-KS | Pregnanetriol |
| Hypoplasia | Severe | No | No | D | D | D | D | D | D | D | D |
| Hemorrhage | Moderate–severe | No | No | D | D | D | D | D | D | D | D |
| P-450$_{scc}$ (STAR) deficiency | Severe | No | Yes | D | D | D | D | D | D | D | D |
| 3β-HSD | Severe | Yes | Yes | D | D | D | I | D | D | I | D |
| P-450$_{c21}$ deficiency | Absent–severe | Yes | No | D | D | I | I | D | D | I | I |
| Aldosterone synthesis block | Severe | No | No | Nl | Nl | Nl | Nl | D | Nl | Nl | Nl |
| Pseudohypoaldosteronism | Severe | No | No | Nl | Nl | Nl | Nl | I | Nl | Nl | Nl |
| P-450$_{c11}$ deficiency | None | Yes | No | D | I | Nl–sl | Nl | D | I | I | Nl–sl I |
| P-450$_{c17}$ deficiency | None | No | Yes | D | Nl–D | D | D | Nl–D | D | D | D |
| Unresponsiveness to ACTH | None | No | No | D | Nl–D | Nl–low | Nl–low | Nl–low | D | D | Nl–low |

* Usually manifested after 5 days of age.
D = decrease; I = increase; Nl = normal; sl = slight; ACTH = adrenocorticotropic hormone; HSD = hydroxysteroid dehydrogenase; 17-KS = 17-ketosteroid; 17-OHCS = 17-hydroxycorticosteroid.

Oelkers W: Adrenal insufficiency. N Engl J Med 335:1206, 1996.

Saenger P: New developments in side-chain cleavage enzyme deficiency and STAR protein. Pediatr Clin North Am 44:397, 1997.

Speiser PW, New MI: Prenatal diagnosis and treatment of congenital adrenal hyperplasia. J Pediatr Endocrinol 7:183, 1994.

# BONE AND MINERAL ENDOCRINOLOGY

## PARATHYROID HORMONE AND VITAMIN D
### (see Chapter 2)

Calcium and phosphate are regulated mainly by diet and three hormones: (1) parathyroid hormone (PTH), (2) vitamin D, and (3) calcitonin. These hormones maintain plasma ionized calcium levels in the normal range. PTH is secreted in response to a decrease in serum ionized calcium level, then acts via adenylate cyclase to mobilize calcium from bone into the serum and to enhance fractional reabsorption of calcium by the kidney while inducing phosphate excretion, all of which help to raise the serum calcium concentration. Because PTH increases renal 1-hydroxylase activity, it also acts indirectly to elevate serum calcium concentration by stimulating the production of 1,25-dihydroxyvitamin D.

1,25-Dihydroxyvitamin D enhances calcium absorption from the gastrointestinal tract, resulting in increased serum calcium levels and increased bone mineralization. Vitamin D derived from sun exposure of the skin or ingestion must be sequentially modified first to 25-hydroxyvitamin D in the liver and then 1α-hydroxylated to the metabolically active form (1,25-dihydroxyvitamin D) in the kidney. The serum concentration of 25-hydroxyvitamin D is considered a better reflection of vitamin D sufficiency.

## HYPOCALCEMIA

The *clinical manifestations* of hypocalcemia (ionized calcium < 4.5 mg/dL; total calcium < 8.5 mg/dL) reflect increased neuromuscular irritability and include muscle cramps, carpopedal spasm (tetany), weakness, paresthesia, laryngospasm, or seizure-like activity (patient is often awake, aware). Latent tetany can be detected by the *Chvostek sign* (facial spasms are produced by lightly tapping over the facial nerve just in front of the ear) or by the *Trousseau sign* (carpal spasms are demonstrated when arterial blood flow to the hand is occluded for 3 to 5 min with a blood pressure cuff inflated to 15 mm Hg above systolic blood pressure). More commonly, total serum calcium concentration is measured, even though serum ionized calcium (~half the total in normal circumstances) is the biologically active form. Albumin is the major reservoir of protein-bound calcium, and the fraction of ionized calcium is inversely related to plasma pH. Therefore, disorders that alter plasma pH or serum albumin concentration must be considered when circulating calcium concentrations are being assessed. *Alkalosis* can precipitate hypocalcemia (i.e., it lowers ionized calcium) in a borderline situation with no change in total serum calcium level. Hypoproteinemia might suggest hypocalcemia, as the serum total calcium level is low but the ionized $Ca^{++}$ remains normal. It is best to avoid all of these considerations by measuring serum ionized calcium in cases of suspected hypocalcemia.

**Primary hypoparathyroidism** causes hypocalcemia. The etiology may be

1. Congenital malformation (e.g., the DiGeorge syndrome) (see Chapters 8 and 13).
2. Surgical procedures (thyroidectomy or parathyroidectomy).
3. Autoimmunity.

Hypoparathyroidism does not cause rickets.

**Pseudohypoparathyroidism** is caused by

1. An abnormality of the G-protein linking the PTH receptor to adenyl cyclase; biologically active PTH is secreted in great quantities but exerts no effect (type Ia).
2. Abnormalities in adenyl cyclase (type Ib).
3. Normal adenyl cyclase but a distal defect (type II).

This is an autosomal dominant condition that may manifest at birth or later. Other clinical features of pseudohypoparathyroidism include short stature, round facies, short 4th and 5th metacarpals, calcification of the basal ganglia, and often developmental delay. **Albright hereditary osteodystrophy** is the term that describes the phenotype.

Hypocalcemia caused by attenuated PTH release is found in infants of mothers with hyperparathyroidism and hypercalcemia; the latter suppresses fetal PTH release, thereby causing **transient hypoparathyroidism** in the neonatal period. During the first 3 days of life, calcium concentrations normally decline in response to withdrawal of the maternal calcium supply so that sluggish PTH response in the neonate results in a transient hypocalcemia.

Normal serum magnesium concentrations also are required for normal parathyroid gland function and action. Thus, **hypomagnesemia** may cause a secondary hypoparathyroidism that will respond poorly to therapies other than magnesium replacement.

**Neonatal tetany** resulting from excessive phosphate consumption classically occurs in the 1-week-old to 1-month-old infant who is fed cow's milk. The resultant hyperphosphatemia drives down the serum calcium level, causing symptomatic hypocalcemia (see Chapter 6). Excessive phosphate retention, as occurs in patients with renal failure, also produces hypocalcemia.

The etiology of hypocalcemia usually can be discerned by combining features of the clinical presentation with determinations of serum total or ionized calcium, albumin, magnesium, phosphate, creatinine, and alkaline phosphatase and with roentgenograms of the hands or wrists and knees. The most important diagnostic test is quantifying the serum PTH at a time when the calcium is low. If the PTH concentration is not elevated appropriately, hypoparathyroidism (transient, primary, caused by hypomagnesemia) is present. Vitamin D stores can be estimated by measuring serum 25-hydroxyvitamin D and renal function assessed with a serum creatinine measurement (Table 17–22).

*Treatment* of severe tetany or seizures resulting from hypocalcemia consists of intravenous calcium gluconate (2 mL/kg of 10% solution) given slowly over 10 min while cardiac status is monitored for bradycardia. Chronic treatment of hypoparathyroidism involves administering vitamin D and calcium. Therapy is adjusted to keep the serum calcium in the lower half of the normal range to avoid episodes of hypercalcemia that might produce nephrocalcinosis and pancreatitis.

### RICKETS

Rickets is defined as decreased or defective bone mineralization in growing children; **osteomalacia** is the same condition in adults. The proportion of osteoid (the organic portion of the bone) becomes excessive. As a result, the bone becomes soft and the metaphyses of the long bones widen. Poor linear growth, bowing of the legs on weight bearing (often painful), thickening at the wrists and knees, and prominence of the costochondral junctions (rachitic rosary) of the rib cage occur. At this stage, the roentgenographic findings are unmistakable.

Rickets develops because of an imbalance in bone mineral metabolism. In **nutritional vitamin D deficiency**, calcium is not adequately absorbed from the intestine (see Chapter 2). Poor vitamin D intake (food fads or poor maternal diet, both affecting breast milk vitamin D) or avoidance of sunlight also may contribute to the development of rickets. Fat malabsorption resulting from hepatobiliary disease (biliary atresia, neonatal hepatitis) or other causes also may produce vitamin D deficiency because vitamin D is a fat-soluble vitamin. Defects in vitamin D metabolism by the kidney (renal failure, autosomal recessive deficiency of 1α-hydroxylation, **vitamin D–dependent rickets**) or liver also can cause rickets. Very-low-birth-weight infants have an increased incidence of rickets of prematurity (see Chapter 6).

In **familial hypophosphatemic rickets**, the major defect in mineral metabolism is failure of the kidney to resorb filtered phosphate adequately. The *diagnosis* of this X-linked disease usually is made within the first few years of life and typically is more severe in males, although it can occur in females. This is now the most common cause of rickets in the United States.

The *etiology* of rickets usually can be determined by assessment of the mineral and vitamin D (25-hydroxyvitamin D < 8 ng/mL suggests nutritional vitamin D deficiency) status as outlined and by analysis of the results in accordance with the clinical presentation and expected laboratory features of the different disorders (see Table 17–22). Further

TABLE 17–22. Important Physiologic Changes in Bone and Mineral Diseases

| Condition | Calcium | Phosphate | Parathyroid Hormone | 25(OH)D |
|---|---|---|---|---|
| Primary hypoparathyroidism | ↓ | ↑ | ↓ | Nl |
| Pseudohypoparathyroidism | ↓ | ↑ | ↑ | Nl |
| Vitamin D deficiency | Nl (↓) | ↓ | ↑ | ↓ |
| Familial hypophosphatemic rickets | Nl | ↓ | Nl (sl ↑) | Nl |
| Hyperparathyroidism | ↑ | ↓ | ↑ | Nl |
| Immobilization | ↑ | ↑ | ↓ | Nl |

Nl = normal; ↑ = high; ↓ = low; sl = slight; 25(OH)D = 25-hydroxyvitamin D.

testing of mineral balance or measuring of other vitamin D metabolites may be required in more difficult cases.

Several chemical forms of vitamin D can be used for *treatment* of the different rachitic conditions, but their potencies vary widely and required dosages depend on the condition being treated (see Chapters 2 and 16). In hypophosphatemic rickets, phosphate supplementation (not calcium) must accompany vitamin D therapy, which is given to suppress secondary hyperparathyroidism. Adequate therapy restores normal skeletal growth and produces resolution of the roentgenographic signs of rickets. Rickets is usually treated with 1,25-hydroxyvitamin D and supplemental calcium. Surgery may be required to straighten legs in long-standing untreated patients.

## HYPERCALCEMIA

Hypercalcemia, rare in children, is due to hyperparathyroidism, immobilization (body casts), hypervitaminosis D (food faddism or incorrectly prepared commercial formula), fat necrosis, maternal hypoparathyroidism with subsequent fetal hypocalcemia, autosomal dominant–familial hypocalciuric hypercalcemia, Williams syndrome, and malignancy. MEN type I combines pseudohypoparathyroidism with pituitary adenomas. MEN type II has the features of medullary carcinoma of the thyroid, parathyroid adenomas, and pheochromocytoma; the hyperparathyroidism initially arises to combat hypocalcemia due to calcitonin secretion and then becomes autonomous. Symptoms include mental disturbances, anorexia, constipation, lethargy, vomiting, weakness, and polyuria. With time, uncontrolled chronic hypercalcemia usually will produce pancreatitis or nephrolithiasis and/or renal insufficiency.

### References

Behrman, RE, Kliegman RM, Arvin AM (eds): Nelson Textbook of Pediatrics, 15th ed. Philadelphia, WB Saunders, 1996, Chapters 525–527.
Carpenter TO: New perspectives on the biology and treatment of X-linked hypophosphatemic rickets. Pediatr Clin North Am 44:443, 1997.
Glorieux FH: Rickets, the continuing challenge. N Engl J Med 325:1875, 1991.
Guise TA, Mundy GR: Clinical review 69: Evaluation of hypocalcemia in children and adults. J Clin Endocrinol Metab 80:1473, 1995.
Mimouni FB, Root AW: Disorders of calcium metabolism in the newborn. In Sperling MA (ed): Pediatric Endocrinology. Philadelphia, WB Saunders, 1996, pp 95–116.

## DIABETES MELLITUS

Diabetes mellitus is characterized by hyperglycemia and glycosuria and occurs as a common endpoint of many disease processes (Table 17–23). The most common type occurring in childhood is **insulin-dependent diabetes mellitus** (IDDM), which is due to autoimmune destruction of the pancreas. Patients with IDDM have severe and usually permanent insulin deficiency and require insulin for survival and prevention of life-threatening episodes of ketoacidosis. **Non–insulin-dependent di-**

**TABLE 17–23.** Classification of Diabetes Mellitus in Children and Adolescents

| Type | Comment |
| --- | --- |
| *Insulin-Dependent (Type I)* | |
| Transient neonatal | Presents immediately after birth; lasts 1–3 mo |
| Permanent neonatal | Other pancreatic defects possible |
| Classic type I | Glycosuria, ketonuria, hyperglycemia, islet cell antibody to glutamic acid decarboxylase positive; definite genetic component |
| *Noninsulin-Dependent (Type II)* | |
| Secondary | Cystic fibrosis, hemochromatosis, drugs (e.g., L-asparaginase) |
| Adult type (classic) | Associated with obesity, insulin resistance; definite genetic component |
| MODY-1 | Early onset, beta cell defect; autosomal dominant—TCF-14 defect |
| MODY-2 | Less severe, early onset; autosomal dominant—GCK defect |
| MODY-3 | Early onset; autosomal dominant—TCF-1 defect |
| Mitochondrial diabetes | Associated with deafness and other neurologic defects, maternal transmission—mtDNA point mutations |
| *Other* | |
| Gestational diabetes | Abnormal glucose tolerance only during pregnancy, which reverts to normal post partum; increased risk for later onset of diabetes |

GCK = glucokinase; MODY = maturity-onset diabetes of youth; mtDNA = mitochondrial deoxyribonucleic acid; TCF = transcription factor.

abetes mellitus (NIDDM) is less common in children. Individuals with NIDDM are not dependent on insulin for survival, but they may require insulin to achieve adequate glycemic control. NIDDM most commonly results from insulin resistance, with inability of the pancreas to maintain adequate compensatory hyperinsulinemia. Less common subtypes of NIDDM result from genetic defects of the insulin receptor or inherited abnormalities in sensing of ambient glucose concentration by pancreatic beta cells (see Table 17–23).

## DEFINITION

A *diagnosis* of diabetes mellitus can be made if a fasting serum glucose concentration is greater than 140 mg/dL or a 2-hr postprandial serum glucose concentration is greater than 200 mg/dL on two separate occasions. A patient is considered *glucose-intolerant* if fasting serum glucose concentrations are greater than 115 mg/dL but less than 140 mg/dL and if 2-hr postprandial values are greater than 140 mg/dL but less than 200 mg/dL. Sporadic **hyperglycemia** occurs in children, usually in the setting of an intercurrent illness. When the hyperglycemic episode is clearly related to an illness or other physiologic stress, the probability that this represents incipient diabetes is small (<5%). Sporadic hyperglycemia occurring without a clear precipitating physiologic stress, however, is of more concern, as diabetes eventually develops in at least 30%.

## INSULIN-DEPENDENT DIABETES MELLITUS

### Epidemiology

IDDM is the most common pediatric endocrine disorder, affecting approximately 1 in 500 children under 18 yr of age. Different ethnic populations vary in their susceptibility to diabetes. The annual incidence in children ranges from a high of 30:100,000 among Scandinavian populations to a low of 1:100,000 in Japan. In the United States, the annual incidence is approximately 10–12:100,000. The prevalence of IDDM in the United States is highest among Caucasian Americans and is lower among African Americans and Hispanic Americans.

Genetic determinants play a role in the susceptibility to IDDM, although the mode of inheritance is complex and likely multigenic. Siblings or offspring of patients with diabetes have a risk of about 5% for development of diabetes; an identical twin has a 50% risk. Because genetic factors do not fully account for susceptibility to IDDM, environmental factors also play a role.

The association of IDDM susceptibility with the human leukocyte antigen (HLA) region on chromosome 6 is the strongest determinant of susceptibility, accounting for approximately 40% of the familial inheritance of IDDM. Individuals with HLA-DR3 or HLA-DR4 alleles have a three- to fourfold increased risk for development of diabetes; individuals with both HLA-DR3 and HLA-DR4 alleles have a 10-fold increase in risk. More than 90% of children with IDDM possess HLA-DR3, DR4 alleles, or both. The insulin gene region on chromosome 11 has also been linked to IDDM susceptibility, and there is some evidence for association of at least 18 other loci with IDDM.

### Etiology

In addition to the presence of diabetes susceptibility genes, an environmental insult must occur to trigger autoimmune destruction of the islet cells. The nature of this environmental insult, however, is unknown. Scandinavian studies have demonstrated an increased incidence of IDDM in children exposed to cow's milk prior to 2 yr of age. These studies lead to theories that cross-reactivity of antibodies to bovine serum albumin (BSA) with islet cell antigens might be involved. Viral infectious agents have also been implicated, including coxsackie B virus, cytomegalovirus (CMV), mumps, and rubella. Possible mechanisms for viral initiation of the autoimmune response include direct beta cell damage through viral infection, antibody cross-reactivity, and polyclonal activation of B-lymphocytes.

Antibodies to islet cell antigens can be demonstrated in the sera of susceptible individuals months to years before the onset of beta cell dysfunction and likely indicate an ongoing destructive process (Fig. 17–10). A number of different antibodies to beta cell antigens can be detected, including islet cell antibodies (ICA), insulin autoantibodies (IAA), and antibodies to glutamic acid decarboxylase (GAD). Studies of family members of patients with IDDM have shown that the risk for diabetes increases with the number of antibodies detected in the serum. In individuals with only one detectable antibody, the risk is only 10–15%; in individuals with three or more antibodies, the risk is 90–100%.

Once initiated, the autoimmune destructive process is thought to continue until 80–90% of the beta cell mass has been destroyed. At that point, the remaining beta cell mass is insufficient to maintain

FIGURE 17–10. Schematic representation of the autoimmune evolution of diabetes in genetically predisposed individuals.

glycemic control and clinical manifestations of diabetes result (see Fig. 17–10).

### Clinical Manifestations

When insulin secretory capacity becomes inadequate to support peripheral glucose uptake and to suppress hepatic glucose production, hyperglycemia results. The initial manifestation of insulin deficiency is postprandial hyperglycemia. Fasting hyperglycemia then develops. Ketogenesis is a sign of severe insulin deficiency. Lack of suppression of gluconeogenesis, glycogenolysis, and fatty acid oxidation contributes to the hyperglycemia and results in the generation of ketone bodies (acetoacetate and β-hydroxybutyrate) and acetone. Protein stores in muscle and fat stores in adipose tissue are broken down to provide substrates for gluconeogenesis and fatty acid oxidation.

Glycosuria occurs when the serum glucose concentration exceeds the renal threshold for glucose reabsorption (at approximately 180 mg/dL). Glycosuria causes an osmotic diuresis (including obligate loss of sodium, potassium, and water) leading to dehydration. Polydipsia occurs as the patient attempts to compensate for the excess fluid losses. Weight loss results from the persistent catabolic state as well as the loss of ingested calories through glycosuria and ketonuria. The classic presentation of IDDM includes polyuria, polydipsia, polyphagia, and weight loss.

**Diabetic Ketoacidosis.** If the clinical features of IDDM are not detected early, diabetic ketoacidosis (DKA) can occur. DKA can also occur in patients with known diabetes if insulin injections are omitted or during periods of intercurrent illness when insulin requirements are increased as a result of elevated concentrations of the counterregulatory hormones, glucagon, cortisol, and catecholamines. In the setting of hyperglycemia, DKA can be considered to be present if (1) the arterial pH is less than 7.25, (2) the serum bicarbonate level is less than 15 mEq/L, and (3) ketones are detected in serum or urine.

*Pathophysiology.* In the absence of adequate insulin secretion, persistent partial hepatic oxidation of fatty acids to ketone bodies occurs. An excess of these organic acids results in a metabolic acidosis with an elevated anion gap. Lactic acidosis can also contribute when severe dehydration results in decreased tissue perfusion. Hyperglycemia causes an osmotic diuresis that is initially compensated for by increased fluid intake. As the hyperglycemia and diuresis worsens, most patients are unable to maintain the large fluid intake required and dehydration occurs. Vomiting due to an ileus, pancreatitis, and so forth and increased insensible losses due to tachypnea worsen the state of dehydration.

Electrolyte abnormalities occur secondary to loss of electrolytes in the urine and transmembrane alterations resulting from acidosis. As hydrogen ions accumulate as a result of ketoacidosis, exchange of hydrogen ions for intracellular potassium occurs. Serum concentrations of potassium rise initially, then decrease as excess serum potassium is cleared by the kidney. Depending on the duration of keto-acidosis, serum potassium concentrations at diagnosis may be increased, normal, or decreased, but intracellular potassium concentrations are depleted. Phosphate depletion can also occur as a result of the increased renal phosphate excretion required for elimination of excess hydrogen ions. Sodium depletion is also common in DKA, resulting from renal losses of sodium due to osmotic diuresis and vomiting (Fig. 17–11).

*Presentation.* Patients with DKA present initially with a history of polyuria, polydipsia, and nausea and vomiting. Abdominal pain occurs frequently and can mimic an acute abdomen. The presence of polyuria, despite a state of clinical dehydration, is indicative of osmotic diuresis and differentiates patients with DKA from those with gastroenteritis or other gastrointestinal disorders. Respiratory compensation for acidosis results in tachypnea with deep (Kussmaul) respirations. The "fruity" odor of acetone can frequently be detected on the patient's breath. The abdomen may be distended secondary to paralytic ileus. An altered mental status can occur, ranging from disorientation to coma. Signs of dehydration may be minimal because increased serum osmolality results in preservation of intravascular volume.

Laboratory studies reveal hyperglycemia, with serum glucose concentrations ranging from 200 mg/dL to greater than 1000 mg/dL. Arterial pH is less than 7.25, and the serum bicarbonate concentration is less than 15 mEq/L. Serum sodium con-

centrations may be elevated, normal, or low, depending on the balance of sodium and free water losses. The measured serum sodium concentration, however, is artificially depressed because of hyperglycemia. A "corrected" sodium concentration can be calculated according to the following formula:

corrected sodium concentration = measured sodium concentration + [1.6 × (serum glucose concentration − 150)/100]

Hyperlipidemia can also contribute to the decrease in measured serum sodium. Potassium concentrations may be elevated, normal, or low, depending on the duration of DKA. Blood urea nitrogen (BUN) can be elevated with prerenal azotemia secondary to dehydration. The white blood cell count is usually elevated and can be left-shifted in the absence of infection. Fever, however, is unusual and should prompt a search for infectious sources that may have triggered the episode of DKA.

*Treatment.* Therapy for patients with DKA involves careful replacement of fluid deficits, correction of acidosis and hyperglycemia via insulin administration, correction of electrolyte imbalances, and monitoring for complications of treatment. The optimal approach to management of DKA is controversial, as the cause of the most serious complication—cerebral edema—is unknown. Therapeutic strategies must strike a balance between adequate correction of fluid losses to avoid complications of severe dehydration and avoidance of

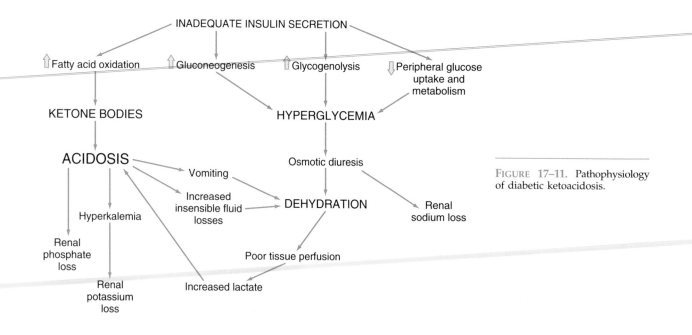

FIGURE 17–11. Pathophysiology of diabetic ketoacidosis.

rapid shifts in osmolality and fluid balance that might precipitate cerebral edema.

*DEHYDRATION.* The patient presenting in DKA can be assumed to be approximately 10% dehydrated. If a recent weight measurement is available, the precise extent of dehydration can be calculated. An initial intravenous fluid bolus of a glucose-free isotonic solution (normal saline, lactated Ringers) at 10–20 cc/kg should be given to restore intravascular volume and renal perfusion. The remaining fluid deficit after the initial bolus should be added to maintenance fluid requirements, and the total should be replaced slowly over 36–48 hr. Ongoing losses due to osmotic diuresis usually do not need to be replaced except if urine output is very large and if signs of poor perfusion are present. Osmotic diuresis is usually minimal when the serum glucose concentration falls below 300 mg/dL. To avoid rapid shifts in serum osmolality, 0.9% NaCl can be used as the replacement fluid for the initial 4 to 6 hr, followed by 0.45% NaCl.

*HYPERGLYCEMIA.* Insulin should be administered intravenously at a dose of 0.1 U/kg/hr. An initial bolus of 0.1 U/kg of regular insulin is sometimes given; use of a bolus is controversial. Proponents of this approach suggest that maximal insulin binding to receptors may occur more rapidly. Opponents argue that use of an insulin bolus may contribute to a rapid decrease in serum glucose, resulting in potentially harmful shifts in serum osmolality.

Optimally, serum glucose concentrations should decrease at a rate no faster than 100 mg/dL/hr. When serum glucose concentrations fall below 250–300 mg/dL, glucose should be added to the intravenous fluids. If serum glucose concentrations fall below 200 mg/dL prior to correction of acidosis, the glucose concentration of the intravenous fluids should be increased but the insulin infusion should not be decreased.

*ACIDOSIS.* Insulin therapy promotes metabolism of ketone bodies, and this process alone is usually sufficient to correct acidosis. Bicarbonate therapy should be avoided unless severe acidosis (pH < 7.0) results in hemodynamic instability. Potential adverse effects of bicarbonate administration include paradoxical increases in CNS acidosis due to increased diffusion of carbon dioxide across the blood-brain barrier, potential tissue hypoxia due to shifts in the oxyhemoglobin dissociation curve, and abrupt osmotic changes. If bicarbonate is given, it should be infused slowly, over several hours.

As acidosis is corrected, urine ketone concentrations may appear to rise. This occurs because beta-hydroxybutyrate, which is not detected in urine ketone assays, is converted to acetoacetate with treatment. Urine ketone concentration, therefore, is not a useful index of the adequacy of therapy.

*ELECTROLYTE IMBALANCES.* Regardless of the serum potassium concentration at presentation, total body potassium depletion is very likely. Potassium concentrations can decrease rapidly, as insulin therapy improves the acidotic state and potassium is exchanged for intracellular hydrogen ions. Once adequate urine output is demonstrated, potassium should be added to the intravenous fluids. Potassium replacement should be given as 50% potassium chloride and 50% potassium phosphate at a concentration of 20–40 mEq/L. This combination provides phosphate for replacement of deficits and avoids excess phosphate administration, which may precipitate hypocalcemia.

*MONITORING.* A flow sheet should be used to monitor fluid balance and laboratory measurements. Initial laboratory measurements should include serum glucose, sodium, potassium, chloride, bicarbonate, BUN, creatinine, calcium, phosphate, and magnesium concentrations as well as arterial or venous pH and a urinalysis. Serum glucose measurement should be repeated every hour during therapy and electrolyte concentrations every 2–3 hr. Calcium, phosphate, and magnesium concentrations should be measured initially and at least once during therapy. Neurologic and mental status should be assessed at frequent intervals, and complaints of headache or deterioration of mental status should prompt rapid evaluation for possible cerebral edema.

*COMPLICATIONS.* Clinically apparent cerebral edema occurs in 1–2% of cases of DKA. Cerebral edema is the most serious complication of DKA, with a mortality rate of 60–80%. The pathogenesis of this complication is incompletely understood. Subclinical cerebral edema is common in patients with DKA, but the factors that exacerbate this process leading to symptomatic brain swelling and possible cerebral herniation are unknown. Cerebral edema typically occurs 6–10 hr after therapy for DKA is begun, often following a period of apparent clinical improvement. Factors that have been found to correlate with increased risk for cerebral edema in some studies include:

- Younger age
- Longer duration of symptoms prior to treatment
- New onset of IDDM
- Higher initial serum glucose
- Higher initial corrected serum sodium
- More rapid and greater decline in serum osmolality with treatment
- Failure of the serum sodium level to rise as glucose concentration falls during treatment

Signs of advanced cerebral edema include obtundation, papilledema, pupillary dilation or inequality, hypertension, bradycardia, and apnea. *Treatment* involves endotracheal intubation, hyperventillation, and the use of intravenous mannitol.

Other complications of DKA include intracranial thrombosis or infarction and acute tubular necrosis caused by severe dehydration. Peripheral edema occurs commonly 24–48 hr after therapy is initiated and may be related to residual elevations in antidiuretic hormone (ADH) and aldosterone.

**Transition to Outpatient Management.** Once the acidosis has been corrected and the patient can tolerate oral feedings, the intravenous insulin infusion can be discontinued and a regimen of subcutaneous insulin injections started. Typical starting doses are approximately 0.5 U/kg/24 hr for prepubertal patients and approximately 0.7 U/kg/24 hr for adolescents; two thirds of the total daily insulin dose should be given as intermediate-acting insulin (NPH or Lente) and one third should be given as short-acting (regular) insulin. The dose should be divided into two daily injections, with two thirds given in the morning, 30 min before breakfast, and one third given in the evening, 30 min before dinner (Fig. 17–12). The first subcutaneous insulin dose should be given 30–45 min before discontinuation of the intravenous insulin infusion. Further adjustment of the insulin dose should be made over the following 1–2 days of the hospitalization.

Another alternative for making the transition to subcutaneous insulin is to begin by giving injections of regular insulin before each meal and NPH at bedtime. This regimen can then be converted to a twice-daily regimen of NPH and regular insulin after the patient is able to tolerate a full diet and serum glucose concentrations stabilize.

Serum glucose concentrations should be assessed before each meal, at bedtime, and at 2–3 A.M. to provide information for adjustment of the regimen. Patients and their families should begin learning the principles of diabetes care as soon as possible. Demonstration of ability to administer insulin injections and test glucose concentrations using a glucometer is necessary prior to discharge, as is knowledge of hypoglycemia management and meal planning.

**Honeymoon Period.** In patients with new onset of IDDM, often the beta cell mass has not been completely destroyed by the autoimmune process. With insulin treatment, the remaining functional beta cells recover from the state of exhaustion and are again able to produce insulin. When this occurs, insulin requirements decrease and there is a period of stable blood glucose control, often with nearly normal glucose concentrations. This phase of the disease, known as the honeymoon period, usually continues for a few months, but can last up to 2 yr.

**Outpatient IDDM Management.** Long-term management of IDDM in children requires a comprehensive approach, with attention to medical, nutritional, and psychosocial issues. Therapeutic strategies should be flexible, with the individual needs of each patient taken into account. Optimal care involves a team of diabetes professionals including a physician, a diabetes nurse educator, a dietitian, and a social worker.

*Goals.* The Diabetes Control and Complications Trial (DCCT) established that intensive insulin therapy, with the goal of maintaining blood glucose concentrations as close to normal as possible, can delay the onset and slow the progression of complications of diabetes, including retinopathy, nephropathy, and neuropathy. In this trial, intensive insulin therapy also resulted in a two- to threefold increase in severe hypoglycemia. One should give careful consideration to the balance of these two features when planning the treatment goals for children with IDDM. Although the risk for diabetic complications increases with duration of diabetes, the rate of increase in risk may be slower in the prepubertal years than in adolescence and adulthood. Thus, the gains from achieving tight control of blood glucose concentrations in childhood appear somewhat less than in adulthood. Furthermore, the adverse effects of hypoglycemia in young children may be significant because the immature CNS may be more susceptible to damage during episodes of glycopenia.

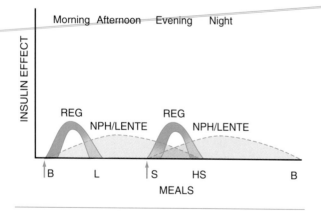

FIGURE 17–12. Representative profile of insulin effect using a twice-daily injection regimen that combines an intermediate-acting insulin (NPH or Lente) with regular (short-acting) insulin. (Reprinted with permission from Schade DS, Santiago JV, Sykler JS: Intensive Insulin Therapy. Excerpta Medica, 1983.)

The goals of therapy will differ, therefore, depending on the age of the patient. For children under 5 yr of age, an appropriate goal would be maintenance of blood glucose concentrations between 100 and 200 mg/dL. For school-aged children, 80–180 mg/dL is a reasonable target range. For adolescents, the goal is 70–150 mg/dL. Goals of therapy should also take into account other individual characteristics, such as a past history of severe hypoglycemia and the abilities of the patient and family.

*Insulin Regimens.* A number of different types of insulin differ in duration of action and time to peak effect (Table 17–24). These insulins can be used in various combinations, depending on the needs and goals of the individual patient. The most commonly used regimen in school-aged children involves two subcutaneous injections per day of intermediate-acting insulin (NPH or Lente) and short-acting insulin (regular) (see Fig. 17–12). This regimen is preferred because it does not require the patient to give an insulin injection at mid-day, during school hours. Patients using this regimen must adhere to a relatively rigid meal schedule, however, and this can be difficult to coordinate with variations in daily activities. Other regimens use multiple injections of short-acting insulin given before meals in combination with a long-acting basal insulin (such as Ultralente) or with an intermediate-acting insulin given at bedtime. These regimens provide more flexibility but require the patient to administer many injections per day and thus are more suitable for adolescents than young children. Pumps that provide a continuous subcutaneous infusion of short-acting insulin are also available and have been used by older children and adolescents who are highly motivated to achieve tight control.

A very short-acting insulin, Lispro, is now avail-able. Lispro is a synthetic human insulin analog in which the amino acids at positions 28 and 29 (lysine and proline) are reversed. This alteration in the insulin structure results in rapid absorption and onset of action (see Table 17–24). Lispro insulin can be substituted for short-acting insulins and may be particularly useful in patients who have problems with postprandial hypoglycemia. Because of the short duration of action, Lispro must be used in combination with an intermediate-acting or long-acting insulin.

Total daily insulin doses will differ, depending on the age and pubertal stage of the patient and the duration of diabetes. Newly diagnosed patients in the honeymoon period may require as little as 0.2–0.4 U/kg/24 hr. Prepubertal patients with a duration of diabetes greater than 1 to 2 yr typically require 0.5–1.0 U/kg/24 hr. During mid-adolescence, when elevated GH concentrations produce relative insulin resistance, insulin requirements increase by 40–50% and doses of 1–2 U/kg/24 hr are typical.

*Nutrition.* Balancing the daily meal plan with the dosages of insulin is critical for maintaining serum glucose concentrations within the target range and avoiding hypoglycemia. The content and schedule of meals will vary according to the type of insulin regimen used; however, it is recommended that carbohydrates contribute 50–65% of the total calories, protein 12–20%, and fat less than 30%. Saturated fat should contribute less than 10% of the total caloric intake, and cholesterol intake should be less than 300 mg/24 hr. High fiber content is recommended. It should be emphasized that these recommendations describe a healthy diet for anyone, regardless of the presence of diabetes. Participation of the entire family is critical to ensure compliance.

Children using a combination of intermediate-acting and short-acting insulins given twice a day need to maintain a relatively strict meal schedule so that peaks of carbohydrate absorption correspond with peaks in insulin action. A typical meal schedule for a patient using this type of regimen involves three meals and three snacks daily. The total carbohydrate content of the meals and snacks should be kept constant. Patients using multiple injection regimens or the insulin pump can maintain a more flexible meal schedule with regard to the timing of meals and the carbohydrate content. These patients give an injection of insulin before each meal, with the total dose calculated according to the carbohydrate content of the meal. Further adjustments in the dose can be made based on the measured serum glucose concentration and plans for exercise during the day.

TABLE 17–24. Insulin Preparations

| Type of Insulin | Onset | Peak Action | Duration |
|---|---|---|---|
| *Very Short-Acting* | | | |
| Lispro | 15–30 min | 30–90 min | 2–4 hr |
| *Short-Acting* | | | |
| Regular | ½–2 hr | 2–4 hr | 6–12 hr |
| *Intermediate-Acting* | | | |
| NPH | 1–4 hr | 4–12 hr | 16–28 hr |
| Lente | | | |
| *Long-Acting* | | | |
| Protamine zinc | 4–6 hr | 8–20 hr | 24–36 hr |
| Ultralente | | | |

*Monitoring.* Routine monitoring of children with IDDM involves daily blood glucose determinations, assessment of long-term glycemic control, screening for complications of diabetes, and evaluation for other disorders that can occur with increased frequency in patients with IDDM.

BLOOD GLUCOSE TESTING. Blood glucose should be routinely monitored (with rapid, portable glucose meters) before each meal and at bedtime. If blood glucose cannot easily be tested at school, the noon test can be omitted on school days. Hypoglycemia during the night or excessive variability in the morning glucose concentrations should prompt additional testing at 2 or 3 A.M. to ensure that there is no hypoglycemia leading to the Somogy effect of rebound hyperglycemia at the 7–8 A.M. sample. During periods of intercurrent illness or when blood glucose concentrations are greater than 240 mg/dL, urine ketones should also be tested.

LONG-TERM GLYCEMIC CONTROL. Measurements of glycohemoglobin or hemoglobin $A_{1c}$ reflect the average blood glucose concentration over the preceding 6–8 wk and provide a means for assessing long-term glycemic control. Glycohemoglobin or hemoglobin $A_{1c}$ should be measured four times a year and the results used for counseling of patients. Table 17–25 summarizes the correlation between hemoglobin $A_{1c}$ or glycohemoglobin and daily blood glucose measurements. Measurements of glycohemoglobin or hemoglobin $A_{1c}$ are inaccurate in patients with hemoglobinopathies. Glycosylated albumin or fructosamine can be used in these cases.

COMPLICATIONS. Routine screening for diabetic complications is not usually recommended for prepubertal patients. After the onset of puberty, patients with IDDM should receive an annual ophthalmologic examination for retinopathy. Urine should be collected for assessment of microalbuminuria; if present, microalbuminuria is suggestive of early renal dysfunction and indicates a high risk of progression to nephropathy. *Treatment* with angiotensin-converting enzyme (ACE) inhibitors may halt the progression of microalbuminuria. In children with IDDM, annual cholesterol measurements and periodic assessment of blood pressure are recommended. Early detection of hypertension and hypercholesterolemia with appropriate intervention can help to limit future risk of coronary disease.

OTHER DISORDERS. Diseases with an autoimmune basis are more prevalent in children with diabetes than in the general population. Chronic lymphocytic thyroiditis is particularly common and can result in hypothyroidism. Because symptoms can be subtle, thyroid function tests should be performed annually. Other disorders that occur with increased frequency in children with IDDM include celiac disease, immunoglobulin A (IgA) deficiency, and peptic ulcer disease.

### Special Problems

*Hypoglycemia.* Iatrogenic hypoglycemia occurs commonly in patients with IDDM. Patients using conventional insulin therapy have an average of one episode per week of symptomatic hypoglycemia, and those on intensive regimens have an average of two episodes per week. Severe episodes of hypoglycemia, resulting in seizures or coma or requiring assistance from another person, occur in 10–25% of these patients per year. Approximately 4% of deaths in patients with IDDM can be attributed to hypoglycemia, usually as a result of accidental trauma.

Hypoglycemia in patients with IDDM results from a relative excess of insulin in relation to the serum glucose concentration. This excess can be caused by alterations in the dose, timing or absorption of insulin, alterations in carbohydrate intake, or changes in insulin sensitivity resulting from exercise. Defective counterregulatory responses also contribute to hypoglycemia. Abnormal glucagon responses to falling serum glucose concentrations develop within the first few years of the disease, and abnormalities in epinephrine release occur after a somewhat longer duration.

Unawareness of hypoglycemia occurs in approximately 25% of patients with diabetes. Recent episodes of hypoglycemia may play a role in the pathophysiology of hypoglycemic unawareness; following an episode of hypoglycemia, autonomic responses to subsequent episodes are reduced. A return of symptoms of hypoglycemia can be demonstrated in these patients after 2 to 3 wk of strict avoidance of hypoglycemic episodes.

Symptoms of hypoglycemia include those resulting from neuroglycopenia (headache, visual changes, confusion, irritability, seizures) and those

TABLE 17–25. Biochemical Indices of Glycemic Control

**Poor Control**
HgbA$_{1c}$ > 10.0%
Average blood glucose >240 mg/dL

**Average Control**
HgbA$_{1c}$ > 8.0–10.0%
Average blood glucose 180–240 mg/dL

**Intensive Control**
HgbA$_{1c}$ 6.0–8.0%
Average blood glucose 120–180 mg/dL

HgbA$_{1c}$ = hemoglobin A$_{1c}$.

resulting from the catecholamine response (tremors, tachycardia, diaphoresis, anxiety; also see Hypoglycemia). Mild episodes can be treated with administration of rapidly absorbed oral glucose (glucose gel or tablets, fruit juices, and non-diet or non–artificially sweetened sodas). More severe episodes that result in seizures or loss of consciousness at home should be treated with glucagon injections. Intravenous glucose should be given in hospital settings.

*Early Morning Hyperglycemia.* A variety of situations can lead to early morning hyperglycemia. The most frequent assumption is that the evening dose of intermediate-acting insulin is inadequate, but this is not always the case. Hypoglycemia that occurs during the night can result in increased secretion of counterregulatory hormones and rebound hyperglycemia, a process known as the *Somogyi phenomenon*. Patients experiencing night-time hypoglycemia also may experience headache on awakening, diaphoresis, and nightmares.

In some children, the evening intermediate-acting insulin is given early and there is waning of the dose by the early morning, resulting in a rise in glucose concentrations. Increased secretion of GH during the early morning hours can also contribute to morning hyperglycemia, particularly during mid-adolescence. This process is known as the *Dawn phenomenon*. Testing of blood glucose concentrations at 2 or 3 A.M. can distinguish between these possibilities. Depending on the results, the evening intermediate-acting insulin dose may need to be decreased or given at bedtime.

## Prognosis

Long-term complications of IDDM include retinopathy, nephropathy, neuropathy, and macrovascular disease. Evidence of tissue damage due to hyperglycemia is rare in patients with a duration of diabetes of less than 5–10 yr, and clinically apparent disease rarely occurs before a duration of 10–15 yr. Therefore, pediatricians encounter these complications infrequently. The eventual morbidity and mortality attributable to these disorders, however, are substantial. Some degree of diabetic retinopathy eventually occurs in nearly 100% of patients with IDDM and is the cause of approximately 5000 new cases of blindness in the United States yearly. Nephropathy eventually occurs in 30–40% and accounts for approximately 30% of all new adult cases of end-stage renal disease. Neuropathy occurs in 30–40% of postpubertal patients with IDDM and leads to sensory, motor, or autonomic deficits. Macrovascular disease results in an increased risk of myocardial infarction and stroke among individuals with diabetes.

The DCCT convincingly demonstrated that intensive control of diabetes, employing frequent blood glucose testing and multiple daily injections of insulin or an insulin pump, can substantially reduce the development or progression of diabetic complications. Intensive management resulted in a 76% reduction of risk for retinopathy, a 39% reduction in microalbuminuria, and a 60% reduction in clinical neuropathy. For pubertal and adult patients, these benefits of intensive therapy likely outweigh the increase in risk for hypoglycemia. For younger patients, in whom the risks for hypoglycemia are greater and the benefits of tight glucose control may be lower, a somewhat less intensive regimen may be appropriate.

Research efforts have focused on prevention of diabetes in patients known to be at risk. In first-degree relatives of patients with IDDM, the future risk for development of IDDM can be determined on the basis of measurements of antibodies to beta cell antigens and insulin responses to stimulation. A preliminary study demonstrated that administration of small doses of subcutaneous insulin to individuals at high risk for development of IDDM may delay or prevent onset of diabetes.

## NON–INSULIN-DEPENDENT DIABETES MELLITUS

### Epidemiology

NIDDM was previously thought to be uncommon in childhood; however, the prevalence of this disorder in children may be increasing, perhaps as a reflection of the increased prevalence of childhood obesity. NIDDM is currently thought to account for approximately 10–15% of cases of diabetes in childhood. The prevalence is highest among children of ethnic groups with a high prevalence of NIDDM among adults, including Native Americans, Hispanic Americans, and African Americans. Obesity and a family history of NIDDM are risk factors.

### Pathophysiology

NIDDM can occur as the result of various pathophysiologic processes; however, the most common form results from peripheral insulin resistance with failure of the pancreas to maintain compensatory hyperinsulinemia (see Table 17–23). The precise defects underlying the insulin-resistant state and the eventual pancreatic failure are complex and poorly understood. Other subtypes of NIDDM can also occur in children. Maturity-onset diabetes of youth (MODY) comprises a group of dominantly inherited forms of relatively mild diabetes. Insulin resistance does not occur in these patients; instead, the primary abnormality is an insufficient insulin secretory response to glycemic stimulation (see Table 17–23). NIDDM in childhood can also result from inherited defects in mitochondrial genes. Other rare subtypes of NIDDM include syndromes of severe insulin resistance due to mutations in the insulin receptor gene and diabetes resulting from the secretion of abnormal forms of insulin.

## Differential Diagnosis

Differentiating NIDDM from IDDM in children can be challenging. The possibility of NIDDM should be entertained in patients who are obese, have a strong family history of NIDDM, have a finding of acanthosis nigricans (excessive axillary pigmentation) on physical examination (a dermatologic manifestation of hyperinsulinism), or have absence of antibodies to beta cell antigens at the time of diagnosis of diabetes. Although ketoacidosis occurs far more commonly in IDDM, it can also occur in patients with NIDDM under conditions of physiologic stress and thus cannot be used as an absolute differentiating factor. The diagnosis of NIDDM can be confirmed by evaluation of insulin or C-peptide responses to stimulation with oral carbohydrate.

## References

Behrman RE, Kliegman RM, Arvin AM (eds): Nelson Textbook of Pediatrics, 15th ed. Philadelphia, WB Saunders, 1996, Section 6.
DCCT Research Group: The effect of intensive treatment of diabetes on the development and progression of long-term complications in insulin-dependent diabetes mellitus. N Engl J Med 329:977, 1993.
DCCT Research Group: Effect of intensive diabetes treatment on the development and progression of long-term complications in adolescents with insulin-dependent diabetes mellitus: Diabetes control and complications trial. J Pediatr 125:177, 1994.

TABLE 17–26.  Classification of Hypoglycemia in Infants and Children

**Abnormalities in the Hormonal Signal Indicating Hypoglycemia**

*Counterregulatory Hormone Deficiency*

Panhypopituitarism
Isolated growth hormone deficiency
ACTH deficiency
Addison disease
Glucagon deficiency
Epinephrine deficiency

*Hyperinsulinism*

Infant of a diabetic mother
Infant with erythroblastosis fetalis
Persistent hyperinsulinemic hypoglycemia of infancy
Beta cell adenoma (insulinoma)
Beckwith-Wiedemann syndrome
Anti-insulin receptor antibodies

**Inadequate Substrate**

Prematurity/small-for-gestational-age infant
Ketotic hypoglycemia
Maple syrup urine disease

**Disorders of Metabolic Response Pathways**

*Glycogenolysis*

Glucose-6-phosphatase deficiency
Amylo-1,6-glucosidase deficiency
Liver phosphorylase deficiency
Glycogen synthase deficiency

*Gluconeogenesis*

Fructose-1,6-diphosphatase deficiency
Pyruvate carboxylase deficiency
Phosphoenolpyruvate carboxykinase deficiency

*Fatty Acid Oxidation*

Long-, medium-, or short-chain fatty acid acyl-CoA dehydrogenase deficiency
Carnitine deficiency (primary or secondary)
Carnitine palmitoyltransferase deficiency

*Other*

Enzymatic defects
  Galactosemia
  Hereditary fructose intolerance
  Propionicacidemia
  Methylmalonic acidemia
  Tyrosinosis
  Glutaricaciduria
Global hepatic dysfunction
Reye syndrome
Hepatitis
Heart failure
Sepsis–shock
Carcinoma/sarcoma (IGF-2 secretion)
Malnutrition–starvation
Hyperviscosity syndrome

**Drugs/Intoxications**

Oral hypoglycemic agents
Insulin
Alcohol
Salicylates
Propranolol
Valproic acid
Pentamidine
Ackee fruit (unripe)
Quinine
Trimethoprim/sulfamethoxazole (with renal failure)

IGF = insulin-like growth factor.

Deary I, Frier B: Severe hypoglycemia and cognitive impairment in diabetes. BMJ 313:767, 1996.

Finberg L: Why do patients with diabetic ketoacidosis have cerebral swelling and why does treatment sometimes make it worse? Arch Pediatr Adolesc Med 150:785, 1996.

Krane E: Diabetic ketoacidosis: Biochemistry, physiology, treatment, prevention. Pediatr Clin North Am 34:935, 1987.

Owerbach D, Gabbay KH: The search for IDDM susceptibility genes: The next generation. Diabetes 45:544, 1996.

Sperling MA: The etiology of insulin-dependent diabetes mellitus. Pediatr Clin North Am 44:269, 1997.

Verge CF, Gianani R, Kawasaki E, et al: Prediction of type 1 diabetes in first-degree relatives using a combination of insulin, GAD, and ICA512bdc/IA-2 autoantibodies. Diabetes 45:926, 1996.

Yki:-Järvinen H: MODY genes and mutations in hepatocyte nuclear factors. Lancet 349:516, 1997.

## HYPOGLYCEMIA

Hypoglycemia in infancy and childhood can result from a large variety of hormonal and metabolic defects (Table 17–26). Hypoglycemia occurs most frequently in the early neonatal period, often as a result of inadequate energy stores to meet the disproportionately large metabolic needs of premature or small-for-gestational-age newborns. Hypoglycemia in the first few days of life in an otherwise normal newborn, however, is less frequent and warrants concern (see Chapter 6). After the initial 2 to 3 days of life, hypoglycemia is far less common and is more frequently the result of endocrine or metabolic disorders.

### DEFINITION

Beyond the early neonatal period, serum glucose concentrations less than 45 mg/dL are considered to be abnormal and require treatment. Serum glucose concentrations less than 55 mg/dL can occasionally occur in normal individuals, especially with prolonged fasting, but should be considered suspect, particularly if there are concurrent symptoms of hypoglycemia (Table 17–27). The *diagnosis* of hypoglycemia should be made on the basis of a low serum glucose concentration, symptoms compatible with hypoglycemia, and resolution of the symptoms after administration of glucose (Whipple triad).

### CLINICAL MANIFESTATIONS

The symptoms and signs of hypoglycemia result from both direct depression of the CNS owing to lack of energy substrate and the counterregulatory response to low glucose via catecholamine secretion (see Table 17–27). The manifestations in infants

**TABLE 17–27.** Symptoms and Signs of Hypoglycemia

| Features Associated with Epinephrine Release* | Features Associated with Cerebral Glucopenia |
|---|---|
| Perspiration | Headache |
| Palpitation (tachycardia) | Mental confusion |
| Pallor | Somnolence |
| Paresthesia | Dysarthria |
| Trembling | Personality changes |
| Anxiety | Inability to concentrate |
| Weakness | Staring |
| Nausea | Hunger |
| Vomiting | Convulsions |
| | Ataxia |
| | Coma |
| | Diplopia |
| | Stroke |

*These features may be blunted if the patient is receiving beta blocking agents.

differ when compared with those in older children. Symptoms and signs of hypoglycemia in infants are relatively nonspecific and include jitteriness, feeding difficulties, pallor, hypotonia, hypothermia, episodes of apnea and bradycardia, and seizures. In older children, symptoms and signs include confusion, irritability, headaches, visual changes, tremors, pallor, sweating, tachycardia, weakness, seizures, and coma.

Failure to recognize and treat hypoglycemia can result in serious long-term morbidity, including mental retardation and seizures. Younger infants and patients with more severe or prolonged hypoglycemia are at greatest risk for adverse outcomes.

### PATHOPHYSIOLOGY

Normal regulation of serum glucose concentrations requires appropriate interaction of a number of hormonal signals and metabolic pathways. An overview of these pathways is presented in Figure 17–13. The components required for glycemic regulation fall into three basic categories:

1. The hormonal signal indicating hypoglycemia.
2. Energy stores adequate to supply substrates for the metabolic pathways.
3. Functioning metabolic-enzymatic pathways for glucose and ketone body generation.

Defects in any of these categories can result in hypoglycemia.

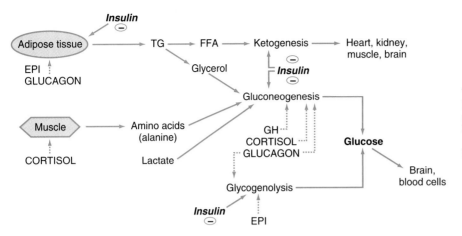

FIGURE 17–13. Regulation of serum glucose. – represents inhibitions. EPI = epinephrine; FFA = free fatty acid; GH = growth hormone; TG = triglyceride.

### The Hormonal Signal

In a normal individual, a fall in serum glucose concentrations will result in suppression of insulin secretion and increased secretion of the counterregulatory hormones (growth hormone, cortisol, glucagon, and epinephrine). This hormonal signal promotes the release of amino acids (particularly alanine) from muscle to fuel gluconeogenesis and the release of triglyceride from adipose tissue stores to provide free fatty acids (FFAs) for hepatic ketogenesis. It also stimulates the breakdown of hepatic glycogen and promotes gluconeogenesis. Failure of any of the components of this hormonal signal can result in hypoglycemia.

**Hyperinsulinemia.** Failure of suppression of insulin secretion in response to low serum glucose concentrations occurs most frequently in infants. In neonates, this situation arises commonly in infants of diabetic mothers who have been exposed to high concentrations of glucose in utero resulting in fetal islet cell hyperplasia. The hyperinsulinemic state is transient, usually lasting hours to days (see Chapter 6). Hyperinsulinism that persists beyond a few days of age can result from a condition previously referred to as "nesidioblastosis" but is more appropriately called **persistent hyperinsulinemic hypoglycemia of the newborn** (PHHN). In these infants, hyperplasia of the islet cells develops in the absence of excess stimulation by maternal diabetes. Some patients with PHHN have genetic abnormalities of the sulfonylurea receptor. Rarely, an islet cell adenoma is responsible. Hyperinsulinism can also occur in the **Beckwith-Wiedemann syndrome,** a condition characterized by macrosomia, macroglossia, omphalocele, visceromegaly, and ear lobe creases.

Regardless of the cause, infants with hyperinsulinism are characteristically large for gestational age. Hypoglycemia is severe and frequently occurs within 1–3 hr of a feeding. Glucose requirements are large, often two to three times the normal basal glucose requirement of 4–8 mg/kg/min. The *diagnosis* of hyperinsulinism is confirmed by the detection of serum insulin concentrations above 5 μU/mL during an episode of hypoglycemia. The absence of serum and urine ketones at the time of hypoglycemia is an important diagnostic feature, distinguishing hyperinsulinism from defects in counterregulatory hormone secretion.

*Treatment* initially involves the use of high intravenous glucose infusion rates and of diazoxide to suppress insulin secretion. If this therapy is unsuccessful, long-acting somatostatin analogs can be tried. Frequent feedings and a low-protein, leucine-free diet are helpful. Often, medical therapy for PHHN is unsuccessful and subtotal (90%) pancreatectomy is required to prevent long-term neurologic sequelae of hypoglycemia.

In children, hyperinsulinemia is rare and usually results from an islet cell adenoma. Children with this condition characteristically have a voracious appetite, obesity, and accelerated linear growth. As in infants, *diagnosis* requires demonstration of insulin concentrations >5 μU/mL during an episode of hypoglycemia. A CT or MRI scan of the pancreas should be attempted, but visualization of an adenoma is usually difficult. Surgical removal of the adenoma is curative.

**Factitious Hyperinsulinemia.** In rare cases, insulin is administered to a child as a form of child abuse or **Munchhausen syndrome by proxy.** This *diagnosis* should be suspected if extremely high insulin concentrations are detected (>100 μU/mL). C-peptide concentrations are low or undetectable, which confirms that the insulin was from an exogenous source.

**Defects in Counterregulatory Hormones.** Abnormalities in the secretion of counterregulatory hormones that produce hypoglycemia usually involve GH, cortisol, or both. Deficiencies in glucagon and epinephrine secretion have been described but are extremely rare. GH and cortisol deficiency occur due to hypopituitarism. Hypopituitarism results rarely from congenital hypoplasia or aplasia of the pituitary or more commonly from deficiency of hypothalamic releasing factors. Clues to this diagnosis in infants include the presence of hypoglycemia in association with midline facial or neurologic defects (such as cleft lip and palate or absence of the corpus callosum), pendular nystagmus (indicating possible abnormalities in the development of the optic nerves and visual impairment which can occur in septo-optic dysplasia), and the presence of microphallus and cryptorchidism in males (indicating abnormalities in gonadotropin or growth hormone secretion). Jaundice and hepatomegaly can also occur, simulating neonatal hepatitis. Despite the presence of GH deficiency, these infants are usually of normal size at birth. Older children with hypopituitarism, however, usually have short stature and a subnormal growth velocity.

Deficient cortisol secretion can also occur in primary adrenal insufficiency resulting from a variety of causes. In infants, primary adrenal insufficiency often results from congenital adrenal hyperplasia, most frequently due to 21-hydroxylase deficiency. Female infants with this disorder have virilized genitalia secondary to increased androgen production in utero; however, male infants usually appear normal (see Disorders of Sexual Differentiation). In older children, primary adrenal insufficiency is most frequently seen in **Addison's disease,** but it can also occur in adrenoleukodystrophy and other disorders (see Adrenal Gland). Addison's disease should be suspected if there is hyperpigmentation of the skin, a history of salt-cravings, hyponatremia, and hyperkalemia.

Confirmation of GH or cortisol deficiency as the cause of hypoglycemia requires the detection of low serum GH and cortisol concentrations during an episode of hypoglycemia or after other stimulatory testing. In contrast to hyperinsulinism, serum and urine ketones are positive at the time of hypoglycemia and FFAs are elevated. Treatment involves supplementation of the deficient hormones in physiologic doses.

### Energy Stores

Sufficient energy stores in the form of glycogen, adipose tissue, and muscle are necessary to respond appropriately to hypoglycemia. Deficiencies in these stores are a common cause of hypoglycemia in neonates who are small for gestational age or premature (see Chapter 6). Beyond the early neonatal period, energy stores are usually sufficient to meet the metabolic requirements. Release of substrate from energy stores, however, is thought to be abnormal in one common form of childhood hypoglycemia, ketotic hypoglycemia.

**Ketotic Hypoglycemia.** This disorder is usually seen in children between 18 mo and 5 yr of age. It is the most common cause of new-onset hypoglycemia in children over 2 yr of age. Typically, these patients present with symptoms of hypoglycemia after a period of prolonged fasting, often in the setting of an intercurrent illness. Children with this disorder are often thin and small and may have a history of being small for gestational age. Defective mobilization of alanine from muscle to fuel gluconeogenesis is thought to be the cause. Because there are no specific diagnostic tests for this disorder, ketotic hypoglycemia is a *diagnosis of exclusion.*

*Treatment* involves avoidance of fasting and frequent feedings of a high-protein, high-carbohydrate diet. Patients may require hospitalization for intravenous glucose infusion if they cannot maintain adequate oral intake during a period of illness. The disorder usually resolves spontaneously by 7–8 yr of age.

**Maple Syrup Urine Disease.** This defect in branched chain amino acid catabolism also results in inadequate release of alanine from muscle. Affected patients present with hypoglycemia along with vomiting, lethargy, seizures, hyperammonemia, and metabolic acidosis. The urine has a characteristic maple syrup odor. Measurement of serum amino acids is required to make the diagnosis.

### Metabolic Response Pathways

Maintenance of normal serum glucose concentrations requires both glucose production via glycogenolysis and gluconeogenesis and the production of alternative energy sources (free fatty acids, ketones) via lipolysis and fatty acid oxidation.

**Glycogenolysis.** Glycogen storage diseases present in a variety of subtypes that differ in severity (see Chapter 5). Among the subtypes that result in hypoglycemia, the most severe form is glucose-6-phosphatase deficiency. This subtype is characterized by severe hypoglycemia, massive hepatomegaly, growth retardation, and lactic acidosis. In contrast, deficiencies in the glycogen phosphorylase enzymes may cause isolated hepatomegaly with or without hypoglycemia.

The *diagnosis* of glycogen storage disease is suggested by a finding of hepatomegaly without splenomegaly. Ketosis occurs with hypoglycemic episodes. Confirmation of the diagnosis requires specific biochemical studies of leukocytes or liver biopsy specimens.

*Treatment* involves frequent high-carbohydrate feedings during the day and continuous feedings at night via nasogastric tube. Feedings of uncooked cornstarch at bedtime are sufficient to maintain serum glucose concentrations in some patients.

**Gluconeogenesis.** Defects in gluconeogenesis are uncommon and include fructose-1,6-diphosphatase deficiency and phosphoenolpyruvate carboxykinase deficiency. Affected patients present with fasting hypoglycemia, hepatomegaly due to fatty infiltration, lactic acidosis, and hyperuricemia. Ketosis occurs and FFA and alanine concentrations are high.

*Treatment* involves frequent high-carbohydrate, low-protein feedings.

**Fatty Acid Oxidation.** These disorders of ketogenesis include the fatty acid acyl-coenzyme A (CoA) dehydrogenase deficiencies; long-chain, medium-chain, and short-chain acyl-CoA dehydrogenase deficiency, and hereditary carnitine deficiency. Of these disorders, medium-chain acyl-CoA dehydrogenase deficiency (MCAD) is both the most common and the least severe. MCAD occurs in 1 in 9,000–15,000 live births. Patients often are well in infancy and can present with the first episode of hypoglycemia at 2 yr of age or older. Episodes of hypoglycemia usually occur with prolonged fasting or during episodes of intercurrent illness. Mild hepatomegaly may be present along with mild hyperammonemia, hyperuricemia, and mild elevations in hepatic transaminases. Ketone concentrations are low or undetected.

The *diagnosis* is confirmed by the finding of elevated concentrations of dicarboxylic acids in the urine. *Treatment* involves avoidance of fasting.

**Other Metabolic Disorders.** A number of metabolic disorders in addition to those just described can lead to hypoglycemia. These include galactosemia, hereditary fructose intolerance, and a number of disorders of organic acid metabolism (see Table 17–26). Hypoglycemia in these disorders is usually a reflection of global hepatic dysfunction secondary to the buildup of hepatotoxic intermediates. Many of these disorders present with low concentrations of ketone bodies because ketogenesis is also affected. The finding of non-glucose reducing substances in the urine suggests a diagnosis of galactosemia or hereditary fructose intolerance. Occurrence of symptoms following ingestion of fructose or sucrose suggests hereditary fructose intolerance. *Treatment* requires dietary restriction of the specific offending substances.

### Medications and Intoxications

Hypoglycemia can occur (1) as an adverse effect of a number of medications, including insulin, oral hypoglycemic agents, and propranolol, and (2) as a result of salicylate intoxication. Valproate toxicity can cause a disorder similar to that seen in the fatty acid oxidation defects. Ethanol ingestion can also cause hypoglycemia, especially in younger children, because the metabolism of ethanol results in the depletion of cofactors necessary for gluconeogenesis.

### Reactive Hypoglycemia

The term "reactive hypoglycemia" has been used to describe hypoglycemia occurring 2 to 3 hr after a meal. This condition can occur in patients who have the *dumping syndrome* as a consequence of gastric surgery. Rapid gastric emptying results in a rapid rise of serum glucose and excess stimulation of insulin secretion. Rarely, transient reactive hypoglycemia can occur in patients who later have IDDM. Delayed insulin secretion in response to elevations in serum glucose concentrations is thought to be responsible for this phenomenon. Except for the patients just described, true reactive hypoglycemia is rare.

### DIAGNOSIS

Because the list of causes of hypoglycemia is long and complex, establishing the *etiology* in a particular patient can be difficult. Frequently, it is not possible to make an accurate diagnosis without obtaining a *critical sample* of blood and urine at the time of the hypoglycemic episode. In a child with unexplained hypoglycemia, a serum sample should be obtained before treatment for the measurement of glucose and insulin, GH, cortisol, and β-hydroxybutyrate. Measurement of serum lactate levels should also be considered. A urine specimen should be obtained for measuring ketones and reducing substances. The results of this initial testing can establish whether endocrine causes are responsible and, if not, provide initial information regarding which types of metabolic disorders are most likely. Whenever possible, additional samples of blood and urine should be frozen for further analysis if necessary.

## EMERGENCY MANAGEMENT

Acute care of the patient with hypoglycemia consists of rapid administration of intravenous glucose (2 cc/kg of 10% dextrose in water is usually sufficient). Following the initial bolus of glucose, an infusion of intravenous glucose should be established to provide approximately one and one half times the normal hepatic glucose production rate (9–11 mg/kg/min in infants, 6–8 mg/kg/min in children). Higher infusion rates may be needed for hyperinsulinemic states. This allows for suppression of the catabolic state and prevents further decompensation in patients with cetain metabolic disorders. If adrenal insufficiency is suspected, stress doses of glucocorticoids should be administered.

## References

Behrman RE, Kliegman RM, Arvin AM (eds): Nelson Textbook of Pediatrics, 15th ed. Philadelphia, WB Saunders, 1996, Chapter 77.

Dunne MJ, Kane C, Sheperd RM, et al: Familial persistent hyperinsulinemic hypoglycemia of infancy and mutations in the sulfonylurea receptor. N Engl J Med 336:703, 1997.

Haymond MW: Hypoglycemia in infants and children. Endocrinol Clin Metab North Am 18:211, 1989.

La Franchi S: Hypoglycemia in infancy and childhood. Pediatr Clin North Am 34:959, 1987.

Service F: Hypoglycemic disorders. N Engl J Med 332:1144, 1995.

Sperling MA, Finegold DN: Hypoglycemia in infants. In Sperling MA (ed): Pediatric Endocrinology. Philadelphia, WB Saunders, 1996, pp 71–96.

Stanley CA: Hyperinsulinism in infants and children. Pediatr Clin North Am 44:363, 1997.

Stanley CA, Hale DE: Genetic disorders of mitochondrial fatty acid oxidation. Curr Opin Pediatr 6:476, 1994.

# Chapter 18

# NEUROLOGY

Michael J. Painter

Ira Bergman

Neurologic disorders include diseases of the central nervous system (CNS), of the peripheral nervous system, of muscle, and of the special senses. These diseases may be localized to one site of the nervous system or may be part of a generalized multisystem disorder (acquired immunodeficiency syndrome–dementia, systemic lupus erythematosus–psychosis, lead poisoning). The pathogenesis of neurologic disorders includes trauma; infections; inborn errors of metabolism and storage diseases; congenital anomalies; metabolic and toxic disturbances; anoxic, ischemic, embolic, and thrombotic complications; primary or metastatic neoplasms; and autoimmunity.

Neurologic diseases become manifest within a narrow range of symptoms and signs, which include pain (headache, paresthesia); altered mental function (encephalopathy, encephalitis, intoxication–poisoning, hypoxia–ischemia, degenerative disorders); altered motor function (cortical, cerebellar, spinal, anterior horn cell, peripheral nerve, neuromuscular junction, or muscle lesion); and/or seizures. These disorders may be congenital or acquired, acute or chronic, progressive or static, and reversible or irreversible.

## DEVELOPMENT OF THE CENTRAL NERVOUS SYSTEM

The precursor of the nervous system is the embryonic ectodermal neural plate, which is present at 18 days of gestation. The neural plate gives rise to the neural tube, which forms the CNS (brain, spinal cord), and the neural crest cells, which give rise to the peripheral nervous system (e.g., the cranial, spinal, and autonomic nerves and ganglia). Neural crest cells thus constitute the cardiac, celiac, mesenteric, and Meissner plexus as well as the chromaffin cells, melanocytes, meninges, and adrenal medulla cells.

The neural tube begins to form on the 22nd day of gestation. The fusion of the neural tube proceeds in a cranial and caudal direction, thus leaving temporary rostral and caudal openings, which close on the 25th and the 27th days of gestation, respectively. The rostral end forms the brain, and the caudal region forms the spinal cord; the lumen of the neural tube forms the ventricles of the brain and the central canal of the spinal cord.

## CONGENITAL ANOMALIES OF THE NERVOUS SYSTEM

Defective closure of the caudal neuropore at the end of the 4th wk of gestation produces defects of the vertebral arches known as *spina bifida* (divided spine). Nonfusion of spinal arches may be isolated to vertebral defects (L5, S1) **(spina bifida occulta)** and is noted in 10% of people, who usually are asymptomatic. A small dimple or tuft of hair may be present over the affected vertebra. **Spina bifida cystica** occurs in 1:1000 births and is a sac-like lesion that has multiple unfused vertebrae and an associated *meningocele* or *meningomyelocele* if the meninges or meninges and spinal cord, respectively, form the sac. Spina bifida with *myeloschisis* is noted when the lesion is an open neural tube without an overlying sac. Spina bifida cystica and myeloschisis produce severe neurologic deficits that correlate to the level of the neural tube defect. Loss of sensation, paralysis, and loss of bowel and bladder control are common and depend on the level of the lesion. Thoracic lesions are associated with the poorest neurologic outcome and vertebral instability. Most patients with any of these lesions have bowel and bladder dysfunction. The bladder dysfunction results in repeated episodes of urinary tract infections, reflux nephropathy, and renal insufficiency. Meningomyelocele usually is accompanied by hydrocephalus that is due to an **Arnold-Chiari malformation**, producing downward displacement of the medulla and cerebellum accompanied by obstruction of the 4th ventricle.

### Meningomyelocele

Treatment of infants with meningomyelocele includes operative skin closure of an open or thin-walled spinal defect, ventricular-peritoneal shunting of hydrocephalus, bracing of the lower extremities to permit ambulation in children with low vertebral lesions, intermittent bladder catheterization to avoid urinary stasis, and physical therapy. Most children have a normal intelligence quotient (IQ), if there are no associated CNS anomalies. *In utero detection* is possible by screening for a high maternal serum alpha-fetoprotein level followed by performing fetal ultrasonography and amniocentesis to confirm elevated amniotic fluid alpha-fetoprotein and acetylcholinesterase levels. *Prevention* is possible by providing supplements of folate early in pregnancy, before neural tube development.

### Diastematomyelia

In diastematomyelia, the spinal cord is divided by bone spicules or by a fibrous band. This diplomyelic condition and a lipomatous tumor (lipomeningocele) may produce a **tethered cord syndrome,** with resultant abnormalities of distal sensation, gait, and bladder or bowel function. The *treatment* is surgery.

### Cranial Defects

Cranial defects may produce anterior or posterior encephaloceles containing either meninges or meninges and brain. Severe malformations resulting from failure of rostral neuropore closure produce exencephaly (exposed brain) or anencephaly. The latter is noted in 1:1000 births in the United States and is uniformly lethal.

Neonates with **anencephaly** have a rudimentary brain stem or midbrain but no cortex or cranium. *Prenatal diagnosis* is possible by detecting elevated maternal serum alpha-fetoprotein levels and by performing fetal ultrasonography. The recurrence risk in subsequent pregnancies for either cranial or spinal neural tube defects is 10%. Within a family,

an anencephalic birth may be followed by the birth of a second child affected with a lumbar-sacral meningomyelocele. The inheritance of neural tube defects is polygenic.

### References

Behrman RE, Kliegman RM, Arvin AM (eds): Nelson Textbook of Pediatrics, 15th ed. Philadelphia, WB Saunders, 1996, Chapter 542.

McCarthy G: Treating children with spina bifida. BMJ 302:65, 1991.

MRC Vitamin Study Research Group: Prevention of neural tube defects: Results of the Medical Research Council Vitamin Study. Lancet 338:131, 1991.

Volpe J: Neurology of the Newborn, 3rd ed. Philadelphia, WB Saunders, 1995.

## NEUROLOGIC EVALUATION

The results and evaluation of the neurologic examination of children vary with chronologic age. The examination of the newborn is unique, whereas examination of the older child approximates that of the adult. Examining the young child is a challenging process because the patient often is uncooperative and has limited ability to assist.

The neurologic evaluation includes a history of the evolution of the illness, its character, and the presence of the illness in similarly affected family members. One attempts to establish the abnormalities as "progressive," "intermittent," "static," or "saltatory." *Static* abnormalities noted in the first few months of life suggest congenital abnormalities or brain injury sustained during the prenatal or neonatal period. *Progressive* disorders suggest degenerative CNS disease, whereas abnormalities that are *intermittent* with return to normal neurologic function indicate paroxysmal disorders. *Saltatory* disorders, characterized by exacerbation and partial recovery, are seen with demyelinating and vascular diseases.

Findings on the general examination often are clues to *diagnosis*. Abnormalities of hair, skin, teeth, and nails, all of neuroectodermal origin, may reflect nervous system lesions. Neurocutaneous lesions, such as *café au lait* spots, neurofibroma, and adenoma sebaceum, occur in several disorders (Table 18–1). The occipital frontal head circumference reflects underlying brain growth and/or the presence of anomalies. The *head circumference* is measured using paper disposable tape and plotted against appropriate standard growth curves (see Chapter 1, Figs. 1–4 and 1–10). A measurement of 3 standard deviations above or below the mean is abnormal and reflects either macrocephaly or microcephaly. Measurements plotted over time

TABLE 18–1.    Differential Diagnosis of *Café au Lait* Spots

Neurofibromatosis
Tuberous sclerosis
Bloom syndrome
McCune-Albright syndrome
Fanconi anemia
Gaucher disease
Russell-Silver dwarf
Ataxia–telangiectasia
Epidermal nevi

may show an accelerating or decelerating pattern of growth indicating hydrocephalus or growth impairment or destruction of brain, respectively.

During infancy, the anterior fontanel is slightly depressed and pulsatile when the infant is placed in the sitting position. When the fontanel is tense or bulging, increased intracranial pressure is suspected. An unusual shape of the head may indicate premature closure of one or more of the sutures **(craniosynostosis)**. Abnormal shape, location, and condition of the ears are found in a number of syndromes (e.g., whether the ears are low set and/or posteriorly rotated). An examination of the eyes should include a search for epicanthal folds, coloboma, conjunctival telangiectasias, or cataracts. Examining the optic fundus with a direct ophthalmoscope helps assess the status of the optic disks and macula. A complete examination of the retina requires dilating the pupil and using an indirect ophthalmoscope. Examining the hands and feet reveals the presence of abnormal creases, polydactyly, or syndactyly (see Chapter 19). An examination of the neck and spine should include searching for *midline defects*, which may be obvious, such as spina bifida with myelomeningocele, or subtle,

TABLE 18–2.    CNS Reflexes of Infancy

| Reflex | Description | Age of Appearance | Age of Disappearance | Origin in Central Nervous System |
|---|---|---|---|---|
| Moro | Sudden head extension causes extension followed by flexion of the arms and legs | Birth | 4–6 mo | Brain stem vestibular nuclei |
| Grasp | Placing a finger in palm results in flexing of the infant's hand, accompanied by flexion at elbow and shoulder | Birth | 4–6 mo | Brain stem vestibular nuclei |
| Rooting | Tactile stimulus about the mouth results in the infant's mouth pursuing the stimulus | Birth | 4–6 mo | Brain stem trigeminal system |
| Trunk incurvation | Infant withdraws from stroking stimulus along the ventral margin | Birth | 9–6 mo | Spinal cord |
| Placing | Infant places foot on examining surface when dorsum of foot is brought into contact with the edge of the surface | Birth | 4–6 mo | Cerebral cortex |
| Crossed extension | One leg held firmly in extension and the dorsum and sole of the foot stimulated results in a sequence of flexion, extension, and adduction, followed by toe fanning of the opposite leg | Birth | 4–6 mo | Spinal cord |
| Tonic neck | With the infant supine, turning of the head results in ipsilateral extension of the arm and leg in a "fencing" posture | Birth | 4–6 mo | Brain stem vestibular nuclei |
| Parachute | With the infant sitting, tilting to either side results in extension of the ipsilateral arm in a protective fashion | 6–8 mo | Never | Brain stem vestibular nuclei |
| Landau | With the infant held about the waist and suspended, extension of the neck produces extension of the arms and legs | 6–8 mo | 15 mo–2 yr | Brain stem |

such as cutaneous dimples, small openings or sinus tracts, or tufts of hair or subcutaneous lipomas, suggesting the possibility of vertebral or spinal cord abnormalities. Kyphosis and scoliosis are important features to note in abnormalities of the central and peripheral nervous systems.

## NEONATAL EXAMINATION

Because the brain is immature, an examination of the neonate is used mainly to assess the function of the subcortical structures.

### Reflexes

A number of primitive reflexes noted at birth (Table 18–2) indicate the functional integrity of the brain stem. As a group, they are symmetric and disappear at 4–6 mo of age, indicating the normal maturation of descending inhibitory cerebral influences. The *Landau* and *parachute* reflexes become apparent after the newborn period, indicating proper maturation of appropriate brain structures. The *grasp* and *rooting* reflexes are inhibited by maturation of frontal lobe structures and may reappear later in life with frontal lobe lesions. Asymmetry of the primitive reflexes often indicates focal brain or peripheral nerve lesions.

### Posture

Posture is defined as the position that the infant naturally assumes when placed supine. An infant at 28 wk of gestation demonstrates total extension, whereas at 32 wk a slight increase in tone of the lower extremities is noted. At 34 wk, the lower extremities are flexed and the upper extremities are extended. At term, the infant flexes both lower and upper extremities. *Recoil* is defined as a liveliness with which an extremity springs back to its original position after passive stretching and release. Recoil is essentially absent in the small premature infant but is very brisk at term.

### Movement/Tone

As gestational age increases, spontaneous movements of the infant change from extensive, generalized, and athetoid to those that are localized and brief. Spontaneous movements of the small premature infant normally are slow, whereas those of the term infant are rapid and jerk-like.

The popliteal angle, heel-to-ear maneuver, scarf maneuver, and head control are utilized in as-

sessing muscle tone and estimating gestational age (see Chapter 6 and Fig. 6–4).

Persistence of the primitive reflexes beyond 4–6 mo of age indicates dysfunction of brain structures responsible for their inhibition. Increased resistance to such maneuvers as the elicitation of the scarf reflex or the popliteal angle in the premature infant may be a manifestation of rigidity or of spasticity, whereas decreased resistance in the performance of these maneuvers in the term infant may be a manifestation of hypotonia. Because CNS maturation is incomplete, one must be cautious in establishing a prognosis based on the newborn neurologic examination alone.

## CRANIAL NERVE EVALUATION

The evaluation of cranial nerve function depends on the stage of maturation of the child's brain and on the ability of the child to cooperate.

### Cranial Nerve I

The child's sense of smell is difficult to assess. Beginning at the age of 2–3 yr, one can discern whether or not the child can smell. Aromatic substances, such as perfumes and ground coffee, should be utilized, not volatile substances (such as ammonia) that irritate the nasal mucosa and do not test smell. Once the child has established speech, it often is possible to assess the ability to perceive and name an odor. Anosmia may be congenital or due to head trauma, fractures, meningitis, diseases of the nose, or brain tumors.

### Cranial Nerve II

Vision can be assessed grossly in the neonate by noting a blinking response to bright light. The visual acuity at birth is approximately 20/150. When visual evoked responses are used, the visual acuity has been found to be 20/20 by 6 mo of age. The examiner can obtain an indication of peripheral vision by noting the infant's detection of objects brought into the visual field from behind. The ability of the child to visually locate and track small objects estimates visual acuity in the infant, whereas in older children standard visual acuity charts and confrontational testing of peripheral vision are utilized. Lesions of the anterior visual pathways, including the optic nerves, chiasm, and tract, are expressed by a reduced pupillary reaction to light, which may be bilateral or unilateral (afferent pupillary defect). Lesions of the posterior visual pathway, involving the occipital cortex, lateral geniculate, and optic radiations, are expressed by loss of visual fields and normal pupillary reactions.

### Cranial Nerves III, IV, and VI

Extraocular movements may be assessed in the neonate by observing eye movements in response to visual stimuli and by noting extraocular movements when stimulating vestibular reflexes by gently spinning the infant. Beyond the newborn period, extraocular movements are observed as the infant follows objects. The pupillary reflex is assessed by a focused bright light. The pupil reacts to light by 30 wk of gestation.

Cranial nerve III innervates the levator palpebrae superioris; the medial, superior, and inferior recti; and the inferior oblique muscles. Cranial nerve IV innervates the superior oblique muscle, which adjusts the globe in the adducted position, and cranial nerve VI innervates the lateral rectus muscle. Because cranial nerve VI has a long intracranial route, sixth cranial palsies may be nonspecific signs of increased intracranial pressure. Cavernous sinus infection affects cranial nerves III, IV, V, and VI. Abnormalities of cranial nerves III, IV, and VI may cause diplopia.

Clinical syndromes may affect cranial nerve III and produce *miosis* (a constricted pupil) or *mydriasis* (a dilated pupil). A constricted pupil may be associated with a **Horner syndrome** (miosis, ptosis, anhidrosis) resulting from a unilateral sympathetic nervous system lesion. Additional causes of miosis include the **Argyll Robertson pupil**, drugs (opiates, cholinergic agents), and pontine lesions (sympathetic paralysis). Mydriasis is seen with drugs (anticholinergic, sympathomimetic), botulism, nerve III compression, and thyrotoxicosis.

### Cranial Nerve V

In newborns and small infants, the examiner can assess the muscles of mastication while watching the infant suck and swallow. The masseter muscles may be directly palpated. In later childhood, as cooperation improves, pterygoid function may be assessed by voluntary jaw deviation. The *corneal reflex* can be tested (cranial nerves V and VII) at any age. Facial sensation of light touch and pain can be determined with cotton gauze and pinprick.

### Cranial Nerve VII

The assessment of facial symmetry at rest and during sucking activity can be utilized in assessment of the small infant. Beyond infancy, the muscles of facial expression are assessed on a voluntary basis.

Complete facial weakness suggests a peripheral lower motor neuron lesion, whereas lower facial weakness suggests an upper motor neuron lesion. Taste to the anterior two thirds of the tongue is difficult to assess, but the ability to discriminate between salt and sugar can be assessed in a cooperative child once language is acquired.

### Cranial Nerve VIII

The neonate demonstrates eye blinking in response to loud noises. At approximately 4 mo of age, an infant will turn to the sound stimulus. The use of spoken words whispered at 2 feet is a more reliable technique and may be used once the child has acquired speech. *Conductive* versus *sensorineural* hearing loss can be differentiated by the fact that air conduction of a tuning fork sound should last twice as long as bone conduction. Symptoms of lesions of cranial nerve VIII include deafness, tinnitus, and vertigo.

Lesions of the vestibular component of the acoustic nerve may produce manifestations such as vertigo, nausea, vomiting, diaphoresis, and nystagmus. Lesions in cranial nerve VIII, the cerebellopontine angle, or the junction of the pons and medulla all may produce these problems. The *differential diagnosis* of vertigo is noted in Table 18–3. Testing of the labyrinth system can be performed by irrigating the ear canal with warm or cold water. Warm calorics stimulate nystagmus toward the irrigated side, whereas cold produces nystagmus to the opposite direction. Nystagmus is defined by the direction of the quick component.

### Cranial Nerves IX and X

The gag reflex is brisk at all ages except in the very immature neonate. Uvula deviation toward the

**TABLE 18–3.  Differential Diagnosis of Vertigo***

**Peripheral Causes**
 Benign positional vertigo
 Acute vestibulopathy (labyrinthitis)
 Ménière syndrome
 Toxic labyrinthopathy
 Motion sickness

**Central Causes**
 Multiple sclerosis
 Cerebrovascular disease
 Cerebellopontine tumors (acoustic neuroma)
 Migraine

*Peripheral vertigo has no other auditory (except Ménière syndrome) or neurologic deficits. Often, an intense sense of severe spinning with nausea, vomiting, a positive Romberg test, past pointing, and rotatory or horizontal nystagmus are present. Vertical nystagmus is often due to brain stem lesions.

stronger unaffected side suggests unilateral palsy of cranial nerves IX and/or X. Nasal speech and vocal cord paralysis (recurrent laryngeal nerve) are additional signs of lesions of cranial nerve X.

### Cranial Nerve XI

The functions of the trapezius and sternocleidomastoid muscles are assessed by observing the infant's posture and spontaneous activity. Head tilt and drooping of the shoulder are suggestive of lesions involving cranial nerve XI. In later childhood, direct examination of these muscles is possible.

### Cranial Nerve XII

Examination of the tongue for atrophy and fasciculation is accomplished at any age. By 1 yr of age, specific tongue movements can be assessed by having the child follow a lollypop with the tongue; by 3–4 years of age, tongue movement to command is possible. The tongue deviates toward the weak side in unilateral lesions.

## MOTOR EXAMINATION

In the neonate and the small infant, the motor examination utilizes the observation of spontaneous activity, primitive reflexes, and muscle tone previously described. When the infant begins to walk, gait is assessed. In early infancy, the gait is broad-based and unsteady. The base narrows with age, so that by the 6th year a child is able to tandem walk. *Pyramidal track* dysfunction results in a stiff, shuffling gait caused by spasticity, whereas a similar gait is noted in *extrapyramidal* motor dysfunction on the basis of rigidity. Abnormalities of the anterior horn cell, peripheral nerve, neuromuscular junction, and muscle (lower motor neuron) result in a wide-based, unsteady gait caused by weakness. Cerebellar dysfunction results in a broad-based, unsteady gait accompanied by difficulty in executing turns. The ability of the child to stand from the supine posture evaluates strength of the back, hip, and proximal leg muscles. The ability of the child to walk on the heels tests the anterior tibial muscles. Toe walking assesses strength of the gastrocnemius and soleus muscles. The examiner assesses dexterity of movements of the upper extremities by having the small infant reach for objects and by having the older child demonstrate the ability to perform finger-to-finger and finger-to-nose maneuvers.

In the toddler, muscle strength is assessed by observation. Arm and shoulder muscle strength is tested by observing the child's ability to raise the arms above the head and by the resistance the examiner feels when lifting the child by placing his or her hands in the infant's axillae.

Muscle weakness of pyramidal origin is spastic, extrapyramidal weakness is rigid, and weakness of lower motor neuron origin is flaccid. Muscle fasciculations suggest denervation.

### Assessment of Muscle Bulk and Tone

Although atrophy eventually is seen in both pyramidal and extrapyramidal lesions, it is most striking in lesions involving the lower motor neuron. Bulk is assessed by observation, palpation, and comparison to contralateral extremities. Excessive muscle bulk is seen in myotonia congenita and pseudohypertrophic muscular dystrophy. Muscle tone is assessed by measuring the extremity's resistance to passive motion. In extrapyramidal disease, an increase in resistance is present throughout passive movement of a joint *(rigidity).* In pyramidal disease, increased resistance to passive movement that suddenly gives way at a critical point *(clasped knife response)* is noted. In lower motor neuron disease, decreased resistance to passive movement is present.

### Evaluation of Deep Tendon Reflexes

Myotactic reflexes (triceps, biceps, knee, ankle) are elicited by sudden tendon stretch and can be obtained at any age. The Babinski response is not helpful in the neonate because the plantar response may be extensor or flexor. The plantar response is consistently flexor (downward) after 2 yr of age.

### Involuntary Movements

See Movement Disorders.

## SENSORY EXAMINATION

Evaluation of the sensory system includes an assessment of pain, touch, hot and cold temperature, and joint position senses. The sensory examination of the newborn and infant is limited to observing the perception of a pinprick by watching for crying, eye closure, facial grimace, or sucking response while feeding. Normal newborns interrupt their continuous sucking activity as they perceive a light pin stimulus. Simple withdrawal of the involved body part may be all that can be observed in the small infant, and without simultaneous facial changes, withdrawal may indicate a spinal cord reflex. In the cooperative child, once language has been achieved, touch, hot and cold, and position sense can be evaluated. Cortical sensation (two-point discrimination, stereognosis, and others) can be assessed reliably only in older children. Properly demarcating a sensory level can help localize a lesion.

## MENTAL STATUS EVALUATION

The assessment of mental status is a critical aspect of the examination. *Alertness* is assessed in the newborn and small infant by observing spontaneous activities, feeding behavior, and the ability of the infant to visually fix and follow the movement of objects. The child's response to tactile, visual, and auditory stimuli is noted. Does the child localize sound, follow objects visually, and verbalize to noxious stimuli? In circumstances of altered consciousness, the response to painful stimuli is noted. Does the child simply withdraw from pain, or is vigorous withdrawal accompanied by vocalization? (See *Glasgow Coma Scale* under Disorders of Consciousness.)

*Language function* is both expressive (involving speech and the use of gestures such as pointing or shaking the head) and receptive (understanding speech or gesture). Abnormalities of language resulting from disorders of the cerebral hemispheres are referred to as *aphasias*. Anterior, expressive, or **Broca aphasia** is characterized by sparse, nonfluent language. Posterior, receptive, or **Wernicke aphasia** is characterized by an inability to understand language. Speech is fluent but nonsensical. **Global aphasia** refers to impaired expressive and receptive language.

The use of a Denver Developmental Standard Screening Test is an efficient means of relating the child's behavior to appropriate age norms (see Chapter 1). Older children should have short-term and long-term *memory* tested with current events and other factors. Orientation to person, place, and time should be assessed, as should cognitive activities, such as mental solution of mathematical problems (e.g., serial subtraction of 7 from 100).

## SPECIAL DIAGNOSTIC PROCEDURES

### Electroencephalography

The electroencephalograph (EEG) records electrical activity generated by the cerebral cortex. EEG rhythms mature throughout childhood. The EEG of the premature infant is discontinuous and accompanied by a predominance of slower frequencies (2–4 Hz) until 36 wk of gestation, when the waking portion of the record is continuous. Sleep is characterized by a discontinuous pattern (trace alternans). In later childhood, the occipital portion of the EEG is characterized by 8–12 Hz activity (alpha), whereas faster rhythms (13–30 Hz) (beta) are seen anteriorly. Theta rhythms (4–7 Hz) are intermixed. Fixed slow-wave foci (1–3 Hz) delta rhythms suggest an underlying structural abnormality. When delta activity is seen diffusely, increased intracranial pressure or other encephalopathy is suspected. Spikes, polyspikes, and spike-and-wave abnormalities indicate an underlying seizure tendency.

### Evoked Responses

Evoked responses are computer-analyzed CNS responses to afferent stimuli. The stimulus (a click for auditory testing, a flash or pattern stimulus for visual testing, and a vibratory stimulus for somatosensory testing) is applied and the CNS response is monitored over the scalp. Repetitive stimuli are computer averaged and a response pattern is obtained. Abnormalities of the components of the response pattern can be localized to specific areas of the CNS. Somatosensory responses are of value in assessing peripheral nerve, spinal cord, and cerebral hemispheric function, whereas visual and auditory responses are of value in assessing hearing, central auditory function, and abnormalities of visual acuity and the visual pathways. Auditory evoked responses also are known as brain stem evoked responses because they assess auditory pathways at the level of the brain stem. Evoked responses are of particular value in small infants and in patients with altered consciousness.

### Electromyography

Electromyography (EMG) is used primarily to assess abnormalities of the lower motor neuron and muscles. Needles inserted into muscles frequently reveal denervation patterns when anterior horn or peripheral nerve disease is present. Normal muscle is electrically silent at rest, and the presence of spontaneous discharge of motor units (fibrillations) or muscle fasciculus (fasciculation) is indicative of denervation. Abnormalities of the motor pattern on muscle contraction are seen in denervation and primary muscle disease. Repetitive nerve stimulation may demonstrate excessive fatigue in **myasthenia gravis**.

Electromyography in conjunction with muscle

biopsy in which tissue is examined histochemically and with electron microscopy frequently is necessary to establish specific diagnoses in neuromuscular disease.

### Neuroradiology

Imaging the brain and spinal cord is accomplished utilizing computed tomography (CT), myelography, cerebral angiography, and magnetic resonance imaging (MRI). Ultrasonography can be used to evaluate the spinal cord as well as the cerebral cortex and ventricles in young infants if the fontanel is patent.

### Reference

Behrman RE, Kliegman RM, Arvin AM (eds): Nelson Textbook of Pediatrics, 15th ed. Philadelphia, WB Saunders, 1996, Chapter 541.

## DISORDERS OF CONSCIOUSNESS

Consciousness is a process by which a person is aware of self and environment. Coma is defined as being unresponsive to stimuli and differs from sleep, in that the person in a coma cannot be aroused. Arousal is impaired either by small lesions involving the reticular activating system (RAS), extensive bilateral cerebral lesions, or unilateral cerebral lesions that distort the upper brain stem (i.e., herniation syndromes). The RAS is a network of neurons located in the core of the brain stem extending from the mid pons through the midbrain and hypothalamus to the thalamus. The RAS projects widely to the cerebral cortex and serves a general arousing function.

Depression of consciousness may be acute, chronic, transitory, or recurring.

### ACUTE DISORDERS OF CONSCIOUSNESS
(see Chapter 3)

*Approach.* Acute changes in consciousness vary in degree from mild lethargy and confusion to deep coma. The *differential diagnosis* of altered consciousness is presented in Table 18–4. An initial approach to the comatose patient is discussed in Chapter 3. In childhood, the most common causes of coma include infections, hypoxia-ischemia (after cardiac arrest, drowning), intoxications, head trauma, and the ictal or postictal state.

Metabolic derangements may require adjustments of certain blood chemistries (glucose, cal-cium, sodium, bicarbonate, blood urea nitrogen [BUN], ammonia) by intravenous infusions or dialysis. Toxic ingestions may necessitate gastric lavage, charcoal administration, forced diuresis, dialysis, or specific antidotes (see Chapter 3). Infections are treated with antibiotics or antiviral agents (see Chapter 10). Structural brain lesions may require surgical excision or medical treatment of raised intracranial pressure (see Chapter 3).

*Clinical Manifestations.* A detailed history and physical examination usually provide sufficient clues to differentiate among the three major diagnostic categories producing coma: metabolic/toxic, infectious, and structural. Fever, petechiae, chills, and sweats suggest infection. Pain on neck flexion, photophobia, and pain on movement of the eyes are symptoms of meningeal irritation. Associated symptoms of abdominal pain, diarrhea, sore throat, conjunctivitis, cough, or rash point to viral encephalitis or a parainfectious syndrome. Neck motion should be avoided in patients with suspected trauma or drowning until the cervical spine films rule out vertebral fracture or subluxation. Headache and severe vomiting can be caused by raised intracranial pressure. A very abrupt loss of consciousness suggests a stroke; stupor progressing to deep, unarousable "sleep" over hours suggests drug intoxication; and a chronic gradual fading of alertness over weeks suggests a growing intracranial mass. Chronic medical conditions or their treatment (e.g., diabetes mellitus, insulin administration, leukemia), head trauma, use of "street drugs," social and emotional difficulties, exposure to sick animals, or travel to areas with known endemic diseases (e.g., Rocky Mountain spotted fever, Lyme disease) all provide specific clues.

*Neurologic examination* begins with observation. Breathing patterns, posture, and spontaneous actions often provide important clues to the depth, localization, and etiology of the depressed consciousness. Important recognizable respiratory patterns include *Cheyne-Stokes respirations*, central neurogenic hyperventilation, and gasping respirations. In Cheyne-Stokes respirations, a period of hyperventilation with a crescendo-decrescendo pattern alternates with a shorter period of apnea. Cerebral, thalamic, or hypothalamic modulation of respirations has been lost, but brain stem control is intact. This pattern also can be observed in patients with heart failure or primary respiratory disease. Midbrain disease yields *central neurogenic hyperventilation,* which consists of sustained rapid deep breathing. Gasping respirations are irregularly irregular. They indicate dysfunction of the low brain stem—medulla and usually are followed by terminal apnea.

**TABLE 18-4.** Diagnostic Approach to Coma

| Cause | Diagnostic Approach |
|---|---|
| *Metabolic Derangements* | $Na^+$, $K^+$, $Cl^-$, $CO_2$, BUN, creatinine, AST, ALT, PT, PTT, blood gas, ammonia, lead level, pyruvate, lactate, urinalysis, and urine amino and organic acids |
|   Hypoglycemia | |
|   Hyponatremia or its correction | |
|   Hypernatremia or its correction | |
|   Hyperosmolarity or its correction | |
|   Hypercapnia | |
|   Uremia | |
|   Hyperammonemia | |
|     Hepatic failure | |
|     Reye syndrome | |
|     Urea cycle enzyme deficiency | |
|     Fatty acid/acyl-coenzyme A dehydrogenase deficiency | |
|     Methylmalonicaciduria | |
|     Propionicaciduria | |
|     Idiopathic of prematurity | |
|   Mitochondrial diseases | |
|   Diabetes mellitus–ketoacidosis or hypoglycemia | |
|   Lead intoxication | |
| *Causes with CSF Abnormalities* | CSF analysis, CT, MRI, angiogram |
|   Bloody CSF | |
|     Subarachnoid hemorrhage | |
|     Subdural hemorrhage | |
|     Intraparenchymal hemorrhage (trauma, vascular malformations, coagulopathy) | |
|   Excess WBCs | |
|     Meningitis | |
|     Encephalitis | |
|     Parainfectious syndrome | |
|     Vasculitis | |
|     Carcinomatosis | |
|     Subacute bacterial endocarditis | |
| *Causes with CT or MRI Abnormalities* | CT, MRI |
|   Infarction | |
|     Global (anoxia) | |
|     Multifocal | |
|     Unilateral, large | |
|     Focal midbrain, hypothalamus or thalamus | |
|     TTP-HUS | |
|   Mass lesion | |
|     Tumor | |
|     Hemorrhage | |
|     Hydrocephalus | |
|     Abscess | |
|     Inflammatory mass | |
|     Cyst | |
|   Postinfectious demyelination processes | |
|   Cerebral edema | |
|     Trauma | |
|     Hypoxia–ischemia | |
|     Rapid correction of hyperosmolarity (hyperglycemia, hypernatremia) | |
|     Infectious–postinfectious | |
|     Toxins–lead | |
| *Causes with Normal CT and CSF* | Blood and urine analyses for toxic substances, EEG |
|   Drug intoxication or withdrawal | |
|   Epilepsy | |
|   Concussion | |
|   Migraine | |
|   Hypoxic-ischemic injury | |

ALT = alanine aminotransferase (formerly SGPT); AST = aspartate aminotransferase (formerly SGOT); BUN = blood urea nitrogen; CSF = cerebrospinal fluid; CT = computed tomography; EEG = electroencephalogram; HUS = hemolytic-uremic syndrome; MRI = magnetic resonance imaging; PT = prothrombin time; PTT = partial thromboplastin time; TTP = thrombotic thrombocytopenic purpura; WBC = white blood cell.

Body posture can indicate the degree of depression of consciousness. Mild depression is manifested by a comfortable "sleeping" posture with limbs slightly flexed, body tilted to one side, and eyes fully closed. Frequent readjustments of position, yawns, and sighs are observed. Deep coma is exhibited by patients who lie in a flat, extended, unvarying position with eyes half-open. An asymmetric posture suggests motor dysfunction of one side.

Observation reveals focal and generalized seizures, tremors, myoclonus, asterixis, choreoathetosis, dystonia, and ballismus. Focal seizures imply focal brain disease but also may be noted in children with meningitis or hypoglycemia. Generalized tremors, myoclonus, and asterixis are seen with metabolic-toxic diseases. Choreoathetosis, dystonia, and ballismus imply basal ganglia dysfunction.

Hallucinations can involve any sensory modality. Typically, olfactory and gustatory hallucinations indicate structural brain disease; visual and tactile hallucinations indicate metabolic-toxic disease; and auditory hallucinations indicate psychiatric illness.

Formal assessment of the degree of unconsciousness is performed utilizing the *Glasgow Coma Scale* (Table 18–5). Unresponsive patients are stimulated with noise, light touch, and pain. The various stages of depression of consciousness are defined in Table 18–6. However, a full description of what is observed should be recorded.

The detailed neurologic examination of the comatose patient focuses on the eyes, patterns of motor movement, tone, and reflexes. Eye movements are observed and then elicited with the *doll's head maneuver* (oculocephalic response) and cold caloric stimulation (oculovestibular response) (Fig. 18–1).

**TABLE 18–6. Stages of Depressed Consciousness**

| Stage | Manifestations |
| --- | --- |
| Lethargy-irritability | Sleepy, poor attention, fully arousable |
| Confusion | Poor orientation |
| Delirium | Agitated confusion, hallucinations, autonomic abnormalities (e.g., excess sweating, tachycardia, hypertension) |
| Obtundation | Arousable only to severe stimuli |
| Stupor | Unarousable, localizes pain |
| Coma | Unarousable, does not localize pain |

Doll's head movement should not be performed until it is clear that the cervical spine has not sustained a fracture or subluxation. People who are awake always can move their eyes whenever and wherever they wish, either by making a quick jumping (i.e., saccadic) eye movement or by slowly following (i.e., pursuing) a target. *Uninhibited eye movements* are seen with an intact brain stem but a poorly functioning cerebrum; the normal oculomotor brain stem reflexes are not controlled or inhibited by the aware brain. There may be no spontaneous eye movements, or the eyes may spontaneously rove slowly side to side. In the doll's head maneuver, the eyes move opposite to the direction of head movement at exactly the same pace, as if they were freely floating "ball bearings" within the orbits. To cold caloric stimulation, the eyes deviate fully and conjugately toward the ear that has been stimulated. Nystagmus is not observed. *Incomplete eye movements* are observed when specific portions of the brain stem, peripheral oculomotor nerves, neuromuscular junctions, or eye muscles are not functioning properly. With complete loss of oculomotor function, the eyes remain in the center of the orbit, as if they are "painted on," regardless of any stimulation.

Certain characteristic postures and tone can define the level or locus of neurologic disability. *Decorticate posturing* consists of rigid extension of the legs and feet, flexion and supination of the arms, and fisting of the hands. It occurs when the midbrain and red nucleus control body posture without inhibition by diencephalon, basal ganglia, and cortical structures. *Decerebrate posturing* consists of rigid extension of legs, arms, trunk, and head with hyperpronation of lower arms. It indicates pontine and vestibular nucleus control of posture without inhibition from more rostral structures. These postures may be exhibited unilaterally or bilaterally, indicating equal or unequal dysfunction of the two

**TABLE 18–5. Glasgow Coma Scale**

| | |
| --- | --- |
| Best motor response | 1. Nil (flaccid) |
| | 2. Extensor response |
| | 3. Abnormal flexion |
| | 4. Withdrawal |
| | 5. Localization of pain |
| | 6. Obeys |
| Best verbal response | 1. Nil |
| | 2. Incomprehensible sounds |
| | 3. Inappropriate words |
| | 4. Confused conversation |
| | 5. Oriented, fluent speech |
| Best eye opening response | 1. Nil |
| | 2. To pain |
| | 3. To speech |
| | 4. Spontaneous |

CONDITION:　　OCULAR REFLEXES IN UNCONSCIOUS PATIENTS

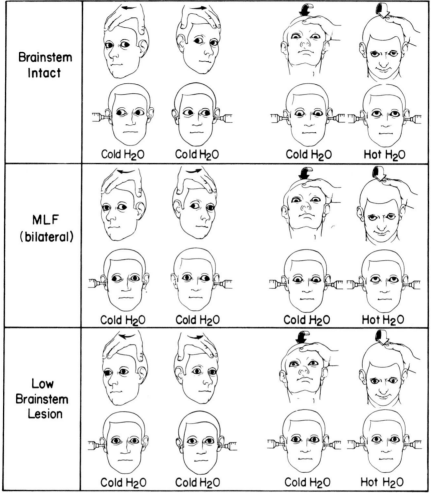

FIGURE 18–1.  Ocular reflexes in unconscious patients.

*Top*, Oculocephalic *(above)* and oculovestibular *(below)* reflexes in an unconscious patient whose brain stem ocular pathways are intact. Horizontal eye movements are illustrated on the left and vertical eye movements on the right: lateral conjugate eye movements *(upper left)* to head turning are full and opposite in direction to the movement of the face. A stronger stimulus to lateral deviation is achieved by irrigating cold water against the tympanic membrane. There is tonic conjugate deviation of both eyes toward the stimulus; the eyes usually remain tonically deviated for 1 min or more before slowly returning to the midline. Because the patient is unconscious, there is no nystagmus. Extension of the neck in a patient with an intact brain stem produces conjugate deviation of the eyes in the downward direction, and flexion of the neck produces deviation of the eyes upward. Bilateral cold water against the tympanic membrane likewise produces conjugate downward deviation of the eyes, whereas hot water (no warmer than 44°C [111.2°F]) causes conjugate upward deviation of the eyes.

*Middle*, Effects of bilateral medial longitudinal fasciculus (MLF) lesions on oculocephalic and oculovestibular reflexes. The left portion illustrates that oculocephalic and oculovestibular stimulation deviates the appropriate eye laterally and brings the eye, which normally would deviate medially, only to the midline, because the medial longitudinal fasciculus, with its connections between the abducens and oculomotor nuclei, is interrupted. Vertical eye movements often remain intact.

*Bottom*, Effects of a low brain stem lesion. On the left, neither oculovestibular nor oculocephalic movements cause lateral deviation of the eyes because the pathways are interrupted between the vestibular nucleus and the abducens area. Likewise, in the right portion, neither oculovestibular nor oculocephalic stimulation causes vertical deviation of the eyes. On rare occasions, particularly with low lateral brain stem lesions, oculocephalic responses may be intact even when oculovestibular reflexes are abolished.

(From Plum F, Posner J: The Diagnosis of Stupor and Coma, 3rd ed. Philadelphia, FA Davis, 1980, p 55.)

sides of the brain. Sometimes stereotyped rigid postures are exhibited that do not fall easily into the category of decerebrate or decorticate positions. These postures also indicate lack of cerebral and diencephalic control of upper brain stem motor reflexes.

*Metabolic* causes of acute coma are suggested by spontaneous fluctuations in the level of consciousness; tremors, myoclonus, and asterixis; visual and tactile hallucinations; and deep coma with preservation of pupillary light reflexes. Acute metabolic or toxic disorders also usually produce a hypotonic limp state, but hypertonia, rigidity, and decorticate and decerebrate posturing sometimes are observed in coma caused by hypoglycemia, hepatic encephalopathy, and short-acting barbiturates. Focal abnormalities on the neurologic examination (i.e., hemiparesis, cortical blindness, choreoathetosis, ataxia) suggest *structural brain disease.*

INTRACRANIAL PRESSURE ELEVATION. Papilledema or cranial nerve III palsies in patients with depressed consciousness are strong evidence of elevated intracranial pressure (ICP), which is a medical emergency. More commonly, progressive loss of consciousness accompanied by a characteristic progression of motor, oculomotor, pupillary, and respiratory signs, as detailed in Table 18–7, warns of incipient transtentorial herniation. Uncal herniation is another sign of severe increased ICP with early unilateral IIIrd nerve palsy and contralateral hemiparesis. Medical therapy must be instituted and emergency cranial CT performed. The initial study is done without contrast material so that blood and calcifications are easily identified. If the patient's condition permits, a study with contrast material follows, to identify inflammatory and neoplastic lesions. Some metabolic derangements give rise to severe elevations of ICP without producing recognizable CT abnormalities. These derangements include hepatic encephalopathy, Reye syndrome, hyponatremia, lead encephalopathy, trauma, treatment of diabetic ketoacidosis, and global or multifocal hypoxic-ischemic injury.

Lumbar puncture increases the risk of transtentorial herniation in patients with raised ICP and should be avoided.

*Differential Diagnosis.* See Table 18–4.

TOXIC OR METABOLIC ABNORMALITIES. Metabolic imbalances associated with depression of consciousness are most severe when the metabolic derangement has developed acutely and rapidly. The neurologic deficits associated with uremia and hypercapnia without hypoxia usually are fully reversible. The other metabolic disorders, however, may produce permanent neurologic disability if they are not treated at an early stage. Pathologic examination of brain tissue has revealed neuronal loss in the presence of hypoglycemia; vascular damage and parenchymal hemorrhages with hypernatremia; cerebral edema with hyponatremia, hepatic failure, Reye syndrome, and lead encephalopathy; and astrocytosis with hepatic failure. Focal deficits are uncommon in metabolic encephalopathy. The presence of asterixis signals hepatic or uremic encephalopathy or hypercapnia. **Reye syndrome** produces an easily recognizable clinical picture consisting of pernicious vomiting, lethargy accompanied by belligerence, hyperventilation, and large pupils.

Systemic acidosis and alkalosis do not significantly depress consciousness but are characteristic features of a number of diseases that produce encephalopathy. Consciousness often is reduced in patients with diabetic ketoacidosis, but the severity of unresponsiveness correlates with the degree of hyperosmolarity, not with the degree of acidosis. Proper treatment results in rapid return of full consciousness (see Chapter 17). In rare instances, patients with diabetes lapse into stupor hours after treatment is begun because of the development of brain swelling and central herniation; mortality is high. Medical therapy to reduce cerebral swelling may be very effective if instituted when consciousness first wanes (see Chapter 3).

The *common drugs* and *toxins* that cause stupor and coma and their effects on pupillary size are

TABLE 18–7. Progression of Stages and Anatomic Levels of Transtentorial Central Herniation

| Signs | Thalamus → | Midbrain → | Medulla* |
|---|---|---|---|
| Consciousness | Confusion; stupor | Coma | Coma |
| Respirations | Sighs; Cheyne-Stokes type | Central neurogenic hyperventilation | Gasping; absent |
| Pupils | Small, reactive | 3–5 mm, fixed | |
| Extraocular movements | Roving; uninhibited | Incomplete, dysconjugate | Absent |
| Motor response | Spastic; decorticate | Decerebrate | Flaccid |

*Uncal herniation with unilateral oculomotor nerve palsy and/or hemiplegia is another sign of severe increased intracranial pressure.

listed in Table 18–8. Delirium can be produced by amphetamines, cocaine, psychedelics, anticholinergics, and withdrawal from alcohol or barbiturates. The clinical profile of depressant drug overdose consists of lethargy, ataxia, dysarthria, and nystagmus, followed by coma in a flaccid state, with diminished stretch reflexes, incomplete extraocular muscle responses, and small reactive pupils.

*CEREBROSPINAL FLUID ABNORMALITIES.* Red blood cells in the cerebrospinal fluid (CSF) indicate primary subarachnoid hemorrhage or parenchymal hemorrhage that has ruptured into the CSF. The former usually is caused by rupture of a **saccular "berry" aneurysm** of one of the major cerebral arteries in the circle of Willis. These aneurysms are presumed to result from localized developmental defects in the arterial walls. Rupture is rare in childhood. The usual *clinical manifestations* are the sudden onset of intense headache followed by collapse and loss of consciousness. Focal neurologic deficits are variable, but nuchal rigidity almost invariably is present. Retinal or subhyloid hemorrhages are common. Some patients have a family history of aneurysms or a personal history of autosomal dominant polycystic renal disease. The patient is treated in an intensive care unit (ICU) with bed rest, sedation, and therapy to eliminate vascular spasm until surgical clipping of the aneurysm is feasible.

Spontaneous parenchymal hemorrhages in children are usually caused by **arteriovenous malformations** (AVMs). These are developmental anomalies consisting of tangled or dilated vessels that form a communication between the arterial and venous systems. The entire complex may enlarge slowly with age. Clinical presentation most commonly occurs between 10 and 40 yr of age with intraparenchymal and subarachnoid hemorrhages, seizures, headaches, or slowly progressive neurologic deficits. The rare AVM that produces a very enlarged "vein of Galen aneurysm" can cause heart failure in infancy as a result of large-volume blood flow through the shunt. In early childhood, these AVMs also can cause hydrocephalus as a result of compression of the aqueduct by the enlarged vein of Galen. A loud cranial bruit, if present, suggests an AVM.

*Treatment* of AVMs consists of surgical ligation of the entire lesion, if possible. Intravascular resins or embolization with particulate matter also has been utilized to halt flow.

Other causes of parenchymal hemorrhages include cerebral trauma, disorders of hemostasis, hypertension, tumors, or hemorrhagic infarctions.

White blood cells in the CSF usually denote infectious meningitis or meningoencephalitis but also may be associated with subacute bacterial endocarditis, vasculitis, carcinomatous meningitis, or a parainfectious syndrome.

**Parainfectious syndromes** (disseminated encephalomyelitis) closely resemble episodes of viral meningoencephalitis but are the consequence of acute multifocal, immunologically mediated demyelination rather than of direct viral invasion of the brain. Fever, stiff neck, depression of consciousness, and focal neurologic deficits occur a few days following a benign systemic viral syndrome. The course is variable, but most children recover without sequelae within a few days to weeks. Systemic viral infection appears to trigger the syndrome by an unknown mechanism. These syndromes were first described following measles, mumps, rubella, and chickenpox and after vaccination against smallpox and rabies.

*CT ABNORMALITIES.* Cerebral CT of a child with an acute disorder of consciousness may disclose either a space-occupying or a destructive lesion. To depress consciousness, unilateral cerebral lesions must directly compress and distort the diencephalon and brain stem, increase intracranial pressure by their bulk and associated edema, or block CSF pathways and produce hydrocephalus with increased ICP. Focal midbrain and diencephalic lesions that impair the RAS also can depress consciousness. Space-occupying lesions include tumors, abscesses, hemorrhages, cysts, and inflammatory masses.

Destructive lesions include infarcts and demye-

TABLE 18–8.   Effect of Coma-Producing Toxins on Pupillary Size

**Pupils Small**
  Narcotics (except meperidine)
  Sedatives
    Barbiturates
    Alcohol
  Major tranquilizers
  Phenothiazines
  Cholinergic agonists
    Organophosphate insecticides
    Nicotine
    Certain plants and mushrooms

**Pupils Large**
  Anticholinergics
    Antihistamines
    Tricyclic antidepressants
    Phenothiazines
  Glutethimide

**Pupils Normal**
  Salicylates
  Acetaminophen

linating plaques. When visible by CT, both appear as low-density areas but the latter are confined to the white matter. Cerebral infarctions can impair consciousness when the lesions are global, multifocal, located in the midbrain, or unilateral and large. The latter create brain swelling and elevations of ICP, which then depress consciousness.

The major diseases that produce demyelinated plaques are multiple sclerosis and the parainfectious (postinfectious) syndromes. The former is a chronic condition that occasionally presents in an acute disseminated manner to produce coma. Parainfectious syndromes, in contrast, usually occur acutely and frequently give rise to multifocal lesions that impair consciousness. Cerebral MRI is the best study to image small infarctions and small demyelinating plaques. Almost all cerebral lesions, except calcifications and acute hemorrhages, are visualized better on MRI than CT. CT remains the preferred imaging technique in emergency situations because it can be performed very rapidly and accurately identifies acute hemorrhages and large space-occupying lesions as well as edema and shifts of the midline.

HYPOXIC-ISCHEMIC INJURY (see Chapter 6). Deprivation of oxygen to the brain, caused by either deficient oxygen in the blood (hypoxemia) or deficient delivery of blood to the brain (ischemia), impairs consciousness (Table 18–9). Severe ischemia produces loss of consciousness within seconds and permanent brain damage within a few minutes. Sometimes progressive deterioration in func-

TABLE 18–9.  Causes of Hypoxia and Ischemia

**Hypoxemia**

$PO_2$ decreased
  Pulmonary disease
  Cardiac disease; right-to-left shunt
  Hypoventilation
    Exogenous (e.g., drowning, choking, suffocation)
    Neuromuscular disease
    Central respiratory drive decreased
$PO_2$ normal; decreased $O_2$ content
  Severe anemia
  Carbon monoxide poisoning
  Methemoglobinemia

**Ischemia**

Cardiac disease (decreased cardiac output)
  Myocardial infarction
  Arrhythmia
  Valvular disease
  Pericarditis
Pulmonary embolism
Hypotension, shock
Hanging, strangulation
Extensive cerebrovascular disease

tioning takes place for several hours after a severe hypoxic-ischemic insult. Some irreversibly damaged cells may continue to function for a brief period of time and then die. Release of metabolites from dead and dying cells may initiate a chemical cascade leading to loss of membrane stability in adjacent cells, intracellular influx of calcium ions, and cell death. In addition, the initial injury may be compounded by the development of circulatory failure from anoxic cardiac injury, disseminated intravascular coagulation (DIC), or cerebral edema.

Rarely, patients undergo delayed *postanoxic encephalopathy.* An initial hypoxic-ischemic event causes stupor or coma. The patients awaken in 24–48 hr, but several days to weeks later they become irritable, apathetic, and confused. Then a spastic quadriplegia accompanied by pseudobulbar palsy develops. Pathologic and radiologic studies reveal severe bilateral leukoencephalopathy. The pathogenesis is unknown. Patients may die, recover completely, or remain in a spastic state.

The *prognosis* of cerebral hypoxic-ischemic injury is extremely variable in children. In general, short duration of coma (hours to 1–2 days) and presence of intact brain stem function on admission to the hospital imply a good prognosis. The most common permanent neurologic sequelae are ataxia, choreoathetosis, parkinsonian syndrome, intention or action myoclonus, memory loss, visual agnosia, and impairments of learning and attention. Improvement can occur for several months to 1 yr following the insult. *Treatment* involves physical therapy, occupational therapy, rehabilitative services, and education.

OCCULT ETIOLOGY. Some causes of coma remain unclear after the entire diagnostic work-up is completed. The most common occult causes are drug or toxin exposure, cranial trauma, seizures, hypoxic-ischemic injury, migraine, and viral encephalitis. Sometimes a diagnosis is verified only as the natural history of the illness unfolds and the results of repeated examinations and testing are known.

**Prognosis.** The outcome of coma relates to many variables, including the etiology (intoxication carries a good prognosis, hypoxia carries a bad prognosis), the duration of coma, the age (children have a better outcome than adults), and the Glasgow Coma Scale on admission. Complete recovery from traumatic coma of several days' duration is possible in children. However, some survivors of severe coma are left in a persistent vegetative state or with severe neuropsychiatric disability.

**Brain Death.** Death of the whole brain (cortex and brain stem) generally is accepted as death of the person. Brain death means irreversible cessation of all functions. Table 18–10 lists the usual guidelines. In addition, total absence of cerebral blood flow on four-vessel intracranial angiography is definitive confirmation of brain death. Application of the criteria of brain death can be very difficult, particularly in newborns.

## TRANSIENT RECURRENT DEPRESSION OF CONSCIOUSNESS

Seizures may cause transient recurrent depression of consciousness.

Basilar artery migraine attacks last hours and may consist of confusion accompanied by agitation, ataxia, cortical blindness, vertigo, or cranial nerve palsies; headache may precede or follow the neurologic signs. Ischemia of the tissues supplied by the basilar artery also can produce amnesia and, infrequently, total loss of consciousness.

Cardiac arrhythmias or an obstructive cardiomyopathy (e.g., septal hypertrophy, left atrial myxoma, critical aortic stenosis) can cause recurrent episodes of syncope. Children with syncope require a cardiac examination, an electrocardiogram, and a tilt test.

Hypoglycemia can give rise to recurrent episodes of lethargy, confusion, seizures, or coma. Attacks often are heralded by anxiety, excess sweating, tremulousness, and hunger. A typical spell usually can be aborted by feeding the child orange juice or other sugar-containing solutions.

Several metabolic disorders cause recurrent bouts of hyperammonemia (see Table 18–4). Symptoms include nausea, vomiting, lethargy, confusion, ataxia, hyperventilation, and coma. Unlike epi-

sodes of hypoglycemia, which evolve over minutes, these spells worsen over hours. They often are precipitated by high-protein dietary intake or systemic viral infections. Early intravenous therapy is required to prevent permanent brain damage or death.

### References

Bannister R: Brain's Clinical Neurology, 6th ed. Cambridge, England, Oxford University Press, 1985.

Behrman RE, Kliegman RM, Arvin AM (eds): Nelson Textbook of Pediatrics, 15th ed. Philadelphia, WB Saunders, 1996, Chapters 549–551.

Plum F, Posner JB: The Diagnosis of Stupor and Coma. Philadelphia, FA Davis, 1980.

Schievink W: Intracranial aneurysms. N Engl J Med 336:28, 1997.

Task Force for the Determination of Brain Death in Children: Guidelines for the determination of brain death in children. Ann Neurol 21:616, 1987.

## CRANIOCEREBRAL TRAUMA

Children with head trauma either may have depression of consciousness and neurologic deficits or may be alert without neurologic deficits. The former require neurosurgical management, and the latter requires neurologic observation. Most serious trauma results from motor vehicle accidents, sports, recreation-related injuries, and violence.

### PATIENTS WITH NEUROLOGIC DEFICITS

Patients with neurologic deficits may have awakened following the injury (lucid interval) and then relapsed into coma or may have remained abnormal from the time of injury. Some patients are stable; others progressively deteriorate, develop acute irreversible loss of brain function, and require immediate neurosurgical care. The circulation must be supported, bleeding controlled, all systemic problems identified, proper intravenous fluids maintained, the neck carefully immobilized in a neutral position, and the cerebral lesions managed immediately. A baseline neurologic evaluation should be followed by intubation, ventilation if indicated, and pharmacologic paralysis or sedation. If consciousness and the neurologic deficits are stable, other life-threatening problems (e.g., an acute abdomen) may take precedence over immediate neurosurgical evaluation or treatment. Skull and cervical spine roentgenograms and cranial CT are obtained as soon as possible. Syndromes of post-traumatic hemorrhage are summarized in Table 18–11.

If surgery is not required, the child should be

**TABLE 18–10.** Guidelines for Determination of Brain Death*

No spontaneous movements, communication, or interaction with the environment

No superspinal response to externally applied stimuli (pain, touch, light, sound)

Absence of brain stem reflexes (including pupillary light, oculocephalic, oculovestibular, corneal, oropharyngeal–gag, and tracheal–cough)

Apnea

Electrocerebral silence on electroencephalogram

*All of the criteria listed should be present on multiple examinations at least 6–24 hr after the onset of coma and apnea. There must be documented absence of drug intoxication (including sedatives and neuromuscular blocking agents), hypothermia, and cardiovascular shock. A cause of coma sufficient to account for the loss of brain function should be established.

TABLE 18–11.  Syndromes of Post-traumatic Intracranial Hemorrhage

| Syndrome | Clinical and Radiologic Characteristics | Treatment |
| --- | --- | --- |
| Epidural | Onset over minutes to hours<br>Uncal herniation with third nerve palsy and contralateral hemiparesis<br>Lens-shaped extracerebral hemorrhage compressing brain | Surgical evacuation or observation<br>Prognosis good |
| Acute subdural | Onset over hours<br>Uncal herniation<br>Focal neurologic deficits<br>Crescentic extracranial hemorrhage compressing brain | Surgical evacuation<br>Prognosis guarded |
| Chronic subdural | Onset over weeks to months<br>Anemia, macrocephaly<br>Seizures, vomiting<br>Crescentic, low-density mass on CT | Subdural taps or subdural shunt as necessary<br>Prognosis good |
| Intraparenchymal | Depressed consciousness<br>Focal neurologic deficits<br>Additional multiple contusions | Supportive care<br>Prognosis guarded |
| Subarachnoid | Stiff neck<br>Late hydrocephalus | Supportive care<br>Prognosis variable |
| Contusion | Focal neurologic deficits<br>Brain swelling with transtentorial herniation<br>CT: Multifocal low-density areas with punctate hemorrhages | Medical treatment of elevated intracranial pressure<br>Prognosis guarded |

CT = computed tomography.

taken to an intensive care unit and followed up (see Chapter 3). If the child's neurologic condition worsens or the child already is comatose, ICP monitoring may be indicated.

Children with cerebral contusion who survive the acute cerebral swelling may improve rapidly or slowly or remain vegetative. Those who show daily improvement starting within days of the injury usually will recover completely. Maximal recovery may take weeks, months, or even a year in some patients. Caution must be used in providing families with a prognosis. Coma lasting for weeks following head trauma still is compatible with an ultimately good outcome, although the risk of late sequelae is increased. Patients who remain in a vegetative state for months following head injury without any clear evidence of improvement are unlikely to improve.

## AWAKE, ALERT CHILDREN WITHOUT NEUROLOGIC DEFICITS WHO HAVE HEADACHES, SLEEPINESS, OR VOMITING

Although the vast majority of children in this category recover fully and uneventfully, a few experience early or late complications that must be recognized and treated.

## Concussion

Concussion is a brief period of unconsciousness, lasting seconds or minutes, that occurs immediately after head trauma, followed by normal arousal. Amnesia often follows concussion. *Retrograde amnesia* is the inability to remember events immediately before the trauma and may extend backward in time for minutes, hours, days, or weeks. Usually, retrograde memory gradually is regained and permanent amnesia lasts only for the few minutes immediately prior to the blow. *Antegrade amnesia* is the inability to form new memories and becomes manifest by the patient incessantly repeating the same questions shortly after they have been answered (e.g., "Where am I?," "Why am I here?"). This state often persists for hours. The period of amnesia, both retrograde and antegrade, usually correlates with the severity of the trauma.

The pathophysiology of concussion is thought to be a shearing lesion of white matter as the brain is shaken within the cranium, resulting in a temporary failure of axon conduction. If loss of consciousness is maintained for longer than an hour or if recovery of consciousness is slow and accompanied by focal neurologic deficits, the pathophysiology is likely to include contusion and laceration, which may lead to focal or generalized *brain swelling*.

## Hemorrhage

See Table 18–11.

## Malignant Post-Traumatic Cerebral Swelling

Occasionally, epidural hemorrhage, other intracranial hemorrhage, or a rapid life-threatening increase in ICP develops unexpectedly in children who appear stable for hours following head trauma. *Diagnosis* and *treatment* proceed as detailed in Table 18–11.

## Syncope

Some patients faint a few minutes after head trauma or on awakening from their initial concussion. These patients complain of "dizzy" lightheadedness and loss of vision and slowly slump to the ground in a sleep-like state. Spontaneous arousal to full orientation occurs within a couple of minutes. Presumably, the psychic trauma produces a vagal discharge resulting in bradycardia and hypotension. *Treatment* consists of keeping the patient lying down until he or she is fully aroused, well perfused, and reassured that all is well.

## Transient Neurologic Disturbance

Transient neurologic disturbances sometimes develop in a few minutes following minor or severe head trauma and last for minutes to hours before clearing. The most common symptoms are occipital blindness and a confusional state, but hemiparesis, ataxia, or any other neurologic deficit may appear. These symptoms may represent migraine precipitated by trauma in susceptible children.

## Post-Traumatic Seizures

See Seizure Disorders later.

## Drowsiness, Headache, and Vomiting

Drowsiness, headache, and vomiting are common following head trauma and are not by themselves of concern if consciousness is preserved and the neurologic examination is normal. Children are especially susceptible to severe sleepiness following head trauma but should be easily arousable to alert wakefulness. If these symptoms persist unabated for more than 1–2 days, CT or MRI is indicated.

## Skull Fractures

Skull fractures may be (1) linear, (2) diastatic (spreading the suture), (3) depressed (an edge displaced inferiorly), or (4) compound (bone fragments breaking the skin surface).

Linear and diastatic fractures require no treatment but indicate severe trauma capable of producing an underlying hematoma.

Small depressed fractures have the same significance as linear fractures, but if the depression is more than 0.5–1 cm, surgical elevation of bone fragments and repair of associated dural tears are recommended.

Compound fractures or penetrating injuries require surgical débridement but not prophylactic antibiotic therapy. Tetanus prophylaxis must be assured. The risk of local brain contusion and early seizures is high.

Clinical *manifestations* of skull fracture include localized bogginess and pain; subcutaneous bleeding over the mastoid process (*Battle sign*) or around the orbit (*raccoon eyes*); blood behind the tympanic membrane (*hemotympanum*); or CSF leak from the nose (*rhinorrhea*) or ear (*otorrhea*).

Rarely, following linear skull fractures, a soft pulsatile scalp mass is palpable within a few weeks to months. Radiographically, the fracture edges are separated by a soft tissue mass that consists of fibrotic and accumulated brain and meningeal tissue and perhaps a leptomeningeal cyst. The recommended *treatment* involves surgical excision of abnormal tissue and dural repair.

## Cerebrospinal Fluid Leak

CSF leak occurs when a skull fracture tears adjacent dura, creating communications between the subarachnoid space and the nose, paranasal sinuses, mastoid air cells, or middle or external ear. Clear fluid that leaks from the nose or ear following head trauma is presumed to be CSF. The presence of air within the subdural, subarachnoid, or ventricular space also indicates a dural tear and open communication between the nose or paranasal sinuses and brain. In most cases, the dura heals spontaneously when the patient's head is kept elevated. If the leak persists or recurs, or if meningitis supervenes, the fracture site is identified and the dura is surgically repaired.

## Cranial Nerve Palsies

Palsies following laceration or contusion resulting from skull fracture may be transitory or permanent. Longitudinal fractures of the petrous bone produce conductive hearing loss and facial palsy, which begin hours after the injury and usually resolve spontaneously. Transverse petrous fractures produce sensorineural hearing loss and immediate facial palsy, with a poor prognosis for spontaneous recovery. Disruption of the ossicular chain is a cause of hearing loss and requires surgery. Permanent loss of olfaction after a head injury is due to a vibrational rupture of the thin olfactory nerves within the cribriform plate. Disruption of cranial nerve III, IV, or VI produces ophthalmoplegia, diplopia, and head tilt.

### Cervical Spine Injuries

Cervical spine injuries should be suspected in any unconscious child, especially if bruises are present on the back. In conscious children, findings of neck or back pain, burning or stabbing pains radiating to the arms, paraplegia, quadriplegia, or asymmetric motor or sensory responses of arms or legs are indications of spinal cord injury. Cervical spine injury (displaced or fractured vertebra) also may result in complete transection with spinal shock, loss of sensation, and flaccid paralysis. A contused cord (without vertebral abnormality) may be exhibited in a similar manner. Any patient with a clinical or radiologic abnormality of the spine requires immediate spine and cardiopulmonary stabilization and neurosurgical consultation. High-dose (30 mg/kg bolus, then 5.4 mg/kg/hr for 23 hr) intravenous methylprednisolone is indicated in cases of spinal cord trauma, and improves the ultimate degree of recovery of function.

### Subdural Fluid

The presence of subdural fluid can be caused either by active accumulation of fluid or by atrophy of adjacent brain tissue. The former process usually begins with a subdural hemorrhage. Vascular membranes arising from dura surround the hemorrhage, and leakage of proteinaceous exudate or small hemorrhages from these membranes may enlarge the subdural collection. Symptoms consist of slowly evolving focal neurologic deficits, focal seizures, or evidence of raised ICP. Treatment may require repeated subdural taps or a subdural-peritoneal shunt.

### Post–Head Trauma Syndrome

Some children complain of headache, dizziness, forgetfulness, inability to concentrate, slowing of response time, mood swings, irritability, and other subtle aberrations of cerebral function for days or weeks following an uncomplicated concussion. These deficits almost always resolve spontaneously. Children may require brief periods of special schooling, home tutoring, and reassurance. Persis-

tent severe headaches often respond to prophylactic therapy with propranolol, 1 mg/kg/24 hr.

### MANAGEMENT

Children who have been unconscious from a head injury or who have amnesia after the event, even if loss of consciousness is not documented, should be observed in an emergency room for several hours following the injury, even if they initially appear to be entirely well. High-risk patients include those with persistent depressed level of consciousness, focal neurologic signs, decreasing level of consciousness, and penetrating skull injury or depressed skull fractures. These patients warrant CT or MRI examination.

The period of observation should increase with the severity of the injury, and there should be no hesitation to admit children without neurologic deficits to the hospital for observation. If the child appears well after several hours and is discharged home, parents should be instructed to call their physician for any change in alertness, orientation, or neurologic functioning or increase in headache or vomiting. The parents should be taught how to test consciousness, orientation, extraocular motions, pupillary reactions, and gait and told to check these functions every 2–4 hr for 1 day following the injury. If conditions at home preclude this type of detailed observation, the child should be admitted to the hospital.

Damage to the brain from trauma occurs immediately and is not treatable. The goal is to prevent secondary brain injury from hemorrhage, cerebral edema, and hypoxia–ischemia.

### PROGNOSIS

Children suffering from concussion without subsequent neurologic deficits do well; late sequelae are rare. Children with contusions are likely to make surprisingly good recoveries, even in the face of relatively persistent neurologic signs that continue for weeks; subtle deficits may persist. Poor memory and slowing of motor skills are most common, but a generalized decrease in cognitive skills, behavioral alterations, and attention deficits also occurs. Language function, especially in the young child, frequently makes a good recovery. Rehabilitation consists of physical therapy, behavior management, and appropriate education. *Poor prognostic features* include a Glasgow Coma Scale score of 3–4 on admission without improvement in 24 hr, absent pupillary light reflexes, and persistent extensor plantar reflexes. Extracranial trauma also contributes to the morbidity of these patients (e.g., adult respiratory distress syndrome, sepsis, emboli).

## References

Behrman RE, Kliegman RM, Arvin AM (eds): Nelson Textbook of Pediatrics, 15th ed. Philadelphia, WB Saunders, 1996, Chapter 551.

Chiles B, Cooper P: Acute spinal injury. N Engl J Med 334:514, 1996.

Duhaime AC, Alario AJ, Lewander WJ, et al: Head injury in very young children: Mechanisms, injury types, and ophthalmologic findings in 100 hospitalized patients younger than 2 years of age. Pediatrics 90:179, 1992.

Lieh-Lai MW, Theodorou AA, Sarnaik AP, et al: Limitations of the Glasgow Coma Scale in predicting outcome in children with traumatic brain injury. J Pediatr 120:195, 1992.

White RJ, Likavec MJ: The diagnosis and initial management of head injury. N Engl J Med 327:1507, 1992.

## INCREASED INTRACRANIAL PRESSURE

Normal ICP measurements vary, depending on the site of determination and the position of the child. In the lateral recumbent position, ICP should be below 170 mm of CSF and is equal in the ventricle, cisterna magna, and lumbar subarachnoid space. Lumbar subarachnoid pressure rises and ventricle pressure falls in the sitting position, and the opposite occurs in the head-down position.

The *diagnosis* and *treatment* of the child with increased ICP constitute a medical emergency. Treatment should be initiated before ICP rises to a level that significantly compromises *cerebral perfusion pressure* (CPP). CPP equals the mean arterial blood pressure minus the ICP. Increased ICP also may result in movement of the brain from normal compartments of the skull across dural structures that divide these compartments (*herniation*). The direction of herniation is dictated by movements from regions of high pressure to regions of lower pressure. Herniation distorts the cortex and brain stem and their vascular supply, resulting in injury and, if not reversed, death.

In infancy, partial compensation for raised ICP is accomplished by spreading the cranial sutures and distending the anterior fontanel. Suture diastasis also may occur in chronically increased ICP and may be detected as late as 10 yr of age. After the sutures close, the intracranial volume is constant, consisting of the volume of the brain tissue, CSF, and blood. Any normal or abnormal (e.g., brain tumor, extravascular blood, inflammation) increase in one component is accompanied by a simultaneous decrease in one or more of the other components. Normally, the brain accounts for 80–85% of the volume, CSF 10–15%, and blood 5–10%. CSF is

displaced readily from the intracranial compartment to the lumbar subarachnoid space and is the first mechanism of normalizing ICP when acute increases occur. Pathologic processes that block the flow of CSF deprive the patient of this compensatory maneuver.

*Clinical Manifestations.* The clinical presentation of increased ICP varies with age (Table 18–12). Hypertension, bradycardia, and irregular respirations (*Cushing triad*) also signify increased ICP. The abducens nerve (cranial nerve VI) has the longest intracranial course and is most susceptible to increased ICP. Therefore, paresis of cranial nerve VI is a false localizing sign when ICP is elevated. Swelling of the optic nerve head **(papilledema)** is one of the most reliable signs of increased ICP. It frequently is absent acutely and in infants, but its absence at any age does not exclude the diagnosis of ICP. Acute papilledema does not affect visual acuity. Swelling of the optic nerve head also may be due to processes other than elevated ICP (e.g., papillitis, optic neuropathy).

*Herniation* of brain tissue from one compartment of the skull to another is a common cause of death in elevated ICP. Herniation of cerebral or cerebellar tissue results in necrosis of the herniated tissue and compression of vital CNS structures. The common herniation syndromes and their clinical characteristics are noted in Table 18–13 (see Table 18–7).

*Etiology.* The most common causes of raised ICP in childhood are cerebral edema, hydrocephalus, pseudotumor cerebri, trauma, infection, and tumors.

CEREBRAL EDEMA. This is the abnormal accumulation of fluid within brain tissue, resulting in volu-

TABLE 18–12.   Frequent Signs and Symptoms of Increased Intracranial Pressure

| Infants | Older Children |
|---|---|
| *Symptoms* | |
| Irritability | Irritability |
| Lethargy | Lethargy |
| Vomiting (initially in morning) | Vomiting (initially in morning) |
| | Headache |
| | Visual obscurations |
| | Diplopia |
| *Signs* | |
| Tense or bulging fontanel | Papilledema |
| Distended scalp veins | Sixth nerve paralysis |
| Head enlargement | Altered mental status |
| Sixth nerve paralysis | Signs of herniation |
| Altered mental status | |
| Signs of herniation | |

TABLE 18–13.  Herniation Syndromes

| Location | Description | Clinical Findings |
|---|---|---|
| *Transtentorial* | | |
| Central | Caudal displacement of cerebral hemispheres, resulting in downward displacement of diencephalon and midbrain | Altered mental status<br>Cheyne-Stokes to central neurogenic hyperventilation<br>Decorticate to decerebrate posturing<br>Loss of oculovestibular reflexes<br>Death |
| Uncal | Temporal lobe displacement into the tentorial opening<br>Third nerve, posterior cerebral artery, and midbrain compression | Unilateral pupillary dilation followed by oculomotor paralysis with or without ptosis<br>Hemiplegia<br>Death |
| *Cerebellar* | | |
| Downward | Cerebellar tonsils displaced through the foramen magnum<br>Compression of medulla, posterior inferior cerebellar artery | Neck stiffness<br>Respiratory, cardiac arrest<br>Lower cranial nerve dysfunction<br>Death |
| Upward | Cerebellar tissue displaced through tentorial opening<br>Compression of midbrain and superior cerebellar arteries | Paralysis of upgaze<br>Pupillary dilation<br>Central hyperventilation<br>Death |
| *Transfalcial* | | |
| (cingulate) | Unilateral cerebral lesions result in displacement of the cingulate gyrus beneath the falx cerebri, compromising the gyrus and the callosal pericallosal arteries | Cingulate gyrus necrosis and ischemia lead to edema and central transtentorial herniation |

metric expansion. Edema is of two varieties. *Vasogenic edema* is due to alterations in the vasculature resulting in increased vessel permeability and fluid escape (e.g., edema surrounding tumors, abscesses, hematomas, or infarcts). *Cytotoxic edema* is due to abnormal cellular function resulting in fluid accumulation, which is primarily intracellular (e.g., edema seen in anoxia, water intoxication, encephalitis, and Reye syndrome). Cytotoxic edema does not respond to steroids but does respond to osmotic agents, whereas vasogenic edema responds to both.

The common causes of cerebral edema in childhood are listed in Table 18–14. Anoxic cerebral edema is seen following neonatal asphyxia and asphyxia with smoke inhalation, near-drowning, and cardiac arrest. Infectious processes can produce a combination of vasogenic and cytotoxic cerebral edema. In brain abscess, the degree of surrounding edema usually is severe. The degree of edema in viral meningoencephalitis is variable. In enteroviral infection and mumps, it usually is mild, but with herpes simplex meningoencephalitis, edema frequently is severe and may lead to herniation.

*PSEUDOTUMOR CEREBRI.* Also known as benign intracranial hypertension, this is a disorder character-ized by markedly elevated ICP without focal neurologic signs or altered mental status. The underlying pathogenesis and the degree to which cerebral edema or subarachnoid fluid accumulation is responsible for the process are unknown. Benign intracranial hypertension is associated with a variety of conditions, among which endocrine

TABLE 18–14.  Common Causes of Cerebral Edema in Childhood

| Vasogenic Edema | Cytotoxic Edema |
|---|---|
| Tumor | Anoxia |
| Abscess | Heavy metal poisoning (lead, mercury, arsenic) |
| Hemorrhage | Infection: bacterial and viral meningoencephalitis |
| Infarct | Pseudotumor cerebri |
| Infection: bacterial and viral meningoencephalitis | Metabolic disorders |
| Trauma |   Methylmalonicacidemia |
| |   Propionicacidemia |
| |   Acyl-coenzyme A dehydrogenase deficiency |
| |   Urea cycle deficiency |
| |   Reye syndrome |
| |   Hepatic coma |
| |   Hypertensive encephalopathy |

**TABLE 18–15.** Abnormalities Associated with Pseudotumor Cerebri

| Endocrine Considerations | Medication Related |
|---|---|
| Obesity | Vitamin A excess |
| Menarche | Vitamin A deficiency |
| Addison disease | Tetracycline (infancy) |
| Adrenal hyperplasia | Steroid therapy (usually |
| Pregnancy | during tapering of |
| Hypoparathyroidism | therapy) |
| Catch-up growth following | Nalidixic acid |
| malnutrition | Oral contraceptives |

**Other Disorders**

Iron-deficiency anemia
Galactosemia
Polycythemia
Middle ear disease
Idiopathic

abnormalities are prominent (Table 18–15). Loss of vision as a result of chronic papilledema may develop.

*TUMORS OF THE BRAIN.* Brain tumors are a common cause of raised ICP (see Chapter 15).

*Diagnosis.* Symptoms of brief duration associated with an altered state of consciousness are ominous. Fever suggests an infectious process. The risk associated with *lumbar puncture* must be weighed against the benefits of obtaining CSF from the lumbar region. Herniation of tissue will occur during lumbar puncture if obstruction of flow within the CSF pathways exists and if the flow of CSF through the lumbar puncture needle or subarachnoid space is faster than at any level in the subarachnoid pathways. If meningitis is suspected but signs of increased ICP are present (other than a bulging fontanel), alternative sources of isolating organisms should be sought (blood culture). Institution of broad-spectrum antibiotics and therapy for elevated ICP before lumbar puncture should be considered, as should the safety and feasibility of obtaining ventricular fluid. Lumbar puncture is contraindicated in patients with brain abscess. *CT* and *MRI* are indicated to assess the degree of cerebral edema or shifting of tissue from the midline (mass effect).

*Laboratory studies* of blood and urine are essential in establishing toxic causes of cerebral edema. Blood ammonia is elevated and partial thromboplastin and prothrombin times are prolonged in Reye syndrome or hepatic failure. Urine samples for amino and organic acids establish the diagnosis of brain edema secondary to propionicaciduria and methylmalonicaciduria as well as to acyl-coenzyme A dehydrogenase deficiency and to certain amino acidopathies. A measurement of blood ammonia and plasma amino acids elucidates disorders of the urea cycle. The EEG usually is diffusely slow in toxic and metabolic cerebral edema irrespective of cause.

*Treatment.* The management of any child with increased ICP should encompass basic mechanisms by which ICP is increased. Hypoxia and hypercapnia increase brain blood flow, brain blood volume, and, thus, ICP. Protection of the airway and proper ventilation are therefore essential. *Hyperventilation* is an effective measure to reduce ICP acutely. The patient should be placed in the head-up position flexed approximately 45 degrees at the waist; constriction of the neck should be avoided to facilitate venous return from the brain. Screaming, thrashing, and seizure activity aggravate increased ICP.

The advantage of *ICP monitoring* is that it provides continuous objective information as a basis for adjusting therapy. The disadvantage is that in the encephalopathic patient, neuromuscular paralysis must be used to obtain satisfactory ICP monitoring and most of the signs and symptoms that must be observed in the neurologic examination are therefore lost. ICP monitoring can be performed by the intraventricular, subarachnoid, epidural, or intraparenchymal route, and in neonates measurements can be obtained from the anterior fontanel (see Chapters 3 and 6).

Systemic hypotension resulting from *intravascular volume depletion*, phenobarbital-induced myocardial depression, or low peripheral vasomotor tone should be corrected with either isotonic crystalloid volume expansion or dopamine to improve CPP. Fluid overload contributes to cerebral edema and should be avoided. Vasodilator therapy should be avoided or used very cautiously in the treatment of systemic hypertension because decreases in mean arterial pressure without concomitant decreases in ICP jeopardize cerebral perfusion. Fluid and electrolyte management should limit the availability of free water, which diffuses rapidly to the brain, adding to cerebral edema. Deficient antidiuretic hormone (ADH) may follow injuries to the hypothalamus or the pituitary tract. Inappropriate ADH secretion may occur in tumor, infection, or trauma or, initially, following neurosurgical procedures. Fluid restriction for inappropriate ADH secretion, and vasopressin therapy in diabetes insipidus, may be indicated.

*CONTROL OF INTRACRANIAL VOLUME.* Normalization of ICP is attempted by correcting the volume-pressure relationships within the cranial cavity. This may be accomplished by hyperventilation; the administration of steroids, osmotic agents, and loop diuretics; removal of CSF; and giving agents to decrease CSF production.

CSF production may be transiently decreased by administration of dexamethasone or acetazolamide. Steroids decrease CSF production by inhibiting the sodium-potassium pump–activated ATP pathways in the choroid plexus, whereas acetazolamide decreases production by inhibiting carbonic anhydrase. In the presence of hydrocephalus or a tumor, a direct surgical approach is appropriate. Steroid therapy is appropriate as an initial measure to reduce peritumor edema.

*Osmotic therapy* requires an intact blood-brain barrier. The administration of an osmotic agent results in free water shifts from brain to the intravascular space. Subsequent renal clearance of free water from the general circulation results in clinically significant reduction of brain edema. Clearance of the osmotic agent from the circulation may result in reversal of the osmotic gradient and rebound intracranial hypertension, especially if a significant leak of the osmotic agent into the extracellular space of the brain has occurred. Mannitol (0.25–1.0 g/kg infused over 10–30 min) is the most commonly employed osmotic agent. Glycerol has the advantages of being effective by the oral route, being metabolized by the liver, and not requiring renal function for elimination. However, it may produce intravascular hemolysis and is used infrequently.

Serum osmolality should be kept below 320 mOsm/L. Levels of 350 mOsm/L may result in progressive renal failure, and osmolality over 375 mOsm/L may result in intracellular dehydration severe enough to produce systemic acidosis. Chronic serum hyperosmolality also may result in neuronal production of intracellular fixed osmoles, which lead to the development of neuronal swelling and damage.

The *treatment of pseudotumor cerebri* includes steroids, repeated lumbar punctures, or, if severe, shunting of CSF.

### References

Behrman RE, Kliegman RM, Arvin AM (eds): Nelson Textbook of Pediatrics, 15th ed. Philadelphia, WB Saunders, 1996, Chapters 548–551, 556.

Miller D: Intracranial pressure monitoring. Arch Neurol 42:1191, 1986.

Schulte FJ: Intracranial tumors in childhood: Concepts of treatment and prognosis. Neuropediatrics 15:3, 1984.

## HEADACHE AND MIGRAINE

The evaluation of children with *headache* is straightforward. If the neurologic examination reveals any abnormalities, cranial CT or MRI is obtained. If neurologic and general physical examinations are negative, the likely diagnoses are either migraine or tension headaches.

Any **space-occupying lesion** within the cranium can cause headache, either by pressure (inflammation, stretching, distortion) on adjacent pain-sensitive structures or by obstruction of CSF circulation and the production of hydrocephalus. Lesions within the posterior fossa usually produce occipital pain, whereas supratentorial lesions produce frontal, temporal, or vertex pain. **Hydrocephalus** usually causes early morning frontal headache that may awaken the child and often is associated with vomiting with or without nausea. **Aneurysms** almost always appear as an acute subarachnoid hemorrhage and are characterized by severe headache, change in consciousness, and stiff neck. **Pseudotumor cerebri** presents with severe daily headaches as well as with signs of raised ICP.

Acute headache also may be caused by hypertension, trauma, lumbar puncture, fever, various drugs, and infection. It is a common symptom in meningitis, encephalitis, sinusitis, pharyngitis, and systemic viral illness. Headache also is associated with a variety of disorders involving the eyes, ears, nose, teeth, and neck.

Many patients with headache visit a doctor only for reassurance that there is no serious underlying disease and thereafter are content to treat the headache symptomatically. An unremarkable history and physical examination are sufficient to provide this reassurance. Sometimes the neurologic examination yields equivocal findings or the history is so compelling for serious intracranial pathology that CT or MRI is required despite a normal examination. Worrisome headaches are those that are most severe on awakening, awaken the patient in the middle of the night, are severely exacerbated by coughing or bending, are acute without a previous history of headache, are present daily and getting progressively more severe in a crescendo pattern, and are accompanied by vomiting with or without nausea.

*Migraine* and *tension headache* are the most common chronic recurrent headaches in both children and adults (Table 18–16). The pathogenesis of migraine is unknown but may involve paroxysmal instability of cell membranes or vasoregulatory elements. There may be release of inflammatory mediators and a phase of intracerebral arterial constriction followed by a phase of extracranial, and sometimes intracranial, arterial dilation. Migraine frequently begins in childhood; infants and toddlers who are unable to verbalize the source of their discomfort may present with spells of irritability, sleepiness, pallor, and vomiting. Young children with migraine frequently lack many of the

TABLE 18–16. Features of Classic Migraine and Tension Headache

| Migraine | Tension |
|---|---|
| Aura | |
|   Flashes of light | |
|   Wavy or zigzag lines | |
|   Enlarging scotoma | |
|     surrounded by luminous | |
|     changes | |
|   Unilateral numbness | |
|   Duration of 10–30 min | |
| Unilateral (hemicrania) | Daily with work or school |
| Throbbing | Present all day with |
| Nausea/vomiting |   worsening in afternoon |
| Photophobia, audiophobia | Moderate band-like or |
| Relief by rest |   boring pain |
| Periodic attacks (lasting hours)* | Multiple somatic |
| Precipitating factors |   complaints (e.g., |
|   Psychologic stresses |   shortness of breath, |
|   Lack of food or sleep |   abdominal pain, |
|   Menses |   dizziness) |
|   Exertion | |
|   Foods or drugs | |
|     Monosodium glutamate | |
|     Cheeses | |
|     Chocolate | |
|     Oral contraceptive pills | |
| Exacerbated by head movement | |
| Family history | |

*Migraines may last as long as 72 hr but usually are less than 24 hr.

typical features. Periodic headaches in children accompanied by nausea or vomiting and relieved by rest are likely to be migraine. Sometimes even the periodic nature of the headache is not appreciated because the children will have frequent mild to moderate headaches between major attacks of severe headaches. The name "common migraine" sometimes is attached to these moderate atypical headaches without other neurologic manifestations or an aura.

The most characteristic symptom of migraine is a visual aura that immediately precedes the headache and persists for 15–20 min. The visual aura consists of spots, flashes, or lines of light that flicker in one visual field. Migraine auras may also consist of brief episodes of unilateral or perioral numbness, unilateral weakness, or vertigo. "Complicated migraine" is a series of transient attacks of neurologic dysfunction that persist for hours but resolve completely. Typically, patients have recurrent episodes of either hemiparesis, amaurosis fugax (monocular blindness), ophthalmoplegia, or confusion. The *diagnosis* is always uncertain during the first attack; therefore, structural lesions of the CNS must be considered.

*Treatment* of migraine includes prophylactic

medications taken daily to reduce the frequency and severity of attacks and symptomatic medications taken during attacks to reduce their intensity and duration (Table 18–17). The first step in migraine prophylaxis is to identify precipitating agents and eliminate as many as possible. Prophylactic medications are utilized when headaches are occurring frequently (more than one per month) and interfering with activities of daily life. Symptomatic therapy requires early administration of analgesic and sedative medication, immediate rest, and sleep in a quiet, dark room. Unfortunately, administration of oral medication often is impossible because of severe nausea and vomiting. Sumatriptan, a serotonin receptor agonist, may abort a migraine following oral or subcutaneous administration. It may produce serious cardiovascular side effects.

Headache frequently is caused by psychologic stresses and diseases. These *tension headaches* have a different clinical profile than that of migraine (see Table 18–16). Tension headaches can be acute and related to environmental stresses or can be chronic and a symptom of underlying psychiatric illness, such as anxiety neurosis, hysterical neurosis, or

TABLE 18–17. Treatment for Migraine

| Nonmedical Treatment | Serotonin Agonists |
|---|---|
| Eliminate precipitating factors | Sumatriptan |
| Reassurance | |
| Biofeedback | |
| Psychotherapy | |
| **Analgesics** | **Prophylactic Agents** |
| Aspirin | Propranolol |
| Acetaminophen | Phenytoin |
| Propoxyphene | Cyproheptadine |
| Codeine | Methysergide |
| Oxycodone | Valproate |
| Meperidine | |
| *Ergotamine (PO, PR, Sublingual, Inhaler, Subcutaneous)* | 1. *NSAID* |
| |   Naproxen |
| *Minor Tranquilizers* | 2. *Calcium Channel Blockers* |
|   Barbiturates |   Nimodipine |
|   Benzodiazepines |   Verapamil |
|   Chloral hydrate | 3. *Tricyclic Antidepressants* |
|   Hydroxyzine |   Amitriptyline |
| *Major Tranquilizers* |   Imipramine |
| **Nonsteroidal Anti-inflammatory Drugs (NSAIDs)** | **Combinations of Medications** |
| | Aspirin, caffeine, barbiturate |
| Ibuprofen | Ergotamine, belladonna, barbiturate |
| Fenoprofen | |
| Sulindac | |

in combination with each other and with generalized tonic-clonic seizures.

*Atypical Absence Seizures.* These seizures appear as episodes of impaired consciousness with automatisms, autonomic phenomena, and/or motor manifestations, such as eye opening, eye deviation, and body stiffening. The EEG does not show the typical absence pattern but is composed instead of several frequencies of epileptiform discharges superimposed on an abnormal background. In children with chronic brain syndromes, the interictal record is abnormal, and during seizure activity, the spike wave discharge is usually slower than 3 Hz frequency, not necessarily symmetric, and often associated with other varieties of epileptiform activity.

**Myoclonus.** Myoclonus is a brief flexion contraction that may be epileptic or nonepileptic. The nonepileptic myoclonus occurs as a normal phenomenon in physiologic sleep jerks as well as in numerous disease states (e.g., spinal cord lesions and disorders of the basal ganglia). Myoclonic seizures almost always are associated with other seizure forms, and the EEG reveals seizure discharges. Progressive myoclonic epilepsy syndromes should be distinguished from more benign forms of myoclonic epilepsy.

*Myoclonic absence* refers to the body jerks that commonly accompany absence seizures and atypical absence seizures. Bilateral massive epileptic myoclonus is symmetric and varies in intensity. It may involve only facial muscles or also limbs in single or repetitive muscle contractions; both types are serious. The peak age of occurrence is within the 1st yr (37%), and status epilepticus is the first ictal manifestation in 77% of patients.

*Astatic-akinetic* or *atonic seizures* have their onset between 1 and 3 yr of age, although they may occur later. The seizures last 1–4 sec and are characterized by a loss of body tone, with falling to the ground, dropping of the head, or pitching forward or backward. A tonic component usually is associated. These seizures frequently result in repetitive head injury if the child is not protected (e.g., with a hockey or football helmet). They are most frequent on awakening and on falling to sleep; 50 or more daily seizures are usual. Children with astatic-akinetic seizures usually have mental retardation and have underlying brain abnormalities. Children without underlying brain damage tend to have later onset of seizures, normal intelligence, and better response to therapy.

*Infantile spasms* **(West syndrome)** are characterized by a brief contraction of the neck, trunk, and arm muscles, followed by a phase of sustained muscle contraction lasting from 2 to 10 sec. The initial phase consists of flexion and extension in various combinations such that the head may be thrown either backward or forward. The arms and legs may be either flexed or extended. As with most seizures, spasms occur most frequently when the child is awakening or falling asleep. Smiling or crying commonly is associated with an attack. The episodes of flexion or extension are followed by relaxation and repetition of the seizure such that these seizures occur in clusters of unpredictable and variable duration. Hundreds of these seizures occur daily. The peak age of onset is 3–8 mo, and 86% of infants experience the onset of seizures before age 1 yr. In circumstances in which flexion of the thighs and crying are prominent, this syndrome often is mistaken for colic.

Mental retardation may accompany or follow the onset of infantile spasms. Approximately 41% of children have no apparent etiology to their seizures (cryptogenic) and respond promptly to treatment; some in this group have a normal outcome. The other 59% have a known etiology (symptomatic) and poor response to therapy, and more than 90% of this group will be developmentally impaired. The *etiology* of infantile spasms is outlined in Table 18–22.

The EEG during the waking state, **hypsarrhythmia**, is dramatically abnormal, consisting of high-voltage slow waves, spikes, and polyspikes accompanied by background disorganization. Commonly, burst suppression patterns are seen during sleep. Hypsarrhythmia is seen in half of the infants with infantile spasms and sometimes is present in infants who do not have spasms. CT scanning is abnormal in 58–75% of infants, most frequently demonstrating intracranial calcifications, congenital anomalies, and atrophy. The most common anomaly is agenesis of the corpus callosum. Regardless of the seizure response to therapy, infants with abnormal CT scans have a poor prognosis, whereas those with normal CT scans, prompt response to therapy, and normal development prior to the onset of their spasms have a good chance for normal outcome.

*Treatment* of infantile spasms includes adrenocorticotropic hormone (ACTH), oral steroids, benzodiazepines, and valproic acid. Vigabatrin, a promising drug available in Europe and Canada, is not yet approved by the Food and Drug Administration (FDA). Hypertension, glycosuria, and severe infections are complications to be anticipated with steroid therapy. Valproic acid and clonazepam may be of value in the treatment of infantile spasms refractory to ACTH.

**Partial Seizures.** Partial seizures constitute 40–60% of the classifiable epilepsies of childhood.

TABLE 18–22. Etiologies of Infantile Spasms

**Metabolic**

Phenylketonuria
Biotinidase deficiency
Maple syrup urine disease
Isovalericacidemia
Ornithine accumulation
Nonketotic hyperglycinemia
Pyridoxine dependency
Hypoglycemia
Lipidosis

**Developmental Malformations**

Polymicrogyria
Lissencephaly
Schizencephaly
Down syndrome and other chromosomal disorders
Aicardi syndrome
Organoid nevus syndrome

**Neurocutaneous Syndrome**

Tuberous sclerosis
Sturge-Weber syndrome

**Congenital Infections**

Toxoplasmosis
Cytomegalovirus
Syphilis

**Encephalopathies**

Postasphyxia
Posthemorrhagic
Trauma
Postimmunization (pertussis)

**Simple partial seizures** arise from a specific anatomic focus, and clinical symptomatology may include motor, sensory, psychic, and/or autonomic abnormalities. Location and direction of spread of the seizure focus determine clinical symptomatology. **Complex partial seizures** have the same array of clinical abnormalities but differ from simple partial seizures in that consciousness is impaired.

The *clinical manifestations* in partial seizures may involve disturbances of olfaction (uncinate seizures), usually characterized by the perception of an unpleasant odor; emotional abnormalities, such as uncontrolled laughing (gelastic epilepsy); the appearance of shivering (pilomotor epilepsy); autonomic phenomena, such as tachycardia, increased gastrointestinal motility, or fever; anterior temporal lobe discharges, resulting in lip smacking; posterior temporal foci, causing episodes of vertigo, macropsia, micropsia, and/or altered depth perception; limbic discharges, resulting in dream-like states (*déjà vu*); simple visual phenomena, like flashing lights and spots; and bizarre combinations of sensory, motor, and psychic abnormalities. Partial seizures may secondarily generalize, and young children may not report sensory experiences.

Fifty to 80% of children with partial seizures have abnormalities on CT scan, and approximately 80% of the abnormalities are focal. The lesions of greatest concern are cerebral hemisphere tumors and arteriovenous malformations (AVMs). Agenesis of the corpus callosum, focal atrophy, medial temporal sclerosis, cortical dysplasia, and hamartomas are additional prominent lesions associated with partial seizures. Children with refractory partial seizures who have normal intelligence, normal neurologic examinations, and a persistence of focally slow EEGs are more likely to harbor a tumor than children with partial seizures who are intellectually impaired and have focal abnormalities on examination, diffusely abnormal EEGs, and known risk factors for seizures. MRI is superior to CT scanning in detecting gliomas in children with partial complex seizures. Although a high incidence of underlying structural brain disease as the cause of partial seizures has been noted, genetic factors also play a role.

*Treatment* is outlined in Table 18–21.

**Benign Focal Epilepsy.** Also known as **rolandic epilepsy**, benign focal epilepsy usually begins between the ages of 5 and 10 (rarely before 2 yr). The incidence may be as high as 21:100,000, comprising 16% of all afebrile seizures in children below the age of 15 yr. The seizures usually are focal motor with generalized spread. In approximately half of the children affected, seizures occur only during sleep or on awakening. When the seizure occurs in the awake state, symptomatology is motor or sensory, involving the tongue, mouth, and face. Speech and swallowing commonly are impaired. A family history is found in 13% of patients. This disorder disappears in adolescence to early adulthood, intelligence is normal, and no associated neurologic or CT scan abnormalities are present.

**Juvenile Myoclonic Epilepsy.** Juvenile myoclonic epilepsy (Janz) occurs in adolescence and is an autosomal dominant disorder with variable penetrance. Myoclonus, predominantly in the morning, with or without generalized seizures characterizes the disorder. Seizures respond only to valproic acid, and *treatment* is lifelong.

**Lennox-Gastaut Syndrome.** This is an epileptic syndrome with variable age of onset, but most children present before age 5 yr. The disorder is characterized by multiple seizure types, including atonic-astatic, partial, atypical absence, and generalized tonic, clonic, or tonic-clonic varieties. Many children have underlying brain injury or malformations (etiology similar to infantile spasms), but a minority have no demonstrable etiology. These seizures as a rule respond poorly to *treatment*, although a significant minority respond well to valproic acid.

**Acquired Epileptic Aphasia.** Acquired epileptic aphasia **(Landau-Kleffner syndrome)** is characterized by language disability related to partial seizures. It appears that the seizures are an epiphenomenon related to underlying acquired brain injury.

**Benign Neonatal Convulsions.** Benign neonatal convulsions are an autosomal dominant syndrome located on chromosome 20, and they are characterized by generalized clonic seizures occurring toward the end of the 1st wk of life. Response to *treatment* is variable, but the outlook generally is favorable.

### Principles of Seizure Therapy

*Treatment* is not considered for benign febrile seizures unless more than three recurrences have occurred. Absence seizures, infantile spasms, atypical absence seizures, and astatic-akinetic seizures are universally recurrent at the time of diagnosis, and therapy is indicated. If the seizure is symptomatic of acute neurologic illness, 23% of patients can be expected to have a recurrence during the illness, and treatment is limited to the acute illness. The overall risk of recurrence for children whose first seizure is generalized tonic-clonic is approximately 50%, and it seems reasonable to wait for recurrence before therapy is instituted.

When treatment is initiated, the goal is to achieve optimal function. Medication risks should be weighed against the risk of seizure type. Initially, a single agent should be chosen, because this reduces cost, improves compliance, and avoids toxicity. Approximately 50% of children obtain satisfactory seizure control with one drug. A second agent is considered only when therapeutic anticonvulsant levels are obtained with the first drug. Anticonvulsant levels are helpful in adjusting medication but should be interpreted in light of the patient's clinical state. Because of phenobarbital's very long half-life, phenobarbital plasma levels can be determined anytime throughout the day; levels of carbamazepine and phenytoin may vary significantly between peak and trough as a result of their shorter half-lives. In disease states in which drug binding is likely to be altered (i.e., hepatic or renal disease), free and bound anticonvulsant determinations can be helpful. Hazardous physical activities are best avoided, and many advise against direct contact sports such as football. Although children with epilepsy have a greater risk of submersion accidents, if anticonvulsant drug levels are maintained in the therapeutic range and the child is afforded appropriate supervision, accidents should be avoidable.

Children with generalized tonic, clonic, and tonic-clonic seizures, absence seizures, and certain partial seizures may not require therapy beyond 4 yr. The risk of recurrence is higher when partial seizures occur. When prophylaxis is used for febrile seizures, the duration need not be longer than 2 yr. Children with myoclonic seizures, progressive myoclonic epilepsy, atypical absence seizures, and the Lennox-Gastaut syndrome require treatment for life. As a rule, children who are neurologically abnormal, have seizures that were initially difficult to control, and have persistently paroxysmal EEGs are at highest risk for recurrence when therapy is discontinued.

### References

Behrman RE, Kliegman RM, Arvin AM (eds): Nelson Textbook of Pediatrics, 15th ed. Philadelphia, WB Saunders, 1996, Chapter 543.

Camfield C, Camfield P, Gordon K, et al: Outcome of childhood epilepsy: A population-based study with a simple predictive scoring system for those treated with medication. J Pediatr 122:861, 1993.

Engel J: Surgery for seizures. N Engl J Med 334:647, 1996.

Holmes GL: Use of EEG in childhood epilepsy. Int Pediatr 7:223, 1992.

Holmes GL: Severe seizures in infancy and early childhood. Int Pediatr 7:237, 1992.

Marson A, Kadir Z, Chadwick D: New antiepileptic drugs: A systematic review of their efficacy and tolerability. BMJ 313:1169, 1996.

Provisional Committee on Quality Improvement, Subcommittee on Febrile Seizures: Practice Parameter: The neurodiagnostic evaluation of the child with a first simple febrile seizure. Pediatrics 97:769, 1996.

Shinnar S, Berg A, Moshe S, et al: The risk of seizure recurrence after a first unprovoked afebrile seizure in childhood: An extended follow-up. Pediatrics 98:216, 1996.

Zupanc M: Update on epilepsy in pediatric patients. Mayo Clin Proc 71:899, 1996.

## ATAXIA

Ataxia is an abnormality of coordination resulting in an impairment of direction, rate, and strength of voluntary movement. A broad-based unsteady gait is termed ataxic, whereas *dysmetria* and *dysdiadochokinesis* refer to ataxic abnormalities of coordination in the extremities. Ataxia may have its origin in lesions of the peripheral nerves, spinal cord, brain stem, cerebellum, thalamus, or cerebral hemispheres. Ataxia may appear suddenly (acute ataxia) or manifest gradually (chronic ataxia). In either circumstance, the condition may be static or progressive.

### ACUTE ATAXIA

Infectious, postinfectious, and toxic etiologic factors are encountered most commonly when ataxia begins abruptly. The former include varicella, Epstein-Barr virus, and encephalitis viruses. Accidental ingestion is most common between the ages of 1 and 4 yr, and the causative agents include barbiturates, other soporifics, alcohol, and antihistamines. Later in childhood, drug ingestion of the same agents as a suicide gesture is encountered. Overdose of phenytoin should be considered in children with epilepsy. Children with ataxia secondary to drug ingestion usually have an altered sensorium. *Treatment* is based on the specific offending agent.

As a group, the metabolic causes of ataxia tend to be episodic; aggravated by intercurrent infections or other stresses, resulting in a catabolic state; and slowly progressive (saltatory progression).

The vascular disorders include migraine, vasculitis (systemic lupus erythematosus), or vasculopathy involving the cerebellum or its pathways. Spontaneous cerebellar hemorrhage seen in coagulopathies and AVMs presents with acute ataxia, nystagmus, and gaze paresis and may be accompanied by an altered sensorium. The hemorrhage is detected readily on CT scan, and therapy consists of clot evacuation and correction of coagulopathy.

Posterior fossa tumors, primarily involving the cerebellum or the brain stem, produce ataxia that may be acute or gradual in onset; however, once present, it follows a progressive course. The ataxia, dysmetria, and titubation (inability to maintain a steady sitting posture) may result from the primary cerebellar lesion or from obstruction of the CSF pathways and resultant hydrocephalus. Hydrocephalus causes ataxia by exertion of pressure on the corticopontocerebellar pathways as they sweep over the lateral ventricles.

### CHRONIC ATAXIA

A number of congenital malformations of the brain result in chronic static or slowly progressive ataxia. Despite the embryologic origin of these conditions, the age of presentation is frequently in infancy or later in childhood (Table 18–23). The hereditary and familial metabolic causes are genetic in origin and have varying ages of presentation (Table 18–24). It is important to consider vitamin E deficiency, as this disorder is approachable therapeutically. Children with chronic ataxia may have episodes of worsening of their disease, resulting in a process exhibiting an apparently static baseline value but with superimposed periods of exacerbation. Some of the causes of acute ataxia also may cause chronic ataxia (brain tumors, toxins, migraine).

### References

Stumpf D: Acute ataxia. Pediatr Rev 8:303, 1987.
Subramony SH: Clinical aspects of hereditary ataxias. J Child Neurol 10:353, 1995.

## PSYCHOMOTOR RETARDATION
(see Chapter 1)

### NONPROGRESSIVE PSYCHOMOTOR RETARDATION

In many children with severe mental retardation, the history and general physical examination are unremarkable. No focal neurologic deficits are present, and laboratory evaluation is unrevealing. Most children with this idiopathic condition probably have microscopic aberrations of CNS development involving the structure of neurons or neuronal organelles, aggregation of neurons, myelinization of white matter, synapse formation, or interneuronal connections. Although *treatment* includes educational programs, such as infant stimulation, no treatment program can increase inherent learning capacity.

#### Congenital Malformations of the Brain

Most brain malformations can be produced by a variety of injuries occurring during a vulnerable period of gestation. These precipitating factors include chromosomal, genetic, and metabolic abnormalities (see Chapters 4 and 5); infections (cytomegalovirus, TORCH;* see Chapters 6 and 10); and exposure to irradiation, certain drugs, and maternal illness during pregnancy.

In all types of **congenital hydrocephalus**, the degree of ventricular enlargement correlates roughly with outcome, but examples of neonates with severe hydrocephalus who receive ventriculoperitoneal shunts and then have normal development are well known. There often are associated defects in the closure of the neural tube.

**Hydranencephaly** is a circumstance in which the brain presumably develops normally but then is destroyed by an intrauterine, probably vascular, insult. The result is a virtual absence of the cerebrum with an intact skull. The thalamus, brain stem, and some occipital cortex are present. The child may have a normal outward appearance but does not achieve developmental milestones.

**Holoprosencephaly** represents varying degrees of failure of the primary cerebral vesicle to divide

*TORCH = *t*oxoplasmosis, *o*ther (syphilis, hepatitis, zoster), *r*ubella, *c*ytomegalovirus, and *h*erpes simplex.

TABLE 18–23. Congenital Causes of Chronic Ataxia

| Disorder | Age of Presentation | Clinical Manifestations | Mechanism of Ataxia, Diagnoses, and Treatment |
|---|---|---|---|
| Cerebellar hypoplasia | Early infancy (occasionally delayed) | Developmental delay, hypotonia, athetosis, chorea, delayed walking, ataxic gait | Absent cerebellar granular cells; CT shows small cerebellum |
| Vermal aplasia Dandy-Walker malformation | Early infancy | Macrocephaly, enlarged occipital region; ataxia | Hydrocephalus and cystic dilation of the fourth ventricle; treatment is by shunting of hydrocephalus and/or the posterior fossa cyst |
| Joubert syndrome | Early infancy | Neonatal episodic hyperpnea and apnea; hypotonia, nystagmus | MRI and CT demonstrate agenesis of the superior cerebellar vermis |
| Arnold-Chiari malformation | Variable | Headache, neck pain, lower cranial nerve dysfunction, nystagmus, ataxia; this variety does not have associated myelomeningocele | MRI and CT demonstrate a caudal fourth ventricle; distortion of the brain stem; treatment is by posterior fossa decompression |
| Hydrocephalus | Variable | Macrocephaly, vomiting, ataxia | CT and MRI demonstrate enlarged lateral ventricles; in aqueductal stenosis, the third ventricle is particularly large, whereas the fourth ventricle is normal or small |

CT = computed tomography; MRI = magnetic resonance imaging.

TABLE 18-24. Hereditary Causes of Ataxia

| Disorder | Usual Age of Onset | Hereditary Pattern | Clinical Characteristics | Etiology and Treatment |
|---|---|---|---|---|
| Friedreich ataxia | 2–16 yr | Recessive | Ataxia, scoliosis, pes cavus, posterior column sensory loss, areflexia, cardiomyopathy | Chromosome 9 trinucleotide repeat expansion; supportive |
| Machado-Joseph disease | 12–15 yr | Dominant | Cerebellar, pyramidal, extrapyramidal degeneration; anterior horn cell disease; Portuguese ancestry | Chromosome 14 trinucleotide repeat expansion; supportive |
| Vitamin E deficiency | 2–16 yr | Recessive | Resembles Friedreich ataxia | Vitamin E |
| Spinocerebellar ataxia 1 | 6–60 yr | Dominant | Nystagmus, dysarthria hyperreflexia, ataxia | CAG-trinucleotide repeat expansion; supportive |
| Spinocerebellar ataxia 2 | 2–65 yr | Dominant | Resembles spinocerebellar ataxia 1 but also oculomotor paresis | Chromosome 12; CAG-trinucleotide repeat expansion |
| Ataxia-telangiectasia | Early infancy (1–2 yr) | Recessive | Ataxia, oculomotor apraxia, sinopulmonary infections, telangiectasia of conjunctiva and skin | B- and T-cell dysfunction; cellular immunity is impaired; supportive |
| Metachromatic leukodystrophy | | | See Psychomotor Retardation | |
| Refsum disease | 4–7 yr | Recessive | Ataxia, neuropathy, retinitis pigmentosa, ichthyosis | Phytanic acid hydroxylase deficiency; phytol-free diet |
| Leigh disease | Infancy to adolescence | Recessive | Ataxia, lactic acidosis, hypotonia, abnormalities of respiration | Some Leigh disorders of pyruvate metabolism; supportive |
| Wilson disease | Infancy to adulthood | Recessive | Hepatic disease, tremor, dystonic, athetosis, chorea | Ceruloplasmin deficiency; penicillamine |
| Abetalipoproteinemia | 5–15 yr | Recessive | Ataxia, dysmetria, fat malabsorption, acanthocytosis, retinitis pigmentosa, sensory loss | Low-fat diet, vitamin E and A supplementation |
| Juvenile gangliosidosis | 3–5 yr | Recessive $GM_1$ or $GM_2$ forms | Ataxia, spasticity, rigidity, dementia | None available |
| Ramsay Hunt syndrome | 7–10 yr | Sporadic | Ataxia, tremor, myoclonus, dementia | Supportive |
| Marinesco-Sjögren syndrome | Infancy to 5 yr | Recessive | Cataracts, ataxia, growth failure, mental retardation | Supportive |
| Juvenile sulfate lipidosis (juvenile MLD) | Infancy to 5 yr | Recessive | Dementia, ataxia, spasticity, aryl sulfidase A deficiency | Supportive |

MLD = metachromatic leukodystrophy.

and expand laterally and often is associated with midline facial defects (e.g., hypotelorism, cleft lip, and cleft palate). This anomaly may occur in an isolated fashion, can be associated with a chromosomal or genetic disorder, and may be mild or severe. The *prognosis* for infants with alobar holoprosencephaly is uniformly poor; for infants with the semilobar form, it is somewhat better.

A number of malformations result from the failure of the normal migration of neurons from the germinal matrix zone at 1–5 mo of gestation. Often, multiple malformations exist in the same patient.

**Schizencephaly** is characterized by symmetric clefts within the cerebral hemispheres that extend from the cortical surface to the ventricular cavity. *Clinical manifestations* include severe mental and motor retardation. Many children with unilateral schizencephaly have hemiparesis and mild motor impairment.

**Lissencephaly** indicates smooth brain with absence of sulcation. The normal six-layered cortex does not develop, and affected children present with seizures and severe developmental delay. This anomaly most commonly is part of a genetic or chromosomal disorder.

In **macrogyria**, the gyri are few in number and too broad, whereas in **polymicrogyria**, the gyri are too many and too small. Sometimes macrogyria and polymicrogyria affect an entire hemisphere, producing enlargement of that hemisphere and a clinical syndrome of severe, medically intractable seizures that begin in early infancy. Hemispherectomy is required to stop the seizures. **Gray matter heterotopias** are abnormal islands of neurons that have never completed the migratory process.

**Agenesis of the corpus callosum** may be partial or complete and may occur in an isolated fashion or in association with other anomalies of cellular migration. Neurologic development with all of these anomalies is variable and depends on the extent of the malformations.

**Megalencephaly**, or large brain, is diagnosed by finding a large head with radiographically normal-appearing intracranial contents. Most often, this is a familial trait of no clinical significance. Sometimes, it is associated with disorders of neuronal migration and a clinical syndrome of developmental retardation.

**Neurofibromatosis** and **Soto syndrome** (cerebral gigantism) are two genetic syndromes associated with megalencephaly and sometimes with mental retardation. Megalencephaly is also a feature of a number of metabolic diseases that produce a progressive degenerative encephalopathy.

**Microcephaly** usually is produced by failure of normal brain growth. Any injury to the brain, intrauterine or postnatal, can retard subsequent brain growth. Autosomal recessive genetic illnesses resulting in microcephaly and mental retardation have been described. Brain malformations often are associated with microcephaly. In general, children with head circumferences more than 3 standard deviations below the mean, regardless of the cause, exhibit retarded intellect.

### Chromosomal Disorders

Chromosomal trisomies (trisomy 21,XXY,XXX) are associated with retardation (see Chapter 4). The most common form of familial mental retardation, affecting 1 in 1250 males, is the **fragile X syndrome**. It is caused by expansion of a trinucleotide repeat, CGG, and abnormal methylation of a CpG island of the *FMR-1* gene at chromosome position Xq27.3. The features are varying degrees of mental retardation, autistic behavior, large ears, macro-orchidism, and an elongated, narrow face. Females may be affected, but usually not as severely as males.

Two other syndromes associated with mental retardation are caused by deletions of the same region of the long arm of chromosome 15. **Angelman syndrome** is caused by the loss of the maternal allele and is manifested by severe mental retardation, severe seizures, tremulousness, a characteristic facies, and a happy external demeanor. **Prader-Willi syndrome** is caused by the loss of the paternal allele and is manifested by severe hypotonia and feeding difficulties in the neonatal period, cryptorchidism, small hands and feet, mild mental retardation, and almond-shaped eyes. The difference in phenotype, depending on loss of the maternal or paternal allele, supports the genetic phenomenon of *imprinting* (see Chapter 4).

## PROGRESSIVE MENTAL RETARDATION

A complete laboratory evaluation is listed in Table 18–25. Degenerative hereditary and metabolic diseases usually are symmetric in their manifestations and slowly progressive over weeks, months, and years. However, some acquired diseases can simulate this clinical picture and must be excluded because they are more likely to be treatable than the degenerative conditions.

### Acquired Illnesses Mimicking Degenerative Diseases

Some children with epilepsy experience **seizures** so frequently that they are continuously in either

TABLE 18–25. Laboratory Evaluation for Degenerative Neurologic Metabolic Diseases

**Blood**
CBC (leukocyte vacuolations)
Blood gas determination
Ammonia
$Na^+$, $K^+$, $Cl^-$, $CO_2$ (anion gap), CPK, uric acid, fasting blood glucose, cholesterol, triglycerides
Lactate, pyruvate
Amino acids
Very-long-chain fatty acids
Acyl-carnitine
Biotinidase level

**Lysosomal Enzymes**
WBC
Serum fibroblasts

**DNA Probes**
Many disorders

**Urine**
Ketones
Screen for inborn errors
Organic acids
24-hr amino acids
24-hr mucopolysaccharides
Carnitine: free, esterified, total
Sialyloligosaccharides

**Imaging**
Skull
Vertebrae
Long bones
CNS, MRI

**Biopsy**
Skin
Bone marrow
Conjunctiva
Rectum
Muscle
Nerve

CBC = complete blood count; CPK = creatine phosphokinase; WBC = white blood cells; CNS = central nervous system; DNA = deoxyribonucleic acid; MRI = magnetic resonance imaging.

an ictal or postictal state and appear stuporous. A treatment program employing high doses of multiple anticonvulsants may compound this problem. The children's decline in alertness arouses suspicion of a progressive illness, but readjustment of medications and amelioration of the seizure disorder return the children to previous levels of functioning.

**Chronic drug overdose** with sedatives, tranquilizers, and anticholinergics as well as anticonvulsants can bring about progressive mental confusion, lethargy, and ataxia. **Lead poisoning** may become manifest as a chronic cause of mental retardation or as irritability, listlessness, anorexia, and pallor leading to fulminant encephalopathy. **Vitamin deficiency** of thiamine, niacin, $B_{12}$, and E can produce encephalopathy as well as peripheral neuropathy and ataxia. Both congenital and acquired **hypothyroidism** impair intelligence and retard movement; congenital hypothyroidism produces irreversible damage if it is not treated immediately after birth. **Structural brain diseases**, such as hydrocephalus and slowly growing tumors, also may mimic dementia.

Certain **indolent brain infections** cause mental and neurologic deterioration over months and years (e.g., syphilitic and fungal infections), but usually many associated clinical manifestations are present. Rubeola (measles), rubella (German measles), and human immunodeficiency virus (HIV) also can cause chronic infection of the CNS, which subsequently results in mental retardation. Measles produces subacute sclerosing panencephalitis, a dementing illness that has a course that can vary from weeks to years. Rubella virus produces a similar panencephalitis accompanied by prominent motor abnormalities, usually in children who have the congenital rubella syndrome. Congenital HIV infection brings about both failure of normal developmental gains and regression of acquired skills.

Severe **psychosocial deprivation** in infancy can give rise to apathy and failure to attain developmental milestones. **Depression** in older children can lead to blunting of affect, social withdrawal, and poor school performance that raise the question of encephalopathy and dementia.

### Hereditary/Metabolic Degenerative Diseases

Degenerative diseases may affect white matter, gray matter, or focal regions of the brain. Many of the white and gray matter degenerative illnesses are specific enzymatic deficiencies in the metabolism of one category of brain lipids, the sphingolipids, or gangliosides. Enzymatic deficiencies are often found in one of the subcellular organelles such as the mitochondria (energy production), peroxisome (structural macromolecules), or lysosomes (structural macromolecules).

Although enzyme deficiencies usually are expressed in classic patterns of disease, such as Niemann-Pick disease, Gaucher disease, and Tay-Sachs disease, the same enzyme deficiencies may produce unusual clinical syndromes that vary in age of onset, rate of progression, and neurologic signs. For any patient with a degenerative neurologic condition of unknown cause, leukocytes or skin fibroblasts should be submitted for measurement of a standard battery of lysosomal enzymes (see Chapter 5).

**Degenerative Diseases with Focal Manifestations.** Ataxia indicates disease of the cerebellum or spinocerebellar pathways. Abnormalities of extraocular movement or respiration indicate disease of the brain stem. Choreoathetosis or dystonia indicates disease of the motor basal ganglia. Paraplegia indicates disease of the spinal cord.

**Friedreich ataxia** is a relentlessly progressive autosomal recessive disorder that becomes manifest in the early teenage years with ataxia, dysmetria, dysarthria, pes cavus, hammer toes, diminished proprioception and vibration sensation, diminished or absent reflexes, upgoing toes, kyphoscoliosis, nystagmus, and a hypertrophic cardiomyopathy. It is caused by a homozygous GAA expansion of 120–1700 trinucleotide repeats of the first intron of the frataxin gene on chromosome 9. The GAA repeats are unstable on transmission. The size of the smaller GAA expansion is associated with the frequency of cardiomyopathy and loss of reflexes in the upper limbs.

**Lesch-Nyhan syndrome** is a sex-linked recessive disorder caused by deficiency of hypoxanthine–guanine phosphoribosyltransferase, leading to the formation of excess uric acid. Infants appear normal until late in the 1st yr of life, when they exhibit psychomotor retardation, choreoathetosis, spasticity, and severe self-mutilation develop. These patients never achieve ambulation. Gouty arthritis and renal calculi with renal failure also occur. The hyperuricemia and renal complications are treated with allopurinol, a xanthine oxidase inhibitor, but no effective treatment for the neurologic disease is available.

**Wilson disease** is an example of a treatable degenerative condition that exhibits signs of both cerebellar and basal ganglia dysfunction. It is an autosomal recessively inherited inborn error of copper metabolism. Serum copper and ceruloplasmin levels are low, and abnormal copper deposition is found in the liver, producing cirrhosis; in the peripheral cornea, producing a characteristic green-brown (Kayser-Fleischer) ring; and in the CNS, producing neuronal degeneration and protoplasmic astrocytosis. Neurologic symptoms characteristically begin in the early teenaged years with dysarthria, dysphasia, drooling, fixed smile, tremor, dystonia, and emotional lability. *Treatment* is with a copper-chelating agent, such as oral penicillamine.

**Subacute necrotizing encephalomyelopathy,** or **Leigh disease**, is a degenerative inherited CNS disease primarily involving the periaqueductal region of the brain stem, caudate, and putamen. Symptoms usually begin prior to 2 yr of age and consist of hypotonia, feeding difficulties, respiratory irregularity, weakness of extraocular movements, and ataxia. Blood pyruvate and lactate levels are elevated. Different disorders of mitochondrial function can produce this clinical syndrome: decreased pyruvate carboxylase or pyruvate dehydrogenase activity, biotinidase deficiency, and cytochrome *c* oxidase deficiency have been identified as causative in some cases. Vitamin therapies have been attempted but with little success.

**Degenerative Diseases of the White Matter.** The prominent signs of diseases affecting primarily white matter are spasticity, ataxia, optic atrophy, and peripheral neuropathy. Seizures and dementia are late manifestations. In general, life expectancy ranges from months to a few years. **Metachromatic leukodystrophy** is an autosomal recessive lipidosis caused by deficiency of the enzyme aryl-sulfatase. Demyelination of the central and peripheral nervous systems occurs, and children present between 1 and 2 yr of age with stiffening and ataxia of gait, spasticity, optic atrophy, intellectual deterioration, absent reflexes, upgoing toes, raised CSF protein, and slowing of motor nerve conduction velocities.

**Krabbe disease** (globoid cell leukodystrophy) presents a similar clinical picture that begins at 6 mo of age and includes irritability, macrocephaly, hyperacusis, and seizures. The same combination of upper and lower motor neuron signs is noted as a result of demyelination of both the central and peripheral nervous systems. Krabbe disease is also an autosomal recessive lipidosis and is caused by a deficiency of the enzyme galactocerebrosidase.

**Adrenoleukodystrophy** is a sex-linked, recessively inherited disorder associated with progressive central demyelination and adrenal cortical insufficiency. It is caused by an impaired capacity of a subcellular organelle, the *peroxisome*, to degrade saturated unbranched very-long-chain fatty acids, particularly hexacosanoate (C26:0). The *diagnosis* is achieved by finding an elevated hexacosanoate level in plasma lipids of the serum and typical abnormalities of neuroimaging. The disease most commonly is exhibited in males in the early school years, with subtle behavior changes and intellectual deterioration followed by cortical visual and auditory deficits and stiff gait. Later, spastic quadriparesis, coma, and seizures supervene. Symptomatic adrenocortical insufficiency with fatigue, vomiting, and hypotension develops in 20–40% of patients, usually at the same time as the neurologic illness.

**Degenerative Diseases of the Gray Matter with Visceromegaly** (see Chapter 5). The prominent signs of gray matter encephalopathy are dementia and seizures. To aid diagnosis, these diseases are divided into those with and without hepatosplenomegaly. All the illnesses discussed next, except for Rett syndrome, are genetic disorders. All are autosomal recessive traits except for Hunter syndrome, which is sex-linked recessive, and the mitochondrial encephalopathies, in which the disease may be transmitted through either nuclear or mitochondrial deoxyribonucleic acid (DNA) defects.

In the **mucopolysaccharidoses**, degradation of mucopolysaccharides (MPS) is defective because of the absence of a variety of lysosomal hydrolases. MPS, important matrix constituents of connective tissue, skin cartilage, bone, and cornea, accumulate

Neurology

within lysosomes and abnormally large amounts are excreted in the urine. The *clinical manifestations* of these disorders are dwarfism, kyphoscoliosis, coarse facies, hepatosplenomegaly, cardiovascular abnormalities, and corneal clouding. Neurologic involvement is seen in MPS types 1H (Hurler syndrome), II (Hunter syndrome), III (Sanfilippo syndrome), and VII. Children with Hurler syndrome, the most severe of these illnesses, appear normal during the first 6 mo of life and then develop the characteristic skeletal and neurologic features. Mental deficiency, spasticity, deafness, and optic atrophy are progressive. Hydrocephalus frequently occurs because of obstruction to CSF flow by thickened leptomeninges.

Mucolipidosis II (I-cell disease), mucolipidosis III, GM₁ gangliosidosis, fucosidosis, and mannosidosis resemble Hurler syndrome clinically but do not exhibit excess excretion of MPS and involve different disorders in lysosomal hydrolases. The *diagnosis* is confirmed by analysis of enzymes in white blood cells, serum, and skin fibroblasts.

Classic **Niemann-Pick disease** is caused by a deficiency of the enzyme sphingomyelinase. Sphingomyelin accumulates in foam cells of the reticuloendothelial system of the liver, spleen, lungs, and bone marrow; it also distends neurons of the brain. Intellectual retardation and regression, myoclonic seizures, hypotonia, hepatosplenomegaly, jaundice, and, sometimes, retinal cherry-red spots are noted within the 1st yr of life. The *diagnosis* is confirmed by finding foam cells in the bone marrow and sphingomyelinase deficiency in leukocytes and skin fibroblasts.

Although the most common form of **Gaucher disease** is an indolent illness of adults, there is a rapidly fatal infantile form featuring severe neurologic involvement caused by deficiency of the enzyme glucocerebrosidase. Glucoceramide accumulates in the liver, spleen, and bone marrow. The characteristic neurologic signs are neck retraction, extraocular movement palsies, trismus, difficulty swallowing, apathy, and spasticity. Gaucher cells are found in bone marrow, and serum acid phosphatase is increased.

### Degenerative Disease of the Gray Matter without Visceromegaly

**Tay-Sachs disease** occurs most commonly in Jewish children of eastern European background. The disease is confined to the CNS. It is caused by deficiency of hexosaminidase A and the accumulation of GM₂ ganglioside in cerebral gray matter and cerebellum. Infants are normal until 6 mo of age, when they develop listlessness, irritability, hyperacusis, intellectual retardation, and a *retinal cherry-red spot*. The ganglion cells of the retina and macula are distended with ganglioside and appear as a large area of white surrounding a small red fovea that is not covered by ganglion cells. Within months, blindness, convulsions, spasticity, and opisthotonos develop.

**Rett syndrome** is a common neurodegenerative disorder affecting only females, with onset at about 1 yr of age. It is characterized by the loss of purposeful hand movements and communication skills; social withdrawal; gait apraxia; stereotypic repetitive hand movements that resemble washing, wringing, or clapping of the hands; and acquired microcephaly. The illness then plateaus for many years before seizures, spasticity, and kyphoscoliosis develop. The etiology, genetic basis, and neurobiologic pathogenesis of the disease are unknown.

Several syndromes of *mitochondrial myopathy* and *progressive encephalopathy* have been described. Skeletal muscle biopsy reveals ragged red fibers representing proliferating abnormal mitochondrial elements. Neurologic signs have included seizures, focal deficits, and dementia in the **MELAS** (*mi*tochondrial myopathy, *e*ncephalopathy, *la*ctic *a*cidosis, and *s*troke-like episodes) **syndrome**, and seizures, dementia, hearing loss, optic nerve atrophy, ataxia, and loss of deep sensation in the **MERRF** (*my*oclonus, *e*pilepsy, and *r*agged *r*ed *f*ibers) **syndrome**. Elevation of creatine phosphokinase, lactic acidosis, and calcification of the basal ganglia suggest this class of disorders. Onset is usually between 5 and 10 yr of age and progression occurs over years.

Many degenerative encephalopathies defy diagnosis despite extensive laboratory analysis. The diagnosis of leukodystrophy usually can be made confidently on the basis of extensive cerebral white matter changes on CT or MRI in the absence of cortical abnormalities. The diagnosis of hereditary/metabolic gray matter encephalopathy without histologic or biochemical confirmation is much less secure. Acquired lesions (infectious, inflammatory, vascular, toxic) are difficult to exclude completely. Unless neuroimaging lesions are demonstrated, brain biopsy is not likely to be helpful.

## References

Behrman RE, Kliegman RM, Arvin AM (eds): Nelson Textbook of Pediatrics, 15th ed. Philadelphia, WB Saunders, 1996, Chapters 542, 546, 548, 552.
Hagberg B: Rett Syndrome: Clinical peculiarities, diagnostic approach and possible course. Pediatr Neurol 5:75, 1989.
Kalter H, Warkany J: Congenital malformations: Etiological factors and their role in prevention. N Engl J Med 308:424, 1983.
Morgan A, Aldag J: Early identification of cerebral palsy using a profile of abnormal motor patterns. Pediatrics 98:692, 1996.
Opitz J: Mental retardation: Biologic aspects of concern to pediatricians. Pediatr Rev 2:41, 1980.

# MACROCEPHALY AND MICROCEPHALY

Abnormalities of head size are among the most common problems encountered by pediatricians. Head circumference varies with race and sex, but measurements greater than 3 standard deviations above the mean constitute **macrocephaly**. Macrocephaly may be due to *macrocrania*, increased skull thickness; *hydrocephalus*, enlargement of the ventricles; or *megalencephaly*, enlargement of the brain. Head circumference measurements more than 3 standard deviations below the mean are termed **microcephaly**. In most circumstances, microcephaly reflects *micrencephaly*, a small brain. With *craniosynostosis* (premature closure of one or more skull sutures), compensatory growth in the vertical or horizontal dimension will result in an altered head circumference measurement, which inaccurately reflects intracranial volume. If brain volume is reduced above the cranial base, as in *microcephaly vera*, in which intracranial content is decreased as a result of deficiency of the frontal lobes, the occipital frontal head circumference may not completely reflect the deficiency. Definitions of microcephaly do not apply to dwarfism, in which head circumference is proportional to body size and intellectual development is normal. As a rule, macrocephaly and microcephaly raise a concern about cognitive ability, but head circumference alone should never be used to establish a prognosis for intellectual development.

## MACROCEPHALY

### Hydrocephalus

Hydrocephalus is an important cause of macrocephaly and is due to increased production, a block in the flow, or impaired absorption of CSF. CSF is an ultrafiltrate of plasma continuously produced by the choroid plexus of the lateral, 3rd, and 4th ventricles. The normal volume of CSF is approximately 50 mL in neonates and reaches the adult volume of 150 mL by late childhood or early adolescence. CSF normally flows from the lateral ventricles through the intraventricular foramen of Monro to the 3rd ventricle. From the 3rd ventricle, it passes through the cerebral aqueduct to the 4th ventricle. CSF exits the 4th ventricle from the single midline foramen of Magendie and the two lateral foramina of Luschka. Subarachnoid flow occurs superiorly to the cisterns of the brain and inferiorly to the spinal subarachnoid space. Absorption of CSF is accomplished by the arachnoid villi, which are microtubular invaginations into the large dural sinuses and are most concentrated along the superior sagittal sinus, and by transependymal absorption. Increased ICP neither effectively facilitates CSF absorption nor inhibits CSF formation.

The *etiology* of hydrocephalus is obstruction of CSF flow anywhere along its course (Table 18–26). **Obstructive** or **internal hydrocephalus** is due to a block before CSF reaches the subarachnoid space. Impairment of CSF flow within the subarachnoid space or impairment of absorption is known by the misnomer **communicating hydrocephalus** (actually extraventricular obstructive hydrocephalus) or **external hydrocephalus**. Hydrocephalus caused by overproduction of CSF without true obstruction is seen in choroid plexus papillomas, which account for 2–4% of childhood intracranial tumors and are exhibited in early infancy.

The *clinical manifestations* of hydrocephalus are caused by ventricular distention and increased intracranial pressure. Dilation of the lateral ventricles results in stretching of the corticopontocerebellar and corticospinal pathways, which sweep around the lateral margins of these ventricles to reach the cerebral peduncles. This stretching results in ataxia and spasticity that initially are most marked in the lower extremities. Distention of the 3rd ventricle may compress the hypothalamic regions and result in endocrine dysfunction. The optic nerves, chiasm, and tracts also are in close proximity to the anterior 3rd ventricle, and visual dysfunction results when these structures are compressed. Dilation of the cerebral aqueduct compresses the surrounding periaqueductal gray matter, a vertical gaze center, causing paresis of upward gaze. Manifestations of increased ICP may evolve slowly in obstructive hydrocephalus when there is time for transependymal absorption of CSF to compensate partially for the obstruction, or they may evolve acutely when compensation is absent. Acute manifestations consist of headache, vomiting, cranial nerve dysfunction, herniation, and coma in rapid sequence. They usually follow acute complete obstruction to CSF flow resulting from tumors, infection, or hemorrhage. Gradually evolving hydrocephalus results in macrocephaly, scalp vein distention caused by obstruction of flow from the bridging veins of the scalp to the sagittal sinus, impairment in upward gaze eventually causing the "sunsetting sign," ataxia, spasticity, papilledema or optic atrophy, and endocrine dysfunction, which most commonly is exhibited as growth failure.

The *treatment* of hydrocephalus is both medical and surgical. Following subarachnoid hemorrhage or meningitis, the flow or absorption of CSF may be transiently impaired. In this circumstance, the use of agents such as acetazolamide, which transiently decreases CSF production, may be of bene-

TABLE 18–26.  Causes of Hydrocephalus

| Obstruction Region | Clinical Characteristics | Etiology |
|---|---|---|
| Intraventricular foramina | Acutely or slowly evolving, unilateral ventricular dilation; can be exhibited at any age | Congenital, parasellar mass, intraventricular tumors |
| Aqueduct of Sylvius (cerebral aqueduct) | May be exhibited in utero or in adults; usually noted in infancy; slowly evolves | Neurofibromatosis, intrauterine toxoplasmosis, post-mumps meningoencephalitis; periaqueductal mass lesions: tumors, vein of Galen malformations; congenital dysplasia; hereditary, sex-linked |
| Impaired flow from the fourth ventricle | | |
| Dandy-Walker malformation | Enlarged occipital shelf; slowly evolving; marked transillumination of the posterior fossa; usually is exhibited in infancy but may be delayed until adult life | Referred to as atresia of the foramina of Luschka and Magendie but actually due to agenesis of the cerebellar vermis, resulting in cystic dilation of the fourth ventricle and aqueductal compression |
| Arnold-Chiari malformation | May or may not be associated with myelomeningocele; may be exhibited in later life with cranial nerve dysfunction, with or without hydrocephalus | Congenital malformation resulting in a small posterior fossa, caudal displacement of the fourth ventricle and cerebellum, and distortion of the brain stem |
| Congenital bone lesions of the cranial base | Slowly evolving hydrocephalus, stiff neck; lower cranial nerve dysfunction | Achondroplasia, rickets, basilar impression; these lesions compress the posterior fossa, preventing CSF flow and distorting the brain stem |
| Extraventricular obstruction (communicating) | Acutely or slowly evolving; is exhibited at any age | Congenital, due to hypoplasia of the arachnoid villi; following infection or hemorrhage due to destruction of arachnoid villi or subarachnoid fibrosis, causing obstruction to CSF flow (following superior sagittal sinus occlusion, preventing absorption of CSF) |

CSF = cerebrospinal fluid.

fit. Surgical management consists of removing the obstructive lesion (tumor, cyst, or aneurysm) or placing a shunt. A shunt consists of polyethylene tubing, with or without a valve, that bypasses the obstruction and diverts CSF to other sites for absorption. The cranial end usually is placed in the lateral ventricles. In the instance of Dandy-Walker malformation, the cranial end may be placed in the posterior fossa cyst. The distal end usually is placed in the peritoneal cavity. Shunts carry the hazards of infection *(Staphylococcus epidermidis, Corynebacterium)* or sudden occlusion with signs and symptoms of acute hydrocephalus.

### Megalencephaly

Megalencephaly may be due to an embryologic proliferative abnormality of the brain and is associated with several rare syndromes (Sotos syndrome, Riley-Smith syndrome, Alexander and Canavan diseases). Megalencephalic brains may be two to three times as large as normal brains. Megalencephaly also may be due to (1) chronic brain edema (i.e., pseudotumor cerebri); (2) tumors (ganglioneuromas, neurocutaneous syndrome); and (3) the accumulation of abnormal metabolic substances. Megalencephaly is seen in achondrodysplasia.

### Macrocrania

Macrocrania refers to a number of processes that directly (abnormalities of bone metabolism) or indirectly (hemolytic processes) result in thickening of the calvaria.

## MICROCEPHALY

Microcephaly is a sign of many heterogeneous disorders. Brain growth is rapid during the perinatal period, and any insult (e.g., infectious, metabolic, toxic, or vascular disorder) sustained during this period or early infancy is likely to impair brain growth and result in microcephaly. In children who have microcephaly vera, endochondral bone formation at the base of the skull is normal but severely deficient membranous bone formation of the calvaria is present secondary to hypoplasia of the frontal regions of the brain. This results in a normal-sized face but a markedly small calvaria that sharply recedes in the frontal regions. Children affected with this condition are free of associated malformations but are severely impaired intellectually. A myriad of syndromic and metabolic disorders are associated with microcephaly, some of which are hereditary (Table 18–27). Although premature closure of all the skull sutures, sometimes associated with hyperthyroidism, is a treatable cause of microcephaly, once a brain insult has resulted in microcephaly, subsequent brain growth is severely limited.

### References

Behrman RE, Kliegman RM, Arvin AM (eds): Nelson Textbook of Pediatrics, 15th ed. Philadelphia, WB Saunders, 1996, Chapters 542, 552, 555.

TABLE 18–27.  Microcephaly

| Etiology | Comment |
| --- | --- |
| **Recognized Chromosomal Disorders** | |
| Partial deletion, trisomy, or ring abnormalities; deletion of the short arm of 5 (*cri du chat* syndrome) | |
| **Genetic Disorders** | |
| *Microcephaly vera* | |
| Microcephaly with lissencephaly, schizencephaly, pachygyria, micropolygyria | Some are autosomal recessive |
| *Agenesis of the corpus callosum* | |
| Male microcephaly | Sex-linked recessive, autosomal dominant |
| Microcephaly with normal intelligence and minor malformations | |
| **Microcephaly with Syndromes** | |
| Prader-Willi syndrome | Hypotonia, cryptorchidism, obesity |
| Smith-Lemli-Opitz syndrome | Cryptorchidism, hypospadias, vomiting, seizures |
| Cornelia de Lange syndrome | Anteverted nostrils, low birth weight, carp mouth, micromelia, synophrys |
| Seckel dwarf syndrome | Bony defects, joint dislocations |
| Cockayne syndrome | Retinal degeneration, cataracts, brain calcifications |
| Leprechaunism | Sunken eyes, low-set ears, absent subcutaneous fat, hypoglycemia |
| Rubinstein-Taybi syndrome | Broad thumbs and toes, narrow nose, maxillary hypoplasia |
| Lowe syndrome | Cataracts, hypotonia, glaucoma, aminoaciduria, X-linked |
| Zellweger syndrome | Hypotonia, high forehead, seizures, absent DTRs, recessive inheritance, paroxysmal disorder |
| Hallermann-Streiff syndrome | Microphthalmia, small nose |
| **Infections** | |
| Congenital rubella | |
| CMV | |
| Herpes simplex | |
| Toxoplasmosis | |
| Syphilis | |
| **Toxic Causes** | |
| Maternal radiation | |
| Maternal alcohol and aminopterin ingestion | |
| Maternal PKU | |
| **Vascular Causes** | |
| Intrauterine or neonatal hypoxia–ischemia | |

CMV = cytomegalovirus; DTRs = deep tendon reflexes; PKU = phenylketonuria.

Jones KL: Smith's Recognizable Patterns of Human Malformation, 5th ed. Philadelphia, WB Saunders, 1997.

Warkany J, Lemire R, Cohen M: Mental Retardation and Congenital Malformations of the Central Nervous System. Chicago, Year Book Medical Publishers, 1981.

# WEAKNESS

## NEUROANATOMY

Voluntary movement is directed by a conscious "will," utilizing a large number of subconscious motor mechanisms. Maintenance of proper tone and coordination of agonist, antagonist, synergistic, and fixating muscle groups involve motor nuclei of the spinal cord, cerebellum, brain stem, thalamus, basal ganglia, and motor cortex of cerebrum.

The corticospinal tract and its neurons that subserve voluntary motor activity are known as the *upper motor neuron*. The *lower motor neuron* includes the anterior horn cells in addition to their motor roots and peripheral motor nerves, the neuromuscular junctions, and the muscles. Destruction of the upper motor neuron causes loss of voluntary control but not total loss of movement. Motor nuclei of the basal ganglia, thalamus, and brain stem have their own tracts that innervate anterior horn cells and produce simple or complex stereotyped patterns of movement. Destruction of the spinal cord leaves intact simple stereotyped reflex movements coordinated by local spinal reflexes below the level of the lesion. Destruction of the lower motor neuron leads to total absence of movement because it is the final common pathway producing muscle activity.

Weakness caused by disease of the lower motor unit is different in quality from weakness produced by central, corticospinal tract lesions. The latter often is not so much an inability to move the limb as a loss of dexterous movements. The corticospinal tract permits fine motor activity, and its function is best tested by asking the patient to perform rapid alternating movements of the distal extremities. Mild dysfunction produces slowed, stiff motions. More severe dysfunction produces stiff, abnormal postures that do not respond to voluntary command. Characteristically, the posture in corticospinal tract disease consists of the forearm being flexed at the elbow and wrist and adducted close to the chest, with the leg extended and adducted. Disease of the lower motor unit produces progressive loss of strength with hypotonia and no abnormality of posture. Function is best tested by measuring the strength of individual muscle groups or, in the young child, by observing the ability to perform tasks requiring particular muscle groups (e.g., walk up or down stairs, arise from the ground, walk on toes or heels, raise the hands above the head, squeeze a ball). Table 18–28 characterizes the findings in weakness of upper and lower motor neuron type.

## DISEASE OF THE UPPER MOTOR NEURON

Stroke is the most common cause of damage to the corticospinal tract. Tumors, trauma, infections, demyelinating syndromes, and metabolic and degenerative diseases also injure the corticospinal tract.

### Stroke in Childhood

Obstruction of blood flow may occur in arteries or veins and may be caused by local thrombosis or embolization from distant sites. Cerebral embolization characteristically occurs without warning, produces its full deficit within seconds, and may be associated with focal seizures, headache, and hemorrhagic infarction. The most common sources of cerebral emboli are the heart and the carotid artery in the neck. Cerebral thrombosis may be preceded by transient ischemic attacks that resolve completely. The deficits themselves evolve over hours in a stepwise or stuttering progression. The sudden emergence of neurologic deficits implies cerebral vascular disease, and the site of occlusion is suggested by the neurologic deficits. If clinical assessment does not reveal the cause of the stroke, a complete laboratory investigation should be undertaken.

Clinical assessment will uncover the most common sources of childhood stroke, which are congenital heart disease, sickle cell anemia (SS), meningitis, and acute and congenital hemiplegias of childhood. Less common causes include hypoxic-ischemic encephalopathy, emboli from the placenta or a dead twin fetus, infections (especially sepsis), disseminated intravascular coagulopathy, congenital disorders of thrombosis and thrombolysis (see Chapter 14), collagen vascular or related inflammatory disease, cerebral vasculitis, accidental air or fat emboli, polycythemia, drugs (amphetamines, birth control pills, cocaine), atlantoaxial dislocation, the syndrome of antiphospholipid-anticardiolipin antibodies associated with systemic lupus erythematosus, spontaneous or traumatic dissection of the carotid artery, moyamoya disease, and rare complications of migraine and metabolic disorders (homocystinuria, mitochondrial myopathy with lactic acidosis).

TABLE 18–28.  Corticospinal (Upper) and Neuromuscular (Lower) Loss of Motor Function

| Clinical Sign | Neuromuscular | Corticospinal |
|---|---|---|
| Posture | Flaccid | Arm flexed, leg extended |
| Tone | Decreased | Increased |
| Reflexes | Decreased | Increased |
| Babinski reflex | Absent | Present |
| Atrophy | Possible | Absent |
| Fasciculations | Possible | Absent |

**Heart disease** and its complications may give rise to thromboses in cerebral arteries or veins or to emboli in cerebral arteries. Cerebral venous and arterial thromboses occur in 1–2% of infants with cyanotic congenital heart disease and probably are related to local congestion of blood flow. Predisposing factors include acute episodes of severe cyanosis, febrile illnesses, dehydration, polycythemia, hyperventilation, and iron-deficiency anemia. Sources of emboli include mural thrombi from dilated poorly contracting cardiac chambers, bacterial endocarditis, nonbacterial endocarditis, valvular disease, atrial myxoma, cardiac catheterization, and cardiac surgery. Septic emboli producing cerebral infarcts occur in 10–20% of patients who develop bacterial endocarditis.

Often, a thorough evaluation of the child with a stroke does not reveal the etiology and angiography may disclose the site of vascular occlusion, but the pathogenetic mechanism remains unknown. This condition has been labeled as **acute hemiplegia of childhood**. Children with this condition suffer a single acute episode, are not at risk for further recurrences, and do not require special treatment.

A similar problem in defining etiology pertains to children with **congenital hemiplegia**. Affected infants typically present at 6–9 mo of age with decreased use of one side of the body. CT reveals an area of encephalomalacia in the contralateral cerebral hemisphere. The details of the child's intrauterine, labor, delivery, and postnatal history often are unremarkable. Some neonates manifest focal seizures. The timing of the injury is unknown.

Completed strokes do not benefit from medical treatment. Strokes in evolution, transient ischemic attacks, or ongoing cerebral embolization may be treated with anticoagulants (intravenous heparin and oral warfarin [Coumadin]), platelet antiaggregants (aspirin and dipyridamole), or surgery to enlarge stenosed channels, excise sources of emboli, or provide alternative sources of intracerebral blood flow.

## DISEASE OF THE LOWER MOTOR NEURON

Each motor neuron in the spinal cord (anterior horn cell) and brain stem gives rise to a single myelinated axon that extends to muscle. After numerous branchings, each axon twig terminates in a synapse with a single muscle fiber. The presynaptic axon terminal releases acetylcholine, which traverses the synaptic cleft, binds to receptors on the muscle membrane, initiates muscle contraction, and is inactivated by acetylcholinesterase. The lower motor unit consists of all of these components.

Neuromuscular disease is illness of any component of the motor unit. The distribution of muscle weakness can point toward specific diseases (Table 18–29). Diseases affecting each component of the motor unit are listed in Table 18–30 and briefly summarized below.

TABLE 18–29.  "Topography" of Neuromuscular Diseases

**Proximal Muscle Weakness**

Dystrophy
    Duchenne
    Limb girdle
Dermatomyositis; polymyositis
Kugelberg-Welander disease (late-onset spinal muscular atrophy)

**Distal Limb Weakness**

Polyneuropathy (Guillain-Barré syndrome, others)
HMSN I
HMSN II
Myotonic dystrophy
Distal myopathy
Transverse myelitis
Spinal trauma, tumors, infarction, or demyelination

**Ophthalmoplegia and Limb Weakness**

Myasthenia gravis
Botulism
Myotonic dystrophy
Congenital structural myopathy
Miller Fisher variant of Guillain-Barré syndrome

**Facial and Bulbar Weakness**

Myasthenia gravis
Botulism
Polio
Miller Fisher variant of Guillain-Barré syndrome
Myotonic dystrophy
Congenital structural myopathy
Facioscapulohumeral dystrophy

HMSN = hereditary motor sensory neuropathy.

TABLE 18–30.   Diseases of the Lower Motor Unit in Infants and Children

| | |
|---|---|
| **Anterior Horn Cell** | **Muscle** |
| Spinal muscular atrophy* | Dystrophy |
| Poliomyelitis (natural or vaccine) | Duchenne |
| Enteroviruses | Becker |
| **Peripheral Nerve** | Limb girdle |
| Guillain-Barré syndrome | Facioscapulohumeral |
| Tick (toxicosis) paralysis | Myotonic* |
| Hereditary* | Congenital* |
| Vitamin E, $B_{12}$, and $B_1$ deficiencies | Myositis (viral, polymyositis) |
| Toxins | Congenital structural myopathy |
| Lead, thallium, arsenic, mercury | Central core |
| Hexane | Nemaline rod |
| Acrylamide | Centronuclear |
| Organophosphates | Congenital fiber type of disproportion |
| Diphtheria | Congenital muscular dystrophy |
| Collagen vascular disease | Miscellaneous types |
| Porphyria | **Metabolic, Endocrine, and Mineral** |
| Paraneoplastic | Glycogen storage disease II (Pompe disease) |
| Drugs | Carnitine metabolism abnormalities |
| Amitriptyline | Mitochondrial abnormalities |
| Dapsone | Thyroid excess or deficiency |
| Hydralazine | Cortisol excess or deficiency |
| Isoniazid | Hyperparathyroidism; calcium excess |
| Nitrofurantoin | Potassium excess or deficiency (familial paralysis) |
| Vincristine | |
| **Neuromuscular Junction** | |
| Myasthenia gravis | |
| Acquired | |
| Neonatal transitory* | |
| Congenital* | |
| Botulism* | |
| Aminoglycosides | |

*Infants.

## Disease of the Spinal Cord

Acute spinal cord disease may produce a flaccid, areflexic paralysis that simulates neuromuscular disease. A child who presents with an acute or subacute flaccid paraparesis is most likely to have either an acute cord syndrome, such as transverse myelitis, a cord tumor, infarction, demyelination, trauma, or a disease of the peripheral nerves, such as the **Guillain-Barré syndrome**. The hallmarks of spinal cord disease are a sensory level, a motor level, disturbance of bowel and bladder function, and local spinal pain or tenderness. Transverse myelitis is treated with high-dose steroids; trauma and tumor require immediate neurosurgical management.

## Diseases of the Anterior Horn Cell

**Werdnig-Hoffmann Disease or Spinal Muscular Atrophy.** Progressive degeneration of anterior horn cells is the sole manifestation of this genetic illness, which may begin in intrauterine life or anytime thereafter and may progress at a rapid or slow pace. In general, the earlier in life that the process starts, the more rapid the progression. Infants who already are affected at birth or who become weak within the first several months of life usually progress to flaccid quadriplegia with bulbar palsy, respiratory failure, and death within the 1st yr of life. This early fulminant form of the illness is called Werdnig-Hoffmann disease. A mild form of the illness, **Kugelberg-Welander syndrome**, begins in late childhood with proximal weakness of the legs and progresses slowly over decades. Between these extremes the illness may be unpredictable: it may begin between 6 mo and 6 yr of age and may progress rapidly, slowly, or rapidly initially and then seemingly plateau. The inheritance of all of these forms is autosomal recessive. It seems highly probable that acute and chronic spinal muscular atrophy generally are due to mutations at the same gene locus, which has been mapped to chromosome 5q13.

The *clinical manifestations* usually are similar in all affected siblings within a single family. Infants present with progressive weakness, especially proximally; decreased spontaneous movement; and floppiness. Atrophy may be marked. Head control is lost. With time, the legs stop moving altogether and the children play only with toys placed in their hands. The range of facial expression diminishes, and drooling and gurgling increase. The eyes remain bright, open, mobile, and engaging. Weakness is flaccid, with early loss of reflexes. Fasciculations sometimes can be seen in the tongue and are searched for best when the child is asleep. The infants have normal mental, social, and language skills and sensation. Breathing becomes rapid, shallow, and predominantly abdominal. In the very weak child, respiratory infections lead to atelectasis, pulmonary infection, and death. Creatine phosphokinase may be mildly elevated. The electromyogram (EMG) shows fasciculations, fibrillations, positive sharp waves, and high-amplitude, long-duration motor units.

No *treatment* for the condition exists. Symptomatic therapy is directed toward minimizing contractures, preventing scoliosis, aiding oxygenation, preventing aspiration, and maximizing social, language, and intellectual skills. Respiratory infections are managed early and aggressively with pulmonary toilet, chest physical therapy, oxygen, and antibiotics. The use or nonuse of artificial ventilation must be individualized for each patient in each stage of the illness.

**Poliomyelitis.** See Chapter 10.

## Peripheral Neuropathy

The principal peripheral nerve diseases in childhood are (1) Guillain-Barré syndrome, (2) hereditary motor sensory neuropathy **(Charcot-Marie-Tooth disease)** and (3) tick paralysis. Peripheral neuropathy produced by diabetes mellitus, alcoholism, chronic renal failure, amyloid, exposure to industrial or metal toxins, vasculitis (often as mononeuritis multiplex), or the remote effects of neoplasms is a common cause of weakness and sensory loss in adults but is rare in infants and children.

**Guillain-Barré Syndrome.** This condition is an idiopathic peripheral neuropathy that often occurs following a respiratory or gastrointestinal *(Campylobacter)* infection; it is exhibited most characteristically by areflexia, flaccidity, and relatively symmetric weakness beginning in the legs and ascending to involve the arms, trunk, throat, and face. Progression can occur rapidly, in hours or days, or more indolently, over weeks.

Typically, the child complains of numbness or paresthesia in the hands and feet and then experiences a heavy weak feeling in the legs, followed by the inability to walk. The examination often reveals complete absence of reflexes even when strength is good. Objective signs of sensory loss usually are minor compared with the dramatic weakness. Meningeal signs frequently are noted. Progression to bulbar and respiratory insufficiency may occur rapidly, and close monitoring of respiratory function is necessary. The loss of arm reflexes, the absence of a sensory level, lack of spinal tenderness, and, usually, normal bowel and bladder function serve to distinguish neuropathy from a spinal cord syndrome. Dysfunction of autonomic nerves can lead to hypertension, hypotension, orthostatic hypotension, tachycardia and other arrhythmias, urinary retention or incontinence, stool retention, or episodes of abnormal sweating, flushing, or peripheral vasoconstriction. A cranial nerve variant (Miller Fisher syndrome) may be isolated or simultaneous with peripheral nerve involvement.

Porphyria and tick paralysis may simulate Guillain-Barré syndrome. Other causes of peripheral neuropathy include vasculitis, heredity, nutritional deficiency (vitamins $B_1$, $B_{12}$, and E), endocrine disorders, infections (diphtheria, Lyme disease), and toxins (organophosphate, lead).

CSF often is normal in the 1st wk of the illness and then shows elevated protein levels without pleocytosis. Nerve conduction velocity and EMG also may be normal early in the disease but then show delay in motor nerve conduction velocity and decreased amplitude and temporal dispersion of the evoked compound motor action potential.

This illness resolves spontaneously, and 75% of patients recover normal function within 1–12 mo. Twenty percent of patients are left with mild to moderate residual weakness in the feet and lower legs. The mortality rate is 5%, and death is caused by autonomic dysfunction (hypertension–hypotension, tachycardia–bradycardia, sudden death), respiratory failure, or complications of mechanical ventilation, cardiovascular collapse, or pulmonary embolism.

Children with moderate or severe weakness or rapidly progressive weakness should receive *treatment* in a pediatric intensive care unit. Endotracheal intubation should be performed electively in patients who exhibit either early signs of hypoventilation, accumulation of bronchial secretions, or obtunded pharyngeal or laryngeal reflexes. Prior to mechanical ventilation, respiratory sufficiency is monitored by frequent spirometric studies, including vital capacity and maximum inspiratory force. Therapy is symptomatic and rehabilitative and directed at hypertension, hypotension, and cardiac arrhythmias; pulmonary embolism; nutrition, fluids, and electrolytes; pain; skin, cornea, and joints; bowel and bladder; infection; psychologic support; and communication. Controlled studies have not supported the efficacy of ACTH or steroids but suggest that plasma exchange and intravenous immunoglobulin (IVIG) may be beneficial in rapidly progressive disease. Most patients are initially treated with IVIG (total dose 2 g/kg given over 4–5 days).

**Hereditary Motor Sensory Neuropathy (Charcot-Marie-Tooth Disease).** Hereditary motor and sensory neuropathy (HMSN), commonly called Charcot-Marie-Tooth (CMT) disease, is a chronic, genetically determined polyneuropathy characterized by weakness and wasting of distal limb muscles and foot deformity. Most often, complaints begin in the preschool years with *pes cavus deformity of feet* and weakness of the ankles with frequent tripping. Examination reveals high-arched feet, bilateral weakness of foot dorsiflexors, and normal sensation despite occasional complaints of paresthesia. Progression is slow, extending over years and decades. Eventually, patients develop weakness and atrophy of the entire lower legs and hands and mild to moderate sensory loss in the hands and feet. Some patients never have more than a mild deformity of the feet, loss of ankle reflexes, and electrophysiologic abnormalities, whereas others in the same family may be confined to a wheelchair and have difficulties performing everyday tasks with their hands in early adult life.

HMSN type I is a demyelinating illness with severely decreased nerve conduction velocity and hypertrophic changes on nerve biopsy. The most common form (CMT 1A) is due to a *duplication* of DNA at 17p11.2–12, a region containing the peripheral myelin protein (PMP). A *deletion* in this region gives rise to a much milder condition, called hereditary neuropathy, with liability to pressure palsies. An X-linked form of CMT is due to mutations of the gap junction protein, connexin 32. HMSN type II is a neuronal form with normal or mildly decreased nerve conduction velocity and no hypertrophic changes. Both type I and type II HMSN are inherited as autosomal dominants with variable expressivity.

Specific *treatment* is not available, but braces such as those that maintain the feet in dorsiflexion can improve function measurably. Early surgery is contraindicated because the progression of the disease destabilizes even good repair.

### Neuromuscular Junction

**Acquired Myasthenia Gravis.** Classic myasthenia gravis may begin in the teenaged years with the acute onset of ptosis; diplopia; ophthalmoplegia, with or without weakness; and fatigability of extremities, neck, face, and jaw. *Clinical manifestations* are least prominent on awakening in the morning and worsen as the day progresses or with exercise. In some children, the disease never advances beyond ophthalmoplegia and ptosis; in others, however, a progressive and potentially life-threatening illness develops that involves all musculature, including that of respiration and swallowing.

Edrophonium chloride (Tensilon) intravenously, but not saline control, usually improves strength and decreases fatigability significantly. Anti-acetylcholine receptor antibodies usually can be detected in the serum, and EMG reveals a decremental response to repetitive nerve stimulation.

*Treatment* includes an acetylcholine esterase inhibitor, such as pyridostigmine (Mestinon), thymectomy, prednisone, plasmapheresis, and immunosuppressive agents. When respirations are compromised, immediate intubation and admission to an intensive care unit are indicated.

**Neonatal Transitory Myasthenia Gravis.** Ten to 20% of neonates born to mothers with myasthenia gravis develop a transitory myasthenic syndrome that persists for 1–10 wk (mean, 3 wk). Almost all infants born to mothers with myasthenia demonstrate anti-acetylcholine receptor antibody, and neither antibody titer nor extent of disease in the mother predicts which neonates will display clinical disease. Symptoms and signs include ptosis, ophthalmoplegia, weak facial movements, poor sucking and feeding, hypotonia, and variable extremity weakness.

The *diagnosis* is made by demonstrating clinical improvement lasting approximately 45 min following intramuscular (IM) administration of neostigmine methylsulfate, 0.1 mg. *Treatment* with oral pyridostigmine (Mestinon) or neostigmine 30 min prior to feeding is continued until spontaneous resolution occurs.

### MUSCLE DISEASE

#### Duchenne Dystrophy

Muscular dystrophy is a common sex-linked recessive trait appearing in 20–30:100,000 boys. Boys present at about 3 yr of age with inability to run properly or keep up athletically with their peers. Some have an antecedent history of mild slowness in attaining motor milestones (walking, climbing stairs). Examination reveals calf hypertrophy and mild to moderate proximal leg weakness exhibited by a hyperlordotic and waddling gait and inability to arise from the ground easily. The child typically arises from sitting by climbing up on his legs and body, the *Gower sign*. Weakness progresses such that arm weakness is evident by 6 yr of age, and most boys are confined to a wheelchair by 12 yr of age. By 16 yr, little mobility of arms remains and respiratory difficulties increase. Death is due to pneumonia or congestive heart failure resulting from myocardial involvement. Patients may develop obesity and mild mental retardation.

Serum creatine phosphokinase levels are always markedly elevated. Muscle biopsy reveals evidence of muscle fiber degeneration and regeneration accompanied by increased intrafascicular connective tissue. This disease results from absence of a large protein called dystrophin. **Becker muscular dystrophy** arises from an abnormality in the same gene locus that results in the presence of dystrophin that is abnormal in either amount or molecular structure. Prenatal *diagnosis* is possible by genetic testing. Approximately one third of cases represent new mutations.

*Treatment* is supportive, with physical therapy, bracing, proper wheelchairs, and prevention of scoliosis. A multidisciplinary approach is recommended.

## Becker Dystrophy

Becker dystrophy is a sex-linked muscular dystrophy that is indistinguishable from Duchenne dystrophy, except that onset is later and progression is slower.

## Limb Girdle Dystrophy

Limb girdle dystrophy is usually an autosomal recessive disease presenting with proximal leg and arm weakness. The *clinical manifestations* are similar to those of Duchenne dystrophy but are seen in an older child or teenager and progress slowly over years. By mid-adult life, most patients are wheelchair-bound and incapacitated. The genetic defect may lie with one of the many muscle proteins that interact with the dystrophin-based membrane cytoskeleton.

## Facioscapulohumeral Dystrophy

This condition is usually an autosomal dominant disease presenting in teenagers with facial and proximal arm weakness. The child has mild ptosis, a decrease in facial expression, inability to pucker the lips or whistle, neck weakness, difficulty in fully elevating the arms, diminished scapular mus-

cle width, and thinness of upper arm musculature. Progression is slow, and most patients retain excellent functional capabilities for decades.

## Myotonic Dystrophy

Myotonic dystrophy is exhibited either at birth with severe generalized weakness or in adolescence with slowly progressive facial and distal extremity weakness and myotonia. The adolescent type is the classic illness and is associated with cardiac arrhythmias, cataracts, male pattern baldness, and infertility in males (hypogonadism). The facial appearance is characteristic, with hollowing of muscles around temples, jaw, and neck; ptosis; facial weakness; and drooping of the lower lip. The voice is nasal and mildly dysarthric.

Some mothers with myotonic dystrophy give birth to children with the disease who are immobile and hypotonic, with expressionless faces, tented upper lips, ptosis, absence of sucking and Moro reflexes, and poor swallowing and respiration. Often, weakness and atony of uterine smooth muscle during labor leads to associated hypoxic-ischemic encephalopathy and its sequelae. The presence of congenital contractures, clubfoot, or a history of poor fetal movements indicates intrauterine neuromuscular disease.

Myotonic dystrophy is an autosomal dominant genetic disease caused by progressive expansion of a triplet repeat, GCT, on chromosome 19q13.2–13.3 in a gene designated myotonin protein kinase (MP-PK) (see Chapter 4).

## Congenital Structural Myopathies

Congenital structural myopathies are a group of congenital, often genetic, either nonprogressive or slowly progressive myopathies characterized by abnormal appearance of the muscle biopsy (see Table 18–30). The *etiology* is uncertain.

The typical *clinical manifestations* consist of a hypotonic infant with moderately diffuse weakness involving limbs and face, often accompanied by congenitally dislocated hips, high-arched palate, clubfoot, and contractures at hips, knees, ankles, or elbows secondary to intrauterine weakness. The attainment of motor milestones is moderately to severely delayed and the illness is either static or slowly progressive. Progressive kyphoscoliosis represents a significant problem in some children. Reflexes are diminished, creatine phosphokinase may be mildly elevated, EMG shows a nonspecific myopathic pattern or is normal, and muscle biopsy demonstrates characteristic changes for each entity.

## Metabolic Myopathies

*Glycogen storage disease type II* (Pompe disease) and *muscle carnitine deficiency* are discussed in Chapter 5.

*Mitochondrial myopathies* are characterized by muscle biopsy specimens that sometimes reveal ragged red fibers, representing collections of abnormal mitochondria. Many of these illnesses involve abnormalities of reactions along the respiratory chain. These syndromes have clinical manifestations that are typical of congenital structural myopathies; the course is generally progressive. Some have both CNS and neuromuscular manifestations, such as the MELAS syndrome. Important clues to this class of disorders are elevations of serum lactate and, in those with cerebral involvement, calcification of the basal ganglia.

*Endocrine myopathies* (hyperthyroidism, hypothyroidism, hyperparathyroidism, and Cushing syndrome), either endogenous or produced by exogenous corticosteroid administration, are all associated with proximal muscle weakness (see Chapter 17).

*Hypokalemia* and *hyperkalemia* produce weakness and loss of tendon jerks but do so in the context of a larger clinical picture that usually is easily recognizable (e.g., gastroenteritis, family history, renal failure). This encompassing picture should be specifically treated.

## Laboratory Evaluation

Laboratory evaluation is required in patients who have a neuromuscular disease but in whom a careful history and physical examination have not revealed a specific diagnosis (Table 18–31). EMG and nerve conduction velocity testing is moderately

TABLE 18–31.   Evaluation of Neuromuscular Disease

---

Examine parents
Complete blood count, differential, ESR, electrolytes, BUN, creatinine, glucose, $Ca^{2+}$, $PO_4^-$ alkaline phosphatase, $Mg^{2+}$, bilirubin, blood gases, CPK, lactate, pyruvate
Chest roentgenogram, ECG
Stool: botulism culture and toxin, *Campylobacter* culture
Cerebral spinal fluid (protein, cells)
Tensilon test, neostigmine test
EMG–NCV
Muscle biopsy
MRI of spinal cord

---

BUN = blood urea nitrogen; CPK = creatine phosphokinase; ECG = electrocardiogram; EMG = electromyogram; ESR = erythrocyte sedimentation rate; MRI = magnetic resonance imaging; NCV = nerve conduction velocity.

painful, and muscle biopsy usually requires general anesthesia.

Patients with Duchenne muscular dystrophy, central core myopathy, and other myopathies are susceptible to the life-threatening syndrome of **malignant hyperthermia** during administration of anesthesia comprised of succinylcholine or of potent inhalation agents such as halothane. Often, a family history of unexplained death during operations is noted. Many patients who develop malignant hyperpyrexia appear normal but have mild ptosis or facial muscle wasting and thus may have subclinical myopathies. Other patients at risk include those with kyphoscoliosis, foot deformity, dislocated hips, hypermobile hips, dislocated patella, and other musculoskeletal anomalies. Children without apparent muscle disease inherit malignant hyperpyrexia as an autosomal dominant trait. Malignant hyperpyrexia is exhibited as a rapid rise of body temperature and $P_{CO_2}$, muscle rigidity, cyanosis, hypotension, arrhythmias, and convulsions.

*Diagnosis* of the patient and family with idiopathic malignant hyperthermia is possible with genetic testing or the in vitro muscle contraction test. Excessive tonic contracture on exposure to halothane and caffeine in vitro indicates susceptibility.

*Treatment* with intravenous dantrolene, sodium bicarbonate, and cooling is helpful.

### Sequelae

The major *complications* of neuromuscular illness are the development of contractures, scoliosis, and pneumonia. *Prevention* and *treatment* of contractures with active range of motion exercises and bracing are important because contractures can be painful or inhibit function even when strength is adequate. Surgery to release contractures or to realign tendons is most helpful in nonprogressive or in very slowly progressive conditions. Kyphoscoliosis produces loss of function, disfigurement, and life-threatening decrease of ventilatory reserve. Vigorous prophylaxis and treatment are achieved by maintaining ambulation for as long as possible, with the provision of a properly fitted wheelchair, bracing, and, eventually, stabilizing surgery. Pneumonia in the weak patient may produce heavy secretions that are difficult to clear, progressive atelectasis, and respiratory failure. Anticipatory treatment with antibiotics, hospitalization, chest physical therapy, oxygen, and ventilatory support helps in most cases.

## NEONATAL AND INFANTILE HYPOTONIA

Neonatal and infantile hypotonia poses certain distinctive diagnostic dilemmas. First, some neuromuscular diseases are exhibited at this age, whereas others rarely or never appear. Second, the distinction between neuromuscular paralysis and cerebral depression is much more difficult in neonates than in older children who, when awake and aware, can communicate. Finally, in some infants a unique syndrome of hypotonia, "floppiness," and hypomotility develop, accompanied by only a small loss of observable strength. This syndrome carries a *differential diagnosis* quite different from that of the definitely weak infant (Table 18–32).

## Neonatal Immobility

The first step in evaluating an infant who does not move spontaneously or in response to stimulation is to determine whether *awareness* is intact. If the child is bright-eyed, able to follow objects with the eyes, and tries to smile but is unable to move, cortical activity is intact. If the face and eyes are immobile and the eyelids are ptotic, the problem is more difficult. Other responses include (1) a reaction to light, tactile stimulation, or a bell; (2) eye movement if the eyelids are lifted (fix on the examiner); (3) the presence of the gag and corneal reflexes; and (4) extremities in a posture that suggests cerebral or neuromuscular disease.

If the arm and hand are positioned above the face and dropped, does the hand strike the face as it would in deep coma or paralysis? Are reflexes increased as in cerebral disease, or are they absent? If clinical examination does not settle the question, an EEG will be helpful; cerebral disease sufficient to suppress all movement produces severe slowing of the EEG. If the EEG is normal or near normal and the infant is immobile, a disease of the neuromuscular unit or spinal cord is present.

If the cause of the child's immobility is depression of consciousness, the *differential diagnosis* is very broad (see Table 18–4). The most common causes of neonatal immobility are severe hypoxic-ischemic encephalopathy (HIE) or endogenous or exogenous intoxication. Severe HIE can result acutely in a flaccid, areflexic infant with complete ptosis, ophthalmoplegia, absent corneal and gag reflexes, and pupillary reactions that may be absent or preserved.

Mothers who, during labor, receive drugs that are cerebral depressants, such as magnesium sulfate, barbiturates, narcotics, benzodiazepines, and inhalation anesthetics, can give birth to children who are transiently floppy, apneic, and unresponsive. Rarely, infants whose mothers received magnesium sulfate and who are themselves treated with an aminoglycoside for suspected sepsis develop neuromuscular weakness because these anti-

---

TABLE 18–32.  Approach to Differential Diagnosis of the Floppy Infant

| Weakness | | No Weakness |
|---|---|---|
| *Awareness Intact* | *Cerebral Depression (Flaccid Encephalopathy)* | |
| *Neuromuscular disease* | *Severe brain illness* | *Acute systemic illness* |
| *Spinal cord disease* | Structural | *Mental retardation* |
| Trauma | Infectious | Specific syndromes |
| Tumor | Metabolic (e.g., anoxia) | Down syndrome |
| Vascular compromise | *Intoxication through mother* | Cerebrohepatorenal (Zellweger peroxisomal disorder) |
| Malformation | Magnesium sulfate | Oculocerebrorenal (Lowe syndrome) |
| Spina bifida | Barbiturates | Kinky hair disease (Menkes syndrome–copper metabolism disorder) |
| Syringomyelia | Narcotics | Neonatal adrenal leukodystrophy |
| | Benzodiazepines | *Prader-Willi syndrome* |
| | General anesthesia | *Connective tissue disorder* |
| | *Metabolic abnormality* | Ehlers-Danlos syndrome |
| | Hypoglycemia | Marfan syndrome |
| | Kernicterus | Congenital laxity of ligaments |
| | | *Nutritional-metabolic disease* |
| | | Rickets |
| | | Renal tubular acidosis |
| | | Celiac disease |
| | | Biliary atresia |
| | | Congenital heart disease |
| | | *Benign congenital hypotonia* |

biotics inhibit acetylcholine release at the neuromuscular junction. Finally, infants who are themselves treated with drugs that are cerebral depressants, who develop severe hyperbilirubinemia accompanied by kernicterus, or who develop hypoglycemia can present with a flaccid encephalopathy. Seizures may occur when the metabolic encephalopathies and HIE are present, but they are unusual with drug intoxication.

## Hypotonia Without Major Weakness

Some infants who appear to move well when supine in their cribs clearly are "floppy" when handled or moved. They often are first perceived as having a problem when gross motor milestones, such as rolling over, sitting, and walking, are delayed. When placed on their backs, most of these children are bright-eyed, have expressive faces, and can lift their arms and legs without apparent difficulty. When they are lifted, however, their heads flop, they "slip through" at the shoulders, do not stand upright on their legs, and form an "inverted U" in prone suspension. When placed prone as neonates, they may lie flat instead of having their arms tucked underneath them and their rumps up in the air. Passive tone is decreased, but reflexes are normal.

When this syndrome is present in the severe form in an infant who appears mentally alert but is having severe feeding problems leading to failure to thrive, the probable diagnosis is the **Prader-Willi syndrome**. Paradoxically, severe hyperphagia and obesity develop in early childhood. The presence of a small penis, small testicles, or cryptorchidism in the male is a useful clue to *diagnosis*; small hands and feet may be seen in either sex. Approximately 60–70% of affected individuals have an interstitial deletion of chromosome 15q11q13, the origin of which is consistently paternal.

*Clinical manifestations* similar to those of Prader-Willi syndrome, with or without feeding difficulties, occur in Down syndrome and in some infants who later prove to have nonspecific **mental retardation**. Infants in whom the combination of severe floppiness with mental dullness or cerebral depression is seen may have one of several syndromes (see Table 18–32).

Children who have a **connective tissue disorder**, such as Ehlers-Danlos syndrome, Marfan syndrome, or familial laxity of the ligaments, may exhibit marked passive hypotonia, "double jointedness," and increased skin elasticity but have normal strength and mentation. They usually achieve motor milestones normally and present to the orthopedist with peculiar postures of their feet or an unusual gait.

Finally, there are children who have **benign congenital hypotonia**. Typically, the child has been well, with an uneventful history, and appears robust, except that motor milestones are delayed. The child usually presents at 9–12 mo, is unable to sit well or achieve a sitting position alone, and is unable to crawl up on hands and knees but has good verbal, social, and manipulative skills and an intelligent appearance. The head may lag a bit when the child is lifted, the child slips through slightly at the shoulders, and the extremities are floppy when shaken, but the child briskly kicks arms and legs when sitting in the mother's lap and can easily bring the toes to the mouth. Parents may remember that the infant has seemed floppy from birth. This *diagnosis* represents a miscellaneous category of unknown causes. Some children may have mild congenital myopathies, and others may have mild cerebellar immaturity or dysfunction, but extensive laboratory investigation is unrevealing and not warranted. Most catch up to their peers and appear normal by 3 yr of age. Often, other family members have exhibited a similar developmental pattern.

## References

Behrman RE, Kliegman RM, Arvin AM (eds): Nelson Textbook of Pediatrics, 15th ed. Philadelphia, WB Saunders, 1996, Chapters 558–566.

Buist NRM, Powell BR: Approaches to the evaluation of muscle diseases. Int Pediatr 7:320, 1992.

Dubowitz V: Evaluation and differential diagnosis of the hypotonic infant. Pediatr Rev 6:237, 1985.

Duggan D, Gorospe J, Fanin M, et al: Mutations in the sarcoglycan genes in patients with myopathy. N Engl J Med 336:618, 1997.

Evans O, Vedanarayqnan V: Guillain-Barré syndrome. Pediatr Rev 18:10, 1997.

Higgins J, Kammerman L, Fitz C: Predictors of survival and characteristics of childhood stroke. Neuropediatrics 22:190, 1991.

Miller G, Wessel HB: Diagnosis of dystrophinopathies: Review for the clinician. Pediatr Neurol 9:3, 1993.

Plasma Exchange Sandiglobulin Guillain-Barré Syndrome Trial Group: Randomized trial of plasma exchange, intravenous immunoglobulin, and combined treatments in Guillain-Barré syndrome. Lancet 349:225, 1997.

Ouvrier R: Correlation between the histopathologic, genotypic, and phenotypic features of hereditary peripheral neuropathies in childhood. J Child Neurol 11:135, 1996.

Sébire G, Hollenberg H, Meyer L, et al: High dose methylprednisolone in severe acute transverse myelitis. Arch Dis Child 76:167, 1997.

Tulinius MH, Holme E, Kristiansson B, et al: Mitochondrial encephalomyopathies in childhood: 11. Clinical manifestations and syndromes. J Pediatr 119:251, 1991.

# NEUROCUTANEOUS DISORDERS

The skin, teeth, hair, and nails have the same embryologic origin from neuroectoderm as the brain, and abnormalities of these structures frequently are clues to neurologic disorders. Neurocutaneous disorders are dysplastic in nature, with varying neoplastic tendencies that share CNS lesions with visceral and cutaneous abnormalities. The term *phakomatosis* refers to tuberous sclerosis and neurofibromatosis and designates the cutaneous lesions as "mother spots" or "birthmarks." Not all of the so-called neurocutaneous disorders, however, have characteristic cutaneous lesions, and not all are of neuroectodermal origin. Von Hippel–Lindau disease does not have characteristic cutaneous lesions, and both von Hippel–Lindau disease and Sturge-Weber disease are of mesenchymal rather than ectodermal origin. More than 40 conditions are referred to as neurocutaneous syndrome, but neurofibromatosis, tuberous sclerosis, Sturge-Weber disease, von Hippel–Lindau disease, and ataxia–telangiectasia are the major disorders.

## NEUROFIBROMATOSIS

This complex and heterogeneous autosomal dominant disorder presents in two distinct fashions, neurofibromatosis (NF) I and NF II. Its frequency is approximately 1:3000. The gene for NF I is located on chromosome 17 and encodes for a probable GTPase tumor suppressor gene called neurofibromin. The gene for NF II is located on chromosome 22.

The major clinical features of NF I are the characteristic pigmented skin lesion referred to as the *café au lait* spot (see Table 18–1), pigmented hamartomas of the iris called Lisch nodules, and neurofibromas of the skin.

*Café au lait* spots eventually are present in more than 90% of patients who have NF I, but they may take a year to appear. More than five spots larger than 5 mm should suggest the possibility of NF I. In addition, freckling commonly is seen in the axillae or other intertriginous areas in NF I. The margins of the spots may be smooth or irregular.

*Lisch nodules* also increase in frequency with age and eventually are present in more than 90% of adults who have NF I. Approximately 25% of children exhibit these iris nodules.

*Neurofibromas* may be discrete or diffuse and are composed of various combinations of Schwann cells, fibroblasts, neurons, and vascular elements. Although benign histologically and almost always involving skin, they may invade and compromise viscera, the spinal cord, or blood vessels, occasionally producing life-threatening airway, neurologic, or vascular compromise. Other manifestations include optic glioma, pheochromocytoma, skeletal dysplasias, macrocephaly, and renovascular hypertension.

Once present, as a rule, the lesions are progressive. Surgical removal of significant approachable tumors is a mainstay of *treatment*. Orthopedic management of scoliosis and pseudoarthrosis is indicated. The response of seizures to anticonvulsants and of attention deficit disorders to medication is unpredictable. Concern for the psychologic burdens of this disorder and attention to genetic counseling should be emphasized.

NF II, or central neurofibromatosis, is not associated with *café au lait* spots, Lisch nodules, or other peripheral manifestations. These children have associated brain tumors. Bilateral acoustic neuromas are diagnostic; other children have other tumors, such as meningiomas or neoplasms of glial origin.

## TUBEROUS SCLEROSIS

Tuberous sclerosis is an autosomal dominant disorder characterized by adenoma sebaceum, mental retardation, and seizures. Like neurofibromatosis, developmental abnormalities of ectoderm result in disorders of segmentation and migration of cells of the brain that frequently are associated with seizures, brain tumor, and/or intellectual impairment. Tuberous sclerosis is a frequent cause of infantile spasms.

The *clinical manifestations* of tuberous sclerosis are quite different when the disorder is encountered in infancy compared with childhood or adolescence. The clinical characteristics of tuberous sclerosis that occurs in infancy include abnormal hair pigmentation, hypopigmented skin (ash leaf) macules, seizures, rhabdomyoma of the heart, mental retardation, and retinal hamartomas.

The lesions of *adenoma sebaceum*, which actually are vascular angiokeratomas (angiofibromas) surrounding sweat glands, usually are not encountered until 2–5 yr of age. These skin lesions predominate in the malar regions and appear as pink or red macules. *Seizures*, particularly mixed astatic-akinetic and generalized tonic-clonic seizures, are prevalent in early childhood as well. In later childhood, *angioleiomyomas* involving the kidney result in hypertension and abdominal masses. *Shagreen patches*, elevated rough plaques of skin with a predilection for the lumbar and gluteal regions, develop in late childhood to early adolescence. Nodules of tissue beneath the nails *(subungual keratomas)* also become evident at this age.

*Intracranial calcifications* typically are subependymal in location, with a predilection for the regions around the intraventricular foramina of Monro. Subependymal lesions have a propensity to enlarge, resulting in significant intracranial masses or obstructive hydrocephalus.

## STURGE-WEBER DISEASE

Sturge-Weber disease is characterized by a unilateral pink-purple vascular nevus (hemangiomata) over the face ("port-wine nevus") and a similar angiomatous malformation involving the meninges over the ipsilateral side of the brain. The *facial nevus* always involves the region between the forehead and eye (the distribution of the first division of the trigeminal nerve) when the meninges are involved but also may involve the face in the distribution of the second and third divisions of the trigeminal nerve in varying combinations. The disease is not hereditary.

The *meningeal nevus* is a slow-flow angioma resulting in hypoxia and encephalomalacia of the developing underlying cortex and is most marked over the occipital and posterior parietal regions of the brain. The vascular lesion and accompanying brain encephalomalacia (cortical atrophy) result in seizures, progressive mental retardation, and contralateral hemiparesis. The seizures as well as the hemiparesis and behavioral abnormalities progress as the child becomes older. Calcium becomes detectable in the gyri of the brain underlying the angioma, and, as the intervening sulci are spared, the radiologic picture of "tram track" or "railroad track" calcifications is seen in about 60% of cases.

The *treatment* of Sturge-Weber disease is controversial. Children treated with successful early surgical resection appear to develop more normally and have better seizure control than those treated with anticonvulsants alone. The degree of hemiparesis also is significantly less in those managed surgically, but significant morbidity and mortality as a result of the hemispherectomy are noted.

The vascular nevus involves the canal of Schlemm in about 25% of children (those with lesions above and below the orbit) and results in obstructive glaucoma. Ophthalmologic evaluations and treatment therefore are mandatory in these children. Laser treatment may improve the cutaneous lesion.

### References

Behrman RE, Kliegman RM, Arvin AM (eds): Nelson Textbook of Pediatrics, 15th ed. Philadelphia, WB Saunders, 1996, Chapter 546.

Gomez MR (ed): Neurocutaneous Diseases: A Practical Approach. Boston, Butterworth, 1987.

Korf BR: Diagnostic outcome in children with multiple café au lait spots. Pediatrics 90:924, 1992.

Riccardi VM: Type 1 neurofibromatosis and the pediatric patient. Curr Probl Pediatr 22:66, 1992.

# MOVEMENT DISORDERS

Movement disorders are due to abnormalities of the extrapyramidal system, which is composed of the basal ganglia and its connections. Disorders of movement may be *bradykinetic*, slowness of movement; *hypokinetic*, paucity of movement; or *hyperkinetic*, excessive involuntary movements. Bradykinesia and hypokinesia describe the agonizingly slow gait, halting speech patterns, apparent inactivity, and paucity of facial expression seen in children with extrapyramidal disorders. The hyperkinetic disorders are associated with many disease states and, as a group, are activated by stress and fatigue but disappear in sleep. *Segmental myoclonic* abnormalities refer to activity in isolated muscle groups (e.g., the palatal myoclonus) that does not disappear in sleep.

## CHOREA

Chorea is a hyperkinetic, rapid, unsustained, irregular, purposeless, nonpatterned movement. Muscle tone is decreased. Choreiform movement abnormalities may be congenital, familial, metabolic, vascular, toxic, infectious, or neoplastic in origin. The movements may occur alone or as part of a more extensive neurologic disorder (e.g., Sydenham chorea, Huntington chorea, cerebral palsy, Wilson disease, reactions to toxins and drugs). Fidgety behavior, inability to sit still, clumsiness, dysarthria, and an awkward gait may occur. The exact site of dysfunction within the extrapyramidal system is unknown.

## ATHETOSIS

Athetosis is a hyperkinetic, slow, coarse, writhing movement that is more pronounced in distal muscles. Muscle tone is increased. Athetosis frequently is seen in combination with chorea (choreoathetosis) and usually is present in conjunction with other neurologic signs. It may be seen in virtually all the disorders mentioned for chorea, but the most prominent cause is encephalopathy. Athetosis is a prominent feature of Hallervorden-Spatz disease, Wilson disease, and Pelizaeus-Merzbacher dystrophy.

## DYSTONIA

Dystonia is a hyperkinetic, sustained, slow, twisting motion (torsion spasm) that may progress to a fixed posture and can be activated by repetitive movement (i.e., action dystonia). It usually begins in the legs when appendicular muscles are involved and in the neck or trunk when axial muscles are involved. Dystonia is a movement disorder with many causes and associated neurologic signs. *Tardive dyskinesia* usually is associated with antipsychotic drug use; darting tongue movements, incessant flexion and extension of the distal muscles, standing and marching in place, and a perception of restlessness are common.

## TREMOR

Tremor is a hyperkinetic, rhythmic, oscillatory movement caused by simultaneous contractions of antagonistic muscles. The amplitude and frequency are regular. In children, tremor is usually of physiologic, familial, or cerebellar origin but may be seen in association with other disease processes (thyrotoxicosis, hypoglycemia, Wilson disease) or drugs (bronchodilators, amphetamines, or tricyclic antidepressants).

## MYOCLONUS

Myoclonus is a hyperkinetic, brief flexion contraction of a muscle group, resulting in a sudden jerk.

Myoclonus may be epileptic or nonepileptic. Nonepileptic myoclonus is distinguished from tremor in that it is a simple contraction of an agonist muscle, whereas tremor is a simultaneous contraction of agonist and antagonist muscles. Myoclonus is seen as a manifestation of various epilepsies as well as of infectious, toxic, and metabolic encephalopathies.

## TIC

Tic movements are similar to myoclonus but are much more stereotyped and involve the face, shoulder, and arm. Motor tics in association with vocal tics are characteristic of Tourette syndrome.

**Tourette syndrome** consists of a chronic tic disorder that begins in early childhood. The severity and form of the tics vary over months and years; vocal tics are common. The pathophysiology underlying the tics is unknown, but a family history of tics is elicited in more than 50% of cases. *Treatment* consists of psychologic support and pharmacologic therapy.

### References

Behrman RE, Kliegman RM, Arvin AM (eds): Nelson Textbook of Pediatrics. 15th ed. Philadelphia, WB Saunders, 1996, Chapter 547.

Pronzatelli M: Advances in the treatment of pediatric movement disorders. Int Pediatr 10:250, 1995.

Chapter

19

# COMMON ORTHOPAEDIC PROBLEMS OF CHILDREN

George H. Thompson

## GENERAL CONSIDERATIONS

Multiple mechanisms produce orthopaedic problems that are specific to childhood; other pathologic mechanisms are common to all age groups (Table 19–1). Most pediatric orthopaedic problems involve the spine and lower extremities, especially the hips and feet. Upper extremity abnormalities, other than trauma, occur less frequently. It is important to have a basic understanding of the various pediatric musculoskeletal system disorders, including diagnosis and nonoperative management. In addition to the challenge of identifying pathologic processes, the necessity of clearly discerning ongoing physiologic, developmental, or matura-

tional changes from abnormal events confronts the pediatrician. What may be physiologic at one age may be pathologic at another.

### IN UTERO POSITIONING

In the neonate, the effect of intrauterine positioning may be evident. The in utero position produces joint and muscle contractures and affects torsional and angular alignment of long bones, especially of the lower extremities (Fig. 19–1). All normal full-term newborns have 20–30 degree hip and knee flexion contractures. These decrease to neutral by 4–6 mo of age. The newborn hip externally rotates in extension 80–90 degrees and has limited internal

TABLE 19–1. Mechanisms of Common Pediatric Orthopaedic Problems

| Category | Mechanism | Example |
|---|---|---|
| *Congenital* | | |
| Malformation | Teratogenesis prior to 12th wk of gestation | Spina bifida |
| Disruption | Amniotic band constriction | Extremity amputation |
| | Fetal varicella infection | Limb scar/atrophy |
| Deformation | Leg compression | Developmental hip dislocation |
| | Neck compression | Torticollis |
| Dysplasia | Abnormal cell growth or metabolism | Osteogenesis imperfecta |
| | | Skeletal dysplasias |
| *Acquired* | | |
| Infection | Pyogenic–hematogenous spread | Septic arthritis, osteomyelitis |
| Inflammation | Antigen–antibody reaction | Systemic lupus erythematosus |
| | Immune mediated | Juvenile rheumatoid arthritis |
| Trauma | Mechanical forces, overuse | Child abuse, sports injuries, accidents, fractures, dislocations, tendonitis |
| Tumor | Primary bone tumor | Osteosarcoma |
| | Metastasis to bone from other site | Neuroblastoma |
| | Bone marrow tumor | Leukemia, lymphoma |

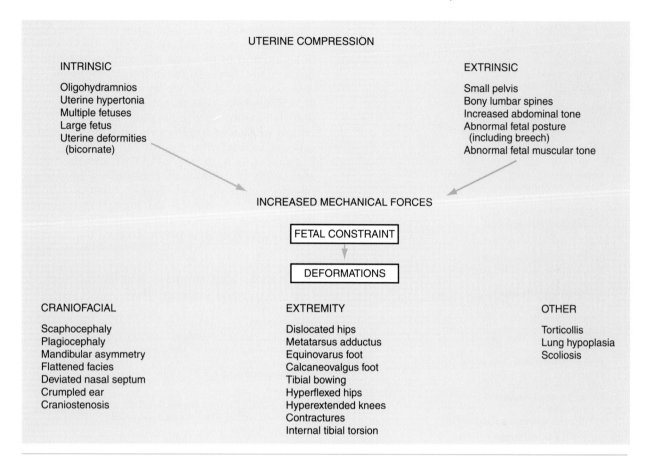

UTERINE COMPRESSION

INTRINSIC

Oligohydramnios
Uterine hypertonia
Multiple fetuses
Large fetus
Uterine deformities
 (bicornate)

EXTRINSIC

Small pelvis
Bony lumbar spines
Increased abdominal tone
Abnormal fetal posture
 (including breech)
Abnormal fetal muscular tone

INCREASED MECHANICAL FORCES

FETAL CONSTRAINT

DEFORMATIONS

CRANIOFACIAL

Scaphocephaly
Plagiocephaly
Mandibular asymmetry
Flattened facies
Deviated nasal septum
Crumpled ear
Craniostenosis

EXTREMITY

Dislocated hips
Metatarsus adductus
Equinovarus foot
Calcaneovalgus foot
Tibial bowing
Hyperflexed hips
Hyperextended knees
Contractures
Internal tibial torsion

OTHER

Torticollis
Lung hypoplasia
Scoliosis

FIGURE 19–1. Deformation abnormalities resulting from uterine compression.

rotation to 0–10 degrees. The normal newborn foot also may reflect the in utero position. Most commonly, in utero the feet are in the tucked-under position, which can be observed after birth. On inspection, the forefoot appears adducted or deviated inwardly with respect to the hindfoot, the heel may be inverted, and the foot tends to be in equinus pointed down at the ankle. If the foot can be positioned so that the lateral border is straight, the heel slightly everted, and the foot dorsiflexed to above a right angle, the clinical diagnosis of normal in utero positioning is validated.

The face also may be distorted, whereas the spine and upper extremities are less affected by in utero positioning. The effects of in utero position, therefore, are physiologic in origin but produce parental concern. The child may be 3–4 yr of age before the intrauterine effects resolve.

## DEVELOPMENTAL MILESTONES AND NEUROLOGIC MATURATION

Neurologic maturation, marked by the passage of motor milestones at the regular intervals, is im-

portant for normal musculoskeletal development (see Chapter 1). A trophic relationship exists between skeletal form and gross motor development. The concept of normal neurologic development, therefore, must be included in the definition of a normal musculoskeletal system. Any process that produces a neurologic abnormality may secondarily cause an aberration of normal skeletal growth. Normal muscle function is necessary for normal skeletal growth. Any disorder that primarily affects skeletal muscle may produce abnormalities of skeletal growth and development.

## GAIT

Disturbances of gait, including *limp*, are common manifestations of pediatric orthopaedic disorders (Tables 19–2 and 19–3). Understanding the normal development aspects of gait is helpful in distinguishing maturational from pathologic processes. Normal gait (walking on level ground) is composed of a stance phase and a swing phase. The gait cycle is the interval between stance phases on

TABLE 19–2.  Differential Diagnosis of Gait Disturbances (Limping)

**Early Walker (1–3 yr)**

*Painful Limp*

Septic arthritis/osteomyelitis
Transient monoarticular synovitis
Occult trauma ("toddler's fracture")
Intervertebral discitis

*Painless Limp*

Developmental dysplasia of the hip
Neuromuscular disorder
  Cerebral palsy
Leg length inequality

**Child (3–10 yr)**

*Painful Limp*

Septic arthritis/osteomyelitis
Transient monoarticular synovitis
Trauma
Rheumatologic disorders
  Juvenile rheumatoid arthritis
Intervertebral discitis
Legg-Calvé-Perthes disease (LCPD)

*Painless Limp*

Developmental dysplasia of the hip
Legg-Calvé-Perthes disease
Leg length inequality
Neuromuscular disorder
  Cerebral palsy
  Muscular dystrophy (Duchenne)

**Adolescent (11 yr–maturity)**

*Painful Limp*

Septic arthritis/osteomyelitis
Trauma
Rheumatologic disorder
Slipped capital femoral epiphysis (SCFE): acute; unstable

*Painless Limp*

Slipped capital femoral epiphysis: chronic; stable
Developmental dysplasia of the hip: acetabular dysplasia
Leg length inequality
Neuromuscular disorder

cluding sepsis), or acquired disorders (see Table 19–3). Stance phase and stride length are shortened in an attempt to spend as little time as possible on the involved limb. Trunk shift to the opposite side also decreases stress while maintaining balance. This is referred to as an **antalgic gait**. A painless limp is characterized by normal stance phase but with a persistent trunk sway. This type of gait is called a **Trendelenburg gait**.

Painless limping (see Table 19–2) may be associated with neuromuscular disorders producing muscle weakness about the hip, especially in the gluteus medius muscle, the major hip abductor. This muscle stabilizes the pelvis during stance phase and prevents a pelvic drop to the opposite

TABLE 19–3.  Mechanisms of Gait Disturbances and Extremity Pain

**Mechanical**

Trauma, fracture, sprain
Sports injury; overuse injury
Child abuse
Hip dysplasia (DDH)

**Osseous**

Legg-Calvé-Perthes disease (LCPD)
Slipped capital femoral epiphysis (SCFE)
Osteomyelitis
Discitis
Osteoid osteoma

**Articular**

Septic arthritis
Toxic synovitis
Rheumatic disease (JRA, SLE)
Hemophilia

**Neurologic**

Guillain-Barré syndrome (other peripheral neuropathies)
Intoxication
Cerebellar ataxia
Brain tumor
Lesion occupying spinal cord space
Myopathy
Hemiplegia
Sympathetic reflex dystrophy

**Hematologic**

Sickle cell pain crisis
Leukemia
Metastatic tumor
Bone tumor
Langerhans cell histiocytosis

**Other**

Kawasaki disease
Conversion reaction
Gaucher disease
Scurvy
Rickets

DDH = developmental dysplasia of the hip; JRA = juvenile rheumatoid arthritis; SLE = systemic lupus erythematosus.

the same limb. The stance phase (60%) is performed when the foot, which bears weight, contacts the ground; it begins with the heel strike and ends with the toe-off. In the swing phase (40%), the foot is off the ground. The early child's or toddler's (12–18 mo) gait is very hesitant and inconsistent. The gait is broad based and characterized by rapid cadence, short steps, flatfoot initial ground contact, not accompanied by the reciprocal arm swing. A 2-yr-old has increased velocity and step length and a diminished cadence. Normal adult gait is achieved by 3–7 yr of age.

*Limping* is either painless or painful (see Table 19–2). A painful limp is characterized by acute onset and usually is due to trauma, infection (inside. Trauma or weakness of this muscle or inflammatory hip disorders are the most common causes of limping. Disorders that have bilateral involvement produce a **waddling gait**.

Knee pathology, usually from trauma, can produce a limp by limiting knee flexion and causing the child to circumduct the leg and elevate the pelvis during swing phase. It also produces a shortened stance phase. Poor dorsiflexion of the foot resulting from weakness (peroneal nerve injury or peripheral neuropathy) or trauma causes increased knee flexion for toe clearance during the swing phase, resulting in a **drop-foot gait**.

Toe-walking, which is common in early walkers, may be due to habit, leg length discrepancy, underlying neuromuscular disorder (cerebral palsy), or a congenital contracture of the gastrocnemius and soleus muscles (Achilles tendon or heel cord).

## GROWTH AND DEVELOPMENT

During the growing years, the ends of long bone contain a much greater proportion of cartilage than after maturity (Fig. 19–2). The high cartilage content (articular and physeal) leads to a unique vulnerability from trauma and metaphyseal infections. The infections may involve the physis and joint space.

Special anatomic features within the child's skeletal system stimulate and support the various kinds of skeletal growth that continuously occur in the immature skeletal (Fig. 19–3). The epiphyseal growth plate, also called the *physis*, provides for longitudinal growth of the bones. Articular cartilage provides for enlargement of the bone ends and also for growth of some of the small bones largely covered by articular cartilage, such as the carpals and tarsals. The perichondrium and the

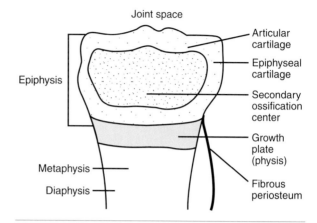

FIGURE 19–3.  Schematic of long bone structure. The shaft, or *diaphysis*, is distal to the *metaphysis*, which is the closest extension of endochondral bone. The epiphyseal growth plate *(physis)* is the avascular cartilage between the articular surface and the metaphyseal bone. The growth plate is the region of longitudinal bone growth. The contribution to eventual bone length varies: 80% for the proximal humerus, 20% for the distal humerus, 75% for the distal radius, 80% for the distal ulna, 70% for the distal femur, 57% for the proximal tibia, and 60% for the proximal fibula. When growth is complete, the epiphyseal growth plate is ossified or closed. The cartilaginous epiphyseal plate is supported by internal interdigitation with the metaphyseal bone and externally by the insertion of the fibrous periosteum. (Modified from Shapiro F: Epiphyseal disorders. N Engl J Med 317:1702, 1987. Used with permission.)

periosteum provide appositional growth or circumferential growth of the cartilage and skeletal structures, respectively. Trauma, infection, nutritional deficiency (rickets), regional soft tissue processes, inborn errors of metabolism (mucopolysaccharidosis, mucolipidosis, Gaucher disease, and disorders of collagen or cartilage synthesis), and other metabolic processes (oxalosis, renal tubular acidosis, uremia, and endocrine excess or deficiencies) may affect each of these processes, producing a distinct aberration in the particular growth function.

## ORTHOPAEDIC TERMINOLOGY

The terminology used in orthopaedics to describe position, motion, and function can be confusing. Some common orthopaedic terms are presented in Table 19–4.

### References

Behrman RE, Kliegman RM, Arvin AM (eds): Nelson Textbook of Pediatrics, 15th ed. Philadelphia, WB Saunders, 1996, Part II.
Thompson GH: Gait disturbances. *In* Kliegman RM (ed): Practi-

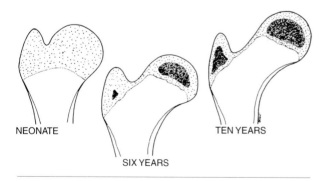

NEONATE                    TEN YEARS

SIX YEARS

FIGURE 19–2.  Lightly stippled areas represent cartilage composition, whereas heavily darkened areas are zones of ossification. (From Tachdjian MO: Congenital Dislocation of the Hip. New York, Churchill Livingstone, 1982, p 104.)

**TABLE 19–4.  Glossary of Orthopaedic Terminology**

| | |
|---|---|
| *Abduction* | Movement away from the midline |
| *Adduction* | Movement toward and possibly across the midline |
| *Anteversion* | Increased angulation of the femoral head and neck with respect to the knee in the frontal plane |
| *Apophysis* | Bone growth center that is not a growth plate and that has a strong muscle insertion (e.g., greater trochanter of femur) |
| *Arthroplasty* | Surgical reconstruction of a joint |
| *Arthrotomy* | Surgical incision into a joint |
| *Calcaneus* | Dorsiflexion of hindfoot |
| *Cavovarus* | High longitudinal or medial arch of foot with plantar-flexed supinated forefoot and hindfoot varus |
| *Cavus* | High longitudinal arch of the foot (usually plantar-flexed forefoot) |
| *Dislocation* | Complete loss of contact between two joint surfaces |
| *Equinus* | Plantar flexion of the forefoot, hindfoot, or entire foot |
| *Extension* | Means to straighten, and is the reverse of flexion |
| *External rotation* | External rotation, away from the midline |
| *Flexion* | Means to bend |
| *Internal rotation* | Inward rotation, toward the midline |
| *Osteotomy* | Surgical division of a bone |
| *Subluxation* | Incomplete loss of contact between two joint surfaces |
| *Valgum* | Angulation of a bone or joint in which the apex is toward the midline; genu valgum or knock-knee |
| *Varum* | Angulation of a bone or joint away from the midline; genu varum or bowleg |

cal Strategies in Pediatric Diagnosis and Therapy. Philadelphia, WB Saunders, 1996, pp 757–778.

Todd FN, Lamoreaux LW, Skinner SR, et al: Variations in the gait of normal children: A graph applicable to the documentation of abnormalities. J Bone Joint Surg 71A:196, 1989.

## THE HIP

The hip is a ball (femoral head) and socket (acetabulum) joint that provides the skeleton with structural balance and stability. The femoral head and acetabulum have a trophic relationship and are interdependent for normal growth and development (Fig. 19–4). When this trophic relationship is interrupted, abnormal hip development follows. Additionally, muscle balance and activity related to appropriate gross motor development are essential to normal development of the hip. The blood supply to the capital femoral epiphysis (CFE) or femoral head is quite unique. The CFE and femoral

neck lie intracapsularly, but the blood supply from the retinacular vessels is extraosseous, lying on the surface of the femoral neck and entering the epiphysis peripherally. This makes the blood supply to the femoral head vulnerable to damage from septic arthritis, trauma, and other vascular insults. *Avascular necrosis* or *osteonecrosis*, either as an idiopathic process or secondary to other disorders, is a common problem in children.

### DEVELOPMENTAL DYSPLASIA OF THE HIP

This disorder represents abnormal development or dislocation of the hip; the hips at birth usually are not dislocated but rather "dislocatable." Dislocations tend to occur following delivery. Because dislocations are not truly congenital in origin, the term developmental dysplasia of the hip (DDH)

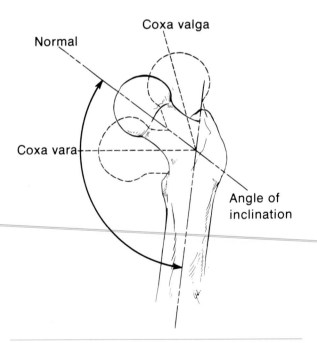

**FIGURE 19–4.** Coxa vara and coxa valga. The neck-shaft angle is measured on an anteroposterior roentgenogram. This angle is formed by a line drawn through the femoral shaft center and one bisecting the head and neck. Normally, the value of this angle decreases with age. A reasonably accurate neck-shaft angle measurement may be made on an anteroposterior pelvic roentgenogram by placing the patient's hips in maximum internal rotation. Otherwise, because of the illusion caused by anteversion or external rotation on a one-plane roentgenogram, the measured neck-shaft angle value may be considerably larger than the true value. Internal femur rotation has a negligible effect on the neck-shaft angle. (From Chung SMK: Hip Disorders in Infants and Children. Philadelphia, Lea & Febiger, 1981, p 85.)

rather than congenital dysplasia or dislocation is suggested. DDH is classified into two major groups: *typical*, in a neurologically normal infant, and *teratologic*, when there is an underlying neuromuscular disorder (myelodysplasia or arthrogryposis multiplex congenita) or syndrome complex. The teratologic type of dislocation occurs in utero. Typical DDH is the most common form and is discussed next.

***Etiology.*** The causes of DDH are multifactorial. *Physiologic* factors include (1) positive family history (20%), (2) generalized ligamentous laxity, (3) maternal estrogen and other hormones associated with pelvic relaxation, and (4) female predominance (9:1). *Mechanical* factors include (1) primigravida (first birth), (2) breech presentation, oligohydramnios, and (3) postnatal positioning. The positive family history and the generalized ligamentous laxity are related factors. Maternal estrogens and other hormones associated with pelvic relaxation also result in further, although temporary, relaxation of the newborn hip joint.

Approximately 60% of children with typical DDH are first born and 30–50% are in a breech position. In this presentation, the fetal pelvis is positioned in the maternal pelvis, which results in extreme hip flexion and limitation of hip motion. Increased hip flexion results in stretching of the already lax capsule and ligament teres. It also produces posterior uncoverage of the femoral head. This position, as well as decreased hip motion, alters the normal trophic relationship of the hip, resulting in abnormal development of the cartilaginous acetabulum.

The sex ratio of infants with DDH who developed in a breech presentation declines to 2:1 (female to male). This decline substantiates the importance of the mechanical factors of the breech position in the development of DDH. There is also an association of congenital muscular torticollis (14–20%) and metatarsus adductus (1–10%) with DDH. The presence of either of these two conditions requires a careful examination of the hips.

*Postnatal* factors also are important determinants in the development of DDH. Maintaining the hips in the position of adduction and extension is a major factor leading to dislocation. Placing the extremities in this position puts the unstable hip under pressure as a result of the normally present hip flexion and abduction contractures. As a consequence, the femoral head can be displaced from the acetabulum over several days, weeks, or perhaps months.

***Clinical Manifestations.*** Common physical findings in infants with DDH include:

- A positive Barlow test (unstable or dislocatable hip)
- A positive Ortolani test (dislocated hip)
- Limitation of hip abduction
- Asymmetric number of thigh skinfolds
- Uneven knee levels (Galeazzi sign)
- Absence of normal knee flexion contracture

The *Barlow test* is the most important maneuver in examination of the newborn hip. This is a provocative test that attempts to dislocate the unstable hip. The examiner stabilizes the infant's pelvis with one hand and then flexes and adducts the opposite hip and applies a posterior force (Fig. 19–5). If the hip is dislocatable, this usually is readily felt. After release of the posterior pressure, the hip will usually relocate spontaneously. It has been estimated that only 1:100 newborns have clinically unstable hips (subluxation or dislocation) but only 1:800–1000 infants eventually develops a true dislocation.

The *Ortolani test* is a maneuver to reduce a recently dislocated hip. The result is most likely to be positive in infants 1–2 mo of age because adequate time must have passed for the true dislocation to have occurred. In this test, the infant's thigh is flexed and abducted and the femoral head is lifted anteriorly into the acetabulum (Fig. 19–6). If reduction is possible, the relocation will be felt as a "clunk," not heard as a "click." After 2 mo of age, manual reduction of a dislocated hip is not usually possible because of the development of soft tissue contractures.

*Limitation of hip abduction* is indicative of soft tissue contractures and may indicate DDH (Fig. 19–7). Conversely, hip abduction contractures may indicate dysplasia of the contralateral hip.

An *asymmetric number of thigh skinfolds* and apparent shortening of an extremity when the supine infant's feet are placed together on the examining table with the hips and knees flexed (positive Galeazzi sign) is suggestive of DDH because these findings indicate proximal displacement of the femoral head. In older or walking children, complaints of limping, waddling (bilateral DDH), increased lumbar lordosis (swayback), toe-walking, and in-toeing may be associated with an unrecognized DDH.

A common concern regarding an unstable hip is the presence of a hip "click." These usually are not pathologic and are secondary to breaking the surface tension across the hip joint, snapping of gluteal tendons, patellofemoral motion, or femorotibial (knee) rotation.

***Roentgenographic Evaluation.*** Ultrasonography is a popular method for initial evaluation and following the results of conservative treatment in newborns and infants (<3 mo) with DDH. Hip stability as well as acetabular development can be assessed accurately by an experienced ultrasonographer, and this modality avoids the use of ionizing radiation.

Roentgenographic evaluation is useful in older infants (>3 mo) and includes an anteroposterior (AP) and Lauenstein (frog) lateral roentgenographs of the pelvis. The ossific nucleus does not appear until 4–6 mo of age and may be further delayed in infants with DDH. Line measurements usually are made in order to determine the relationship of the femoral head to the acetabulum. Arthrography, computed tomography (CT), and magnetic resonance imaging (MRI) may be beneficial in select or difficult cases.

***Treatment.*** The treatment of DDH is individualized and depends on the child's age at diagnosis. The goal is a concentric and stable reduction that results in normal growth and development of the hip.

When an unstable hip is recognized at birth, maintenance of the hip in the position of flexion and abduction ("human" position) for 1–2 mo usually is sufficient. This position maintains reduction of the femoral head and allows for tightening of the ligamentous structures as well as for stimulation of normal growth and development of the acetabulum. Usually, double or triple diapers are sufficient in neonates. Treatment usually is continued until there is clinical stability of the hip and the radiographic or ultrasonography measurements are within normal limits. Between 1 and 6 mo of age, the Pavlik harness is indicated. It places the hips in the human position by flexing the hips more than 90 degrees (preferably 100–110 degrees) and providing gentle abduction. This redirects the femoral head toward the acetabulum. Usually, spontaneous relocation of the femoral head occurs within 3–4 wk. The Pavlik harness is approximately 95% successful in dysplastic or subluxated hips and 80% in true dislocations.

If a reduction does not occur, a surgical closed reduction is attempted. This consists of preliminary skin traction for 1–3 wk to stretch the soft tissue contractures, percutaneous adductor tenotomy,

**FIGURE 19–6.** Ortolani (reduction) test. With the infant relaxed and content on a firm surface, the hips and knees are flexed to 90 degrees. The hips are examined one at a time. The examiner grasps the infant's thigh with the middle finger over the greater trochanter, and lifts the thigh to bring the femoral head from its dislocated posterior position to opposite the acetabulum. Simultaneously, the thigh is gently abducted, reducing the femoral head into the acetabulum. In a positive finding, the examiner senses reduction by a palpable, nearly audible "clunk." (From Robert N, Hensinger MD: Congenital dislocation of the hip. Clin Symp 31[1]:5, 1979. Copyright 1979. CIBA-GEIGY Corporation. Reproduced with permission from Clinical Symposia by Frank H. Netter, M.D. All rights reserved.)

closed reduction, and application of a hip spica cast in the "human" position. In the older infant (6–18 mo), surgical closed reduction is the major method of treatment. If, at the time of closed reduction, the hip shows significant residual instability, an open reduction may be indicated. Beyond 18 mo of age, the dysplastic changes are so advanced that open reduction followed by pelvic or femoral osteotomy, or both, is usually necessary.

*Complications.* The most important and severe complication of DDH is avascular necrosis (osteonecrosis) of the capital femoral head or CFE. This is an iatrogenic complication. Reduction of the femoral head under pressure produces cartilaginous compression, and this can result in occlusion of the intra-articular, extraosseous epiphyseal vessels and produce partial or total CFE infarction. Revascularization follows, but abnormal growth and development may occur, especially if the physis is severely damaged. The hip is most vulnerable to this complication prior to the development of the ossific nucleus (4–6 mo).

## SEPTIC ARTHRITIS AND OSTEOMYELITIS

See Chapter 10.

## TRANSIENT MONOARTICULAR SYNOVITIS

Transient synovitis of the hip is a common cause of limping in young children and is characterized by acute onset of pain, limp, and mild restriction of hip motion, especially abduction and internal rotation. This is a diagnosis of exclusion because septic arthritis or osteomyelitis of the hip must be excluded.

*Etiology.* The etiology of transient synovitis remains uncertain. Possible causes have included active or recent infection, especially viral syndromes; trauma; and hypersensitivity. Approximately 70% of involved children have a nonspecific viral upper respiratory infection 7–14 days prior to the onset of hip symptoms.

*Diagnosis.* Biopsy specimens from the hip joint of patients with transient synovitis have demonstrated synovial hypertrophy secondary to nonspecific inflammatory reaction. Hip joint aspirations, if necessary, will be negative, although a small synovial effusion is common.

*Clinical Manifestations.* The mean age of onset is 6 yr, with most patients being 3–8 yr of age. The acute onset of pain is felt in the groin, anterior thigh, or knee. It must be remembered that any child with nontraumatic anterior thigh or knee pain must be evaluated carefully for hip pathology because this is the site of referred pain. Patients usually are ambulatory and the hip is not held in the flexed, abducted, and externally rotated position typical of infection unless a significant effusion is present. Children are usually afebrile and the white blood cell count and erythrocyte sedimentation rate (ESR) are normal or slightly elevated.

*Roentgenographic Evaluation.* AP and frog lateral roentgenographs of the pelvis are usually normal. Occasionally, ultrasound examination of the hip may be useful in demonstrating the hip joint effusion. Bone scans help differentiate a septic process.

*Treatment.* Bed rest (~7 days) and non–weight

## ABDUCTION TEST

1) 90° — Normal at birth to 1 month of age

2) 70° — Often normal, 1 to 9 months of age

3) 60° — Suspected significant limitation

4) 50° — Definite limitation

FIGURE 19–7. Hip abduction test. Place the infant supine, flex the hips 90 degrees, and fully abduct. While the normal abduction range is quite broad, one can suspect hip disease in any patient who lacks more than 35–45 degrees of abduction. (From Chung SMK: Hip Disorders in Infants and Children. Philadelphia, Lea & Febiger, 1981, p 69.)

bearing until the pain resolves, followed by limited activities (1–2 wk) thereafter, are the treatments of choice. This sometimes is difficult because children want to return to normal activities when their symptoms resolve. If the child returns to normal activities too early, exacerbation of symptoms can occur. Nonsteroidal anti-inflammatory agents (NSAIDs) may be helpful.

## LEGG-CALVÉ-PERTHES DISEASE

Legg-Calvé-Perthes disease (LCPD) is idiopathic avascular necrosis (osteonecrosis) of the CFE and the associated complications in a growing child. This disorder is caused by an interruption of the CFE blood supply. It is more common in males (4–5:1) and is bilateral in approximately 20% of patients. Children with LCPD have delayed bone ages, disproportionate growth, and mild short stature.

*Clinical Manifestations.* The clinical onset occurs between the ages of 2 and 12 yr (mean age of 7 yr). There is mild or intermittent pain in the anterior thigh, limp, or both. The classic presentation has been described as a "painless" limp. The pertinent early physical findings include antalgic gait; muscle spasm and mild restriction of motion, especially abduction and internal rotation; proximal thigh atrophy; and mild shortness of stature.

*Roentgenographic Evaluation.* Roentgenographic assessment is necessary to determine the disease progression, sphericity of the femoral head, possibility of CFE collapse and extrusion, and the response to treatment. AP and frog lateral pelvic roentgenographs usually are adequate, but occasionally additional procedures such as arthrography, bone scans, and MRI may be useful. Bone scans and MRI are helpful in recognizing early LCPD but are of limited value in assessing the extent of CFE involvement or following the disease progression.

*Prognosis.* The short-term prognosis concerns femoral head deformity at the completion of the healing stage. The long-term prognosis involves the potential for osteoarthritis of the hip in adulthood. The six prognostic factors for the short-term prognosis are:

- Sex
- Age at clinical onset
- Extent of CFE involvement
- Femoral head containment
- Hip range of motion
- Premature CFE closure

The prognostic factors for the development of late degenerative arthritis include femoral head deformity and age at clinical onset. Older children with significant residual femoral head deformity are at risk for development of degenerative arthritis. The incidence is essentially 100% in children who are 10 yr of age or older at onset. This rate is in contrast to a negligible risk in children 5 yr or younger and 38% when onset occurs between 6 and 9 yr.

*Treatment.* LCPD is a local, self-healing disorder. Prevention of femoral head deformity and secondary osteoarthritis are the only justifications for treatment. There are four basic treatment goals:

- Elimination of hip irritability
- Restoration and maintenance of a good range of hip motion
- Prevention of CFE collapse, extrusion, or subluxation
- Attainment of a spherical femoral head at healing

Treatment utilizes the concept of containment; the femoral head is contained within the acetabulum so the latter acts as a mold for the reossifying CFE. Containment is indicated for children 6 yr of age (perhaps 5 yr in females) or older in whom more than one-half the CFE is involved. This is accomplished by nonsurgical containment using abduction casts and orthoses or by surgical containment with proximal femoral varus osteotomy, with or without derotation, and pelvic osteotomies to redirect the acetabulum and thereby contain the femoral head in the position of weight bearing. The long-term results of surgical containment treatment are 75–90% satisfactory (round or oval femoral head).

## SLIPPED CAPITAL FEMORAL EPIPHYSIS

Slippage of the capital femoral epiphysis (SCFE) is the most common adolescent hip disorder.

*Etiology.* The etiology of SCFE is unknown. An endocrine basis has been suggested because SCFE frequently occurs in adolescents who are either obese and have delayed skeletal maturation or tall and thin, following a recent growth spurt. In obese children, a low level of sex hormones has been postulated; in tall, thin children, an overabundance of growth hormone is implicated. It is known that both sex hormones and growth hormones alter the rate of proliferation of the cartilage cells in the physis and the rate of skeletal growth. SCFE also can occur as a complication of an underlying endocrine disorder, such as hypothyroidism, pituitary disorders, pseudohypoparathyroidism, and treatment with recombinant growth hormone. When a SCFE occurs prior to puberty, a hormonal abnormality or systemic disorder should be suspected. Nonetheless, the histopathology of SCFE indicates mechanical factors as the ultimate cause of slippage. Obesity produces high shear forces across the weakened and obliquely oriented growth plate.

*Roentgenographic Evaluation.* AP and frog lateral roentgenographs of the pelvis are used for assessment of the hips. The earliest sign of SCFE is widening of the physis without slippage. This is considered a preslip condition. As slippage occurs, the CFE stays in the acetabulum and the femoral neck rotates anteriorly and occasionally superiorly, resulting in a varus, retroverted femoral head and neck (Fig. 19–8). The degree of slippage between the CFE and the femoral neck can be classified into mild (0–33%), moderate (34–50%), and severe (>50%) by roentgenographic measurement techniques. Slippage resulting in a valgus deformity is rare except in metabolic disorders, such as renal osteodystrophy and Marfan syndrome, and as a sequela to irradiation therapy.

*Classification.* SCFE is classified into four distinct clinical groups. It may also be classified as stable or unstable.

*PRESLIP.* The physis is wide, but slippage has not occurred. There may be mild discomfort but the physical findings are usually normal. Preslips frequently are seen in the opposite hip of an adolescent with a previous SCFE.

*ACUTE.* Usually, there are no or only mild ante-

Normal          Slipped capital femoral epiphysis

FIGURE 19–8. Klein's line extends along the lateral femur neck and normally passes through a small part of the lateral femoral head. In slipped capital femoral epiphysis (SCFE), the line will not pass through the head or may just touch its lateral margin. A frog-leg lateral, rather than an anteroposterior, projection gives the clearest view of SCFE. (From Chung SMK: Hip Disorders in Infants and Children. Philadelphia. Lea & Febiger, 1981, p 85.)

cedent symptoms, such as pain and limp for less than 3 wk. Slippage occurs suddenly, with or without significant trauma; the pain is so severe that the child usually is unable to stand or bear weight. The CFE is *unstable*.

*ACUTE-ON-CHRONIC.* The epiphysis slips acutely on an existing chronic slip. These adolescents have had previous symptoms (pain, limp, out-toed gait) for several months. Trauma is a potential underlying factor that results in the sudden slippage. The CFE is *unstable*.

***Chronic.*** Chronic SCFE is the most common type. There is usually a several-month history of the previously described symptoms. The symptoms typically worsen as the slip progresses. However, because there is continuity between the femoral neck and CFE, the symptoms are not severe and the child is able to walk, albeit with a mildly antalgic, externally rotated gait. The CFE is *stable*.

***Clinical Manifestations.*** The physical findings in SCFE depend on the degree of slippage and the classification. In unstable acute or acute-on-chronic SCFE, the physical examination is limited by pain with any attempted hip motion. In stable chronic SCFE, the patient will have an antalgic gait and the affected extremity is externally rotated. Hip range of motion will demonstrate a lack of internal rotation and increased external rotation. Also, as the hip is flexed, it will become progressively externally rotated. Limitation of flexion and abduction also may be present as a result of a varus deformity of the proximal femur. Adolescents, especially those who are obese, with nontraumatic knee pain (referred pain) should be evaluated carefully for SCFE.

***Treatment.*** The goals of treatment for SCFE are to prevent further slippage and to minimize complications. This is accomplished by epiphysiodesis of the CFE. The technique selected depends on the classification and the severity of the slippage. The current methods include (1) in situ internal fixation with pins or screws (single or multiple), (2) open bone graft epiphysiodesis, (3) closed bone graft epiphysiodesis, (4) osteotomies of the femoral neck or subtrochanteric regions to realign the proximal femur, and (5) hip spica cast immobilization.

***Complications.*** The two serious complications in SCFE are avascular necrosis and chondrolysis. Avascular necrosis occurs as a result of injury to the retinacular vessels. This can be due to forced manipulation of an acute slip, compression from intracapsular hematoma, or direct injury during surgery. Partial forms of avascular necrosis also may occur following internal fixation as a result of disruption of the intraepiphyseal blood vessels. Chondrolysis occurs when there is destruction of the articular cartilage of the hip joint. The etiologic mechanism of this complication is unclear but has been demonstrated to be associated with more severe slips, black race, pins or screws protruding out of the femoral head, and female gender.

## References

Aronsson DD, Goldberg MJ, Kling TF Jr, et al: Developmental dysplasia of the hip. Pediatrics 94:201, 1994.

Behrman RE, Kliegman RM, Arvin AM (eds): Nelson Textbook of Pediatrics, 15th ed. Philadelphia, WB Saunders, 1996, Chapters 627.1–627.4

Gabuzda GM, Renshaw TS: Current concepts review: Reduction of congenital dislocation of the hip. J Bone Joint Surg 74A:624, 1992.

Harcke HT: Imaging in congenital dislocation of the hip. Clin Orthop 281:22, 1992.

Hauseisen DC, Weiner DS, Weiner SD: The characterization of "transient synovitis of the hip" in children. J Pediatr Orthop 6:11, 1986.

Herring JA: Current concepts review: The treatment of Legg-Calvé-Perthes disease: A critical review of the literature. J Bone Joint Surg 76A:448, 1994.

Loder RT, Richards BS, Shapiro PS, et al: Acute slipped capital femoral epiphysis: The importance of physeal stability. J Bone Joint Surg 75A:1134, 1993.

# THE LOWER EXTREMITIES

Torsional (in-toeing and out-toeing) and angular (physiologic bowlegs and knock-knees) variations of the lower extremities are common reasons parents seek medical attention for a child. Most of these complaints do not require active treatment because they will resolve with normal growth. It is important to understand the natural history to reassure a concerned family.

## ANGULAR VARIATIONS

There are both physiologic (variations) and pathologic (deformities) reasons for angular deformities. The physiologic or angular variations, fortunately, are the most common and occur predominantly in the tibia. The femur is much less frequently involved.

### Physiologic Bowlegs (Genu Varum)

The lower extremities of newborns and infants (<1 yr of age) commonly have mild to moderate bowing and internal rotation (Fig. 19–9). This is due to in utero positioning in which the hips are flexed, abducted, and externally rotated; the knees flexed and lower legs internally rotated; and the feet in slight equinus, supination, and contact with the posterolateral aspect of the opposite thigh. This

FIGURE 19–9.    *A*, Bowleg deformity. Bowlegs are referred to as varus angulation (genu varum) because the knees are tilted away from the midline of the body. *B*, Knock-knee or valgus deformity of the knees. The knee is tilted toward the midline. (From Scoles P: Pediatric Orthopedics in Clinical Practice, 2nd ed. Chicago, Year Book Medical Publishers, 1988, p 91.)

position produces hip flexion, abduction, and external rotation contractures; knee flexion contractures and internal tibial torsion; and mild supination of the feet. The bowed appearance is actually a torsional combination from the external rotation of the hip (tight posterior capsule) and the internal tibial torsion. With the onset of standing and independent walking, the bowing spontaneously corrects over a 6–12 mo period. Significant improvement does not occur during the 1st yr of life. The typical infant has 15 degrees of genu varum or bowleg configuration. This decreases to approximately 10 degrees by 1 yr of age. By 2 yr of age, the majority of children have straight or neutrally aligned lower extremities. *Treatment* is indicated for children older than 2 yr in whom there has been no documented improvement with growth.

### Physiologic Knock-Knees (Genu Valgum)

As the spontaneous correction of physiologic bowlegs continues, there is typically an overcorrection, of variable degree, into mild genu valgum or knock-knee (see Fig. 19–9). This physiologic angular variation commonly is seen between 3 and 4 yr of age but resolves spontaneously between 5 and 8 yr. As with physiologic bowlegs, *treatment* rarely is indicated.

## TORSIONAL VARIATIONS

The common causes of in-toeing and out-toeing are delineated in Table 19–5.

### In-Toeing

**Internal Femoral Torsion.** Internal femoral torsion is the most common cause of in-toeing in children 2 yr of age or older. It occurs more commonly in females than males (2:1). Most children with this condition have generalized ligamentous laxity. The *etiology* of femoral torsion is controversial; it may be congenital (persistent infantile femoral anteversion) or acquired secondary to abnormal sitting habits.

*Clinical Manifestations.* The primary clinical feature of internal femoral torsion is an in-toed gait. While watching the undressed child walk, the examiner notes the entire lower leg to be internally rotated. There is 80–90 degrees of internal rotation of the hip in the extended position; as a result, external rotation is limited to 0–10 degrees. Generalized ligamentous laxity, including elbow and finger hyperextension, knee recurvatum, and hypermobile flatfeet (pes planus), are present. These children sit almost exclusively in the "television" or "W" position. This position may allow the lower leg to act as a lever, thereby producing the torsional change in the "biologically plastic" femur. Although this condition is also called *femoral anteversion*, which implies an abnormality of the proximal femur, it is actually a torsional abnormality throughout the femoral shaft that results in a change in the normal alignment between the hip and knee.

*Roentgenographic Evaluation.* Roentgenography for internal femoral torsion is not routinely necessary. Clinical measurements usually are quite accurate. CT of the hip and knee can be used to precisely measure the degree of torsion roentgenographically.

*Treatment.* Management consists primarily of observation. It was previously believed that internal femoral torsion was associated with bunions,

TABLE 19–5.    Common Causes of In-Toeing and Out-Toeing

| In-Toeing | Out-Toeing |
| --- | --- |
| Internal femoral torsion | External femoral torsion |
| Internal tibial torsion | External tibial torsion |
| Metatarsus adductus | Calcaneovalgus feet |
| Talipes equinovarus (clubfoot) | Hypermobile pes planus (flatfoot) |

back pain, degenerative osteoarthritis of the hip and knee, and difficulty with athletic ability; however, this idea is no longer accepted. Correction of abnormal sitting habits usually allows this torsional variation to resolve with normal growth and development. However, it can take 1–3 yr for complete correction to occur. Children over 10 yr of age and young adolescents may not have enough remaining musculoskeletal growth for spontaneous correction to occur. After these children have been followed up for 1–2 yr without improvement, and if there is significant cosmetic or functional disability, surgical correction may be necessary.

**Internal Tibial Torsion.**  Internal or medial tibial torsion is the most common cause of in-toeing in children younger than 2 yr of age and is secondary to in utero positioning. This condition may be associated with metatarsus adductus. It also is the major component of physiologic bowlegs.

*Clinical Manifestations.*  The degree of tibial torsion can be measured by the supine or prone thigh-foot angle. In both tests, the child's knee is flexed to 90 degrees to neutralize the normal tibiofemoral rotation and the foot is placed in a neutral or simulated weight-bearing position. The long axis of the foot is compared to the long axis of the thigh (prone test) or tibia (supine test). An inwardly rotated foot is assigned a negative value and represents internal tibial torsion. The measurements must be recorded on each visit to document improvement. Roentgenographic measurements usually are of no value in assessment of medial tibial torsion.

*Treatment.*  Internal tibial torsion is a physiologic condition, and spontaneous resolution with normal growth and development can be anticipated. If there has been no documented improvement by 2 yr of age, a nighttime orthosis, such as a Denis-Browne splint, may be considered. Rarely, persistent internal tibial torsion in an older child or adolescent may necessitate surgical derotation.

## Out-Toeing

**External tibial torsion** is common and always is associated with a calcaneovalgus foot (see The Foot). External tibial torsion is due to a variation in normal in utero position. When these two conditions are combined with the normally externally rotated hip (tight posterior hip capsule), it produces a very externally rotated or out-toed appearance. Fortunately, both conditions undergo spontaneous resolution after a clinical course similar to that of internal tibial torsion.

## PATHOLOGIC GENU VARUM

### Tibia Vara (Blount Disease)

Idiopathic tibia vara, or Blount disease, is the most common pathologic disorder producing a progressive genu varum deformity. It is characterized by abnormal growth of the medial aspect of the proximal tibial epiphysis, resulting in a progressive varus angulation below the knee. Tibia vara can occur at any age in a growing child. It is classified according to the age at clinical onset: infantile (1–3 yr), juvenile (4–10 yr), and adolescent (11 yr or older). The infantile group is the most common; the juvenile and adolescent forms are combined as late-onset tibia vara and occur less frequently.

*Etiology.*  Although the exact cause of tibia vara remains unknown, it appears to be secondary to growth suppression from increased compressive forces across the medial aspect of the knee.

*Clinical Manifestations.*  The characteristics of infantile tibia vara include predominance of black race and female gender, marked obesity, approximately 80% bilateral involvement, a prominent medial metaphyseal beak, internal tibial torsion, and leg length inequality. Characteristics of the juvenile and adolescent (late-onset) form include black race, predominance of males, marked obesity, normal or above-normal height, approximately 50% bilateral involvement, slow progressive genu varum deformity, pain rather than deformity as the primary initial complaint, no palpable proximal medial metaphyseal beak, minimal internal tibial torsion, mild medial collateral ligament laxity, and mild leg length inequality.

*Roentgenographic Evaluation.*  Standing AP and lateral roentgenographs of the lower extremities are necessary to assess pathologic genu varum deformities. Roentgenographically, fragmentation with a protuberant step deformity and beaking of the proximal medial tibial metaphysis are considered the major features of infantile tibia vara. The changes of the proximal medial tibia are less conspicuous in the late-onset forms and are characterized by wedging of the medial portion of the epiphysis, a mild posteromedial articular depression, a serpiginous cephalad curved physis of variable width, and mild or no fragmentation or beaking of the proximal medial metaphysis. The differences between the three tibia vara groups appear to be due primarily to the age at clinical onset, the amount of remaining growth, and the magnitude of the medial compression forces on the involved side. Thus, the infantile-onset group has the potential for the greatest deformity and the adolescent-onset group, the least.

The major deformity that must be differentiated from infantile tibia vara is the physiologic genu varum deformity. It is difficult to differentiate roentgenographically between these two disorders in children younger than 2 yr of age.

*Treatment.* Once the roentgenographic findings confirm the diagnosis, treatment should begin immediately. Orthotic management may be considered for children 3 yr of age or younger with a mild deformity. Approximately 50% of children with this criterion may achieve adequate correction using orthoses. Conservative management in the late-onset forms of tibia vara is contraindicated. The children are too large, compliance is poor, and the remaining growth too small to allow for adequate correction.

The indications for surgical treatment in infantile tibia vara include 4 yr of age or older, failure of orthotic management, and moderate to severe deformity. Proximal tibial valgus osteotomy and associated fibular diaphyseal osteotomy is the procedure of choice.

## LOWER EXTREMITY LENGTH DISCREPANCIES

Length discrepancies in the femur, tibia, or both are common problems. The *differential diagnosis* is extensive, and some of the common causes are presented in Table 19–6.

### Normal Growth and Development

Approximately 65% of the growth of the entire lower extremity comes from the distal femoral (38%) and proximal tibial (27%) physeal plates. Thus, growth disturbances about the knee can have

TABLE 19–6.  Common Causes of Leg Length Inequality

| Congenital | Infectious |
|---|---|
| Proximal femoral focal deficiency | Pyogenic osteomyelitis with physeal damage |
| Coxa vara | **Trauma** |
| Hemiatrophy/hemihypertrophy (anisomelia) | Physeal injury with premature closure |
| **Developmental** | Overgrowth |
| Developmental dislocation of the hip | Malunion (shortening) |
| Legg-Calvé-Perthes disease | **Tumor** |
| **Neuromuscular** | Physeal destruction |
| Polio | Radiation-induced physeal injury |
| Cerebral palsy (hemiplegia) | Overgrowth |

the most adverse effect on lower extremity length, depending on the amount of remaining growth.

### Methods of Limb Length Measurement

*Clinical Measurements.* The available clinical methods are less accurate than the roentgenographic techniques. The most common clinical measurement is from the anterior superior iliac spine to the medial malleolus. This minimizes measurement error secondary to pelvic obliquity. It also is possible to measure limb length by leveling the pelvis. Blocks of various thickness may be placed beneath the foot on the involved side until the iliac crests are level. The thickness indicates the amount of discrepancy.

*Roentgenographic Measurements.* Roentgenographic evaluations are the most accurate method of assessment of leg length. The *teleoroentgenogram* is a single exposure of both lower extremities. Its primary indication is for young children, usually under 5 yr of age. There is a small amount of magnification error present but it has the advantage of showing angular deformities.

The *orthoroentgenogram* consists of three separate, slightly overlapping exposures of the hips, knees, and ankles on a long cassette. Bone length is measured directly on the roentgenograph. Less magnification is present, and angular deformities are demonstrated. It has the disadvantage of being bulky and difficult to handle.

The *scanogram* is the most accurate method and consists of three narrow exposures of the hips, knees, and ankles on a standard cassette with a roentgenographic ruler next to the extremity. Minimal magnification is present and accurate measurements can be made. However, angular deformities cannot be visualized fully, which may lead to errors in interpretation. Currently, *CT scanogram* techniques are being used with the best accuracy.

The measured discrepancy is followed with the Moseley and Green-Anderson graphs. An AP roentgenograph of the left hand and wrist for bone age determination is necessary to assess maturation.

*Treatment.* Issues in management include etiology of the discrepancy, skeletal age, ultimate discrepancy, anticipated adult height, neuromuscular status of the extremities, joint involvement, and psychologic aspects of the child and parents. Discrepancies of greater than 2 cm at maturity usually require treatment. Equalization can be achieved by nonsurgical and surgical methods. The nonsurgical methods include orthotic and prosthetic devices; surgical methods include shortening of the longer extremity, lengthening of the shorter extremity, or a combination of both. Discrepancies of 2–5 cm are treated by epiphyseodesis (surgical physeal closure) of the affected side and discrepancies greater than 5 cm by lengthening.

## References

Behrman RE, Kliegman RM, Arvin AM (eds): Nelson Textbook of Pediatrics, 15th ed. Philadelphia, WB Saunders, 1996, Chapters 624.1–624.7, 625.

Greene WB: Infantile tibia vara. J Bone Joint Surg 75A:130, 1993.

Heath CH, Staheli LT: Normal limits of knee angles in white children: Genu varum and genu valgum. J Pediatr Orthop 13:359, 1993.

Kling TF, Jr: Angular deformities of the lower limbs in children. Orthop Clin North Am 18:513, 1987.

Moseley CF: Leg length discrepancy. Orthop Clin North Am 18:529, 1987.

Staheli LT: Rotational problems of the lower extremities. Orthop Clin North Am 18:503, 1987.

Thompson GH, Carter JR: Late-onset tibia vara (Blount's disease): Current concepts. Clin Orthop 255:24, 1990.

## THE KNEE

The knee joint is unique because the movement of the tibiofemoral articulation is constrained only by soft tissues rather than by the usual geometric fit between the ends of articulating bone (Fig. 19–10). Paramount among these constraints are the medial and lateral collateral ligaments, the anterior and posterior cruciate ligaments, and the medial and lateral menisci. Weight is transmitted by load path that includes both the points of articular cartilage and the menisci. A second clinically important area, the patellofemoral joint, is part of the knee and a common site of problems, especially in adolescents.

Accumulation of fluid (effusion) in the knee is common during childhood and adolescence. When fluid accumulates rapidly following an injury, blood is usually in the joint (hemarthrosis); this may indicate an occult fracture or an injury to one of the ligaments or menisci. If there has been repeated trauma, an accumulation of synovial fluid may indicate a chronic internal derangement, usually a tear of a meniscus. Unexplained accumulation of fluid may occur with arthritis (septic, viral, postinfectious, juvenile rheumatoid arthritis, systemic lupus erythematosus), in association with ligamentous laxity (hypermobile joint syndrome), and with overactivity. In addition to the evaluation of other systemic manifestations and the clinical history (e.g., fever, hemophilia, rash, trauma), an analysis of an aspiration of fluid from the joint generally is indicated and expedites precise diagnosis (see Chapter 10).

### DISCOID LATERAL MENISCUS

Each meniscus is semilunar in shape, but occasionally the lateral meniscus persists as a solid disk of fibrocartilage, an entity referred to as *discoid lateral meniscus*. A normal meniscus is attached about its periphery and glides anteriorly and posteriorly with knee motion, but a discoid meniscus is less mobile and may become torn. Occasionally, there is no peripheral attachment about its posterolateral aspect. During knee flexion, the entire discoid meniscus may suddenly displace anteriorly to produce a loud click or clunk. Most commonly, the patient comes to clinical attention during the late childhood years and early adolescence (11–15 yr). AP roentgenographs may show widening of the lateral aspect of the knee joint. Arthroscopy, arthrography, and MRI are diagnostic.

*Treatment* in most cases involves excision of tears and reshaping of the meniscus arthroscopically. Peripheral reattachment is performed when possible.

### POPLITEAL CYST

A popliteal cyst ("Baker cyst") is commonly seen during the middle childhood years (Fig. 19–11). The cause is distention of the gastrocnemius and semimembranosus bursa along the posteromedial aspect of the knee by synovial fluid from the tendon sheaths. In childhood, the cysts usually are benign and resolve with time, even though several years may be required. Knee roentgenographs are

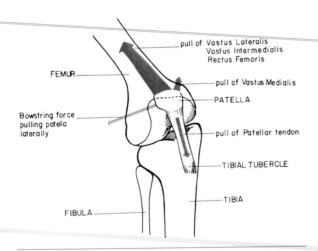

FIGURE 19–10. Diagram of the knee extensor mechanism. The major force exerted by the quadriceps muscle tends to pull the patella laterally out of the intercondylar sulcus. The vastus medialis muscle pulls medially to keep the patella centralized. (From Smith JB: Knee problems in children. Pediatr Clin North Am 33:1443, 1986.)

FIGURE 19–11. Diagram of popliteal cyst location—posterior and medial aspect of knee, usually inferior to knee crease. (From Ferguson A: Orthopedic Surgery in Infancy and Childhood, 5th ed. Baltimore, Williams & Wilkins, 1981, p 261.)

normal; the *diagnosis* is confirmed by ultrasound or aspiration. *Treatment* should be directed at reassurance because surgery usually is rarely indicated.

## OSTEOCHONDRITIS DISSECANS

Osteochondritis dissecans commonly involves the knee and occurs when an area of bone adjacent to the articular cartilage becomes avascular and separates from the underlying bone. In the older child or young adolescent, this condition usually affects the lateral portion of the medial femoral condyle. AP, lateral, and "tunnel" roentgenographs of the knee are diagnostic and are used to follow the course of the disease. In the young patient, the overlying articular cartilage usually remains intact and the area of avascular necrosis revascularizes and heals spontaneously. With increasing age, the risk increases for fracture of the articular cartilage and separation of the bony fragment. MRI is helpful in determining the integrity of the articular cartilage. In the young adolescent, one must decide whether to follow the lesion expectantly or to attempt to stimulate healing surgically. Once cartilage fracture takes place, surgical treatment is necessary. This may consist of arthroscopic excision,

drilling of the lesion to promote revascularization and healing, and possible internal fixation.

## OSGOOD-SCHLATTER DISEASE

The portion of the patellar ligament inserted into the tibial tubercle is vulnerable to fibrocartilage microfracture during late childhood and early adolescence. This condition, Osgood-Schlatter disease, is more common in males. The natural history almost always is benign, with activity-related pain persisting for 12–24 mo. Physical examination demonstrates swelling and prominence of the tibia tubercle and exquisite local tenderness. Roentgenograms are necessary to rule out other lesions. Frequently, bony enlargement of the tibial tubercle will be a residual manifestation of the proliferative healing response. Rest, restriction of activities, and occasionally a knee immobilizer may be necessary, combined with an isometric exercise program. Anti-inflammatory medications may also be beneficial.

## PATELLOFEMORAL DISORDERS

The patellofemoral joint depends on a subtle balance among restraining ligaments, muscle forces, alignment, and articular anatomy for normal function (see Fig. 19–10). On its deep surface, the patella has a V-bottom shape; it moves through a matching groove in the distal femur called the *trochlea*. The force of the muscle pulling through the quadriceps tendon and the patellar ligament does not act in a straight line because the patellar ligament inclines in a slightly lateral direction with respect to the line of the quadriceps tendon. This lateral movement, coupled with the movement of the restraining ligaments, tends to move the patella in a lateral direction. The vastus medialis muscle functions to counteract the laterally acting forces. An abnormality of any one or a group of these factors makes the patellofemoral joint function abnormally; the usual clinical manifestation is knee pain.

Idiopathic anterior knee pain is common in adolescents. It was previously called **chondromalacia patellae,** but this term was incorrect because the joint surfaces of the patella are normal. Abnormal mechanics and variables associated with puberty are possible etiologic factors. The condition is easily assessed by directly palpating the extended knee and also by compressing the patellofemoral joint. To elicit the latter sign, one merely exerts manual pressure against the patella as the knee is extended. Crepitus may be elicited. Roentgenograms are rarely helpful. Running and climbing stairs elicit pain when the knee is flexed. With early articular damage, pain usually is perceived maximally as the knee comes to within 15–20 degrees of full extension (crepitance also may be felt by the examiner). Although it may be reasonable to treat recent or mild cases empirically with anti-inflammatory medication and an exercise program aimed at developing strength and bulk in the vastus medialis muscle, persistent or refractory cases should be referred to an orthopaedist. Patellofemoral pain is particularly prevalent among young athletes (participating in running, basketball, soccer) and in adolescent women.

Recurrent *patellar subluxation* and *dislocation* resulting from similar muscle imbalance also can occur in late childhood and early adolescence. There are several other predisposing factors, including generalized ligamentous laxity, internal femoral torsion, genu valgum, and lateral femoral condyle hypoplasia. Acute traumatic dislocations also occur in a normal knee.

Initial *treatment* is nonoperative, with a vigorous physical therapy program to strengthen predominantly the quadriceps muscles. If this fails, surgical correction is necessary.

### References

Behrman RE, Kliegman RM, Arvin AM (eds): Nelson Textbook of Pediatrics, 15th ed. Philadelphia, WB Saunders, 1996, Chapters 626.1–626.6.
Bentley G, Dowd G: Current concepts of etiology and treatment of chondromalacia patellae. Clin Orthop 189:209, 1984.
Dinham JM: Popliteal cysts in children: The case against surgery. J Bone Joint Surg 57B:69, 1975.
Krause BL, Williams JPR, Catterall A: Natural history of Osgood-Schlatter disease. J Pediatr Orthop 10:65, 1990.
Stanitski CL: Anterior knee pain syndromes in the adolescent. J Bone Joint Surg 75A:1407, 1993.

## THE FOOT

In the newborn and nonambulatory infant, it is helpful to remember the difference between posturing and deformity. Posturing is the habitual position in which the infant holds the foot but still allows a normal range of motion so that the examiner can position the foot in a normal shape. Deformity produces an appearance similar to posturing, but the deformed foot cannot be manually repositioned to a normal shape. Most pediatric foot disorders are painless. However, foot pain does occur, especially in older children. The *differential diagnosis* of foot pain in children is presented in Table 19–7.

### METATARSUS ADDUCTUS

*Congenital* metatarsus adductus is a common problem of infants and young children. It also is known as *metatarsus varus* if the forefoot is supinated as well as adducted. It occurs equally in males and females and is bilateral in 50% of patients. Metatarsus adductus has hereditary tendencies and is more common in firstborn than in later children because of the molding effect from the primigravida uterus and abdominal wall. Approximately 10% of children with metatarsus adductus will have DDH. Thus, careful examination of the hips is necessary.

*Clinical Manifestations.* The forefoot is adducted and occasionally supinated. The hindfoot and midfoot are normal. The lateral border of the foot is convex and the base of the fifth metatarsal appears prominent. The medial border of the foot is concave. There is usually an increased interval between the first and second toes, with the great toe being held in a greater varus position. Ankle dorsiflexion and plantar flexion are normal. Forefoot flexibility can vary from flexible to rigid. To perform an assessment, the examiner stabilizes the

TABLE 19–7.  Differential Diagnosis of Foot Pain by Age

| 0–6 yr | 6–12 yr | 12–20 yr |
|---|---|---|
| Poor-fitting shoes | Poor-fitting shoes | Poor-fitting shoes |
| Foreign body | Sever disease | Stress fracture |
| Fracture | JRA | Foreign body |
| Osteomyelitis | Foreign body | Ingrown toenail |
| Juvenile rheumatoid arthritis (JRA) | Accessory tarsal navicular | Metatarsalgia |
| Leukemia | Tarsal coalition | Plantar fasciitis |
| Puncture wound | Ewing sarcoma | Avascular necrosis of metatarsal (Freiberg infarction) or navicular bone (Köhler disease) |
| Dactylitis | Hypermobile flatfoot | Sever disease |
|  | Trauma (fractures; sprains) | Achilles tendinitis |
|  | Puncture wound | Trauma (fractures; sprains) |
|  |  | Plantar warts |

hind and midfoot in a neutral position and applies pressure over the first metatarsal head. In the walking child with an uncorrected metatarsus adductus deformity, an in-toed gait is noted. Abnormal shoe wear is also commonly seen.

*Roentgenographic Evaluation.* Routine roentgenographs of the foot usually are not necessary for metatarsus adductus. AP weight-bearing roentgenographs demonstrate adduction of the metatarsals at the tarsometatarsal articulation and an increased intermetatarsal angle between the first and second metatarsals.

*Treatment.* The feet may be classified into three groups, depending on forefoot flexibility.

*Type I* deformities concern flexible feet that can be actively positioned into the overcorrected (abducted) position. Voluntary correction usually can be elicited by stimulating the peroneal musculature by stroking the lateral border of the foot. Usually, no treatment is needed.

*Type II* deformities concern feet that can be corrected to the neutral position both passively and actively. These feet may benefit from a trial of corrective shoes, such as straight or reversed last shoes. These shoes are worn full time (22 hr/day), and the child is re-evaluated in 4–6 wk. If the condition has improved, treatment can be continued. If no improvement occurs, serial plaster casts are necessary.

*Type III* deformities are rigid and cannot be corrected. These feet are treated with serial casts that are changed at 1–2 wk intervals. Usually, complete correction can be obtained in 4–6 wk, depending on the child's age and the severity of deformity. The best results are obtained when casting is initiated before the child is 8 mo of age.

For metatarsus adductus deformities persisting or presenting after 4 yr of age, usually surgical intervention is required. Children 4–6 yr of age with a fixed deformity usually are considered for soft tissue release. Children 7 yr of age or older usually do not benefit from the soft tissue release and require metatarsal osteotomies.

## CALCANEOVALGUS FEET

The calcaneovalgus foot is a relatively common finding in the newborn and appears to be secondary to in utero positioning. This condition is manifested by a hyperdorsiflexed foot with forefoot abduction and heel valgus and usually is associated with external tibial torsion. These variations usually are unilateral but may be bilateral. In utero, the plantar surface of the foot was against the wall of the uterus, forcing it into a hyperdorsiflexed,

abducted, and externally rotated position. When calcaneovalgus feet and external tibial torsion are combined with the normal newborn external rotation of the hip (tight posterior capsule), it results in an excessively externally rotated lower extremity.

*Clinical Manifestations.* The infant typically presents with an externally rotated extremity. The dorsum of the foot can be brought into contact with the anterior aspect of the tibia and the forefoot will have an abducted appearance.

The most common condition that must be distinguished from the calcaneovalgus foot is a congenital vertical talus. The differentiation usually can be made clinically because a vertical talus is a rigid deformity.

*Roentgenographic Evaluation.* Simulated weight-bearing AP and lateral roentgenographs of the feet may be necessary to differentiate between the calcaneovalgus foot and a congenital vertical talus. In a calcaneovalgus foot, the roentgenographs either are normal or show a slight increase in hindfoot valgus. In congenital vertical talus, the hindfoot is in equinus and the midfoot dorsally displaced (**rocker bottom deformity**).

*Treatment.* The typical calcaneovalgus foot requires no treatment. The hyperdorsiflexion of the foot resolves during the first 3–6 mo of life. The external tibial torsion, however, persists and follows the same natural history as internal tibial torsion. Spontaneous improvement does not occur until the child begins to pull to stand and walk independently. Most involved infants will have normally aligned feet and lower extremities by 2 yr of age.

## TALIPES EQUINOVARUS (CLUBFOOT)

A clubfoot represents a deformity of not only the foot but also the entire lower leg. Clubfoot can be congenital, teratologic, or positional. The congenital clubfoot is usually an isolated abnormality, whereas the teratologic form is associated with a neuromuscular disorder, such as myelodysplasia, arthrogryposis multiplex congenita, or a syndrome complex. Positional clubfoot is a normal foot that has been held in a deformed position in utero.

*Etiology.* The cause of clubfoot is unknown. There are inheritance factors that may be multifactorial with a major influence from a single autosomal dominant gene. Recent biopsy studies of the extrinsic muscles of the calf have suggested a nonprogressive neuromuscular etiology.

*Clinical Manifestations.* The congenital form of clubfoot, which constitutes 75% of cases, is characterized by the absence of other congenital abnormalities, variable rigidity of the foot, mild calf atrophy, and mild hypoplasia of the tibia, fibula, and bones of the foot. It occurs more commonly in males (2:1) and is bilateral in 50% of cases. The probability of random occurrence is approximately 0.1%, but within involved families the probability is approximately 3% for subsequent siblings and 20–30% for offspring of involved parents.

Examination of the infant clubfoot demonstrates hindfoot equinus, hindfoot varus, forefoot adduction, and variable rigidity. All are secondary to the medial dislocation of the talonavicular joint. In the older child, the calf and foot atrophy are more obvious than in the infant regardless of how well corrected or functional the foot. These findings are due to the neuromuscular etiology of clubfoot.

**Roentgenographic Evaluation.** AP and lateral standing or simulated weight-bearing roentgenographs are used in the assessment of clubfoot (Fig. 19–12). Useful measurements in assessing clubfoot include the AP talocalcaneal angle, the lateral talocalcaneal angle, and the talocalcaneal overlap. The navicular, which is the primary site of deformity, does not ossify until 3 yr in the female and 4 yr in the male. Thus, line measurements are necessary in order to determine the position of the unossified navicular.

*Treatment*

CONSERVATIVE MANAGEMENT. Conservative methods of treatment include taping, malleable splints, and serial plaster casts. Taping and malleable splints are particularly useful in premature infants until they attain an appropriate size for casting. Serial plaster casts are the major method of treat-

ment. Failure to achieve clinical and roentgenographic correction by 3 mo of age is an indication for surgical treatment. Further attempts at conservative management may result in articular damage and a midfoot breech (rocker-bottom deformity).

SURGICAL MANAGEMENT. The most common method of initial surgical treatment is a complete soft tissue release simultaneously correcting all components of the clubfoot deformity. Satisfactory long-term results can be expected in 75–90% of these cases. Those feet with unsatisfactory results requiring additional treatment usually are secondary to extrinsic muscle imbalance (neuromuscular etiology) rather than incomplete correction.

## HYPERMOBILE PES PLANUS (FLEXIBLE FLATFEET)

Hypermobile or pronated feet are common sources of parental concern. The child is usually asymptomatic and has no limitations of activities. Flexible flatfeet are common in neonates and toddlers as a result of associated ligamentous laxity and fat in the area of the medial longitudinal arch; significant improvement is noted by 6 yr of age. In the older child, flexible flatfeet usually are secondary to generalized ligamentous laxity.

**Clinical Manifestations.** In the non–weight-bearing position in the older child with a flexible flatfoot, the normal medial longitudinal arch is present, but in the weight-bearing position, the foot becomes pronated with varying degrees of pes planus and heel valgus. Subtalar motion is normal

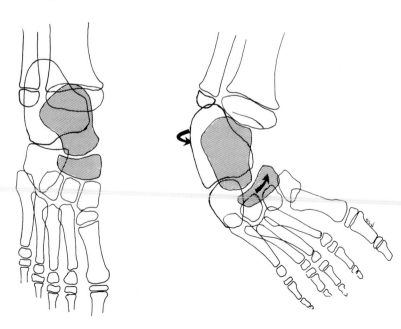

FIGURE 19–12. Diagram of anteroposterior roentgenogram of a normal foot and talipes equinovarus. (From Tachdjian MO: Pediatric Orthopedics. Philadelphia, WB Saunders, 1972, p 1283.)

or slightly increased. Loss of subtalar motion may indicate a rigid flatfoot. Common causes of rigid flatfeet include tight Achilles tendon (heel cord), tarsal coalitions, and neuromuscular abnormalities (cerebral palsy). Rigid flatfeet also may be a familial trait.

*Roentgenographic Evaluation.* Roentgenograms of asymptomatic flexible flatfeet usually are not indicated.

*Treatment.* The treatment of flexible flatfeet is conservative; the diagnosis is not possible until after 6 yr of age. Treatment is indicated only for persistent symptoms not attributable to other causes or abnormal shoe wear. Feet that are symptomatic with vigorous physical activities usually respond readily to the use of a commercially available medial longitudinal arch support.

## PERONEAL SPASTIC FLATFOOT

Peroneal spastic flatfoot is a common disorder characterized by a painful, rigid valgus deformity of the mid and hindfoot (flatfoot) and peroneal (lateral calf) muscle spasm but without true spasticity. Peroneal spastic flatfoot usually is synonymous with tarsal coalition, a congenital fusion or failure of segmentation between two or more tarsal bones. However, any condition that alters the normal gliding and rotatory motion of the subtalar joint may produce the appearance of a peroneal spastic flatfoot. Thus, congenital malformations, arthritis or inflammatory disorders, infection, neoplasms, and trauma can be potential, although uncommon, causes.

The most common tarsal coalitions occur at the medial talocalcaneal (subtalar) facet and between the calcaneus and navicular bones. Coalitions can be fibrous, cartilaginous, or osseous. Peroneal spastic flatfoot is bilateral in approximately 50% of involved children.

*Clinical Manifestations.* The onset of symptoms usually occurs during the 2nd decade of life. Although mild limitation of subtalar motion and a valgus deformity are present since early childhood, the onset of symptoms varies with the age at which the fibrous or cartilaginous bar begins to ossify and further decrease motion. The talonavicular coalitions ossify between 3 and 5 yr; the calcaneonavicular coalitions, between 8 and 12 yr; and the middle-facet talocalcaneal coalitions, between 12 and 16 yr of age. The pain typically is felt laterally in the hindfoot and radiates proximally along the lateral malleolus and distal fibula (peroneal muscle spasm). Symptoms frequently are aggravated by sports or by walking on uneven ground. The foot is pronated in both the weight-bearing and the non–weight-bearing positions. Subtalar or mid-tarsal joint motion is diminished or absent, and attempts at motion produce pain.

*Roentgenographic Evaluation.* The diagnosis of tarsal coalition is confirmed roentgenographically by AP, oblique, and lateral weight-bearing roentgenographs of the foot. Beaking of the anterior aspect of the talus on the lateral view suggests a tarsal coalition. Axial views through the posterior and middle talocalcaneal joints can be useful in the diagnosis of the middle-facet talocalcaneal coalition. However, CT is the procedure of choice in the evaluation of tarsal coalitions, especially those involving the middle facet.

*Treatment.* The treatment of symptomatic tarsal coalition varies according to the type of coalition, the age of the patient, the extent of the coalition, the presence or absence of degenerative osteoarthritis, and the degree of disability. Nonoperative treatment consists of cast immobilization, shoe inserts, or orthotics. When this fails, excision of the coalition and soft tissue interposition to prevent hematoma formation and reossification of the coalition is very effective in relieving pain, improving subtalar motion, and allowing resumption of normal activities.

## CAVUS FEET

Cavovarus foot, an exaggerated medial longitudinal arch associated with a varus alignment of the hindfoot, often appears during the middle childhood years (Fig. 19–13). Both idiopathic and neuromuscular types may be seen; in either instance, cavovarus is usually a progressive deformity leading to considerable compromise of foot function. In hypermobile pes planus, the foot rotates externally; in high arch or cavovarus posture, however, the foot rotates internally. The cavovarus foot also tends to be rigid. Aggressive treatment is warranted and usually involves reconstructive surgery. Special shoes and shoe modifications are not helpful but sometimes may be warranted for symptomatic treatment. Because a neuromuscular etiologic mechanism is possible whenever such a deformity of the foot exists, careful assessment of the patient's neurologic function is mandatory. Spinal cord pathology, poliomyelitis, and peripheral neuropathy (Charcot-Marie-Tooth disease) always are to be considered.

## OSTEOCHONDROSES

Both the tarsal navicular (Köhler disease) and the head of the second metatarsal (Frieberg disease)

FIGURE 19–13.   The normal muscular balance of the foot is demonstrated on the left. A right triangle of muscle forces is generated by the gastrocnemius-soleus muscle group posteriorly, the plantar muscles inferiorly, and the tibialis anterior muscle. Weakness, as demonstrated in the diagram on the right, causes imbalance in the foot with resultant pes cavus. (Redrawn from Chuinard E, Baskin M: Clawfoot deformity. J Bone Joint Surg 55A:351, 1973.)

may undergo idiopathic avascular necrosis. These conditions are relatively uncommon, and both produce pain in the affected site on activity or weight bearing. The pathologic process involves infarction and subsequent revascularization, resorption, and reformation of the affected bone. Symptomatic treatment based on the severity of the child's complaints is appropriate.

As the child enters the pubescent growth spurt, the fibrocartilaginous insertion of major muscle groups to bone is vulnerable to microfracture through the fibrocartilage, resulting in inflammatory and healing responses. The usual site of microfracture in the foot is at the attachment of the triceps surae to the os calcis, producing **Sever disease**. Symptoms wax and wane, depending on the level of activity, until skeletal maturity is achieved. The usual residual manifestation, if any, is some bony enlargement at the tendon insertion site when the cartilage, which proliferated as part of the healing response, undergoes its normal maturation to become bone. *Treatment* is symptomatic and includes the use of anti-inflammatory agents.

The major cause of adolescent heel pain is a tight Achilles tendon (heel cord) caused by rapid growth. A stretching exercise program is usually effective in relieving symptoms.

## ADOLESCENT BUNIONS

Bunions or hallux valgus deformities are common in adolescents, and there is typically a positive family history. The deformity is usually bilateral and occurs predominantly in females. Most commonly, there is a congenital malalignment of the first metatarsal (metatarsus primus varus). The hallux valgus deformity, enlargement of the medial aspect of the first metatarsal head, and symptoms usually begin in early adolescence.

*Roentgenograms* of the feet are necessary to assess the deformity; the AP and lateral weight-bearing views are selected.

*Treatment* is directed toward relief of symptoms. Initially, this consists of appropriate fitting shoes with a wide toe box and, occasionally, orthotics if there is associated pes planus. If this measure fails, surgical realignment will be necessary. Surgery is very effective in relieving symptoms, although it usually does not restore the appearance of the foot to normal.

## TOE DEFORMITIES

Extra toes **(polydactyly)** usually are recognized at birth, and it is appropriate to decide on a management strategy at that time. When the extra toe is attached to the foot by only a tag of skin and soft tissue, as commonly occurs adjacent to the fifth toe, simple amputation or ligation through the stalk is effective. When the abnormality involves the great toe or the intercalary toes or when there is some rudiment of cartilage or bone connecting it with the foot proper, delayed surgical treatment targeted at the specific abnormality is indicated. Malformation syndromes may be associated with polydactyly (Table 19–8).

Fusing of the toes **(syndactyly)** is usually a benign cosmetic problem that does not warrant treat-

TABLE 19–8.   Syndromes Associated with Polydactyly

| | |
|---|---|
| Carpenter syndrome | Trisomy 13 |
| Ellis–van Creveld syndrome | Orofaciodigital syndrome |
| Meckel-Gruber syndrome | Rubinstein-Taybi syndrome |
| Polysyndactyly | |

## TABLE 19–9. Syndromes Associated with Syndactyly

| | |
|---|---|
| Apert syndrome | Fetal hydantoin syndrome |
| Carpenter syndrome | Laurence-Moon-Biedl syndrome |
| de Lange syndrome | Fanconi pancytopenia |
| Holt-Oram syndrome | Trisomy 21 |
| Orofaciodigital syndrome | Trisomy 13 |
| Polysyndactyly | Trisomy 18 |

ment. Syndromes also may be associated with syndactyly (Table 19–9).

### PUNCTURE WOUNDS

Puncture wounds of the foot are common and generally trivial. For most of these injuries, cleaning the wound, ensuring prophylaxis for tetanus infection, and administering broad-spectrum oral antibiotic prophylaxis are all that is needed. When infection occurs despite these measures, *Pseudomonas aeruginosa* and *Staphylococcus aureus* are the offending organisms in most cases of osteomyelitis, supposedly because these organisms normally colonize the skin surface of the foot as a result of the moist environment in an athletic shoe.

Treatment of these infections includes débriding the wound to remove necrotic tissue, which invariably is present, and administering parenteral antibiotics, initially with methicillin and gentamicin. Subsequent antibiotic treatment should be based on culture and sensitivity studies. Following surgery, parenteral antimicrobial therapy is required for 10–14 days.

### References

Behrman RE, Kliegman RM, Arvin AM (eds): Nelson Textbook of Pediatrics, 15th ed. Philadelphia, WB Saunders, 1996, Chapters 623.1–623.12.

Crawford AH, Gabriel KR: Foot and ankle problems. Orthop Clin North Am 18:649, 1987.

Farsetti P, Weinstein SL, Ponseti IV: The long-term functional and radiographic outcomes of untreated and non-operatively treated metatarsus adductus. J Bone Joint Surg 76A:257, 1994.

McClusky WP, Lovell WW, Cummings RJ: The cavovarus foot deformity: Etiology and management. Clin Orthop 247:27, 1989.

Mosca VS: Flexible flatfoot and skewfoot. J Bone Joint Surg 77A:1937, 1995.

Thompson GH: Bunions and deformities of the toes in children and adolescents. J Bone Joint Surg 77A:1924, 1995.

Thompson GH, Cooperman DR: Peroneal spastic flatfoot. *In* Gould JS (ed): Operative Foot Surgery. Philadelphia, WB Saunders, 1994, pp 858–877.

Thompson GH, Simons GW III: Congenital talipes equinovarus (clubfeet) and metatarsus adductus. *In* Drennan JC (ed): The Child's Foot and Ankle. New York, Raven Press, 1992, pp 97–133.

## THE SPINE

A simplified classification of the common spinal abnormalities is presented in Table 19–10.

### CLINICAL EXAMINATION

A complete physical examination is necessary for any child or adolescent with a spinal deformity because it may indicate an underlying disease process. The back is examined with the patient in the standing position and viewed from behind (Fig. 19–14). The levelness of the pelvis is assessed first.

### TABLE 19–10. Classification of Spinal Deformities

**Scoliosis**
  *Idiopathic*
    Infantile
    Juvenile
    Adolescent
  *Congenital*
    Failure of formation
      Wedge vertebrae
      Hemivertebrae
    Failure of segmentation
      Unilateral bar
      Bilateral bar
    Mixed
  *Neuromuscular*
    Neuropathic diseases
      Upper motor neuron
        Cerebral palsy
        Spinocerebellar degeneration
          Friedreich ataxia
          Charcot-Marie-Tooth disease
        Syringomyelia
        Spinal cord tumor
        Spinal cord trauma
      Lower motor neuron
        Myelodysplasia
        Poliomyelitis
        Spinal muscular atrophy
      Myopathic diseases
        Duchenne muscular dystrophy
        Arthrogryposis
        Other muscular dystrophies
  *Syndromes*
    Neurofibromatosis
    Marfan syndrome
  *Compensatory*
    Leg length inequality
**Kyphosis**
  Postural roundback
  Scheuermann disease
  Congenital kyphosis

Adapted from the Terminology Committee of the Scoliosis Research Society, 1975.

Anterior superior iliac spine    Umbilicus

Medial
malleolus

Measurement of leg length for
determination of pelvic obliquity
AB = actual leg length;
A'B = apparent leg length

Gauging
trunk
alignment
with plumb
line

Measurement of
rib hump with
straight edge

Estimation of rib hump
and evaluation of curve
unwinding as patient
turns trunk from side
to side

Older sister,
severe curve

Younger sister,
mild curve

FIGURE 19–14.   Clinical evaluation of the scoliosis patient. (From Hugo A, Keim MD: Scoliosis. Clin Symp 30[1]:16, 1978. Copyright 1978. CIBA-GEIGY Corporation. Reproduced with permission from Clinical Symposia by Frank H. Netter, M.D. All rights reserved.)

Leg length inequality results in pelvic obliquity and can produce the appearance of *scoliosis*. When the pelvis is level or has been leveled with wood blocks placed under the foot, the spine is examined for symmetry. The back is observed for areas of deformity, spinal curvature, and areas of tenderness.

Next, the patient is asked to bend forward with the hands directed between the feet. A tangential view of the spine while standing behind (thoracic area) and in front (lumbar area) allows the observer to determine the symmetry of the back. The presence of a hump is the hallmark of a scoliotic deformity. The corresponding area opposite the hump typically is depressed. The reason for these "humps and valleys" is *spinal rotation*. Scoliosis represents a rotational malalignment of one vertebra on another. This results in rib rotation when the curve is in the thoracic area and paravertebral muscle rotation when the curve is in the lumbar region. When the trunk is viewed from the side with the patient still in the forward flexed position, the degree of roundback can be ascertained. A sharp, abrupt forward angulation in the thoracic or thoracolumbar region is indicative of a *kyphotic deformity*.

In a scoliosis patient, other areas of the body also must be examined, including the skin (hairy patches, nevi, and lipomas for *spinal dysraphism* and *café-au-lait* spots for neurofibromatosis), the extremities (skeletal dysplasia), the heart (murmurs for Marfan syndrome), and the neurologic system, to determine whether the scoliosis is truly idiopathic or possibly secondary to an underlying neuromuscular disorder.

## ROENTGENOGRAPHIC EVALUATION

Initial roentgenograms of the spine include a posteroanterior (PA) and lateral standing roentgenogram of the entire spine. This allows assessment for scoliosis, kyphosis, lordosis, congenital malformations, and, if the iliac crests are visible, the skeletal maturity of the patient. The degree of curvature is measured from the most tilted or end vertebra of the curve superiorly and inferiorly using the *Cobb method* (Fig. 19–15).

## SCOLIOSIS

Alterations in normal spinal alignment that occur in the AP or frontal plane are termed scoliosis. Most scoliotic deformities are idiopathic (unknown causation). Others, however, can be congenital, secondary to an underlying neuromuscular disorder, or compensatory from a leg length inequality.

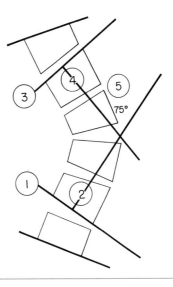

**FIGURE 19–15.** Scoliosis; measurement of a curve by the Cobb (roentgenographic) method. 1, Bottom vertebra: lowest one whose bottom tilts to concavity of curve. 2, Erect perpendicular from bottom of bottom vertebra. 3, Top vertebra: highest one whose top tilts to concavity of curve. 4, Drop perpendicular from top of top vertebra. 5, Measure intersecting angle. This is the accepted method of measurement of a curve according to the Scoliosis Research Society. Curves of 0–20 degrees are mild, 20–40 degrees are moderate, and above 40 degrees are severe. (From Ferguson A: Orthopaedic Surgery in Infancy and Childhood, 5th ed. Baltimore, Williams & Wilkins, 1981, p 856.)

### Idiopathic Scoliosis

The most common form of scoliosis occurs in healthy, neurologically normal children; its *etiology* is unknown. The incidence is only slightly higher in females, but females are more likely to progress and require treatment. Hereditary tendencies occur; approximately 20% of patients have other family members with the same condition.

Idiopathic scoliosis is classified into three age groups: infantile (birth to 3 yr), juvenile (4–10 yr), and adolescent (11 yr and older). *Idiopathic* adolescent scoliosis (80% of cases) is the most common cause of spinal deformity. The right thoracic curve is the most common pattern. *Infantile* scoliosis is very rare in the United States but is common in England. *Juvenile* scoliosis is not common, but many children with the diagnosis of adolescent scoliosis actually had the juvenile-onset type but the diagnosis was not made until later.

***Clinical Manifestations.*** Idiopathic scoliosis is a painless disorder. Any child with scoliosis and back pain requires a careful neurologic examination. Left thoracic curves and back pain are associated with an increased incidence of intraspinal pathology, such as a syrinx or tumor. These children should be evaluated by MRI.

*Treatment.* Treatment of idiopathic scoliosis is based on the skeletal age of the patient and whether the curve is progressive or nonprogressive. No treatment is necessary for nonprogressive deformities. The possibility for progression varies with several factors: sex, skeletal age, curve location, and curve magnitude. The risk for progression is much higher for females (5:1). The younger the child, the higher the risk for progression. The treatment of progressive idiopathic adolescent scoliosis is by an orthosis or surgery; exercises alone are ineffective. Typically, progressive curves between 25 and 45 degrees in a skeletally immature patient are managed by an orthosis. Curves greater than 45 degrees generally require surgery.

## Congenital Scoliosis

Abnormalities of vertebral formation during the 1st trimester result in structural deformities of the spine that are evident at birth or in early childhood. Congenital scoliosis can be classified as (1) partial or complete failure of vertebral formation (wedge vertebrae or hemivertebrae), (2) partial or complete failure of segmentation (unsegmented bars), or (3) mixed (Fig. 19–16). It may occur as a single anomaly or in combination with other bone, neural, or soft tissue abnormalities of the axial or appendicular skeleton. Congenital genitourinary malformations occur in 20% of children with congenital scoliosis. Unilateral renal agenesis is the most common abnormality, but 6% may have a silent, obstructive uropathy.

Renal ultrasonography is performed in all patients to assess for possible genitourinary problems. Congenital heart disease may be found in 10–15%. Spinal dysraphism occurs in approximately 20% of patients with congenital scoliosis. These include tethered spinal cord, intradural lipomas, and diastematomyelia. These abnormalities frequently are associated with cutaneous lesions of the back (such as hairy patches, skin dimples, and hemangiomas) and abnormalities of the feet and lower extremities (such as cavus feet, calf atrophy, asymmetric foot size, and neurologic changes). MRI is the procedure of choice for evaluation of possible spinal dysraphism. Congenital scoliosis also occurs in association with syndromes (such as Klippel-Feil and VATER) and spinal dysraphism disorders such as myelodysplasia.

The risk of progression of spinal deformity in a child with congenital scoliosis is variable, depending on the growth potential of the malformed vertebra. Defects such as a block vertebra have little growth potential, whereas unilateral unsegmented bars produce progressive deformities. Sev-

enty-five percent of involved patients will demonstrate some progression that continues until skeletal growth stops; approximately 50% will require treatment. Rapid progression can be expected during periods of rapid growth, before 2 yr and after 10 yr of age.

Early *diagnosis* and prompt *treatment* of progressive curves are essential elements in the care of congenital spinal deformity. Orthotic treatment is of limited value because these curves tend to be rigid. A spinal fusion without instrumentation is the most common procedure.

## Neuromuscular Scoliosis

Progressive spinal deformity is a common and potentially serious abnormality associated with many neuromuscular disorders, such as cerebral palsy, Duchenne muscular dystrophy, spinal muscular atrophy, and myelodysplasia. Progression is usually continuous once scoliosis begins. The magnitude of the deformity depends on the severity and pattern of weakness and whether the disease process is progressive. In nonambulatory patients, the curves tend to be long and sweeping, produce pelvic obliquity, involve the cervical spine, and alter pulmonary function, producing restrictive lung disease. As these curves progress, sitting balance can be lost and the affected individuals must use their arms to support an upright position. Spinal alignment must be part of the routine examination of a child with a neuromuscular disorder. Ambulatory patients have a much lower incidence of spinal deformity than nonambulatory or more severely involved patients. The standing or sitting forward bending test can be used in assessing the symmetry of spinal alignment.

Any asymmetry is an indication for *roentgenographic evaluation*, which should include a PA and lateral standing or sitting view of the entire spine. If the child or adolescent cannot sit unsupported, a supine AP radiograph may be necessary.

The goal of *treatment* is to prevent progression and loss of function. Nonambulatory patients usually are most comfortable, more independent, and have better respiratory function when they are able to sit erect without external support. Orthotic management or bracing is not usually effective; surgery will be necessary in most cases. The current instrumentation systems are sufficiently strong and distribute the corrective forces such that postoperative immobilization is not usually necessary.

## Compensatory Scoliosis

Adolescents with leg length inequality may have a positive screening examination for scoliosis. With

## Congenital Scoliosis

### Closed vertebral types
(MacEwen classification)

**A.** Partial unilateral failure of formation (wedge vertebrae)

**B.** Complete unilateral failure of formation (hemivertebra)

**C.** Unilateral failure of segmentation (congenital bar)

**D.** Bilateral failure of segmentation (block vertebra)

FIGURE 19–16. *A–D,* Types of closed vertebral and extravertebral spinal anomalies that result in congenital scoliosis. (From Hugo A, Keim MD: Scoliosis. Clin Symp 30[1]:16, 1978. Copyright 1978. CIBA-GEIGY Corporation. Reproduced with permission from Clinical Symposia by Frank H. Netter, M.D. All rights reserved.)

a pelvic obliquity, the patient will stand erect and curve the spine in the same direction. The magnitude of the leg length discrepancy can be measured radiographically by a scanogram of the lower extremities. It is important to distinguish between a structural and a compensatory spinal deformity.

### KYPHOSIS

The term "kyphosis" refers to a roundback deformity or to an increased angulation in the thoracic or thoracolumbar spine in the sagittal plane.

Roundback deformities can be either postural or structural; the latter is termed **Scheuermann's kyphosis.** Kyphosis also can be congenital in origin.

### POSTURAL ROUNDBACK

Postural kyphosis is secondary to bad posture and is a common concern of parents. Postural kyphosis is voluntarily corrected in both the standing and prone positions. Radiographically, no vertebral abnormalities are present. There may be some increase in the normal kyphosis of the thoracic region, but a supine hyperextension film will show complete correction. The child is responsible for correcting posture. Active *treatment* is not indicated.

## Scheuermann Disease

Scheuermann disease is common and second only to idiopathic scoliosis as a cause of spinal deformity. It occurs equally among male and female adolescents. Its *etiology* is unknown; hereditary factors are present but with no definite pattern of inheritance. The differentiation between postural kyphosis and Scheuermann disease is determined by clinical and roentgenographic evaluation.

***Clinical Manifestations.*** A patient with Scheuermann disease cannot correct the kyphosis either in the standing position or in the prone, hyperextended position. When viewed from the side in the forward flexed position, patients with Scheuermann disease usually show an abrupt angulation in the mid to lower thoracic region (Fig. 19–17). A patient with a postural roundback shows a smooth symmetric contour. In both conditions, there is an increase of the normal lumbar lordosis. Approximately 50% of patients with Scheuermann disease have apical back pain, especially with thoracolumbar kyphosis.

The classic roentgenographic findings of Scheuermann kyphosis include narrowing of disc space; loss of the normal anterior height of the involved vertebra, producing wedging of 5 degrees or more in three or more vertebrae; irregularities of the end plates; and Schmorl nodes.

***Treatment.*** Treatment of Scheuermann kyphosis is similar to that for scoliosis and is dependent on the skeletal age of the patient, the degree of deformity, and the presence or absence of pain in the apical region. Nonoperative treatment consists of a corrective plaster cast followed by an orthosis. Permanent correction of the kyphotic deformity can be achieved with nonoperative management. Surgical treatment in Scheuermann disease rarely is necessary and is indicated for those patients who have completed growth, who have a severe deformity, or who have chronic pain in the apical region.

## Congenital Kyphosis

Congenital kyphosis includes congenital failure of formation of all or part of the vertebral body, but with preservation of the posterior elements, and failure of anterior segmentation of the spine (anterior unsegmented bar). The more severe deformities usually are recognized at birth and rapidly progress thereafter. The less obvious deformities may not appear until years later. Once the progression begins, it does not cease until the end of growth. The most important factor regarding congenital kyphosis is that a progressive deformity in the thoracic spine can result in *paraplegia*. This usually is associated with the failure of vertebral body formation.

*Treatment*, when necessary, is operative. Orthotic management is ineffective.

## SPONDYLOLYSIS AND SPONDYLOLISTHESIS

*Spondylolysis* is a defect in the pars interarticularis without forward slippage of the involved vertebra on the one below. *Spondylolisthesis* refers to the forward slippage or displacement of the involved vertebra. The lesions are not present at birth but occur in 5% of children by 6 yr of age. Children involved in certain sports, such as gymnastics, have an even higher incidence of spondylolysis. This has been attributed to repetitive hyperextension stresses.

Spondylolisthesis is classified according to the degree of slippage of one vertebra on the other: grade 1, less than 25%; grade 2, 25–50%; grade 3, 50–75%; grade 4, 75–100%; and grade 5, complete displacement. The most common location of spondylolisthesis is the fifth lumbar vertebra on the sacrum (first sacral vertebra).

***Clinical Manifestations.*** Physical examination for spondylolysis or spondylolisthesis is similar to that for any disorder of the spine. A palpable "step-off" at the lumbosacral area and a vertically ori-

FIGURE 19–17. Note the sharp break in the contour in the child with kyphosis. (From Behrman RE [ed]: Nelson Textbook of Pediatrics, 14th ed. Philadelphia, WB Saunders, 1992, p 1715.)

ented sacrum indicate severe spondylolisthesis. A neurologic examination must be performed because nerve root involvement can occur, especially with severe displacement.

*Roentgenographic  Evaluation.* Roentgenographic evaluation should include standing PA and lateral views of the entire spine with an oblique radiograph of the lumbar spine. Myelography and MRI may be required in patients with neurologic findings.

*Treatment.* Children and adolescents with asymptomatic spondylolysis require periodic evaluation during growth to assess for possible slippage; treatment rarely is required. Painful spondylolysis may benefit from orthotic management. If this does not relieve pain, surgical intervention with an in situ posterior spinal fusion may be required.

Adolescents with spondylolisthesis may require treatment, which depends on age, type of defect, degree of the slippage, and associated malalignment in the involved area.

- *Grade 1*: Usually, no treatment is required unless there is chronic pain. Conservative management may be tried initially; if this fails, surgical intervention may be necessary.
- *Grade 2*: Usually, a spinal fusion is required because of the high risk for further progression.
- *Grade 3* and *grade 4*: Usually, fusion is required to prevent further injury.

## DISC SPACE INFECTION

A disc space infection is usually regarded as an osteomyelitis of the vertebral end plates that secondarily invades the disc without producing an acute osteomyelitis of the vertebral body. The most common organism is *S. aureus*. The infection can occur at any age. Children may present with back pain, but they also may present with abdominal or pelvic pain, irritability, and refusal to walk.

*Clinical Manifestations.* The child typically maintains the spine in a straight, stiff, or splinted position and refuses to flex the lumbar spine. The normal lumbar lordosis is reversed, and there may be paravertebral muscle spasms. However, in comparison with other forms of osteomyelitis, there are few systemic symptoms, such as fever and an elevated white blood cell count. The ESR typically is elevated.

*Roentgenographic Evaluation.* The roentgenographic features will vary according to the interval between the onset of symptoms and delay in diagnosis. AP, lateral, and oblique radiographs of the lumbar spine or thoracic spine, depending on the location of symptoms, usually are necessary to make the diagnosis. There is narrowing of the disc space with irregularity of the adjacent vertebral body end plates. In very early cases, bone scan or MRI studies may be helpful because they may be positive before routine roentgenographic changes are present.

*Treatment.* The treatment of disc space infection usually is antibiotic therapy. Blood cultures may be helpful in establishing a precise organism. Aspiration needle biopsy of the disc space is reserved for children who do not respond to initial treatment with antistaphylococcal antibiotics. Immobilization of the spine may be used on a symptomatic basis. In most children, however, symptoms rapidly resolve with intravenous antibiotics. Intravenous antibiotics are continued for 1–2 wk and followed by oral antibiotics for an additional 4 wk.

## TORTICOLLIS

The literal definition of torticollis is twisted neck, but the traditional definition is shortening of one sternocleidomastoid muscle. Shortening and secondary contractures can be a primary abnormality of the sternocleidomastoid muscle (muscular torticollis) or secondary to central nervous system or upper cervical spine abnormalities.

Infants and young children with muscular torticollis present with the ear pulled down toward the clavicle on the ipsilateral side. The face looks upward toward the contralateral side. Early in childhood, a "tumor" is palpated in the midportion of the sternocleidomastoid muscle. This represents swelling or fibrosis of the central portion of the muscle and often is a precursor of the subsequent contracture.

*Etiology.* In infants, in utero malposition, birth trauma, sternocleidomastoid muscle compartment syndrome, and heredity have been implicated as etiologic factors. In acquired torticollis in children, central nervous system mass lesions, abnormalities of the cervical spine, and local head and neck infections are more likely. Psychiatric causes may occur during adolescence.

*Diagnosis.* A thorough neurologic examination should be performed and AP and lateral radiographs of the cervical spine obtained. A CT scan or MRI of the head and neck is necessary for any patient with persistent neck pain or other neurologic signs and symptoms.

*Treatment.* Treatment goals include ruling out an underlying disorder, increasing range of motion of the neck, and correcting the cosmetic deformity.

Some infants with muscular torticollis may respond to nonoperative measures, which include range of motion exercises of the head and neck, stretching the restrictive muscles several times daily. General indications for nonoperative management include age younger than 1 yr, positive response to stretching exercise over several weeks, and no underlying cervical spine abnormalities or central nervous system findings.

Principles of surgical management of patients with muscular torticollis include identifying and releasing all restricting bands involving the sternocleidomastoid muscle and other neck structures, moving the head through a full range of motion prior to completion of the surgery, and resuming physical therapy within 2 wk of operation to prevent recurrent contracture.

## BACK PAIN IN CHILDREN

Back pain in children is unusual and should be viewed with concern. In contrast to adults, in whom back pain frequently is mechanical or psychologic in origin, back pain in children is usually due to organic causes, especially in the preadolescent. Back pain lasting more than a few days requires careful investigation. Approximately 85% of children with back pain of more than 2 mo have a specific lesion: 33% post-traumatic (occult fracture, spondylolysis), 33% developmental (kyphosis, scoliosis), and 18% infection or tumor. In the remaining 15% the diagnosis will be undetermined.

*Clinical Manifestations.* The history should include the onset and duration of symptoms; antecedent factors; general health; family history; location, character and radiation of pain; and neurologic symptoms such as muscle weakness, sensory changes, and bowel or bladder dysfunction. Physical examination should include a complete musculoskeletal and neurologic evaluation. Spinal alignment, mobility, muscle spasm, and areas of tenderness should be evaluated and recorded. Muscle strength, sensory assessment (such as pain and light touch), deep tendon reflexes, and pathologic reflexes (such as the Babinski sign are tested). The danger signs in childhood back pain include persistent or increasing pain; systemic symptoms such as fever, malaise, or weight loss; neurologic findings; bowel or bladder dysfunction; young age, especially under 4 yr (suspect tumor); and painful left thoracic spinal curvatures.

*Roentgenographic Evaluation.* The first diagnostic procedure is PA and lateral standing films of the entire spine with right and left oblique views of the involved area. Other roentgenographs may be necessary, depending on the location of the pain

and the differential diagnoses. These include bone scans, CT scan, laminograms, myelography, and MRI. MRI is especially useful when intraspinal pathology is suspected.

*Laboratory Evaluation.* Laboratory studies such as complete blood count, erythrocyte sedimentation rate, and tests for the juvenile forms of arthritis (juvenile rheumatoid arthritis and ankylosing spondylitis) may be necessary. Cerebrospinal fluid should be evaluated if myelography is performed.

*Differential Diagnosis.* The differential diagnosis in pediatric back pain is extensive (Table 19–11).

*Treatment.* The treatment of back pain is based on an accurate diagnosis.

### References

Behrman RE, Kliegman RM, Arvin AM (eds): Nelson Textbook of Pediatrics, 15th ed. Philadelphia, WB Saunders, 1996, Chapters 628.1–628.9.

TABLE 19–11.    Differential Diagnosis of Back Pain

**Inflammatory Diseases**

  Discitis (common before 6 yr)
  Vertebral osteomyelitis (pyogenic, tuberculous)
  Spinal epidural abscess
  Pyelonephritis
  Pancreatitis

**Rheumatologic Diseases**

  Pauciarticular juvenile rheumatoid arthritis
  Reiter syndrome
  Juvenile ankylosing spondylitis
  Psoriatic arthritis

**Developmental Diseases**

  Spondylolysis
  Spondylolisthesis
  Scheuermann syndrome
  Scoliosis (especially left thoracic)

**Mechanical Trauma and Abnormalities**

  Hip/pelvic anomalies
  Herniated disc
  Overuse syndromes (common with athletic training and in gymnasts and dancers)
  Vertebral stress fractures
  Upper cervical spine instability

**Neoplastic Diseases**

  Primary vertebral bone tumors (osteogenic sarcoma)
  Metastatic tumor (neuroblastoma)
  Primary spinal tumor (neuroblastoma, astrocytoma)
  Malignancy of bone marrow (ALL, lymphoma)
  Benign tumors (eosinophilic granuloma, osteoid osteoma)

**Other**

  After lumbar puncture
  Conversion reaction
  Juvenile osteoporosis

ALL = acute lymphocytic leukemia.

Davids JR, Wenger DR, Mubarak SJ: Congenital muscular torticollis: Sequela of intrauterine compartment syndrome. J Pediatr Orthop 13:141, 1993.

Hensinger R: Current concepts review: Spondylolysis and spondylolisthesis in children and adolescents. J Bone Joint Surg 71A:1098, 1989.

Lonstein JE: Adolescent idiopathic scoliosis: Screening and diagnosis. Instr Course Lect 38:105, 1989.

Lonstein JE, Carlson JM: The prediction of curve progression in untreated idiopathic scoliosis during growth. J Bone Joint Surg 66A:1061, 1984.

Lowe TG: Current concepts review: Scheuermann disease. J Bone Joint Surg 72A:940, 1990.

McMaster MJ, Ohtsuka K: The natural history of congenital scoliosis: A study of 251 patients. J Bone Joint Surg 68B:588, 1986.

Ring D, Johnston CE II, Wenger DR: Pyogenic infectious spondylitis in children: The convergence of discitis and vertebral osteomyelitis. J Pediatr Orthop 15:652, 1995.

Scoles PV: Back pain in children and adolescents. *In* Kliegman RM, et al (eds): Practical Strategies in Pediatric Diagnosis and Therapy. Philadelphia, WB Saunders, 1996, pp 779–791.

Thompson GH: Back pain in children. J Bone Joint Surg 75A:928, 1993.

Weinstein SL: Adolescent idiopathic scoliosis: Problems and natural history. *In* Weinstein SL (ed): The Pediatric Spine: Principles and Practice. New York, Raven Press, 1994, pp 463–478.

# THE SHOULDER

The shoulder joint has minimal geometric stability because of the relatively small glenoid fossa that articulates with a proportionately large hemispheric humeral head. A large range of motion is gained at the expense of intrinsic stability; consequently, the musculature about the shoulder, particularly the muscles of the rotator cuff, must function with normal glenohumeral contact. Scapulothoracic movement greatly expands the range of motion possible at the shoulder area, and the scapula, just as is the case with the glenohumeral joint, requires strong coordinated musculature to function with stability.

## SPRENGEL DEFORMITY

Failure of the upper extremity to descend to its normal location is Sprengel deformity, which occurs with varying degrees of severity. The scapula is located abnormally high with respect to the child's neck and thorax. Webbing of the neck or skin of the neck and a low posterior hair line may be associated findings. In the severe form, a bone (omovertebral) may connect the scapula with the lower cervical spine and virtually no scapulothoracic movement may be possible; often, associated muscle anomalies are present as well that further limit strength and stability of the shoulder girdle. In the mild form, the scapula is slightly high ri-

ding, with less than normal motion. Association with congenital cervical vertebral anomalies, particularly the **Klippel-Feil anomaly,** occurs and suggests the possibility of significant problems in other organ systems. The best outcome in severe Sprengel deformities is achieved in early childhood by surgically repositioning and occasionally partially resecting the scapula. This improves cosmesis and motion, especially shoulder abduction.

## BRACHIAL PLEXUS (OBSTETRIC) PALSY

See Chapter 6.

## DISLOCATION OF THE SHOULDER

Dislocation of the shoulder is uncommon in childhood but becomes more frequent in adolescence. The younger the individual at the time of the initial dislocation, the more likely recurrent dislocation is to develop. The chances of redislocation are so high that many orthopaedic surgeons now favor early reconstruction rather than instituting conservative treatment and awaiting further dislocations.

## EPIPHYSIOLYSIS OF THE PROXIMAL HUMERAL EPIPHYSIS

The youngster who engages regularly in a throwing sport is at risk for traumatic epiphysiolysis of the proximal humeral physis. This disorder is a fatigue fracture through the physis; it heals with rest and avoidance of repetitive throwing. Pain about the shoulder is the usual presenting complaint.

## OVERUSE SYNDROMES

Overuse syndromes, inflammatory responses in tendons and bursae subjected to repetitive mild trauma, are uncommon in childhood but may be seen in the adolescent. Subacromial **bursitis,** for example, occurs in tennis players and swimmers. Bicipital **tendinitis** is uncommon in the young but may produce a sensation of something snapping in the shoulder or shoulder pain when the bicipital groove is shallow and the tendon can sublux from it. In these types of inflammatory responses, direct tenderness over the involved anatomic structure is diagnostic.

### References

Behrman RE, Kliegman RM, Arvin AM (eds): Nelson Textbook of Pediatrics, 15th ed. Philadelphia, WB Saunders, 1996, Chapters 630.1–630.2.

Wagner KT, Lyne ED: Adolescent traumatic dislocations of the shoulder with open epiphyses. J Pediatr Orthop 3:61, 1983.

## THE ELBOW

The elbow joint consists of three articulations: the ulna and the humerus, the radius and the humerus, and the proximal radius and the ulna. Collectively, they provide for a hinge-type joint that allows for a palm-up (supination) and a palm-down (pronation) positioning of the wrist and hand. The elbow has great geometric stability, and the musculature moving the joint primarily motors flexion and extension at the elbow joint, but there are smaller muscles that primarily serve to rotate the radius about its long axis.

### NURSEMAID'S ELBOW

The radial head is not as bulbous in the infant as in older children. During infancy, the circular ligament that passes around its base can partially slip off the head with traction across the elbow. When the ligament slips, the entity is known as nursemaid's elbow, or subluxation of the annular ligament (Fig. 19–18). The subluxation is initiated by a jerk on the extended elbow when a child falls with the hand being held or when a child is forcefully lifted by the hand. When the subluxation occurs, the hand typically is held in a palm-down position, and the child may refuse to use the hand or may cry when the elbow is moved. Moving the hand to a palm-up position with pressure over the radial head usually reduces the ligament subluxa-

FIGURE 19–18.   The pathology of pulled elbow. The annular ligament is torn when the arm is pulled. The radial head moves distally and, when traction is discontinued, the ligament is carried into the joint. (From Rang M: Children's Fractures, 2nd ed. Philadelphia, JB Lippincott, 1983, p 193.)

tion and restores full normal use of the extremity. The parents should be educated about the mechanism of injury and should be encouraged to avoid picking the child up by holding the hand or forearm. Once subluxation has occurred, there is a propensity for subsequent episodes. Generally, the problem resolves with maturation.

### PANNER DISEASE

Panner disease is an osteochondrosis that involves the ossific nucleus of the capitellum, the lateral portion of the distal humeral epiphysis. It is most common in adolescents, especially those involved in throwing activities. They complain of pain and may have crepitation and loss of motion. AP, lateral, and oblique roentgenographs, tomograms, or CT may be helpful. In the absence of a loose osteocartilaginous body, *treatment* is conservative; if such a body is present, surgery is indicated.

### THROWING INJURIES

The elbow is especially vulnerable to throwing injuries in the skeletally immature child. The most common pathology results from abnormal compressive forces acting across the radial side of the joint. In addition to Panner disease, the ossific nucleus of the radial head may become asymmetric compared with the opposite side or may be fragmented. Some irregularity in shape of the cartilaginous radial head is present. Additionally, there may be irregularity of the ossific nucleus of the capitellum or compressions in the normally rounded articular cartilage of the capitellum. Rarely, small pieces of cartilage from the capitellum or radial head may shed into the joint, producing loose bodies. Before the problem becomes established or severe, the child complains of an aching pain about the elbow, which generally is worse after throwing than during the time spent at the throwing activity. On physical examination, an early loss of supination (the palm-up position of the hand) can be detected. Children in whom these lesions develop generally have a high emotional investment in their particular sport, most commonly baseball, and nonparticipation is a difficult option for them to accept. Avoidance of pitching until the elbow is normal on physical examination and follow-up roentgenogram is the best solution. Often, switching the baseball player to another position allows the child to avoid pitching. Behind such highly motivated youngsters is usually an overzealous parent or coach in need of appropriate counseling.

## References

Behrman RE, Kliegman RM, Arvin AM (eds): Nelson Textbook of Pediatrics, 15th ed. Philadelphia, WB Saunders, 1996, Chapters 630.3–630.4.
Bora FW: The Pediatric Upper Extremity: Diagnosis and Management. Philadelphia, WB Saunders, 1986.

## THE HAND

Multiple small joints, a delicately balanced intrinsic muscle system, a powerful extrinsic muscle system, dense sensory innervation, and specialized skin combined to make the hand a highly mobile, sensitive, delicate yet powerful anatomic part.

The extrinsic muscles, those whose muscle origin is in the forearm and that motor the hand via tendons that pass to it, provide great power, whereas the intrinsic muscles, those that are located in the hand itself, modulate the effects of the powerful extrinsic musculature and provide for delicate coordinated movement. Simply asking the patient to open the hand, extending and spreading the fingers and thumb, and, subsequently, clenching the hand to a fist yields much insight, because these maneuvers require coordinated function of both the intrinsic and extrinsic musculature as well as full range of motion in the small joints of the hand. After this maneuver, simply having the individual squeeze the examiner's fingers gives further information about the strength of the hand.

### FINGER ABNORMALITIES

Extra digits (polydactyly) occur as both simple and complex varieties (see Table 19–8). Those skin tags and digit remnants typically seen near the metacarpophalangeal joint of the small finger or of the thumb that do not have palpable bone in their base or possess voluntary movement may simply be excised while the child is still in the nursery. Varieties of polydactyly more complex than this should be referred for amputation.

**Syndactyly** also occurs in both simple and complex patterns (see Table 19–9). There always is concern about the sharing of common important structures between the digits and about the tethering effect of the syndactyly on the growth of the affected digits. Referral for delineation of the specific pathology and development of a treatment strategy is indicated when the condition is recognized.

### GANGLION

A synovial fluid-filled cyst about the wrist, a *ganglion*, is common in childhood. The usual site is the dorsum of the wrist near the radiocarpal joint, and a secondary site is over the volar radial aspect of the wrist. The essential pathology is a defect in one of the joint capsules; with wrist use, synovial fluid is pumped into the soft tissue, where it becomes walled off by reactive fibrous tissue. Often, in the skeletally immature child, the process is benign and tends to disappear with the passage of time. In the event that a ganglion is sufficiently large to cause pain or interfere with normal tendon function, aspiration and injection of the cyst are sometimes helpful; in refractory cases, surgical excision of the cyst accompanied by removal of the tract that extends into the joint is curative.

## References

Behrman RE, Kliegman RM, Arvin AM (eds): Nelson Textbook of Pediatrics, 15th ed. Philadelphia, WB Saunders, 1996, Chapters 630.5–630.9.
Bora FW Jr: The Pediatric Upper Extremity: Diagnosis and Management. Philadelphia, WB Saunders, 1986.
Satku K, Ganesh B: Ganglia in children. J Pediatr Orthop 5:513, 1985.

## MUSCULOSKELETAL TRAUMA

Fractures in children have been estimated to account for 10–15% of all childhood injuries. Children are not small adults; their skeletal systems have anatomic, biomechanical, and physiologic differences from those of adults. These result in different fracture patterns, including epiphyseal injuries, problems of diagnosis, and variation in management techniques.

The anatomic differences in the pediatric skeleton include the presence of preosseous cartilage, physes, and thicker, stronger periosteum that produces callus more rapidly and in greater amounts. Biomechanically, the pediatric skeletal system can absorb more energy prior to deformation and fracture than adult bone can. This has been attributed to lower ash content and the greater porosity of young bone. As maturation occurs, the porosity decreases and the cortical bone becomes thicker and stronger. The thick periosteum of a child is a major determinant in whether a fracture becomes displaced. The thick periosteum also can act as an impediment to closed reduction because of the hinging phenomenon. Conversely, it can help stabilize a fracture following reduction.

### UNUSUAL FEATURES

#### Fracture Remodeling

Remodeling occurs by a combination of periosteal resorption and new bone formation. Thus, anatomic alignment in certain pediatric fractures is not always necessary. The major factors affecting fracture remodeling include (1) the child's age, (2) the proximity of the fracture to a joint, and (3) the relationship of the fracture to the plane of joint motion. The amount of remaining musculoskeletal growth provides the basis for remodeling; the younger the child, the greater the remodeling potential. Certain physes also have a relatively greater growth potential than others. Fractures adjacent to a physis undergo the greatest amount of remodeling, provided that the residual deformity is in the plane of motion of that joint. Fracture remodeling is not effective in displaced intra-articular fractures, diaphyseal fractures, malrotation, and fracture displacement or deformity not in the plane of joint motion. The amount of remodeling will be significantly diminished as a child approaches skeletal maturity.

### Overgrowth

Overgrowth, especially in long bones such as the femur, is due to the increased blood flow associated with fracture healing. Femoral fractures in children under 10 yr of age frequently overgrow 1–3 cm. This accounts for the concept of *bayonet apposition* to compensate for the overgrowth that may occur over the next 1–2 yr. After 10 yr of age, overgrowth is less of a problem and end-on alignment is recommended.

### Progressive Deformity

Injuries to a physis can result in complete or partial closure. As a consequence, angular deformity, shortening, or both can occur. The magnitude depends on the bone involved and the amount of remaining growth. Growth arrest most commonly occurs in the distal femur, distal tibia, and proximal tibia.

### Healing Rate

Fractures heal more quickly in children than in adults. This effect is due to their growth potential and thicker, more metabolically active periosteum. As the older child and adolescent mature, the rate of healing slows and approaches that of an adult.

## PEDIATRIC FRACTURE PATTERNS

### Nonepiphyseal Fractures

**Complete.** Complete fractures occur when both sides of the bone are fractured. This is the most common fracture type. These fractures may be classified as spiral, transverse, oblique, or comminuted, depending on the direction of the fracture line.

**Buckle or Torus Fracture.** Compression of bone produces a buckle or torus fracture. These fractures typically occur in the metaphyseal areas in young children, especially the distal radius. They are inherently stable and usually heal in 2–3 wk with simple immobilization.

**Greenstick.** When a bone is angulated beyond the limits of plastic deformation, a greenstick fracture may occur. This represents bone failure on the tension side and compression or bend deformity on the opposite side. The energy has been insufficient to result in a complete fracture.

**Bowing or Bend Fractures.** Traumatic bowing or bend deformities are due to plastic deformation of bone. The bone was angulated beyond its limit of plastic deformation but did not fracture. Thus, no fracture line is visible roentgenographically.

### Epiphyseal Fractures

Fractures involving the physes are common and comprise 15–20% of all children's fractures. There is a male-to-female ratio of 2:1, and the upper extremity is involved twice as frequently as the lower. The peak incidence in males is 13–14 yr and in females 11–12 yr. The distal radius is the most common site, followed by the distal tibia.

Ligaments frequently insert into epiphyses. As a consequence, traumatic forces supplied to an extremity may be transmitted to the physis. The strength of the physes is enhanced by their shape and perichondrial ring. However, the physis still is not as strong biomechanically as the metaphyseal or diaphyseal bone. The physis is most resistant to traction and least resistant to torsional or angular forces.

*Classification.* Salter and Harris have classified epiphyseal injuries into five groups (Fig. 19–19):

- *Type I,* epiphyseal separation through the physis
- *Type II,* fracture through a portion of the physis but exiting across the metaphysis
- *Type III,* fracture through the physis but exiting across the epiphysis into the joint
- *Type IV,* a fracture line extending across the metaphysis, physis, and epiphysis
- *Type V,* a crush injury to the physis

This classification allows generalized prognostic information regarding the risk for premature physeal closure and the indications for treatment. A *type VI* injury (injury to the perichondrial ring that often

FIGURE 19–19. The types of growth plate injury as classified by Salter and Harris. (From Salter RB, Harris WR: Injuries involving the epiphyseal plate. J Bone Joint Surg 45A:587, 1963.)

results in a peripheral bony bridge and rapid angular deformities) has also been suggested.

*Treatment.* Types I and II fractures usually can be managed by closed reduction techniques and do not require perfect alignment. A major exception are type II fractures of the distal femur. Fractures in this location carry a poor prognosis unless almost anatomic alignment is obtained by either closed or open methods. Types III and IV epiphyseal fractures require anatomic alignment because of displacement of the physis and the articular surfaces. Type V fractures usually are recognized in retrospect and invariably result in premature growth plate closure.

### MANAGEMENT OF PEDIATRIC FRACTURES

#### Closed Treatment

Most pediatric fractures can be managed by closed methods.

#### Operative Treatment

Certain pediatric fractures have been demonstrated to have better prognosis if the fractures are reduced, by either open or closed techniques, and then internally fixed. Approximately 3–4% of pediatric fractures require internal fixation. The common indications for internal fixations in children and adolescents with open physes include:

- Displaced epiphyseal fractures
- Displaced intra-articular fractures
- Unstable fractures

- Fractures in the multiply injured child
- Open fractures

In children, the goals of surgery and type of internal fixation device used are different. The goals of surgery are not rigid internal fixation but, rather, attainment and maintenance of anatomic alignment. Thus, simple fixation with the use of Steinmann pins, Kirschner wires, and small cortical screws is indicated. Fractures subsequently are protected with external immobilization, usually a plaster cast, until satisfactory healing has occurred. All internal fixation devices are removed following fracture healing to prevent incorporation into the callus formation and bone and to prevent physeal damage if a physis has been transgressed by a smooth wire or pin.

External fixation also has been very successful for certain pediatric fractures. The major indications have been pelvic and open extremity fractures, especially those with extensive soft tissue loss, burns, or vascular and nerve repairs.

### SPECIAL PROBLEMS

#### Neurovascular Injuries

The most common sites of neural or vascular injuries are the distal humerus, in which supracondylar fractures occur, and the knee, in which dislocations and physeal fractures or dislocations occur. Careful neurovascular examination is necessary for all fractures and should be documented in the patient's medical record.

## Compartment Syndromes

Hemorrhage and soft tissue swelling within tight fascial compartments may result in muscle ischemia and neurovascular compromise unless decompressed surgically. This condition is called compartment syndrome. The forearms and lower legs are the major sites, and these syndromes tend to occur following supracondylar fractures at the distal humerus and tibial shaft fractures. The common findings are tense compartments, severe pain, decreased sensation in the nerves that transverse the involved compartment, and pain with passive stretch (fingers or toes) of involved muscles. In addition, once an injured extremity is placed in a cast, it is possible that a cast-induced compartment syndrome may develop. It is the responsibility of the treating physician to ensure that parents understand the signs of ischemia and appreciate that it is an emergency. The parents must contact the physician or return to the hospital immediately.

## Toddler's Fracture

An oblique fracture of the distal one third of the tibia without a fibula fracture can occur with minimal trauma in children 1–3 yr of age and occasionally up to 6 yr of age. Limping or inability to bear weight is a common complaint. These fractures

TABLE 19–12.  Benign Bone Tumors and Cysts

| Disease | Characteristics | Roentgenography | Treatment | Prognosis |
|---|---|---|---|---|
| Osteochondroma (osteocartilaginous exostosis) | Common; distal metaphysis of femur, proximal humerus, proximal tibia; painless, hard, nontender mass | Bony outgrowth, sessile or pedunculated | Excision, if symptomatic | Excellent; malignant transformation rare |
| Multiple hereditary exostoses | Osteochondroma of long bones; bone growth disturbances | As above | As above | Recurrences |
| Osteoid ostoma | Pain relieved by aspirin; femur and tibia; predominantly found in boys | Dense sclerosis surrounds small radiolucent nidus, <1 cm | As above | Excellent |
| Osteoblastoma (giant osteoid osteoma) | As above, but more destructive | Osteolytic component; size greater than 1 cm | As above | Excellent |
| Enchondroma | Tubular bones of hands and feet; pathologic fractures, swollen bone; Ollier disease if multiple lesions are present | Radiolucent diaphyseal or metaphyseal lesion; may calcify | Excision or curettage | Excellent; malignant transformation rare |
| Nonossifying fibroma | Silent; rare pathologic fracture; late childhood adolescence | Incidental roentgenographic finding; thin sclerotic border, radiolucent lesion | None or curettage with fractures | Excellent; heals spontaneously |
| Eosinophilic granuloma | Age 5–10 yr; skull, jaw, long bones; pathologic fracture; pain | Small, radiolucent without reactive bone; punched out lytic lesion | Biopsy, excision rare; irradiation | Excellent; may heal spontaneously |
| Brodie abscess | Insidious local pain; limp; suspected as malignancy | Circumscribed metaphyseal osteomyelitis; lytic lesions with sclerotic rim | Biopsy; antibiotics | Excellent |
| Unicameral bone cyst (simple bone cyst) | Metaphysis of long bone (femur, humerus); pain, pathologic fracture | Cyst in medullary canal, expands cortex; fluid-filled unilocular or multilocular cavity | Curettage; steroid injection into lesion | Excellent; some heal spontaneously |
| Aneurysmal bone cyst | As above; contains blood, fibrous tissue | Expands beyond metaphyseal cartilage | Curettage, bone graft | Excellent |

may not be visible roentgenographically, but occasionally oblique roentgenographs may be helpful. A physical examination may show minimal soft tissue swelling, pain, and slight warmth.

### Child Abuse

Fractures attributable to child abuse constitute a special issue that constantly must be considered in trauma assessment of the infant and younger child, especially those 3 yr of age or less (see Chapter 1). Multiple fractures that are visible roentgenographically at different stages of healing are a classic sign. If a child has been shaken, frequently there will be areas adjacent to the epiphysis on the metaphyseal side that will fracture, producing the appearance of metaphyseal "corner" fractures. Long bone fractures, especially spiral fractures of the humeral, tibial, or femoral shaft, suggest that someone has forcefully twisted the extremity. When there is any suspicion of abuse, the child should be admitted to the hospital for full assessment. Roentgenographs of a specific area are appropriate, but a bone scan may be more helpful in identifying other fractures, old and new. A thorough physical examination focusing on soft tissues, the skeletal system, and the cranium, along with a careful examination of the retina for hemorrhage or detachment, is very important.

### References

Behrman RE, Kliegman RM, Arvin AM (eds): Nelson Textbook of Pediatrics, 15th ed. Philadelphia, WB Saunders, 1996, Chapters 632.1–632.10.
King J, Kiefendorf D, Apthorp J, et al: Analysis of 429 fractures in 189 battered children. J Pediatr Orthop 8:585, 1988.
Peterson HA: Partial growth plate arrest and its treatment. J Pediatr Orthop 4:246, 1984.
Rockwood CA Jr, Wilkens KE, King RE: In Fractures in Children, 3rd ed. Philadelphia, JB Lippincott, 1991.
Tenenbien M, Reed MH, Block GB: The toddler's fracture revisited. Am J Emerg Med 8:208, 1990.
Thompson GH, Wilber JH, Marcus RE: Internal fixation of fractures in children and adolescents: A comparative analysis. Clin Orthop 188:10, 1984.

## METABOLIC BONE DISEASE

Metabolic bone disease may occur from disorders that primarily affect bone, cartilage, and collagen or that indirectly affect bone mineralization. Primary bone disorders often occur in the fetus or young infant, such as the skeletal dysplasias–dwarf-like syndromes (e.g., achondroplasia, Kneist dysplasia, osteogenesis imperfecta).

Patients with metabolic disorders that produce indirect effects may appear normal at birth and later develop signs of bone disease. The signs of bone disease may occur after or concomitant with the manifestations produced by the underlying metabolic disorder (e.g., homocystinuria, Marfan syndrome, Gaucher disease, renal rickets). The *treatment* of primary disorders of bone is limited, and therapy of inborn errors of metabolism must be tailored to the specific disease (see Chapter 5).

## BONE TUMORS AND CYSTIC LESIONS

Benign bone tumors and cystic lesions are common in childhood. Some represent fibrous dysplasia and others are benign tumors, whereas subacute osteomyelitis **(Brodie abscess)** or eosinophilic granuloma represent lesions unrelated to abnormal osseous or cartilage growth (Table 19–12). Many of these lesions produce pain, pathologic fractures, or limp; others may be incidental findings on roentgenographic examination. The *prognosis* usually is excellent. *Treatment* is summarized in Table 19–12. Malignant bone tumors are discussed in Chapter 15.

### References

Behrman RE, Kliegman RM, Arvin AM (eds): Nelson Textbook of Pediatrics, 15th ed. Philadelphia, WB Saunders, 1996, Chapters 454.1–454.2.
Gitelis S, Wilkins R, Conrad EU III: Benign bone tumors. J Bone Joint Surg 77A:1756, 1995.

# Appendices

**TABLE AP–1.** Drug Doses* (Drugs Listed Alphabetically by Generic Name)

| KEY: | | | | |
|---|---|---|---|---|
| NB | newborn (birth to end of 1st mo) | † | available as generic preparation | |
| IN | infant (1–12 mo) | ‡ | available also under other brand name(s) | |
| CH | child (1–12 yr) | | | |
| AD | adult | g | gram | |
| caps | capsules | mg | milligram $= 10^{-3}$ g | |
| div | divided | $\mu$g | microgram $= 10^{-6}$ g | |
| DW | dextrose in water | | (sometimes abbreviated "mcg") | |
| IM | intramuscular | ng | nanogram $= 10^{-9}$ g | |
| inj | injection | kg | kilogram $= 10^{3}$ g | |
| IV | intravenous | mL | milliliter $= 10^{-3}$ liter $\simeq$ cm$^3$ $=$ cc (cubic centimeter) | |
| LO | linguo-occlusal | Rx | prescription | |
| ointm | ointment | | | |
| PO | per os, oral | | | |
| PR | per rectum | | | |
| SC | subcutaneous | | | |
| SL | sublingual | | | |
| sol | solution | | | |
| susp | suspension | | | |
| tabl | tablets | | | |

## I. ANTIBIOTICS

**Acyclovir;** antiviral agent against herpes simplex and varicella-zoster virus by selective inhibition of viral DNA synthesis

Rx in clinical herpes simplex infection in neonates: NB = IV (over 60 min): 10 mg/kg/dose every 8 hr, for 10–14 days
Dosing interval should be increased to 24 hr if renal function is less than 25% of normal

Rx in immunocompromised individuals with herpes simplex or varicella-zoster virus infection: CH = IV (over 60 min): 7.5 mg/kg per dose every 8 hr for 7 days. PO: 7.5–20 mg/kg per dose administered 4–5 times per day. AD = IV (over 60 min); PO: 800 mg 5 times/day for 7–10 days

Rx mucocutaneous herpes simplex virus (HSV) infection: CH = IV (over 60 min) 5 mg/kg per dose every 8 hr for 7 days; HSV encephalitis: 10 mg/kg per dose every 8 hr for 10–14 days; varicella-zoster infection: 5 mg/kg per dose every 8 hr for 7 days

Rx IV prophylaxis in bone marrow transplant recipients: HSV seropositive 4.5–5 mg/kg ev-

---

*No attempt has been made to reproduce a comprehensive list of adverse side effects or of formulations available for the drugs listed. For these, the reader again is referred to standard textbooks of pharmacology, to the package inserts accompanying the commercial preparations of each drug, and to *Physician's Desk Reference*, distributed annually in the United States by Physician's Desk Reference, Box 210, Westwood, NJ 07675.

Dosages listed in the table are not specifically intended for premature and newborn infants unless so indicated.

All doses are average doses and are approximate. Variability of individual response may require alteration of dosage upward or downward. Doses based on different criteria (e.g., body weight, surface area) frequently do not correspond. Surface area may be calculated from Figure AP–1.

Doses generally are expressed as grams or milligrams per kilogram of body weight per 24 hours (g or mg/kg/24 hr), even for drugs ordinarily administered on a p.r.n. (as needed or indicated) basis.

For teratogenic effects of drugs, see Chapter 6, package inserts, and *Physician's Desk Reference*.

Because of the multiplicity of proprietary names and formulations of the drugs listed, only a few representative examples have been given of the many proprietary preparations available in most instances. We have intended no bias in selecting the proprietary names used, and we make due apology to any manufacturers and distributors whose products may appear to have been slighted.

**See KEY to abbreviations, above; for further information about drugs, see package inserts.**

TABLE AP–1.    Drug Doses* (Drugs Listed Alphabetically by Generic Name) *Continued*

ery 8–12 hr; CMV seropositive 15 mg/kg per dose every 8 hr; in markedly symptomatic patients, consider ganciclovir

℞ in severe first episode of herpes genitalis: CH, AD = LO: 5% ointm

**Caution:** Acyclovir dosing should be adjusted for patients with renal insufficiency (i.e., glomerular filtration rates <50 mL/min in patients >6 mo of age).

ZOVIRAX; inj, ointm, caps, susp, tabl

**Amikacin sulfate;** antimicrobial aminoglycoside effective primarily against gram-negative microorganisms

NB <7 days: <28 wk = IM, IV (over 20–30 min): 7.5 mg/kg once daily; 28–34 wk, 7.5 mg/kg every 18 hr; >34 wk, 7.5 mg/kg every 12 hr

NB >7 days: <28 wk, 7.5 mg/kg every 18 hr; 28–34 wk, 7.5 mg/kg every 12 hr; >34 wk, 7.5 mg/kg every 8 hr

IN, CH = IM, IV 15–25 mg/kg/24 hr. AD = IM, IV 15 mg/kg/24 hr every 12 hr.

Serum concentrations should be monitored; therapeutic peak concentration 25–35 mg/L, trough concentration <10 mg/L

AMIKIN: inj

**Amoxicillin;** acid-resistant ampicillin congener

IN, CH = PO: 20–50 mg/kg/24 hr, div, every 8 hr

†, AMOXIL, LAROTID, ‡: caps, oral susp, pediatric drops

**Amoxicillin + clavulanic acid;** combination of a β-lactam antibiotic with a β-lactamase (penicillinase) inhibitor.

℞ for otitis media, sinusitis, lower respiratory tract, skin, soft tissue, and urinary tract infections: CH = PO: amoxicillin 20–40 mg/kg/24 hr + clavulanic acid 5–10 mg/kg/24 hr, div, every 8 hr

*Note:* Many cause diarrhea, abdominal pain, urticaria and other rashes, possibly due to clavulanic acid alone.

Amoxicillin is available as single component.

AUGMENTIN: tabl of 2 strengths: 250 mg amoxicillin + 125 mg clavulanic acid, and 500 mg amoxicillin + 125 mg clavulanic acid; oral susp with amoxicillin 125 mg + clavulanic acid 31.25 mg/5 mL, or amoxicillin 250 mg + clavulanic acid 62.5 mg/5 mL

**Ampicillin;** acid-resistant penicillin congener

NB (≤7 days old) = IV (over 15–30 min), IM: 50 mg/kg/24 hr, div, every 12 hr

℞ for meningitis: IV: 100 mg/kg/24 hr, div, every 4 hr

NB (>7 days old) = IV (over 15–30 min), IM: 100 mg/kg/24 hr, div, every 8 hr

℞ for meningitis: IV: 200 mg/kg/24 hr, div, every 4 hr

℞ for septicemia: IV (over 15–30 min), IM: 100–200 mg/kg/24 hr, div, every 4 hr (IV) or every 6 hr (IM)

℞ for meningitis: IV (over 15–30 min): 300–400 mg/kg/24 hr, div, every 4 hr

ampicillin sodium, for injection, OMNIPEN-N, PEN-BRITIN-S, ‡: inj

ampicillin trihydrate, †, OMNIPEN, PEN-BRITIN, ‡: caps, oral susp, pediatric drops

**Azithromycin;** macrolide antibiotic indicated for the treatment of mild to moderate upper and lower respiratory tract infections and infections of the skin caused by susceptible bacteria. *Chlamydia trachomatis, Haemophilus influenzae, Moraxella catarrhalis, Mycoplasma pneumoniae, Staphylococcus aureus, Streptococcus pneumoniae.* Less gastrointestinal distress than associated with erythromycin

CH = PO, 10 mg/kg day 1 followed by 5 mg/kg/day administered once daily for 5 days. AD = 500 mg/day 1 followed by 250 mg once daily for 5 days

**Caution:** Coadministration with aluminum- and/or magnesium-containing antacids may decrease azithromycin peak serum concentrations by 25%.

ZITHROMAX, caps

**Carbenicillin** disodium; semisynthetic penicillin susceptible to destruction by penicillinase

℞ for systemic use: NB = IV (over 15–30 min), IM: initial dose 100 mg/kg, followed by maintenance therapy according to the following criteria:

≤2000 g + ≤7 days old: 225 mg/kg/24 hr, div, every 8 hr

≤2000 g + >7 days old: 400 mg/kg/24 hr, div, every 6 hr

>2000 g + ≤7 days old: 300 mg/kg/24 hr, div, every 6 hr

>2000 g + >7 days old: 400 mg/kg/24 hr, div, every 6 hr

**See KEY to abbreviations, p. 783; for further information about drugs, see package inserts.**

TABLE AP–1.    Drug Doses* (Drugs Listed Alphabetically by Generic Name) *Continued*

IN, CH = IV (over 15–30 min), IM: 400–600 mg/kg/24 hr, div, every 4 hr (IV) or every 6 hr (IM)
   GEOPEN: inj; 1 g carbenicillin disodium contains 6.5 mEq Na$^+$
℞ for treatment of urinary tract infection only: CH = PO: 10–30 mg/kg/24 hr, div, every 6 hr carbenicillin indanyl sodium; GEOCILLIN: tabl

**Cephalosporins;** semisynthetic derivatives of 7-amino-cephalosporanic acid, structurally related to penicillins
a. **First-generation cephalosporins:** active against most gram-positive cocci (excluding enterococci and methicillin-resistant *S. aureus*), some strains of *Escherichia coli, Klebsiella pneumoniae,* and *Proteus mirabilis*
*Note:* First-generation drugs do not cross the blood-brain barrier and therefore are ineffective for treatment of infections within the central nervous system.
*Cefadroxil:* relatively resistant against β-lactamases; absorption appears unaffected by food intake; minimal inhibitory concentrations for *E. coli, P. mirabilis, Klebsiella* species may be maintained in urine for about 20 hr after single dose
   ℞ CH = PO: 30 mg/kg/24 hr, div, every 12 hr
   DURICEF, ULTRACEF: caps, powder for oral susp
*Cefazolin sodium:* NB = IV (over 15–30 min), IM: 40 mg/kg/24 hr, div, every 12 hr; IN, CH = IV (over 15–30 min), IM: 50–100 mg/kg/24 hr, div, every 6 hr
   ANCEF, KEFZOL: inj
*Cephalothin:* NB = IV (over 15–30 min), IM: <7 days old: 40 mg/kg/24 hr, div, every 12 hr; >7 days old: 60 mg/kg/24 hr, div, every 8 hr; IN, CH = IV: 80–160 mg/kg/24 hr, div, every 4 hr
   KEFLIN; inj
   ANSPOR, VELOSEF; caps, oral susp, inj
b. **Second-generation cephalosporins:** more active against gram-negative bacteria such as *H. influenzae* type b, *Neisseria gonorrhoeae,* and enteric gram-negative bacilli
*Cefaclor:* effective against some β-lactamase–producing, ampicillin-resistant strains of

*H. influenzae*; absorption not affected by food intake
℞ for treatment of otitis media and infections of the upper and lower respiratory tracts, urinary tract, skin, and soft tissues with susceptible organisms: IN, CH = PO: 20–40 mg/kg/24 hr, div, every 8 hr
   CECLOR: powder for oral susp, caps
*Cefoxitin:* IN (>3 mo old), CH = IV, IM: 80–160 mg/kg/24 hr, div, every 4–6 hr
*Note:* May cause renal impairment and cross-reaction with penicillin.
   MEFOXIN: vials, infusion bottles, inj
c. **Third-generation cephalosporins:** less active against gram-positive cocci than older cephalosporins but more active against most strains of enteric gram-negative bacilli, moderately active against *Pseudomonas aeruginosa,* highly active against *H. influenzae* and *N. gonorrhoeae*
*Ceftriaxone sodium:* biliary and renal excretion
   ℞ misc. infection 50–75 mg/kg/24 hr (not to exceed 2 g), div, every 12 hr; meningitis 100 mg/kg/24 hr (not to exceed 4 g) divided every 12 hr
*Cefotaxime:* IN, CH = IV, IM: 100–150 mg/kg/24 hr, div, every 4–6 hr
   ℞ in meningitis: NB = IV 200 mg/kg/24 hr, div, every 6 hr
*Note:* May cause hypersensitivity reactions in penicillin-sensitive patients. Adjust dose with renal failure. Nephrotoxicity may develop with combined use of a cephalosporin and an aminoglycoside.
   CLAFORAN: vials, inj
*Ceftazidime:* possesses antipseudomonal activity
   NB = IV, IM: <7 days <2000 g, 100 mg/kg/24 hr, div, every 12 hr; >2000 g, 100 mg/kg/24 hr, div, every 8 hr; >7 days, 100–150 mg/kg/24 hr, div, every 8 hr
   IN, CH = IV, IM: 100–150 mg/kg/24 hr, div, every 8 hr (meningitis, 150 mg/kg/24 hr, div, every 8 hr)
   FORTAZ, TAZIDIME: inj

**Chloramphenicol;** derivative of dichloracetic acid combined to a structure containing a nitrobenzene ring
   NB = IV (over 15–30 min), (PO):

**See KEY to abbreviations, p. 783; for further information about drugs, see package inserts.**

TABLE AP–1.    Drug Doses* (Drugs Listed Alphabetically by Generic Name) *Continued*

≤14 days old, irrespective of weight: 25 mg/kg/24 hr, div, every 4 hr

15–30 days old and ≤2000 g: 25 mg/kg/24 hr, div, every 4 hr

15–30 days old and >2000 g: 50 mg/kg/24 hr, div, every 4 hr

IN, CH = PO: 50–100 mg/kg/24 hr, div, every 6 hr; IV (over 15–30 min): 100 mg/kg/24 hr, div, every 4 hr

**Caution:** Newborn infants susceptible to development of high blood levels and gray-baby syndrome on usual doses; therefore, careful monitoring of blood levels, if available, mandatory. Dose-duration–related suppression of erythrocyte production universal; weekly hematocrit or hemoglobin and reticulocyte count mandatory. Idiosyncratic aplastic anemia occasionally occurs without warning and may be lethal. **Use only when specifically indicated.**

CHLOROMYCETIN: caps

chloramphenicol palmitate, CHLOROMYCETIN palmitate: oral susp

chloramphenicol sodium succinate, CHLOROMYCETIN sodium succinate: inj

**Chloroquine;** a 4-aminoquinoline antimalarial agent; drug of choice for the treatment of attacks of malaria caused by *Plasmodium vivax, Plasmodium ovale, Plasmodium malariae,* and susceptible strains of *Plasmodium falciparum.* Not advised for use in treatment of juvenile rheumatoid arthritis.

℞ oral treatment of uncomplicated attacks (excluding those caused by chloroquine-resistant *P. falciparum*):

*Chloroquine diphosphate:* CH = PO:

  **first day:** 25 mg/kg/first 24 hr (equivalent to base: 15 mg/kg/first 24 hr), div in initial dose of 16.5 mg/kg (equivalent to base 10 mg/kg) and subsequent dose of 8.5 mg/kg (equivalent to base 5 mg/kg) 6 hr later;

  **second and third days:** 8.5 mg/kg/24 hr (equivalent to base 5 mg/kg/24 hr), as single daily dose

℞ intramuscular treatment of severe illness (excluding malaria caused by chloroquine-resistant *P. falciparum*):

*Chloroquine dihydrochloride:* CH = IM: 6 mg/kg/dose (equivalent to base 5 mg/kg/dose), every 12 hr, until clinical response is obtained

and treatment can be completed by the oral route

℞ clinical prophylaxis of malaria (prevention of clinical manifestations from infection with any of the *Plasmodium* species):

*Chloroquine diphosphate:* CH = PO: 8.5 mg/kg/dose (equivalent to base 5 mg/kg/dose) once every 7 days, beginning 2 wk before entering the malarious area and continuing for 8 wk after return. For eradication of *P. vivax* and *P. ovale,* treatment for 14 days wtih primaquine should be considered on leaving malarious area.

Chloroquine diphosphate, ARALEN diphosphate, (RESOCHIN) diphosphate: tabl

chloroquine dihydrochloride, ARALEN dihydrochloride: inj

(1 mg chloroquine base is equivalent to 1.65 mg chloroquine diphosphate or 1.2 mg chloroquine dihydrochloride)

**Caution:** Irreversible retinal damage may occur with prolonged use; frequent ophthalmologic examination necessary to detect early changes. *Note:* Chloroquine does not cause hemolysis in individuals with G-6-PD deficiency.

**Chlortetracycline:** see Tetracyclines

**Clarithromycin;** macrolide antibiotic indicated for the treatment of mild to moderate upper and lower respiratory tract infections and infections of the skin structure caused by susceptible bacteria, *C. trachomatis, H. influenzae, M. catarrhalis, M. pneumoniae, S. aureus, S. pneumoniae, Legionella* spp. Less gastrointestinal distress than associated with erythromycin.

CH = PO 15 mg/kg/24 hr, div, every 12 hr.

AD = PO 500–1000 mg/24 hr, div, every 12 hr

*Note:* Dose adjustment is necessary with renal disease, creatinine clearance <30 mL/min. May interfere with the hepatic metabolism of certain drugs (e.g., carbamazepine, theophylline).

BIAXIN, tabl

**Clindamycin:** semisynthetic derivative of lincomycin

NB <7 days <2000 g, 10 mg/kg/24 hr, div, every 12 hr

**See KEY to abbreviations, p. 783; for further information about drugs, see package inserts.**

TABLE AP–1.  Drug Doses* (Drugs Listed Alphabetically by Generic Name) *Continued*

NB >7 days <2000 g, 15 mg/kg/24 hr, div, every 8 hr
NB <7 days >2000 g, 15 mg/kg/24 hr, div, every 8 hr
NB >7 days >2000 g, 20 mg/kg/24 hr, div, every 6 hr
IN, CH: 20–45 mg/kg/24 hr, div, every 6–8 hr
*Note:* Therapy may be associated with the development of pseudomembranous colitis.
clindamycin hydrochloride, CLEOCIN hydrochloride: caps
clindamycin palmitate hydrochloride, CLEOCIN pediatric: oral susp
clindamycin phosphate, CLEOCIN phosphate: inj

**Cloxacillin sodium monohydrate;** penicillinase-resistant penicillin
IN, CH = PO: 50–100 mg/kg/24 hr, div, every 6 hr (expressed in terms of the base)
TEGOPEN: caps, oral susp

**Demeclocycline:** see Tetracyclines

**Dicloxacillin sodium monohydrate;** penicillinase-resistant penicillin
IN, CH = PO: 12.5–25 mg/kg/24 hr, div, every 6 hr
DYNAPEN: caps, oral susp

**Doxycycline;** see Tetracyclines

**Erythromycin;** macrolide antimicrobial agent
IN, CH = PO: 30–50 mg/kg/24 hr, div, every 6 hr; IV: 15–20 mg/kg/24 hr, div, every 6 hr
erythromycin, †, ILOTYCIN, ‡: tabl
erythromycin estolate, ILOSONE: tabl, oral susp
erythromycin ethylsuccinate, PEDIAMYCIN, ‡: tabl, oral susp, drops
erythromycin glucceptate, ILOTYCIN glucceptate IV: inj
erythromycin lactobionate, ERYTHROCIN lactobionate IV: inj
erythromycin stearate, ERYTHROCIN stearate, ‡: tabl

**Ethambutol hydrochloride;** antituberculous agent used concomitantly with isoniazid
℞ in the treatment of tuberculosis as part of multiple drug regimen. Conditions for safe use in children not firmly established. In adults: 15–25 mg/kg/24 hr, as single daily

dose, for course of treatment or retreatment. *Because of rare side effects of optic neuritis and decreased visual acuity,* eye examinations are indicated before inception of treatment and at monthly intervals thereafter.
MYAMBUTOL: tabl

**Fluconazole;** synthetic broad spectrum *bis*-triazole antifungal drug. Selective inhibitor of fungal cytochrome $P_{450}$ sterol C-14 α-demethylation; limited data in pediatrics available.
℞ for the treatment of fungal infections; CH = PO, IV: 3–6 mg/kg/24 hr, div, every 12–24 hr
DIFLUCAN: tabl, inj

**Fluoroquinolones;** antimicrobial agents that inhibit the action of microbial DNA gyrase (topoisomerase 2). Drugs in this class include ciprofloxacin, enoxacin, norfloxacin, ofloxacin, and so on. Many of these drugs possess potent activity against a wide range of pathogens, including *P. aeruginosa,* and are available for oral administration. The use of these drugs in pediatrics, primarily for the treatment of children with cystic fibrosis, has been limited owing to concern about possible fluoroquinolone-induced joint damage. Toxicity studies in animals have shown destructive lesions of growing cartilage following administration of these agents. Reports of arthropathy in teenage patients with cystic fibrosis have appeared in the literature, suggesting caution in the use of this class of compounds in patients whose skeletal growth is incomplete.
*Ciprofloxacin:* CH = PO 20–30 mg/kg/24 hr, div, every 8–12 hr. Usual maximum dose 1.5 g/24 hr. IV (over 60 min) 4–15 mg/kg/24 hr, div, every 8–12 hr. Dose should be adjusted in patients with creatinine clearance <20 mL/min.

**Gentamicin sulfate;** antimicrobial aminoglycoside
NB = IV (30–60 min), IM: <7 days <34 week <1500 g, 3 mg/kg every 24 hr; <34 wk >1500 g, 2.5 mg/kg every 18 hr; >34 wk >1500 g, 2.5 mg/kg every 12 hr; >7 days and term NB, 5 mg/kg/24 hr, div, every 12 hr
IN, CH = IM, IV (30–60 min): 5–7.5 mg/kg/24 hr, div, every 6–8 hr
Serum concentrations should be monitored, therapeutic peak concentration 5–10 mg/L,

**See KEY to abbreviations, p. 783; for further information about drugs, see package inserts.**

TABLE AP–1.    Drug Doses* (Drugs Listed Alphabetically by Generic Name) *Continued*

trough <2 mg/L. Dosage and interval may require modification for treatment of patients with cystic fibrosis.
GARAMYCIN: inj
**Caution:** Ototoxic, nephrotoxic

**Griseofulvin;** antifungal agent
℞ against deep-seated mycotic infections (skin, hair, nails) with organisms of the species *Microsporum, Trichophyton, Epidermophyton:* CH = PO (microcrystalline): 10–15 mg/kg/24 hr for 4–6 wk (4–6 mo for fingernails, 6–12 mo for toenails)
*Note:* "Ultramicrosize" form is an ultramicrocrystalline suspension for which 125 mg is biologically equivalent to 250 mg of a "microsize" preparation. The daily dose of an ultramicrosize preparation is reduced to 5 mg/kg/24 hr and offers comparable efficacy without additional advantages.
griseofulvin, microcrystalline, †, FULVICIN-U/F, GRIFULVIN V, ‡: tabl, oral susp
griseofulvin, ultramicrocrystalline, GRIS-PEG: tabl

**Isoniazid** (INH), isonicotinic acid hydrazide; tuberculostatic agent
℞ in the treatment of active tuberculosis, in combination with other antituberculous drugs: IN, CH = PO, IM: 10–20 mg/kg/24 hr, div, every 8–12 hr; maximum daily dose: 500 mg/24 hr. AD = PO, IM: 5–10 mg/kg/24 hr, div, every 8–12 hr; maximum daily dose: 300 mg/24 hr
℞ for prophylaxis of complications in recent conversion to positive tuberculin reaction (primary tuberculosis), or after suspected exposure: IN, CH = PO: 5–10 mg/kg/24 hr, as single dose, or div, every 12 hr; maximum daily dose: 300 mg/24
*Note:* "Slow" acetylators (homozygous) need only about 0.20–0.50 of this dose to reach therapeutically effective plasma concentrations achieved by "rapid" acetylators (homozygous and heterozygous). Higher than necessary plasma concentrations of unmetabolized isoniazid seem not to be associated with risk of isoniazid hepatotoxicity.
†, INH: tabl, syrup, inj
**Caution:** Formation of toxic metabolite in some patients may lead to hepatic necrosis with usual doses (rare under 20 yr of age).

**Kanamycin sulfate;** antimicrobial aminoglycoside
NB = IM, IV (over 20–30 min):
≤2000 g and ≤7 days old: 15 mg/kg/24 hr, div, every 12 hr
≤2000 g and >7 days old: 20 mg/kg/24 hr, div, every 12 hr
>2000 g and ≤7 days old: 20 mg/kg/24 hr, div, every 12 hr
>2000 g and >7 days old: 30 mg/kg/24 hr, div, every 8 hr
IN, CH = IM, IV (over 20–30 min): 6–15 mg/kg/24 hr, div, every 8–12 hr. Usual duration therapy: 7–10 days; not indicated in long-term therapy because of ototoxic hazard.
**Caution:** Ototoxic, nephrotoxic
KANTREX: inj

**Ketoconazole;** imidazole antifungal agent used for prophylaxis and treatment of a variety of mild to moderate fungal infections. Is not effective against infections arising within the central nervous system as the drug does not penetrate the blood-brain barrier.
CH = PO 5–10 mg/kg/24 hr, div, every 12–24 hr. Usual max 800 mg/24 hr.
AD = PO 200–400 mg/24 hr administered once daily.
*Note:* Gastric acidity is necessary for best oral absorption; thus, avoid drug administration with antacids or $H_2$ receptor antagonists. Numerous potential drug interactions, including ketoconazole-induced increases in serum drug concentrations of astemizole, cyclosporine, phenytoin, terfenadine, theophylline, warfarin. Use may be associated with hepatotoxicity.
NIZORAL; tabl, susp, topical cream/shampoo

**Mebendazole;** antihelmintic agent that blocks glucose uptake by the susceptible parasites and interferes with their survival
℞ against pinworms (*Enterobius vermicularis;* cure rate 90–100%): CH = PO: 100 mg/dose, as single dose; against whipworms (*Trichuris trichiura;* cure rate 61–75%), roundworms (*Ascaris lumbricoides;* cure rate 91–100%), and hookworms (*Ancylostoma duodenale, Necator americanus;* cure rate 96%); alternative method = PO: 200 mg/24 hr, div, every 12 hr, for 3 consecutive days. If patient is not free of parasites 3 wk after treatment, a 2nd course is indicated.

**See KEY to abbreviations, p. 783; for further information about drugs, see package inserts.**

TABLE AP–1.    Drug Doses* (Drugs Listed Alphabetically by Generic Name) *Continued*

*Note:* Not extensively studied in children under 2 yr of age.
VERMOX: chewable tabl

**Methicillin sodium;** semisynthetic penicillinase-resistant penicillin
NB = IM, IV (over 15–30 min):
  ≤2000 g and ≤14 days old: 50 mg/kg/24 hr, div, every 12 hr
  ≤2000 g and 15–30 days old: 75 mg/kg/24 hr, div, every 8 hr
  >2000 g and ≤14 days old: 75 mg/kg/24 hr, div, every 8 hr
  >2000 g and 15–30 days old: 100 mg/kg/24 hr, div, every 6 hr
IN, CH = IV (over 15–30 min), IM: 200–400 mg/kg/24 hr, div, every 4 hr (IV) or every 6 hr (IM)
CELBENIN, STAPHCILLIN: inj

**Metronidazole hydrochloride;** synthetic antibacterial agent highly active against most obligate anaerobes, including *Bacteroides* species such as *B. fragilis,* and *Clostridium* and *Peptostreptococcus* species. The drug also is effective in the treatment of amebiasis, *Giardia,* and *Trichomonas.*
℞ for amebiasis: CH = PO: 35–50 mg/kg/24 hr, div, every 8 hr
℞ for the treatment of anaerobic infections: IV
  NB <2000 g, 15 mg/kg/24 hr, div, every 12 hr
  NB >2000 g, <7 days: 15 mg/kg/24 hr, div, every 8 hr
  NB >2000 g, >7 days: 30 mg/kg/24 hr, div, every 8 hr
℞ for giardiasis: CH = PO: 15 mg/kg/day, div, every 8 hr
℞ for trichomonas vaginitis: CH = PO: 15 mg/kg/24 hr, div, every 8 hr, for 7 days
Topical therapy: Apply and rub in thin film twice daily to affected area. May be administered as vaginal suppositories.
**Caution:** Patient should not ingest alcohol for 24 hr after receiving a dose of this drug (disulfiram-type reaction). Drug interactions possible; may prolong anticoagulant effect of warfarin-type anticoagulants.
†, FLAGYL: tabls, inj

**Miconazole;** synthetic antifungal imidazole derivative effective against systemic infections with *Coccidioides immitis, Candida albicans, Crypto-*

*coccus neoformans, Paracoccidioides brasiliensis.* IV infusion alone is inadequate for the treatment of fungal meningitis and urinary bladder infection; intrathecal administration and bladder instillation also must be carried out.
℞ for treatment of proved coccidioidomycosis, candidosis, cryptococcosis, or paracoccidioidomycosis: CH = IV (after dilution with isotonic saline or 5% D/W and over 30–60 min): 20–40 mg/kg/24 hr, div, every 8 hr, until clinical and laboratory tests no longer indicate activity of fungal infection. Dose may vary with type of fungus involved; MONISTAT IV; ampules for IV inj

**Minocycline:** see Tetracyclines

**Nafcillin sodium;** semisynthetic penicillinase-resistant penicillin
NB = IM, IV (over 15–30 min); ≤7 days old: 40 mg/kg/24 hr, div, every 12 hr; >7 days old: 60 mg/kg/24 hr, div, every 8 hr
IN, CH = PO: 50–100 mg/kg/24 hr, div, every 6 hr; IM, IV (over 15–30 min): 100–200 mg/kg/24 hr, div, every 6 hr (IM) or every 4 hr (IV)
UNIPEN: caps, tabl, oral susp, inj

**Nystatin;** antifungal agent; 1 mg = 2000 units; seems to be active by altering permeability of cell membrane of yeasts
℞ for topical treatment of candidosis of the buccal cavity (thrush) and the gastrointestinal tract. Very poorly absorbed. In oral candidosis, spread nystatin suspension into recesses of mouth:
  NB (<2000 g) = PO: 200,000–400,000 units/24 hr, div, every 4–6 hr
  NB (>2000 g), IN = PO: 400,000–800,000 units/24 hr, div, every 4–6 hr
  CH = PO: 800,000–2,000,000 units/24 hr, div, every 4–6 hr
†, MYCOSTATIN, NILSTAT: oral susp, tabl

**Oxacillin sodium;** semisynthetic penicillinase-resistant penicillin
NB = IV (over 15–30 min), IM: for dosage same criteria apply as for methicillin in newborns; *see* Methicillin sodium
IN, CH = PO: 50–100 mg/kg/24 hr, div, every 6 hr; IV (over 15–30 min), IM: 100–200 mg/kg/24 hr, div, every 4 hr (IV) or every 6 hr (IM)

**See KEY to abbreviations, p. 783; for further information about drugs, see package inserts.**

TABLE AP–1.   Drug Doses* (Drugs Listed Alphabetically by Generic Name) *Continued*

BACTOCILL, PROSTAPHLIN: caps, oral susp, inj

**Penicillin G, benzylpenicillin;** potassium penicillin G (1 mg = 1595 units); sodium penicillin G (1 mg = 1667 units). One million units of these salts of penicillin contain either 1.68 mEq $K^+$ or $Na^+$; in other terms, 1 g contains either 2.7 mEq $K^+$ or 2.8 mEq $Na^+$.

NB = IV (over 15–30 min), IM:
  <2000 g: 50,000 units/kg/24 hr, div, every 12 hr
    ℞ for meningitis: 100,000 units/kg/24 hr, div, every 12 hr
  >2000 g: 75,000 units/kg/24 hr, div, every 8 hr
    ℞ for meningitis: 150,000–200,000 units/kg/24 hr, div, every 8 hr
IN, CH = PO, IM, IV (15–30 min): 100,000–250,000 units/kg/24 hr, div, every 4–6 hr
    ℞ for meningitis: 200,000–300,000 units/kg/24 hr, div, every 4 hr
(The higher doses should be chosen for meningitis caused by group B streptococci.)
IN, CH = PO, IM, IV (over 15–30 min) (minor infections): 25,000–50,000 units/kg/24 hr, equivalent to 15.5–31 mg/kg/24 hr, div, every 4–6 hr; if given PO, administer penicillin G 0.5 hr before or 2 hr after the meal
    ℞ for prophylaxis of rheumatic fever; PO: 200,000 units/dose, equivalent to 125 mg/dose, twice daily, spaced from meals

**Penicillin G benzathine,** for injection; combination of 1 mole of dibenzylethylenediamine with 2 moles of penicillin G; 1 mg = 1211 units
  ℞ for prophylaxis of rheumatic fever: CH = IM: 600,000–1,200,000 units, equivalent to 500–1000 mg penicillin G, once a month
  †, BICILLIN L-A, PERMAPEN, ‡: susp for inj
  †, PENTIDS, PFIZERPEN G, ‡: tabl, caps, oral susp, inj (IV)

**Penicillin G procaine,** for injection; combination of penicillin G with procaine, mole for mole (1 mg = 1009 units)
  NB = IM: 50,000 units/kg/24 hr, equivalent to 50 mg/kg/24 hr, in single daily dose
  IN, CH = IM: 25,000–50,000 units/kg/24 hr, equivalent to 25–50 mg/kg/24 hr, in single daily dose

†, CRYSTICILLIN, DURACILLIN A.S., ‡: susp for IM inj

**Penicillin V, penoxymethyl penicillin;** acid-resistant penicillin; 1 mg = 1695 units
  IN, CH = PO: 25,000–50,000 units/kg/24 hr, equivalent to 15–30 mg/kg/24 hr, div, every 6–8 hr. *Note:* 400,000 units = 250 mg (approx.)
  †, PEN-VEE K, VEETIDS, ‡: tabl, oral susp, drops

**Primaquine;** 8-aminoquinoline antimalarial agent, used for prophylaxis against *P. vivax, P. ovale,* and *P. malariae* and for "radical" cure for *P. vivax* and *P. ovale.*
  IN, CH = PO: 0.55 mg/kg/24 hr (equivalent to 0.3 mg/kg/24 hr of base), as single daily dose, for 14 days
  *Note:* Degree of intravascular hemolysis in individuals with G-6-PD deficiency is related to dosage and particular variant of the deficiency.
PRIMAQUINE DIPHOSPHATE: tabl

**Pyrantel pamoate;** antihelmintic agent effective by means of neuromuscular paralysis of the parasite
  ℞ against pinworms (*E. vermicularis*), roundworms (*A. lumbricoides*), and hookworms (*N. americanus, A. duodenale*): pyrantel pamoate has not been extensively studied in infants and children below 2 yr of age, hence particular attention should be given to children of this age group during treatment of parasitic infestation with pyrantel. CH = PO: 11 mg/kg/dose, as single dose and without regard to food intake or time of day; purging not necessary prior to, during, or after therapy
  *Note:* In pinworm infestation, in which possibility of reinfection with eggs from the host exists, a 2nd treatment 2–3 wk after the 1st might be indicated.
ANTIMINTH: oral susp

**Pyrimethamine;** inhibitor of dihydrofolate reductase, antimalarial agent; for use in treatment of toxoplasmosis
  ℞ for clinical prophylaxis of malaria, especially effective against *P. falciparum:* IN, CH = PO: 0.5–0.75 mg/kg/dose, once every 7 days. Begin prophylaxis 2 wk before entering malarious area and continue for 8 wk after leaving.

**See KEY to abbreviations, p. 783; for further information about drugs, see package inserts.**

**TABLE AP-1.   Drug Doses\* (Drugs Listed Alphabetically by Generic Name) *Continued***

To eradicate *P. vivax* and *P. ovale* infections, treatment for 14 days with primaquine should be considered immediately on leaving malarious area while pyrimethamine prophylaxis is still in effect.

*Note:* Hematologic abnormalities (anemia, thrombocytopenia, leukopenia) secondary to folic and folinic acid depletion can be prevented or reversed by IM administration of folinic acid (leucovorin) without affecting the efficacy of pyrimethamine.

DARAPRIM: tabl

**Quinacrine hydrochloride,** mepacrine hydrochloride; acridine derivative formerly used as antimalarial agent and against infestation with tapeworms, presently regarded as drug of choice against giardiasis

℞ against *Giardia lamblia:* CH = PO: 6 mg/kg/24 hr, div, every 8 hr, for 5 consecutive days; maximum daily dose: 300 mg/24 hr

ATABRINE: tabl

**Ribavirin;** synthetic nucleoside antiviral drug, Ribavirin possesses antiviral inhibitory activity in vitro against respiratory syncytial virus (RSV), influenza virus, and herpes simplex virus. Various protocols exist for the use of this compound; the drug usually is reserved for use in the treatment of severe lower respiratory tract infections due to RSV. Ribavirin is administered by the aerosol route as a continuous aerosolization for 12–18 hr daily for 3–7 days. Aerosol solution usually is prepared in sterile water, without preservatives, to a final concentration of 20 mg/ml.

VIRAZOLE: aerosol

**Rifampin;** macrocytic antimicrobial and antimycobacterial agent, interfering with RNA-polymerase of infecting organisms

℞ in treatment of tuberculosis, in conjunction with at least 1 other antituberculous agent (isoniazid) and

℞ in carriers of *Neisseria meningitidis* resistant to sulfonamide; treatment course of 4 consecutive days (possibility of rapid emergence of resistance); IN, CH = PO: 10–20 mg/kg/24 hr, in single daily dose (1 hr before or 2 hr after meal): maximum daily dose: 600 mg (= adult dose)

RIFADIN, RIMACTANE: caps

**Sulfonamides;** analogs of *para*-aminobenzoic acid, interfering with the synthesis of tetrahydrofolic acid in sensitive bacteria

*Sulfadiazine, sulfisoxazole,* and trisulfapyrimidines: IN, CH = PO: initial dose 75 mg/kg/1st dose, followed by 120–150 mg/kg/24 hr, div, every 4–6 hr; IV (over 30 min), SC: 100–110 mg/kg/24 hr, div, every 4–6 hr

Sulfadiazine, †: tabl

sulfadiazine, sodium, †: inj

sulfisoxazole, †, GANTRISIN: tabl

sulfisoxazole acetyl, GANTRISIN acetyl: oral susp, syrup

sulfisoxazole diolamine, GANTRISIN diolamine: inj

trisulfapyrimidines (equal parts of sulfadiazine, sulfamerazine, and sulfamethazine), †, ‡: tabl, oral susp

*Sulfamethoxazole:* IN, CH = PO: initial dose 50–60 mg/kg/1st dose, followed by 50–60 mg/kg/24 hr, div, every 12 hr GANTANOL: oral susp, tabl

*Trimethoprim/sulfamethoxazole* (combination of TMP + SMX): IN (>2 mo old), CH = PO: 6–12 mg TMP + 30–60 mg SMX/kg/24 hr, div, every 12 hr

℞ in severe urinary tract or *Shigella* infection: CH = PO, IV: 8–10 mg TMP + 40–60 mg SMX/kg/24 hr, div, every 6–8 hr

℞ against *Pneumocystis carinii:* CH = PO, IV: 15–20 mg TMP + 75–100 mg SMX/kg/24 hr, div, every 6–8 hr

**Caution:** Do not use in infants less than 2 mo old. Reduce dose in severe renal insufficiency. May cause bone marrow depression.

BACTRIM, SEPTRA: susp: 40 mg TMP + 200 mg SMX/5 mL; tabl: 80 mg TMP + 400 mg SMX/tabl or 160 mg TMP + 800 mg SMX/tabl; ampule: 80 mg of TMP + 400 mg SMX/5 mL

**Tetracyclines;** a group of derivatives of polycyclic naphthacenecarboxamide

*Chlortetracycline hydrochloride:* CH = PO: 25–50 mg/kg/24 hr, div, every 6 hr

AUREOMYCIN: caps, inj (IV)

*Demeclocycline* and *demeclocycline hydrochloride:* CH = PO: 7–13 mg/kg/24 hr, div, every 6–12 hr

DECLOMYCIN: pediatric drops, syrup

DECLOMYCIN hydrochloride: caps, tabl

**See KEY to abbreviations, p. 783; for further information about drugs, see package inserts.**

TABLE AP–1.  Drug Doses* (Drugs Listed Alphabetically by Generic Name) *Continued*

*Doxycycline monohydrate* and *doxycycline hyclate:*
CH = PO: 5 mg/kg/24 hr, div, every 12 hr
†, VIBRAMYCIN monohydrate: oral susp
†, VIBRAMYCIN hyclate: caps, inj (IV)
*Methacycline hydrochloride:* CH = PO: 7–13 mg/kg/24 hr, div, every 6–12 hr
RONDOMYCIN: caps, syrup
*Minocycline hydrochloride:* CH = PO, IV: initial dose 4 mg/kg, followed by 4 mg/kg/24 hr, div, every 12 hr
MINOCIN, VECTRIN: caps, syrup, inj (IV)
*Oxytetracycline, oxytetracycline hydrochloride, oxytetracycline calcium:* same dosage as tetracycline hydrochloride, below TERRAMYCIN: tabl, inj (IM)
TERRAMYCIN hydrochloride, †: caps, inj (IV, IM)
TERRAMYCIN calcium: pediatric drops, syrup
*Tetracycline hydrochloride:* CH = PO: 25–50 mg/kg/24 hr, div, every 8 hr; IM (often very painful): 15–25 mg/kg/24 hr, div, every 8–12 hr; IV: 10–20 mg/kg/24 hr, div, every 12 hr
†, ACHROMYCIN V, PANMYCIN, ‡: caps, inj (IV, IM); sol for IM inj contains local anesthetic. Pediatric drops, oral susp, and syrup prepared with tetracycline base
*Note:* Tetracyclines have limited indications in infancy and childhood because of their accumulation in bone and teeth and their potential to interfere with growth. Their use should be avoided insofar as possible until formation of dental enamel is complete in most permanent teeth (at about 8 yr), to avoid unsightly discolored, pitted teeth. Tetracyclines may cause increased intracranial pressure in infants (pseudotumor cerebri).

**Ticarcillin disodium;** semisynthetic penicillin susceptible to penicillinase; each gram of drug contains 5.2 mEq of sodium.
NB = IV (over 20–30 min), IM:
<7 days <2000 g; 150 mg/kg/24 hr, div, every 12 hr;
<7 days >2000 g: 225 mg/kg/24 hr, div, every 8 hr;
>7 days <2000 g: 225 mg/kg/24 hr, div, every 8 hr;
>7 days >2000 g: 300 mg/kg/24 hr, div, every 8 hr
IN, CH = IV (over 20–30 min), IM: 200–300 mg/kg/24 hr, div, every 4–6 hr. IM injection is painful.
TICAR: IV and IM inj

**Ticarcillin + clavulanic acid;** combination of a β-lactam antibiotic (ticarcillin) with a β-lactamase (penicillinase) inhibitor (clavulanic acid). The addition of clavulanic acid extends the activity of ticarcillin to include β-lactamase–producing strains of *H. influenzae* and other drug-resistant pathogens. Doses administered as either IM or IV are the same as those for ticarcillin noted above.

**Tobramycin sulfate;** antimicrobial aminoglycoside
NB = IV (30–60 min), IM: <7 days <34 wk <1500 g: 3 mg/kg every 24 hr; <34 wk >1500 g: 2.5 mg/kg every 18 hr; >34 wk >1500 g: 2.5 mg/kg every 12 hr; >7 days and term NB: 5 mg/kg/24 hr, div, every 12 hr
IN, CH = IV (30–60 min), IM: 5–7.5 mg/kg/24 hr, div, every 6–8 hr. Serum concentration should be monitored; therapeutic peak concentration 5–10 mg/L, trough <2 mg/L. Dosage and interval may require modification for the treatment of patients with cystic fibrosis.
**Caution:** Ototoxic, nephrotoxic
†, NEBCIN: inj

**Vancomycin;** complex glycopeptide that inhibits synthesis of cell wall in gram-positive bacteria and is effective against methicillin-resistant staphylococci; in oral application effective in pseudomembranous colitis caused by toxin-producing bacteria such as *C. difficile* and *S. aureus;* excreted mainly by kidneys
NB = IV (slow over 1 + hr) <7 days, <1200 g, 15 mg/kg/24 hr administered once daily; <7 days, >1200 g, 30 mg/kg/24 hr, div, every 12 hr; >7 days, <1200 g, 15 mg/kg/24 hr administered once daily; >7 days, >1200 g, 30–45 mg/kg/24 hr, div, every 8–12 hr
IN, CH (<12 yr of age) 45–60 mg/kg/24 hr, div, every 6–8 hr
AD = IV 0.5 g every 6 hr to 1 g every 12 hr
℞ for *C. difficile*–associated pseudomembranous colitis in CH = PO: 40–50 mg/kg/24 hr, div, every 6–8 hr.
**Caution:** Combined administration with an aminoglycoside enhances nephrotoxic potential of both drugs.
*Note:* Reduced dosage in renal insufficiency.

**See KEY to abbreviations, p. 783; for further information about drugs, see package inserts.**

TABLE AP–1.  Drug Doses* (Drugs Listed Alphabetically by Generic Name) *Continued*

Therapy may be associated with ototoxicity and renal impairment, skin rashes ("red man" syndrome), and hematologic side effects. Serum concentration should be monitored, therapeutic peak concentration 30–40 mg/L, trough 5–10 mg/L.

†, VANCOCIN: inj

**Vidarabine;** antiviral agent used for treatment of neonatal herpes simplex infections

IN = IV: 15–30 mg/kg infused over 12 hr every 24 hr for 14–21 days

*Note:* May rarely cause hepatic and hematologic toxicity.

VIRA-A: 200-mg/mL vial inj

## II. DRUGS OTHER THAN ANTIBIOTICS

**Acetaminophen,** paracetamol, APAP, NAPAP

℞ antipyretic, analgesic: IN, CH = PO: 60 mg/kg/24 hr, div, every 4–6 hr, prn

†, LIQUIPRIN, TYLENOL, ‡: tabl, liquid preparations

**Caution:** Massive overdose may cause hepatic necrosis through formation of a toxic metabolite. Lesser overdoses frequently cause reversible jaundice.

**Acetylcysteine;** mucolytic agent; detoxifying agent in acetaminophen overdose

℞ in acetaminophen overdose: CH, AD = PO: 140 mg/kg/1st dose, followed by 70 mg/kg/dose every 4 hr for a total of 72 hr

MUCOMYST: vials 10% (100 mg/mL) or 20% (20 mg/mL)

**Acetylsalicylic acid (ASA)**

℞ antipyretic, analgesic, anti-inflammatory: IN, CH = PO: 30–65 mg/kg/24 hr, div, every 4–6 hr, prn. This dosage corresponds to 27–58 mg salicylate sodium/kg/24 hr, or 20–50 mg salicylic acid/kg/24 hr

℞ antirheumatic: CH = PO: 65–130 mg/kg/24 hr, div, every 4–6 hr

†, ASPIRIN, BUFFERIN, ‡: tabl; also contained in many combination products

**Caution:** Acute or chronic overdose may cause life-threatening poisoning syndrome. Use in children <16 yr with varicella or a flu-like illness is associated with Reye syndrome.

**Activated charcoal;** adsorbent for treatment of oral drug overdose PO: 10 times (by weight) estimated quantity of drug ingested or 1 g/kg orally; may repeat every 4 hr when necessary

**Adenosine;** endogenous nucleoside; treatment of choice to terminate supraventricular tachycardia; causes acute transient AV nodal conduction block

NB, IN, CH = IV; 0.10 mg/kg/dose rapid injection (1–2 sec), increase to 0.20 mg/kg/dose if prior dose is ineffective (in 1–2 min)

**Albuterol;** catecholamine analogue; β-adrenergic receptor agonist with preferential effect on β₂-adrenergic receptors

℞ bronchodilator: CH = PO: 0.1 mg/kg, div, every 8 hr; 6–12 yr; 2 mg 3–4 times/24 hr; nebulization: 0.01–0.03 mL/kg of 5 mg/mL solution.

VENTOLIN, PROVENTIL: tab, liquid, inhalation

**Atropine sulfate,** *dl*-hyoscyamine; anticholinergic agent used mainly in premedication for anesthesia, as antiarrhythmic agent, and as antispasmodic. Dosage varies according to indications and sensitivity of patients. On the average for IN, CH = SC, PO (IV): 0.01 mg/kg/dose, to be repeated p.r.n. after 2 hr until desired effect is obtained or adverse effects preclude further increase; for continued ℞: PO: 0.04 mg/kg/24 hr, div, every 6 hr, preferably with meals

†: inj, tabl

**Betamethasone;** long-acting anti-inflammatory corticosteroid with little to no sodium retention potential. CH = IM: 0.0175–0.2 mg base/kg/24 hr, div, every 6–12 hr; PO: 0.0175–0.25 mg/kg/24 hr div every 6–8 hr. AD = IM: 0.6–9 mg/24 hr, div, every 12–24 hr; PO: 2–5 mg/24 hr, div, every 12–24 hr

*Note:* For more information on steroid medications, see Corticosteroids.

CELESTONE, VALISONE, inj, syrup, tabl, topical cream, gel, lotion, ointm

**Captopril,** competitive inhibitor of angiotensin I–converting enzyme, antihypertensive agent, congestive heart failure

℞ for cardiovascular response:

NB = PO: 0.1–0.4 mg/kg/dose administered every 6–24 hr

**See KEY to abbreviations, p. 783; for further information about drugs, see package inserts.**

TABLE AP–1.    Drug Doses* (Drugs Listed Alphabetically by Generic Name) *Continued*

IN = PO: 0.5–0.6 mg/kg/24 hr, div, every 6–12 hr

CH = PO: 0.15 mg/kg every 4–8 hr; dose may be slowly increased to desired effect: max pediatric dose 6 mg/kg/24 hr

AD = PO: 6.25–12.5 mg/dose every 8–12 hr; usual AD max 450 mg/24 hr.

*Note:* May cause renal impairment, neutropenia, immunodeficiency, rashes, disturbances of taste. Adjust dose with renal failure.

CAPOTEN: tabl

**Carbamazepine,** anticonvulsant agent; structurally related to tricyclic antidepressants

IN, CH = PO: initially 5–10 mg/kg/24 hr, div, every 8–12 hr; to be increased progressively, if needed, to 20 mg/kg/24 hr, div, every 12 hr or as a single daily dose, if tolerated. Usual maintenance dose range 20–30 mg/kg/24 hr

CH (>12 yr), AD = PO: initially 200 mg every 24 hr, titrated as needed, max 800–1200 mg/24 hr

*Note:* Carbamazepine is a potent inducer of hepatic microsomal metabolizing enzymes that may stimulate the metabolism of numerous other drugs metabolized via the liver.

TEGRETOL: tabl, chew tabl, susp

**Chloral hydrate;** trichloro derivative of acetaldehyde; tolerance to its hypnotic effect may develop

℞ for sedation: IN, CH = PO: 25 mg/kg/24 hr, div, every 6–8 hr

℞ for sleep: IN, CH = PO, (PR): 25–75 mg/kg/dose, to be repeated p.r.n. after 12–24 hr

†, NOCTEC, SOMNOS, ‡: elixic, syrup, suppos

**Chlorothiazide;** saluretic, inhibiting sodium reabsorption and interfering with dilution of urine

IN, CH = PO: 20–40 mg/kg/24 hr, div, every 12 hr

†, DIURIL: tabl, oral susp

**Chlorpromazine;** phenothiazine with aliphatic side chain

℞ for sedation: CH = PO: 2 mg/kg/24 hr, div, every 4–6 hr, p.r.n.; IM: 2 mg/kg/24 hr, div, every 6–8 hr, p.r.n. THORAZINE: suppos

chlorpromazine hydrochloride, THORAZINE hydrochloride: tabl, syrup, inj

**Caution:** Overdose may produce parkinsonian syndrome. Diphenhydramine may be antidotal.

**Cimetidine,** $H_2$-receptor antagonist competitively inhibits secretion of gastric acid

℞ for treatment of duodenal and gastric ulcers and for relief of symptoms caused by gastroesophageal reflux: compatible with concomitant treatment with oral antacids (which should be administered at frequent intervals and in adequate doses) or other therapeutic modalities

NB = PO, IM, IV: (15–20 min) 5–10 mg/kg/24 hr, every 8–12 hr;

IN, CH = IV, PO: 20–40 mg/kg/24 hr, div, every 4–6 hr

*Note:* Cimetidine may compete with hepatic metabolism of other hepatically metabolized drugs. Many possible drug interactions. May cause gynecomastia, rash, and neutropenia. Reduce dose in renal insufficiency.

TAGAMET; tabl, inj, syrup

**Clonazepam;** benzodiazepine with selective anticonvulsant effect

CH = PO: start with 0.01–0.05 mg/kg/24 hr, div, every 8 hr, and progressively increase up to 0.3 mg/kg/24 hr, div, every 8 hr, if needed.

**Caution:** Concomitant use of clonazepam and valproate sodium may lead to petit mal status.

CLONOPIN: tabl

**Codeine phosphate** or **sulfate;** narcotic analgesic

℞ as antitussive: CH = 1–1.5 mg/kg/24 hr, div, every 4 hr p.r.n.

℞ against moderately severe pain: CH = PO: 4 mg/kg/24 hr, div, every 4–6 hr, p.r.n.; SC: 3 mg/kg/24 hr, div, every 4–6 hr, p.r.n.

†: tabl, oral susp, inj; mostly in combination with other drugs

**Corticosteroids**

℞ physiologic replacement

*Cortisone:* PO 1 mg/kg/24 hr, div, every 8 hr; IM: 0.5 mg/kg/24 hr, every 24 hr. *Note:* "Increased demand" under stressful situation (e.g., in children with congenital adrenogenital syndrome, receiving replacement therapy, for stressful situation in which 2 mg/kg/24 hr of cortisol may be safer)

**See KEY to abbreviations, p. 783; for further information about drugs, see package inserts.**

TABLE AP–1.   Drug Doses* (Drugs Listed Alphabetically by Generic Name) *Continued*

℞ use in pharmacologic doses (leukemia, lymphoma, nephrosis, rheumatic carditis, certain types of tuberculosis, immunologic reactions, and other types of autoimmune disease): adjust dosage to the specific situation

*Cortisone:* PO: 10 mg/kg/24 hr, div, every 6–8 hr; IM: 3–6 mg/kg/24 hr, div, every 12 hr

*Prednisone:* PO: 2 mg/kg/24 hr, div, every 6–8 hr (or analog in equally effective dosage; see Table)

(For continued treatment after initial response, adjust dosage, frequency of administration, and duration of treatment according to type of disease and side effects to be avoided.)

℞ in status asthmaticus refractory to other types of treatment: methylprednisolone IV: 2–4 mg/kg/dose every 4–6 hr

**Relative Potencies of Corticosteroids**

| Drug | Anti-Inflammatory Effect (mg) | Sodium-Retaining Effect (mg) |
|---|---|---|
| Hydrocortisone (cortisol) | 100 | 100 |
| Cortisone | 80 | 80 |
| Prednisolone | 20 | 100 |
| Prednisone | 20 | 100 |
| Methylprednisolone | 16 | 0 |
| Triamcinolone | 16 | 0 |
| Dexamethasone | 2 | 0 |
| Desoxycorticosterone | 0 | 2 |

*Dexamethasone,* DECADRON, GAMMACORTEN, ‡: tabl; elixir dexamethasone sodium phosphate, DECADRON phosphate

*Hydrocortisone,* †, CORTEF, HYDROCORTONE, ‡: tabl, oral susp; hydrocortisone sodium phosphate, †, HYDROCORTONE phosphate: inj; hydrocortisone sodium succinate, †, SOLUCORTEF: inj

*Methylprednisolone,* MEDROL: tabl; methylprednisolone sodium succinate, SOLU-MEDROL: inj

*Prednisone,* †, DELTASONE, METICORTEN, ‡: tabl

*Prednisolone,* †, DELTA-CORTEF, METICORTELONE, ‡: tabl

*Triamcinolone,* ARISTOCORT, KENACORT: tabl, syrup

**Caution:** May inhibit clinical signs of infection.

**Cromolyn sodium**

℞ topical prophylaxis of bronchial asthma, allergic rhinitis: not useful in the treatment of acute asthmatic attack because it is not a bronchodilator. CH (≥5 yr) = inhalation of 20 mg every 6 hr; nebulize contents of one ampule (2 mL) every 6–8 hr; aerosol inhaler, 1–2 puffs 4 times daily.

AARANE, INTAL: inhalation with Spinhaler, sol, nasal spray

**Cyproheptadine hydrochloride;** piperidine; serotonin and histamine antagonist with mild anticholinergic and mild sedative effect

℞ antiallergic effect: CH = PO: 0.25 mg/kg/24 hr, div, every 6 hr

PERIACTIN: tabl, syrup

**Deferoxamine;** chelating agent for treatment of iron intoxication; may cause hypotension; contraindicated in renal failure or acute anuria unless concomitant hemodialysis is used.

IV: 10–15 mg/kg/hr infusion

DESFERAL: 500 mg/vial inj

**Desmopressin acetate;** synthetic analogue of vasopressin indicated as replacement therapy in the management of central diabetis insipidus. Toxicities include headache, abdominal cramping, excessive water retention. Nasal insufflation: 0.03–0.05 mL, div, b.i.d. or t.i.d. dose determined by patient response.

DDAVP: 0.1 mg/mL for nasal insufflation

**Dexamethasone:** see Corticosteroids

**Diazepam;** benzodiazepine with anxiolytic and muscle-relaxant effects

℞ in status epilepticus: NB, IN, CH = IV (slowly as controlled "push" injection): 0.1–0.5 mg/kg/dose; may be repeated 2 times after intervals of 5 min; give IM if impossible to give IV (efficacy diminished)

℞ for symptomatic relief of anxiety: CH = PO: 0.1–0.3 mg/kg/24 hr, div, every 6 hr; adjust dosage according to response

VALIUM: tabl, inj

**Caution:** Confusion and prolonged extreme drowsiness may follow overdose or concurrent ingestion of alcohol in any form.

**Digoxin;** cardiac glycoside with rapid onset of action and half-life of approximately 48 hr

**See KEY to abbreviations, p. 783; for further information about drugs, see package inserts.**

TABLE AP–1.   Drug Doses* (Drugs Listed Alphabetically by Generic Name) *Continued*

℞ for digitalization: 0.5 × digitalizing dose initially, 0.25 × digitalizing dose 8 and 16 hr later.
(Digitalizing dose: NB = IV, IM: 0.010–0.030 mg/kg, div in fractions, or PO: 0.040 mg/kg, div in fractions. IN = IV, IM, PO: same doses as indicated for NB)

℞ for maintenance: begin maintenance dosage 24 hr after 1st fraction of digitalizing dose. NB = PO: 0.010 mg/kg/24 hr, div, every 12 hr. IN, CH = PO: 0.015 mg/kg/24 hr, div, every 12 hr

*Note:* Digitalizing and maintenance doses must be adjusted to the condition of the patient.

†, LANOXIN: tabl, elixir, inj

**Caution:** Fatal arrhythmia may follow overdose.

**Diphenhydramine hydrochloride;** ethanolamine; antihistamine with mild anticholinergic, sedative, antiemetic, and antitussive effects
℞ antiallergic effect; sometimes used as sedative. IN, CH = PO, IM, IV: 5 mg/kg/24 hr, div, every 6–8 hr

†, BENADRYL: caps, elixir, inj

**Edetate calcium disodium (EDTA),** a heavy metal–chelating agent with greatest affinity for lead. Used in the diagnosis and treatment of lead poisoning. EDTA-lead chelate excreted from the body via the kidney. Drug has affinity for calcium, which is the reason for administering the drug as the calcium (disodium) salt.
℞ for lead poisoning. Many regimens have been suggested; CH = IM, IV (over 1 hr to continuous 24-hr infusion): 50–75 mg/kg/24 hr, div, every 4–6 hr or by continuous IV infusion

℞ as a diagnostic test for lead body burden. CH = IM, IV: 500 mg/m² and collect all urine excreted over the next 8–24 hr to determine EDTA : lead ratio.

*Note:* Painful on IM injection. For comfort, may add 1 mL of 1% lidocaine with each 1 mL of EDTA injection. Dose must be adjusted for patients with renal disease.

**Epinephrine racemic;** inhalation treatment of acute spasmodic croup
Inhalation: 0.25–0.5 mL of 2.25% solution diluted in 3 mL of saline given via nebulizer
VAPONEPHRINE: inhalation 2.25% solution

**Furosemide;** saluretic with a duration of action of about 2 hr when given IV; inhibits chloride and sodium reabsorption and interferes with concentration of urine

IN, CH = PO: start with 2 mg/kg/dose; if needed, increase progressively to 3–6 mg/kg/dose, at intervals of 6–8 hr; IV: start with 1 mg/kg/dose; if needed, increase progressively to 6 mg/kg/dose, with an interval of at least 2 hr between doses

LASIX: tabl, oral sol, inj

**Hydralazine hydrochloride;** phthalazine derivative; causes relaxation of vascular smooth muscles, especially of arterioles
℞ as antihypertensive in long-term treatment: CH = PO: initially 0.75 mg/kg/24 hr, div, every 6 hr; increase progressively until desired response or daily maximum dose of 7.5 mg/kg/24 hr is reached

℞ for emergency reduction of hypertension: IV (immediate onset of action), IM (onset of action after 15–20 min): 0.15 mg/kg/dose; repeat p.r.n. every 30–90 min up to daily dose of 1.7–3.6 mg/kg/24 hr; switch to oral administration if conditions permit

*Note:* Hydralazine may produce sodium retention and usually increases plasma renin activity.

**Caution:** May induce lupus erythematosus–like syndrome: frequency related to dosage.

†, APRESOLINE, ‡: tabl, inj

**Hydrochlorothiazide;** saluretic, inhibiting sodium reabsorption and interfering with dilution of urine
IN, CH = PO: 2 mg/kg/24 hr, div, every 12 hr

†, ESIDRIX, HYDRODIURIL, ‡: tabl

**Hydroxyzine hydrochloride;** neuroleptic agent of the piperazine type, with sedative and antihistamine effects
℞ for sedation and/or antihistamine effect: CH = PO: 2 mg/kg/24 hr, div, every 6–8 hr, p.r.n.
ATARAX: tabl, syrup
VISTARIL IM: inj (IM)
hydroxyzine pamoate, VISTARIL: caps, oral susp

**Ibuprofen;** nonsteroidal anti-inflammatory agent of the propionic acid class that possesses analgesic and antipyretic activities. The drug's mechanism of action remains to be described

**See KEY to abbreviations, p. 783; for further information about drugs, see package inserts.**

TABLE AP–1.    Drug Doses* (Drugs Listed Alphabetically by Generic Name) *Continued*

but may involve prostaglandin synthetase inhibition. Pharmacologic effect appears to be equivalent to that of equipotent doses of acetaminophen or aspirin.

℞ as antipyretic or for mild analgesia: CH = PO: 10–15 mg/kg/dose at intervals of 4–6 hr

℞ for juvenile rheumatoid arthritis: CH = PO: 30–70 mg/kg/24 hr, div, every 4–6 hr

*Note:* Complete scope of associated adverse reactions in infants and children remains to be described. Adverse effects appear to be similar to those associated with aspirin administration, including gastritis, platelet dysfunction, and possible compromise in renal function. Drug should be used cautiously in patients with renal insufficiency.

†, ADVIL, MEDIPRIN, MOTRIN, NUPRIN: tabs, caps, susp

**Ipecac;** emetic agent used in the adjunctive management of poisoning or intoxication. Active ingredient emetidine produces local gastric irritation and central effect, resulting in emesis, which usually occurs within 15–35 min of drug administration

℞ to induce vomiting:

IN >8 mo of age, CH = PO: 15–30 mL/dose; if no effect occurs same dose may be repeated in 30 min

N <8 mo of age = PO: 1 mL/kg single dose

*Note:* Children usually vomit 3–5 times within 1 hr of receiving Ipecac. Ipecac should be available in all households with young infants and children but should not be administered except on the advice of a physician or a poison control center.

**Iron preparations**

℞ Daily maintenance iron requirement, as elemental iron: PO: 0.5–1 mg/kg/24 hr, in single dose or divided

℞ In iron deficiency anemia, as elemental iron: PO: 6 mg/kg/24 hr, div, with meals

*Note:* Iron supply at this dosage level ought to be continued for 2–3 mo to compensate for the deficits in erythrocytes and iron stores. Only iron in the ferrous form ($Fe^{2+}$) is absorbed from the gastrointestinal tract. The content of elemental iron in different preparations varies. The percentage of dry weight as elemental iron of ferrous choline citrate is 20;

ferrous fumarate, 33; ferrous gluconate, 12; ferrous lactate, 19; ferrous sulfate, 20; and iron-dextran complex (ferric hydroxide), 2.

℞ Dose calculation for parenteral iron administration: elemental Fe deficit = 2.5 mg/kg × deficit of hemoglobin concentration (in g/dL) in blood. (The deficit of the hemoglobin concentration is obtained as the difference between the measured and the desirable value, expressed in g/dL.) When iron must be supplied by the parenteral route, deep IM injection is preferable to IV administration. In either case, a test dose of approximately 25 mg elemental Fe in the form of the dextran complex should precede the administration of the total dose. If the total dose is large, it should be divided in separate daily doses of which none should exceed 5 mg/kg/24 hr of elemental iron.

*Note:* An additional 20–30% of the calculated deficit is needed to restore the tissue iron reserves.

**Caution:** Acute overdose may lead to shock, CNS depression, death.

**Ketorolac tromethamine;** nonsteroidal anti-inflammatory drug (NSAID) available for oral or parenteral administration; possesses analgesic and antipyretic activities; mechanism of action most likely inhibition of prostaglandin synthesis via antagonism of cyclooxygenase activity

CH = PO, IM: 2 mg/kg/24 hr, div, every 6 hr; many centers have administered the IM formulation via the IV route over 15–20 min

*Note:* As with all NSAIDs, the use of these drugs may be associated with gastritis, reversible antiplatelet activity, and possible compromised renal function; should be used cautiously in NB and other patients with decreased renal function.

TORADOL; inj, tabl

**Lidocaine hydrochloride;** anesthetic agent used systemically for its antiarrhythmic effects: delayed slow diastolic depolarization, diminished automaticity. Does not affect normal conduction but seemingly improves conduction velocity in damaged areas of myocardium. In therapeutic doses does not depress myocardial contractility or atrioventricular conduction.

**See KEY to abbreviations, p. 783; for further information about drugs, see package inserts.**

TABLE AP–1.   Drug Doses* (Drugs Listed Alphabetically by Generic Name) *Continued*

℞ against ventricular tachyarrhythmia: IN, CH = IV (slowly, as 20 mg/mL sol): 1 mg/kg/dose, to be repeated p.r.n. after 20 min, or continuous IV infusion as 1 mg/mL sol: 0.020–0.050 mg/kg/min, to a maximum total dose of 5 mg/kg/24 hr

XYLOCAINE HYDROCHLORIDE IV: inj

**Caution:** Excessive depression of cardiac conductivity may occur; ECG monitoring indicated during treatment.

**Mannitol;** osmotic diuretic

℞ test dose for oliguria: CH = IV: 0.2 g/kg/dose, injected within 3–5 min

℞ in cerebral edema: CH = IV: 1–2.5 g/kg/dose, injected as 15–25% sol over 30–60 min

†, OSMITROL, ‡: IV inj

**Meperidine hydrochloride;** synthetic narcotic analgesic agent; addictive

℞ against severe pain: CH = PO, SC, IM: 6 mg/kg/24 hr, div, p.r.n. every 4–6 hr (maximum single dose: 100 mg)

†, DEMEROL hydrochloride, ‡: tabl, elixir, inj

**Caution:** May produce respiratory depression, seizures, coma in some sensitive patients. Test dose advisable. Naloxone is antidote.

**Metaproterenol sulfate;** catecholamine analogue; β-adrenergic receptor agonist with relatively selective effect on $β_2$-adrenergic receptors

℞ bronchodilator: IN, CH (<6 yr of age) = PO: 1.3–2.6 mg/kg/24 hr, div, every 6–8 hr; >6 yr of age: 10–20 mg/dose administered 3–4 times daily

†, ALUPENT; METAPREL; syrup, tabl, inhalation

**Methylphenidate hydrochloride;** piperidine derivative structurally related to amphetamine; CNS stimulant with more prominent effects on mental than on motor activities

℞ in minimal brain dysfunction (MBD): drug treatment of MBD not recommended below the age of 3 yr or in nonstructured therapeutic situation. CH (over 3 yr) = PO: initiate treatment with 5 mg dose given at the onset of daytime activities and again 4–6 hr later; if needed, increase the dose at weekly intervals by increments of 5 mg/dose and adjust the size of the respective doses (early morning and mid-day) according to the response in

the patient; daily dose usually should not exceed 2 mg/kg/24 hr. To avoid insommia, do not administer closer than 6 hr before bedtime.

**Caution:** Reduction of growth rate and weight gain might accompany prolonged use. Chronic abuse can lead to tolerance.

℞ in narcolepsy: PO: proceed for dosage adjustment as in MBD, with correction of the abnormal symptomatology as the end point.

RITALIN: tabl

**Metoclopramide hydrochloride;** gastrointestinal prokinetic agent that increases lower esophageal sphincter pressure and rate of gastric emptying, and augments gastrointestinal peristaltic activity. Use of this drug for the treatment of symptomatic gastroesophageal reflux in infants and children remains controversial. Drug is also used for the treatment of diabetic gastroparesis and as an adjunctive measure facilitating small bowel intubation when the tube does not pass the pylorus with conventional maneuvers. High-dose metoclopramide therapy has been shown to be an effective aid in the adjunctive management of nausea and vomiting associated with cancer chemotherapy.

℞ for gastroesophageal reflux or gastrointestinal dismotility: CH = PO: 0.1 mg/kg/dose administered 4 times a day

℞ for prevention of chemotherapy-induced emesis: 2–3 mg/kg/dose administered before and after chemotherapeutic drug; timing of dose and actual regimen are dependent on the specific chemotherapeutic agent administered.

**Caution:** Metoclopramide possesses dopamine receptor antagonist activity; thus, acute dystonic reactions may occur and are relatively frequent with high-dose therapy. Diphenhydramine may be used to treat metoclopramide (or phenothiazine)-induced acute dystonic reaction. It may be appropriate to coadminister diphenhydramine with high-dose metoclopramide to prevent dystonic reactions in patients receiving this therapy for nausea and vomiting associated with cancer chemotherapy.

†, REGLAN: tabs, syrup, inj

**Mineral oil;** indigestible liquid hydrocarbon with limited absorbability; lubricant

**See KEY to abbreviations, p. 783; for further information about drugs, see package inserts.**

TABLE AP–1. Drug Doses* (Drugs Listed Alphabetically by Generic Name) *Continued*

R mild laxative: PO: 0.5 mL/kg/dose
†, liquid petrolatum: plain liquid or emulsion

**Morphine sulfate;** narcotic analgesic agent; addictive
R against severe pain: CH = SC: 0.6–1.2 mg/kg/24 hr, div, p.r.n. every 4 hr, equivalent to 0.1–0.2 mg/kg/dose, to be repeated p.r.n. every 4 hr
†: inj
**Caution:** Overdose produces severe respiratory depression, hypothermia, coma. Naloxone antidotal.

**Naloxone hydrochloride;** opioid antagonist; nonaddictive
R in respiratory depression due to opioids: NB, IN, CH = IV, IM, SC: 0.01 mg/kg/dose, to be repeated p.r.n. after 2–3 min, up to 3 times. After satisfactory response, the dose must be repeated every 1–2 hr as long as opioid depression persists.
NARCAN, NARCAN neonatal: inj

**Phenobarbital,** central nervous system depressant of barbiturate class with long duration of action; initially, hypnotic effect of 8–12 hr; tolerance to hypnotic effect may develop on continued use
R for sedation: IN, CH = PO, IM: 2–3 mg/kg/24 hr, div, every 8–12 hr
R for sleep: IN, CH = PO, IM: 2–3 mg/kg/dose, repeat p.r.n. after 12–24 hr
R as anticonvulsant. Status: IV (rate <1 mg/kg/min or 50 mg/min for patients weighing >60 kg). Loading dose: NB = 15–20 mg/kg in single or div dose; IN, CH, AD = 15–18 mg/kg in single or div dose. Maintenance dosing NB = PO, IV: 3–4 mg/kg/24 hr, div, every 12–24 hr; IN, CH: 5–8 mg/kg/24 hr, div, every 12–24 hr. CH (>12 yr of age), AD = PO, IV: 1–3 mg/kg/24 hr
R hyperbilirubinemia: CH (<8 yr of age) = PO 3–8 mg/kg/24 hr, div, every 8–12 hr
*Note:* Dosing may be guided by serum concentration monitoring, therapeutic values 15–40 mg/L.
**Caution:** All barbiturates, including phenobarbital, are respiratory depressants. Serum concentrations should be monitored.
†, LUMINAL, elixir, tabl; phenobarbital sodium, †, LUMINAL sodium, inj

**Phenytoin,** diphenylhydantoin; anticonvulsant agent; effective also in certain types of cardiac arrhythmias; antiarrhythmic effects similar to those of lidocaine; delayed slow diastolic depolarization, diminished automaticity; may facilitate conduction in damaged myocardial areas; does not depress myocardial activity
R as anticonvulsant. Status: IV (rate <1–3 mg/kg/min or 50 mg/min), PO loading dose NB = 15–20 mg/kg in single or div dose; IN, CH, AD = 15–18 mg/kg in single or div dose. Maintenance dosing IV, PO = NB: 5 mg/kg/24 hr, div, every 8–12 hr; IN, CH: 5–10 mg/kg/24 hr, div, every 8–12 hr; CH (>12 yr of age): 5 mg/kg/24 hr, div, every 12 hr
R for arrhythmias. CH, AD = IV: 1.25 mg/kg IV (over 1–3 min) every 5 min p.r.n., up to total loading dose of 15 mg/kg
*Note:* Anticonvulsant effects may be guided by monitoring serum phenytoin concentrations, therapeutic 10–20 mg/L.
*Note:* Phenytoin disposition is most often characterized by nonlinear (Michaelis-Menten) pharmacokinetics. Phenytoin is highly protein-bound (>90%) and may be associated with protein-binding displacement interaction; therapy is associated with unpredictable effects on the activity of hepatic drug-metabolizing enzymes. Caution should be used in generic substitution because all generic preparations may not be bioequivalent.
**Caution:** Imbalance in phenytoin protein binding reflected by abnormally low but therapeutic free serum phenytoin concentrations in patients with renal dysfunction and critically ill with acute head trauma.
†, DILANTIN; oral susp; phenytoin sodium, †, DILANTIN sodium; caps, inj

**Procainamide hydrochloride;** antiarrhythmic agent with general cardiodepressant effects; diminished myocardial excitability (decreased threshold potential, prolonged refractory period), reduced conduction velocity, diminished automaticity; decreases myocardial contractility; effects similar to those of quinidine
R for ventricular tachyarrhythmia: IN, CH = IM: 20–30 mg/kg/24 hr, div, every 4–6 hr; IV loading dose 10–15 mg over 30 min followed by continuous IV maintenance infusion of

**See KEY to abbreviations, p. 783; for further information about drugs, see package inserts.**

Table AP–1.  Drug Doses* (Drugs Listed Alphabetically by Generic Name) *Continued*

20–80 µg/kg/min; PO: 15–50 mg/kg/24 hr, div, every 3–6 hr. Serum concentration should be monitored for both procainamide and its active metabolite *N*-acetyl procainamide (NAPA).

†, PRONESTYL: tabl, caps, inj

**Promethazine hydrochloride;** phenothiazine with aliphatic side chain

℞ for sedation, prevention or treatment of motion sickness, and as antihistamine: CH = PO: 1 mg/kg/24 hr, divided into half dose at bedtime and quarter doses every 6 hr of the remaining daytime

†, PHENERGAN: syrup, tabl, suppos

**Propranolol hydrochloride;** β-adrenergic blocking agent (β$_1$ and β$_2$); racemic mixture of D- and L-propranolol, of which only L form has adrenergic blocking activity

℞ against selected forms of supraventricular and ventricular tachycardia: IN, CH = IV: 0.01–0.10 mg/kg/dose given slowly; repeat every 6–8 hr p.r.n. PO: 0.5–4 mg/kg/24 hr, div, every 6–8 hr

℞ as antihypertensive in long term therapy. CH = PO: initially 1 mg/kg/24 hr, div, every 6 hr, and progressive increase of dosage, if needed up to 5 mg/kg/24 hr, div, every 6 hr. Combination with diuretic and/or hydralazine indicated, because propranolol blocks physiologic compensatory mechanisms such as adrenergic inotropic and chronotropic responses, as well as renin activity.

℞ for prevention of migraine attack in severe cases and to combat the manifestations of thyrotoxicosis: Propranolol requirements vary widely from patient to patient because of individual differences in severity of underlying disease, endogenous sympathetic neuronal activity, sensitivity of β-adrenergic receptors to blockade, degree of protein binding, hepatic blood flow. For comparable effect, oral dose 6–10 times higher than intravenous dose in spite of good absorption from the gut because of inactivation of important fraction of propranolol in liver after entrance through portal vein.

Measures in case of exaggerated response: against bradycardia, atropine, if no response, isoproterenol, *cautiously;* against cardiac failure, digitalization, and diuretics; against hypotension, epinephrine; against bronchospasm, isoproterenol, theophylline (aminophylline)

INDERAL: tabl, inj

**Spironolactone;** aldosterone antagonist and potassium-sparing diuretic, which interferes with sodium reabsorption

℞ as diuretic in selected cases (with normal renal function), most effective in combination with a potassium-wasting diuretic: CH = PO: 1.5–3 mg/kg/24 hr, div, every 4–8 hr

*Note:* Monitoring of serum concentration of potassium, of potassium intake, and of renal function is indicated during treatment with spironolactone.

ALDACTONE: tabl

**Terbutaline sulfate,** catecholamine; β-adrenergic receptor agonist with preferential effect of β$_2$-adrenergic receptors

℞ bronchodilator: Dosage in pediatric age group not firmly established. PO: 0.10–0.15 mg/kg/24 hr, div, every 8 hr. β$_2$-selectivity is reduced with increasing dosage or on parenteral administration. SC: 0.005 mg/kg/dose, to be repeated p.r.n. after 20 min, once only

BRETHINE, BRICANYL: tabl, inj

**Theophylline;** methylxanthine commonly used in acute and chronic management of reversible airways disease (asthma), and neonatal apnea, bronchopulmonary dysplasia, among others. Cellular mechanism of action originally believed to be a result of phosphodiesterase inhibition; however, pharmacologic effect is most likely a result of adenosine receptor antagonism.

℞ in neonatal apnea: IV, PO: initial loading dose 5 mg/kg followed by maintenance therapy depending on age: preterm NB (<36 wk): 1–2 mg/kg/24 hr, div, every 8–12 hr; term infants (>36 wk): 2–4 mg/kg/24 hr, div, every 8–12 hr

℞ in status asthmaticus: Initial loading dose IV: 4–7 mg/kg/dose, infused after dilution in equal volume of intravenous fluid over 20–30 min, followed by maintenance IV: 20 mg/kg/24 hr, div, every 4–6 hr, or by continuous IV drip; switch to PO maintenance as soon as possible. Daily theophylline dose adjustment

**See KEY to abbreviations, p. 783; for further information about drugs, see package inserts.**

TABLE AP–1.  Drug Doses* (Drugs Listed Alphabetically by Generic Name) *Continued*

necessary relative to patient age and hepatic and cardiac function.

℞ oral maintenance: PO: 20 mg/kg/24 hr, div, every 6 hr; as conditions permit, taper to lowest effective dosage, usually around 10 mg/kg/24 hr, div, every 6 hr. Time-release theophylline preparations permit extension of the dosage interval (i.e., administration every 8–12 hr).

*Note* the content of theophylline in the following formulations: theophylline (anhydrous), 100%; aminophylline, 85%; theophylline monoethanolamine, 75%; dihydroxypropyltheophylline, 70%; oxtriphylline, choline salt, 64%; theophylline sodium glycinate, 50%; theophylline calcium salicylate, 48%. Serum concentration should be monitored; therapeutic range for neonatal apnea, 7–13 mg/L; in the management of bronchospasm, 10–20 mg/L.

theophylline, †, ELIXOPHYLLIN elixir, ELIXICON oral susp, SLOPHYLLIN caps, oral susp, SOMOPHYLLIN caps, ‡; component of many combination products

aminophylline, †, SOMOPHYLLIN oral liquid, ‡: inj, oral preparations

**Caution:** Circulatory collapse, seizures, coma may result from acute or chronic overdose.

**Valproate sodium,** dipropylacetate sodium; anti- convulsant agent with singular mode of action (effective probably by increasing γ-aminobutyric acid in brain tissues)

℞ in the treatment of simple petit mal and of complex absence seizures, either alone or in combination with other drugs (see reservation below) according to the results: CH = PO: start with 15 mg/kg/24 hr, div, every 8–12 hr; if needed, dosage increased by weekly increments of 5–10 mg/kg/24 hr up to a maximum recommended dose of 30 mg/kg/24 hr, div, every 8 hr

**Caution:** Concomitant use of valproate sodium and clonazepam might result in petit mal status. Blood concentrations of phenobarbital and phenytoin may be affected by addition of valproate sodium to the regimen.

DEPAKENE: caps (valproic acid), syrup (valproate sodium)

**Verapamil;** calcium channel blocker; toxic effects include allergic reactions, urticaria, bronchospasm, hypotension, decreased cardiac output, and asystole. Cardiac monitoring should be used during administration.

IN = IV: 0.1–0.2 mg/kg infused over 2 min
CH = IV: 0.1–0.3 mg/kg infused over 2 min
Maintenance dose = 1–2 mg/kg every 8 hr
CALAN, ISOPTIN: IV 2.5 mg/mL vial inj, PO tabs: 80, 120 mg

Modified from Behrman RE, Kliegman RM, Arvin AM (eds): Nelson Textbook of Pediatrics, 15th ed. Philadelphia, WB Saunders, 1996, pp 2058–2078.

**See KEY to abbreviations, p. 783; for further information about drugs, see package inserts.**

TABLE AP–2.  Drug Interactions of Potential Importance in Pediatric Practice (Partial Listing)*

| Interacting Drug | Adverse Effect | Interacting Drug | Adverse Effect |
|---|---|---|---|
| **Acetaminophen** | | **Barbiturates** | |
| Alcohol | Hepatotoxicity | Anticoagulants (oral) | ↓ Anticoagulation |
| Oral anticoagulants | ↑ Anticoagulation | Beta-adrenergic blockers | ↓ Beta-blockade |
| Probenecid | ↑ Acetaminophen toxicity | Carbamazepine | ↑ Production of carbamazepine epoxide |
| Zidovudine | Granulocytopenia | Chloramphenicol | ↑ Barbiturate toxicity |
| **Acyclovir** | | Contraceptives (oral) | ↓ Contraception |
| Narcotics | ↑ Narcotic toxicity? | Corticosteroids | ↓ Steroid effect |
| Zidovudine | Lethargy | Influenza vaccine (viral) | ↑ Barbiturate toxicity |
| **Alcohol** | | Rifampin | ↓ Barbiturate effect |
| Antidepressants (tricyclic) | ↑ Toxicity | Theophylline | ↓ Theophylline effect |
| Barbiturates | ↑ CNS depression (acute) | Valproate | ↑ Barbiturate toxicity |
| Benzodiazepines | ↑ CNS depression | **Bleomycin** | |
| Cephalosporins (not all) | Disulfiram effect | Oxygen | ↑ Pulmonary toxicity |
| Chloral hydrate | ↑ CNS depression | **Captopril** | |
| Doxycycline | ↓ Antibiotic effect | Allopurinol | ↑ Cutaneous hypersensitivity |
| Isoniazid | ↑ Hepatotoxicity | Aspirin | ↓ Antihypertensive effect |
| Metronidazole | Disulfiram effect | Cimetidine | Neuropathy |
| Phenothiazines | Impaired coordination | Nonsteroidal anti-inflammatory agents | ↓ Antihypertensive effect |
| Phenytoin | ↑ Phenytoin toxicity | Potassium | Hyperkalemia |
| **Allopurinol** | | Spironolactone | Hyperkalemia |
| Aluminum hydroxide | ↓ Allopurinol absorption | **Carbamazepine** | |
| Ampicillin | Rash | Anticoagulants (oral) | ↓ Anticoagulation |
| Anticoagulants (oral) | ↑ Anticoagulant effect | Antidepressants (tricyclic) | ↑ Both toxicities |
| Azathioprine | ↑ Azathioprine toxicity | Cimetidine | ↑ Carbamazepine toxicity |
| Captopril | ↑ Cutaneous hypersensitivity | Contraceptives (oral) | ↓ Contraception |
| Cyclophosphamide | ↑ Cyclophosphamide toxicity | Corticosteroids | ↓ Steroid effect |
| Theophylline | ↑ Theophylline toxicity | Cyclosporine | ↓ Cyclosporine effect |
| Thiazide diuretics | ↑ Allopurinol toxicity | Erythromycins | ↑ Carbamazepine toxicity |
| **Aminoglycoside Antibiotics** | | Influenza vaccine (viral) | ↑ Carbamazepine toxicity |
| Amphotericin B | ↑ Nephrotoxicity | Isoniazid | ↑ Both toxicities |
| Bumetanide | ↑ Ototoxicity | Phenytoin | ↓ Carbamazepine effect |
| Cisplatin | ↑ Nephrotoxicity | Theophylline | ↓ Theophylline effect |
| Cyclosporine | ↑ Nephrotoxicity | Valproate | ↓ Valproate effect |
| Furosemide | ↑ Nephrotoxicity and ototoxicity | **Cimetidine** | |
| Magnesium | ↑ Neuromuscular blockade | Alcohol | ↑ Alcohol effect |
| | | Antacids | ↓ Cimetidine effect |
| Neuromuscular blocking agents | ↑ Blockade | Anticoagulants (oral) | ↑ Anticoagulation |
| | | Antidepressants (tricyclic) | ↑ Antidepressant toxicity |
| Vancomycin | ↑ Nephrotoxicity? | Benzodiazepines | ↑ Benzodiazepine toxicity |
| | | Beta-adrenergic blocking agents | ↑ Beta-blockade toxicity |
| **Antacids** | | Captopril | Neuropathy |
| Beta-adrenergic blockers | ↓ Absorption | Carbamazepine | ↑ Carbamazepine toxicity |
| Captopril | ↓ Absorption | Digoxin | ↑ Digoxin toxicity |
| Cimetidine | ↓ Absorption | Ketoconazole | ↓ Ketoconazole absorption |
| Corticosteroids | ↓ Absorption | | |
| Digoxin | ↓ Absorption | Metoclopramide | ↓ Cimetidine effect |
| Iron | ↓ Absorption | Phenytoin | ↑ Phenytoin toxicity |
| Isoniazid | ↓ Absorption | Theophylline | ↑ Theophylline toxicity |
| Ketoconazole | ↓ Absorption | **Contraceptives (Oral)** | |
| Nonsteroidal anti-inflammatory agents | ↓ Absorption | Anticoagulants (oral) | ↓ Anticoagulation |
| Phenytoin | ↓ Absorption | Antidepressants (tricyclic) | ↑ Antidepressant toxicity |
| Salicylates | ↓ Absorption | Barbiturates | ↓ Contraception |
| Tetracycline | ↓ Absorption | Carbamazepine | ↓ Contraception |
| Theophylline | ↑ Toxicity | Griseofulvin | ↓ Contraception |
| **Aspirin** | | Penicillins (ampicillin, oxacillin) | ↓ Contraception? |
| Anticoagulants (oral) | ↑ Bleeding | Phenytoin | ↓ Contraception |
| Captopril | ↓ Antihypertensive effect | | |

TABLE AP–2.    Drug Interactions of Potential Importance in Pediatric Practice (Partial Listing)* *Continued*

| Interacting Drug | Adverse Effect | Interacting Drug | Adverse Effect |
|---|---|---|---|
| **Contraceptives (Oral)** *Continued* | | **Methotrexate** | |
| Rifampin | ↓ Contraception | Blood transfusion | ↑ Toxicity |
| Theophylline | ↑ Theophylline toxicity | Cisplatin | ↑ Methotrexate toxicity |
| | | Etretinate | ↑ Hepatotoxicity |
| **Cyclosporine** | | Nonsteroidal anti-inflammatory agents | ↑ Methotrexate toxicity |
| Alkylating agents | ↑ Nephrotoxicity | | |
| Aminoglycosides | ↑ Nephrotoxicity | Trimethoprim/sulfamethoxazole | Megaloblastic anemia |
| Amphotericin B | ↑ Nephrotoxicity | | |
| Carbamazepine | ↓ Cyclosporine effect | **Metoclopramide** | |
| Erythromycins | ↑ Cyclosporine toxicity | Carbamazepine | Neurotoxicity |
| Furosemide | Gout | Cimetidine | ↓ Cimetidine effect |
| Ketoconazole | ↑ Nephrotoxicity | Cyclosporine | ↑ Cyclosporine toxicity |
| Metoclopramide | ↑ Cyclosporine toxicity | Digoxin | ↓ Absorption |
| Nafcillin | ↓ Cyclosporine effect | Narcotics | ↑ Sedation |
| Phenytoin | ↓ Cyclosporine effect | | |
| Rifampin | ↓ Cyclosporine effect | **Nifedipine** | |
| | | Beta-adrenergic blockers | Heart failure, A-V block |
| **Digoxin** | | Cyclosporine | ↑ Gingival hyperplasia |
| Antacids | ↓ Absorption | Phenytoin | ↑ Phenytoin toxicity |
| Anticholingergics | ↑ Digoxin toxicity | Prazosin | Hypotension |
| Cholestyramine | ↓ Absorption | Quinidine | ↓ Quinidine effect |
| Cimetidine | ↑ Digoxin toxicity | | |
| Diuretics (hypokalemia) | ↑ Digoxin toxicity | **Phenytoin** | |
| Phenytoin | ↓ Digoxin effect | Alcohol | ↑ Toxicity (acute) |
| Quinidine | ↑ Digoxin toxicity | Antacids | ↓ Phenytoin effect |
| Verapamil | ↑ Digoxin toxicity | Anticoagulants (oral) | ↑ Phenytoin toxicity, ↑ ↓ Anticoagulation |
| **Erythromycins** | | Antidepressants (tricyclic) | ↑ Phenytoin toxicity |
| Anticoagulants (oral) | ↑ Anticoagulation | Carbamazepine | ↓ Carbamazepine effect |
| Astemizole (Hismanal) | ↑ Astemizole toxicity: arrhythmias | Chloramphenicol | ↑ Toxicity (both) |
| | | Cimetidine | ↑ Phenytoin toxicity |
| Carbamazepine | ↑ Carbamazepine toxicity | Contraceptives (oral and implant) | ↓ Contraception |
| Cyclosporine | ↑ Cyclosporine toxicity | | |
| Phenytoin | ↓ Phenytoin effect | Corticosteroids | ↓ Corticosteroid effect |
| Terfenadine (Seldane) | ↑ Terfenadine toxicity: arrhythmias | Cyclosporine | ↓ Cyclosporine effect |
| | | Digoxin | ↓ Digoxin effect |
| Theophylline | ↑ Theophylline toxicity | Dopamine | Hypotension |
| | | Folic acid | ↓ Phenytoin effect |
| **Fluoroquinolones** | | Isoniazid | ↑ Phenytoin toxicity |
| Antacids | ↓ Antibiotic effect | Miconazole | ↓ Phenytoin effect |
| Theophylline | ↑ Theophylline toxicity | Neuromuscular blocking agents | ↓ Blockade |
| **Griseofulvin** | | Nifedipine | ↑ Phenytoin toxicity |
| Anticoagulants (oral) | ↓ Anticoagulants | Quinidine | ↓ Quinidine effect |
| Contraceptive (oral) | ↓ Contraceptive | Rifampin | ↓ Phenytoin effect |
| | | Theophylline | ↓ Effects (both) |
| **Isoniazid** | | Valproate | ↑ Phenytoin toxicity |
| Alcohol | Hepatitis | | |
| Antacids | ↓ INH absorption | **Quinidine** | |
| Carbamazepine | ↑ Toxicity (both) | Amiodarone | ↑ Quinidine toxicity |
| Ketoconazole | ↓ Ketoconazole effect | Anticoagulants (oral) | ↑ Anticoagulation |
| Phenytoin | ↑ Phenytoin toxicity | Barbiturates | ↓ Quinidine effect |
| Rifampin | ↑ Hepatotoxicity | Cimetidine | ↑ Quinidine toxicity |
| Valproate | ↑ Hepatic and CNS toxicity | Digoxin | ↑ Digoxin toxicity |
| | | Metoclopramide | ↓ Quinidine effect |
| **Ketoconazole** | | Phenytoin | ↓ Quinidine effect |
| Antacids | ↓ Absorption | Procainamide | ↑ Procainamide toxicity |
| Anticoagulants (oral) | ↑ Anticoagulation | Rifampin | ↓ Quinidine effect |
| Cimetidine | ↓ Ketoconazole effect | Verapamil | Hypotension |
| Cyclosporine | ↑ Nephrotoxicity | | |
| Isoniazid | ↓ Ketoconazole effect | | |
| Phenytoin | Altered metabolism of both drugs | | |
| Rifampin | ↓ Effects of both drugs | | |

TABLE AP–2.    Drug Interactions of Potential Importance in Pediatric Practice (Partial Listing)* *Continued*

| Interacting Drug | Adverse Effect | Interacting Drug | Adverse Effect |
|---|---|---|---|
| *Rifampin* | | *Theophylline* Continued | |
| Anticoagulants (oral) | ↓ Anticoagulation | Interferon | ↑ Toxicity? |
| Barbiturates | ↓ Barbiturate effect | Marijuana smoking | ↓ Theophylline effect |
| Beta-adrenergic blockers | ↓ Beta-blockade | Phenytoin | ↓ Effect (both) |
| Chloramphenicol | ↓ Chloramphenicol effect | Rifampin | ↓ Theophylline effect |
| Contraception (oral) | ↓ Contraception | Tobacco smoking | ↓ Theophylline effect |
| Corticosteroids | ↓ Corticosteroid effect | Troleandomycin | ↑ Theophylline toxicity |
| Cyclosporine | ↓ Cyclosporine effect | | |
| Isoniazid | ↑ Hepatotoxicity | *Trimethoprim/* | |
| Ketoconazole | ↓ Effects (both) | *Sulfamethoxazole* | |
| Phenytoin | ↓ Phenytoin effect | Anticoagulants (oral) | ↑ Anticoagulation |
| Quinidine | ↓ Quinidine effect | Antidepressants (tricyclic) | Depression |
| Theophylline | ↓ Theophylline effect | Mercaptopurine | ↓ Antileukemia effect |
| Verapamil | ↓ Verapamil effect | Methotrexate | Megaloblastic anemia |
| *Theophylline* | | *Valproate* | |
| Barbiturates | ↓ Theophylline effect | Barbiturates | ↑ Phenobarbital toxicity |
| Beta-adrenergic blockers | ↑ Theophylline toxicity | Benzodiazepines | ↑ Diazepam toxicity |
| Carbamazepine | ↓ Theophylline effect | Carbamazepines | ↓ Valproate effect |
| Cimetidine | ↑ Theophylline toxicity | Cimetidine | ↑ Valproate toxicity? |
| Erythromycins | ↑ Theophylline toxicity | Ethosuximide | ↑ Ethosuximide toxicity? |
| Fluoroquinolones | ↑ Theophylline toxicity | Phenytoin | ↑ Phenytoin toxicity |
| Influenza vaccine (viral) | ↑ Theophylline toxicity | | |

Modified from Rizack M, Hillman C: The Medical Letter Handbook of Adverse Drug Interactions. New Rochelle, The Medical Letter, 1989.
*When possible, an alternate drug combination should be given. If not possible, drug levels *and* signs of toxicity must be monitored.
A-V = atrioventricular; CNS = central nervous system; INH = isoniazid; ? = possible effect.

**FIGURE AP–1.** Nomogram for estimation of surface area. The surface area is indicated where a straight line that connects the height and weight levels intersects the surface area column; or the patient is roughly of average size, from the weight alone *(enclosed area)*. (Modified from data of E. Boyd by C. D. West.)

# Index

Note: Page numbers in *italics* indicate illustrations; those followed by t refer to tables.

Thyroid gland *(Continued)*
  medullary carcinoma of, 668
  physiology of, 663–664
  tumors of, 668
Thyroid hormones, excess, 647
  growth effects of, 74t, 651
  synthesis of, in iodine deficiency, 87
Thyroid storm, 667
Thyroiditis, Hashimoto, 665–666
  lymphocytic, 665–666
Thyroid-stimulating hormone, 647
  in iodine deficiency, 87
  measurement of, 650t
  release of, 663
Thyrotoxicosis, 647
Thyrotropin-releasing hormone, in
    pituitary thyroid-stimulating
    hormone release, 663
Thyroxine (T₄), synthesis of, 663
Thyroxine-binding globulin, disorders
    of, 663, 663t
Tibia, external torsion of, 758
  internal torsion of, 757–758
Tibia vara, 758–759
Tic, 745
Ticarcillin, 347t
  dosages for, 792t
Tick bites, 114t
  Lyme disease from, 377
Tick paralysis, vs. Guillain-Barré
    syndrome, 737
Tidal volume, 461
Time-out procedures, for behavioral
    problems, 33
Tine test, 358
Tinea capitis, 409t
Tinea corporis, 409t
Tinea cruris, 409t
Tinea pedis, 409t
Tinea unguium, 409t
Tinea versicolor, 409t
Tissue factor, 573
Tissue factor pathway inhibitor, *572,*
    *573*
Toads, envenomation by, 115t
Tobacco, abuse of, 256t, 258t
Tobramycin, 348t
  dosages for, 792t
Tocopherol, deficiency of, 79
  serum concentration of, diet and, 79
Toddler's diarrhea, 427
Toddler's fracture, 780–781
Toe(s), deformities of, 766–767, 766t,
    767t
Toe-walking, 749
Toilet training, 36, 36t
Tone, neonatal, 697
Tongue, evaluation of, 699
  geographic, in allergic rhinitis, 288
Tonsillitis, 343
Tonsils, abscess of, 471t–472t
  adenoidal, hypertrophy of, 474–475
  diphtheria of, 353
Tooth (teeth), caries of, 436
  delayed eruption of, 434, 436
  enamel of, fluoride in, 87
    hypoplasia of, 434
  eruption timing of, 434, 436t
  primary (deciduous), 434

Tooth (teeth) *(Continued)*
  secondary (permanent), 434
TORCH syndrome, 218–219, 220t–221t,
    387–388
  vs. idiopathic hepatitis, 455
Torticollis, 773–774
  neonatal, 189
Torus fracture, 778
Total anomalous pulmonary venous
    connection, 530–531
Total parenteral nutrition, 90–92
  central, 91–92
  cholestasis in, 91–92
  complications of, 91–92, 91t
  hepatobiliary dysfunction in, 91–92
  indications for, 90
  peripheral, 90–91
Tourette syndrome, 745
Toxemia, 565
Toxic shock syndrome, 372
  streptococcal, 374
Toxic syndromes, 105t
Toxicity, nutrient, 80t
  poisoning and, 105–106, 106t
  vitamin, 80t
Toxicology assays, in poisoning, 109,
    *111, 112*
Toxins, acute consciousness disorders
    from, 705–706, 706t
  circulating, hemolysis from, 565
  red urine from, 629
*Toxocara canis,* 417
*Toxocara catii,* 417
*Toxocara leonina,* 417
Toxocariasis, 417
Toxoplasmosis, 415
  acquired, 415
  congenital, 415
Toxoplasmosis, other, rubella,
    cytomegalovirus, herpes simplex
    (TORCH). See *TORCH syndrome.*
Trace elements, deficiency of, 85–88
  in neonate, 212
Trachea, 459
  compression of, 476
  encirclement of, 476
Tracheitis, bacterial, 471t–472t, 482
Tracheobronchial tree, anatomic defects
    in, 264t
  foreign bodies in, 493–494
Tracheoesophageal fistula, *437,* 437–438,
    476
Tracheomalacia, 476
Tracheostomy, for respiratory disorders,
    468
Trachoma, *Chlamydia trachomatis* and,
    378
Transaminase, metabolism of, *149*
Transcription, 129
Transcuprein, in copper transport, 85
Transfusion, 581
  cytomegalovirus infection in, 387
  exchange, for indirect hyperbilirubi-
    nemia, 206
    for polycythemia, 207
  products for, 580t, 581
  reactions to, 581, 581t
Transient tachypnea of newborn, 197
Translation, 129

Transplantation, fever in, 328
Transport, disorders of, pathogenesis
    of, 147, 148t
Transposition of great arteries, 505, 513,
    524–527, *525*
  fetal effects of, 512
  treatment of, 517t, 518t
  with intact ventricular septum, 525–
    526
  with ventricular septal defect, 526–
    527
Transtentorial herniation, stages of, 705,
    705t
Trauma, abdominal, 97–98, 98t
  accidental, prevention of, 95
  assessment of, 93–128
  biliary, 99
  epidemiology of, 95
  evaluation of, 95–97, 97t, 98t
    primary survey in, 96–97, 97t, 98t
    secondary survey in, 97
  fatalities from, 95
  head. See *Craniocerebral trauma.*
  hepatic, 99
  intestinal, 99–100
  laboratory evaluation of, 97, 98t
  major, 95–100
  nutrition in, 56, *57*
  pancreatic, 99
  prehospital care in, 95, 96t
  renal, 99
  scoring system for, 95, 96t
  splenic, 98–99
  synovial fluid findings in, 334t
  to specific organs, 97–100
  trauma center care in, 95, 96t
Trauma center, children requiring, 95,
    96t
Trauma score, pediatric, 95, 96t
Traveler's diarrhea, 423, 426
Trematodes, infections by, 417–418
Tremor, 745
  vs. seizure, 220–221
*Treponema pallidum,* syphilis from,
    375–377
Triage, 93
Trichobezoars, 440
Trichomoniasis, 249t, 250–251
Tricuspid atresia, treatment of, 517t,
    518t
Tricuspid valve, atresia of, 528–529, *529*
Triiodothyronine (T₃), synthesis of, 663
Trimethoprim/sulfamethoxazole, 349t
Trisomy 13, 138, 139t
Trisomy 18, 138, 139t
Trisomy 21, 137–138
  cancer in, 585t
  clinical manifestations of, 138, 138t
  cytogenetics of, 137–138
  endocardial cushion defect of, 518–
    519
Trousseau sign, 215
  in hypocalcemia, 677
Truancy, 260–261
Truncus arteriosus, 529–530
Trunk, growth in, 56
  rhabdomyosarcoma of, 605
*Trypanosoma cruzi,* 413